Occupational Musculoskeletal Disorders

Function, Outcomes, and Evidence

Occupational Musculoskeletal Disorders
Function, Outcomes, and Evidence

Editors

Tom G. Mayer, M.D.
Clinical Professor
Department of Orthopedic Surgery
University of Texas Southwestern Medical School
Medical Director
Productive Rehabilitation Institute of Dallas for Ergonomics (PRIDE)
Dallas, Texas

Robert J. Gatchel, Ph.D.
Elizabeth H. Penn Distinguished Professor of Clinical Psychology
Department of Psychiatry and Rehabilitation
University of Texas Southwestern Medical School, Dallas, Texas

Peter Barth Polatin, M.D.
Associate Clinical Professor
Department of Anesthesiology and Pain Management
University of Texas Southwestern Medical School
Associate Medical Director
Productive Rehabilitation Institute of Dallas for Ergonomics (PRIDE)
Dallas, Texas

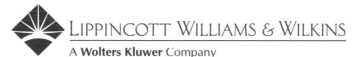

LIPPINCOTT WILLIAMS & WILKINS
A **Wolters Kluwer** Company
Philadelphia · Baltimore · New York · London
Buenos Aires · Hong Kong · Sydney · Tokyo

Acquisitions Editor: Elizabeth Greenspan
Developmental Editor: Maureen Iannuzzi
Production Editor: Rakesh Rampertab
Manufacturing Manager: Tim Reynolds
Cover Designer: Mark Lerner
Compositor: Lippincott Williams & Wilkins Desktop Division
Printer: Maple Press

Library of Congress Cataloging-in-Publication Data
Occupational musculoskeletal disorders : function, outcomes, and evidence / edited by Tom G. Mayer, Robert J. Gatchel, Peter B. Polatin.
    p. cm.
Includes bibliographical references.
ISBN 0-7817-1735-3
1. Musculoskeletal system—Wounds and injuries. 2. Orthopedic disability evaluation. I. Mayer, Tom G. II. Gatchel, Robert J., 1947– . III. Polatin, Peter B.
[DNLM: 1. Musculoskeletal Diseases. 2. Occupational Diseases.
WE 140 O149 1999]
RD680.O27 1999
616.7—dc21
DNLM/DLC

For Library of Congress

10 9 8 7 6 5 4 3 2 1

Contents

Part III: Prevention

Part IV: Acute Occupational Musculoskeletal Disorders

Part V: Postacute Occupational Musculoskeletal Disorders

Contributing Authors

Gunnar B. J. Andersson, M.D., Ph.D.
Professor and Chairman
Department of Orthopaedic Surgery
Rush Medical College
600 South Pauline Street; and
Senior Attending
Department of Orthopaedic Surgery
Rush-Presbyterian-St. Luke's Medical Center
1653 West Congress Parkway, 1471 Jelke
Chicago, Illinois 60612

Peter S. Barth, Ph.D.
Professor
Department of Economics
University of Connecticut
341 Mansfield Road
Storrs, Connecticut 06269-1063

Robert J. Benz, M.D.
Clinical Instructor
Department of Orthopaedics
University of California, San Diego
200 West Arbor Drive
San Diego, California 92103

A. Kim Burton, Ph.D., Eur Erg
Director
Spinal Research Unit
University of Huddersfield
Queensgate
Huddersfield, HD1 3DH
United Kingdom

Richard J. Butler, Ph.D.
Professor
Industrial Relations Center
University of Minnesota
312 19th Avenue South
Minneapolis, Minnesota 55455

Allard E. Dembe, Sc.D.
Assistant Professor
Center for Health Policy and Health Services
  Research
University of Massachusetts Medical School
222 Maple Avenue
Shrewsbury, Massachusetts 01545

Martin Deschner, Ph.D.
Assistant Professor
Departments of Psychiatry and Anesthesiology and
  Pain Management
Eugene McDermott Center for Pain Management
University of Texas Southwestern Medical School
5323 Harry Hines Boulevard
Dallas, Texas 75235-9068

James W. DeVocht, DC, Ph.D.
Assistant Professor
Palmer Center for Chiropractic Research
Davenport, Iowa 52803; and
Adjunct Assistant Professor
Iowa Spine Research Center
JPP–Ortho
University of Iowa
Iowa City, Iowa 52242

David F. Fardon, M.D.
Associate Clinical Professor
Department of Orthopaedics
University of Tennessee, Knoxville; and
Staff Surgeon
Knoxville Orthopaedic Clinic
Southeastern Orthopaedics
1128 Weisgarber Road
Knoxville, Tennessee 37909

David W. Florence, M.D., M.P.A.
Associate Physician
Department of Occupational Medicine
Marshfield Clinic
1000 North Oak Avenue
Marshfield, Wisconsin 54449

Noor M. Gajraj, M.D., F.R.C.A.
Assistant Professor
Department of Anesthesiology and Pain
  Management
University of Texas Southwestern Medical Center
5323 Harry Hines Boulevard; and
Medical Director
Pain Clinic
Parkland Memorial Hospital
5201 Harry Hines Boulevard
Dallas, Texas 75235-9068

Steven R. Garfin, M.D.
Professor and Chair
Department of Orthopaedics
University of California, San Diego
200 West Arbor Drive
San Diego, California 92103-8894

Robert J. Gatchel, Ph.D.
Elizabeth H. Penn Distinguished Professor of
*   Clinical Psychology*
Department of Psychiatry and Rehabilitation
University of Texas Southwestern Medical School
5323 Harry Hines Boulevard
Dallas, Texas 75235-9044

Michael E. Goldsmith, M.D.
Clinical Instructor
Department of Orthopaedics
Georgetown University Medical Center
3800 Reservoir Road
Washington, D.C. 20007

Mark D. Grabiner, Ph.D.
Staff Scientist
Department of Biomedical Engineering
Learner Research Institute
The Cleveland Clinic Foundation
9500 Euclid Avenue, ND-2
Cleveland, Ohio 44106

Judith Greenwood, Ph.D., M.P.H.
Clinical Associate Professor
Department of Community Medicine
Institute of Occupational and
*   Environmental Health*
University of West Virginia
Morgantown, West Virginia 26506; and
Assistant Director
Workers' Compensation Research
Research, Information, and
*   Analysis Division*
West Virginia Bureau of
*   Employment Program*
112 California Avenue
Charlestown, West Virginia 25305

Thomas T. Haider, M.D.
Clinical Professor
Department of Orthopaedics
University of California
Riverside, California; and
Chief
Division of Spine Surgery
Riverside County Regional Medical Center
Riverside, California 92501

Andrew J. Haig, M.D.
Assistant Professor
Physical Medicine and Rehabilitation and Surgery
University of Michigan; and
Director
The Interdepartmental Spine Program
University of Michigan Health Center
325 East Eisenhower
Ann Arbor, Michigan 48108

Scott Haldeman, D.C., M.D., Ph.D.
Clinical Professor
Department of Neurology
University of California, Irvine
1125 East 17th Street, Suite W-127
Santa Ana, California 92701

Thomas R. Hales, M.D., M.P.H.
Senior Medical Epidemiologist
National Institute for Occupational Safety and
*   Health (NIOSH)*
4676 Columbia Parkway, R-9
Cincinnati, Ohio 45226

Robert H. Haralson III, M.D., M.B.A.
Associate Clinical Professor
Department of Surgery
University of Tennessee Center for the Health Sciences
Knoxville, Tennessee 37902; and
Department of Surgery
Blount Memorial Hospital
1203 South Heritage Drive
Maryville, Tennessee 37804

Sharona Hoffman, J.D.
Assistant Professor
Case Western Reserve University School of Law
11075 East Boulevard
Cleveland, Ohio 44106–7148

Paul D. Hooper, D.C.
Chair
Department of Principles and Practice
Los Angeles College of Chiropractic
16200 East Amber Valley Drive
Whittier, California 90609

Susan J. Isernhagen, P.T.
President
Isernhagen and Associates
1015 East Superior Street
Duluth, Minnesota 55802

Malcolm I.V. Jayson, M.D., F.R.C.P.
Professor
Rheumatic Diseases Centre
University of Manchester; and
Consultant Rheumatologist
Rheumatic Diseases Center
Hope Hospital
Salford, M6 8HD
United Kingdom

John H. Jones, Jr., Esq.
Nationwide Insurance Companies
P.O. Box 8017
Wausau, Wisconsin 54402-8017

Eric M. Kennedy, M.S., CPE
Senior Ergonomist
Occupational Health Services
Healthsouth Corporation
2825 Randolph Road
Charlotte, North Carolina 28211

Nancy D. Kishino, OTR, CVE
Director
West Coast Spine Restoration Center
6177 River Crest Drive, Suite A
Riverside, California 92507

David R. Lord, M.S.
Graduate Student
Department of Mechanical Engineering
Case Western Reserve University
10900 Euclid Avenue
Cleveland, Ohio 44106-1712; and
Research Assistant
Department of Biomedical Engineering
The Cleveland Clinic Foundation
9500 Euclid Avenue
Cleveland, Ohio 44195

Chris J. Main, Ph.D.
Professor
School of Medicine
University of Manchester
Oxford Road, Manchester; and
Head
Department of Behavioural Medicine
Hope Hospital
Scott Lane
Salford, M6 8HD
United Kingdom

Barton G. Margoshes, M.D.
Clinical Instructor
Family and Community Medicine
University of Massachusetts Medical Center
Worcester, Massachusetts 01655; and
Vice President
National Medical Director
Liberty Mutual Insurance Group
175 Berkeley Street
Boston, Massachusetts 02117

Tracy K. Marker, M.S., AEP
Interlogics, Inc.
700 Inverness Avenue, Suite 204
Nashville, Tennessee 37204

Leonard N. Matheson, Ph.D.
Program in Occupational Therapy
Washington University School of Medicine,
*   St. Louis; and*
Occupational Therapy
4444 Forest Park Avenue
St. Louis, Missouri 63108

Tom G. Mayer, M.D.
Clinical Professor
Orthopedic Surgery
University of Texas Southwestern Medical School
5323 Harry Hines Boulevard; and
Medical Director
Productive Rehabilitation Institute of Dallas for
Ergonomics (PRIDE)
5701 Maple Avenue, Suite 100
Dallas, Texas 75235

Donald R. McIntyre, Ph.D.
President and Chief Executive Officer
NDX, Inc.
6429 Mount Mitchell Road
Efland, North Carolina 27243

J. Mark Melhorn, M.D.
Clinical Assistant Professor
Section of Orthopaedics, Department of Surgery
University of Kansas School of Medicine—Wichita
The Hand Center, P.A.
625 North Carriage Parkway, Suite 125
Wichita, Kansas 67208-4510

Vert Mooney, M.D.
Clinical Professor of Orthopaedics
Department of Orthopaedics
University of California, San Diego
200 West Arbor Drive
San Diego, California 92103; and
Medical Director
San Diego Spine Center
3444 Kearny Villa Road, Suite 205
San Diego, California 92123

Carl Edward Noe, M.D.
Medical Director
Eugene McDermott Center for Pain Management
University of Texas Southwestern Medical Center
5323 Harry Hines Boulevard
Dallas, Texas 75235; and
Medical Director
Baylor Center for Pain Management
Baylor Medical Center
3600 Gaston, Suite 360
Dallas, Texas 75246

Takuma Ozaki, M.D.
Department of Biomedical Engineering
The Cleveland Clinic Foundation
9500 Euclid Avenue
Cleveland, Ohio 44106

Manohar M. Panjabi, Ph.D.
Professor
Department of Orthopaedics and
* Rehabilitation*
Yale University School of Medicine
P.O. Box 208071
New Haven, Connecticut 06520-8071

Mohamad Parnianpour, Ph.D.
Associate Professor
Department of Industrial, Welding &
* Systems Engineering*
Ohio State University
1971 Neil Avenue
Columbus, Ohio 43210

Alejandro Pérez, M.D., M.P.H.
Research Fellow
Department of Physical Medicine and
* Rehabilitation*
University of Michigan Hospitals
325 East Eisenhower
Ann Arbor, Michigan 48108

Bendt P. Petersen III, M.D.
Old Shell Orthopaedic Associates
Mobile, Alabama 36608

Peter Barth Polatin, M.D.
Associate Clinical Professor
Department of Anesthesiology and Pain
* Management*
University of Texas Southwestern Medical School;
* and*
Associate Medical Director
Productive Rehabilitation Institute of Dallas for
Ergonomics (PRIDE)
Dallas, Texas 75235

Malcolm H. Pope, MedSc, Ph.D.
Professor
Department of Environmental & Occupational
* Medicine*
University of Aberdeen; and
Grampian University Hospitals NHS Trust
Foresterhill
Aberdeen, AB25 2ZD
Scotland, United Kingdom

Glenn S. Pransky, M.D., M.Occ.H.
Associate Professor
Department of Family and Community Health
University of Massachusetts Medical School
Worcester, Massachusetts 01655; and
Director
Occupational and Environmental Health Program
University of Massachusetts Medical Center
Worcester, Massachusetts 01655

J. Matthew Prescott, M.Ed., C.R.C
Senior Medical Case Manager
Department of Case Management Services
Productive Rehabilitation Institute of Dallas for
* Ergonomics (PRIDE)*
5701 Maple Avenue, Suite 100
Dallas, Texas 75235

James Rainville, M.D.
Clinical Assistant Professor
Department of Physical Medicine and Rehabilitation
Harvard Medical School
Boston, Massachusetts; and
Chief
Department of Spine Physiatry
The Spine Center
New England Baptiste Hospital
125 Parker Hill Avenue
Boston, Massachusetts 02120

Mohammed I. Ranavaya, M.D., M.S.,
* **FAADEP***
Director
Appalachian Institute of Occupational and
* Environmental Medicine*
West Virginia
State Route 10 North, RR4 Box 5C
Chapmanville, West Virginia 25508

Lori Rectanus, M.A.
Senior Project Manager
U.S. General Accounting Office
Health, Education, and Human Services Division
441 G Street NW
Washington, D.C. 20548

Peter N. Rogers, J.D.
Rogers, Bookers & Treviño, P.C.
901 Waterfall Way, Suite 105
Richardson, Texas 75080

Jeffrey A. Saal, M.D. F.A.C.P.
Associate Clinical Professor
Department of Functional Restoration
Stanford University School of Medicine
SOAR, Physiatry Group
2884 Sand Hill Road, Suite 110
Menlo Park, California 94025

Joel S. Saal, M.D.
Assistant Clinical Professor
Department of Functional Restoration
Stanford University School of Medicine
SOAR, Physiatry Group
2884 Sand Hill Road, Suite 110
Menlo Park, California 94025

William S. Shaw, M.D.
Integrated Health Management
1221 South Clarkson Street, Suite 300
Denver, Colorado 80210

Alfred Taricco, M.D.
Consultant
113 Kimberly Drive
Manchester, Connecticut 06040

Dennis C. Turk, Ph.D.
John and Emma Bonica Professor
Department of Anesthesiology
University of Washington
Box 356540
Seattle, Washington 98195

Akshay S. Vakharia, M.D., M.S.
Assistant Professor
Department of Anesthesiology and Pain Management
University of Texas Southwest Medical Center
5323 Harry Hines Boulevard
Dallas, Texas 75235

William Charles Watters III, M.D.
Clinical Associate Professor
Department of Orthopedic Surgery
Baylor College of Medicine
6550 Fannin, Suite 2625; and
Attending
Department of Orthopedic Surgery
St. Luke's Episcopal Hospital
6720 Bertner
Houston, Texas 77030

Barbara S. Webster, RPT, PA-C
Researcher
Liberty Mutual Research Center
71 Franklund Road
Hopkinton, Massachusetts 01748

A. LaVonne Wesley, Ph.D.
Assistant Professor
Department of Psychiatry
University of Texas Southwestern Medical School
5323 Harry Hines Boulevard
Dallas, Texas 75235-9044

Augustus A. White III, M.D.
Department of Orthopedics
Beth Israel Deaconess Hospital
330 Brookline Avenue
Boston, Massachusetts 02215

Sam W. Wiesel, M.D.
Professor and Chairman
Department of Orthopaedics
Georgetown University Medical Center
3800 Reservoir Road, NW
Washington, D.C. 20007

David A. Wong, M.D., MSc.,
 F.R.C.S.C.
Assistant Clinical Professor
Department of Orthopedics
University of Colorado
1601 East 19th Avenue, Suite 5000
Denver, Colorado 80218

Joseph P. Zeppieri, M.D.
Senior Surgeon
Department of Orthopaedic Surgery/Plastic Hand
Lawrence & Memorial Hospital
365 Montauk Avenue
New London, Connecticut 06320

Preface

In the United States alone the annual cost associated with the diagnosis and care of musculoskeletal trauma amounts to tens of billions of dollars. Moreover, these costs are continuing to increase at an alarming rate. Indeed, occupational musculoskeletal disorders are the leading causes of work disability in the United States today. Changes in health care policy and demands for improved allocation of health resources have recently placed great pressure on health care professionals to provide the most cost-effective treatment for these disorders, as well as to validate treatment efficacy. As a result, treatment-outcome monitoring has assumed new importance in medicine. It is particularly vital in musculoskeletal care, which is currently targeted for attention by health planners because of its high cost and perceived inefficient care. A variety of health policy initiatives are undergoing pilot implementation, such as second surgical opinion programs, fee-schedule "reforms" (with variable multiplier modifications to favor utilization of specific modalities), and "24-hour coverage" (rolling group health and workers' compensation benefits into a single package).

With the above dramatic changes in the medical/health care environment as a background, it was deemed important to develop an updated, state of the art text for many of the important issues that occupational medicine health care providers need to be aware of in dealing with musculoskeletal disorders. The present text has been developed for use by the practicing occupational medicine provider. These providers span a number of medical and allied health disciplines, including occupational medicine, orthopedics, physical medicine and rehabilitation, chiropractic care, physical and occupational therapies, psychology/psychiatry, ergonomics-biomechanics, etc. The text is designed to serve as a comprehensive reference for these disciplines, as well as for health care administrators, lawyers, insurance carriers, etc., who all interface with the practice of occupational medicine. The most recent "cutting edge" material in the primary areas of occupational musculoskeletal medicine will be provided.

One of the major threads running through the fabric of this text is the importance of emphasizing the utilization of objectively quantified functional outcomes, such as return to work, subsequent health care utilization, etc., in order to address cost-effectiveness issues which remain an important issue in health care today. Moreover, the significance of psychosocial factors in the evaluation, treatment, and prevention of musculoskeletal disorders is also emphasized. The contributors are internationally recognized for their extensive background in the area of disability management and treatment outcome evaluation, so the most recent, scientifically acceptable methods and approaches will be presented. Indeed, these contributors were carefully selected on the basis of their being at the forefront of the field in providing the most effective methods for the care and management of musculoskeletal trauma. We, the editors of this text, are internationally recognized for our work relating to musculoskeletal disorders and pain. Altogether, we have been working in the field for over 60 years and have contributed extensively to its literature—publishing approximately 350 papers in journals and scholarly texts. In addition, we have edited or authored 17 other books. This provided us with a great advantage in our efforts to recruit the best contributors because we have crossed paths with these contributors many times in the past.

The new technology of functional evaluation and restoration is revolutionizing the field of musculoskeletal medicine. No longer does the clinician have to rely solely on the less-than-adequate self-report and structural measures, originally designed to identify only the small percentage of musculoskeletal disorder sufferers requiring surgery. The recent advances that are being embraced throughout this country and the world, in emphasizing the objective measure of function, are presented in this text.

Overall, this text will provide the reader with important, everyday clinical concerns and issues that arise when dealing with occupational musculoskeletal disorder patients. The reader will receive a balanced mixture of material on basic theory, assessment, treatment, and specific practical issues. The material has been written with the primary care and general practitioner in mind, though it should also be of great interest to orthopedic specialists, physical and occupational therapists, psychologists/psychiatrists, and pain treatment specialists in general. We are cognizant of the fact that the readers will have different levels of expertise in these areas. The material, therefore, is presented in clear, understandable language without introducing overly technical and complicated jargon or, conversely, oversimplifying basic concepts and issues.

Of course, a comprehensive text of this type is not possible without the help from many gifted people. All of the contributors were quite diligent in providing outstanding state of the art chapters in a timely manner. We would also like to thank and acknowledge the help and support we received from the staff of Lippincott Williams & Wilkins, particularly Elizabeth Greenspan and Maureen Iannuzzi. Finally, preparation of this text and the timeliness in bringing it to fruition were greatly aided by the efforts of Carol Gentry.

Tom G. Mayer
Robert J. Gatchel
Peter Barth Polatin

Occupational Musculoskeletal Disorders

Function, Outcomes, and Evidence

PART I

Occupational Injury Concepts

Occupational Musculoskeletal Disorders
edited by T. G. Mayer, R. J. Gatchel, and P. B. Polatin.
Lippincott Williams & Wilkins, Philadelphia © 2000.

1

Occupational Musculoskeletal Disorders: Introduction and Overview of the Problem

Robert J. Gatchel and *Tom G. Mayer

*Department of Psychiatry and Rehabilitation; *Department of Orthopedic Surgery,
University of Texas Southwestern Medical School, Dallas, Texas 75235*

Musculoskeletal disorders involve the musculoskeletal system, the 90% of the human body devoted to interacting with the external environment. Although linked to all other systems, the musculoskeletal system is less concerned with issues of homeostasis, sensory input, and problem solving. The bones and joints provide the frame, with ligament connectors and muscle/tendon pulleys providing the motor power. The peripheral nerves and nerve roots, providing the communication links from the central nervous system, may be included in the paradigm, especially in the upper extremity. Occupational injuries represent an important cost to industry and therefore to the productive capacity of every developing nation. An occupational musculoskeletal disorder provides the most significant component of occupational injury in frequency, disability, loss of productivity, and cost.

Statistics on the prevalence of work-related musculoskeletal disorders may vary from one reference source to another, primarily due to variations in the diagnostic criteria used for such disorders and variations among different jurisdictions. Such disorders can range from well-defined ones such as disc herniation, tendinitis, and carpal tunnel syndrome, to those less well-defined such as facet syndrome, to nondefined or nonspecific disorders, such as cumulative trauma disorder or fibromyalgia. In Chapter 15, Melhorn provides a comprehensive review of such definitions and other issues, considering the epidemiology of these disorders.

There can be no doubt, though, that the prevalence of such disorders, regardless of the vagaries of definition, is strikingly high in the United States and other developed countries. Data from the U.S. Department of Labor reveal that occupational musculoskeletal disorders are the leading cause of work disability in the United States. Moreover, a 1995 report of the Bureau of Labor Statistics revealed that there were 705,800 cases of lost work days that were attributed to overexertion or pain from repetitive motion (1). In addition, it has been estimated that the costs associated with lost work days and compensation claims associated with such disorders range from $13 billion to $20 billion each year (2,3). Although growing more rapidly than other types of musculoskeletal disorder, repetitive motion disorders still represent a small minority of occupational musculoskeletal disorders. Moreover, costs are attributable not only to lost work days but also to the indemnity paid for temporary and permanent disability, medical costs designed to restore preinjury function, and system-friction costs (despite the "no-fault" nature of the vast majority of administrative workers' compensation systems). These costs are continuing to escalate at an alarming rate. In addition, recent trends in health care policy and the demand for improved allocation of health resources have placed a great deal of pressure on health care professionals to provide the most cost-effective evaluation and treatment for these disorders, as well as to validate treatment outcomes. Indeed, treatment-outcome monitoring has assumed a new importance in medicine. Such outcome monitoring is particularly vital in musculoskeletal disorder care because it is currently targeted for attention by health planners due to the high cost and perceived inefficient care.

WHAT WE NEED TO KNOW ABOUT WORK-RELATED MUSCULOSKELETAL DISORDERS

The critical nature of occupational musculoskeletal disorders is further highlighted by the fact that in 1998 the National Institutes of Health (NIH) requested that the National Academy of Sciences/National Research Council convene a panel of experts (from the fields of orthopedic surgery, occupational medicine, epidemiology, human factors and ergonomics, statistics, and risk-assessment analysis) to carefully examine seven major questions raised by the U.S. Congress concerning occupational musculoskeletal disorders (4):

- Which conditions affecting humans are considered to be work-related musculoskeletal disorders?
- What is the status of medical science with respect to the diagnosis and classification of such disorders?
- What is the state of scientific knowledge, characterized by the degree of certainty or lack thereof, with regard to occupational and nonoccupational activities causing such conditions?
- What is the relative contribution of any causal factors identified in the literature to the development of such conditions in (a) the general population, (b) specific industries, and (c) specific occupational groups?
- What is the incidence of such conditions in (a) the general population, (b) specific industries, and (c) specific occupational groups?

- Does the literature reveal any specific guidance to prevent the development of such conditions in (a) the general population, (b) specific industries, and (c) specific occupational groups?
- What scientific questions remain unanswered and may require further research to determine which occupational activities in which specific industries cause or contribute to work-related musculoskeletal disorders?

As is readily apparent, either there remains a significant lack of information regarding occupational musculoskeletal injuries, or data have not recently been concisely summarized or categorized to permit evidence-based conclusions and solutions. The concern at the national level, combined with the dramatic changes in the medical/health care environment occurring in this country, dictates the importance of developing an updated, state of the art, scientific, and clinically meaningful approach to the many important issues that health care providers need to be aware of when dealing with work-related musculoskeletal disorders.

As further evidence of the growing worldwide concern about musculoskeletal disorders, an inaugural consensus meeting was convened in April 1998 by the World Health Organization in Sweden (5). During this conference, a large number of international scientific journals and societies were represented in discussing the significant problem of musculoskeletal disorders and the burden on patients and society that it has created. Major concerns included the following:

- Back pain as the second leading cause of sick leave,
- Joint diseases accounting for 50% of all chronic conditions in patients 65 years and older,
- Anticipation that 25% of health care expenditures in developing countries will be spent on musculoskeletal trauma-related care by the year 2010.

This recognition prompted a proposal for declaring the years 2000 to 2010 as the

"Decade of the Bone and Joint System." This initiative was based on the earlier successful project declaring the decade 1990 to 2000 as the "Decade of the Brain." On a worldwide basis, this project led to increased awareness of the impact of brain disorders and to significant scientific achievements. It is hoped that the musculoskeletal decade will similarly raise awareness and result in improvement in health-related quality of life for individuals with bone and soft tissue disorders throughout the world. Thus, the problem of occupational musculoskeletal disorders is perceived as extremely significant at both the national and international level.

ORGANIZATION OF THIS BOOK

The chapters in this text have been designed to provide a comprehensive reference for health care providers on these prevalent occupational musculoskeletal disorders, as well as for health care administrators, lawyers, insurance carriers, and other stakeholders, who all interface with the issues of occupational injury and medicine. The most recent cutting-edge material in the areas of occupational musculoskeletal medicine is presented. As will become evident, many factors can affect the etiology, progression, and chronicity of occupational musculoskeletal disorders. These include factors such as workplace characteristics (physical work factors, equipment, and other work-environment risk factors), work organizational factors, physical and psychologic factors of individuals, and social factors (Fig. 1). All of these potentially important contributory factors are reviewed in this text. Moreover, one of the major threads running through the fabric of this volume is the importance of emphasizing the utilization of objectively quantified functional outcomes (e.g., return to work, subsequent health care utilization, etc.) to address cost-effectiveness issues, which remain an important issue in health care policy today. In addition, the long

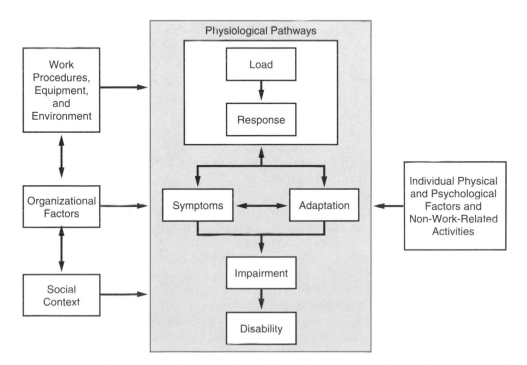

FIG. 1. A conceptual framework of proposed physiological pathways and factors that may potentially contribute to musculoskeletal disorders. (From ref. 4, with permission.)

neglected significance of psychosocial factors in the evaluation, treatment, and prevention of these disorders is emphasized.

Several important dimensions are to be considered in occupational musculoskeletal disorders. The major parts of this book cover these dimensions in separate sections. In Part I, epidemiologic perspectives of these disorders are reviewed, as well as the importance of a biopsychosocial approach to develop a more comprehensive understanding of the processes of pain perception and disability/illness development. The biopsychosocial-model approach views dysfunction and occupational illness as a complex interaction of biologic, psychologic, and social variables (6). The diversity of disability/illness expression (including its severity, duration, and consequences for an individual) is accounted for by the complex interrelationships among many factors: host, predisposition, physiology, psychology (e.g., genetic and prior learning experiences), and the sociocultural contexts that help shape a person's perceptions and reactions to an adverse external or internal environment. According to this model, now being widely embraced by the medical community, occupational disability cannot be narrowly conceptualized and treated by merely physicochemical techniques. This concept leads in directions different from the high-technology public fascination with the products and delivery system of the medical/industrial complex. Instead, the biopsychosocial model involves prevention, evaluation, and treatment that fall into the realm of an older type of medicine: one of human interaction, education and counseling, personal responsibility, and plain detective work. The nuances of different workers' compensation systems based on a Bismarckian model are carefully discussed, and in these discussions the reader is made aware of the compromise at the core of all of these systems, that is, the employer's relief from the obligation for negligence in the workplace in return for "no-fault" wage replacement, medical benefits, and permanent injury or death compensation. These systems provide predictability but lead

to a series of both mutual and adversarial interests that drastically changes the medical care paradigm for the 4% to 5% of total medical care provided under these systems. Differing perspectives of injured workers and employers, as well as their representatives and health care providers, are presented in this section of the volume. The various incentives and disincentives for different behaviors are highlighted by the authors.

The above leads naturally into a discussion of practical issues, such as how to better navigate through the managed care system in the treatment of these disorders—practical issues of utmost interest to clinical practitioners. In Part II, a review of the anatomy, physiology, and biomechanics of the major musculoskeletal systems is presented. Indeed, much research is needed concerning biologic responses of tissues and the musculoskeletal system to biomechanical stressors, as well as a better understanding of the basic biomechanics of work stressors that lead to excessive internal loads. The most recent medical advances in understanding these systems are reviewed. A discussion of these factors leads directly into Part III, which provides a summary of some of the most recently developed and potentially efficacious approaches to prevention. Intervention to prevent or mitigate occupational musculoskeletal disorders is a very important issue because of the obvious implications for financial savings that would occur by preventing chronicity. Issues such as preemployment screening, fitness programs to prevent injury, workplace safety, and ergonomic issues are highlighted. Indeed, in the Human Capital Initiative Coordinating Committee (7) report, sponsored by the NIH, a high priority area of clinical research and practice to be supported by the NIH is the early detection and prevention of chronic disability, especially including musculoskeletal disorders.

Part IV of this volume is dedicated to issues involved in acute injuries, followed by postacute disorders (Part V) and finally chronic disorders (Part VI). In each of these three parts, diagnostic clarity through objective testing is highlighted. Diagnostic uncertainty and controversy are discussed in detail relative to each of the anatomic areas. Evidence for certain treatments and areas where little evidence exists are covered in detail. Advancing chronicity as a factor in developing physiologic change is explained, along with the quantification of function needed to help clinicians identify deconditioning and physical inhibition. In addition, the most recent significant advances in the assessment of psychosocial issues involved in disabling musculoskeletal disorders, and how these issues might be integrated into the overall treatment process, are delineated. Moreover, recent novel work on surgical decision-making processes, as well as a review of new alternative interventions, is presented. It is our belief that it is important for clinicians working with musculoskeletal-disorder patients to be aware of both basic and applied science, as well as the various methodologies for evaluating the efficacy of assessment and treatment outcomes, to better understand the best way of dealing with the costly musculoskeletal-disorder crisis occurring in this country, as well as in the rest of the world.

FOOD-FOR-THOUGHT ISSUES

Finally, there are other important issues that readers should consider when reviewing the various topics presented here. These issues, which require additional future clinical research, include the following:

- Is there a solution for the inherent adversarial nature of the workers' compensation system, or might it be better to scrap it entirely for a concept of "24-hour coverage" that separates short- and long-term disability coverage from medical treatment?
- What proof is there of the relationships between loading or repetitive motion and injury? Do biomechanical defects such as posttraumatic arthritis or scar tissue cause pain in all circumstances, and, if not, what are the cofactors?
- How can one best develop and evaluate prevention strategies for quantifying risks in a multifactorial injury model?

- Should the emphasis in acute injury be on pain relief or recovery of function?
- How does strategy change when pain persists beyond a normal "healing period" and/or patients appear to resist recovery?
- How can we improve diagnostic specificity?
- Should we target interventional treatments based on known mechanisms or newer outcomes evidence?
- Should rehabilitation be oriented toward socioeconomic outcomes, such as return to work, or toward patient satisfaction and pain relief, when those goals may be at odds with one another?
- Should chronicity be the primary defining factor for treatment determinations in occupational musculoskeletal disorders as suggested by the Quebec Task Force a decade ago, or are other factors important in determining eligibility for surgical, interventional, or rehabilitation approaches?
- What happens to patients who fail to respond to all treatments? Should they become lifelong financial dependents on a disability welfare system that both takes their productivity away from society and compensates them for it? Should resources for "permanent" musculoskeletal disability be equivalent to those for more defined disabilities, or for those who have retired after a lifetime of work?
- What is the role of psychologic assessment in understanding the multivariate nature of musculoskeletal disorders? Is mental health assessment and treatment, as part of the rehabilitation process, more deserving of reimbursement than in general health?
- What are the best methods for determining permanent impairment and disability, and should they be compensated through a "no-fault" or a tort system?
- What is the role of vocational rehabilitation and retraining in occupational musculoskeletal disorders? Is it possible to develop effective musculoskeletal treatment guidelines? What is the role for managed care in medical delivery in occupational injury?

• How does one define an ideal system? What role do system administrators play in simplifying or complicating tasks and behaviors of the other stakeholders?

Insofar as possible, we have tried to bring together an international team of experts familiar not only with the system of managing occupational musculoskeletal disorders in the United States but also with international perspectives. The multidisciplinary viewpoints of medical providers and nonmedical specialists lead to a comprehensive yet concise perspective on this growing medical and socioeconomic crisis. Although the authors present the answers as we know them today, they all raise as many questions as they answer. However, once the human mind is focused on in-depth analysis of a problem, who can say how quickly the solutions will follow? Indeed, we must have continued exposure to *both* empiric research data/information and clinical experience to guide the significant advancement of knowledge of a phenomenon such as occupational musculoskeletal disorders. The subsequent chapters of this book were written by an array of professionals who provide both and have helped us better grasp the importance of the complexity often inherent in taking an appropriate biopsychosocial approach to understanding medical pain disabilities such as oc-cupational musculoskeletal disorders. Rather than trying to overly simplify the gestalt of such disorders by taking a purely biomechanical or psychochemical orientation, we must embrace a more comprehensive perspective. Thus, as noted by Albert Einstein: "Everything should be made as simple as possible, but not simpler." A biopsychosocial approach embraces this maxim.

REFERENCES

1. Bureau of Labor Statistics. *Workplace injuries and illnesses in 1994.* Washington, DC: U.S. Department of Labor, 1995. U.S. Department of Labor publication 95-508.
2. AFL-CIO. *Stop the pain.* Washington, DC: AFL-CIO, 1997.
3. U.S. Department of Health and Human Services, Public Health Service, Centers for Disease Control and Prevention, National Institute for Occupational Safety and Health. Washington, DC: Department of Health and Human Services, 1996. National Institute for Occupational Safety and Health publication 96-115.
4. National Research Council. *Work-related musculoskeletal disorders:* a review of the evidence. Washington, DC: National Academy Press, 1998.
5. Bone and joint decade 2000–2010. *Acta Orthop Scand* 1998;69:219–220.
6. Turk DC. Biopsychosocial perspective on chronic pain. In: Gatchel RJ, Turk DC, eds. *Psychological approaches to pain management:* a practitioner's handbook. New York: Guilford Publications, 1996, pp. 3–32.
7. Human Capital Initiative Coordinating Committee. *Doing the right thing:* a research plan for healthy living. Washington, DC: American Psychological Association.

Occupational Musculoskeletal Disorders
edited by T. G. Mayer, R. J. Gatchel, and P. B. Polatin.
Lippincott Williams & Wilkins, Philadelphia © 2000.

2

Workers' Compensation Concepts and Economics

Richard J. Butler

Industrial Relations Center, University of Minnesota, Minneapolis, Minnesota 55455

WORKERS' COMPENSATION AND ACCIDENT COSTS

Workers' compensation laws in each state require employers to provide cash benefits, medical care, and rehabilitation services to their employees for injury or illness arising out of or in the course of employment. Provision of coverage is mandatory in 48 states. In the other two states (New Jersey and Texas), employers opting out of the workers' compensation system forgo their right to common defenses against negligence, and their potential liability is not limited, as it is for employers choosing coverage. As a consequence, relatively few employers opt out of the workers' compensation system.[1] The "no-fault" trade-off in workers' compensation is that employers provide insurance coverage in exchange for which employees agree to forgo their rights to sue when such injuries occur. The cash payment for lost wages is not "full" in the sense of replacing all lost wages. Typically, two-thirds of weekly wages are replaced for those whose wages are between specific minimum and maximum amounts. These minimums and maximums, as well as the waiting periods (the number of days since the injury that must elapse before a worker is eligible to receive cash benefits for lost wages), are determined separately in each state.

A primary objective of workers' compensation laws is the efficiency objective of reducing accident costs, broadly defined. Accident costs include the following:

- Losses suffered by the victims of accidents, both monetary losses (in particular, loss of income, medical expenses, and rehabilitation expenses) and nonmonetary losses (i.e., pain and suffering, loss of enjoyment of life, etc.);
- Effect of the accident on workplace productivity (the production process may slow down or stop because of the injury; skilled labor that is difficult to replace may be unavailable because of the injury, etc.);
- Costs incurred to prevent accidents, including money spent on accident prevention and output forgone in order to reduce the risk of accidents;
- Cost of administering workers' compensation laws, including the costs incurred by all participants in that system.

Many workers' compensation laws and institutions can be viewed as attempts to achieve economic efficiency by minimizing the sum of these costs as the workers' compensation system has evolved over time. Examples of some of these cost-minimizing insurance arrangements include waiting periods, partial reim-

---

[1] While virtually no employers in New Jersey opt out of the workers' compensation system, almost 40% of Texas employers (mostly smaller employers) opt out of workers' compensation. For an analysis of the Texas market, including a comparison of costs between the two systems in Texas, see Butler (1).

bursement for wage loss, and experience rating of the firm so as to link injury costs with insurance costs. These costs are discussed below.

Cost minimization in the workers' compensation system is complex, since a reduction in one type of cost can often only be made by increasing other types of cost. Cash benefits (called *indemnity payments* in the workers' compensation system) that replaced all of an injured worker's lost wages would achieve the objective of minimizing wage loss to the worker but would likely affect many workers' incentives to return to work as soon as they were able. Hence, the increase in indemnity payment may also increase the duration of claims and hence the cost of insurance and productivity losses. So it is necessary to trade one type of cost off against others. Yet many of these costs are difficult to measure, and even where the data exist to measure them, relatively little reliable research has been done on the nature tradeoffs. This research is reviewed below.

Workers' compensation law is complex. While there is substantial variation in benefits among states, workers' compensation laws in all states establish liabilities among the parties. The allocation of these liabilities is most efficient when it (a) creates appropriate incentives for those involved in the workers' compensation program, (b) allocates the risk to those who are most willing and able to bear it, and (c) results in lower transactions costs. *Transactions costs* are the resources forgone in order to administer the *liability rules* in workers' compensation. Transactions costs therefore include the value of all time and goods devoted to establishing, interpreting, administering, and enforcing the (legal, administrative, and "common practice") laws. For example, most legal expenses represent transactions costs of administering the system of liability rules.

Liability laws allocate specified accident costs. For example, employers are required to provide workers' compensation claimants with two-thirds of their wages lost due to a workplace injury (subject to a waiting period and statewide maximum and minimum payments). In workers' compensation, the liability is conditional: The injury must be employment-related. Specifically, to be compensable, the injury must arise out of and in the course of work. This work-related requirement generates most of the legal controversies in workers' compensation: Is the back pain or sprained ankle really the result of working at the current worksite? Is a given "cumulative trauma" or mental stress claim really work-related?

LIABILITY RULES AFFECT BEHAVIOR

People vary in their potential to take action affecting accidents. Workers and firms make decisions and take action that affect accident risk. For example, workers' may choose not to use safety devices and procedures provided by employers, and employers may choose not to purchase safety devices if they do not perceive them to be cost-effective.

Sometimes, only one party can influence the risk of an accident's occurring: A self-employed professional working out of his or her own home controls the accident risk that he or she faces, for example. In workers' compensation, however, usually both the worker and the firm can take steps to reduce the risk of accident. This situation, known as *bilateral precaution*, is the most difficult to address through liability rules. Because both parties can affect risk and changes that improve the allocation of risk for one party usually make it worse for the other party, empiric research is necessary to help define an optimal workers' compensation policy.

Hence, in some workplaces, employees may be more able to take precaution against accidents than firms. Whether or not they take appropriate precaution will, however, depend on the incentives that they have to do so, including the extent to which they will bear the cost of failing to take care. This is one reason that workers' compensation benefits do not fully replace lost wages. Since a claimant bears some of the lost-wage costs, he or she has a greater incentive to take care before an accident occurs and to return to work once an accident has taken place. Incentives are important because return-to-work capability for many workers' compensation claimants is difficult to observe directly—sometimes the injured worker knows more about his or her health condition than does the firm or even the treating physician. The extent of back pain, for example, is generally accessed through the worker's self-report of pain.

A socially efficient liability law satisfies the marginal-expenditure-equals-marginal-cost rule: If an additional dollar of safety effort results in more benefits than costs, then the dollar so spent increases social welfare. In other words, keep on spending as long as the additional benefits exceed the additional costs. Expenditures on safety precautions should proceed until the additional benefits no longer exceed the additional costs, that is, until the point at which additional benefits (or marginal benefits) just equal additional costs (or marginal costs).

The marginal-cost-equals-marginal-benefit rule has a corollary: If $100 in accident costs can be saved by providing either safety training at $75 or better equipment at $110, then safety training should be provided because the marginal benefit, namely the $100 reduction in costs, is greater than the marginal cost ($75) (whereas the marginal cost of the equipment is greater than the marginal benefit and hence should not be employed). The efficient outcome is to use the least-cost means available to avoid the liability costs. An important

economic result known as the *Coase theorem* says that if bargaining between a firm and its workers were costless and everyone had full information concerning accident risk, then the efficient level of safety would be achieved regardless of liability rules. The Coase theorem is illustrated in Table 1 with reference to the safety example.

In Table 1, the effect of different liability arrangements on the optimal provision of safety is examined: In cases 1 and 3, the worker is the least-cost safety provider, and in cases 2 and 4 the firm is the least-cost safety provider. For all the examples in Table 1, it is assumed that taking care on the part of the worker or providing a safety device on the part of the firm reduces accident costs equally (by $10 in each case). Hence, the optimal outcome in case 1 and 3 is to have the worker take care (so the marginal cost of safety prevention is less than the marginal gain), while in cases 2 and 4 the optimal safety outcome is to have the firm provide the safety device.

With or without bargaining, the optimal safety outcome is achieved in cases 1 and 4 because the least-cost safety provider also happens to be liable for the accident costs. Without bargaining, in cases 2 and 3, the accident would occur, even though it would be possible to (cost-) effectively prevent the accident. The problem in cases 2 and 3 is that the party that is liable is not the least-cost safety provider: In case 2, for example, the worker is liable for the injury and can only prevent it if he or she takes care. In case 2, taking care is

TABLE 1. *Efficient safety precautions and the Coase theorem*

Case	Liability rule A: worker is liable for accident costs		Liability rule B: firm is liable for accident costs	
	1	2	3	4
Outcomes when	Worker has least cost	Firm has least cost	Worker has least cost	Firm has least cost
Worker takes care	$8	$12	$8	$12
Firm provides device	$12	$8	$12	$8
Outcome when no bargaining allowed	Worker will take care	No care—accident	No device—accident	Firm provides device
Outcome when bargaining allowed	Bargaining not necessary	Worker pays firm between $8 and $10 to provide device	Firm pays worker between $8 and $10 to take care	Bargaining not necessary

assumed to cost $12, which is more than the cost of the accident. Hence, care is not taken, and the accident occurs. For an analogous reason, the firm does not provide the safety device in case 3, and the accident occurs, since bargaining between the firm and worker is not allowed.

Bargaining changes the outcomes. In case 2, the worker is liable for $10 in accident costs but finds that he or she cannot cost-effectively take care: Taking care costs more than the cost of the accident. But the worker could offer the firm $9 if the safety device is installed. This saves the worker money because, instead of the $10 in accident costs, the worker now has to pay the firm only $9, and the accident is prevented. The firm is glad to take the $9 because that is a dollar more than it costs to provide the safety device. In fact, the worker could offer any amount between $8 and $10, and both the worker and the firm would be better off having the worker pay the firm to install the safety device. Moreover, the optimal safety outcome given the costs—namely, the installation of the safety device—would occur, even though the high-cost safety provider is liable.

Similarly, in case 3, even if the high-cost provider (the firm) is liable for the accident costs, the firm will pay the worker between $8 and $10 for the worker to take care. Again, this makes both the firm and the worker better off. Thus, bargaining between the firm and the worker ensures that the optimal result is achieved: The low-cost provider prevents the accident. This is the Coase theorem.

The Coase theorem has implications for optimal safety outcomes even where bargaining is so difficult that side deals like those described immediately above cannot be made: Efficient safety outcomes can be achieved by assigning the liability to the part that can prevent accidents at least costs. Pre–workers' compensation liability laws, the common law, has been interpreted to have operated in roughly this way. Under common law, the duty of employers was to provide their employees the safety that a prudent person would provide. This meant providing appropriate tools for the work, safety rules, and qualified coworkers.

However, even when employers did not meet these standards, they would not be considered negligent if they could claim one of three defenses:

- Fellow-servant defense: The employer was not liable if the injury was caused by a fellow worker;
- Assumption-of-risk defense: The employer was not liable if the workplace was known to be especially risky, and the worker took a job despite this knowledge;
- Contributory-negligent defense: The employer was not liable if the worker could have avoided the consequences of the accident by taking ordinary precautions.

These common law defenses can be viewed as an attempt to assign liability on the basis of the Coasian least-cost safety-provider rule discussed above. Such an interpretation is offered by Richard Posner (2):

> The fellow-servant rule...provides, in principle at least, a powerful instrument for industrial safety when combined with the rule making the employer liable for injuries inflicted on an employee through the negligence of a fellow employee if the employer was on notice of the fellow employee's habitual neglect or incompetence. The effect of the two rules [the fellow-servant rule plus the duty to provide qualified coworkers] is to give employees a strong incentive to report careless fellow workers to their supervisors [since presumably they can do so at less cost].

Posner argued that the contributory-negligence rule more directly encourages those who can most cheaply provide safety with an incentive to do so. He suggested that the assumption-of-risk rule is to allow those workers with greater tastes for risk the chance to market those tastes.

A substantial downside to the common law environment, however, was that the application of these principles in real life meant that juries were often left with the task of interpreting the law in specific situations. The transaction costs from this system, namely, the resources devoted to resolving legal disputes, were relatively high. To reduce those costs, the "no-fault" tradeoff discussed earlier was established when workers' compensation laws were passed at the beginning of the twentieth century: All medical care and limited, lost-work time disability payments were provided by the firm to the worker, in exchange for which these payments became the worker's exclusive remedy—that is, a worker could no longer sue the firm for additional payments. The determination of fault was no longer relevant; the accident need only have occurred on the job and be work-related. For example, workers would receive roughly two-thirds of their lost wages (subject to a maximum benefit) whether or not they "caused" the accident, but they could no longer sue their employer for additional compensation for pain and suffering even if the employer was wholly at fault.

PASSING THE COSTS ALONG: BENEFIT COSTS AND THE COST OF RISK

Workers' compensation that the law provides made employers strictly liable (i.e., liable without proof of fault) for all medical costs and some of the lost-wage costs associated with workplace accidents. That is, the law assigns the risk and costs of workplace accidents initially to employers. Employers have three ways to satisfy their obligation to provide for workers' compensation coverage: They may self-insure if they are large enough; They may buy insurance from private insurance carriers; They may buy insurance from a state fund.

The cost of the liability is passed on by the insurance contract, the premium on average being equal to the actuarial cost of the liability plus administrative expenses.

Since an insurer has no direct control over the risk, several mechanisms have been put in place to give firms an incentive to monitor workers' compensation costs, as well as allocating the cost of workplace injuries through their pricing mechanisms. These pricing mechanisms include the following:

- Partial coverage: Deductible insurance policies, in which employers pay the first $250,000 of claims out of their own expenses, are a popular recent example;
- Risk categorization: Employers are lumped together according to their risks, and insurance rates are set within each group, based on a group's historical costs;
- Experience rating: An individual firm's insurance premium is adjusted upward or downward, depending on whether its costs are lower or higher than its risk groups' costs.

Experience rating—required for larger firms—was especially designed to provide firms with incentives to increase workplace safety as a means of lowering their insurance costs. Experience rating remains controversial with the labor movement because it is believed that it provides firms with an incentive not so much to improve safety as to fight (legitimate) claims. Although the evidence is somewhat mixed, on net it appears that experience rating (and insurance pricing mechanisms in workers' compensation generally) has effectively contributed to greater workplace safety over time (3). Small firms that are not experience-rated have insurance premiums that depend only on their groups' average costs and not directly on their own individual safety efforts.

Besides these three traditional methods for providing incentives to firms, an insurer may also require additional precautions to be taken by an employer and condition the firm's insurance premiums on meeting such requirements. For example, it is not uncommon for an insurer to provide some lost prevention services with the workers' compensation insurance policy. An insurer may also have informal medical guidelines or policies that the firm is suggested to follow. An insurer may provide safety advice and may monitor the employer's compliance with these and other practices specified in the insurance policy.

Firms can pass some of their workers' compensation liability cost on to employees (through lower wages, see Chelius and Burton [4]). In a competitive market for labor with full information about risks and costs, this ability to pass on some workers' compensation costs does not affect a firm's incentives to provide safety, following the same line of argument developed for the Coase theorem above. The firm's incentives to provide safety are reduced only to the extent that risk (rather than cost) is passed on to some other party. The evidence reviewed in Chelius and Burton (4), though not unambiguous in terms of the magnitude of the effect, suggests that a substantial proportion of the cost of the program is shifted onto the workers.

Shifting of costs is not just a one-way street, however. Some workers' costs associated with their *residual risk* (not covered by the workers' compensation benefit structure) are shifted back onto the firm. The workers' compensation system is designed so that the workers bear some of the risks of the accident. There is a waiting period (usually 3 to 7 days, depending on the state) during which no lost-wage payments are received. Once disability payments begin, only a fraction of lost wages is reimbursed, and there are no payments for pain or suffering. For the family of a fatally injured worker, the weekly survivor benefits are usually the same or less than the benefits to a temporarily injured worker, are often of limited duration, and are frequently offset by social security benefits. This means that workers retain some of the risk of workplace injuries, even with workers' compensation.

The lost-wage risk that injured workers retain after they receive their workers' compensation benefits varies by state because of the differences in waiting periods, maximum and minimum benefits, and claim duration caps. The risk also varies within a state from employer to employer. Some workplaces are much safer than others. Given two otherwise equal employment opportunities, an informed worker would demand higher compensation from the employer at the riskier workplace. This extra pay for extra workplace risk is called the *compensating wage premium for risk*. There is good evidence that compensating wages for injury risk exists, especially for fatal injury risk, although compensation may

or may not be fully adequate.[2] Since providing a riskier workplace leads to higher wage demands (or a lower quality of worker, or both), the firm has an incentive to reduce accident risk to minimize the compensating wage premium. In this sense, some of the cost of a worker's residual risk under the workers' compensation system is passed back to the employer in the form of higher wages.

The workplace-risk exposure of workers' and the firm affects their behavior. In a fully competitive, fully informed, costless-bargaining Coase world, the initial assignment of liability will not matter in terms of the optimal levels of safety. In this case, the cost-effective outcomes are reached because the least-cost provider of safety will have an incentive to take care either because they are liable themselves for the risk or because those who are liable will bargain with them to take the appropriate behavior. In the workplace, bargaining costs between workers' and firms (who already bargain over wages) may be low enough to achieve an efficient (Coase) outcome. But, especially for medium sized and larger firms, they are not insignificant, and there may still be large enough bargaining costs to preclude the Coase outcomes. So rather than assign the workplace risks solely to either firms or workers, the workers' compensation solution is to make both employers and employees bear some of the risk of the accidents, while reducing the legal (transaction) costs by explicitly indicating which costs are borne by which party, regardless of fault.

MORAL HAZARD: BEHAVIOR CHANGES WITH INSURANCE COVERAGE

There is some litigation in workers' compensation, including issues involving the work origins of an injury or "occupational" illness and the determination of permanent-

---

[2]Since the effective risk, after workers' compensation payment, is much higher for fatal than for nonfatal injuries, it is not surprising that the strongest evidence on compensating wages is for fatal injury risk. For evidence on compensating-wage mechanisms and especially compensating differentials for fatal injuries, see Moore and Viscusi (5).

impairment benefits. However, the low legal (transaction) costs (relative to a tort system in which an employee would have to sue the firm for each workplace-injury claim) have long been recognized as one of the main virtues of the workers' compensation system. This virtue is in better repair in some states than in others because of differences in ambiguity of some of the liability rules associated with workplace injuries and diseases.

Another virtue of the workers' compensation system, aside from the historically low level of attorney involvement, is that it is insurance: Workers enjoy the reduction in risk associated with workplace-injury insurance. Risk-averse workers are better off with insurance, even when it reduces their expected total compensation, as long as the reduction in risk compensates workers for the lowered average level of compensation. However, after the initiation of an insurance plan, workers or health care providers may change their behavior for personal gain. Such changes in behavior are known as moral hazard, and examples of it were mentioned above.

Moral hazard is a technical term used in the economics of insurance and health care to indicate that workers (or firms or health care providers) can change the size or probability of a loss by changing their behavior relative to a situation in which there was no insurance coverage. Workers, for example, may change their safety precautions or their reported health status as insurance coverage changes. This can occur in a number of different ways. Workers' compensation law specifies that the only disabilities covered are those arising from injuries while on the job. Hence, a worker may claim that a given condition arose from a job injury and seek temporary total-disability benefits because his or her real health condition (broadly defined) does not qualify as a workers' compensation claim. Or, perhaps, a worker has a recurring health condition, such as low back pain, that, in the absence of insurance, he or she has simply tolerated because treatment would impose personal costs. When insured, however, the worker may choose not to work and incur

health services cost and draw disability because others are paying much or all of the bill. An extreme case of behavioral change might be overt fraud in which a worker facing a pending layoff claims injury benefits when no injury or health condition was incurred either on or off the job.

The workers' compensation system has long recognized that moral hazard is potentially costly. If firms could make the health-benefits claim process entirely "objective" such that participants in the insurance contract would not change their behavior, they would do so. But completely monitoring the behavior of all participants in an insurance contract is a costly activity, with the costs of such monitoring generally exceeding the benefits. Workers and health care providers know this, and because they often have some latitude to change their behavior to enhance their short-run well-being under the workers' compensation system, some will do so. Therefore, the root of the moral-hazard problem is insurance contracts that cannot preclude such behavior, often because of an information asymmetry among workers, health care providers, and employers that makes it impossible to monitor all the participants in the system. Bridging this information/monitoring gap is usually costly.

Hence, workers and health care providers can exploit this information asymmetry to their advantage. Such information asymmetries will always be a problem with insurance contracts, but opportunistic behavior will be greatest where the ability to monitor is most difficult and the benefits are the largest.

DEALING WITH MORAL HAZARD IN WORKERS' COMPENSATION

Insurers try to handle moral hazard by having workers (and firms) retain some of the accident risk either through partial insurance or experience rating. *Partial insurance* for employees means that not all of their workplace costs are reimbursed by insurance. There is a waiting period in all states before wage-loss benefits begin. Once they begin, they usually cover only two-thirds of the lost wages up to a maximum, and total benefits are often capped. For firms, partial insurance takes the form of new deductible policies in which they pay the first, usually large deductible before the insurer begins to pay the remaining costs. *Experience rating* is an adjustment to firms' insurance premiums made whenever their actual costs are better or worse than the expected group costs. The effect of experience rating can come in more than one form: Positively, if a firm increases its safety efforts as its insurance costs become aligned with its safety outcomes; or negatively, if the experience rating induces a firm to deny otherwise legitimate claims to save costs.

Again, there are always tradeoffs to be considered. Raising the replacement rate in workers' compensation increases its value as insurance to employees, but also increases the moral-hazard potential facing firms and workers. First-dollar medical coverage in workers' compensation makes it more likely that workers will seek medical care for their injuries (and hence perhaps reduce future medical costs), but it may increase utilization of medical services beyond the efficient point at which marginal cost equals marginal benefits, since the worker has no out-of-pocket expenses for medical services at the time that they are received. The marginal benefit to a worker of an extra x-ray examination or office visit will likely be less than the marginal cost that the firm pays for these. The form of medical reimbursement may affect doctors' behavior as well: Fee schedules may limit unit prices but result in greater quantities of health care services delivered; reimbursement on a capitation rather than a fee-for-service basis may result in more health conditions being classified as compensable under workers' compensation; and so on.

The size of the moral-hazard response is inferred from behavioral changes as system incentives change. The best evidence on these changes comes from analyses of how increases in statutory benefits change claim frequency and duration. In the absence of moral hazard, increases in benefits should affect neither claim frequency nor claim duration. Studies in workers' compensation that examine the impact of benefits on claims utilization have fallen into two groups:

- Examination of claimant behavior where responses are identified from benefit variations across individual observations: *wide-benefit-variation* studies such as those regressing claim duration on individual worker's expected benefits;
- Examination of claimant behavior where responses are identified by a before-and-after comparison from a single change in maximum benefits in a given state: *natural-experiment* studies.

The wide-benefit-variation type of study is by far the larger source of estimated workers' compensation benefits' effects.

Among studies that use the wide-benefit-variation approach, claim duration has been found to be positively correlated with benefit increases. This positive duration response has been estimated in studies employing individual insurance claim data (6–8), insurance data for individual firms (9), and sample survey data (10–12). In addition, claim frequency increases with higher benefits in studies using aggregate data (7,13–20), as well as those using microeconomic data (21–25).

Butler and Appel (26) showed that changes in the statutory maximum payment in recent years effectively account for all of the changes in the expected workers' compensation benefits. The natural-experiment studies have exploited the close relationship between workers' compensation statutory maximum payment and expected benefits to identify the benefits-utilization response. The focus of these articles is on claims within a single state, comparing average severity before and after a large benefit increase has been enacted. Natural-experiment studies are easy to present and interpret but have been limited to using insurance-claims data rather than information on individual workers. Hence, most have not been able to estimate changes in claim frequency or the average costs per worker as benefit maximums change.

Moreover, existing natural-experiment estimates of the benefit/duration response vary widely. Krueger (27), using data from Minnesota's workers' compensation system, found a very large positive response, as moral-hazard response would predict; but Currington (28), using data from New York, and Meyer et al. (29), using data from Kentucky and Michigan, found much smaller but still positive and statistically significant responses.

In a recent study using data from one type of worker for one firm, Butler et al. (30) reported that in states where benefits increased substantially, claim frequency and average cost rose, whereas in states where benefits decreased substantially, claim frequency and average cost fell. This suggests that moral-hazard responses are symmetric: Decreases in benefits lower frequency just as increases in benefits tend to raise frequency. The results were robust with respect to controls for other confounding influences, although the estimated claim duration response was relatively small.

Moral-hazard responses have been found for health care providers as well. Physicians are generally paid either on a fee-for-service basis if self-employed or by an employer such as a health maintenance organization (HMO). HMOs at the plan level have capitated payment programs and contract to meet all the health care needs of an individual (or family) for an annual fee. In the absence of a moral-hazard response, one would not expect to see any differences in the number of workers' compensation claims between employees covered by a HMO and those covered by fee-for-service physicians. The form of compensation of the treating physician (fee for service or capitated payment) is not likely to affect inherent risk in the workplace.

However, HMO physicians are differentially influenced by the fee-for-service payment practice of all workers' compensation programs. Fee-for-service doctors are paid the same for treating a broken bone arising from an accident at home as they are for the same type of fracture occurring on the job. The fact that the latter injury is compensable in the workers' compensation system makes no difference to them.[3] It does make a difference to an HMO, however, because treating an injury compensable under workers' compensation insurance represents a net increase in its income. Because the HMO is paid on a fee-for-service basis for workers' compensation injuries, on top of the capitation amount, it is financially better off if more treatments are classified as work-related.[4]

This suggests that doctors in HMOs have an incentive to classify workers' health conditions that might otherwise only be marginally work-related or nonwork-related as having arisen "in the course of or out of their employment"—and therefore compensable un-

---

[3] In fact, workers' compensation is viewed in some states as a more reliable and speedy form of coverage, and, to that extent, fee-for-service physicians would also have an incentive to classify as many health conditions as "possible" as workplace-related to qualify for workers' compensation. However, their incentives are certainly much weaker than physicians in HMOs. This implies that our estimates are lower bounds on the true effects that HMO doctors have on workers' compensation costs.

[4] These data on HMOs come from the national HMO census (see Butler et al. [32] for details). It includes only those HMOs licensed by the state or federal government and so excludes such groups as preferred provider organizations (PPOs), in which physicians accept discounted fees. Even so, HMOs vary widely in the way in which they reimburse physicians. However, even in "staff"-type HMOs, where physicians are employees who are not directly remunerated on a fee-for-service basis for treating work-related injuries, physicians may still have incentive to classify marginal cases as work-related. HMO management will wish to bill as many claims as possible to workers' compensation to increase revenues and may therefore pressure physicians to at least raise the issue of work-relatedness with their patients.

An important question is why employers do not make HMOs treat all sources of injuries for a fixed fee, regardless of work-relatedness. One answer is that workers' compensation laws in all states require fee-for-service reimbursement. Another answer is that many HMOs only reimburse for injuries and illnesses not covered by workers' compensation (and so contractual costs to the firm might be reduced as cost-shifting to workers' compensation increases). But in the presence of asymmetric information and higher reimbursement under workers' compensation than group health insurance, the incentives to encourage claim migration to workers' compensation will still be significant. Moreover, empiric results indicate that the consequence of this migration is not cost-neutral, because even if group health costs fall dollar for dollar with the increase in indemnity costs (and if this were the case, then there would be no incentive for claims migration), the amount of indemnity claims (i.e., lost work-time claims) has risen as HMOs have expanded.

der workers' compensation. This is especially true for "cumulative trauma" conditions, which may have a long latency period and be difficult to monitor as to whether or not they are work-related. Ducatman (31) was the first analyst to record and explain the fact that HMO-covered employees had higher workers' compensation costs than fee-for-service-covered employees. Ducatman reported on the per capita costs of federal civilian employees working at eight shipyards in 1983 and 1984, finding a strong positive correlation between average workers' compensation costs and the proportion of workers covered by an HMO. He suggested that fee-for-service payments made to HMO providers creates "a favorable climate for zealous attribution of health problems to workplace causes."

Butler et al. (32) reported that HMO coverage significantly increased workers' compensation costs, analyzing both aggregate state trends during the 1980s and individual companies. In particular, they found physician fees, price controls effects, and HMO enrollment effects indicate that there is also health care provider moral hazard. States with price controls on physicians services experienced 3.5% more workers' compensation medical claims (but not more group health medical claims) than states without such controls. Absent any change in health care provider behavior, effective price ceilings on workers' compensation treatments should have no effect on frequency but should lower medical claims severity. In fact, in multivariate analysis of medical claims severity, Butler et al. found that medical claims costs rise when there are controls on physician fees.

That severity and frequency are both higher in states with medical fee schedules suggests that physicians may be providing more complex procedures (33) or more frequent but lower duration modes of care. These "volume offsets" are discussed in Barer et al. (34) and Reinhardt (35). Roberts and Zonia (36) found that after workers' compensation medical fee schedules were implemented in Michigan, physicians provided more complex procedures in a shorter period of time, in accord

with the findings here.[5] That is, when physicians find their fees limited by law, they tend to increase the frequency of health care visits. They also found that workers' compensation medical claim frequency is 4% higher for HMO doctors, controlling for everything else, consistent with moral-hazard response.

One implication of these results is that not only should the number of medical claims filed increase with the expansion of HMOs but those medical claims should disproportionately fall into those categories that are most difficult to determine objectively. This expectation follows directly from the hypothesis that doctors in HMOs have an incentive to classify health conditions that might otherwise only be marginally work-related as compensable in workers' compensation, since this increases HMO revenue. This "work-related" reclassification is especially applicable for more subjective injuries, such as sprains and strains, whose work origin is difficult to ascertain, as well as for other so-called "cumulative trauma" diseases.

Indeed, during the 1980s when HMOs were expanding rapidly, the proportion of soft tissue injuries rose from 44.7% of all claims in 1980 to 50.6% of all claims in 1989. At the same time, the relative cost share attributable to soft tissue injuries rose from 41% to 48.8%. In a multivariate analysis of these trends using a 15-state national data base (with 400,000 claims), Butler et al. (39) were able to reject other explanations of the increase: Neither additional safety incentives nor the movement away from heavy manufac-

---

[5]This study differs from all previous studies because we employ individual data from a single firm operating in all 50 states, thus holding constant not only industry demand factors but also overall employee benefit alternatives and policies. Roberts and Zonia (36) examined data spanning several firms from a single insurer in Michigan in their unmatched before-and-after analysis. Pozzebon (37) and Boden and Fleischman (38) used data spanning several insurance carriers and several firms as well. The former two did not find any evidence that fee schedules lowered medical costs (indeed, Pozzebon found a positive effect similar to that in Butler et al. [32]), while the latter study pointed out many of the problems encountered when estimating fee schedule effects is attempted.

turing seems to account for the change. Instead, consistent with the results reported above for the other two samples, the expansion of HMOs has had a statistically positive impact on soft tissue injuries. Indeed, most of the 30% increase in the proportion of soft tissue injuries during the 1980s was the result of the expansion of HMOs.[6]

ECONOMIC RESEARCH FINDINGS BESIDES MORAL HAZARD

The empiric evidence cited above suggests that workers and health care providers are not passive with respect to the incentives generated by the workers' compensation system. Private practice and public policy in workers' compensation that ignore these responses—that assume physicians objectively treat well defined health conditions and injured workers appropriately respond to physicians' prescriptions regardless of the financial incentives of either the physicians or the workers—are bound to work imperfectly, at best.

A more appropriate framework (than that of passive participants) is the human-capital approach. In its labor-market context, *human capital* means the stock of potential productivity embodied in a worker. This stock is augmented by educational, training, and health investments that typically increase wages over the working life of an employee. Thus, investments in maintaining the health of a company's workforce and in preventing or curing workers' illnesses and injuries are potentially productivity-enhancing, and could be considered "value-added" to the extent that these investments achieve this goal. Skilled, productive employees are a firm's most valued asset, and the impact of workers' compensation on the value of those assets should be carefully considered. The discussion in this chapter argues that liability for risk and the incentives that workers' compensation generates affect behavior: They influence claims-filing by workers, as well as medical practice by health care providers. Workers' compensa-

tion should be aligned (and to a large extent it has been aligned) to promote and protect workers' human capital. Other research lessons from economic analyses would include the following:

1. *"Cumulative trauma" claims are different from other types of claims.* The workers' compensation system arose in response to injuries whose work origins were clear and undisputed: fractures, lacerations, amputations, and so on. In the last 20 years, the importance of these claims with well defined incidences has fallen as more and more "cumulative trauma" claims whose work origin is little understood (e.g., low back pain, carpal tunnel syndrome, etc.) have been filed (39). While claims for low back pain account for roughly one-third of workers' compensation disability costs, the work origin of such claims is still subject of considerable controversy. One of the most important concerns to come out of the American Academy of Orthopaedic Surgeons' (AAOS) workshop on musculoskeletal symptoms in the workplace (40) was that

> Terms such as "cumulative trauma," "repetitive trauma," "repetitive motion," and "repetitive strain injury" are medically meaningless; they suggest a work-caused injury, but frequently cannot be documented as such.

Not only are the work origins of claims involving "cumulative trauma" symptoms often subjective, such claims typically involve very different return-to-work outcomes than other types of workers' compensation claims. Johnson et al. (41) found that low-back and carpal-tunnel claimants were very much alike with respect to incentive response and socioeconomic profiles, but exhibit claim behaviors statistically distinct from those with other types of claims: "Cumulative trauma" claimants were more sensitive to economic incentives and job accommodations than other claimants and exhibited significantly different postinjury employment patterns than other claimants.

2. *Set the appropriate expectations: It is not a "disability;" it is a "temporary work intolerance."* Early in the communication

---

[6]Butler, Durbin, and Helvacian (39).

process, it is also imperative that appropriate expectations be set for the claim. Especially if an injury is severe or of the "cumulative-trauma" variety, employers do not want their valued workers viewing themselves as suddenly "disabled." In workers' minds at least, a disability may denote a serious impairment with some unknown "recovery" bar that they must leap over before they are ready to return to work. Rather, they have a temporary work intolerance. As the AAOS noted in its workshop report (40):

> Terminology pertaining to upper-extremity musculoskeletal pain should be changed. "Work-related upper extremity symptoms" should be replaced with "upper-extremity symptoms that interfere with activity." The second phrase does not indicate causality.

Treating physicians must effectively and sincerely communicate the importance of returning to productive activity as soon as possible, including being careful of the kind of language used to describe the injury symptoms.

3. *Return-to-work failures are frequently management failures.* Many workers regarded as return-to-work failures, added to workers' compensation and disability costs, are really management failures. Physicians need to be sensitive to this. Workers' responses to the symptoms that they experience are influenced as much by job satisfaction as by work capability. Here too incentives can play a role. If supervisors are compensated solely on the basis of payroll and output from their units (with no consideration of health-benefit and disability costs generated by their workers), then they have every incentive to channel their less productive or disgruntled workers into the disability system. Gardner and Butler (42) found in one company that workers with job productivity warnings (unrelated to health conditions) were twice as likely to subsequently end up in the disability program as those with no warnings.

4. *The first episode of workers' compensation is the most important.* Firms analyzing the return-to-work outcomes of their workers frequently find that some workers file disability claims at a much higher rate than others.

From a statistical perspective, many more claims are filed by relatively fewer workers than would be expected if such claims were strictly random events. Alternative explanations for the nonrandom nature of some claims include the following:

a. Some workers are intrinsically more inclined to use the system than others, perhaps due to differences in the employability values associated with terms such as *work ethic* and *company loyalty*.

b. Many injuries are residual in nature, involving several episodes.

c. Participation in the disability insurance system leads to a "claimant-learning" effect that increases the filing of subsequent claims quite apart from health status and the innate values of the employee.

To answer this question, Butler et al. (43) analyzed individual blue-collar employee data from a large private firm, using two analytic devices: (a) tests that analyze patterns of claim-filings and compare these with what would be expected if the filings were random or just a matter of individual employability values ("a" above) as opposed to the alternatives that there are residual health ("b" above) problems or claimant learning ("c" above); and (b) a standard analysis that regresses the number of claims made in a given year against several demographic, socioeconomic, and workplace characteristics, including indicators of whether claims had been made in prior years.

The pattern tests indicated that claims were neither purely random nor fully explained by the employability values of the workers, although employability values contributed much to return-to-work outcomes. Therefore, health status ("b" above) and/or claimant-learning effects ("c" above) obviously were also important contributors to the observed patterns. To distinguish between these two explanations, Butler et al. (43) looked at how often repeaters filed the same type of claim when there were only six broad injury types (back strains, other strains, cuts and lacerations, fractures, contusions and concussions, and all others). They found that roughly 25% of repeat claims were of the same type, suggesting that residual impairments do not explain the patterns of repeat claimants. If residual impairments associated with the same injury were driving these repeat claims, then a much higher percentage of repeat claimants would be expected to be reporting repeat health conditions. This suggests that claimant learning is very important in workers' compensation, so that past claims contribute significantly to the likelihood that future claims will be filed.

Statistical analysis confirms this and allows several important attributes of this process to be quantified. Not only does the previous filing of a claim significantly increase claim-filings in future years, but also the impact of that experience does not diminish for at least 5 full years after a claim is filed. Moreover, the effect of prior experience with the system is substantial: If a worker has filed two claims in any of the last 5 years, then he or she is twice as likely to file a claim this year as a year with no prior claimant experience. If the worker has filed claims in 4 of the last 5 years, he or she is three times as likely to file a claim. Moreover, economic incentives (as measured by workers' increased willingness to file claims when benefits rise) mattered a get deal to workers' filing their first claim, but once they had been in the system, economic incentives mattered a great deal less. This suggests that after a worker has been in the system for a while he or she is much less likely to respond to incentives to leave the system.

Butler et al. (43) also presented evidence indicating that the results presented here cannot simply be the result of residual impairments, that is, recurrence of the same injuries. The claimant-learning effect appears to be significant, and it also appears to diminish workers' responses to other economic incentives in the program.

These findings have important implications for employer and public policy. It would appear that resources invested in reducing claimant-learning effects, as well as improving the health status of employees, would have large payoffs in reducing insurance costs and productivity losses. This is especially true since claimant-learning effects not only are significant but also do not depreciate during the first 5 years after the claim. So early intervention in workers' first-claim experience offers the best opportunity to help steer them back into productive employment and maintain their human capital.

5. *Initial return to work is not necessarily a good measure of success for serious injuries.* Most return-to-work research in workers' compensation assumes that the initial return to work is the end of the limiting condition and that the initial return to work is the appropriate measure of program effectiveness. This is a reasonable assumption for lost-day claims for which there is no residual impairment, such as cuts, lacerations, and fractures. However, for many injuries and certainly for the most expensive injuries (the permanent partial-disability injuries), focusing exclusively on the initial return to work can be misleading.

Butler et al. (11) and Baldwin et al. (44) analyzed 10,500 workers with permanent partial impairments, finding that the effects of injuries on employment are more enduring than previously assumed. The rate of successful return-to-work employment, measured by the first return to work, was 85%, but fully 40% of those reporting an initial successful return ultimately reported being jobless because of their impairment; hence, the true rate of success over a longer time is only 50%. Moreover, the authors found that the variables that were statistically significant in explaining first return to work were not generally the same as the variables explaining ultimate employment outcomes. Clearly, the effectiveness of any return-to-work protocol for workers with serious injuries needs to follow them beyond the initial return to work.

REFERENCES

1. Butler RJ. Economic determinants of workers' compensation trends. *J Risk Insur* 1994;61: 383–401.

2. Posner R. A theory of negligence. *J Legal Studies* 1974;1:24–50.

3. Durbin D, Butler RJ. Prevention of disability from work-related sources. In: Thomason T, Burton JF, Hyatt D, eds. *Disability in the workplace: prevention, compensation, cure.* Madison, WI: Industrial Relations Research Association, 1998, pp. 63–86.

4. Chelius JR, Burton JF. Who actually pays for workers' compensation? *Workers' Comp Monitor* 1992;5:25–35.

5. Moore MJ, Viscusi WK. *Compensating mechanisms for job risk: wages, workers' compensation and product liability.* Princeton, NJ: Princeton University Press 1990.

6. Worrall JD, Butler RJ. Heterogeneity bias in the estimation of the determinants of workers' compensation loss distributions. In: Borba PS, Appel D, eds. *Benefits, costs, and cycles in workers' compensation.* Boston, MA: Kluwer Academic Publishers, 1990, pp. 23–44.

7. Butler RJ, Worrall JD. Workers' compensation: benefit and injury claims rates in the seventies. *Rev Econ Stat* 1983;65:580–589.

8. Butler RJ, Worrall JD. Gamma duration models with heterogeneity. *Rev Econ Stat* 1991;73:161–166.

9. Butler RJ, Worrall JD. Labor market theory and the distribution of workers' compensation losses. In: Appel D, Borba PS, eds. *Workers' compensation insurance pricing: current programs and proposed reforms.* Boston: Kluwer Academic Publishers, 1988, pp. 19–34.

10. Johnson WG, Ondrich JI. The duration of post-injury absences from work. *Rev Econ Stat* 1990;72:578–586.

11. Butler RJ, Johnson WG, Baldwin M. Managing work disability: why first return to work is not a measure of success. *Ind Labor Relat Rev* 1995;48:452–469.

12. Johnson WG, Butler RJ, Baldwin M. First spells of work absences among Ontario workers. In: Thomason T, Chaykowski R, eds. *Research in Canadian workers' compensation.* Kingston, Ontario: Industrial Relations Centre, Queen's University, 1995, pp. 72–84.

13. Butler RJ. Wage and injury rate response to shifting levels of workers' compensation. In: Worrall JD, ed. *Safety and the work force: incentives and disincentives in workers' compensation* Ithaca, NY: ILR Press, 1983, 61–86.

14. Chelius JR. The influence of workers' compensation on safety incentives. *Ind Labor Relat Rev* 1982;35:235–242.

15. Ruser JW. Workers' compensation insurance, experience rating, and occupational injuries. *Rand J Econ* 1985;16:487–503.

16. Worrall JD, Appel D. The wage replacement rate and benefit utilization in workers' compensation insurance. *J Risk Insur* 1982;49:361–371.

17. Lanoie P. Safety regulation and the risk of workplace accidents in Quebec. *South Econ J* 1992;58:950–965.

18. Lanoie P. The impact of occupational safety and health regulation on the risk of workplace accidents: Quebec, 1983–1987. *J Hum Resources.* 1992;27:643–660.

19. Butler RJ. Economic determinants of workers' compensation trends. *J Risk Insur* 1994;61:383–401.

20. Lanoie P, Streliski D. L'impact de la reglementation en matiere de sante et securite du travail sur le rissque d'accident au Quebec: de nouveaux resultats. *Ind Relat* 1996;51:778–801.

21. Leigh JP. Analysis of workers' compensation laws using data on individuals. *Ind Relat* 1985;24:247–256.

22. Krueger AB. Incentive effects of workers' compensation insurance, *J Public Econ* 1990;41:73–99.

23. Ruser JD. Workers' compensation and occupational injuries and illnesses. *J Labor Econ* 1991;9:325–350.

24. Dionne G, St-Michel P. Workers' compensation and moral hazard. *Rev Econ Stat* 1991;73:236–244.

25. Hirsch BT, Macpherson DA, Dumond JM. Workers' compensation recipiency in union and nonunion workplaces. *Ind Labor Relat Rev* 1997;50:213–236.

26. Butler RJ, Appel D. Benefit increases in workers' compensation. *South Econ J* 1991;56:594–606.

27. Krueger AB. *Workers' compensation insurance and the duration of workplace injuries.* Cambridge, MA: National Bureau of Economic Research, 1990. Working paper number 3253.

28. Currington WP. Compensation for permanent impairment and the duration of work absence. *J Hum Resources* 1994;29:888–910.

29. Meyer BD, Viscusi WK, Durbin DL. Workers' compensation and injury duration: Evidence from a Natural Experiment. *Am Econ Rev* 1995;85:322–340.

30. Butler RJ, Gardner HH, Gardner BD. Workers' compensation costs when maximum benefits change. *J Risk Uncertainty* 1997;15:259–269.

31. Ducatman AM. Workers' compensation cost-shifting: a unique concern of providers and purchasers of prepaid health care. *J Occup Med* 1986;28:11–16.

32. Butler RJ, Hartwig RP, Gardner HH. HMOs, moral hazard and cost shifting in workers' compensation. *J Health Econ* 1997;16:191–206.

33. Feldman R, Sloan F. Competition among physicians, revisited. *J Health Politics Policy Law* 1988;13:19–32.

34. Barer ML, Evans RL, Labelle RJ. Fee controls as cost control. *Milbank Q* 1988;66:1–64.

35. Reinhardt U. The theory of physician-induced demand: reflections after a decade, *J Health Econ* 1985; 4:187–193.

36. Roberts K, Zonia S. Workers' compensation cost containment and health care provider income maintenance strategies. *J Risk Insur* 1994;61:117–131.

37. Pozzebon S. Health care cost containment in workers' compensation. In: *Proceedings of the 1990 spring meeting of the Industrial Relations Research Association.* Madison, WI: Industrial Relations Research Association, 1991:546–550.

38. Boden L, Fleischman C. *Medical costs in workers' compensation: trends and interstate comparisons.* Cambridge, MA: Workers' Compensation Research Institute, 1994.

39. Butler RJ, Durbin DL, Helvacian NM. Increasing claims for soft tissue injuries in workers' compensation: cost shifting and moral hazard. *J Risk Uncertainty* 1996;13:73–87.

40. American Academy of Orthopaedic Surgeons. *Workshop on musculoskeletal symptoms in the workplace.* Rosemont, IL: AAOS Occupational Health Committee, 1997.

41. Johnson WG, Baldwin ML, Butler RJ. Back pain and work disability: the need for a new paradigm. *Ind Relat* 1998;37:9–34.

42. Gardner HH, Butler RJ. A human capital perspective for cumulative trauma disorders: moral hazard effects in disability compensation programs. In: Sauter SL,

Moon SD, eds. *Beyond biomechanics: psychosocial aspects of cumulative trauma disorders*. London: Taylor and Francis Publishers, 1996, pp. 231–250.

43. Butler RJ, Gardner BD, Gardner HH. *Claimant learning in workers' compensation:* do past claims cause future claims? Minneapolis, MN: Industrial Relations Center, University of Minnesota, 1997.

44. Baldwin M, Johnson WG, Butler RJ. The error of using returns to work to measure the outcomes of health care. *Am J Ind Med* 1996;29:632–641.

Occupational Musculoskeletal Disorders
edited by T. G. Mayer, R. J. Gatchel, and P. B. Polatin.
Lippincott Williams & Wilkins, Philadelphia © 2000.

3

Employers' and Insurers' Perception of Doctors: Societal Reactions and Consequences

Joseph P. Zeppieri

*Department of Orthopaedic Surgery/Plastic Hand, Lawrence and Memorial Hospital,
New London, Connecticut 06320*

William Haggar, president of the National Council of Compensation Insurers, referred to doctors and their patients as "parasites" when he spoke before the International Association of Industrial Accident Boards and Commissions (IAIABC) in 1991.

Society has had a love-hate relationship with its physicians throughout history. Hippocrates (460 to 370 BC) founded medicine with astute observations and interventions in the course of diseases and injuries. The Romans refused to recognize medicine as a profession for centuries after Hippocrates because "...they refused to pay fees to profiteers in order to save their own lives" (1). Archagathus was the first Greek physician who emigrated to Rome in 219 BC. Initially, his treatments were successful, and he was heralded and subsidized with public funds. He had some later failures with his surgery, and he and his profession became objects of loathing. Cato wrote:

> Greeks are a worthless people.... when that race gives us its literature it will corrupt all things, and even the more if it sends hither its physicians. They have conspired together to murder all foreigners with their physic, but this very thing they do for a fee, to gain credit and destroy us easily (1).

Voltaire personifies the dichotomy, saying at one time, "The art of medicine consists in keeping the patient entertained while his disease runs its inevitable course," and at another time:

> Men who are occupied in the restoration of health to other men, by the joint exertion of skill and humanity, are above all the great of the earth. They even partake of divinity, since to preserve and renew is almost as noble as to create.

Mr. Haggar's sentiments echo through history. His perception is shared by much of the insurance and business community. This abject view of physicians arose from several causes. Costs in workers' compensation, as well as in social security disability, had risen at a double-digit inflation rate for 20 years (2). That rate far exceeded the growth in population or any combination of risk factors in the two decades preceding Mr. Haggar's speech. Figure 1 shows the dramatic rise in workers' compensation premiums paid by employers nationally. Every individual receiving disability benefits has to be certified as disabled by a physician.

This disparaging view of doctors is further fueled by a refusal of the medical community to properly address the needs of the insurance and legal professions as they process disability claims. Few physicians recognize the need to return patients to work. Published research cites workers' compensation as a cause for failed medical treatment, without ever exploring the causes for the negative influence of

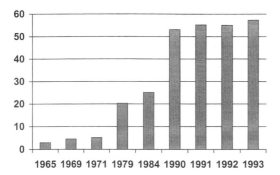

FIG. 1. Workers' compensation costs in billions of dollars, 1965 to 1993. (From ref. 5, with permission.)

workers' compensation. Authors leave their readers to surmise that there is a sinister motivation for workers' compensation patients for whom treatment fails. Finally, the repeated assertion of medical failures provide a diversion of public attention from the failures and frauds of the insurance and business communities. The medical community all but volunteered to be the scapegoat for the commercial interests that control the workers' compensation system.

Government and private insurers paid $120 billion in disability claims in 1987. That amounted to 5% of the total payroll for the year and did not include indirect losses in lowered productivity and the cost of retraining replacement workers (3). In 1990, 12.8 million people had a work-related disability (4). The total workers' compensation premium was $5.2 billion in 1971 and $57.3 billion in 1993 (5). In 1986, more than 11 million people had low back impairments, and more than 5.6 million of them were disabled by their back injuries (6). Of all expenses for back pain, 14% came from workers' compensation, while only 1.25% of all other medical care and disability payments came from workers' compensation (7).

Employers and insurers see themselves as bearing a disproportionate share of the nation's health care costs. Medicare and Medicaid reimbursements fall below the level of costs in providing health care. Providers attempt to cover the losses by charging more to

private insurers and by shifting patients from Medicare and Medicaid into private coverage. When patients are personally uninsured, the only alternative for private insurance coverage is the workers' compensation system. A physician needs only to say that an injury or disease arose from a patient's employment to shift the costs onto workers' compensation. The vagaries of "repetitive strain injury" and "cumulative trauma" provide a broad avenue for access to funding through workers' compensation. The incidence of work-related "repetitive strain injury" or "cumulative trauma disease" rose from 23,800 in 1972 to 332,000 in 1994. "Cumulative trauma" accounted for 62% of work-related disease 1997, and this excluded spine-related complaints that are considered injuries (8). Workers' compensation insurers have complained about cost-shifting for years.

"Repetitive strain" and "cumulative trauma" account for more than 50% of all workers' compensation claims. There is no single demonstrable event causing an injury in "repetitive strain injury" and "cumulative trauma disease." There is only an insidious slow accumulation of events, each of which would not produce a significant injury but in combination result in disabling back pain, tendinitis, or nerve compression. Carpal tunnel syndrome can result from a number of avocational activities, as well as from keyboard activities at work. The injury is attributed to "cumulative trauma" at work when a person engages in keyboard activity at work and develops carpal tunnel syndrome, regardless of whether or not the patient also plays the piano, crochets, or sculpts when not at work.

The only scientific support for the conclusion that "repetitive strain" or "cumulative trauma" causes injury or disease lies in statistical studies that show a marked increase in risk for people engaged in such work (8). Many of these studies are criticized for their design. There are no known thresholds or specific pathogenic mechanisms. The lack of scientific data leaves this category of injury open to broad interpretation, abuse, and litigation. The extremely rapid increase in the use of work-related "repetitive strain" leads to a reasonable insurance complaint of abuse. Yet there is no way to identify the individual claim as legitimate or not.

Health care providers have not responded to the needs of insurers and employers. Medical training is focused on the biologic and technical issues relevant to disease and injury treatment. The workers' compensation system needs physicians' opinions on causation, disability, and impairment. Without these medical opinions, insurers and the compensation commission cannot initiate benefits for injured workers. The reporting requirements of workers' compensation systems are not taught in the course of training in medical schools and residency programs, and physicians frequently forget to address them. Some physicians feel that judgments concerning causation, disability, and ultimate impairment are not scientifically justifiable. Many physicians shy away from them.

Insurers and the employers require medical opinions regarding causation, disability, impairment, point of maximum medical improvement, and residual abilities to meet the requirements of the individual statutes in the various states. Physicians know more about injury mechanisms and biologic responses to injuries than any other persons associated with claimants in the workers' compensation system. They are the best qualified to make judgments as to whether or not a given injury is consistent with the injury mechanism claimed by a patient, as well as to the time when no further recovery can be expected, the extent of loss of function to any body part, and the residual abilities of a patient to function with an impairment at work. The science is less than exact, but these judgments are necessary to process any claim. Physicians must work with the scientific data available to make the best judgments possible for their patients, their employers, and the payers. The frequent failure of doctors to meet these requirements has led to legitimate criticism of the medical community.

Physicians routinely fail to take an adequate work history. They do not gain an un-

derstanding of what an injured worker usually does in a normal workday. Thus, when a doctor indicates that the medical condition is due to "repetitive strain" or "cumulative trauma," he or she is making more of a guess than a reasonable judgment. Further, when the same patient's condition progresses, the doctor cannot adequately judge when the patient can return to his or her prior employment or whether job accommodations or a change of employment are necessary.

Doctors make no attempts to familiarize themselves with the requirements of the statutes that control the flow of benefits to their patients. A physician's statement that a patient has reached maximum medical improvement means that benefits cease in some states. The same statement in other states may mean simply that the patient is entitled to a separate permanency award while partial- or total-disability payments continue.

Insurers complain that they rarely see the specific terms that they need to make their case dispositions:

- No disability,
- Temporary partial disability,
- Temporary total disability,
- Maximum medical improvement,
- Permanent partial disability,
- Permanent total disability,
- Impairment rating.

The statement that there is *no disability* means that the patient can continue to work at his or her usual job and no accommodation is necessary for that person to work. It also means that the patient will not receive any financial support or wage replacement from the insurer. *Temporary partial disability* means that the patient's injury or disease is in a state of flux. It also means that the patient can do some work but needs to be excused from certain tasks or that he or she will need special accommodation with assistive devices to complete those tasks. For instance, a patient recovering from a meniscectomy can do some work but cannot kneel, crawl, climb a ladder, or squat. Light bench work or assembly-line work could be well within that patient's capability. A patient may be forced to seek employment elsewhere if his or her employer is unable or unwilling to provide work within his or her residual abilities. Financial support for patients varies from state to state, depending on the statutes governing the given jurisdiction. Frequently, a patient is supported as *temporarily totally disabled* until he or she finds work within the restrictions prescribed. When work is found but the new job pays less than the patient's usual wage, most jurisdictions provide that the insurer will pay the injured worker approximately two-thirds of the difference between the new wage and the preinjury income. Recovery is expected to continue, and restrictions will change with the recovery when the patient is temporarily disabled. Temporary total disability means that a patient is not capable of any work or is not able to travel to and from work. An example is a patient recovering from a femoral fracture or a spine fusion. Most jurisdictions require that insurers replace two-thirds of an injured worker's lost wages when he or she is temporarily totally disabled.

Maximum medical improvement means that the healing process is essentially complete, and no significant change in the patient's condition or abilities can be expected. When stating that the patient has reached maximum medical improvement, the doctor should assign a *permanent impairment rating* and discuss the effect of that impairment on the patient's ability to work. The doctor should rate the patient for permanent impairment according to the statutes of the jurisdiction that apply to the patient.

Some doctors rate permanent impairment "based on years of personal experience." Unfortunately, the knowledge derived from years of experience for one doctor can differ greatly from the lessons of experience for another doctor. Insurers and claimants' attorneys know which doctors are very liberal or very conservative. They enlist the assistance of the doctors with attitudes that fit their needs. The situation that develops is called "dueling doctors." Insurers and lawyers blame the medical community for the conflicts, but they have

chosen those very doctors to create the discrepancy of opinion.

Monetary awards for impairments are totally arbitrary because it is impossible to reasonably determine the monetary value of an arm, a leg, or any other body part. The wide disparity between ratings made by different doctors for the same condition in the same patient leads to litigation and expensive delays in disposition of the case. Impairment ratings should be made using a guide. Appropriate and consistent use of the guides required by specific jurisdictions will minimize the disparity in ratings assigned to the same condition by different doctors. The American Medical Associations's *Guides to the Evaluation of Permanent Impairment* is required for making impairment ratings in 38 states (9).

A patient can have a permanent impairment and still have no disability. For instance, a plumber with an amputation of the fifth finger has a 10% permanent impairment of the hand but no disability insofar as his or her trade as a plumber is concerned. He or she should be rated for the impairment of the finger loss and certified for work with no restrictions. However, a plumber with a lumbar disc herniation may not be able to return work at all. He or she should be rated for the lumbar disc herniation and recommended for vocational rehabilitation. The reasonable limits to patients' work abilities should be defined at the time that a rating is assigned.

Second-injury funds were established in many states at the end of World War II. They were intended to encourage employers to hire veterans who returned home with impairments from war wounds. Employers were concerned that a relatively minor injury at work would result in sufficient additional impairment that such workers would not be able to return to work at all. Employers would then be liable for all the expenses of the veterans' disability for a lifetime. The second-injury funds assumed the liability of prolonged disability in such cases. They continued long after the war because there were many other causes for impairments in people seeking work. Second-injury funds limited the liability for employers in hiring people with physical limitations. They usually require that a doctor make a judgment that a patient's degree of permanent disability is "materially and substantially greater" as a result of the combination of two or more injuries than it would be from any of the single injuries alone. The terms *materially* and *substantially greater* have been interpreted with great latitude. Second-injury funds have been abused, and many are closing. States and insurers blame doctors for the abuse of these funds. In fact, state agencies administering these funds have not defended or administered them effectively. The abuse was invited by administrative neglect.

The impediment to hiring impaired workers is thought to be covered by the Americans with Disabilities Act (ADA). The ADA has so many exemptions for employers that it does not adequately replace second-injury funds. Abuse of second-injury funds cannot occur without a doctor's statement regarding the disabilities arising from multiple work injuries.

The doctor–patient relationship makes doctors patient advocates. This relationship is based on trust. A patient ordinarily comes to a doctor with a health problem that concerns him or her. The doctor relies heavily on the patient's history to assess the problem. There is an implicit contract between the two: The patient seeking the doctor's assistance will tell the truth, and the doctor will use that information to formulate a diagnosis and treatment plan. The history will be correlated with physical examination, laboratory testing, and imaging data. The history is still the most important part of the formula. The doctor must consider the patient's view of the illness and its effect on the patient's life in making treatment plans. The relationship between doctor and patient is established the instant that the physician accepts the patient for treatment. The doctor accepts a number of obligations to the patient. The patient rightly expects the doctor to be his or her advocate. This relationship naturally expands with the progress of time and multiple personal encounters.

Every physician can recall patients whose progress affected his or her own feelings. Doctors become their patients' friends and allies in sharing the experience of their injuries. While treating the patient, the doctor hears only the patient's view of how he or she is being treated by the workers' compensation insurer, the employer, and the commission.

Treating physicians are vulnerable to the retribution of angry patients. A patient who is not satisfied with the doctor's actions or stated opinions will look for a reason to sue regardless of the quality of the care. Juries hearing medical malpractice cases also expect treating physicians to be patient advocates. Treating physicians' natural advocacy for their patients and their vulnerability to retribution from angry patients can prejudice them in rendering any judgments with economic impact for their patients. Thus, a treating physician is less likely to make the "hard call" that might lessen or end a patient's workers' compensation benefits.

Independent medical examiners have a very different relationship with patients. They are paid to review the records, take a patient history, and examine the patient and all other laboratory and imaging studies. They must then make a judgment as to the extent that objective data support a patient's claim for impairment and disability benefits. There is no doctor–patient relationship with independent examiners. However, once an independent examiner treats a patient, objectivity is lost. A traditional doctor–patient relationship is established, and the doctor becomes a patient advocate. Despite this change in roles, many doctors initiate treatment for examinees who have been referred for an independent examination.

Insurers make more money when losses are high than when they are low. Table 1 shows a trend of increasing benefits paid to injured workers and their health care providers for selected years from 1952 through 1991. Comparison to Fig. 1 shows that a great deal of money paid to insurers was not disbursed in benefits for injured workers but remained within the insurance companies. In 1952,

TABLE 1. *Workers' compensation benefit payments in millions for selected years*

1952	$785	1982	$16,407
1957	$1,062	1987	$27,318
1962	$1,489	1988	$30,733
1967	$2,189	1989	$34,316
1972	$4,061	1990	$38,238
1977	$8,630	1991	$42,179

From ref. 2, with permission.

workers' compensation indemnity and medical benefit payments totaled $785 million (3). In 1990, insurers paid $38.238 billion in benefits, but employers paid $53.1 billion in premium (5). Insurers claimed a loss ratio of 0.84 in 1990. The loss ratio is the loss and loss adjustment expense divided by total premium. That means that their losses were 84% of $53.1 billion or $44.6 billion. The $44.6 billion was $6.362 billion more than the total benefit payments. The 0.84 loss ratio claimed was not a lie. Insurers reserve money to cover a claim as soon as the claim is received. Conservative insurance companies reserve for a worst-case scenario. They also reserve for a category called "losses incurred but not reported." When money is reserved, it is considered a loss. The loss in reserves is factored into the rate setting for the following years' premiums. Later, when cases result in lower total benefit payments than the amount reserved, the excess reserve remains in the insurer's reserve pool. The reserve pool remains invested returning interest for the insurer. If the investments returned a meager 6% interest, the interest returned on the $6 billion that premium exceeded benefits paid in 1992 would be $375 million per year. The $6 billion would remain in the reserves and be added to the surplus reserves produced from previous and subsequent years. In just 2 years, the interest earned from the surplus premium collected in 1990 would equal the total benefits paid in 1972 ($4.061 billion). It would be impossible to accrue surplus reserves at that rate if paid benefits remained at the 1952 level of $785 million.

Insurers reported a combined loss ratio of 1.17 in 1990 (3). The combined loss ratio is the sum of losses, loss adjustment expenses, underwriting expenses, and dividends divided by premium. Considering that insurers were claiming a combined loss ratio of 1.17 in a year in which they took in $53.1 billion, one can infer that their total cost of losses, loss adjustment expenses, underwriting expenses, and dividends was $62.1 billion. Since the losses and loss adjustment expenses were $44.6 billion, the underwriting expenses and dividends came to $17.5 billion. In 1991, when costs were up, medical payments amounted to only $17 billion (2). In other words, the cost of operating the insurance industry exceeds the cost of providing medical care for the same workers' compensation population covered. Nonetheless, insurers blame the medical community for inefficiencies that supposedly drive up the cost of workers' compensation.

Insurers, employers, and legislatures responded to the rapid escalation in costs of the 1970s and 1980s by reducing wage-replacement and permanent-impairment awards and denying injured workers access to benefits.

Referring to a report of the Workers' Compensation Research Institute, Ed Welch reported on recent history in Oregon (10). Oregon was a high-cost state in 1980s and experienced a double-digit drop in losses through the 1990s. One-third to one-half of the reduction was attributed to the action of a single Oregon workers' compensation carrier. The State Accident Insurance Fund established a fraud and abuse department and simply denied a large number of claims. The fund was the largest workers' compensation carrier in Oregon. The overall rate of denial in the state rose to 28.5% in that period, while the average rate of denial for other carriers was only 12.9%.

Restriction of injured workers' access to compensation benefits and reduction in benefit payments resulted in great savings to insurers through the 1990s. Figures 2, 3, and 4 show trends in the measures for insurance profitability. Profits for workers' compensation insurers are now at the highest levels in recorded history.

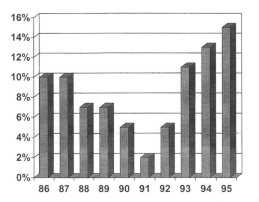

FIG. 2. Insurers' broad measure of profitability. The darker shade of gray represents the return on net worth.

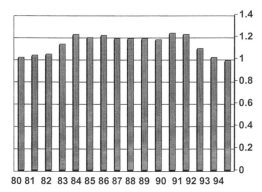

FIG. 4. Combined loss ratio: sum of losses, loss adjustment expenses, underwriting expenses, and dividends divided by premiums. The gray shade represents a combined ratio.

Michael Clingman, president of the IA-IABC, listed a series of trends for cost reduction in August 1995 (11). He indicated that state legislatures will continue to limit employers' liability for injuries, especially those that have significant causal connection to factors outside the workplace. Since "repetitive motion" and "cumulative trauma" injuries are easily the fastest growing type of workers' compensation claim, attempts to restrict compensability to "single-event" injuries will continue. There will be more attempts to apportion impairment ratings so that only the impairment due to the work injury is compensated. There will be more attempts to introduce thresholds so that the injured employee will have to prove that the work injury was the major cause of his or her disability. Managed

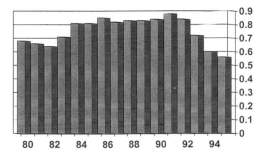

FIG. 3. Loss ratio: sum of losses and loss adjustment expenses divided by premiums. The gray shade represents a loss ratio.

care in workers' compensation will continue to increase, with fee schedules and medical treatment protocols being increasingly prevalent (12). Basically, the trends are to deny access to treatment and compensation, to reduce the level of benefits, and to artificially cap costs for medical treatment for all injured workers.

The trends show some backlash that may result in increased costs. There is an increase in litigation. In 1978 in California, the total cost of workers' compensation litigation was about $150 million. In 1992, it was $2.2 billion, rising 25% per year since 1978 (13). Litigants are escaping the exclusive-remedy restriction of workers' compensation and suing in the tort system for larger awards than those available in the workers' compensation system (14). More injured workers are denied treatment and benefits under the compensation system, and more of them are seeking compensation through suits for negligence (11,14). The reductions in workers' compensation losses experienced in the early 1990s may produce new heights of losses as the legal backlash takes greater toll.

Insurers can show a short-term reduction in losses by denying the compensability of any given injury. Claims management tends to focus on reducing medical expenses by limiting and delaying medical treatment once an injury is admitted to the workers' compensation system. The method appears to be successful overall on a quarterly report but is counterproductive for the premium payer in the long run. When insurers delay paying benefits and deny medical treatment, injured workers are forced to either accept the financial losses that come with their injury or seek legal assistance to contest an insurer's action. Significant amounts of money are at risk for injured workers. They tend to litigate more often. Litigation results in greater delays in return to work, greater losses in temporary disability payments, and greater expense in the litigation process. Each of these costs is factored in to determine future and higher premiums. Whenever possible, the fault for the delays and increased costs is laid at the feet of the treating physician.

The business community would have it believed that all of the excessive costs in the workers' compensation system are due to the failings of the medical community. In fact, all of the parties bearing on injured workers contribute to the excessive costs. Commissions, insurers, labor unions, employers, and lawyers act as if they are the major controlling force to whom all others report. There is no spirit of cooperation to achieve a common goal.

Once lawyers are involved, injured workers will be coached in ways to demonstrate the most severe aspects of their injury. Disability is protracted (6). The two opposing sides dig in. Patients cannot give up their disability and illness behavior until their case passes through a long legal process to settlement. The underlying injury goes untreated, and the illness behavior establishes a pattern. The probability for return to work diminishes as time progresses. If a patient is out of work for 2 years, there is virtually no chance of his or her ever returning to work (15,16). If he or she returns to work early, this shows evidence that the injury was not all that bad. Protracted disability because of long legal proceedings produces a lifestyle change for patients. They become mentally and physically deconditioned for work. The longer the period of the disability lifestyle, the more difficult it becomes to return to work.

Current trends to reduce access and benefits result in increased indemnity costs for a protracted disability, and the medical expenses for multiple tests, consultations, and independent medical examinations also rise. Both sides seek to prove or disprove the severity of the injury. Insurers would reduce total losses by ensuring prompt appropriate treatment and early return to work.

Individual employers have the greatest opportunity to reduce losses in the workers' compensation system. Injury prevention is key to reducing losses. Once a disabling injury has occurred, many factors within the control of management can alter the course of a worker's disability. Job satisfaction is the foremost factor correlating with an early return to work (5). Persons with high levels of discretion are more than two times as likely to be working as those with less autonomy. Those with high demands and little discretion to deal with them are far less likely to return to work after a disabling injury (17–19). Considering that psychologic comorbidity plays an important role in predisposing patients to prolonged disability, it must be recognized that an unpleasant and stressful work environment will greatly reduce the probability for their return to work. As depression and a need for support are common accompaniments of disability, it should be realized that a single supportive phone call from a patient's employer would be a strong force in motivating a return to work.

Unfortunately, most people are employed by small firms that are not individually experience-rated by their insurers. Therefore, they see little gain in premium reductions from efforts to reduce losses (3). Too often, employers take the attitude that they can let the insurance company handle all contact with injured workers following an injury. They give up the greatest opportunity to reduce disability losses. Some respond angrily to injured workers and refuse to file an initial report of injury. Thus, not even the insurer has the opportunity to deal with the injured worker. Occasionally, employers are simply happy to be rid of injured workers and do as little as possible to promote their return to work. Considering the prevalence of psychiatric comorbidity, one could understand that attitude. Depressed, anxious, or substance-abusing people do not make the most desirable and productive employees.

Employers who are willing to be supportive to injured workers do more to reduce workers' compensation costs than any other initiative within the system. Employers should call injured workers to express concern for their condition and reassure them of their value to the company. Employers should provide for return to work with limitations or decreased hours. They should communicate with the insurer not only to report an injury but to request prompt treatment and benefits for injured workers. Employers who call treating physicians to assure them that limited work is available for the specific injured worker will assert a force that will promote return to work. Employers have introduced programs to monitor performance of the health care team, create provider profiles, contract for discounted fees, and employ managed care. They should turn some of their attention to their compensation insurers to be sure that their injured workers are receiving prompt and appropriate treatment.

Unions with rigid seniority policies that assign the easier jobs to workers with more seniority instead of to those with limited abilities also hamper return-to-work efforts. Unions with strict rules prohibiting a worker from crossing trades can also hinder return to work. Unions can promote safety and return to work as specific contract issues in negotiating a labor contract.

Treating physicians should understand the system, establish return to work as a priority in the treatment plan, and report the diagnosis, treatment plan, disability status, and expected period of disability following each patient encounter. Treating physicians should recognize that disability itself is pathogenic, and should make return to work a treatment goal. They should try to engage employers in assisting to return a patient to work and must provide consistent permanency ratings. Most important, treating physicians should expand their view beyond the diagnosed injury to the whole patient and all of the factors affecting that patient, and then beyond to the societal impact of the patient's disability.

When patients are disabled for longer periods of time, they suffer more because of the morbidity associated with disability. Insurers, employers, and society suffer the economic losses of that disability. The key to turning a lose-lose situation into win-win situation lies in prompt treatment and return to work. This goal can be accomplished with improved communication among all parties concerned and with dedication to the goal of return to work. Antagonism between payers and providers must end and communication and cooperation begin. Truly, the best interests of injured workers, the financial interests of employers, and the intended fairness of the system would be best served by a joint effort of all parties to reduce the period of disability and promote return to work. Across the board cuts in benefits, restriction of access to the system, and delaying of medical treatment all promote conflict among patients, employers, health care providers, and insurers. Conflicts lead to litigation, prolonged disability, greater illness, and greater expense.

REFERENCES

1. Pliny; Rackham H, Jones WHS, Eicholz DE, trans. *Natural history.* Cambridge, MA: Loeb Classical Library, 1991; cited in Majino G. *The healing hand.* New York: Gryphon Editions 1991.
2. Nelson W. Workers' Compensation: Coverage Benefits, and Costs, 1990–91. *Social Security Bull* 1993;56: 68–74.
3. Drury D. Disability management in small firms. *Rehabil Couns Bull* 1991;34:243–256.
4. Engelberg AL. Disability and workers' compensation. *Occup Health* 1994;21:275–289.
5. Burton JF. Workers' compensation, twenty-four-hour coverage, and managed care. *John Burton's Workers' Comp Monit* 1996;Jan/Feb:11–22.
6. Lumbar spine. In: *Orthopaedic knowledge update 3.* Park Ridge, IL: American Academy of Orthopaedic Surgeons, 1990, pp. 455–468.
7. Hogan AJ, Welch EM. Who pays for bad backs? *Ed Welch on Workers' Compen* 1996;6:81–84.
8. Bernard BP, ed. *Musculoskeletal disorders and work-*

place factors. Washington, DC: NIOSH, U.S. Department of Health and Human Services, 1997.

9. Doege TC, Houston TP, eds. *Guides to the evaluation of permanent impairment*, 4th ed. Chicago: The American Medical Association, 1993.

10. Oregon explained. *Ed Welch on Workers' Comp* 1996;6: 104–105.

11. Clingman M. *Summary of recent trends in workers' compensation.* International Association of Industrial Accident Boards and Commissions, August 1995.

12. Employers take charge. *Ed Welch on Workers' Comp* 1996;6:117.

13. Hughson WG. Work-related disabilities. In: *Proceedings of the annual meeting of the medical section of the American Council of Life Insurers.* San Diego, CA: University of California, San Diego, 1994:53–65.

14. Trading compensability for the exclusive remedy. *Ed Welch on Workers' Comp* 1996;6:104–105.

15. Hazard RG, Fenwick JW, Kalisch SM, et al. Functional restoration with behavioral support. *Spine* 1989;14:157–161.

16. Lanes RC, Gauron EF, Spratt KF, Wernimont TJ, Found EM, Weinstein JN. Long-term follow-up of patients with chronic back pain treated in a multidisciplinary rehabilitation program. *Spine* 1995;7: 801–806.

17. Yelin E. Displaced concern: the social context of the work-disability problem. *Milbank Q* 1989;67: 114–165.

18. Cheadle A, Franklin G, Wolfhagen C, et al. Factors influencing the duration of work-related disability: a population-based study of Washington State workers' compensation. *Am J Public Health* 1994;84:190–196.

19. Yelin E. The myth of malingering: why individuals withdraw from work in the presence of illness. *Milbank Q* 1986;64:622–649.

Occupational Musculoskeletal Disorders
edited by T. G. Mayer, R. J. Gatchel, and P. B. Polatin.
Lippincott Williams & Wilkins, Philadelphia © 2000.

4

Injured Workers and Medical Evidence: A Judge's Perspective

Peter N. Rogers[1]

Rogers, Booker & Treviño, P.C., Richardson, Texas 75080

A doctor's care of a patient in the occupational medicine setting does not end with the provision of treatment for the presenting complaint. By necessity, doctors today are also tasked with the preparation of various documents for insurance companies, employers, agencies, and patients, as well as their own records. The following discussion provides a pragmatic approach to the preparation of medical reports. Its purpose is to provide some guidance for health care providers who are probably not thinking ahead to a time when their progress notes may become medical evidence and they are called on to explain them. It is important when a doctor treats an injured worker and prepares medical reports concerning him or her that the doctor be aware of how those reports will be perceived by state agency officials responsible for making decisions in workers' compensation cases.

This discussion centers on four main considerations in the evaluation of doctors' medical reports: the injured worker, claimant and carrier doctors, medical reports as evidence, and the law.

The first consideration is the worker's injury and the worker's reaction to the injury. Also considered under the same topic is the tendency of state agency personnel to place injured workers into categories. Treating doctors must know, anticipate, and react to such categorizations. Second, doctors are themselves categorized by the state agency, and they must be aware that their reputations for fairness and impartiality will determine whether or not their medical reports are accepted at face value. Third, medical reports, which are at the heart of any workers' compensation claim and serve as the basis for decision making concerning that claim, are discussed in detail. Doctors must understand which issues are decided based on medical reports and what information to include in a report to make it effective. Fourth, doctors must know the law. Too often, a case is decided based on an inadvertent statement in a medical report.

---

[1]Peter N. Rogers served as an administrative law judge for 4 years with the Texas Workers' Compensation Commission, the agency charged by the Texas legislature with the administration of the injured workers' comprehensive and exclusive system of remedies for work-related injuries. As an administrative law judge with the official title of a hearing officer, he worked with approximately 30 other judges and 40 mediators throughout Texas. This group's sole function is to hear disputes, weigh evidence, and prepare written decisions on cases. Communication among the members of this group is frequent and occurs through various channels. More formal methods include conferences and continuing education courses for the judges and mediators. Less formal methods consist of direct communication among the judges and through a central office. This discussion among peers tends to create a normative approach to evaluating medical evidence. Thus, Mr. Rogers' observations are not merely the perceptions of one individual but rather the perceptions of a group, a group with the authority to make decisions based on medical evidence. This group's analysis of medical reports therefore becomes highly relevant because it represents the prism through which medical reports are viewed and evaluated. The information presented is not purported to adhere to any scientific method of analysis. Rather, it is a discussion of the mindset of the decision makers in an administrative agency, the forum in which health care providers must operate if their practice includes patients with work-related injuries.

THE INJURED WORKER

Strains and Sprains

Most workers' compensation cases are simple and relatively straightforward. The typical work-related injury is a back strain that will heal over time, with or without medical treatment. Cases involving strains and sprains do reach the litigation stage and often involve a question of disability. A doctor who has maintained an injured worker in an "off work" status after normal healing time should be aware that workers' compensation judges will doubt disability beyond 2 months in a case of simple back strain and will discount evidence of disc bulges unless there is nerve impingement. Judges will have the experience of hundreds of cases, as well as published treatment guidelines, to back up their decisions in these cases. At the same time, however, liberal treatment guidelines will support a claim of continued disability while an injured worker is in a treatment program such as a secondary care or a tertiary rehabilitation program. Judges will generally not make a disability finding that is contrary to treatment guidelines. These guidelines create a presumption that certain treatment is reasonable, and the presumption is not easily rebutted.

Psychological Aspects of an Injury

Chronic pain and inactivity often accompany an injury and may lead to depression. The depression must then be addressed, and both the physical and the psychologic effects of a work-related injury must be treated. Having read the medical reports and treatment guidelines, and having heard testimony on psychological problems, the agency official is aware of the possible emotional and psychological effects of a work-related injury. The problems confronting judges in cases involving a disability issue and psychological problems are complex because not only will conflicting medical evidence be presented, but judges will also be influenced by viewpoints derived from other cases over which they presided.

For instance, one viewpoint is that it is better for injured workers to achieve closure on their workers' compensation case because the body has the ability to heal itself when it has no alternative but to do so. Judges will be influenced by cases in which an injured worker is said to have developed the "sick person syndrome," in which an injury is prolonged because being incapacitated yields "secondary-gain" benefits. Specifically, the injured worker receives secondary gain in the form of indemnity benefits, sympathy from family members, and regular physical therapy from a doctor. An injured worker is thus rewarded financially, emotionally, and physically for being sick and has no incentive for improving. A judge, cognizant of this phenomenon and adhering to this belief, may determine an end date for disability based on objective data only. For the judge with this mindset, the objective data in the medical reports are most important in the decision making.

Indirect Psychological Factors

Psychological stressors are not limited to chronic pain and feelings of worthlessness based on incapacity. Indirect stressors also add to depression. In any workers' compensation system, an injured worker may experience feelings of frustration and powerlessness caused by the insurance carrier's denial or delay of medical treatment and indemnity benefits. He or she is then faced with having to process a dispute through a confusing impersonal bureaucratic system, thus adding to the stress. Workers' compensation judges who deal with many insurance carriers and adjusters will have some understanding of which adjusters and insurance carriers regularly deny and delay benefits in an effort to keep costs down. They will recognize that denial and delay may be standard responses to any claim from some carriers, but the injured worker whose claim is denied will be greatly stressed. In these situations, the injured worker would be well advised to obtain the assistance of an attorney both to obtain denied benefits and to alleviate to some extent the feeling of frustration and powerlessness.

Long-term Injury

When injured workers remain disabled for an extended period of time, the injury will become the focal point of their lives. They will often make repeated telephone calls to adjusters, attorneys, doctors, and state agencies, asking the same questions and making the same demands. Unfortunately, any legitimate points that they may have will fall on increasingly unsympathetic ears. These workers will often fare poorly in litigation because they are perceived as whiners and complainers. The frequency and multitude of the complaints diminishes their import.

The Injured Worker's Anger

Employers, not injured workers, pay workers' compensation insurance premiums, unlike other insurance such as disability and homeowner's insurance. Insurance carriers will respond to the whims of employers and give employers' interests priority over injured workers' interests. If an employer takes a tough stand on work-related injuries, the insurance carrier will also take a hard line to keep its client satisfied. Fairness often takes a back seat to the employer's interests, and this results in anger from the injured worker who, understandably, believes that the insurance carrier is there to provide full and appropriate coverage for the worker's claim.

Another cause of injured workers' anger is lack of sympathy and understanding by employers. In the context of a workers' compensation claim, the interests of the injured employee and the interests of the employer are in conflict. A previously good relationship with supervisors can instantly change to one of intense hostility after a claim is filed. If there were any conflicts between the employer and the employee before the injury, the insurance company may use those conflicts to assert that the reported injury is a "spite" claim, an injury reported in retaliation for some personnel action taken by the employer. The medical provider who documents in the progress notes problems at work reported by the injured worker may find those notes used as evidence of a spite claim. Such information can and does influence hearing officers in assessing the validity of a claim.

CLAIMANT AND CARRIER DOCTORS

Credibility

Doctors who treat work-related injuries and prepare medical reports that become evidence in workers' compensation cases will very quickly develop reputations. These reputations are based on countless medical reports that contain similar language, even though they relate to different cases. Most doctors use the same stationery and font for every medical report, so judges will know before reading the report who wrote it and what it says to some extent. Administrative judges will not be limited to personal observations and experience in forming their opinions of some doctors. States conduct statistical studies that have been used as evidence for determining the credibility of certain doctors.

For example, statistics are available on second opinions in spine surgery cases and impairment ratings. Second-opinion statistics set forth the number of times that (a) each practicing orthopedic surgeon in Texas was selected to provide a second opinion on the advisability of spine surgery; (b) the doctor was selected by the insurance carrier; (c) the doctor was selected by the injured worker; and (d) the doctor concurred that spine surgery was necessary (1). These statistics bore out what was already thought to be true: The more "liberal" surgeons agreed that spine surgery was necessary in nearly every case, and insurance carrier doctors rarely agreed spine surgery was necessary.

As demonstrated by Tables 1 and 2, the statistics on impairment ratings were equally revealing. Ratings from treating doctors were high, while ratings from carriers' independent medical evaluation (IME) doctors were low (2).

TABLE 1. *Distribution of differences in impairment ratings between different types of medical examiners*

Difference between ratings	Mean difference	Percentiles								
		1st	5th	10th	25th	50th	75th	90th	95th	99th
Designated doctor[a] and insurance doctor	3.7	−11	−5	−2	0	+3	+7	+11	+15	23
Treating doctor and insurance doctor	3.6	−14	−7	−4	0	+2	+7	+13	+17	+29
Treating doctor and designated doctor	0.5	−18	−11	−7	−4	0	+4	+9	+13	+23
Treating or other and insurance doctor	3.3	−13	−6	−3	0	+1	+7	+12	+16	+28
Treating or other and designated doctor	0.2	−18	−11	−7	−4	−0	+4	+9	+12	+22

This table shows that insurance doctors tend to provide lower ratings than treating doctors when a claim has a rating from both a treating doctor and an insurance doctor. Insurance doctors also tend to provide lower ratings than designated doctors do when a claim has a rating from each of these types. Ratings assigned by treating and designated doctors tend to be close, although treating doctors on average show a slight tendency toward higher impairment ratings than designated doctors. The percentile distribution shows that both the direction and size of the difference vary a good deal. In many cases, the insurance doctor gave higher ratings than treating or designated doctors.

[a]A designated doctor is a neutral doctor appointed by the Texas Workers' Compensation Commission (TWCC) to resolve a dispute over impairment ratings.

From TWCC Forms Database; *Texas Monitor*, Vol. 1, November 7, 1996, p. 8.

The Problem of Carrier Doctors

When an insurance carrier hires a doctor to perform an IME of an injured worker, that doctor will have been made aware of the legal effect of his or her report. In many cases, insurance carriers will have a special arrangement with doctors and will provide a high percentage of their revenues. There is no need for the insurance company adjuster to ask for a given result or to express any opinion about an injured worker because experience has shown that these doctors' reports will be "conservative." They are financially motivated to keep their opinions "conservative" and realize that any trend in the other direction would eradicate their IME business.

The Problem of Claimant Doctors

Doctors who treat high numbers of injured workers also develop their own particular image. State agency officials expect claimant-oriented doctors to overtreat, to keep injured workers "off work" for an indefinite amount of time, and to assess high impairment ratings. These doctors are also perceived as being motivated by their own financial incentives and the realization that their business is based on a "liberal" perspective. Injured workers in large companies provide word-of-mouth marketing to the effect that a doctor is highly sympathetic to injured workers, and new patients from that company will supply a never-ending source of revenue.

TABLE 2. *Distribution of differences in impairment ratings between different types of medical examiners for claims with one rating from each of the three doctor types*

Computed differences between doctor types	Mean difference	Cases (no.)
Treating and insurance	5.8	986
Treating and designated	1.6	986
Designated and insurance	4.2	986
Treating/other and insurance	5.2	1,270
Treating/other and designated	1.0	1,270
Designated and insurance	4.2	1,270

This table shows average differences between ratings from different types of examiners when the same injury had been rated by all three types of examiners. Only cases with one rating from a treating doctor, one from an insurance doctor, and one from a designated doctor are used in these comparisons. The average differences tend to be larger than those in Table 1 because these injuries tended to have higher ratings.

From TWCC Forms Database; *Texas Monitor*, Vol. 1, November 7, 1996, p. 8.

Treating Doctors

Most doctors want to assist an injured worker to get back to work by practicing good medicine. Often, doctors in this group will be less familiar with the law than insurance carrier doctors or claimant doctors. To be effective, it is important to know the law and to recognize the legal effect of statements and opinions contained in medical reports. Often, a doctor who is not knowledgeable of the law will attempt to assist an injured worker but may instead cause harm through inadvertent statements in medical reports.

Reports from treating doctors who do not have a reputation as a claimant doctor will be accorded more weight by the administrative agency when there is a contradictory report by a doctor hired by the insurance company. In many cases, the injured worker's attorney will not have to prove the bias of the insurance carrier's doctor because that doctor's reputation will be well known to the administrative agency officials. In situations where it is necessary to prove that a doctor is fair and neutral, statistical studies such as the ones mentioned above support an argument that the doctor is fair and the reports are accurate.

Accessibility

Doctors' accessibility greatly affects their professional reputations and the weight given their opinions. Doctors who are willing to testify either by telephone or by attending hearings provide hearing officers with additional support for making decisions based on their credibility. In testifying before a hearing officer, a doctor's credibility is enhanced by the citation of learned treatises that support an opinion and by a reasoned basis for his or her position. On the other hand, a doctor who appears to take the same approach to every case is not as credible. The key to a positive professional reputation is a willingness to provide testimony that demonstrates attention to a patient's particular circumstances and treatment.

Written responses to agency inquiries are also important and should be handled accordingly. Disputes frequently arise between injured workers and insurance carriers over the interpretation of a medical report or the certification of an impairment rating. The administrative agency may try to resolve the issues by writing a letter of clarification to the doctor. A prompt, forthright response by the doctor to the questions asked increases the doctor's credibility, while evading a question or refusing to acknowledge an obvious error diminishes credibility. Doctors should telephone for clarification when questions from an agency official are not clear.

MEDICAL RECORDS AS EVIDENCE

Hearings

Most workers' compensation hearings are low-budget affairs. The amount of money involved generally does not permit medical testimony, and the parties to hearings recognize that a doctor with a busy practice cannot take the time to testify at a hearing. One alternative is telephone testimony, by which the doctor is permitted to testify over a speakerphone set up in the hearing room. Generally, speakerphone testimony will take approximately 15 to 30 minutes and will not overly inconvenience the doctor. Another alternative is a written or oral deposition. The usual procedure would permit the doctor's testimony to be taken at his or her office. A transcription of the testimony would substitute for live evidence.

While live testimony, telephone testimony, and depositions are used in workers' compensation hearings, the most common form of evidence by far is the medical record. Office notes, narratives, reports, and medical letters will be assembled by the attorney for the insurance carrier and by the attorney for the injured worker and offered into evidence in support of their respective positions.

Simple Reports

State workers' compensation agencies are extremely busy places, and it is impossible for judges to read numerous medical reports in each case. Attorneys on both sides of a workers' compensation issue will place complete sets of medical records into evidence without reading them, without removing duplicates, and without any consideration for relevance. Time constraints make judges look for summaries in the records that set forth the issue and the opinion. The key to preparing a simple and effective report is to prepare a thorough report that contains a summary. Only the summary will be read when a case is litigated. Thus, doctors' ability to write concise reports, as well as their reputation and accessibility, will determine whether their opinion will be accepted by fact-finders as persuasive.

Medical Information

As stated earlier, treating doctors' function is twofold: they act as medical providers and information providers. Once an insurance carrier receives written notice of an injury, it has a limited amount of time to investigate the claim. Therefore, the injured worker's medical records are the insurance carrier's roadmap for determining whether or not to accept workers' compensation claims and what body parts to include as part of the compensable injury. It is extremely important for doctors to provide the insurance carrier as much information as possible when drafting a medical report.

The primary focus in the litigation of workers' compensation claims is the information contained in medical reports. Doctors' medical notes and narratives and the results of objective testing are the evidence that will most often determine:

- Whether the injured worker sustained an injury,
- Extent of the injury,
- Disability,
- Whether maximum medical improvement has been attained,
- Degree of impairment,
- Whether the impairment has resulted in the unemployment or underemployment of the injured worker.

The Treating Doctor's Initial Report

The initial medical report is one of the most important medical reports submitted to carriers by treating doctors. In the initial medical report, an insurance carrier will look for a date of injury, the nature of the injury, the body parts affected by the injury, the cause of the injury, and whether the injured worker suffers disability as a result of the injury. If a dispute arises, judges will also scrutinize the initial medical report for pertinent evidence. Great weight is placed by agency officials on the information contained in the initial report, and inaccuracies can create serious problems for injured workers.

Date of Injury

The first matter to determine when completing an injured worker's initial medical report is the date of injury. It is very important to be as accurate as possible about the date of injury because it will most likely be the date used by the injured worker, the insurance carrier, and the administrative agency at the benefit starting date. The date of injury is also important because it often triggers the injured worker's requirement to report the injury. If the injured worker sustained an injury as a result of trauma such as lifting a box at work at a known time and place, then the notice requirement is straightforward. The injured worker is charged with the obligation to report an injury within a specified time from the date of injury.

Date of Injury: "Repetitive Trauma"

It is more difficult to determine the date of injury if the injured worker is diagnosed as having or manifesting symptoms of a "repetitive trauma" injury such as carpal tunnel syndrome. In Texas, the date of injury for a repetitive trauma injury or occupational disease is the date on which the injured worker knew or should have known that his or her injury may be work-related (3). When an injured worker knew or should have known that the injury was work-related is liberally construed by the Texas Workers' Compensation Commission (TWCC) Appeals Panel. The recognized factual test is when a reasonably prudent person would have recognized the nature, seriousness, and work-related nature of the disease (4–6).

When an injured worker first comes to a treating doctor's office, the doctor should provide him or her with a form to fill out or have a discussion to ascertain what body parts are the source of the injured worker's complaint of pain. Further, the injured worker should provide an accurate description of the accident and injury, and the development of pain subsequent to it. If the complaint is what the doctor recognizes as a repetitive trauma injury, then the injured worker should provide a job-duty description, the average number of hours he or she performs those duties each day, and how long he or she has been employed doing those repetitive activities. Proof that the injured worker's duties are repetitive in nature is a necessary prerequisite for successfully presenting a claim for a repetitive trauma injury.

Extent of Injury

After determining the date of injury, the doctor must, of course, determine the nature of the injury and, if possible, provide a diagnosis. It is important to include in the initial medical report every complaint of pain the injured worker is experiencing and every diagnosis that the doctor thinks is appropriate for each body part. Remember that insurance carriers will only accept as compensable those injuries that are documented.

Causation

Causation is one of the most important elements to include in an initial medical report. Even if an injury exists, the doctor must clearly link the diagnosis to the injury reported. For example, the doctor must explain that the diagnosed back sprain resulted from the lifting incident at work on the reported

date of injury. If the injury is rather complex, as with an occupational disease, the doctor must explain how the injury developed as a result of the activities at work. The more information the doctor provides in a medical report regarding how the injury was caused by the work activity or incident, the more information the insurance carrier has, and the more difficult it will be to rebut a claim that an injury or incident happened at the job site. Further, the earlier the doctor prepares a medical report that explains the work-related cause of the injury, the more credible the doctor's opinion will be, because it will probably be given prior to the insurance carrier's or the injured worker's attorney asking for this information. It is also important to remember that any expert medical opinion regarding causation must be within a reasonable medical *probability*, not *possibility*.

Disability

Finally, the doctor should indicate in the initial medical report whether or not the injured worker has disability as a result of his or her injury. If the injury has resulted in a disability, the doctor must clearly explain why the injured worker has a disability and how long the injured worker will be disabled. Not only should the doctor include disability information in the medical report, he or she should also provide the injured worker with a disability statement that the injured worker can forward to the employer and the insurance carrier. If the doctor believes that the injured worker can return to work with some limitations, those limitations must be clearly stated in the medical report and explained to the injured worker.

Subsequent Medical Reports

Subsequent medical reports are normally provided by treating doctors to the workers' compensation administrative agency and insurance carriers. Subsequent medical reports are important because they allow the parties to review the progress of the injured worker's compensable injury. Often, new symptoms will manifest themselves during the course of treatment. For example, an injured worker initially diagnosed as having a lumbar sprain or strain may begin experiencing radiculopathy that results in the doctor's ordering a magnetic resonance imaging (MRI) examination. MRI imaging may reveal disc bulges or herniations in part of the lumbar spine. Once a new diagnosis is established, the doctor must immediately record the diagnosis or probable diagnosis in a medical report and explain the progression of the symptomatology. The doctor must further remember to link the previously undiagnosed medical condition to the original work-related injury.

The injured worker may also present new complaints of pain in a body part that the doctor had not examined previously as part of the compensable injury. It is vital that injured workers' complaints, no matter how minor, be recorded in the medical report. A medical report acts as a roadmap. If an injury or complaint is not contained in the medical report, then no evidence exists regarding the complaint or injury. In addition, the medical report must always make links back to the original injury. Therefore, even if a doctor is focusing on treating a knee injury and the injured worker begins complaining of low back pain, a prudent doctor should make a note of the low-back-pain complaints. Injury to the low back may be ruled out in the future, but if the work-related accident did cause a back injury, the early medical reports will be the key to receiving payment for treatment involving the back.

Often, an insurance adjuster will inform the treating doctor that a body part is not included in the injury and that it must not be included in medical reports. This instruction should be ignored if the treating doctor either believes the compensable injury includes that body part or is uncertain as to whether the worker sustained an injury to that body part. If the extent-of-injury issue is litigated, the insurance carrier's attorney will assert that the omission of a body part from the medical report is evidence that the injury did not include that body

part. In a typical scenario involving litigation of that issue, the injured worker will argue that the treating doctor was informed that the injury included a body part but that the doctor failed to mention that body part in the reports. The judge hearing this argument will not be convinced by what may have been said and will focus on the written reports.

Reasonable and Necessary Medical Care

One of the most important aspects of treating injured workers is, of course, obtaining payment from insurance carriers for the treatment prescribed. Again, the more information contained in the medical records, the better will be the treating doctors' chances of collecting medical fees. In Texas, insurance carriers must only pay for reasonable and necessary medical care (7). An injured worker is entitled to medical care that "cures or relieves the effects naturally resulting from the compensable injury; promotes recovery; or enhances the ability of the employee to return to or retain employment" (8). Therefore, treating doctors must explain to insurance carriers why the treatment that they are prescribing is medically necessary for the type of injury sustained by the injured worker. They must further explain how the type of treatment promotes the injured worker's recovery. Further, the medical records must document the injured worker's progress and must illustrate whether or not the treatment prescribed is benefiting the injured worker. If the injured worker's condition is improving because of the given treatment, it is a good indication that the treatment is reasonable and necessary and promotes recovery.

Disability Statements

The information most often requested from treating doctors is information regarding injured workers' disability status. The term *disability* has many definitions. Short-term disability insurance policies normally define disability as the inability to return to the job that the employee was doing at the time of the injury. Long-term disability policies normally define disability in terms of whether the worker can return to any job. The Social Security Administration defines disability as the inability to return to any work that the employee has ever done or ever been trained to do.

The treating doctor must indicate in the initial medical report that the injured worker's compensable injury is such that he or she is unable to return to the type of work he or she was doing, or the doctor must indicate what limitations, if any, the injured worker has sustained as a result of his or her compensable injury. The doctor should address the question of the injured worker's disability status periodically.

In Texas, there are several stages of "disability" in the life of a workers' compensation claim. Disability is defined as the inability because of a compensable injury to obtain or retain employment at wages equivalent to the preinjury wage (9). Depending on the stage of the claim, an injured worker's disability will be analyzed using a different definition and standard. For example, after impairment income benefits have expired, the injured worker is entitled to receive supplemental income benefits (SIBs). To be eligible to receive SIBs, an injured worker must have an impairment rating of 15% or greater, have not returned to work or returned to work earning less than 80% of his or her average weekly wage as a direct result of the impairment, have not elected to commute any portion of the impairment income benefits, *and* have attempted in good faith to obtain employment commensurate with his or her ability to work (10).

SIBs are different from other types of indemnity benefits under the workers' compensation system. They are applied for quarterly, and each quarter covers a 90-day period or 13 weeks. The 90-day period prior to the quarter is called the qualifying or filing period. To receive SIBs, the injured worker must demonstrate a good faith effort to obtain or retain employment commensurate with the ability to work during the filing period for the SIBs quarter. Eligibility for each SIBs quarter is determined on an individual basis. Therefore, the injured worker must meet the requirement for each quarter for which application is made.

If an injured worker has not looked for work during the filing period because his or her doctor has not given a release to return to work, the doctor must indicate the basis for not providing a return to work. To qualify for SIBs when there has been no job search, the burden is on the injured worker to show that there is *absolutely no ability to work because of the compensable injury*. This standard for disability is stricter than any other standard. For the injured worker to show no ability to work, the doctor must indicate in the medical report that the injured worker cannot return to work in any capacity because of the impairment. Further, the doctor must fully explain why the injured worker cannot return to work in any capacity and must clearly explain the injured worker's physical limitations. The doctor should also list the medications prescribed for the injured worker and any effects they may have on the injured worker's ability to drive, concentrate, or focus in a daily setting.

The secret to writing a good medical report for workers' compensation purposes is accuracy and detail. Treating doctors' medical reports are the parties' main source of information on the treatment and progression of injured workers' conditions. The more information given to the parties involved, the smoother the path will be for injured workers' claim, and fewer complications will arise throughout the life of the claim.

THE LAW

Medical Letter

State administrative judges who hear workers' compensation cases will view medical letters to attorneys, adjusters, or whomever it may concern with some degree of skepticism. This is true because the motivation to write these letters probably came from the injured worker, an attorney, or an adjuster. Administrative judges will infer that the contents of the letter were discussed with, dictated by, or written by a party to the case. Presumably, the party was aware of the disputed issue in the workers' compensation case and obtained a medical letter to assist in proving a medicolegal point.

Medical letters between treating and referring doctors are not viewed with the same cynicism. Administrative judges will normally view correspondence between doctors with an understanding that the motivation was an honest desire to diagnose and treat the patient. These letters are not normally written with a view toward making a point in an administrative hearing.

There are, however, problems with medical letters between doctors and with medical reports written without an understanding of the law. While medical letters written for a party to a dispute may be viewed with some skepticism, it at least will not inadvertently damage the injured worker's case. This is true because the doctor will be aware of the law on the issue before drafting the letter. This same statement cannot be made about medical letters between doctors and other medical records that are used as evidence in workers' compensation cases. These other records and letters often inadvertently create problems for injured workers because the authors of the reports did not know or anticipate the legal effect of the statements or terms used in the reports.

Definition of Disability

In Texas cases, the best example of doctors who try to be helpful but fail because they do not know the law occurs in SIBs cases. As noted above, a worker with no ability to work because of impairment from a compensable injury is entitled to SIBs if other criteria are satisfied. When the injured worker who feels he or she has no ability to work submits a quarterly application for SIBs, he or she typically asks his or her treating doctor for a release-from-work statement to attach to the

SIBs application. Doctors unfamiliar with the pertinent law are often surprised to learn that the medical statements were not only discounted by the hearing officer but actually harmful to the injured worker's case.

In a review of several of these work-release forms, the TWCC Appeals Panel stated that using terms such as *disabled* or *unemployable* or phrases such as "cannot perform meaningful work" or "not capable of gainful employment" does not satisfy the requirement that injured workers provide medical evidence of no ability to work (11–13). The TWCC Appeals Panel over the last 4 years has clearly reiterated what a medical report must specifically contain in order to support an argument of no ability to work. Yet, reports are still being drafted with definitions of ability to work in terms of "gainful" or "meaningful' work or whether any employer would hire the injured worker. If these reports are the only evidence of no ability to work, the outcome of the case is certain: Benefits will be denied.

Aggravation Injuries

Another example of using words or phrases that will ensure a denial of benefits occurs in cases of reinjury. Under Texas law, an aggravation injury is defined as one involving a worsening or exacerbation of an original injury (14,15). The most common kinds of aggravation injuries involve the back and carpal tunnel syndrome. It is quite common for a worker to return to work after a long period of disability and then sustain a reinjury. When treating a patient with an aggravation injury, the doctor has a choice. He or she may decide that there is no new damage, simply a continuation of a previous injury. Alternatively, the doctor may decide that prior to the new injury the worker was able to return to work but now cannot work because there is a new injury and there must be new damage. It is important for the doctor to make a clear choice in these aggravation injury cases and to recognize the legal standards. Clearly, if the doctor uses the old date of injury in workers' compensation billing and reporting forms, this will cause a loss or reduction in indemnity benefits. In addition, using words such as "flare-up" will create an impression that there is no new injury (16). Judges will focus on and be influenced by language that carries specialized meanings within the context of the workers' compensation system.

Mean versus Median Values

Another category of medical report that may inadvertently damage an injured worker's case is an impairment rating report written by a doctor who has not kept up with the latest developments, training, and interpretations of impairment rating guidelines. Doctors who blindly use computer-generated impairment rating reports can also do inadvertent damage. Computer-generated ratings are susceptible not only to programming errors but also to outdated or incorrect rule interpretations.

The Texas workers' compensation statute (17) states that doctors must use the American Medical Association's (AMA) *Guides to the Evaluation of Permanent Impairment* (18). Each impairment rating point is worth 3 weeks of indemnity benefits (19). Under the third edition of the AMA *Guides,* and under the range of motion model contained in the fourth edition, range-of-motion deficit is combined with other components to reach a whole-person rating, but the measurements must be consistent to be considered valid. Consistency is determined by taking three consecutive measurements and determining whether they are within plus or minus five degrees from each other. The issue and problem involve the wording of the AMA *Guides.* Paragraph 3.3a.A.3 states that the measurements must be within plus or minus 5 degrees of the maximum or median motion values. A computer program used by a large number of doctors interprets this paragraph as stating that three consecutive measurements must be within plus or minus 5 degrees of each other. That means that lateral flexion measurements of 17, 19, and 23 degrees would be invalidated by the computer program. The TWCC

Appeals Panel considered this issue and decided that the measurements are valid only if they are within plus or minus 5 degrees of the median number. The median number is the middle number when the numbers are arranged in ascending order (20).

This variance in interpreting the AMA *Guides* results in discrepancies in ratings. Doctors who have taken training courses and use hand-held inclinometers will validate the measurements and provide a rating for range-of-motion deficit, while the untrained doctors who blindly use computer systems will cheat injured workers.

Improper Rounding of Measurements

Another computer error occurring in range-of-motion cases involves inappropriate rounding of numbers. The TWCC Appeals Panel stated that if an injured worker does not reach the "normal" angle on range-of-motion tests, he or she has impairment (21). That means that a program that rounds 23 degrees to 25 degrees, because 23 is closer to 25 than it is to 20, will provide an incorrect impairment rating. Again, doctors who have received training and use hand held inclinometers ensure that injured workers receive the correct rating.

CONCLUSION

Doctors who treat patients with work-related injuries must be cognizant of the potential impact that medical reports have on their patients' workers' compensation claims. It is not enough that a doctor's records are accurate and thorough, because they may be used as medical evidence, a purpose for which they were never intended when they were produced. However, in today's litigious society, that possibility cannot be overlooked. Doctors who are aware of the possible ramifications of their medical reports are in a better position to serve injured workers and take affirmative steps to enhance their professional reputation with the agency responsible for adjudicating workers' compensation claims.

In conclusion, many factors under doctors' control contribute to the administrative and legal consequences of occupational injuries. In general health, doctors are usually free of nonmedical concerns, except those associated with reimbursement. When factors of causation, disability status, permanent impairment or disability, mechanism of injury, and compensable body parts are thrown into the mix, many doctors become confused, frustrated, and avoidant. Doctors who intend to be relevant in the workers' compensation system, whether as a primary care physician at the early phase of injury, a surgeon, or a rehabilitation specialist, must become reasonably conversant with the critical factors involved in workers' compensation administrative law. Although the system is "no fault," physician documentation and case management are critical to the ultimate outcomes of cases and the achievement of societally desirable goals. This chapter has used the experience of a workers' compensation judge and the Texas workers' compensation environment to illustrate many of the factors that are generic to the federal and all state systems. Details may change from state to state, but the general principles illustrated in this chapter are similar, if not identical.

REFERENCES

1. Texas Workers' Compensation Commission. Spinal surgery system second-opinion doctor performance summary from 11/01/94 to 04/01/98. Texas Workers' Compensation Commission, 4000 South IH-35, Austin, Texas, 79704.
2. Discrepancies in impairment ratings by types of doctors. *Texas Monitor*, Vol. 1, no. 4, 1996, p. 8.
3. Texas Labor Code §409.001(a)(2).
4. Texas Workers' Compensation Commission appeal no. 960323.
5. Texas Workers' Compensation Commission appeal no. 952127.
6. Texas Workers' Compensation Commission appeal no. 951870.
7. Texas Labor Code §408.021.
8. Texas Labor Code §408.021(a).
9. Texas Labor Code §401.011(16).
10. Texas Labor Code §408.142.
11. Texas Workers' Compensation Commission appeal no. 971368.
12. Texas Workers' Compensation Commission appeal no. 970890.
13. Texas Workers' Compensation Commission appeal no. 970290.
14. Texas Workers' Compensation Commission appeal no. 960304.
15. Texas Workers' Compensation Commission appeal no. 951313.
16. Texas Workers' Compensation Commission appeal no. 951123.
17. Texas Labor Code §408.124(b).
18. Doege TC, Houston TP, eds. *Guides to the evaluation of permanent impairment*, 4th ed. Chicago: The American Medical Association, 1993.
19. Texas Labor Code §408.121(a)(1).
20. Texas Workers' Compensation Commission appeal no. 980985.
21. Texas Workers' Compensation Commission appeal no. 980894.

Occupational Musculoskeletal Disorders
edited by T. G. Mayer, R. J. Gatchel, and P. B. Polatin.
Lippincott Williams & Wilkins, Philadelphia © 2000.

5

Why Do Occupational Injuries Have Different Health Outcomes?

Barton G. Margoshes and *Barbara S. Webster

Liberty Mutual Insurance Group, Boston, Massachusetts 02117;
*Liberty Mutual Research Center, Hopkinton, Massachusetts 01748

The belief is widespread that cases involving the workers' compensation system have worse outcomes than similar cases not involving workers' compensation. This belief is supported by studies comparing workers' compensation cases with those covered by other insurance systems. Most of these studies examined patients with chronic low back pain who had undergone surgery or were involved in a chronic pain or rehabilitation program. In general, they found that workers' compensation cases incurred higher medical costs and had prolonged disability durations and a poorer response to treatment.

What is not clear, however, is why these differences exist. Some authors conclude that the workers' compensation system itself has inherent characteristics, dynamics, and incentives that promote increased utilization of resources and prolong disability. Others believe that the differences are a result of the patient population, physician behavior, or workplace issues. Another theory is that the sense of entitlement to "benefits" after a workplace injury is a factor. On closer evaluation of more recent studies that included multivariate analysis, it becomes apparent that several factors affecting the outcomes measured must be considered. This chapter reviews the results of selected studies reporting different outcomes for workers' compensation cases, including explanation of their findings.

First, it is important to define the scope of the problem in financial terms. It has been estimated that the cost for occupational injuries and illnesses is $171 billion (1). This estimate includes both direct costs ($65 billion) for medical and lost-wage payments and indirect costs ($106 billion) including administrative costs and costs for lost productivity and retraining. Up to 75% of all workers' compensation claimants' problems resolve readily, either losing no time from work or not meeting the waiting-period requirements to receive payments for lost time (2). Those patients who go on to be chronically disabled are of great concern to both employers, compensation carriers, and medical providers. Two studies on disability duration for workers' compensation claims reported that a small percentage of longer disability duration claims represented the highest percentage of total disability days and costs. The first study of low back pain disability duration found that the 7% of claims with greater than 1 year of disability accounted for 84.2% of the total disability days and 75.1% of the cost (3). The second study of work-related musculoskeletal disorders of the upper extremity reported that the 6.8% of claims with a length of disability greater than 1 year accounted for 75% of the total disability days and 59.9% of the cost (4). It is the high cost, chronically disabled cases that are most often studied in regard to treatment outcomes.

HOW WORKERS' COMPENSATION DIFFERS FROM GROUP HEALTH AND DISABILITY INSURANCE

Many studies examining workers' compensation outcomes compared cases covered under the workers' compensation system with those covered under the group health system. One problem with these studies is that the amount and level of coverage are not defined. This makes accurate direct comparisons between the two systems difficult. To understand the differences between the workers' compensation system and the group system of medical and disability benefits, it is helpful to review the distinctive characteristics of the two systems.

Workers' compensation insurance was first established in the United States in 1911 as a "no-fault" system. The main objectives of workers' compensation insurance are to provide wage replacement and medical, rehabilitation, and vocational services for those injured in workplace accidents; encourage workplace safety; and provide effective benefit delivery. The type and level of benefits are defined by law. Each state or jurisdiction has its own unique set of laws, including insurance requirements, types of employment covered, coverage of injuries and illnesses, benefits provided (income replacement and medical benefits), waiting periods (number of disability days that must pass before initiation of compensation payments), and administrative requirements and safeguards. All employees, with few exceptions, are covered under the workers' compensation system and coverage is mandated by state legislation.

Workers' compensation insurance is designed to make injured employees as whole as possible after a workplace injury. Therefore, both medical expenses and lost wages are covered. These are covered (paid) by one entity. The medical and wage-replacement (indemnity payments) coverage in workers' compensation, in general, continues for the duration of the claim, which may be lifelong. Coverage in the workers' compensation system for medical care requires no copay or de-

ductible. Wage-replacement benefits are tax free and are paid from the first day of disability or after a short waiting period. There are provisions for permanency awards, meaning that injured workers are eligible to receive compensation for a permanent disability resulting from a workplace accident.

In workers' compensation, the claim appeal process involves an administrative law process and possibly litigation. Coverage is usually determined by legally defined parameters and may differ from state to state. The usual standard for compensability is that the injury "arises out of and in the course of employment." That is, the injury is causally related to work activities and occurred while engaged during work activities. Many states provide coverage under the workers' compensation system for an aggravation of an existing injury or if the workplace accident contributed to a condition but was not the sole reason for that condition.

It is important to understand that workers' compensation is a single system designed to cover both the medical and lost-wage costs, whereas medical expenses and lost wages in the group insurance system are covered and administered by different entities. Group medical coverage is a voluntary benefit, and employers are not required by law to provide this coverage. Benefits are defined by the specific wording of the policy (contract), as opposed to workers' compensation benefits' being defined by state law. Many, though not all, employers, provide some level of group health coverage. Employees are frequently required to pay some of the premium out of pocket, as well as a copay or deductible. Frequently, group health policies contain clauses excluding coverage for preexisting conditions or stipulating a waiting period before coverage takes effect. The appeal process is administered by the health care plan through a nonlegal process. There are no permanency awards.

Short-term disability (STD) and long-term disability (LTD) plans are the nonoccupational or group equivalent of the indemnity portion of workers' compensation. There are significant differences compared with workers' compensation, however. STD and LTD are voluntary benefits, and employees are frequently required to pay part or all of the premium. Fewer employers provide coverage for STD and LTD than for group health. The eligibility and extent of wage replacement is defined by the policy contract and not by law. The appeal process is administered by the insurers through a nonlegal process.

WHAT IS A HEALTH OUTCOME?

In general terms, a *health outcome* is the result of a medical intervention or series of interventions. Health outcomes can be viewed by:

- Health care setting in which the care is delivered,
- Health care system in which it occurs,
- Time frame under consideration,
- Type of intervention,
- Perspective of the individual or entity interested in the outcome.

The choice of the outcome to be measured depends on the viewpoint of the examiner. For example, the outcomes studied in clinical asthma research differ significantly than those studied in low-back-pain investigations. Asthma researchers may be more interested in clinical indicators of success, such as peak flow or revisits to the emergency room, while low-back-pain investigators may be interested in the duration of disability after various therapeutic interventions. The setting of the medical care also influences what outcomes are measured. Studies in inpatient settings may measure the length of hospitalization (length of stay) as the endpoint, while duration of treatment or number of treatments may be significant in an ambulatory care setting. The time frame being considered can be different in that short-term endpoints such as revisits to the emergency department after treatment of an asthmatic episode are not the same as the long-term functional outcomes after rehabilitation of chronic low back pain. Finally, the health care system influences what is measured. The outcomes in workers' compensation research differ significantly from group health outcomes.

Outcomes research in workers' compensation emphasizes functional outcomes such as return to work and financial outcomes such as cost, while group health outcomes generally focus more often on the clinical outcomes of care such as morbidity, mortality, and symptom resolution. Over the past several years, however, this disparity of focus has narrowed, and outcomes such as function, symptom relief, disability, quality of life, and cost are now being studied in both the workers' compensation and group health areas. Low back pain, its treatment, and its outcomes have been extensively studied in the workers' compensation literature, as well as the group health literature. The reason for this is clear: Low back pain is one of the most common complaints and diagnoses encountered in both the occupational and nonoccupational setting, and its financial and social impact are felt regardless of the system that administers its treatment. The lifetime prevalence for low back pain is 60% to 80%, and it is the second most frequent symptom-related reason why people seek medical attention (5,6).

WHAT OUTCOMES ARE SIGNIFICANT?

As mentioned, workers' compensation outcomes differ in focus from group health outcomes. In general, workers' compensation outcomes focus more on how patients recovered in relation to their employment and the combined costs associated with the medical care and lost wages. Therefore, there is a greater emphasis on functional and financial outcomes as related to return to work and the total cost of care. It is helpful to group outcomes relevant in workers' compensation medical care into five categories (7) (Table 1).

Some important observations deserve attention in the comparison of the workers' compensation outcomes literature with the group health outcomes literature.

The workers' compensation literature is replete with studies measuring vocational status

TABLE 1. *Important outcomes in workers' compensation medical care*

1. Resolution of the condition
   a. Symptoms, especially pain
   b. Function in daily activities compared with preinjury levels
      1. Household and family responsibilities
      2. Transportation/driving
      3. Sexual activity
      4. Sleep
      5. Social and recreational activities
   c. Health perceptions and self-esteem
   d. Mood
   e. Ongoing medical care requirements—number of visits per case
2. Vocational status
   a. Work status (full-/part-time, same/different job employer)—lost time per case, restricted duty days
   b. Quality of work (psychosocial and other aspects of work)
      1. Quality of work life
      2. Function at work—physical and psychosocial dimension
      3. Interpersonal relationships
      4. Conflicts-late decision to retain attorney
   c. Comparison of the postinjury job with the previous job-preinjury function, tasks (physical and mental tasks) versus postdischarge job function, requirements, etc.
   d. Short-term and long-term job retention
   e. Productivity, quality, and flexibility at work
   f. Appropriate advancement and skill acquisition
3. Total costs (by cases, by diagnosis, by company)
   a. Direct: workers' compensation payments for indemnity and medical care
   b. Indirect:
      1. Employer's additional costs—retraining, accommodations
      2. Patient: financial burden (income change, health care, and other costs)
      3. Cost shifting to other systems, especially short-term
      4. Disability plans and group health
4. Patient and employer satisfaction
   a. Communication and explanations
   b. Appropriateness of care
   c. Opportunity for input in decisions; perception of control over outcome
5. Prevention
   a. How the job where the injury was noted was changed to reduce risk of injury to workers: include level of exposure prior to injury
   b. Modifications to decrease injury risk for coworkers

as an outcome endpoint. This is not common in the group health literature except in the study of low back pain. Vocational status refers to what job a patient returned to after or during treatment. This can be divided into full duty or restricted duty, part time or full time, regular job or modified job, and same employer or different employer. The specific vocational status outcome has tremendous significance to the employer, the employee, and the insurer. The vocational status has productivity implications for the employer, and the type of disability payment (e.g., temporary total disability or temporary partial disability) determines the amount of wage replacement afforded to the injured worker.

Another area where workers' compensation outcomes research differs from group health research is cost outcomes. Group health cost outcomes focus primarily on the cost of medical and rehabilitation treatment, whereas workers' compensation research considers the total cost of care as the relevant outcome. The total cost of care includes medical, physical, and vocational rehabilitation, wage replacement, and litigation expenses. Group health researchers generally do not measure the financial impact of lost time associated with an illness or injury. This is a critical element of workers' compensation outcomes research, since indemnity costs (disability payments) make up approximately 60% of the total cost associated with a workplace injury. The employer or workers' compensation insurer is responsible for covering both medical and indemnity costs. In the group health system, these expenses are usually covered and managed by two separate and distinct processes and systems (i.e., group health medical and STD).

Common areas of interest and study in workers' compensation and group health outcomes research are resolution of symptoms, quality of life, patient satisfaction, and prevention. There is increasing interest in studying outcomes such as patient satisfaction and quality-of-life issues. These are usually measured by survey tools such as questionnaires or telephone sampling. While these studies are fraught with the usual problems encountered with survey tools, such as reliability and subjectivity, the information obtained may reveal interesting trends and findings.

The SF-36 tool has been used in both workers' compensation and group health outcomes research. The SF-36 is a self-administered questionnaire that assesses the functional status and well-being of individuals (8). These measures assess quality-of-life outcomes that are affected by disease (or injury) and treatment. The SF-36 survey assesses both physical and mental status by function, well-being, disability, and personal perceptions of status. There are 36 questions grouped into eight scales: physical functioning, role-physical, bodily pain, general health, vitality, social functioning, role-emotional, and mental health (7) (Table 2). The SF-36 questionnaire is well suited to explore the physical and mental outcomes associated with treatment in workers' compensation and group health.

A problem associated with measuring health outcomes, particularly in a workers' compensation context, is that multiple confounders may influence the outcome (8) (Table 3). Due to these confounders or "moderators," it is frequently difficult to compare the results of one study with those of another

TABLE 2. *Meaning of SF-36 scores*

Concepts	Items (no.)	Levels (no.)	Meaning of scores	
			Low	High
Physical functioning	10	21	Limited a lot in performing all physical activities, including bathing or dressing due to health	Performs all types of physical activities, including the most vigorous without limitations due to health
Role-physical	4	5	Problems with work or other daily activities as a result of physical health	No problems with work or other daily activities as a result of physical health
Bodily pain	2	11	Very severe and extremely limiting pain	No pain or limitations due to pain
General health	5	21	Evaluates personal health as poor and believes it is likely to get worse	Evaluates personal health as excellent
Vitality	4	21	Feels tired and worn out all the time	Feels full of pep and energy all the time
Social functioning	2	9	Extreme and frequent interference with normal social activities due to physical or emotional problems	Performs normal social activities without interference due to physical or emotional problems
Role-emotional	3	4	Problems with work or other daily activities as a result of emotional problems	No problems with work or other daily activities as a result of emotional problems
Mental health	5	26	Feelings of nervousness and depression all the time	Feels peaceful, happy, and calm all the time
Reported health transition	1	5	Believes general health is much better now than 1 year ago	Believes general health is much worse now than 1 year ago

TABLE 3. *Factors related to return-to-work success and other outcomes in workers'*
compensation medical care

1. **Demographic**
   a. Age
   b. Education
   c. Length of employment in job at time of injury
   d. Ease of changing occupations and availability of suitable jobs
   e. Geographic variations
2. **Illness**
   a. Physical examination measures—limited predictive value
   b. Severity, especially pain intensity and previous history
   c. Daily functional activities (inconsistent correlation with functional-capacity testing)
   d. Comorbid conditions and fitness
   e. Treatment (e.g., surgery)
   f. Length of time out of work prior to enrollment
   g. Prior injury, especially workers' compensation injury
3. **Psychosocial factors**
   a. Perception of fault
   b. Health locus of control
   c. Hysteria
   d. Somatic focus
   e. Readiness to return to work
   f. Other stresses
4. **Job factors**
   a. Physical demands
   b. Ergonomic risks
   c. Job satisfaction
   d. Employee–supervisor relations
   e. Workplace accommodations
   f. Compensation issues, especially conflicts and attorney representation
   g. Job strain
5. **System factors**
   a. Access—unrestricted vs. managed care
   b. Provider—experience, incentives
   c. Insurers—resource reallocation, support
6. **Treatment factors**
   a. Type of program
   b. Length and intensity of program
   c. Range and quality of services
   d. Communication with workplace

or determine which variable affects the outcome (9). It is also difficult at times to successfully compare the outcomes studied in a group-health setting with those in a workers' compensation setting. This is primarily because moderators and confounders studied as variables in the workers' compensation literature are frequently not mentioned in the group health literature. For example, a workplace issue such as job satisfaction is generally considered more of a confounder in studies examining workers' compensation. It is becoming increasingly recognized that many of the same incentives, dynamics, and moderators influencing workers' compensation outcomes also affect group health outcomes.

Geographic variability is another significant confounder. Each state has its own specific laws and regulations regarding workers' compensation. These have a significant effect on outcomes. States with a more generous benefit structure have prolonged disability and higher medical costs. Boden (10) summarized many of the studies that have reported on the effects of changes in worker's compensation benefits on the rate of injury-reporting, duration of disability, and average cost per claim. It has been reported that a 10% increase in benefit payments will increase the frequency of claims-reporting by 4% to 10%, the average claim cost by 2% to 5%, the disability duration, and the chance for a claim to become permanent. It has also been shown that a decrease in the waiting period results in an increase in both claim frequency and claim severity.

Other confounders have particular influence in the workers' compensation setting. These include job tenure, prior injuries, perception of fault, readiness to return to work, job demands, employee–supervisor relations, report lag time (time from date of injury to date of report to insurer), and workplace accommodations.

OUTCOME STUDIES

Cost

Several studies have looked at cost outcome differences between workers' compensation and noncompensation cases. All found that medical expenses are higher for cases covered by workers' compensation insurance than for cases covered by other insurance systems. The study most often cited was done by the Minnesota Department of Labor and Industry (11). It compared treatment charges matched by injury type, billed (rather than the actual amount paid) to a workers' compensation carrier (Liberty Mutual) and a group health carrier (Blue Cross of Minnesota) during the first 6 months of 1987. The study found that the charges for treatment for all injuries covered by the compensation claims carrier were twice the charges for cases covered by the group carrier. The differences were even higher for certain injury types with less definitive diagnoses, such as soft tissue injuries. For example, medical charges for back sprains and strains were 2.3 times higher for workers' compensation cases than for those covered by the group carrier. More definitive injuries such as fractures had more equivalent costs for the two insurance carriers.

Zaidman (11) attributed these cost differences to higher service utilization and higher charges per service for the workers' compensation cases. It was felt that greater utilization of services and higher charges occurred as a result of a wider selection of treatment options for those less definitive diagnoses for

which there is little agreement by providers as to a standard course of treatment. In further analysis of the Minnesota study, Baker and Krueger (12) suggested that the differences in costs between the two systems was a result of "price discrimination" by providers and lack of cost controls in the workers' compensation system.

Johnson et al. (13) studied claims in California covered by a workers' compensation carrier (Zenith Insurance Company) and a group health carrier (CalFarm Life Insurance Company), looking at both charges and actual payments made. They found an even greater differential in health costs (specifically payments) than was seen in the Minnesota study for cases with less definitive diagnoses such as low back pain (4.8 in California versus 2.5 in Minnesota). The differential for fractures, a more definitive diagnosis, was also greater in California (2.1) than in Minnesota (1.3), but less so than for back pain.

Durbin et al. (14), using National Commission on Compensation Insurance data from 1988 to 1991, compared medical costs from four states (Florida, Illinois, Oregon, and Pennsylvania) covered by 15 of the largest workers' compensation carriers with a control group of group health claims involving injuries that were likely to have occurred at work. Results of descriptive and multivariate analyses found that costs were significantly higher for the workers' compensation group for the three outcomes studied: total payments, total service per episode duration, and number of outpatient dates of service. Workers' compensation cases had twice the number of outpatient procedures, more dates of outpatient service, and three to four times longer duration of service. In another study of this sample, Durbin (15) reported little difference in utilization of high-cost, more invasive procedures (e.g., surgery) between the workers' compensation and noncompensation groups.

These studies suggest that cost differences between the two systems are due to service utilization rather than price discrimination (13–15). Johnson et al. (13) found the cost differences to be the result of greater utilization of services and more providers. They suggested that the uncertainty of treatment options offered "revenue-maximizing providers the opportunity to overutilize services." Durbin et al. (14) attributed the higher workers' compensation costs to a higher utilization of services and the mix of providers such as physical therapists, radiologists, orthopedists, and chiropractors. There was no evidence that workers' compensation claims were charged more for procedures. That Durbin (15) found little difference in utilization of high-cost, more invasive procedures between the workers' compensation and noncompensation groups also reinforces that cost differences were the result of a higher volume of procedures in the workers' compensation group. Durbin suggested that a major contributing factor for the higher cost of treatment for workers' compensation claims is the "moral-hazard" incentive of the lack of a copay requirement in the compensation system.

Function and Return to Work

Several studies have looked at the differences in functional outcomes for workers' compensation and noncompensation populations. Some have looked at return to work (either frequency of return to work or disability duration), while others have measured patient's self-assessment of function utilizing various questionnaires. Different conditions have also been studied, including low back pain, surgical treatment outcomes for carpal tunnel syndrome, and other diagnostic groups. The findings have been mixed, depending on the outcomes studied, whether uni- or multivariate statistical analyses were utilized, and the length of follow-up.

Several studies of low back pain patients receiving workers' compensation reported worse functional outcomes than in a noncompensation comparison group, based on different outcomes measured. Atlas et al. (16) found that low back pain sciatica patients receiving workers' compensation had less functional improvement based on the Roland back disability scale and the SF-36 at 6-month follow-up. Workers' compensation recipients were also less likely to return to work than those not receiving compensation, unless they had received surgical intervention. Sander and Meyers (17) examined the effect of compensation on disability duration for railroad workers with low back pain. Workers with work-related injuries had statistically significant longer periods of disability than workers with nonwork-related injuries, even when the patients were matched for age, type, and severity of injury.

The worse outcomes seen by Atlas et al. (16) for the workers' compensation sciatica patients were associated with different characteristics found between the two groups. The workers' compensation group was younger and more likely to be male, and had a lower level of education and less surgery than the noncompensation group. The workers' compensation group also had worse symptoms and functional status measured at baseline and worse general and mental health perceptions.

Other studies found mixed results for low back pain patients participating in functional restoration programs. Tollison (18) included return-to-work status as one outcome measured in a study of the effect of compensation status on low back pain patients participating in a comprehensive functional restoration treatment program. Return-to-work outcomes measured at the end of the treatment program found a statistically significant worse outcome for compensation patients, but no differences were found at 6-month follow-up. Another study of low back pain patients in a highly structured functional restoration program found similar outcomes for return to work and increased function for both workers' compensation and noncompensated patients (19). The authors attributed the similar return to work and functional outcomes to the interdisciplinary and goal-focused approach of the program that encourages improved communication between involved parties.

Several studies found that patients' employment status had an effect on the outcome of rehabilitation, rather than compensation status for chronic pain patients. On univariate analysis, Dworkin et al. (20) found that both compensation and employment status had an effect on treatment response. When multivariate analysis was performed, only employment status had an effect for both short-term effects rated by research assistants and long-term effects based on patient self-reports. Catchlove and Cohen (21) studied the return-to-work rate for pain clinic patients. All patients received the same treatment, but one group was given specific instructions to return to work, while the other did not receive these instructions. No significant differences were found in age, sex, duration of pain or treatment, and pain location between the compensated and noncompensated groups. The better return-to-work rate was found for the group that was given specific instructions to return to work.

In a prospective study, Higgs et al. (22) evaluated return to work and need for job change for compensated versus noncompensated surgically treated carpal tunnel syndrome populations. Statistically significant fewer workers' compensation patients had returned to work and more had changed jobs due to carpal tunnel symptoms than in the noncompensated group. Attempts to perform fully stratified analysis to elucidate the impact of physical job demands on ability to return to the same job could not be done because of the small subset size and imprecision of job classification. The authors suggested several reasons for the outcome differences, including the requirement of work-relatedness for an injury to be covered by workers' compensation. This requirement results in workers' attributing fault to their employer, which may then lead to employees' accepting only complete resolution of symptoms before returning to work. The authors also suggested that "unrealistic employer expectations for prompt return to preoperative work levels and inflexibility in altering job demands may contribute to patient discomfort, frustration, and ultimately job performance failure" (22).

Functional status was an outcome for carpal tunnel release surgery evaluated by Atroshi et al. (23), based on two patient questionnaires: the SF-36 and the Carpal Tunnel Syndrome Instrument (CTSI). While univariate analysis found surgically treated carpal tunnel syndrome patients receiving workers' compensation had significantly worse scores for part of the SF-36, multivariate analysis failed to verify these findings. Neither uni- nor multivariate analysis could find significant differences in functional status based on the CTSI between workers' compensation and noncompensation patient groups. This study demonstrates that multivariate analysis is important to adjust for possible confounding variables. Although Atroshi et al. (23) found no difference in patient-measured functional outcomes, they acknowledged that there are other factors unrelated to function that influence actual return to work. These include lack of modified duty, union work rules, and workers' compensation regulations.

Bessette et al. (24) evaluated patient's preferences, including functional improvement, for specific health outcomes in carpal tunnel surgery. Workers' compensation patients assigned more importance to achieving improved function than noncompensation patients and had a lower return-to-work rate 6 months postsurgery. The compensation population in this study had more severe functional impairment at baseline than the noncompensated population, which may explain their higher preference for improved function and worse return-to-work rate. These findings point out the need to also obtain pretreatment measurements to better understand posttreatment outcomes. Higgs et al. (22) acknowledged that a major weakness of their study was its retrospective nature and the small subset sample size that made it impossible to fully evaluate the reasons for poorer outcomes. Studies of other diagnoses had mixed results regarding return to work or disability duration between workers' compensation and noncompensation populations. Choi et al. (25) included long-term employment status as part of their study of surgical treatment for brachial plexus injury. Fifty-four percent of those that were employed at the time of injury were able to return to work. Employment status was not found to be significantly affected by workers' compensation coverage or quality of functional recovery.

Noyes and Barber-Westin (26) assessed the mean number of days of lost time both pre- and postoperatively for compensated and noncompensated patients undergoing anterior cruciate ligament (ACL) reconstruction. While there was no significant difference for other measures of factors that normally affect reconstruction results for ACL repairs, there were differences in the duration of both pre- and postoperative periods, with the compensation group incurring significantly longer disability durations. The authors hypothesized that other factors may have affected the long disability duration for the workers' compensation group. These factors included "wage systems that support workers' compensation injuries long-term, inability of employers to modify job requirements, inability of employees to receive job retraining, or lack of immediate diagnosis and treatment of the injury" (26).

Satisfaction

The effect of compensation status on satisfaction has not been extensively studied. Satisfaction has usually been considered as a function of recovery either by the relief of symptoms or improved function. Greenough et al. (27) and Penta and Fraser (28) studied patient satisfaction after anterior lumbar fusion. Satisfaction outcomes were based on patients' subjective report of relief from symptoms. Greenough et al. (27) found that 2 years postoperatively compensation status and psychologic disturbance at presentation were significant prognostic factors. In addition, satisfaction after anterior lumbar fusion was negatively influenced by compensation status; that is, satisfaction was less. Penta and Fraser (28) confirmed Greenough et al.'s findings of a negative effect of compensation on patient satisfaction at 2 years, but this effect dissipated over time by 10 years' follow-up.

Clinical

The effect of compensation on clinical outcomes has demonstrated mixed results. Clinical outcomes often overlap with functional outcomes. Residual symptoms and pain intensity are the usual clinical outcomes measured. Greenough et al. (27) and Penta and Fraser (28), however, looked at radiographic evidence of lumbar fusion after anterior lumbar fusion procedures in compensated and noncompensated patients. Greenough et al. (27) found that compensated patients had a statistically significant lower rate of fusion than noncompensated patients. Also of interest was that fusion success did not correlate with functional improvement. Patients with radiologic fusion were not improved as measured by pain, satisfaction, or function, compared with those with a pseudarthrosis. The authors explained these findings by the observation that noncompensated patients may mobilize more vigorously, thereby promoting fusion. Compensated patients, on the other hand, may be more prone to straining their backs early in the rehabilitation period by falling, lifting, or bending, so that mobilization is compromised, thereby delaying healing. Penta and Fraser (28), using similar outcome measures to those of Greenough et al. (27), found the opposite result: no statistical difference in fusion rates after anterior lumbar fusion between compensated and noncompensated patients.

Tomaras et al. (29) studied patients who underwent outpatient surgical treatment for cervical radiculopathy. They found that in cases where workers' compensation claims were not involved, 92.8% of patients reported an excellent or good outcome and returned to work or comparable duties at a mean of 2.9 weeks postoperatively. In cases in which workers' compensation claims were involved, 77.8% of patients reported an excellent or good outcome and returned to work at a mean of 7.6 weeks postoperatively. They offered no explanation for the worse outcomes for compensated patients undergoing outpatient cervical surgical treatment; however, because the patients were selected on the basis of their willingness to undergo outpatient surgery and were not matched in the compensated and noncompensated groups, selection factors may play a significant role.

In a study of patients undergoing arthroscopic ACL reconstruction Noyes and Barber-Westin (26) found no significant difference between compensation and noncompensation groups with regard to anteroposterior displacements, functional limitations with daily or sports activities, patient perception of the knee condition, overall rating score, or complications. They concluded based on these findings that workers' compensation benefits had no apparent influence on the subjective, objective, or functional results after ACL reconstruction. They recommended that individuals who sustain work-related ACL injuries should not be treated differently from other patients in terms of selection criteria for operative intervention.

In their carpal tunnel release surgery study, Higgs et al. (22) found that residual symptoms were significantly more common in patients receiving workers' compensation than those not receiving workers' compensation. They were careful to point out that their study demonstrated an association between workers' compensation and poor outcomes, but not a causal relationship. The poor outcomes were hypothesized to include the result of the adversarial situation that develops when a worker believes the employer to be at fault for the accident: a higher expectation of recovery in the compensated population, legal representation, and unrealistic employer expectations for prompt return to preoperative work levels.

In Tollison's (18) study of injured patients participating in a nonsurgical treatment program for low back pain, compensated patients rated their pain intensity significantly higher than those in the noncompensation group at admission, discharge, and follow-up. Tollison stated that "it is entirely possible that group differences may be attributable to compensation status," and suggested that secondary gain and the workers' compensation laws that reinforce slow recovery may be also be operable.

While there is a belief among many that compensated patients have worse clinical outcomes, these studies indicate that there is no clear consensus. Patient factors, patient selection factors, employer factors, or factors inherent in the compensation system all contribute to the mixed results.

OTHER FACTORS AFFECTING OUTCOMES IN WORKERS' COMPENSATION

Workers' compensation laws have been shown to affect the decisions and behaviors of patients/employees, employers, providers, and insurers (30). Before compensation is conferred, a causal relationship must be determined. Patients must "prove" a work-related history for their injury or illness, which providers are then asked to substantiate. If the doctor questions the relationship of the symptoms to a work activity or believes the patient is seeking secondary gain, it may result in a "compromised ethical state of mind" for the provider. This has the potential to establish an adversarial relationship between patients and providers, resulting in compromised treatment and poorer outcomes (31,32).

Some employers, providers, and insurers believe that employees are malingerers, who intentionally fake an injury to defraud the compensation system. In reality, there are very few actual instances of malingering (33). But the perception persists, resulting in "social labeling," stereotyping, and observer bias on the part of examiners. Ogden-Niemeyer (33) provided a model that demonstrated the dynamics of this belief on the interactions between providers and injured workers. A practitioner reacts to a patient's "illness behaviors" (those behaviors that are magnified responses to a physical injury), and following the biomedical model, attributes these behaviors to malingering and withholds treatment, resulting in a threat to the patient's integrity and increased distress and illness behavior. This behavior unfortunately serves to confirm the provider's bias. Several studies have found a negative bias on the part of providers toward patients receiving compensation (34–36). This dynamic may lead to worse outcomes in workers' compensation.

More enlightened providers follow a biopsychosocial model and respond to a patient's illness behaviors by providing appropriate treatment or rehabilitation (33). Hazard et al. (37) showed that models looking at disability exaggeration were unable to predict poor outcomes for chronic low back pain patients in a multidisciplinary treatment program. This may be because the program studied provided counseling that addressed those factors that led to disability exaggeration, including "fear of re-injury, overly protective spouses, physician warnings against painful activity, anxiety, depression, and other personality features" (37). It is therefore recommended that rehabilitation programs include counseling to address these factors.

Another bias held by providers is the concept of "compensation neurosis." This was first recognized in the 1880s as part of industrial accident litigation. It was thought that individuals with work-related disability exaggerated their complaints and suffered from psychiatric disorders such as depression and neuroticism only until they received a "curative" financial settlement, at which time they were able to return to work (38). Many early studies supporting this concept were descriptive in nature (39–42), but more recent studies have refuted this concept (9,43).

Some believe that workers' compensation patients have a greater incidence of psychologic disturbance than those not receiving compensation. Leavitt et al. (44) found that compensation patients were similar clinically in relation to the relative frequency of psychologic disturbance and nonorganic findings, compared to noncompensated patients.

Over the past 10 years, workers' compensation managed care has become more prevalent. Administrative controls, such as utilization management and direction to specific providers, are employed to reduce costs and, in theory, improve quality. Limiting patients' access to care has the potential to set up an adversarial relationship between employees and

providers, thus affecting treatment outcome. Restrictions to care may also create a hostile relationship between employees and employers. These adversarial factors in the workers' compensation managed care system may lead to an injured employee's hiring a lawyer to deal with these issues through a litigated process.

Once a compensation claim has been accepted, there may be few restrictions of services and there are no deductibles for employees to pay. Employees may access more medical services as a result of not having to pay out of pocket expenses. As more treatment is provided, patients may become reluctant to discontinue ineffective treatments. The compensation system also leads to the "medicalization" of disability by requiring claimants to be under active treatment to maintain their benefits (45). This concept was supported by Engel et al. (46) in a study that described health care utilization of high-cost primary care back patients in a health maintenance organization setting. Back pain disability compensation was one predictor for high back pain costs and was an independent predictor of higher utilization of health care services. The authors suggested that the continuation of compensation for pain-related treatments "set up incentives for patients receiving disability to initiate more health-care visits" (46). In another study of compensated and noncompensated low back pain patients, Leavitt (47) found that patients with work-related injuries had longer disability durations irrespective of the physical job demands and pain intensity. He suggested that this prolonged disability was associated in part with the provision of medical services under the compensation system. Others have described this as an "operant conditioning" effect of workers' compensation (48,49).

Indeterminate diagnoses, such as nonspecific low back pain, can lead to "catastrophizing" by claimants with increased levels of pain and distress. Without a diagnosis to validate their pain, these claimants have no clear expectations for prognosis, pain relief, appropriate treatment options, or, in the case of workers' compensation, continued compensation benefits. This may lead to further unnecessary diagnostic testing either at the patient's insistence or that of the insurer as part of an independent medical examination to set indemnity benefits (13). Despite negative diagnostic findings, excessive testing has the potential to lead patients to believe that their problem is more serious than it is (45).

On the other hand, a specific initial diagnosis was found to be highly predictive of chronic disability for back pain patients, especially for older patients (50). While certain diagnoses, such as sciatica, are likely to result in prolonged disability due to a poorer prognosis, Abenhaim et al. (50) noted that the "labeling effect" has consequences for both physicians' approaches to management and patients' responses to diagnoses. A physician may focus on the investigation and treatment of the pain-producing lesion. The time spent on performing diagnostic and pain reduction procedures often prolongs disability, and functional rehabilitation efforts may be ignored until a time when they have less chance for success. With a diagnostic label, the patient believes that a cure in the form of pain reduction is possible, even though few cures for low back pain exist. As a result, patients become dependent on their practitioner for pain management and fail to accept responsibility for their own functional recovery.

Studies have found that patients receiving workers' compensation have different expectations regarding relief of symptoms. Bellamy (51) suggested that patients are compelled to guard against getting well in order to maintain their benefits. Patients fear that they may be without lost-wage coverage if they have a recurrence of their symptoms once their claim is closed. As a result, they may resist efforts to return to work before they feel 100% recovered—"just in case." Hazard et al. (37) suggested that patients may also unconsciously overreport symptoms and perform poorly on functional testing because they fear discrimination and dismissal if they return to work.

In a study of patients' expectations for specific outcomes following surgery, Bessette et al. (24) found that patients receiving compensation assigned higher expectations to pain relief and functional improvement. Perhaps, this is true because employers often require that injured employees be 100% recovered before returning to work. The interpretation of "100% recovered" includes being free of pain. Often, pain does persist, although the patient is functionally able to work. Studies of low back pain by Von Korff et al. (52) and Wahlgren et al. (53) found that approximately 70% of patients experiencing low back pain for the first time still had pain 1 year later but few were disabled from work at that point. Requirements for 100% recovery should be eliminated. Management as well as unions should be educated in the benefits of modified work, alternative work schedules, job redesign, job placement, and other incentives for early return to work (54,55).

Based on a review of studies, Nachemson (56) provided indirect scientific support that treatment should include early, gradual, biomechanically controlled return to activity and work. Early return to work is therapeutic by inhibiting the development of illness behaviors and psychologic dependence, as well as limiting the development of decreased mobility and strength that occurs as a result of inactivity. These recommendations are also part of several different diagnostic and treatment guidelines on the management of low back pain published over the last decade (57–60).

The concept of encouraging early return to work finds support in a study by Catchlove and Cohen (21), who found an improved return-to-work rate when patients were given specific instructions to return to work, and in a study by Dworkin et al. (20), who found that employed chronic pain patients had better treatment outcomes. Dworkin et al. (20) concluded their study with a statement by White (41) made in the late 1960s but still relevant today:

> Perhaps effective placement of these unfortunate workmen in jobs which are within the limitations imposed by the pain would maintain morale, avoid concentration of their attention on their complaints and, while keeping up reasonable bodily activities, allow passage of sufficient time for the condition to subside.

Employers can facilitate return to work through a number of efforts. These include administrative procedures to provide injured workers with modified duty and allow them to recover while at work. This can be facilitated through performing an ergonomic job assessment and job redesign. These interventions help accommodate injured workers, encouraging them either to stay on the job or, if disabled, return to work sooner.

CONCLUSION

The findings of the studies cited for workers' compensation cases versus group health cases are not conclusive in showing that the workers' compensation system alone is directly associated with worse outcomes. These studies do suggest, however, that cases covered by the workers' compensation system have quantitatively and qualitatively worse outcomes for cost and duration of disability. The specific reasons why this occurs are unclear; however, there are indications that multiple variables other than compensation influence outcomes. These variables include "clinical, economic, psychosocial, and work organizational determinants" (61). Unfortunately, most studies to date have not successfully controlled for these multiple variables and confounders. In addition, it is important to note that many of these variables exist in both systems. The studies to date have not matched medical and disability benefit coverage for the two systems to adequately compare outcomes. It is possible that the health care and disability utilization profiles are similar for both systems in an adequately controlled study sample. Future studies must adequately control for these complex variables and better match the group health and workers' compensation systems.

REFERENCES

1. Leigh JP, Markowitz SB, Fahs M, Shin C, Landrigan PJ. Occupational injury and illness in the United States: estimates of costs, morbidity, and mortality. *Arch Intern Med* 1997;157:1557–1568.
2. Webster BS, Snook SH. The cost of 1989 workers' compensation low back claims. *Spine* 1994;19:1111–1116.
3. Hashemi L, Webster BS, Clancy EA, Volinn E. Length of disability and cost of workers' compensation low back pain claims. *J Occup Environ Med* 1997;39:937–945.
4. Hashemi L, Webster BS, Clancy EA, Courtney TK. Length of disability and cost of work-related musculoskeletal disorders of the upper extremity. *J Occup Environ Med* 1998;40:261–269.
5. Frymoyer JW, Cats-Baril WL. An overview of the incidences and costs of low back pain. *Orthop Clin North Am* 1991;22:2147–2152.
6. Cypress BK. Characteristics of physician visits for back symptoms: a national perspective. *Am J Public Health* 1983;73:389–395.
7. Pransky G, Himmelstein J. Evaluating outcomes of workers' compensation medical care. In: Kimpan K, ed. *Workers' compensation medical care: effective measurement of outcomes.* Cambridge, MA: Workers' Compensation Research Institute, 1996:11–32.
8. Ware JE, Snow KK, Kosinski M, Gandek B. *SF-36 health survey: manual and interpretation guide.* Boston, MA: Nimrod Press, 1993:3–5.
9. Burns JW, Sherman ML, Devine J, Mahoney N, Pawl R. Association between workers' compensation and outcome following multidisciplinary treatment for chronic pain: roles of mediators and moderators. *Clin J Pain* 1995;11:94–102.
10. Boden LI. Workers' compensation in the United States: high costs, low benefits. *Annu Rev Public Health* 1995;16:189–218.
11. Zaidman B. Industrial-strength medicine: a comparison of workers' compensation and Blue Cross Health Care in Minnesota. A background report for the Minnesota legislature. St. Paul, MN: Department of Labor and Industry, 1990.
12. Baker LC, Krueger AB. Twenty-four hour coverage and workers' compensation insurance. *Health Affairs* 1993;12(suppl):271–281.
13. Johnson WG, Baldwin MJ, Burton JF. Why is the treatment of work-related injuries so costly? New evidence from California. *Inquiry* 1996;33:53–65.
14. Durbin DL, Corro D, Helvacian N. Workers' compensation medical expenditures: price vs. quantity. *J Risk Insur* 1996;65:13–33.
15. Durbin D. Workplace injuries and the role of insurance: claims costs, outcomes, and incentives. *Clin Orthop* 1997;336:18–32.
16. Atlas SJ, Singer DE, Keller RB, Patrick DL, Deyo RA. Application of outcomes research in occupational low back pain: the Maine lumbar spine study. *Am J Ind Med* 1996;29:584–589.
17. Sander RA, Meyers JE. The relationship of disability to compensation status in railroad workers. *Spine* 1986;11:141–143.
18. Tollison CD. Compensation status as a predictor of outcome in nonsurgically treated low back injury. *South Med J* 1993;86:1206–1209.
19. Ambrosius FM, Kremer AM, Herkner PB, DeKraker M, Bartz S. Outcome comparison of workers' compensation and noncompensation low back pain in a highly structured functional restoration program. *J Sports Phys Ther* 1995;21:7–12.
20. Dworkin RH, Handlin DS, Richlin DM, Brand L, Vannucci C. Unraveling the effect of compensation, litigation, and employment on treatment response in chronic pain. *Pain* 1985;23:49–59.
21. Catchlove R, Cohen K. Effect of a directive return to work approach in the treatment of workmans' compen-

sation patients with chronic pain. *Pain* 1982;14: 181–191.

22. Higgs PE, Edwards D, Martin DS, Weeks PM. Carpal tunnel surgery outcomes in workers: effect of workers' compensation status. *J Hand Surg [Am]* 1995;20: 354–360.

23. Atroshi I, Johnsson R, Nouhan R, McCabe SJ. Use of outcome instruments to compare workers' compensation and non-workers' compensation carpal tunnel syndrome. *J Hand Surg [Am]* 1997;22:882–888.

24. Bessette L, Keller RB, Liang MH, Simmons BP, Fossel AH, Katz JN. Patients' preferences and their relationship with satisfaction following carpal tunnel release. *J Hand Surg [Am]* 1997;22:613–620.

25. Choi PD, Novak CB, Mackinnon SE, Kline DG. Quality of life and functional outcome following brachial plexis injury. *J Hand Surg* [Am] 1997;22:605–612.

26. Noyes FR, Barber-Westin SD. A comparison of results of arthroscopic-assisted anterior cruciate ligament reconstruction between workers' compensation and non-compensation patients. *Arthroscopy* 1997;13:474–484.

27. Greenough CG, Taylor LJ, Fraser RD. Anterior lumbar fusion: a comparison of noncompensation patients with compensation patients. *Clin Orthop* 1994;300:30–37.

28. Penta M, Fraser RD. Anterior lumbar interbody fusion: a minimum 10-year follow-up. *Spine* 1997;22: 2429–2434.

29. Tomaras CR, Blacklock JB, Parker WD, Harper RL. Outpatient surgical treatment of cervical radiculopathy. *J Neurosurg* 1997;87:41–43.

30. Beals RK. Compensation and recovery from injury. *West J Med* 1984;140:233–237.

31. Martin RD. Secondary gain, everybody's rationalization. *J Occup Med* 1974;16:800–801.

32. Carron H, DeGood DE, Tait R. A comparison of low back pain patients in the United States and New Zealand: psychosocial and economic factors affecting severity of disability. *Pain* 1985;21:77–89.

33. Ogden-Niemeyer L. Social labeling, stereotyping, and observer bias in workers' compensation: the impact of provider–patient interaction on outcome. *J Occup Rehabil* 1991;1:251–269.

34. Melzak R, Katz J, Jeans ME. The role of compensation in chronic pain: analysis using a new method of scoring the McGill Pain Questionnaire. *Pain* 1985;23: 101–112.

35. Krusen EM, Ford DE. Compensation factors in low back injuries. *JAMA* 1958;166:1128–1133.

36. Simmonds M, Kumar S. Does the knowledge of patients' workers' compensation status influence clinical judgments? *J Occup Rehabil* 1996;6:93–107.

37. Hazard RG, Bendix A, Fenwick JW. Disability exaggeration as a predictor of functional restoration outcomes for patients with chronic low-back pain. *Spine* 1991;16:1062–1067.

38. Gallagher RM, Williams RA, Skelly J, et al. Workers' compensation and return-to-work low back pain. *Pain* 1995;61:299–307.

39. Miller H. Accident neurosis. *BMJ* 1961;XX:919–925.

40. Thompson GN. Post-traumatic psychoneurosis: a statistical survey. *Am J Psych* 1965;121:1043–1048.

41. White AWM. Low back pain in men receiving workmen's compensation. *Can Med J* 1966;95:50–56.

42. Sternbach RA, Wolf SR, Murphy RW, Akeson WH. Traits of pain patients: the low back "loser." *Psychosomatics* 1973;14:226–229.

43. Mendelson G. Not "cured by a verdict:" effect of legal settlement on compensation claimants. *Med J Aust* 1982;2:132–134.

44. Leavitt F, Garron DC, McNeill TW, Whisler WW. Organic status, psychological disturbance, and pain report characteristics in low-back-pain patients on compensation. *Spine* 1982;7:398–402.

45. Himmelstein JS, Feuerstein M, Stanek EJ, et al. Work-related upper-extremity disorders and work disability: clinical and psychosocial presentation. *J Occup Environ Med* 1995;37:1278–1286.

46. Engel CC, Von Korff M, Katon WJ. Back pain in primary care: predictors of high health-care costs. *Pain* 1996;65:197–204.

47. Leavitt F. The physical exertion factor in compensable work injuries: a hidden flaw in previous research. *Spine* 1992;17:307–310.

48. Block AR, Kremer E, Gaylor M. Behavioral treatment of chronic pain: variables affecting treatment efficacy. *Pain* 1980;8:367–375.

49. Brena SF, Chapman SL, Bradford LA. Conditioned responses to treatment in chronic pain patients: effects of compensation for work-related accidents. *Bull Los Angeles Neurol Soc* 1980;44:48–52.

50. Abenhaim L, Rossignol M, Gobeille D, Bonvalot Y, Fines P, Scott S. The prognostic consequences in the making of the initial medical diagnosis of work-related back injuries. *Spine* 1995;20:791–795.

51. Bellamy R. Compensation neurosis: financial reward for illness as nocebo. *Clin Orthop* 1997;336:94–106.

52. Von Korff M, Deyo R, Cherkin D, Barlow W. Back pain in primary care: outcomes at 1 year. *Spine* 1993;18: 855–862.

53. Wahlgren DR, Atkinson JH, Epping-Jordan JE, et al. One-year follow-up of first onset low back pain. *Pain* 1997;73:213–221.

54. Snook SH. Approaches to the control of back pain in industry: job design, job placement and education/training. *Spine: State Art Rev* 1987;2:45–59.

55. Snook SH. The control of low back disability: the role of management. In: Kroemer KHE, McGlothlin JD, Bobick TG, eds. *Manual materials handling: understanding and preventing back trauma*. Akron, OH: American Industrial Hygiene Association, 1989:97–101.

56. Nachemson A. Work for all: for those with low back pain as well. *Clin Orthop* 1983;179:77–85.

57. Bigos S, Bowyer O, Braen G, et al. *Acute low back problems in adults. Clinical practice guideline no. 14.* Rockville, MD: Agency for Health Care Policy and Research, Public Health Service, U.S. Department of Health and Human Services, 1994. AHCPR publication 95-0642.

58. Spitzer WO, LeBlanc FE, Dupuis M. Scientific approach to the assessment and management of activity-related spinal disorders. *Spine* 1987;12:S1–S60.

59. Rosen M. *Back pain: report of a Clinical Standards Advisory Group (CSAG) committee on back pain.* London: Her Majesty's Stationer's Office. (HMSO), 1994.

60. American College of Occupational and Environmental Medicine. Low back complaints. In: Harris JS, ed. *Occupational medicine practice guidelines: evaluation and management of common health problems and functional recovery in workers*. Beverley, MA: OEM Press, 1997:14-1–14-30.

61. Katz JN, Keller RB, Fossel AH, et al. Predictors of return to work following carpal tunnel release. *Am J Ind Med* 1997;31:85–91.

PART II

Biomechanics and Ergonomics

Occupational Musculoskeletal Disorders
edited by T. G. Mayer, R. J. Gatchel, and P. B. Polatin.
Lippincott Williams & Wilkins, Philadelphia © 2000.

6

The Thoracolumbar Spine

Malcolm H. Pope, *James W. DeVocht, †Donald R. McIntyre,
and ‡Tracy K. Marker

*Department of Environmental & Occupational Medicine, University of Aberdeen,
Foresterhill, Aberdeen AB9 2ZD, Scotland, United Kingdom; *Palmer Center for Chiropractic
Research, Palmer College of Chiropractic, Davenport, Iowa, 52803; †NDX, Inc.,
Efland, North Carolina 27243; and ‡Interlogics, Inc., Nashville, Tennessee 37204*

Musculoskeletal injuries either are acute or can be classified as *cumulative trauma disorders* (CTDs). This latter category includes the most disabling and costly health problems in both the United States and in all industrialized countries. Of these low back pain (LBP) and carpal tunnel syndrome (CTS) are the most prevalent; however LBP is by far the most common and costly.

In the United States, administrative records (e.g., worker's compensation) frequently are used to estimate incidence rates, but the data are extremely difficult to interpret because of varying decision rules. Chronic LBP and upper (cervical) back pain are the most pervasive health problems during the peak years of productivity. LBP severely restricts the activities of 20% of older adults and is a particular problem of a rural community because of the high prevalence and the relative lack of rehabilitative and diagnostic service providers. According to the National Center for Health Statistics, back and spine impairments are the third leading cause of impairment in the United States. More than four million Americans are now permanently disabled by LBP, and 25% of all disabling injuries are back or spine injuries. In fact, disabling chronic LBP (CLBP) is more common, if less visible, than any other disability. Often it presents few outward, visible manifestations, and yet it can be profoundly disabling. LBP frequently eludes precise diagnosis. In at least 50% of cases, objective physical findings cannot be specified even by the most sophisticated diagnostic methods. CLBP can have devastating effects on emotional as well as physical well-being, severely reducing personal independence and quality of life.

EPIDEMIOLOGY AND COST

Between 1971 and 1985, the number of people who have back or spine disabilities increased by 168%, whereas the U.S. population increased by only 12.5%. The vast majority of those with LBP impairment or disability are reported to be between 17 and 64 years of age. In fact, about 80% of adults experience LBP that impairs activity sometime in their lives. Epidemiologic studies (1,2) report a lifetime prevalence of 60% to 90% and an annual incidence of 5% (3–5). Most of these people recover within 4 to 6 weeks, but about 10% develop CLBP (constant or intermittent pain that lasts for months, years, or for life). About 50% of those with CLBP become *disabled*, that is, unable to work, to carry out the tasks of normal daily living, or to participate in recreational and leisure activities. The rate of CLBP disability continues to increase dramatically (6).

Only 50% of persons who have LBP receive a definite diagnosis, although many disorders can be identified. The most common diagnoses for LBP are lumbosacral strain and sprain, which are nonspecific. Numerous studies attest to a high failure rate in rehabilitation when disability extends longer than 6 months. The duration of disability has been related directly to the likelihood of successful treatment and rehabilitation. Only about 40% of those whose disability persists for 6 months or longer are able to return to work eventually, only about 20% of those disabled for a year or more return to work, and those whose disability persists for 2 years or longer rarely ever work again (7).

The seemingly small percentage of people who are disabled with CLBP accounts for 80% to 90% of the tremendous costs associated with low back disorders. Estimates of cost vary widely, depending on how they are computed. The longer a person is away from work after a work-related injury, the lower the probability of ever returning to work. As time away from work increases, the costs of care and compensation accumulate rapidly. In the United States, the combined costs of medical expenses, compensation, lost earnings, and lost productivity for LBP is approaching 100 billion dollars a year. Longer duration of disability is related to reduced chances of recovery. Compensation awards in the Social Security Disability program increased by 2,800% between 1957 and 1976, reflecting a growth rate 14 times that of the population.

IMPLICATIONS FOR INDUSTRY

The effects of LBP are especially marked in the workplace and they represent the second most common cause of absences from work. The highest rates of back injuries occur in occupations that require heavy manual labor, repeated lifting, long-term exposure to vehicle vibration, and static positions, especially when the worker is required to be in awkward or unsupported postures. CLBP is most common among workers in agriculture, construction, mining, transportation, sedentary work, and aviation. Office workers who sit for most of the workday also report high levels of back discomfort and fatigue, which may predispose them to CLBP. The U.S. Public Health Service reports that LBP represents 32% of compensable injuries and 42% of costs. LBP disability claims have increased dramatically in the last three decades, growing at a rate 14 times that of population growth. According to the U.S. Equal Employment Opportunity Commission, 87,942 charges concerning employment discrimination were filed under Title I of the Americans with Disabilities Act (ADA) during fiscal year 1993; more than 20% of these dealt with back impairment (8).

Repetitive work is still an important component of our industrial economy. In many cases, workers can do the job better and cheaper than machines, particularly true when there are variations in the process, materials, or parts. Some companies have shifted from automation back to manual work, and for the foreseeable future, manual work will be an important part of our industrial economy.

Considering the usual course of LBP and the source of the high costs, it is clear that some logical points for intervention exist. The most responsible public health strategy is to involve all vested parties in preventing LBP (i.e., *primary prevention* through ergonomic intervention). The most effective cost reduction, however, may be *secondary prevention*, by helping back injured employees return to work as soon as possible through appropriate, timely treatment and worksite accommodations. The development of such strategies depends on continued research. It is critical to address primary, secondary, and tertiary prevention measures, meaning that workplace and environmental factors that contribute to LBP must be identified and changed so that persons whose back pain is likely to become episodic, chronic, or disabling also can be identified; thus, it will be possible to identify and implement appropriate prevention strategies. The increased awareness that psychosocial factors are of critical importance in CLBP *disability* is noteworthy.

Because CLBP costs so much in lost productivity, compensation payments, and human suffering, occupational rehabilitation has become critical; however, returning injured or impaired workers to their jobs requires concerted efforts on the part of employees, employers, supervisors, unions, rehabilitation professionals, and others to modify specific tasks and to provide workers with requisite accommodations. This is particularly challenging with the older worker.

The cost of work-related injuries and illnesses is overwhelming the workers' compensation system. Too many workers are getting injured, they cost too much to compensate, employers feel that they cannot spend any more on compensation, and workplace injuries and illnesses continue to occur. In addition, the American workforce is suffering the loss of many skilled people who are no longer able to contribute because they are injured or ill. Almost all LBP injuries can be identified as resulting from a mismatch between the worker and the workplace.

Epidemiologic studies make it clear that some occupations are more hazardous than others in terms of LBP and present some of the most difficult obstacles for returning injured workers to their jobs. The most critical workplace risk factors appear to be heavy manual labor, repetitive lifting, twisting, and other motions (9). This association between awkward work postures and LBP has been well documented (10,11). Simultaneous lifting and twisting also constitute a high-risk factor for prolapsed lumbar intervertebral discs (12). Back-injured workers most often attribute their injuries to excessive lifting (13). Other risk factors include sudden, unexpected maximal efforts, stretching and reaching, exposure to whole-body vibration, prolonged sitting, and years of employment (9). A high incidence of accidents in the workplace are due to manual materials handling (MMH) (14). Workers whose primary tasks involve heavy lifting are, thus, at high risk of LBP (11). Several studies demonstrated that heavy work contributes to LBP more than any other stressor. Medical and work histories of employees about to retire from the Eastman Kodak Company were reviewed by Rowe (15), who categorized jobs associated with heavy, moderate, or light work. Of those who worked with heavy loads, 65% report having had LBP.

Magora (11) found a positive correlation between heavy lifting and LBP. In this study, four different occupations were evaluated: heavy-industry workers, light-industry workers, bus drivers, and bank clerks. Of the four occupations, the heavy-industry workers ranked highest in LBP reports. In another study, Jensen (16) compared occupations and categorized them in terms of annual incidence ratio. Of the 24 ranked-ordered occupations, the top five were nursing aides, orderlies, attendants, construction laborers, and truck drivers. The work required from these occupations typically involves frequent MMH.

PREVENTION OF OCCUPATIONAL LBP

Efforts to prevent occupational LBP have become increasingly important because diagnostic and therapeutic approaches have proved inadequate to curb the soaring incidence and cost of this problem (17,18). Most such methods can be classified as primary, secondary, CTDs. This classification comprises several distinct elements, including preemployment or preplacement testing of workers, training workers in safe and effective performance of job tasks, ergonomic job design or job modification, and employee fitness programs. Secondary prevention strategies aim to identify employees who have experienced an injury and are at high risk for becoming disabled and to intervene appropriately and early enough to change the predicted outcome (i.e., to prevent disability). Such interventions may take many forms, such as treatment, education, ergonomic counseling, and job accommodation and modification. Tertiary prevention includes treatment and rehabilitation strategies to minimize the consequences of injury, reduce the duration of chronicity or disability, restore function, and return people to work. Overexertion injuries, two thirds of which are attributed to MMH, are incurred by 500,000 workers per year in the United States (about 1 in 20 workers), and such injuries account for 25% of all reported occupational injuries. Additionally, fewer than one third of LBP injured workers with significant time lost from work ever return to their previous jobs. These facts make it imperative to develop strategies that will enable employers to accommodate workers with low back injuries. The National Institute of Occupational Safety and Health (NIOSH) guide cites evidence that injury rates, as well as severity rates, increase significantly when (a) heavy objects are lifted, (b) the object is bulky, (c) an object is lifted from the floor, or (d) objects are lifted frequently (14).

Occupational risk factors include heavy repetitive lifting, particularly in forward-flexed or twisted postures (19), lifting demands that exceed workers' physical capacities (20), prolonged sitting (1,11), and vehicle vibration (4,21). High-risk occupations typically involve one or more of the following: MMH, awkward postures, prolonged sitting, or vibration. Some occupations with the highest injury rates are warehousing, nursing, trucking, construction, mining, aviation, and transportation (16). Among such occupations, the annual incidence of back pain may be as high as 20% (22). As for workers themselves, the least physically fit are more likely to sustain acute back injuries; paradoxically, however, the more physically fit workers may incur the most costly injuries (23).

Workers and work tasks must be appropriately matched; this means both accommodation and adaptation. In general, little consideration has been given to what injured workers are expected to do on the job or how intervention at the workplace might be implemented. The "medical model" focuses primarily on treatment of the patient and usually does not include any analysis of workplace demands. Current approaches to rehabilitation stress the need for those who have been injured to resume normal activities as soon as possible. It also seems prudent to identify ergonomic mismatches in the workplace as soon as possible during rehabilitation to reduce injury recurrence (24).

The identification of risks, especially in the context of the essential functions of the job, is the first step in providing accommodations and minimizing the risks of CTDs. Integration of various methods of data collection on CTDs is probably the most effective way to identify the risk factors. Accident reports alone are not sufficient for risk estimates, because they provide only information associated with injuries that result in sick leave. Identifying risks generally begins by reviewing health and safety records and identifying those tasks with the highest incidence of CTDs. Interviewing workers is also a major source of information. Checklists have been used to assist in identifying specific tasks that may present an increased risk of CTDs (25) and have proved to be an effective method for communicating ergonomic concepts in a clear and concise format. We recently developed (in partnership with Interlogics) a workplace analysis system based on a systems approach to the ubiquitous problem of occupational LBP.

RISK IDENTIFICATION

Once high-risk tasks are identified, specific risk factors can be objectively quantified using currently available tools. Then, and only then, is there the opportunity to recommend controls to ameliorate the risks of LBP and, indeed, any CTD. Such controls can be either accommodations for workers or changes in the nature of the task or process by which it is carried out. Although many risk factors are well recognized, considerable need remains for information about the biomechanical stresses that lead to back pain and injury and the ways in which specific work tasks impose these stresses. This information is invaluable for the proper workplace and job design. Returning injured or disabled workers to the workforce through accommodations and redesign of the work environment and tasks is possible only with sufficient information on the physical and cognitive requirements of the tasks.

MMH entails the exertion of muscles to move or maintain the position of the body and to effect the lift or transfer. Thus, both posture and load are of import. In the United States, work commonly is performed for 8 hours per day and 5 days per week, but 10- and 12-hour days and 6 days per week are not uncommon. Developing nations frequently have longer working hours. MMH work exposes the body to physical stressors that may produce physiological and biomechanical tissue injuries. These disturbances may result in pain, impaired work performance, and other adverse health effects. In most cases, these disturbances subside with time. If, however, time is too short for complete recovery between successive work periods, these disturbances may begin to accumulate, thus increasing pain and impairment. In extreme cases, the pain and impairment can be disabling and can persist for days, weeks, months, or even years.

LBP is caused by one of two injury mechanisms: CTD and single overexertion. Traditional safety practices should be sufficient to prevent trauma to the low back. Preventing and accommodating overexertion and cumulative trauma injuries require information about the biomechanical factors experienced by the low back. Indications of overexertion activity can be determined by knowing how much weight is being lifted or carried and how much force is being applied while pushing or pulling. Variables, such as postures assumed while lifting or exerting forces, can contribute significantly to stresses experienced by the low back. The time histories of the forces exerted and the postures held are important in understanding the mechanisms of cumulative trauma.

Numerous techniques are available to quantify the physical parameters that involve biomechanical stress, such as awkward pos-

tures. Systems such as Priel's "Posturegram" (26), Corlett and Bishop's "Posture Targeting" (11), Keyserling's posture menus (27), the *NIOSH Guidelines for Manual Lifting* (14), and the ISO (International Standard Organization) 2631 vibration exposure limits have proved useful in quantifying biomechanical variables. None of these techniques is ideal, however, and the behaviors or conditions to be assessed are constantly changing. For example, almost all workers change their posture frequently, even when their jobs require more or less static positions (e.g., sitting). During real-time analysis, the analyst must focus constantly on the operator. The analyst must simultaneously observe and record body positions. Recording the work tasks on video is helpful; however, using video to record activity involves many other problems.

All posture-assessment systems involve some degree of tradeoff between time required to perform the analysis and the level of detail obtained. The more convenient a system, the less specific its information. Additionally, currently available systems require continuous tracking or shadowing of workers, which may affect behavior. Furthermore, observations of more than one worker at a time requires more observers. According to Corlett and Bishop (10), the ideal method should be easy to learn, easy to use, and reliable (providing repeatable results across technicians). It is also important, for epidemiologic applications, that data be easily coded for computer storage and analysis. The B-Tracker (Fig. 1) is an example of a new commercially available system that internally records postural data about the low back.

The Taskworks system we developed in conjunction with Interlogics has proven effectiveness and ease of action. The job description (JD) module is a software program within that system that assists technicians in collecting information to generate functional job descriptions. The JD runs on a portable, palmtop personal computer (PC) and provides a systematic method for recording all the neces-

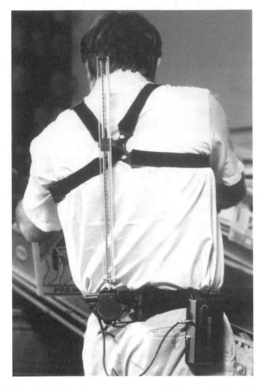

FIG. 1. B-Tracker: a commercially available (Interlogics, Inc.) device to take and internally store low back postural data.

sary information about a job. Each unit is capable of storing approximately 80 to 100 sessions with each session containing several thousand pieces of information.

This module helps the job analyst to identify and document specific aspects of a job while at the work site. This task can be cumbersome, especially considering all the different types of environments the job analyst must be prepared to document.

The organization of the JD program is based on the simplified breakdown of a job into its component parts. This software organizes a job into a series of actions or events. The first level of hierarchy within a job is *essential function*, the fundamental job duties of the position. The next level within a job is *activity*. A series of different activities constitute a specific essential function. Activities describe the physical movements performed within each essential function, such as lift,

push, pull. Figure 2 illustrates this hierarchical breakdown of a job used in the JD module of the Taskworks system.

In addition to static postures and the range of motion required to perform a task, dynamic characteristics (e.g., velocity and acceleration) of work demands are also important. The influence of speed on spinal loads has been shown to be important during lifting a small load (28). Ferguson and colleagues (29) found an increase in the sagittal peak acceleration for lifting with increasing task asymmetry, whereas the sagittal peak acceleration decreased and then increased as a function of increasing task asymmetry for lowering.

High levels of muscular exertions in the back place workers at risk for back injury (30). Numerous attempts have been made to correlate back pain and muscle forces to electromyographic (EMG) activity of back muscles. When dealing with static postures, EMG amplitude muscle correlates with the force of the contraction. Use of EMG to analyze dynamic activity is more complicated; however, it is clear that excursions of the EMG signal do represent the ability of muscle to exert force. The onset of fatigue provides critical information for assessing risk factors in the workplace. We found that spectral measures, such as the downward shift of the median frequency of the EMG power spectrum with fatigue, is a more reliable indicator than amplitude measurements (31,32). We recently found wavelet analysis to be helpful in analyzing EMG signals in the frequency and frequency domains.

Sitting is the most common posture in today's workplace, particularly in industry and business. Three quarters of all workers in industrial countries have sedentary jobs. An estimated 45% of all American workers are employed in offices, and this number is projected to grow significantly through the year 2000. Occupational LBP has been long associated with sedentary work. Rowe (33) showed that in slightly longer than 10 years, 35% of the sedentary workers visited the medical department for back pain. The esti-

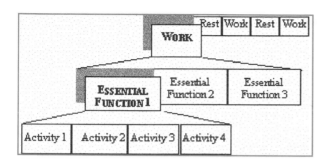

FIG. 2. Hierarchical breakdown of job components.

mated time lost was 4 hours per person per year. Wood and McLeich (34) reported a significant rate of intervertebral disc disorders in insurance and bank workers, who spend long periods of sitting at work. Bergquist-Ullman also reported a high rate of sick leave resulting from acute low back pain among workers who must sit for prolonged periods. LBP has been closely associated with sitting for prolonged periods (1,11). In a study conducted by Damkot and colleagues (19), the activities of people with severe and moderate LBP were compared. Those who reported severe LBP engaged in fewer seated activities than those with moderate pain. Those with severe LBP also reported fewer instances of twisting while in a seated posture. Severe LBP patients twisted 1.9 times per hour, moderate LBP patients 2.9 times per hour, and no LBP patients 6.8 times per hour. Clinical observations of patients with LBP also reveal that many display poor postural habits and report increased pain when sitting (35). People with LBP frequently report intolerance for sitting, and their pain severity is related inversely to their ability to change posture while seated (19,36). Even people without clinical histories of back pain report pain with prolonged static sitting (37).

As society moves toward more information processing and industrial automation, sitting will become even more prevalent. Workplace alterations have been made to increase productivity, sometimes at the expense of the worker's health. Today the workplace is optimized by setting up the workstation within easy reach of the seated individual. The need to get up and move, for example, to a filing cabinet or to receive memos, has been replaced by simply accessing a computer. Tasks that previously required moving from one location to another have been modified, presumably to increase productivity. Prolonged immobility can have deleterious effects on the spine, however.

Holm and Nachemson (38) found that spinal movement alters spinal loads and produces variations in nourishment. They reported that the flow of nutrients transported in and out of the disc improves with lumbar movement. Adams and Hutton (39) also found that alternating periods of activity and rest and posture changes further boost the fluid exchange and that fluid flow plays a supplementary role in nourishing the intervertebral discs. In addition, these investigators state that sitting postures that entail flexion of the lumbar spine cause more fluid to be expressed from the lumbar discs than do erect postures. Alternately loading and unloading the spine (through movement) is ergonomically beneficial, because the process pumps fluid in and out of the discs, thereby improving nutritional supply. Good seating should allow a worker to maintain a relaxed, but supported, posture and should allow for freedom of active motion over the course of the day. Johnson and colleagues (40) state that seat design should allow free vertical motion of the backrest to decrease the strain on the spinal column. Excessive contouring and padding can be detrimental if they restrict motion. Thus, active movement and postural changes are inevitable and, in fact, desirable throughout the day. Many researchers agree that motion should be incorporated in seating while the body is being supported in different postures.

Repetition and LBP, as noted, have been associated in several studies. Probably these adverse health effects will follow a dose-response relationship in which prevalence asymptotically approaches zero with a decreasing dose and asymptotically approaches 100% with an increasing dose. More work is needed to quantify this relationship. In practice, there will be some background level resulting from other factors; so the prevalence is almost never zero. Similarly, situations in which the dose is so great that 100% of the workforce is affected are rare. Consequently, most studies only examine part of the dose-response relationship. Dose-response models are potentially useful for designing jobs that entail an acceptable level of risk. Unfortunately, sufficient data are not available to determine a dose response relationship for LBP disorders and all of their possible factors.

Vibration is a vector quantity with properties of amplitude and frequency, both of which are important in defining the LBP risk. The adverse effects of whole-body vibration (WBV) exposure are multifactorial and result from the interaction of vibration variables, work attributes, other workplace stressors, and physiologic responses and individual attributes. The complex reactions of the musculoskeletal system to WBV arise from the physical movement of body parts and the responses of the musculoskeletal system. The human body does not behave like a passive system, but it reacts to vibratory stimulus in many ways. These responses contribute to the multiple mechanisms by which CLBP occurs. Thus, WBV has been identified as a significant risk factor for LBP and one that must be controlled to enable workers with LBP to resume their jobs. Epidemiologic work (4,41) indicates a significant association of the LBP reports with exposure to both industrial and nonindustrial (particularly vehicular) vibration. Heliovaara (42) and Kelsey and associates (21) found a relationship between the incidence of herniated discs and long-term vibration exposure in automobiles and trucks. In a study of 3,920 patients, Frymoyer and associates (2) determined that LBP reports were more common among workers exposed to vibration, for example, in truck and tractor driving and heavy construction equipment operation, than among those in other occupations. Johanning et al. (43), in a study of workers in the New York City subway system, found lateral vibration to be associated with a high incidence of back pain. Recently, Magnusson and colleagues (44,45) studied bus and truck drivers in both Sweden and the United States and found a significant correlation between LBP and a history of WBV exposure.

The seated vibration environment is particularly associated with LBP. Several mechanical factors contribute to stressing the posterior portion of the intervertebral disc in the lumbar spine during sitting. This position causes a flattening of the normal lumbar lordosis (curvature in the lumbar region of the spine), shifting the line of force of the spine to a point posterior to the effective pivot point of the ischial tuberosities. The ischial tuberosities are offset anteriorly relative to the spine. Consequently, in a vibration environment, there is a moment arm associated with the force transmitted through the structures connecting the ischial tuberosities to the spine which may cause that force to induce a rocking motion in the pelvis, which can amplify the vibration motion transmitted to the spine. Sitting also causes an increase in the posterior disc height, which can mechanically strain the posterior and posterolateral collagen fibers of the annulus fibrosus where they are thinner and fewer (46–48). Additional strains are created in forward-flexed motion segments because the facets disengage and allow an increase in the anterior–posterior translation compliance (49–50). Lumbar intradiscal pressures are significantly greater in seated postures, resulting in a tension-increasing effect on the disc collagen fibers that is analogous to increasing the tension in a taut wire by pushing on it from the side (51,53). Polymers such as rat and human medial collateral ligaments become softer and weaker after vibration loading, an indication of fatigue (54,55). Physical changes and disc herniations have been caused in motion segments by exposure to cyclic and vibration loading (39,56).

WBV studies have established that the seated human has a resonant frequency close to the frequencies produced in common working and vehicle environments. A structure or mechanism vibrating at its resonant frequency is more likely to fail (57–61). *In vitro* lumbar motion segment studies (57) and *in vivo* WBV studies have established the motion characteristics of the lumbar region during vibration exposure (62,63).

A vehicle driver is also at increased risk for disc damage when unloading the vehicle after driving, because back muscles fatigue with vibration (64). The lumbar "balance point" locations shift posteriorly following sustained sitting, thereby decreasing the erector spinae moment arm, increasing the stabilizing load requirements of the erectors, and increasing the imposed loads on the disc (65–67). Trunk fatigue (68) results in increased coupled (out of plane) torques (69), and muscles overcompensate for unexpected loads (70). All these changes increase the tendency of the motion segment to buckle after exposure to seated vibration (66,67). The ISO 2631 vibration guidelines are commonly used as a reference for vibration limits; however, these were compiled from task performance data, and mounting evidence shows that these limits are not conservative enough to protect the lumbar spinal system from damaging fatigue and biomechanical strain (67,71).

MODEL FOR REDUCING AND MANAGING OCCUPATIONAL LOW BACK PAIN

Traditional approaches for cost containment attempt either to manage the treatment of the injured worker or to prevent injuries from occurring in the first place. Although both approaches have yielded reports of cost reductions, greater savings can be realized if there is a sharing of information about the healthy worker, the injured worker, and the workplace. It has been proposed that the integration of prevention programs and patient management programs increases efficiency by minimizing redundant, inconsistent, and irrelevant information and facilitates communication between affected entities and persons.

In an integrated program, the cost of workplace injuries is reduced by both decreasing lost workdays and by decreasing medical expenditures. These reductions in turn may be considered the result of decreased replacement and training costs, increased successful return to work, reduced injury incidence, and reduced injury severity. Further economic gains may be realized from improved employee morale and productivity. Additional benefits result from the efficiencies associated with sharing objective and meaningful information, targeting interventions, and the imposition of program consistency.

Injury prevention in the workplace should begin with an understanding of the nature of the problems in the workplace, which should result in the formulation of strategies to address those problems. Following the implementation of the chosen strategies and the passage of sufficient time for the prevention programs to cause measurable changes in the incidence, severity, and cost of the workplace injuries, the outcomes of the chosen prevention and management paths should be examined. A failure to achieve the desired outcomes should initiate a reexamination of the chosen strategies and implementation procedures and possibly the outcome measures.

A common method used to determine the nature of the problem is to review the OSHA 200 records of injuries and illnesses. Ideally, this information should be in the form of electronic records, which can be readily subjected to statistical analysis. The most that can be expected from such an analysis, however, is a ranking of those jobs according to incidence, body part involved, and type of injury or illness. Although a measure of severity can be obtained, the calculation is based on lost work time and thus only indirectly reflects severity in terms of the nature of the injury or illness and associated costs. In addition, the analysis provides little reliable information that can be used to gain insight into the cause of the injury. For example, it may be learned that there were many injuries of the low back at a particular job, but the cause of the injury is generally not well documented in any accompanying written commentary. At best, the analysis indicates, for example, that a group of workers experienced a large number of low-back injuries. For a more complete understanding, the analysis should include a comparison with the records of comparable industries. Such information is readily available from the Bureau of Labor Statistics. Even with all of this information, however, it is still difficult to formulate a targeted prevention strategy without gathering more detailed information about the job.

Data can be collected in many ways to accumulate sufficient information to form an accurate and meaningful description of each job, but it is often not obvious as to exactly what information is appropriate or what methods of data collection are most efficient. Some businesses find it helpful to use commercially available systems, such as the Taskworks component of the BSafe module from Interlogics. These types of systems typically have well-developed protocols to enable quick and easy collection of vital job information. As the data are collected, the information is used to develop a database of all functional job descriptions. Once the database has been developed, the information can be easily accessed to perform tasks such as generating reports or identifying risk factors.

A well-constructed database also can serve as a platform from which a comprehensive training protocol can be developed. In many jobs, the employee is trained in the operation of equipment and generalized techniques, but ergonomic aspects of safety are neglected. A training program based on specific job information can be tailored to teach workers safe techniques, encourage productive noninjurious workplace behaviors, and teach workers how to recognize potentially hazardous situations. Benefits of this training method include constant interaction and attention by the trainer, which creates a positive environment for the new or transferred worker; the ability of the trainer, employer, or employee to pinpoint potential problem areas and address them appropriately; and exposure of inefficient practices early on so that they can be corrected before problems arise.

An additional capability of using such databases is the ability to assist in the identification of hazardous jobs, not to be confused with the concept of identifying and addressing the hazardous tasks within a job. Analysis of the job descriptions should include identification and assignment of the potential severity to any hazardous job characteristics. Examples of hazardous characteristics include lifting a heavy object, pushing or pulling an object at knee level or below, and using vibrating tools. This listing of "red flags" for each job and identifying jobs that historically have reported a high incidence of severe workplace injuries and illnesses can direct the prevention program toward those jobs that are candidates for an ergonomic assessment.

It is possible that some hazardous jobs could be modified to reduce the level of risk. An in-depth ergonomic assessment of the hazardous jobs serves as the process for identifying the aspects of a job and job tasks that may not be physically or psychologically compatible with the human body. This knowledge provides the investigator with the necessary information to design a safer, more productive work environment and to remedy unsafe worker behavior.

The ergonomic assessment is task specific and should include the gathering of company and workforce demographics, a time and motion study of the tasks, a posture analysis for each task, and a risk-factor analysis for each task. Employee pain surveys can be used to correlate worker experiences of discomfort during the performance of specific tasks with the risk factors associated with these tasks. Depending on the complexity of the task, it may be appropriate to use instrumentation attached to the worker to document task characteristics fully, such as awkward and prolonged static postures or asymmetric repetitive movements of, say, the low back and wrist joints. Subsequent assessments can be used to evaluate the efficacy of the ergonomic interventions and recommended engineering and administrative controls. Despite the provision of a safe and "ergonomically correct" workstation, the concern remains that a worker may not have the necessary skills, training, and physical attributes required to perform the essential functions of a job or task.

The data constituting each job description can be analyzed to create a description of the essential functions of each job; in turn, this description can be used to create a battery of functional capability tests. A prospective employee then can be tested, after an offer but preplacement, to determine whether he or she can perform the essential functions of a job safely. Such testing is in compliance with the requirements of the ADA as long as the test items faithfully replicate the essential job functions, in contrast to a screening program that provides a comparison of the individual to a standard population using dependent measures such as joint flexibility and trunk strength as components of a generic physical fitness test. Job-specific screening programs do not, however, provide opportunities for identifying existing medical concerns that may make the individual a candidate for a proactive intervention program.

The injury incidence and severity review should serve not only to identify the hazardous jobs but also to indicate which workers are at risk for a particular injury involving a particular body segment or joint. Baseline data can be collected on these individual workers to determine the functional status of the body part of concern. Ideally,

this type of evaluation should be administered quickly at the work site, pose no risk to the person being tested, use a standard protocol, comprise tests that have documented validity and reliability, and provide comparisons with standard healthy and symptomatic populations. Although the preventative purpose of such testing is to identify those persons who would benefit from a proactive treatment program, the records also should serve as a baseline for that person if an injury does occur.

The functional deficits associated with a musculoskeletal injury can be assessed by two methods: (a) a comparison of the injured worker's performance with both normal healthy and injured populations and (b) a comparison with the individual subject's own healthy performance profile. The former comparison yields the most useful information if the comparison with a similarly injured population includes diagnostic categories. If the intent is to use the test results for a determination of injury-induced functional deficits, however, then the assessment will fall short because of an inability to document preinjury-to-postinjury changes. For such documentation to occur, the analysis must involve a comparison with the individual's baseline profile. It follows that the injury evaluation protocol and the tools used to obtain the performance data should be identical to those used to collect the baseline data. In addition to measures of the injured worker's functional ability, assessments also should be made of the subject's perception of his or her severity and location of pain and, if the instruments are available, the presence of nonphysiological factors.

The efficacy of the injured worker's clinical treatment and, if appropriate, the assignment of any disability or impairment should be determined using exactly the same tools and protocols as those used during collection of the baseline and acute-injury evaluations. Furthermore, comparisons should be made with the individual serving as his or her own control. Ultimately, an analysis should be conducted to determine optimum treatment regimens and possibly to develop algorithms to predict individual outcomes. For any of these comparisons and analyses to occur most efficiently, the data should be electronically stored and readily available to the clinician.

Once the injured worker has achieved functional stability with respect to the standardized protocol, further rehabilitation may be required according to the functional demands of the job to which the injured worker is to return. A functional rehabilitation program ensures that the worker, once clinically stabilized, is placed on a path designed specifically to return to the job, in contrast to a general fitness rehabilitation protocol. A functional rehabilitation process teaches the worker to perform essential functions of the job safely and enhances rehabilitation by focusing on returning the worker to work. It also follows that the tools used in this phase of treatment must allow for a safe simulation of the actual job tasks.

A database of job descriptions also can be helpful in developing an effective return-to-work program. Ultimately, a clinician must determine whether the injured worker can return to his or her previous job. If this determination is negative, either appropriate modifications must be made to the job or appropriate alternative work opportunities provided.

The determination of an injured worker's ability to perform a job or job task satisfactorily is dependent on the availability of a useful description of the essential functions of the job, the existence of valid and reliable measurement tools, and the use of an efficient and safe test protocol. The pool of company job descriptions that have been collected as a component of the prevention program should serve as the primary information source.

The process should begin with a standardized physical examination of the capabilities of the injured worker. The specific items in the physical examination should be generalizations of the physical examination and the observations recorded with each job description. For example, the job descriptions may require documentation of any manual-dexterity requirements. In the return-to-work appli-

cation, the clinician would be required to record the manual dexterity capabilities of the injured worker without any reference to the specific manual-dexterity requirements of a particular job. Ideally, the results of this clinical examination should be electronically stored and comparisons made with the data constituting the pool of company job descriptions. The results of this comparison should be a listing of those jobs the worker may be able to perform; based on the results of the standardized physical examination, a description of the objectively determined functional requirements of each of the jobs that have passed this preliminary filtration process should be included. The resulting report then can be used to create a battery of job-specific tests that can be administered to the injured worker. The test equipment used by the clinician can be those tools that are commonly available in clinical facilities, although the protocols inevitably will require modification for valid task simulation. The resultant evaluations can be used by clinicians to determine whether the injured worker can return to his or her original job; or, if not, what alternative jobs or temporary work assignments he or she can perform; or what modifications need to be made to the job. Figure 3 illustrates an algorithmic approach to the use of job descriptions for training, rehabilitation, screening, and return-to-work applications.

As can be seen from the preceding discussion, further opportunities exist for reducing the high cost of workplace injuries by integrating the concerns of both risk control/loss prevention and patient treatment/claims management by using common data sets for multiple applications. Figure 4 summarizes how a pool of functional job descriptions can be used for screening, training, functional rehabilitation, and making return-to-work decisions. The job descriptions also can be used with historical records of the nature, incidence, and severity of the workplace injuries to target those jobs that would benefit from an in-depth ergonomic assessment and possible intervention. The injury records also indicate those populations who are candidates for

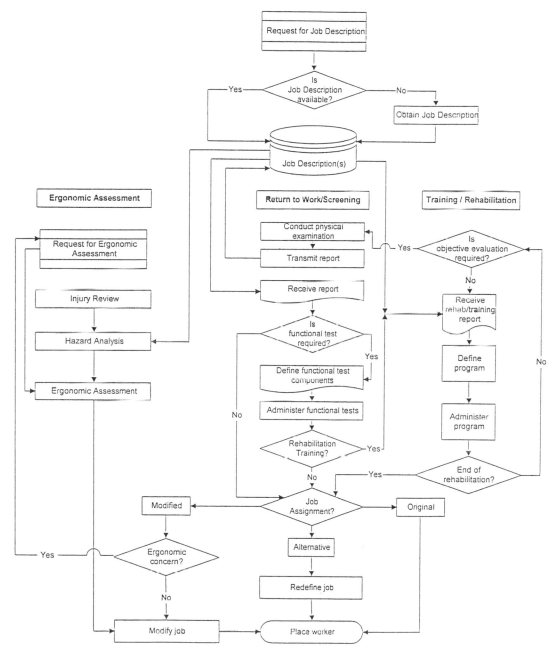

FIG. 3. Algorithmic approach to the use of job descriptions for training, rehabilitation, screening, and return-to-work applications.

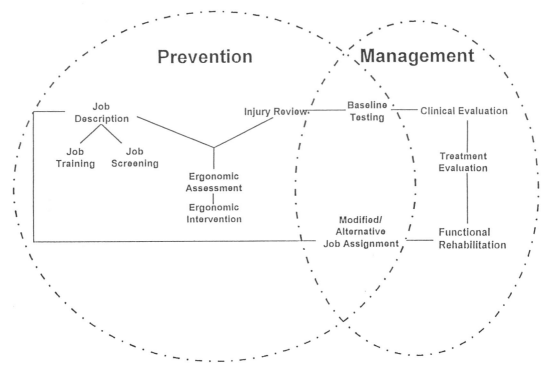

FIG. 4. Integrating prevention and patient management.

baseline testing. In the event of an injury, comparisons with the baseline evaluations serve to document functional changes that have occurred as a result of the injury and the effectiveness of the rehabilitation program. Although each component of the integrated program has been shown to reduce the cost of workplace injuries, greater cost savings can be realized by combining prevention and patient-management programs.

CONCLUSIONS

The ADA and pending amendments to the Rehabilitation Act provide a clear mandate to the public. People who have disabilities will no longer be segregated or denied access to ordinary freedoms of activity for lack of reasonable accommodations. Back disabilities are more common, if less visible, than most other disabilities, and people who have back disabilities must be accommo-

dated appropriately, including appropriate seating in the workplace, public buildings, and public transportation. This also means access to more jobs through the redesign of workplaces and work tasks. Besides the mandates of the ADA, the shrinking of a skilled workforce also means that now, more than ever, it is important to prevent occupational injuries, to encourage the employment of people with disabilities, and to enable injured workers to return to work as soon as possible.

Accommodating people with back disabilities currently requires much more research-based knowledge, the application of research findings, and the training of people who can apply those findings. Information about back disabilities is important not only to health care providers but also to employers, insurance companies, and manufacturers of the many goods and services used by people with and without back pain. Surveys of people with LBP have reported the need for information about preventing pain and injury and about treatment modalities and program. People want to know how to remain maximally active while protecting against reinjury.

Research on injury risk factors in the workplace should be undertaken to establish the importance of, and interactions among, ergonomic, psychosocial, and demographic factors. Different types of workplaces should be taken into account as well as different kinds of workers. Special emphasis should be given to the workplace needs of women, older adults, and persons with disabilities, who are joining the American workforce in increasing numbers. Mechanisms of injury should be studied and means of prevention specified. In addition, systems, methods, and equipment for workplace analyses should be developed and tested. Perhaps most important to current and future generations of older adults is rehabilitation engineering research aimed at minimizing and accommodating functional limitations and promoting independent living through product and device design and accommodations in the home and workplace.

We believe the ADA should be regarded as an opportunity and not a burden. The algorithmic approach outlined herein has the best chance of dealing with the problem of occupational chronic LBP.

REFERENCES

1. Kelsey JL. An epidemiological study of acute herniated lumbar intervertebral discs. *Rheumatol Rehabil* 1975; 14:144-59.
2. Frymoyer JW, Pope MH, Costanza MC, Rosen JC, Goggin JE, Wilder DG. Epidemiologic studies of low-back pain. *Spine* 1980;5:419–423.
3. Svensson HO, Andersson GB. Low-back pain in 40- to 47-year-old men: work history and work environment factors. *Spine* 1983;8:272–276.
4. Frymoyer JW, Pope MH, Clements JH, Wilder DG, MacPherson B, Ashikaga T. Risk factors in low-back pain: an epidemiological survey. *J Bone Joint Surg Am* 1983;65:213–218.
5. Biering-Sorensen F. Physical measurements as risk indicators for low-back trouble over a one-year period. *Spine* 1984;9:106–119.
6. Andersson GBJ, Pope MH, Frymoyer JW, Snook S. Epidemiology and Cost. In: Pope MH, Andersson GBJ, Frymoyer JW, Chaffin DB, eds. *Occupational low back pain: assessment, treatment and prevention.* St. Louis: Mosby–Year Book, 1991:95–113.
7. Beals RK, Hickman NW. Industrial injuries of the back and extremities. Comprehensive evaluation: an aid in prognosis and management: a study of one hundred and eighty patients. *J Bone Joint Surg Am* 1972;54: 1593–1611.
8. *Disability compliance bulletin.* Palm Beach Gardens, FL; LRP Publications, 1994:3.
9. Kelsey JL, Golden AL. Occupational and workplace factors associated with low back pain. *Occup Med* 1988;3:7–16.
10. Corlett EN, Bishop RP. A technique for assessing postural discomfort. *Ergonomics* 1976;19:175–182.
11. Magora A. Investigation of the relation between low back pain and occupation. 3. Physical requirements: sitting, standing and weight lifting. *Industrial Medicine Surgery* 1972;41:5–9.
12. Kelsey JL, Githens PB, White AAD, et al. An epidemiologic study of lifting and twisting on the job and risk for acute prolapsed lumbar intervertebral disc. *J Orthop Res* 1984;2:61–66.
13. Bigos S, Spengler D, Martin N, et al. Back injuries in industry, a retrospective study, III: employee-related factors. *Spine* 1986;3:252–256.
14. *Work practices guide for manual lifting.* Cincinnati, Ohio: NIOSH (National Institute for Occupational Safety and Health) Division of Biomedical and Behavioral Science, 1981. Report No. 81–122.
15. Rowe ML. Low back disability in industry: updated position. *J Occup Med* 1971;13:476–478.
16. Jensen RC. Epidemiology of work related back pain. *Topics in Acute Care Trauma Rehabilitation* 1988;2:1–15.
17. Frymoyer JW, Mooney V. Occupational orthopaedics. *J Bone Joint Surg Am* 1986;68:469–74.
18. Chaffin D. Functional assessment for heavy physical labor. *Occup Health Saf* 1981;1:24–64.
19. Damkot DK, Pope MH, Lord J, Frymoyer JW. The relationship between work history, work environment and low-back pain in men. *Spine* 1984;9:395–399.
20. Chaffin DB, Herrin GD, Keyserling WM. Preemployment strength testing: an updated position. *J Occup Environ Med* 1978;20:403–408.
21. Kelsey JL, Githens PB, O'Conner T, et al. Acute prolapsed lumbar intervertebral disc: an epidemiologic study with special reference to driving automobiles and cigarette smoking. *Spine* 1984;9:608–613.
22. Snook SH. Low back pain in industry. In: White AAI, Gordon S, eds. *Symposium on idiopathic low back.* St. Louis: Mosby; 1982:23–28.
23. Cady LD Jr, Thomas PC, Karwasky RJ. Program for increasing health and physical fitness of fire fighters. *J Occup Med* 1985;27:110–114.
24. Buckle P, Stubbs D. The contribution of ergonomics to the rehabilitation of back pain patients. *Journal of the Society of Occupational Medicine* 1989;39:56–60.
25. Lifshitz Y, Armstrong K. A design checklist for control and prediction of acculative trauma disorders in hand intensive manual jobs. In: *30th Meeting of the Human Factors Society*, 1986:837–841.
26. Priel VZ. A numerical definition of posture. *Hum Factors* 1974;16:576–584.
27. Keyserling WM. Postural analysis of the trunk and shoulders in simulated real time. *Ergonomics* 1986;29: 569 583.
28. Tsuang YH, Schipplein OD, Trafimow JH, Andersson GB. Influence of body segment dynamics on loads at

the lumbar spine during lifting. *Ergonomics* 1992;35: 437–444.

29. Ferguson SA, Marras WS, Waters TR. Quantification of back motion during asymmetric lifting. *Ergonomics* 1992;35:845–859.

30. Chaffin DB, Park KS. A longitudinal study of low-back pain as associated with occupational weight lifting factors. *Am Ind Hyg Assoc J* 1973;34:513–525.

31. Hakkinen K, Komi PV. Electromyographic and mechanical characteristics of human skeletal muscle during fatigue under voluntary and reflex conditions. *Electroencephalogr Clin Neurophysiol* 1983;55:436–444.

32. Lindstrom L, Kadefors R, Petersen I. An electromyographic index for localized muscle fatigue. *J Appl Physiol* 1977;43:750–754.

33. Rowe ML. Low back pain in industry: a position paper. *J Occup Environ Med* 1969;11:161–169.

34. Wood PHN, Mc Leich CL. Statistical appendix: digest of data in the rheumatic diseases. 5. Morbitity in industry and rheumatism in general practice. *Ann Rheum Dis* 1974;33:93–105.

35. Bergquist-Ulman M, Larsson U. Acute low back pain in industry: a controlled prospective study with special reference to therapy and confounding factors. *Acta Orthop Scand* 1977;170:1–117.

36. Majeske C, Buchanan C. Quantitative description of two sitting postures: with and without a lumbar support pillow. *Phys Ther* 1984;64:1531–1535.

37. Andersson G. Evaluation of muscle function. In: Frymoyer JW DT, Hadler NM, Kostiuk JP, Weinstein JN, Whitecloud TS, eds. *The adult spine.* New York: Raven Press, 1991:241–274.

38. Holm S, Nachemson A. Variations in the nutrition of the canine intervertebral disc induced by motion. *Spine* 1983;8:866–874.

39. Adams MA, Hutton WC. The effect of fatigue on the lumbar intervertebral disc. In: *Proceedings of the International Society for the Study of the Lumbar Spine,* Cambridge, England, 1983.

40. Johnson DA, Samin JC, Neve M. A new design of vehicle seat intended to alleviate lower back pain. *J Biomech Eng* 1989;111:261–262.

41. Hushof C, van Zanten B. Whole body vibration and low back pain; a review of epidemiologic studies. *Int Arch Occup Environ Health* 1987;59:205–220.

42. Heliovaara M. Occupation and risk of herniated lumbar intervertebral disc or sciatica leading to hospitalization. *Journal of Chronic Diseases* 1987;40:259–264.

43. Johanning E, Wilder DG, Landrigan PJ, Pope MH. Whole-body vibration exposure in subway cars and review of adverse health effects. *J Occup Environ Med* 1991;33:605–612.

44. Magnusson M, Almqvist M, Broman H, Pope M, Hansson T. Measurement of height loss during whole body vibrations. *J Spinal Disord* 1992;5:198–203.

45. Magnusson M, Wilder D, Pope M, Hansson T. Investigation of the long-term exposure to whole-body vibration: a two country study. *European Journal Physical Medicine and Rehabilitation* 1993;3:28–34.

46. Galante JO. Tensile properties of the human lumbar annulus fibrosus. *Acta Orthop Scand* 1967;100(Suppl):1–91.

47. Krag MH, Seroussi RE, Wilder DG, et al. Internal displacement distribution from in vitro loading of human thoracic and lumbar spinal motion segments: experi-

mental results and theoretical predictions. *Spine* 1987; 12:1001–1007.

48. Panjabi M, White A. *Physical properties and functional biomechanics of the spine:* clinical biomechanics of the spine. Philadelphia: JB Lippincott Co, 1978:74–77.

49. Panjabi MM, Krag MH, White AA, Southwick WO. Effects of preload on load displacement curves of the lumbar spine. *Orthop Clin North Am* 1977;8:181–192.

50. Tencer AF, Ahmed AM, Burke DL. Some static mechanical properties of the lumbar intervertebral joint, intact and injured. 1982;104:193–201.

51. Nachemson A, Morris J. *In vivo* measurements of intradiscal pressure. *J Bone Joint Surg* 1964;46A: 1077–1092.

52. Okushima H. Study on hydrodynamic pressure of lumbar intervertebral disc. *Nippon Geka Hokan* 1970;39: 45–57.

53. Belytschko T, Kulak RF, Schultz AB, Galante JO. Finite element stress analysis of an intervertebral disc. *J Biomech* 1974;7:277–285.

54. Weisman G, Pope MH, Johnson RJ. Cyclic loading in knee ligament injuries. *Am J Sports Medicine* 1980;8: 24–30.

55. Hertzberg R, Manson J. *Fatigue of engineering plastics.* New York: Academic Press, 1980:64.

56. Wilder DG, Pope MH, Frymoyer JW. Cyclic loading of the intervertebral motion segment. In: *Proceedings of the Tenth Northeast Bioengineering Conference,* 1982; Hanover, NH: Dartmouth College, 1982.

57. Wilder D. *On the loading of the human lumbar intervertebral motion segment* [PhD dissertation]. Burlington, Vermont: University of Vermont, 1985.

58. Wilder DG, Woodworth BB, Frymoyer JW, Pope MH. Vibration and the human spine. *Spine* 1982;3: 243–254.

59. Seroussi RE, Wilder DG, Pope MH. Trunk muscle electromyography and whole body vibration. *J Biomech* 1989;22:219–229.

60. Seidel H, Bastek R, Brauer D, et al. On human response to prolonged repeated whole-body vibration. *Ergonomics* 1980;23:191–211.

61. Pope MH, Wilder DG, Jorneus L, Broman H, Svensson M, Andersson G. The response of the seated human to sinusoidal vibration and impact. *J Biomech Eng* 1987;109:279–284.

62. Panjabi MM, Andersson GB, Jorneus L, Hult E, Mattsson L. *In vivo* measurements of spinal column vibrations. *J Bone Joint Surg Am* 1986;68:695–702.

63. Pope M, Wilder D, Donnermeyer D. Muscle fatigue in the static and vibrational seating environment. AGARD-CP-378 Pozzuoli, Naples, 1986.

64. Wilder D, Donnermeyer D, Wong J, Pope M. Paravertebral muscle fatigue in static and fore-aft vibration seating environments. *Orthopaedic Transactions* 1984; 8:423–424.

65. Wilder D, Pope M, Seroussi R, Dimnet J. The effects of cyclic loading on the balance point of the lumbar motion segment. In Proceeding of the: *International Society Study Lumbar Spine.* Rome, Italy; 1987.

66. Wilder DG, Pope MH, Frymoyer JW. The biomechanics of lumbar disc herniation and the effect of overload and instability. *J Spinal Disord* 1988;1:16–32.

67. Wilder D, Pope M, Seroussi R, Dimnet J. Buckling or "giving way" in the lumbar spine following prolonged exposure to sitting. In Proceeding of the: *Orthopaedic*

Research Society, 1988. Atlanta, Georgia: Orthopaedic Transactions; 1988:383–384.

68. Pope MH, Andersson GB, Broman H, Svensson M, Zetterberg C. Electromyographic studies of the lumbar trunk musculature during the development of axial torques. *J Orthop Res* 1986;4:288–297.

69. Parnianpour M, Nordin M, Kahanovitz N, Frankel VH. The triaxial coupling of torque generation of trunk muscles during isometric exertions and the effect of fatiguing isoinertial movements on the motor output and movement patterns. *Spine* 1988;13:982–992.

70. Marras WS, Rangarajulu SL, Lavender SA. Trunk loading and expectation. *Ergonomics* 1987;30:551–562.

71. Bovenzi M, Zadini A. Self-reported low back symptoms in urban bus drivers exposed to whole-body vibration. *Spine* 1992;17:1048–1059.

Occupational Musculoskeletal Disorders
edited by T. G. Mayer, R. J. Gatchel, and P. B. Polatin.
Lippincott Williams & Wilkins, Philadelphia © 2000.

7

Functional Cervical Biomechanics in the Ergonomic Environment

Bendt P. Petersen III, *Augustus A. White III, and †Manohar M. Panjabi

*Old Shell Orthopaedic Associates, Mobile, Alabama 36608; *Department of Orthopedics,
Beth Israel Deaconess Hospital, Boston, Massachusetts 02215; and
†Department of Orthopaedics and Rehabilitation, Yale University School of Medicine,
New Haven, Connecticut 06520-8071*

The functional range of motion and load demands placed on the cervical spine over the course of a workday vary greatly among occupations and individuals. All loads and motions, however, as varied as their ergonomic circumstances may dictate, result in reproducible and defined responses from the functional spinal units and their supporting musculature. Within the physiologic range, repetitive motions, prolonged loading and lengthy static or dynamic muscular contractions may lead to overuse, fatigue and ultimately neck or cervical spine related discomfort. Ergonomic related injuries or discomfort are usually the result of phenomena that may in their apparent simplicity go unnoticed, but with the cumulative effect of time become symptomatic. It is the timely interruption of this evolutionary cycle, before causally related subjective or objective symptoms develop that is most effective in the treatment of ergonomic injuries. An understanding of the basic biomechanics of applied loads and their corresponding response in the intevertebral discs, surrounding musculature, and capsuloligamentous structures is integral to both timely intervention and effective design of a workplace free of excessive demands placed on our fellow humans as they perform their workplace tasks.

KINEMATICS

Terms and Definitions

Kinematics: Kinematics involves the study of motion on rigid bodies without consideration of the forces involved.

Kinetics: Kinetics is concerned with the study of motion and the weights, moments, and muscle forces acting on the spine.

Degrees of freedom: Vertebrae have six degrees of freedom, translation along, and rotation about each of the three orthogonal axes. Translation is expressed in meters or inches and rotation is expressed in degrees.

SPINAL MOTION

The motion segment of functional spinal unit (FSU) is composed of two adjacent vertebrae and their intervening soft tissues. The most representative values for rotatory ROM at different levels of the spine are presented in Table 1.

The muscles are located anterior, posterior, and lateral to the spine. They provide for motion and stabilize the spine to carry physiologic loads. The anterior muscles flex the spine. If an anterior muscle runs a little obliquely and contracts independently of the corresponding muscle on the opposite side, it

TABLE 1. *Summary of cervical and lumbar spine rotations (comprehensive references)*

Cervical spine ranges of motion

Flexion plus extension

Dvorak, 1988 Spine 13/7:748 — In vivo/active

	Mean	Lower	Upper
C2–3	12.0	5.0	20.0
C3–4	10.0	5.0	15.0
C4–5	15.0	7.0	23.0
C5–6	19.0	13.0	26.0
C6–7	20.0	13.0	28.0
C7–T1	19.0	11.0	26.0

Panjabi, 1988 Spine 13/7:728 — In vitro/whole spine

	Mean	Lower	Upper
C0–1	5.5	1.7	13.3
C1–2	6.7	0.8	16.5

Dvorak, 1988 Spine 13/7:748 — In vivo/passive

	Mean	Lower	Upper
C2–3	15.0	8.0	22.0
C3–4	12.0	6.0	17.0
C4–5	17.0	10.0	24.0
C5–6	21.0	14.0	28.0
C6–7	23.0	16.0	31.0
C7–T1	21.0	13.0	29.0

Panjabi, 1988 Spine 13/7:728 — In vitro/whole spine

	Mean	Lower	Upper
C0–1	24.5	9.9	37.4
C1–2	22.4	3.0	41.3

Penning, 1978 AJRoentig 130:317, 1978 — In vivo/active

	Mean	Lower	Upper
C0–1	30.0	25.0	45.0
C1–2	30.0	25.0	45.0
C2–3	12.0	5.0	16.0
C3–4	18.0	13.0	26.0
C4–5	20.0	15.0	29.0
C5–6	20.0	16.0	29.0
C6–7	15.0	6.0	25.0

White and Panjabi, 1978

	Mean	Lower	Upper
C0–1	13.0		
C1–2	10.0		
C2–3	8.0	5.0	23.0
C3–4	13.0	7.0	38.0
C4–5	12.0	8.0	39.0
C5–6	17.0	4.0	34.0
C6–7	16.0	1.0	29.0
C7–T1	6.0	4.0	17.0

Lateral bending (one side)

Moroney, 1988 J BIOM 21/9:769,88 — In vitro/FSU

	Mean	Lower	Upper
C2–3	4.7		
C3–4	4.7		
C4–5	4.7		
C5–6	4.7		
C6–7	4.7		
C7–T1	4.7		

Penning, 1978 AJR 130:317, 1978 — In vivo/active

	Mean	Lower	Upper
C0–1	5.0		
C2–3	6.0		
C3–4	6.0		
C4–5	6.0		
C5–6	6.0		
C6–7	6.0		
C7–T1	6.0		

White and Panjabi, 1978

	Mean	Lower	Upper
C0–1	8.0		
C1–2	0.0		
C2–3	10.0	11.0	20.0
C3–4	11.0	9.0	15.0
C4–5	11.0	0.0	16.0
C5–6	8.0	0.0	16.0
C6–7	7.0	0.0	17.0
C7–T1	4.0	0.0	17.0

Axial rotation (one side)

Penning, 1987 Spine 12/8:732, 1987 — In vivo/active

	Mean	Lower	Upper
C0–1	1.0	−2.0	5.0
C1–2	40.5	29.0	46.0
C2–3	3.0	0.0	10.0
C3–4	6.5	3.0	10.0
C4–5	6.8	1.0	12.0

Dvorak, 1987 Spine 12/8:726, 1987 — In vivo/passive

	Mean	Lower	Upper
C0–1	4.0		
C1–2	41.5	38.0	44.0
C2–3	3.0	−2.7	8.7
C3–4	6.5	1.2	11.8
C4–5	6.7	1.3	12.1

Panjabi, 1988 Spine 13/7:728 — In vitro/whole spine

	Mean	Lower	Upper
C0–1	7.3	3.8	11.2
C1–2	38.9	27.1	49.0

White and Panjabi, 1978

	Mean	Lower	Upper
C0–1	0.0		
C1–2	47.0		
C2–3	9.0	6.0	28.0
C3–4	11.0	10.0	28.0
C4–5	12.0	10.0	26.0

TABLE 1. *Continued.*

	Mean	Lower	Upper	Mean	Lower	Upper	Mean	Lower	Upper
C5–6	7.0	1.3	12.7	6.9	2.0	12.0	10.0	8.0	34.0
C6–7	5.4	0.0	10.8	5.4	2.0	10.0	9.0	6.0	15.0
C7–T1	2.1	-2.8	7.0	2.1	-2.0	7.C	8.0	5.0	13.0

Lumbar spine ranges of motion

Flexion plus extension

	Yamamoto, 1989 ISSLS, Kyoto *In vitro*			Hayes, 1989 *Spine* 14/3:327–331 *In vivo/active*			Pearcey, 1984 *Spine* 9/3:294–297 *In vivo/active*			Dvorak, 1989 ISSLS, Kyoto *In vivo/passive*			White and Panjabi, 1978		
	Mean	Lower	Upper	Mean	Lower	Upper	Mean	Lower	Upper	Mean	Lower	Upper	Mean	Lower	Upper
L1/2	10.7	5.0	13.0	7.0	1.0	14.0	13.0	3.0	23.0	11.9	8.6	17.9	12.0	9.0	16.0
L2/3	10.8	8.0	13.0	9.0	2.0	16.0	14.0	10.0	18.0	14.5	9.5	19.1	14.0	11.0	18.0
L3/4	11.2	6.0	15.0	10.0	2.0	18.0	13.0	9.0	17.C	15.3	11.9	21.0	15.0	12.0	18.0
L4/5	14.5	9.0	20.0	13.0	2.0	20.0	16.0	8.0	24.0	18.2	11.6	25.6	17.0	14.0	21.0
L5/S1	17.8	10.0	24.0	14.0	2.0	27.0	14.0	4.0	24.0	17.0	6.3	23.7	20.0	18.0	22.0

Lateral bending (one side)

	Yamamoto, 1989 ISSLS, Kyoto *In vitro*			Pearcey, 1984 *Spine* 9/6:582–587 *In vivo/active*			Dvorak, 1989 ISSLS, Kyoto *In vivo/passive*			White and Panjabi, 1978		
	Mean	Lower	Upper	Mean	Lower	Upper	Mean	Lower	Upper	Mean	Lower	Upper
L1/2	4.9	3.8	6.5	5.5	4.0	10.0	7.9		14.2	6.0	3.0	8.0
L2/3	7.0	4.6	9.5	5.5	2.0	10.0	10.4		16.9	6.0	3.0	9.0
L3/4	5.7	4.5	8.1	5.0	3.0	8.0	12.4		21.2	8.0	5.0	10.0
L4/5	5.7	3.2	8.2	2.5	3.0	6.0	12.4		19.8	6.0	5.0	7.0
L5/S1	5.5	3.9	7.8	1.0	1.0	6.0	9.5		17.6	3.0	2.0	3.0

Axial rotation (one side)

	Yamamoto, 1989 ISSLS, Kyoto *In Vitro*			Pearcey, 1984 *Spine* 9/6:582–587 *In vivo/active*			White and Panjabi, 1978		
	Mean	Lower	Upper	Mean	Lower	Upper	Mean	Lower	Upper
L1/2	2.1	0.9	4.5	1.0	-1.0	2.0	2.0	1.0	3.0
L2/3	2.6	1.2	4.6	1.0	-1.0	2.0	2.0	1.0	3.0
L3/4	2.6	0.9	4.0	1.5	0.0	4.0	2.0	1.0	3.0
L4/5	2.2	0.8	4.7	1.5	0.0	3.0	2.0	1.0	3.0
L5/S1	1.3	0.6	2.1	0.5	-2.0	2.0	5.0	3.0	6.0

rotates and bends the spine laterally as well as flexes it. The muscles posterior to the spine provide extension. If a posterior muscle runs a little obliquely and contracts independently of the corresponding muscle on the opposite side, it rotates and bends the spine laterally as well as extends it. The muscles on the side bend the spine laterally.

The coordinated action of the muscles stabilizes the spine to resist compressive loads. These muscle actions are important, because the normal loads on the spine (lumbar) by body mass alone in standing are about two to three times body weight (140 to 210 kg)

Motion and load-bearing capabilities are determined by the contours, dimensions, and relationship of the vertebrae, discs, and facet joints. The ligaments, joint capsules, and discs provide constraints to motion in a checkrein manner. In general, for flexion/extension movements, ligaments that are located posterior and the bony structures located anterior to the IAR resist flexion. Ligaments located anterior and bony structures located

posterior to the IAR resist extension. In lateral bending and axial rotation, the ligament functions are often more complex.

UPPER CERVICAL SPINE (OCCIPITALATLANTOAXIAL COMPLEX)

Both joints of this complex (CO–1 and C1–2) significantly contribute to the total motion of this area. The amount of flexion and extension at the two joints is roughly equal, and most of the rotation occurs at C1-2. The ligament and muscle stabilizers for C0-1 and C1-2 are given in Table 2.

For the C0–1 articulation, the IAR in flexion/extension (x-axis) passes through the centers of the mastoid processes. Flexion movement is checked by skeletal contact between the anterior margin of the foramen magnum and the tip of the dens. Extension is checked by the tectorial membrane. With flexion of the C0–1 joint beyond neutral, the tectorial membrane becomes taut and limits forward flexion

TABLE 2. *Atlanto-occipital range of motion (C0–1)*

Type of Motion	Passive constraints	Muscles responsible for action
Flexion (+Θx)	Tectorial membrane	Longus capitis
	Posterior atlantooccipital membrane	Rectus capitis anterior
	Articular capsule between occipital condyles and superior atlantal facets (posterior)	Ligamentum nuchae
	Anterior margin of the foramen magnum and the tip of the dens[a]	
Extension (−Θx)	Anterior atlantooccipital membrane	Rectus capitis posterior major
	Articular capsule between occipital condyles and superior atlantal facets (anterior)	Rectus capitis posterior minor
	Anterior longitudinal ligament	Obliquus capitis superior (both acting simultaneously)
	Apical dental ligament	Splenius capitis
		Semispinalis capitis
Lateral bending (Θz) (one side)	Lateral atlantooccipital ligament	Obliquus capitis superior
	Alar ligaments	Splenius capitis
	Occipital condyle and atlantal facet[a]	Sternocleidomastoid
		Trapezius
Axial rotation (Θy) (one side)	Alar ligaments	Sternocleidomastoid
	Articular capsule between occipital condyles and superior atlantal facets	Semispinalis capitis
		Splenius capitis

[a]Skeletal (nonligamentous) constraint.

at the C1-C2 joint. Similarly, with extension of the C0–1 joint, the tectorial membrane again becomes taut and limits extension between C1 and C2.

In lateral bending (z-axis rotation), the IAR is located at a point 2 to 3 cm above the tip of the dens. The motion involves 5 degrees to one side at C0-1 and C1-2 and is controlled by both components of the alar ligaments. During left lateral bending, the right upper portion of the alar ligament, which is connected to the ring of C1, checks the motion. The opposite is true for right lateral bending.

Axial rotation at C0-C1 involves about 5 (degrees) to one side and is limited by the ligaments and osseous anatomy of the C0-C1-C2 complex. The joint surfaces are cup-shaped, with the arcuate occipital articulation fitting into the cup of C1. At C1-C2, roughly 40 (degrees) of axial rotation to one side occurs, and the IAR is located in the dens. During left axial rotation, motion is checked by the right alar ligament; the opposite is true for right axial rotation. The C1-C2 articulation is biconvex and has been described as a "double-threaded screw" joint. This biconvexity gives rise to a coupling pattern of motion where there is translation along the axis of the dens so that alternating rotations produce a pistonlike cephalocaudal movement. Radiographic evaluation may reveal apparent translation because of a shift in the projection of the lateral masses of C1 in relation to the dens. Kinematic studies, however, confirm that there is insignificant lateral translation (x-axis) of the C1-C2 joint because of the snug fit of the anterior ring of C1 and transverse ligament around the dens.

MIDDLE AND LOWER CERVICAL SPINE (C2-T1)

Rotation ranges for the middle and lower cervical spine are shown in Table 3. The C5-C6 FSU has the largest range. There may be a causal relationship between this relative increased range and the higher incidence of cervical spondylosis at this interspace. In lateral bending and axial rotation, there is smaller range in the more caudal segments.

Flexion and extension motion involves a strong coupling of rotation (x-axis) and translation (x-axis). The uncovertebral joints guide flexion and extension and prevent lateral (x-axis) translation. In extension, the cervical vertebrae are positioned in series and form a smooth curve. As flexion occurs, the vertebrae translate forward in a slight stair-step pattern of motion. The anterior vertebral disc heights decrease, and the posterior heights increase. The facet joints glide anteriorly and superiorly, and the posterior interspinous space widens. The upper limit of normal translation radiographically is 3.5 mm, which takes into account at 25% magnification. The same motion pattern occurs in reverse when going from flexion to extension. Lysell coined the term

TABLE 3. *Limits and representative values of ranges of rotation of the middle and lower cervical spine*

Interspace	Combined flexion/extension (±x-axis rotation)		One-side lateral bending (z-axis rotation)		One-side axial rotation (y-axis rotation)	
	Limits of ranges (degrees)	Representative angle (degrees)	Limits of ranges (degrees)	Representative angle (degrees)	Limits of ranges (degrees)	Representative angle (degrees)
Middle						
C2–3	5–16	10	11–20	10	0–10	3
C3–4	7–26	15	9–15	11	3–10	7
c4–5	13–29	20	0–16	11	1–12	7
Lower						
C5–6	13–29	20	0–16	8	2–12	7
C6–7	6–26	17	0–17	7	2–10	6
C7–T1	4–7	9	0–17	4	0–7	2

top angle to indicate the steepness of the arch that is described by the vertebra while moving from full extension to full flexion. The arch is almost flat at C2 and the steepest at C6. The cephalocaudal decrease in the top angle (decrease in the arch) indicates a greater amount of translation occurring in the middle cervical spine than in the lower, where more tilting motion of the vertebral body occurs.

Lateral bending (z-axis rotation) is coupled with axial rotation (y-axis) such that the spinous processes go in the opposite direction of the lateral bending (-z-axis is coupled with -y-axis, and -z-axis is coupled with-y-axis). About 50% of head rotation occurs through the middle and lower cervical spine. The annulus and facet joints are the major limiting structures to axial rotation. The amount of axial rotation coupled with lateral bending varies by level. At C2, there are 2 degrees of coupled axial rotation for every 3 degrees of lateral bending, a ratio of 2:3 or 0.67. At C7, lateral bending of around 7.5 degrees is coupled with 1 degree of axial rotation, a ration of 1: 7.5 or 0.13. Between C2 and C7, there is a gradual cephalocaudal decrease in the amount of axial rotation that is associated with lateral bending, which may be related to the orientation of the facet joints in the frontal plane. Left lateral bending in this region of 0.75 degree is associated with 1 degree of axial rotation for a ratio of 0.75 (Fig. 1).

A SYSTEMATIC APPROACH TO CLINICAL INSTABILITY

Clinical instability of the spine is a controversial term, and there is significant disagreement even among experts (1). Clinical instability can occur as a result of trauma, disease, surgery, or some combination of the three. However, certain underlying observations relate the mechanical derangement to clinical problems of pain and neurologic deficit. These various considerations have been combined in the form of a definition (2). Clinical instability of the spine is defined as "the loss of the ability of the spine under physiologic loads to maintain relationships between vertebrae in such a way that there is neither initial nor subsequent damage to the spinal cord or nerve roots, and in addition, there is neither development of incapacitating deformity nor severe pain."

In this definition, physiologic loads are those incurred during normal activity of the particular patient being evaluated. Incapacitating deformity is defined as gross deformity that the patient finds intolerable. Incapacitating pain is defined as pain that cannot be controlled by nonnarcotic analgesic medications.

To systemize the evaluation of clinical instability, we have proposed the use of a checklist (2). This approach ensures that all perti-

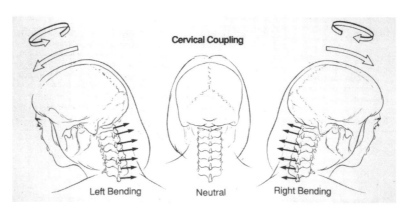

FIG. 1. Shows left lateral bending at approximately 0.75 degree is associated with 1 degree of axial rotation for a ratio of 0.75.

nent factors, such as clinical and biomechanical, are considered and reasonably balanced. As in the earlier two sections of this chapter, we separate the cervical spine into three regions: upper, middle and lower.

The anatomic and biomechanical characteristics of the occipitoatlantal (C0-C1-C2) joint complex and its specific patterns of instability are very different from those of the middle and lower cervical spine. Presently, no checklist is available for this region of the spine.

OCCIPITOATLANTAL JOINT: OCCIPUT-C1

Stability Evaluation

Anatomy

The anatomic structures that provide stability for articulation of occiput-C1 include the cup-shaped configuration of the occipitoatlantal joints and their capsules, along with the anterior and posterior atlantooccipital membranes. Additional anatomic stability is gained through the ligamentous connections between the occiput and the axis: the tectorial membrane, alar ligaments, and apical ligament (3). We believe that because of its structural characteristics, the occipitoatlantal joint is relatively unstable, at least in children. Its stability may increase in adult life because of a decrease in elasticity of the ligaments.

Biomechanics

Weisel and Rothman showed that the normal range of sagittal plan translation in flexion-extension does not exceed 1 mm. This measurement is made between the basion of the occiput and the tip of the odontoid. The findings of more than 5 mm between the tip of the dens and the basion of the occiput or more than 1mm of translation in flexion-extension are important and useful criteria for instability.

The presence of symptoms of weakness of the limbs, with or without associated neck and occipital pain, provide additional indications of instability. The criteria are shown in Table 4. When any criterion shown in Table 4

TABLE 4. *Criteria for C0–1–2 instability*

>8 degrees	Axial rotation C0–C1 to one side
>1 mm	C0–C1 translation
>7 mm	Overhang C1–C2 (total right and left)
>45 degrees	Axial rotation C1–C2 to one side
>4 mm	C1–C2 translation
<13 mm	Posterior body C2–posterior ring C1
Avulsed transverse ligament	

is present, one should make a comprehensive analysis of the C0-C1-C2 complex for possible clinical instability.

ATLANTOAXIAL JOINT: C1-2

Stability Evaluation

Anatomy

The most important anatomic structures affecting the clinical stability of articulation C1-2 are transverse ligaments, dentate ligaments, the apical and alar ligaments, and joint capsules (3–5). The dentate, alar, and apical ligaments are considered secondary stabilizers of the C1-2 complex. The cruciate ligament, the most well-developed portion of which is the transverse ligament, is the major stabilizing ligament. The atlantooccipital membrane also plays a role in the stabilization of these joints. The importance of the mutual dependence of these major ligaments and an intact normal dens is apparent. If the dens is hypoplastic, congenitally not intact, or fractured, the ligaments cannot provide stability.

Biomechanics

Studies of horizontal translation showed that an anterior dislocation of C1 on C2 can occur with an insufficiency of the transverse ligament only. The alar ligaments and the tectorial membrane did not prevent dislocation after the transverse ligament was transected. The biomechanical studies of Fielding and coworkers on the transverse ligament showed that the structure, although very weak in some subjects, prevented more than 3 mm of anterior translation of C1 on C2 when present (6). They also showed that the alar ligaments deform readily and are not capable of preventing additional displacement under loads that would rupture the transverse ligament.

MIDDLE AND LOWER CERVICAL SPINE: C2-T1

A checklist for the middle and lower cervical spine has been developed (7) based on

biomechanical studies (8,9). Some factors important for the evaluation of clinical instability are presented below.

Anatomic and Biomechanical Considerations

A schematic of the anatomy of the middle and lower cervical spine is shown in Fig. 2. At

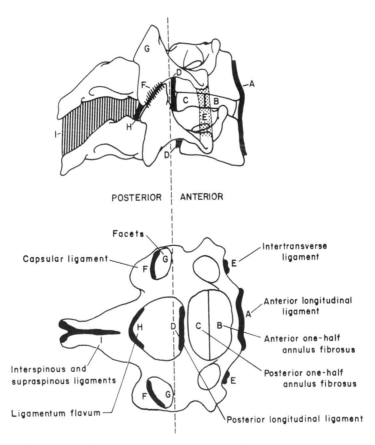

FIG. 2. Schematic illustration of the ligamentous structures that participate in the stabilization of the middle and lower cervical spine. The components are divided into *anterior* and *posterior* elements. Anatomic components posterior to the posterior longitudinal ligament and all the anatomic components anterior to it are defined as the *anterior* elements. In the experiments on clinical stability, ligaments were cut in the alphabetical order indicated in the diagram from anterior to posterior and in reverse alphabetical order from posterior to anterior. (Reprinted with permission from White AA, Panjabi MM. *Clinical Biomechanics of the Spine*, 2nd edition. Philadelphia: JB Lippincott, 1990:321.)

the level of the intervertebral disc the annulus fibrosis appears to be the crucial stabilizing structure (7). Bailey (10) has emphasized the importance of this structure. Munro performed experimental studies on cadaver spines and concluded that cervical spine stability derives mainly from the invertebral discs and the anterior longitudinal ligaments and PLL (11).

Checklist Considerations

White, Panjabi, and colleagues (8,9) performed experiments on cervical spine functional spine units in high-humidity chambers using physiologic loads to simulate flexion and extension. They defined the anterior elements as the posterior longitudinal ligament and all structures anterior to it. The posterior elements were defined as all structures behind the PPL. On the basis of these studies, it was suggested that if a functional spinal unit (FSU) has all its anterior elements plus one additional structure, or all its posterior elements plus one additional structure, it will probably remain stable under physiologic loads. Therefore, in the checklist, to provide for some clinical margin of safety, we suggest that any FSU in which all the anterior elements or all the posterior elements are either destroyed or unable to function should be considered potentially unstable. Two points in the checklist are given for the loss of each of these anatomic elements.

Controlled, monitored axial traction (the stretch test) may be helpful to evaluate the integrity of the ligamentous structures of the middle and lower cervical spine. An abnormal test is indicated by differences either greater than 1.7 mm of interspace separation or greater than 7.5 of change in angle between vertebrae, comparing the prestretch condition with the condition after application of axial traction equivalent to one third body weight. This is based on a biomechanical study simulating the stretch test in fresh cadaveric cervical spines (12). Two points in the checklist are given for a positive stretch test.

One final anatomic consideration should be noted. If all other considerations are the same,

patients with the anterior elements destroyed or unable to function are more clinically unstable in extension, whereas patients with the posterior elements destroyed or unable to function are more unstable in flexion. These factors should be considered during the patient transfers and when a patient's neck is immobilized after injury.

Radiographic Criteria

The measurement of translation and displacement is shown in Fig. 3. This method takes into account variations in magnification and should be useful when there is a tube-to-film distance of 72 inches. Sagittal plane displacement or translation greater than 3.5 mm on either static (resting) or dynamic (flexion-extension) lateral radiographs should be considered potentially unstable. This value was determined from an experimentally obtained value of 2.7 mm and an assumed radiographic magnification of 30% (7). If the x-ray magnification is not known, the 3.5-mm measurement is equivalent to a translation or displacement of 20% of vertebral body A-P diameter. Two points in the checklist are given for abnormal sagittal plane displacement or translation.

Angular measurements are shown in Fig. 4. There is no magnification problem in measuring rotation or angulation. More than 20 degrees of sagittal plane rotation on dynamic (flexion-extension) radiographs should be considered abnormal and potentially unstable. This value was based on a review of the literature of *in vitro* and *in vivo* cervical spine ROM (7). When dynamic radiographs cannot be obtained (i.e., in an acute traumatic setting), a static (resting) latreal radiograph that shows more than 11 degrees of relative sagittal plane angulation should be considered potentially unstable. This value is based on a biomechanical study. Note that 11 degrees of relative angulation means 11 degrees more than the amount of angulation at the presumed intact FSU above or below the one in question. This standard of comparison takes into account the normal angulation between FSU (i.e., normal cervical lordosis). Two points in the checklist are given for abnormal sagittal plane rotation or abnormal relative sagittal plane angulation.

Note that a total of four points in the cervical checklist is given for the above radi-

ographic measurements; either dynamic (flexion-extension) or static (resting) radiographs are used in the checklist, not both. When both dynamic and static radiographs have been obtained, the measurements should be made on

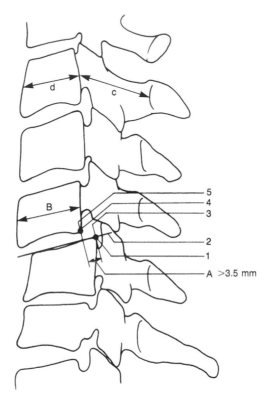

FIG. 3 The method for measuring translatory displacement is as follows: (1) A point is marked at the posterosuperior angle of the projected image of the vertebral body below the interspace of the functional spinal unit(FSU) being evaluated. (2) A line is drawn along the upper vertebral end plate of the vertebra below the interspace of the FSU under analysis. (3) At the point where this intersects the mark, at the posterior portion of the end plate, a short perpendicular line is drawn. (4) Next, a mark is made at the posteroinferior angle of image of the vertebral body above the interspace of the FSU being evaluated. (5) A short line through the second mark and perpendicular to the line on the subjacent vertebral end plate is drawn. the linear distance between the two perpendicular lines is measured. This can be called distance A. The anteroposterior sagittal plane diameter at the midlevel of the supraadjacent vertebra is measured. This distance is called B. If distance A is more than 20% of distance B instability is considered to exist, and should be so entered on the checklist. An alternate method is to simply measure the linear distance A; if this is more than 3.5 mm, it is considered suggestive of instability, and two points are entered onto the checklist. Pavlov's ratio is a reliable, accurate method for recognizing a developmentally narrow canal without the variables involved in linear measurements. The measurement c is the distance between the midlevel of the posterior aspect of the vertebral body and the nearest point on the corresponding spinolaminar line. The measurement d is apparent on lateral radiograph as the anteroposterior distance from the front to the back of the vertebral body measured at the midlevel. The ratio c/d is considered normal if 1 or greater and abnormal if less than 0.8. (Reprinted with permission from White AA, Panjabi MM. *Clinical Biomechanics of the Spine*, 2nd edition. Philadelphia: JB Lippincott, 1990: 316.)

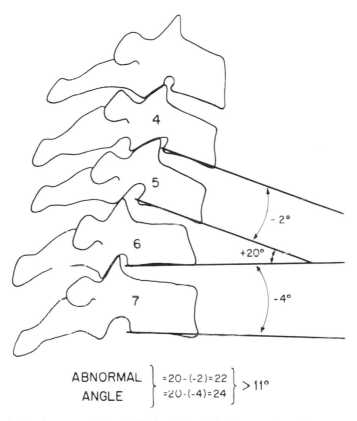

ABNORMAL $\left.\begin{array}{l} =20-(-2)=22 \\ =20-(-4)=24 \end{array}\right\}$ > 11°
ANGLE

FIG. 4. The angulation between C5 and C6 is 20°, which is more than 11° greater than that at either adjacent interspace. The angle at C4 and C5 measures-2, and that at C6 and C7 measures -4. This finding of abnormal angulation is based on a comparison of the interspace in question with either adjacent interspace, which allows for the angulation present due to the normal lordosis of the cervical spine. We interpret a difference of 11° or greater as evidence of clinical instability. These measurements are to be used in conjunction with the checklist. (Reprinted with *permission* from White AA, Panjabi MM. *Clinical Biomechanics of the Spine*, 2nd edition. Philadelphia: JB Lippincott, 1990:316.)

the dynamic films. Static radiographs should be used in the cervical checklist only when flexion-extension films cannot be obtained.

The radiographic interpretaion in general, especially for sagittal plane translation and displacement, is decidedly different in children to age 7 years. It is risky to interpret radiographs of patients in this age group without knowledge of some of the normal findings that may appear to be pathologic to an inexperienced physician.

Two final radiographic considerations should be noted. First, Bailey (13) remarked, and we have observed, that in the traumatized spine there may be narrowing of the disc at

the damaged FSU (10). In patients aged less than 35 years, we submit that posttraumatic disc narrowing is suggestive of disruption of the annulus fibroses of possible instability. Second, if all other considerations are the same, patients with a developmentally narrow spinal canal are moreapt to develop neurologic deficit because less space is available for the spinal cord. A developmentally narrow canal is defined as measuring less than 13 mm in AP dimension on a lateral radiograph (14) or with Pavlov's ratio of less than 0.8 (15–17). The 13-mm absolute value accounts for some radiographic magnification, whereas the Pavlov's ratio need not consider magnification since it is the ratio of the AP diameter of the canal of AP diameter of the vertebral body. One point each in the checklist is given for abnormal disc narrowing or a developmentally narrow canal.

Clinical Considerations

Is the presence of distinct medullary or root damage associated with spinal trauma or disease evidence of clinical instability? This consideration deserves some discussion. We have suggested that clinical instability concerns the prediction of subsequent neurologic damage. What is the significance of the presence of initial neurologic damage to the probability of subsequent neurologic damage? We believe that if the trauma is severe enough to cause initial neurologic damage, the support structures probably have been altered sufficiently to allow subsequent neurologic damage and that the condition is thus clinically unstable. However, Gosch and colleagues showed that in animals with intact supporting structures it is possible to produce medullary damage. In general, we believe that neurologic deficit is an important consideration of the evaluation of clinical instability. Evidence of root involvement is a weaker indicator of clinical instability. For example, a unilateral facet dislocation may cause enough foraminal encroachment to result in root symptoms or signs but not enough ligamentous damage to render the FSU unstable. Two points in the checklist are given for spinal cord damage and one point is given for nerve root damage.

The final consideration involves the important individual variation in physiologic load requirements. The clinician uses judgment in an attempt to anticipate the magnitude of loads that the particular patient's spine is expected to maintain after injury. Anticipating dangerous loads can be helpful. One point in the checklist is given if dangerous loading is anticipated. A total of five points is suggestive of instability.

BIOMECHANICAL RESPONSE TO LOAD-FUNCTIONAL SPINAL UNIT

In general, the cervical spine displays the most intersegmental motion of all spinal segments, if all parameters of motion are considered. However, the loads are relatively low in this region. A biomechanical analysis of the incidence of pain in the different regions of the spine suggests a relationship between loads and motion. While the degree of motion is highest in the cervical spine, its loads are the smallest. It ranks second among spinal segments in incidence of pain. There is relatively little motion in the thoracic spine, and the loads in this region are moderate. It ranks third in incidence of pain. The lumbar spine undergoes a moderate degree of motion and very high loads. It ranks first in incidence of pain (Table 5).

The specific response of the cervical spine to applied loads and motion is a complex interaction between supporting musculotendinous units, restraining capsuloligamentous structures, loaded intervertebral discs and the vertebral bodies. The ultimate response of these tissues in the dynamic in vivo environment has yet to be fully determined, but sufficient studies exist to establish broad parameters for behavior of various components of the functional spinal unit [FSU].

Goel and Clausen (18) have recently studied the role of the spinal elements in the transmission of applied loads. They have developed a three-dimensional finite element

TABLE 5. *Relationship between motion, loads, and pain in regions of the spine*

	Degree of motion (Rank)	Magnitude of loads (Rank)	Incidence of pain (Rank)
Cervical	1st	3rd	2nd
Thoracic	3rd	2nd	3rd
Lumbar	2nd	1st	1st

model of a C5–6 motion segment inclusive of the facet and unconvertebral articulations, intervertebral disc and capsuloligamentous tissues. The model has an ability to predict biomechanical responses to complex loading modes throughout the cervical spine's physiologic range of motion. Coupled motions are not reproduced. Initially, a simulated load of 73.6N compressive force was applied to a cervical segment in a neutral posture. Load transmission was purely through the disc and facet articulations, with the calculated ligamentous strain near zero. 88% (65.2N) of the load was transferred through the disc and the remaining 12% (4.2N) shared equally by the facet articulations. The addition of a 1.8NM flexion movement showed 116% (05.6NM) of the compressive load to be carried through the disc, with the facets being relieved of all loading. This flexion moment produced the highest predicted tensile strain in the interspinous ligament (25.9%) followed by the ligamentum flavum (LF)(19%) and posterior longitudinal ligament (PLL) (6.6%). The capsular ligament strain was 2.8%. The converse was shown with extension where compression was seen to shift load from the disc (14%–10.4NM) posteriorly to the facet joints (102%–37.6NM shared equally). Predicted strain was highest in the anterior longitudinal ligament (10.1%), followed by the capsular ligaments (3.4%). Lateral bending in compression loaded the disc (68%–50.1NM) and ipsilateral facet (41%–29.9NM). Ligamentous strain was 3.4% in the contralateral capsular ligaments and LF, 3.2% in the ipsilateral capsules ligament and 2.8% in the interspinous ligament. Axial rotation in compression displayed 75% (54.9NM) of load transmitted through the disc and 37% (27.56NM) through the contralateral facet. Strain was calculated at 13.0% for the ipsilateral capsular ligament and 1.6% for the contralateral capsular ligament. Throughout broad parameters of general motion, there is a reproducible pattern of load sharing among the structures of the FSU. Structures are loaded in varying fashion and subject to a unique stress dependent upon the particular cervical spine posture.

An *in vivo* study calculating cervical spine loads was conducted by Harms-Ringdahl (19) carrying a healthy, asymptomatic cohort through an experimentally directed flexion-extension arc. Five postures about the sagittal axis of motion for the atlanto-occipital articulation and the C7-T1 motion segment were studied; maximal flexion, slight flexion, neutral, neutral with the chin tucked in and maximal extension. Measurements were taken both of load moments and surface electromyographic activity in the erector spinae musculature. Load moments in neutral exhibited the lowest values at both C0-C1 (1.3NM) and C7-T1 (1.2 NM). The magnitude of the load moment at the atlanto-occipital joint showed little variation throughout the range of tested motions. A value of close to zero was achieved in maximal extension and with maximal flexion a value of 1.5 times the neutral value was recorded. As the spine was carried through the positions of flexion, values at C7-T1 were found to be 3.7NM with slight flexion and 4.3NM with extreme flexion. Extension values for C7-T1 were 0.4NM with the chin tucked in and 1.7NM in maximal extension.

Electromyographic activity was recorded for each of the five examined positions in the cervical erector spinae musculature. Recorded measurements were low for positions of neutral and for those of extreme flexion and extension. The median level of activity ranged from 0-6% of prior recorded levels of maximum muscular activity. These low activity values confirmed the earlier work of Fountain (20) and Takabe (21), where similar low postural paraspinal musculature activity levels were recorded. These results led the authors to conclude that in maximal positions of flexion and extension, the restraints required in counterbalancing the movement provided by the weight of the head are the supporting passive capsuloligimteous tissues. Working in these postural extremes places these tissues under considerable stress.

Schuldt (22) studied biomechanical cervical muscular functions in eight sitting postures during electromechanical assembly work. Measurements were compared with normalized quantified values from the same cohort. The lowest level of electromyographic activity occurred with the trunk inclined slightly backward and the neck vertical, or in neutral posture as the heads center of mass is coincident with the weight bearing axis of the spine. Slight flexion led to higher levels of activity in the cervical erector spinae. The erector spinae are posterior to the instantaneous axis of rotation of the cervical spinae. As the cervical spinae assumes a flexed posture, the erector spinae are required to lengthen in a controlled, eccentric fashion to control forward progression of the head. This eccentric musculature contraction is recorded as an increase in EMG activity. These studies show that at neutral positions, muscular activity is low. As the neck falls forward into a flexed posture, there is a commensurate increased level of activity seen in the erector spinae musculature as they contract while lengthening to control and counterbalance the movent of the head. Isometric contraction of the posterior cervical musculature is involved with lateral bending and extension, with a consequent increase in electromyographic activity. As full flexion and extension are achieved, muscular activity deceases as the flexion and extension movement is counterbalanced by the passive capsuloligametous tissues of the cervical spine.

In general, the purpose of a muscles mechanical output a force is to produce torque or movement across one or more joints. This muscular force or torque also generates compressive forces across the facet joints or discs across which the muscle works (23). This compressive reaction force is equal in magnitude to the vectorial sum of all the tensile muscle forces across the segment. Moroney and Schultz (24) studied maximal values for movement in fourteen males resisting maximal loads applied to the head while in a seated position. The observed movements were highest in extension, at 30NM. Flexion and lateral bending yielded values of 12-14NM while axial rotation yielded a mean maximal voluntary movement of 10NM. The values for movement calculated by Harms-Ringdahl are approximately 10% of these maximum values (19). The investigators also calculated compressive reaction forces across the C4-5 segment for these maximal voluntary movements. Compression force in extension was found to be 1,100 N. Flexion, rotation and lateral bending reaction forces were from 500-700 N. Force calculations were also exhibited to be representative of recorded electromyographic activity in this study.

Measurements of intradiscal pressure as indicators of spinal compressive load have been validated with fresh cadaveric specimens (25). Biomechanical studies in vivo by Hattori and associates (26) have determined intradiscal pressures in various cervical spine postures. Eighty discs in 48 patients were examined. Maximal cervical disc pressure is developed with neck extension (910 N). A supine neutral posture showed recorded values of 410 N which rose to 440N upon the assumption of a standing posture with the cervical spine in neutral. As the cervical spine was flexed, intradiscal pressure rose to 590N, as shown in Fig. 5. These findings have been confirmed in an *in vitro* study by Pospiech and associates (27). These authors showed that simulation of muscular force led to a marked increase in intradiscal pressure. Certain members of the current work force have undergone successful cervical fusion procedures. This study also demonstrated that anterior cervical fusions have a significant influence on increasing intradiscal pressure in both the immediately cephalad and caudad adjacent segments. This finding implies that in the post-fusion setting, less tolerance of equitable load application may be expected in this particular population than in their nonfused coworkers.

Conclusions

1. In seated postures, cervical intradiscal pressure and electromyographic activity are lowest in the neutral position.

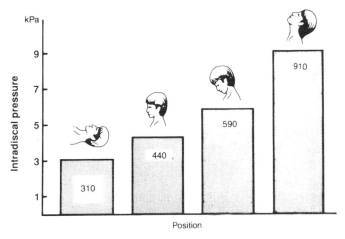

FIG. 5. A schematic of the anatomy of the middle and lower cervical spine.

2. Cervical spine flexion results in increasing levels of intradiscal pressure and eccentric muscular lengthening, with increased EMG activity, until full flexion is achieved. At this point, the passive capsuloligamentors restraints serve to counterbalance the forward weight of the head.

3. Cervical spine extension results in the highest levels of intradiscal pressure. Increases in isometric erector spinae contraction may be observed by electromyography. The compressive loads across the facet joints are also seen to increase.

4. Cervical segments adjacent to fused segments experience increased levels of load compared to nonfused speciments.

BIOMECHANICAL RESPONSE TO LOAD-CERVICAL MUSCULATURE

The cervical musculature has several biomechanical functions. Through their activity they produce body movements by generating bending movements and torques. Through the same mechanism they also perform tasks and resist external loads. Most important, they provide dynamic stability to the spine where very little exists. The spine, with its ligaments intact but devoid of muscles, is an extremely unstable structure. First, the muscles must generate force isometrically as well as with changing length. Second, they must increase the stiffness of the spine, thus inereasing stability.

Muscles may generate force through voluntary contracture with no change in length (isometric contracture), by shortening (concentric contracture) or by lengthening as it contracts (eccentric contracture). Force generation is a function of the resting length of a muscle at the initiation of contraction. Maximum force is developed at about 120–130% of the resting length of a muscle, or eccentric posture, while at about 50% of its resting length, the muscle produces very little force. A muscle produces force also in direct relationship to its cross-sectional area. The maximum force per unit area of the muscle has been determined by several researchers with results ranging from 29-93N/CM for different muscles of the extremities (7). With the use of strength testing machines and magnetic resonance images, the maximum stress that the erector spinae can develop has been determined to be 48N/CM.

The stiffness characteristics of a muscle are a crucial determinant in the maintenance of spinal stability. The active stiffness of a muscle increases rapidly at small force levels and then saturates at higher levels of the force. One may hypothesize that, while resting, the spinal column is quickly stabilized when subjected to reasonable physiologic loads. As the load continues to increase, there is a threshold that is reached beyond which there is no further increase in the stiffness of the muscles. In effect, this mechanism sets an upper load limit for spinal column muscular stabilization. Beyond this limit, stability is achieved through capsuloligamentors and structural vertebral body support.

Muscle contraction will ultimately result in fatigue. The time of a muscle to its fatigue level is known as the endurance time and is a function of the contraction force. Carpenter and colleagues (28) have shown a relationship between muscle fatigue and subsequent decrements in joint position sense. The authors stated that this decreased proprioceptive sense may play a role in decreasing athletic performance and in fatigue-related shoulder dysfunction. Yoshikawa and associates (29) subjected ten adult foxhounds to fatiguing exercise and found through correlative analysis a significant increase in bone strain with decreasing levels of myoelectric activity after 20 minutes of exercise. Arresting muscular activity prior to fatigue and possible dysfunction and pain is implicit in its possible benefit. Important to preventive ergonomic biomechanics is the relationship of the endurance time of a muscle to its exertion or percent of maximal muscle force level. Maintained static contracture of a muscle, before exceeding its endurance time, or fatigue limit, may be associated with the production of neck pain. Static muscular workload has been examined and found to display a more consistent association with musculoskeletal morbidity than dynamic muscular work. Tension placed upon a muscle during static loading is often expressed in terms of a percentage of the muscle's maximum voluntary contraction (MVC). The critical value for endurance in static loading beyond which fatigue and pain develop has been estimated by Hamilton to be below 10% of MVC (30). A load for at least 10 minutes may be sustained comfortably at or below this level. Jensen recommended a level for maintained static work at 2% MVC (31). Veiersted and co-workers analyzed muscular activity during stereotyped work requiring static contracture and its relationship to muscular dis-

comfort. Complaints from workers of muscle fatigue, soreness and pain were found to occur at levels of 1.6% MVC (32). It is important to remember that muscular tension in the spine cannot be measured directly, but as in the studies above is measured indirectly by electromyography using bipolar surface and needle electrodes. These studies are also limited in their scope by using live human volunteers, where perceptions of pain vary from individual to individual. They do, however, serve as a set of defined reproducible measurements across a broad section of the work force for which general data may be accumulated and recommendations made. By electromyographic measurement, the acceptable limit for sustained static muscular contraction should be less than 5% of maximum voluntary contracture.

BIOMECHANICAL BASIS OF SPINE PAIN

Muscular response to sustained contraction is quite complex and multifactoral. Eccentric muscular contracture is associated with greater possible force generation and at the same time a predisposition to both fatigue and possible pain. Acute and chronic fatigue may have a basis in decreased blood flow and reduced tissue oxygenation. The lack of local metabolite clearance efficacy may potentiate muscular pain. Microstructural muscular damage may occur in association with an inflammatory response which is provocation of pain. Edema, reflective of tissue injury/inflammation is seen in exercised muscles 24-72 hours after exercised periods and may bear a causal relationship or be reflective of other causal entities responsible for delayed muscular soreness.

The initiation or provocation of a painful stimulus from the cervical erector spinae musculature has several theoretical etiologies. Tissue loading (muscular contracture) may occlude the vasculature; depriving muscles, tendons and nerves of nutrition. The relative ischemia of this condition diminishes the physical tissue repair rate, allowing repetitious activity to produce structural trauma and pain. Murthy and associates (33) employed an infrared spectroscopy technique to examine tissue oxygenation levels in the extensor carpi radialis brevis (ECRB) at low levels of isometric contraction. Contractions at 5%, 10%, 15% and 20% of MVC were sustained for one minute each and followed by a 3-minute recovery period. Mean tissue oxygenation levels were found to decrease during the contraction phase to 89%, 81%, 78%, and 47%, respectively, of resting levels. Tissue oxygenation was shown to decrease during brief, low levels of static musculature and found to be statistically significant at levels of 10%, 15% and 50% of MVC. Larrson and colleagues (34) examined the relationship between blood flow and chronic pain in the cervical spine. Microcirculatory blood flow in the trapezius muscle was measured by laser-doppler flowometry while levels of sustained static muscular contracture were recorded by EMG. Thirteen tested patients had chronic unilateral neck pain as a result of soft tissue injury to the neck, while 12 tested patients had chronic bilateral symptoms. Muscle blood flow on the painful sides was found to be impaired with increasing levels of tension and fatigue as compared to the "uninjured" sides. Biopsies from patients with chronic trapezius muscle pain have displayed low capillary density. Increased capillary density has been associated with greater endurance and resistance to fatigue. These studies suggest the presence of vascular ischemic mechanism at work in sustained muscular contractions casally related to chronic pain.

The posterior cervical erector spinae musculature is frequently placed in a lengthened or eccentric posture. Muscles are at greater risk for injury when loaded in an eccentric posture and when their action is imposed across two or more joints as occurs in the cervical spine. Clarkson and Newham (35) have recently reported eccentric contraction to result in muscle soreness, strength, ROM and structural integrity loss. Strength loss of up to 50% in affected muscle groups has been shown immediately post-exercise.

Also, fatigue of greater magnitude and longer duration was shown to occur with eccentrically exercised musculature as compared to muscles exercised in isometric and concentric fashion. The level of active strain during eccentric contractions suggested by the author creates an initial muscular insult which increases over the next 2 to 3 days. This structural injury is accompanied by edema and delayed muscle soreness and followed by regenerative repair. Friden and associates (36) looked directly at delayed muscular soreness in eccentric and concentric muscular contractures. They observed 400 submaximal eccentric anterior compartment contractions in 8 healthy males and compared them to 400 opposite leg submaximal concentric contractions. Needle biopsies taken 48 hours later showed in the eccentric group a significantly higher water content which displayed a direct association with the development of delayed muscle soreness. The authors found "scant" evidence of muscle necrosis or inflammation.

Hasselink and colleagues (37) evaluated muscular damage and strength after eccentric and isometric contractions. They exercised the tibialis anterior muscles in an animal model subjected to increasing numbers of isometric and eccentric contractions. They found evidence of histologic changes in exercised muscle inclusive of an inflammatory response, z-line streaming and decreased muscular function as reflected in a prolonged decline in maximal isometric muscular strength. These findings were more pronounced in the eccentric than in the isometrically exercised group. While a relationship was displayed between the percentage of histologic muscle damage and decreasing isometric torque generation after eccentric contractures, the authors concluded that the correlation was not sufficiently strong enough to preclude factors other than muscle damage resulting in the decline of muscle force.

Conclusions

1. The cervical musculature may be implicated along with the intevertebral disc

and supporting osseo-capuloligamentous structures, as a source of spinal pain.

2. Eccentric muscular contractions place the muscle in a more demanding environment than do isometric and concentric contractures. This may bear a causal relationship to muscular soreness, fatigue and pain.

FUNCTIONAL POSTURAL BIOMECHANICS

Flexion

Cervical extensor muscle activity is intimately related to postural adaptation in the ergonomic environment. The lowest level of paraspinal muscular activity is exhibited when the spine is held in a neutral or vertical posture with the head's center of mass coincident with the weightbearing axis of the spine. Cervical spine flexion increases the length of the movement arm from the head's center of mass to the motion axis of the vertebral axis of motion. This causes an increase in load as has been exhibited by Harms-Ringdahl and increases the counteracting muscular load required of the cervical extensor musculature through a functional range of motion. Neck extensor strength and relative load has been studied for different levels of postural flexion. Approximately 10% of muscular strength is needed to maintain the neck in a 20 degree flexed position. At 50 degrees of flexion 17% of muscular strength is needed (38). Chaffin found that neck musculature fatigued from cervical flexion exceeding 15 degrees (39). The more the head and neck is tilted forward, the earlier pain develops. He also found a correlate between the degree of cervical flexion and the average time to fatigue. Increasing levels of flexion are associated with less average time to fatigue. Ohlsson and associates (40) investigated female industrial assembly line workers exposed to repetitive tasks with short cycles (< 30 sec) and made measurements of neck flexion angles. This cohort was compared to age and sex matched referents without such exposure. A diagnosis of neck pain was found to have a significant association with flexion angles > 15 degrees as well as time spent in flexion.

Serratos-Perez studied the incidence of musculoskeletal pain in male sewing machine operators (41). Flat machine operators, where sustained cervical flexion is required, displayed a significantly higher incidence of neck pain over column machine operators, where a neutral posture is allowed. Maintained cervical flexion has also been shown to result in an increased incidence of pain and discomfort in dentists (42). Kilbom (43) studied female electronic workers in highly repetitive tasks with static postured loads to the neck. These workers were followed over a three year period and compared with workers who, through workplace intervention, decreased their number of repetitive tasks. A statistically significant association (P <0.05) was found between neck symptoms and cervical flexion > 20(43). The authors concluded that relocation to more varied work tasks, with decreased static loading and increased patterns of movement was a strong predictor for symptomatic alleviation.

Extension

Yoo and colleagues (22) have noted significant decreases in neuroforaminal size with extension. Farmer and Wisneski (44) have taken C5-7 neuroforaminal pressure measurements in fresh (<48 HRS) cadaveric specimens in neutral, 20 and 40 flexion, and 20 and 40 degrees extension. Measurements were also taken with the arm in neutral and abduction. Increasing neck extension led to consistent and significant pressure increases over neutral positioning. With 20 degrees of cervical extension, pressures from 22.6 to 36.9 mmhg were recorded. With 40 degrees of cervical extension, pressures range from 38.9 to 41.0 mmhg. Muckley and colleagues (45) used an intervertebral occlusion transducer in cadavers and measured changes in the geometry of the cervical intervertebral foramen. They showed cervical extension to create a decrease in intervetebral foramen area which relates linearly with the angle of extension. External pressures of 30-50 mm Hg have been shown to cause an alteration in blood flow, vascular permeability and axonal transport. Garfin and colleagues (46) have reviewed the pathophysiology of spinal nerve root compression. Compression has been shown to alter the chemical and metabolic nerve root environment which can lead to an inflammatory response. Varying degrees of compression coupled with local inflammation can result in the provocation of pain from the nerve root. Similar increases in intradiscal pressure may incite inflammation and pain from the intervertebral disc (7,47). Sakakibara and associates (48) have studied the effects of overhead work requiring cervical extension in pear and apple baggers. Pears grow at heights of 170-190 cm, requiring almost constant neck extension and arm elevation for cultivation (75% of total work time). Apples grow at various heights both above and below eye level, so inconstant extension and arm elevation are required (40% work time). Fifty-two female farmers were studied bagging both pears and apples. Neck/shoulder pain was found to be much more prevalent when bagging pears than apples. Other musculoskeletal complaints showed no difference. Eklund (49) studied forklift drivers with goods handled high above ground. This forced the workers into a position of "substantial extension in combination with rotation" which was perceived by the drivers as their most strenuous work posture. Arm elevation, as with the orchard workers, is not a confounding variable. Therefore, it follows that maintenance of extreme cervical extension may be provocative of cervical discomfort.

AXIAL ROTATION/LATERAL BENDING

Axial rotation loads the contralateral facet, the ipsilateral facet with its capsuloligamentous supports, and the intevertebral disc. Axial rotation less than 35 degrees does not require great muscular force. Axial rotation greater than 35 degrees causes a fast increase in muscle reactiono and joint reaction forces (50). Lateral bending loads the ipsilateral facet and disc. The most potentially injurious uniplanar motion to the posterolateral annular fibers of the disc is axial rotation (51). The combined motion pattern most provocative of injury is a coupling of axial rotation and lateral bending. The flexibility characteristics (ability of a structure to deform under the application of load) of axial rotation are markedly different from those seen with other motions. In the cervical spine, the spine is only 37% as flexible in torsion as compared with flexion. The spine is more flexible in lateral bending than axial rotation, but more stiff than seen in pure flexion. Increasing activity is seen in the paraspinal musculature with axial rotation and lateral bending (52).

Side bending and rotation more than 15 degrees during the greater part of a work day have been suggested to be injurious to the vertebral column (53). Rundcrantz and colleagues (42) evaluated occupational cervicobrachial disorders in dentists and compared them to a similar professional cohort without clinical symptoms. They found those dentists working with a direct view of specific upper tooth surfaces required to hold their neck in varying postures of axial rotation and lateral bending. Dentists with cervical pain kept their head side bent (>15) degrees, rotated or in combination (35) to a greater extent than dentists without symptoms. All dentists maintained cervical flexion of 15 degrees. They also found that significantly more dentists without symptoms were both aware of and utilized natural pauses in their work. Dentists without pain employed the use of a mirror, which allowed for the substitution of indirect vision for posture and reduced loads on the neck.

Eklund and associates (49) reviewed the incidence of cervical pain in operators of fork lifts, cranes and forestry machines. They employed an electric goniometer measurement system (Nickometer, SE-Ergonomic Products, Goteberg, Sweden) and recorded sagittal plane flexion, lateral plane flexion and rotation in the transverse plane. The fork lifts were fitted with sideway sitting seats, requiring head rotation to the left for driving and to the right for material handling. Little time was spent with head straight. The drivers rotated their heads exceeding 70% of their maximal voluntary movement for the work day or between 150 and 550 times per hour. The mean arc of head rotation was in the 15-45 degrees arc with a mean of 38 degrees. Smaller females bent strongly backward and sideways to see because the chairs had been shifted forward to allow them to reach the pedals. Several of the forklifts were fitted with forward facing seats. These workers spent comparatively little of the work day in the 15-45 degrees rotation arc with the majority of measured rotation being <15 degrees. Cranes were fitted with a conventional fixed or rotatable cabin. Those workers in the conventional cabin were required to employ cervical rotation for observation of the worksite, with a mean rotation angle of 33 degrees. The implementation of a rotating cabin decreased the mean angle to 14 degrees. The forestry machine gave less head rotation compared to the other machines, with a mean rotation angle of 7 degrees. There was a correlate found by the authors between head rotation and the incidence of cervical discomfort.

The authors noted that in seats with high backrests, larger degrees of rotation are required of the cervical spine. Less rotation thru the trunk is possible with the limiting backrest. This results in more neck discomfort as larger degrees of rotation are shifted from the trunk to the neck. Rotatable driver seats decreased the need for head rotation. They concluded that viewing angles with less than 15 degrees of required cervical rotation was optimal in decreasing cervical complaints. For larger fields of vision, rotatable seats or cabins avoid adverse head postures. Also important for vision was the use of larger windows and narrower frames, so that postural adjustments were limited. Low light or scratches and dirt on windows should be minimized. With rotating seats, steering wheels and controls should follow seat movements to decrease postural restrictions. Backrests should not be so high as to limit rotation of the upper trunk.

EXTERNAL LOADS

Cervical spine loads are significantly affected by loads borne by the head. The influence of axial load on the development of cervical degenerative change has been studied in a population of porters who use their heads as a means of carrying packages. A population of 35 asymptomatic porters was compared to an age and sex matched control cohort who had never carried weights on their heads. The prevalence of radiographic degenerative change was 88.6% in the carriers and 22.9% in the noncarriers. For each cervical segment evaluated (C3-7) there was a higher prevalence of degenerative change in the carrier group, with the highest values obtained at the C5-6 segment (54). Jumah and Nyame (55) studied 305 porters in Ghana and found 63.6% of carriers to exhibit radiographic degenerative change, compared to 36% of those who carried no weight. A study of headloading in rural Zimbabwe has shown a change in the pattern of spondylosis. Carrying heavy loads on the head was found to create a shift in the incidence in spondylosis from the 5th intervertebral disc to more cephalad levels. Risk of early or accelerated degenerative change has also been shown in meat carriers. In placing large weights of meat partially on the side of the head and neck and partially on the shoulders high loads are transferred to the cervical spine (56,57). Rugby players are also subjected to an increase in axial cervical force transmission during participation in scrums (58). The increased weight of a helmet has also been hypothesized as contributing to the increased incidence of spondylosis seen in miners. Diving from a board has been shown to have an association with acute prolapse of cervical intervertebral discs.

Levy demonstrated by lateral radiographs a straightening of the physiologic cervical lordosis and narrowing of the intervertebral space when 90-kg weights were axially loaded onto the head (59). Maiman and colleagues found (60) cadavers loaded at neutral in axial compression sustained much greater loads to failure (33567N) than those loaded in flexion or extension (means 1023N and 1089N). Hodgson and Thomas (61) recorded cervical spine vertebral body strains for various cervical postures. The highest vertebral body strains were seen with axial loading at the crown of the head with relative flexion of the neck sufficient to straighten the cervical lordosis. Thus, the straightened cervical spine will sustain and withstand the highest axial compressive loads. As the cervical spine is straightened, the loaded weight is borne progressively anteriorly by the vertebral bodies and discs. This increased load over time becomes manifest as spondylotic change through disc space degeneration, narrowing and the formation of ventral, dorsal, uncovertebral and facet articulation osteophytes. These radiographic findings may become clinically relevant in the form of neck/shoulder pain, radiculopathy, radiculitis or myelopathy.

SHOULDER POSITIONING

Spurling noted that "raising the arm above the head sometimes brings relief" to symptomatic extradural root compression (62). Possible etiologies for this finding are (a) decreasing nerve root transitting distance; (b) decreasing dural ligament tension on the nerve root; (c) opening of the intervertebral foramen. Davidson and coworkers (63) described shoulder abduction as providing relief in cervical monoradiculopathies and coined the shoulder abduction test as a reliable clinical indicator of nerve root compressive phenomena. Measurements taken from the transverse process of C5 to the coracoid decrease by 3.1 cm or 24% with shoulder abduction. The authors concluded that nerve roots traversing this shorter distance could be under less tension. Farmer has recently shown in cadaveric specimens that movement of the arm from a neutral to an abducted position consistently lowered neuroforaminal pressure (44). The converse of this test may present clinically as neck/shoul-

der/arm pain. Patients will sometimes report exacerbations of arm pain after carrying a briefcase, shoulder bag or lap-top computer, etc. When a ten-pound weight is added to the hand, the C5 transverse process to coracoid distance was found to ignore 4 mm or 31% (63). Load carrying with a symptomatic upper extremity should be avoided.

While shoulder abduction may relieve the pain from neural compressive phenomena, prolonged or repetitive shoulder elevation in the ergonomic environment is associated with the production of neck and shoulder discomfort. Work with the arms abducted or elevated, rather than kept by the sides, leads to increasing EMG activity and signs of fatigue in the trapezius, the cervical and thoracic erector spinea, the rhomboids and the shoulder musculature (38). Placing the hands above shoulder level has been shown to significantly increase both the risk of muscular fatigue and postural discomfort in the setting of light work where postural exertions are small (22). Neck/shoulder pain was reviewed in 1773 construction workers. The one year prevalence of neck/shoulder pain was 12% with the predominant physical risk factor being working with hands above shoulder level (64). Static, rather than dynamic muscular workload displayed the most consistent positive association for symptom production. Holmstrom found a clear dose-response relationship between prolonged work with hands above shoulder level and neck/shoulder pain. Tichauer showed that the metabolic cost of packing groceries increases while performance level decreases if the work height is such that the arms have to be abducted greated than 20 degrees (65).

Desk height and forearm support play a significant role in workplace cervical musculoskeletal discomfort. A workstation that requires shoulder elevation and abduction may cause the trapezius and deltoids to sustain contractions of 20% of their maximum potential (66). High levels of trapezius load have also been recorded in the data entry workers working without forearm support. Supporting the forearms led to significantly decreased trapezial loads in both sitting and standing postures (67). Arm rests have also been shown to decrease pressure in the lumbar intervertebral disc (11). Schuldt and associates (22) have shown in skilled female workers performing standardized work assembling circuit boards a reduction in neck and shoulder muscular activity obtained with the use of elbow supports in the seated position. The elbow supports worked more efficiently when the trunk was inclined slightly backward. The height of a work surface 5 cm below the elbow is optimal for light work and 5-10cm above the elbow for precision work. Bendiz and colleagues suggested that for both seated and standing postures that all work 5 cm above elbow level should be accompanied by elbow supports.

Conclusions

1. Maintained cervical flexion greater than 15-20 degrees is associated with neck pain.
2. Cervical extension increases neuroforaminal pressure and maintained cervical extension may be provocative of neck pain.
3. Axial rotation coupled with lateral bending is potentially injurious to the posterolateral annular fibers of the intevertebral disc. Axial rotation greater than 35 degrees should be avoided on a repetitive or sustained basis. Lateral bending greater than 15 degrees should be avoided on a repetative or sustained basis. Rotation or flexibility of the workstation (chairs, etc.) should substitute for required cervical motion
4. Axial loads lead to an increase in potentially symptomatic cervical spondylosis.
5. Repetitive shoulder abduction is associated with neck/shoulder/arm pain. Work should be kept below neutral (<90) degrees other than for short intervals.

Placing weights in the hands or across the shoulder may result in neck/shoulder/arm pain. Briefcases should be alternated and carrying straps placed across asymptomatic shoulders.

SITTING

The modern work environment is becoming increasingly saturated with the use of computers and their video display terminals. Frequently, prolonged periods involving a static work posture are required. Sitting offers the advantage of stability for executing fine motor tasks such as typing with less overall energy expenditure. Sustained postures require static muscular contracture which will result in local fatigue and cervical discomfort. This may be further exacerbated by maintenance of a posture that is ergonomically suboptimal. Sitting postures is under the influence of variables from the eyes to the lumbar spine. All must be considered and their environmental influence recognized in order to minimize the incidence and prevalence of musculoskeletal disorders in the workplace.

Seated posture is determined initially by the position of the lumbar spine. The work of Anderson shows, in seated positioning, lower intervertebral pressures with slight (90–110) degrees posterior inclination (2). Cervical positioning is under the influence of lumbar posture. With the visual gaze maintained at a fixed object, video screen, etc., increasing degrees of lumbar extension lead to compensatory cervical flexion and vice versa. This has recently been validated by Black and associates (62). The authors sought to attempt in this study a defined set of reproducible sagittal plane compensatory motions in both the upper and lower cervical spines for given changes in lumbar posture. The degree and location of cervical adaptation, upper or lower, were found to show considerable variability among tested subjects. This study does remind us of the respect needed for individual variation in the workplace and the design of the workplace around and for the worker, rather than fitting people into prefit space.

Cervical spine position as is dictated by the line of sight required for the particular task at hand. The normal visual angle in the sagittal plane is from 15-22 degrees (69). A person cannot accurately estimate size or the relative distance of objects without binocular vision, which takes place (without head movement) only within a visual cone of 60 degrees. This means that there is little necessity for cervical flexion within this range as the eyes will shift comfortably. Aaras (70) recently studied the relationship between head flexion and movement of the eyes as contributors to the sightline angle. When the sightline to a video display screen was fixed at 15 degrees, the observed median head angle was 3–5 degrees. The corresponding downward gaze of the eyes was approximately 11 degrees. During typing, the document source was the primary sightline focus and approximately 30 below the horizontal. The median neck flexion was from 10–22 degrees which again, corresponded to a downward gaze of the eyes of 0–12 degrees. For sightlines below 15–30 degrees of horizontal, the authors concluded the eyes downward gaze to be approximately 10 degrees, with compensatory increases of cervical flexion to maintain gaze.

Kumar and Schaife (71) found reports of neck discomfort related to neck inclination angle. Postural discomfort and worker neck strain are produced if a source document is located flat on a work surface, as opposed to being held by a document holder. Chaffin (39) found the endurance time of five young asympotmatic females to be greatly decreased when the neck inclination exceeded 30 degrees. Trapezius load does not change appreciably for a sightline between 15 degrees and 30 degrees below horizontal (69). For the most comfortable work posture, the angle of head flexion should not exceed 20–30 degrees. The field of vision determines the sightline angle and should not exceed 20, with little rotation. This requires a screen that is adjustable for height, distance and angle. Document holders should be placed at the same height and distance from the eyes as the monitor. The angle of the head should not exceed 20–30 degrees of flexion or the potential for cervical spine symptom provocation increases. Apart from sagittal angulation, depth of focus is important. For tasks requiring typing or reading, a monitor or document source should be placed 10–25 inches from the view-

ers face. This will help avoid "craning" of the neck and possible symptom provocation. Eye and muscular strain may also be relieved by focusing on objects from 10–20 feet away intermittently.

Cervical extension muscle force values are 50% higher for a 30-degree flexion inclination angle from neutral (vertical). EMG activity is lowest at vertical. Even slight forward inclination, therefore, is reflected by an increase in cervical extension musculature activity.

Conclusions

1. The elbow should be supported in static sitting or standing postures. While individual variation exists, the work surface should be 5 cm below the elbow for light (assembly) work and 5–10cm above the elbow for precision work.
2. Video display terminals should have (a) adjustable screens; (b) be placed within a sightline angle of 20 degrees; and (c) be 10–25 inches from the viewers face.
3. Documents should be placed in a holder the same height and distance, from 10–25 inches, from the viewers face as the VDT. Little cervical rotation (<10 degrees) should be required for visualization.
4. Frequent breaks help to decrease both visual and muscular fatigue.
5. Fit the workplace to the worker, rather than the worker to the workplace.

TIME

Frequent relaxation intervals from prolonged, repetitive, static muscular work have been described as "crucial" to aid in the mitigation of muscular fatigue and pain (72–74). A study of dentists with and without neck discomfort showed that significantly more dentists without pain and discomfort took advantage of small subtle breaks during their work schedules, such as shrugging their shoulders during intervals in which the nurse mixed amalgam or the patient rinsed their mouth (42). Haag (75) studied the load pattern and pressure pain threshold in medical secretaries. They found that secretaries with complaints of neck pain displayed a monotonous muscular load pattern at 1-5% of MVC. The secretaries without complaints of pain had more frequent pauses and more frequent episodes with totally relaxed musculature. Carter and Banister (72) have suggested that workers stand from seated postures and move about during a break. They suggested that the area set aside for coffee breaks be at some distance from work areas, up or down a flight of stairs, for example,to encourage a "physiologic break" from work. This type of "active pause" changed muscular activity patterns. They also supported the alternation on an hourly basis between VDT work and another, more active and less statically repetitive and demanding task. Westgaard and Jansen (76) have found that groups with more varied work tasks have less reported neck discomfort. A helpful strategy to decrease ergonomic complaints would be to allow for frequent, active breaks and/or allow for the performance of varied rather than more monotonous tasks during the work day.

Conclusions

Frequent pauses result in less static muscular contracture and decreasing complaints of neck pain. "Active" pauses may be more beneficial than more "passive" pauses.

UNIQUE OCCUPATIONAL RISKS

The range of occupations and/or vocations available at this point in history are as varied as the people who pursue them. With this expansive range of opportunity comes a variety of stresses and challenges to the physiologic integrity of the cervical spine. Injuries may be a result of cumulative unnoticed events only becoming naggingly symptomatic after decades or violent, sudden and with terrible consequence. Numerous patterns of injury fill a middle ground between these two extremes. A brief survey of some of these unique occupational disorders follows.

Perhaps the most extreme example of chronic, occupational, low-grade trauma was recently presented by Kelkar and colleagues (77). The authors recently presented the cases of two patients who had been serving as railway porters for 25 years. They had begun at ages 14 and 15. Clinical examination revealed the obvious presence of severe cervical deformity, noticed by the patients prior but asymptomatic. Magnetic resonance imaging revealed a gross kypkoscoliosis in one patient and a grossly lordotic deformity in the second patient. Associated vertebral subluxations were also present. Cervical spine radiographs as pre-employment tests taken 25 years prior in both patients were normal, ruling out congenital osseous deformity. There was no prior surgery, tuberculosis, tumor, spondyloarthropathy, or any other form of known pathologic etiology. The conclusion of the authors was that chronic low grade vertebral trauma from carrying heavy loads on their head resulted in the extreme deformities presented.

At the other end of the spectrum from the asymptotic, chronic low grade deformity is the violent application of extreme axial loads to the spine. Spinal injuries in sports constitute only 3% of all athletic injuries. However, it is thought that 50–75% of the fatal injuries involve the head and neck, with cervical spine trauma accounting for 25% of those injuries (78). Tackling with the crown of the helmet in American football is associated with significant axial loads and buckling/flexion movements which may result in cervical spine failure and quadriplegia. Rugby, hockey and gymnastics are other sports which carry a similar risk.

In the middle category are those activities which may not stress the spine to failure, but may be of sufficient stress to result in a painful stimulus. Competitive swimming has been associated with a variety of strains on the cervical spine due to the repetitive, functional demands of various strokes. A case report recently was presented of an adolescent competitive swimmer who developed neck pain and suboccipital headache related to a congenital atlanto-occipital fusion and associated intevertebral disc degeneration (79). This may be a consideration in patients with cervical spondylosis who wish to engage in aggressive swimming programs. The cervical extension and axial rotation involved with a tennis serve may initiate or aggravate cervical symptoms. The use of a standard telephone receiver is often associated with exaggerated lateral bending which may in cumulative fashion be associated with discomfort or pain. For this reason, when telephone usage is a significant part of the work day, headsets may be of benefit.

Vibration

Vibrations are applied to the spine most frequently through motor vehicles and heavy vibrating equipment. Animal and human studies have shown that vibration causes creep and muscular fatigue, resulting in increased intradiscal pressures (80). A study by Magnusson (81) has shown in humans that seated whole body vibrations at 5 Hz and 0.1 g root mean square corresponds to a lumbar axial load of 1,200 N. It is known that the resonating frequency of the spine is about 4–5 Hz both *in vitro* and *in vivo* (7). This is the vibration frequency of all automobiles that are not of Swedish or Japanese manufacture. Drivers of Swedish and Japanese automobiles have a lower incidence of herniated discs than drivers of other vehicles.

Erector spinae musculature respond synchronously to sinusoidal vibration (82,83) with the highest levels of activity seen with increased vibration amplitudes at the resonant frequency of the trunk. Muscle fatigue follows, and has been suggested as an etiology in fatigue injuries. Fatigue injury has also been hypothesized in the annulur fibers of the discs (84). Other hypothesis relate to vascular mediation, with vasospasm and nutritional changes resulting in disc failure and/or inflammation. Another consideration is vibration induced accumulation of metabolites which leads to a more accelerated development of degenerative changes in the discs. This equates low back pain with discogenic

pain, but could be from muscles, facet capsules, etc.

Most vibrational studies have centered in the lumbar spine, where causality between disc disease and pain is being supported by a growing body of epidemiological data. The cervical data is less clear. A multicenter epidemiologic study of acute prolapsed cervical intevertebral discs by Kelsey (85) and colleagues found driving or riding in automobiles or motorcycles, or operating or driving vibrating equipment as presenting risk factors. In general, though, these associations were not statistically significant. Viikari-Juntura and associates (86) studied machine operators exposed to static work and whole-body vibration compared to carpenters exposed to dynamic physical work and no vibration. The studies showed a significant difference due to vibration progressing from no neck pain to moderate to severe neck pain. However, the study did not measure vibration exposure and did not control for neck-twisting or static loads. Bjurvald et al. (87) found that a rotated spinal posture while seated caused increased vibration transmission from the seat to the head. Vibration exposure from hand held tools has been related to neck and shoulder pain in forestry workers. It is unclear from this study, whether vibration was a primary etiology for pain or a cofounding variable. A recent epidemiologic review conducted by the National Institute for Occupational Safety and Health found insufficient current evidence as a result of too few studies to support an association between vibration and cervical musculoskeletal disorders.

Conclusion

The cervical spine has significant demands placed upon its functional spinal units and supportive musculature over the course of the workday. Demands which exceed "normal" physiologic limits may be productive of significant and limiting discomfort. These demands may occur with a single large force application, but are more commonly the result of repetitive motion or sustained maintenance of a given posture. Significant strides are being made with continued, dedicated cervical ergonomic and biomechanical research. Muscular and nerve physiology is becoming increasingly defined. The importance of the successful implementation of this research into the workplace cannot be understated in the mitigation of work-related neck pain. Fitting the workplace to the individual worker rather the the worker to a generically designed workplace poorly suited to their particular habitus is a significant contribution. Attention should be given to possible vibrational exposure, time spent over the course of the day in static postures, the cumulative effects of loads, etc. Further research should continue to refine the understanding of these basic principles and allow for further improvement in the ergonomic environment.

REFERENCES

1. Nachemson A. Lumbar spine instability: a critical update and symposium summary. *Spine* 1985;10:290–291.
2. Anderson GBJ, Ortengren R. Lumbar disc pressure and myoelectric activity during sitting III: studies on an office chair. *Scand J Rehab Med* 19974;3:122–177.
3. Hecker P. Appareil ligamenteux occipito-atloido-axiodien: etude d'anatomie comparee. *Arch Anat Hist Embryol* 1923;2:57–95.
4. Crisco JJ, Takenori O, Panjabi MM, Bueff HU, Dovrak J. Grob D. Transections of the C1-C2 joint capsular ligaments in the cadaveric spine. *Spine* 1991;16: S474–S479.
5. Panjabi M, DvorakJ, Crisco JJ, Oda T, Wang P, Grob D. Effects of alar ligament transection on upper cervical spine rotation. *J Orthop Res* 1991; 9:584–93
6. Fielding JW, Cochran GVB, Lansing JF, Hohl M. Tears of the transverse ligament of the atlas: a clinical biomechanical study. *J Bone Joint Surg Am* 1974;56:1683.
7. White AA, Panjabi MM, *Clinical biomechanics of the spine,* 2nd edition, Philadelphia: JB Lippincott, 1990.
8. Panjabi MM, White AA, Johnson RM. Cervical spine mechanics as a function of transection of components. *J Biomech* 1975;8:327.
9. White AA, Panjabi M. *Spinal kinematics in the research status of spinal manipulative therapy.* Washington, D.C.: U.S. Dept. of Health, Education and Welfare, 1975.
10. Bailey RW. Fractures and dislocations of the cervical spine: orthopedic and neurosurgical aspects. *Postgrad Med* 1964;35:588.
11. Munro D. Treatment of fractures and dislocations of the cervical spine complicated by cervical cord and root injuries: a comparative study of fusion vs non fusion therapy. *N Engl J Med* 1961;264:573.
12. Panjabi MM, White AA, Keller D, Southwick WO, Friedlander, G. Stability of the cervical spine under tension. *J Biomech* 1978;11:189–197.
13. Bailey RW. Observations of cervical intervertebral disc lesions in fractures and dislocations. *J Bone Joint Surg [Am]* 1963;
14. Ferguson RJL, Caplan LR. Cervical spondylitic myelopathy. *Neurol Clin* 1985;3:373.
15. Torg J, Sennett B, Vegso J, Pavlov H, Lehmann R. Axial loading injuries to the middle cervical spine segment: an analysis and classification of twenty-five cases. Cervical Spine Research Society, 1986.
16. Torg JS, Pavlov H, Genuario SE, et al. Neuropraxia of the cervical spinal cord with transient quadriplegia. *J Bone Joint Surg [Am]* 1986;68:1354
17. Torg JS. Pavlov's ratio: determining cervical spinal stenosis on routine lateral roentgenograms. *Contemp Orthop* 1989;18:153.
18. Goel VK, Clausen JD. Prediction of load sharing among spinal components of a C5-C6 motion segment using the finite element approach. *Spine* 1998;23:684–91.
19. Harms-Ringdahl K. On assessment of shoulder exercise and load elicited pain in cervical spine. *Scand J Rehab Med* (Suppl 14) 1986.
20. Fountain FP, Minear WL, Allison RD, Function of longus colli and longissimus cervicis muscles in man. *Arch Phys Med* 1996;47:665.
21. Takabe K, Vitti, M., Basmajian JV. The funcions of semispinalis capitas and splenius capitas muscles: an electromyographic study. *Anat Rec* 1974;179:477.
22. Schuldt K. On neck muscle activity and load reduction in sitting postures. *Scand J Rehab Med Suppl* 19,1988.
23. Wilke HJ, Wolf S, Claes LE, Arand M, Wiesend A. Influence of varying muscle forces on lumber inradiscal pressure: an in-vitro study. *J Biomech* 1996;29: 549–555.
24. Moroney SP, Schultz AB. Analysis and measurement of loads on the neck. *Trans Ortho Res Soc* 1985;10:329.
25. Nachemson A. Lumbar intradiscal pressure. *Acta Orthop Scand Suppl* 43, 1960.
26. Hattori S, Oda H, Kawai S. Cervical intradiscal pressure in movements and traction on the cervical spine. *J Orthop* 119:568, 1981.
27. Pospiech J, Wilke HJ, Claes LE, Stolke D. In-vitro measurements of cervical intra-discal pressure in different situations. *Langenbecks Arch Chir* 381:303–308, 1996.
28. Carpenter JE, Blasier RB, Pellizzon GC. The effects of muscle fatigue on shoulder position sense. *Am J Sports Med* 26:262–5, 1998.
29. Yoshikawa T, Mori S, Santiestaben AJ, et al. The effects of muscle fatigue on bone strain. *J Exp Biol* 1994;188: 217–233.
30. Hamilton N. Source document position as it affects head position and neck muscle tension. *Ergonomics* 39: 593–610, 1996.
31. Jensen BR, Schibye B, Sogaard K, Simonsen EB, Sjogarrd G. Shoulder muscle load and muscle fatigue among industrial sewing machine operators. *Eur J Applied Physiology* 67:467–475, 1993.
32. Veiersted KG, Westgaard RH.: Work related risk factors for trapezius myalgia. International scientific conference on prevention of work-related musculoskeletal disorders Premus, Sweden, 1992. *Arbeteoch Halsa* 17; 307–309.
33. Murthy G, Kahan NJ, Hargens AR, Remper DM. Forearm muscle oxygenation decreases with low levels of voluntary contraction. *J Ortho Res* 15:507–11, 1997.
34. Larsson SE, Bengtsson A, et al. Muscle changes in

work-related chronic myalgia. *Acta Orthop Scand* 59: 552–556, 1988.

35. Clarkson PM, Newham DJ. Associations between muscle soreness, damage and fatigue. *Adv Exp Med Biol* 384:457–69, 1995.

36. Friden J, Sfakianos PN, Hargens AR, Akeson WH. Residual muscle swelling after repetitive eccentric contractions. *J Ortho Res* 6:493–498, 1988.

37. Hasselink MK, Kuipers H, Geurten P, Vanstraaten H. Structural muscle damage and muscle strength after incremental number of isometric and forced length contractions. *J Muscle Res Cell Motil* 17:335–41, 1996.

38. Harms-Ringdahl K. Schuldt K. Maximum neck extension strength and relative neck muscular load in different cervical spine positions. *Clinical Biomechanics* 4: 17–24, 1988.

39. Chaffin DB. Localized muscle fatigue-definition and measurement. *J Occup Med* 15:346–354, 1993.

40. Ohlsson K, Attewell R, et al. Repetitive industrial work and neck and upper limb disorders in females. *Am J Ind Med* 27:731–747, 1995.

41. Serratos-Perez, JN, Mendoza-Anda C. Musculoskeletal disorder among male sewing machine operators in shoemaking. *Ergonomics* 36:793 800, 1993.

42. Rundcrantz B, Johnsson B, Moritz U. Occupational cervico-brachial disorders among dentists. *Swed Dent J* 15: 105–115, 1991.

43. Kilbom A, Horst R, Kemfert K, Richter A. Observation methods for reduction of load and strain on the human body—a review. *Abetarskyoosstyrelsen Publikation Service* 171:92, 1986.

44. Farmer JC, Wisneski RJ. Cervical spine nerve root compression. *Spine* 19:1850–1855, 1994.

45. Muckley DJ, Raynack GC, Mirza SK, Ching RP. Cervical spine intervertebral foramen stenosis resulting from quasistatic normal ranges of motion. Presented at the CSRS annual meeting, Westin Mission Hills Resort, Rancho Mirage, CA 1997.

46. Garfin SR, Rydevik B, Lind B, Massie J. Spinal nerve root compression. *Spine* 20:1810–1820, 1995.

47. Saal JS. The role of inflammation in lumbar pain. *Spine* 20:1821–1827, 1995.

48. Sakibara H, Miyao M, Kondo T, Yamada S. Overhead work and shoulder-neck pain in orchard farmers harvesting pears and apples. *Ergonomics* 38:700–706, 1995.

49. Eklund J, Odenrick P, Zettergren S, Johansson H. Head posture measurements among work vehicle drivers and implications for work and workplace design. *Ergonomics* 37:623–639, 1994.

50. Snijders CJ, Hoek Van Dijke GA, Roosch ER. A biomechanical model for the analysis of the cervical spine in static postures. *J Biomech* 24:783–792, 1991.

51. Farfan HF. *Mechanical disorders of the low back.* Philadelphia, Lea & Febiger, 1973.

52. Lu WW, Bishop PJ. Electromyographic activity of the cervical musculature during dynamic lateral bending. *Spine* 21:2443–2449, 1996.

53. Andersson G, Bjurvald M. Modell for bedomning av skador pa halsrygg och axelled i enlighet med arbetsskadeforsakring. *Kakartidningen* 1993;36: 3186–3188.

54. Jager HJ, Harris LG, Mehring UM, Goetz GF, Mathias KD. Degenerative change in the cervical spine and load carrying on the head. *Skel Radiol* 26:475–481, 1997.

55. Jumah KB, Nyame PK. Relationship between load carrying on the head and cervical spondylosis of Ghanians. *West Afr J Med* 13:101–102, 1994.

56. Bolm-Audroff U. Intervertebral disc disorders due to lifting and carrying heavy weights. *Med Orthop Tech* 1992;112:293–296.45:461.

57. Hagberg M, Wegman DH. Prevelance rates and odds ratios of shoulder-neck diseases in different occupational groups. *Br J Ind Med* 44:602–610, 1987.

58. Scher AT. Serious cervical spine injury in the older rugby player: An indication for routine radiological examination. *S Afr Med J* 1983;64:138–140.

59. Levy L. Porters neck. *BMJ* 2:16–19, 1968.

60. Maiman DJ, Sances A, Myklebust JB, Larson SJ, et al. Compression injuries of the cervical spine: A biomechanical analysis. *Neurosurgery* 13: 254, 1983.

61. Hodgson VR, Thomas LM. Mechanism of cervical spine injury during impact to the protected head. *Proceedings of the 24th STAPP Conference,* p.17, Society of Automotive Engineers, Warrendale, PA, 1980.

62. Spurling RG. *Lesions of the cervical intervertebral disc.* Springfield, Charles C. Thomas, 1956.

63. Davidson RI, Dunn EJ, Metzmaker JN. The shoulder abduction test in the diagnosis of radicular pain in cervical extradural compressive monoradiculopathies. *Spine* 6:441–446, 1981.

64. Wilker SF, Chaffin DB, Langolf GD. Shoulder posture and localized muscle fatigue and discomfort. *Ergonomics* 1989;32:211–237.

65. Tichauer ER. Potential of biomechanics for solving specific hazard problems. *Proceedings of ASSE 1968 Conference,* Amer. Soc. Safety Eng., Park Ridge, IL.1968. 149–187.

66. Gassett RS, Hearne B, Keelan B. Ergonomics and body mechanics in the work place. *Ortho Clin North Am* 27: 861–879, 1996.

67. Aaras A, Fostervold KI, Thoresen M, Larsen S. Postural load during VDU work: a comparison between various work postures. *Ergonomics* 1997;40:125–60.

68. Black KM, McClure P, Polansky M. The influence of different sitting positions on cervical and lumbar support. *Spine* 21:65–70, 1996.

69. McCormick EJ, Sanders MS. *Human factors in enginering and design,* 5th ed: McGraw-Hill, New York.

70. Aaras A, Horgen G, Bjorset HH, Ro O, Thoresen M. Musculoskeletal visual and psychosocial stress in VDU operators before and after multidisciplinary ergonomic interventions. Submitted.

71. Kumar S, Shaife WGS. A precision task, posture and strain. *J Safety Research* 11:28–36, 1979.

72. Carter JB, Banister EW. Musculoskeletal problems in VDT work. A review. *Ergonomics* 37:1623–1648, 1994.

73. Harms-Ringdahl K, Schuldt K, Ekholm. Principles of prevention of neck and shoulder pain. *Scand J Rehab Med Supp* 32:87–96, 1995.

74. Mathiassen SE. The influence of exercise, rest schedule on the physiological and psychophysical response to isometric shoulder-neck exercise. *Eur J Applied Phys* 67:528–539, 1993.

75. Haag GM, Astrom A. Load pattern and pressure pain threshold in the upper trapezius muscle and psychosocial factors in medical secretaries with and without shoulder/neck disorders. *Int Arch Occup Environ Health* 69:423–32, 1997.

76. Westgarrd RH. Measurement and evaluation of postural

load in occupational work situations. *European Journal of Applied Physiology* 1988;57;291–304.

77. Kelkar P, O'Callaghan B, Lovblad K. Asymptomatic grotesque deformties of the cervical spine. *Spine* 23: 737–740, 1998.

78. Liedholdt JD. Spinal injuries in sports. *Surg Clin North Am* 43:351, 1963.

79. Hill, J.M., Phillips, E.D.: Cervical pain due to atlanto-occipital fusion in a swimmer. *Orthopedics* 20:270–272, 1997.

80. Magnusson NL, Pope MH, Wilder DG, Areskoug B. Are occupational drivers at an increased risk for developing musculoskeletal disorders? *Spine* 21:710–717, 1996.

81. Magnusson ML. *Effect of seated whole body vibrations. An experimental study in man.* Goteberg: University of Goteberg, Sweden, 1991.

82. Cursiter MC, Harding RH. Electromyographic recordings of shoulder and neck muscles of seated subjects exposed to vertical vibrations. Proceedings of Physiology Society: I *Physiology* 239: 117–118, 1974.

83. Serooussi RE, Wilder DG, Pope MH. Trunk muscle electromyography and whole body vibration. *J Biomech* 22:219–29, 1989.

84. Hanson T, Keller T, Spengler D. Mechanical behavior of the human lumbar spine. II Fatigue strength during dynamic compressive loading. *J Ortho RES* 5:479–87, 1987.

85. Kelsey JL, Githens PB, Walter SD, et al. An epidemiological study of acute prolapsed cervical intervertebral discs. *JBJS* 66A:907–914, 1984.

86. Viikari-Juntura E, Riihimaki H, Tola S. Videman T, Mutanen P. Neck trouble in machine operating, dynamic physical work and sedentary work: a prospective study on occupational and individual risk factors. *J Clin Epidemiol* 47:1411–1422, 1994.

87. Bjurvald M, Carlson S, Hansson JE, Sjoflot L. Whole body vibrations: a mechanical-physiologic study of work postures and drivers seats. *Arbete Och Halsa,* 37, *Arbetarskyddsstyrelsen,* Stockholm, 1973.

Occupational Musculoskeletal Disorders
edited by T. G. Mayer, R. J. Gatchel, and P. B. Polatin.
Lippincott Williams & Wilkins, Philadelphia © 2000.

8

Biomechanics and Ergonomics of the Upper Extremity

J. Mark Melhorn, *Thomas R. Hales, and †Eric M. Kennedy

*Section of Orthopaedics, Department of Surgery, University of Kansas School of Medicine—Wichita, Wichita, Kansas 67208-4510; *National Institute for Occupational Safety and Health, Cincinnati, Ohio 45226; and †Occupational Health Services, Healthsouth Corporation, Charlotte, North Carolina 28211*

Work-related musculoskeletal disorders (MSD), commonly described as cumulative trauma disorders (CTD), are a major cause of worker impairment and disability. In the American workplace "sprains and strains" are typically the largest category of claims in workers' compensation, representing more than half of claims and dollar costs (1,2). In 1996, the U.S. Bureau of Labor and Statistics (2,3) released its most current data for 1996 in its annual survey of lost work time for all injuries and illnesses. It reported a total of nearly 1.9 million injuries and illnesses in private-industry workplaces that required recuperation away from work beyond the day of the incident. In 1997, the cost of workplace health and safety was estimated at more than 418 billion dollars in direct costs, and (using the lower range of estimates) indirect costs were 837 billion dollars (4). Although the pathogenesis of these disorders is not fully understood, the need for reduction and prevention by employees, employers, insurance systems, health care systems, and government is clear.

Given the multifactorial etiology for MSD and its association with individual and workplace risk factors, their reduction and prevention will require a multidisciplinary effort. The sciences of ergonomics, biomechanics, epidemiology, and medicine are being used to understand more fully the interdependence of MSD. *Ergonomics* (Greek "ergon" = work and Greek "nomos" = law) (5) is the study of the problems of people in adjusting to their environment, especially the science that seeks to adapt work or working conditions to suit the worker (i.e., the study of work) (6). *Biomechanics* (Greek "bios" = life or living organisms and "mechanics" = of or pertaining to machines or tools or acting like a machine) (5) is the study of how the living organism performs activities (i.e., the study of how work is performed) (7). Biomechanics uses laws of physics and engineering to describe the motion of various body segments and the forces that act on these body parts during normal daily activities. By this definition, biomechanics is a multidisciplinary science. *Epidemiology* (Latin "epidemia" = of people and "ology" = the study of) (5) is the medical science that focuses on the distribution and determinants of disease frequency in human populations and the application of the study to the control of the disease (8). *Medicine* (Latin "medicus" = doctor or mederi = to heal) (5) is the science of diagnosing, treating, or preventing disease and other damage to the body or mind.

The implementation of a successful ergonomics program can benefit the employer and employee by (a) reducing the number and severity of work-related injuries and illnesses, (b) reducing employee turnover, (c) increasing productivity, (d) increasing product quality, and (e) increasing employee morale. The study of biomechanics and ergonomics is further defined by terms such as *human factors*, *anthropometry measurements*, *individual risk factors* (age, gender, inherited genetic characteristics), *workplace risk factors* (methods, materials, machines, environment, and physical stressors), *psychological factors*, *economic concerns*, and *return-to-work issues* (9). Each of these group headings will be defined in this chapter (Fig. 1).

Review of the injuries and illnesses in the American workplace reveals two points of view (see Chap. 15 for more about causation versus association). Realizing the limitations and considering the concerns regarding causation, the two points of view are not mutually exclusive but often seem to be at odds. These apparent differences may be more related to (a) the multiple factors involved in the devel-

opment of work-related musculoskeletal pain, (b) the individual's unique response to musculoskeletal pain, (c) the lack of valid measures for many MSD, (d) the lack of valid measures for ergonomic risk factors, (e) how the injury and illness data are collected and reported, (f) how the analysis and conclusions from the data are applied to the employee and workplace, and (g) potential disease misclassification resulting from the motivation of the employee, reporter, and applier (6,10–22).

The ergonomist is fully aware of the multifactorial nature of MSD but chooses to focus on the factors that can be evaluated and changed (workplace conditions) rather than on factors that cannot be changed (age, gender, inherited genetics) or that cannot be treated (medical conditions). Therefore, the workplace becomes the primary focus for the development of a MSD. Too many repetitions, high forces, awkward positions, direct pressure, vibration, cold temperature, contact stress, and unaccustomed work activities are

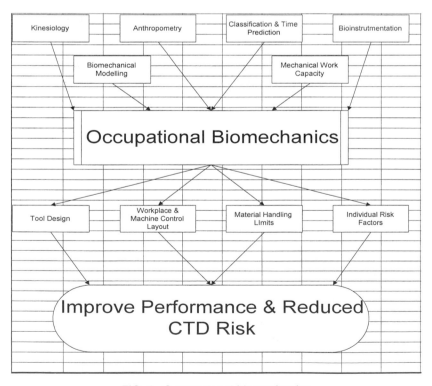

FIG. 1. Occupational biomechanics.

the causative factors. The basis for this approach is supported by epidemiologic studies that industries with high occupational risk factors, such as meatpacking and textiles, routinely have the highest rates (1,23–31). The ergonomist, therefore, would attempt to reduce repetition and force, avoid awkward postures, isolate vibration, modify temperature, and eliminate direct pressure to eliminate or reduce the risk. Where possible, the ergonomist would consider prevention programs for employees, wellness tips, biomechanics training, and redesign of tools and workstations.

Many health care providers believe the etiology of MSD is multifactorial but choose to focus on what they can evaluate and change (medical conditions) rather than on what cannot be changed (e.g., age, gender, inherited genetics) or affected (e.g., workplace conditions). Therefore, some health care providers believe the individual's medical history largely determines whether a person will develop MSD. The proof is that employees can and do perform identical jobs; only some will develop a MSD, whereas others never experience a symptom (14,19,32–35). From an epidemiologic viewpoint, this is illogical. For example, fewer than half of cigarette smokers develop lung cancer. Does this mean, therefore, that cigarette smoking is not a risk factor for lung cancer? Health care providers easily relate to the clinically defined disorders in which the criteria for the epidemiologist's case definition are similar to the physician's diagnostic criteria. Health care providers often attempt to fit MSD into a specific medical model.

The conversion required from individual medical treatment to population-based epidemiology can be challenging, as seen in heart disease. For example, a chain-smoking stockbroker in his third marriage who drinks a lot and is 40 pounds overweight is viewed as a high risk for a heart attack, stroke, and other such conditions. On the other hand, the librarian who eats a low-fat diet, does not drink or smoke, and does aerobics three times a week is at low risk. The challenge for the health care provider comes when the emphasis shifts from diagnostic criteria to the more inclusive

surveillance case definitions to identify high-risk industries and occupations for prevention activities. For example, Vender and associates (17) selectively reviewed the medical literature for articles that they considered to represent acceptable clinical criteria to assess the relationship between upper-extremity disorders and work activities. Their conclusions were that the medical literature currently fails to incorporate sound medical diagnostic criteria in defining and identifying MSD and does not establish a causal relationship between distinct medical disorders and work activities. This article has been criticized for lack of defining medical diagnostic criteria and for not addressing interexaminer and intraexaminer reliability for various MSD. Bernard and colleagues (1), using epidemiologic evidence, provided the most comprehensive manuscript on the biomechanical hazards in the workplace. Epidemiological evidence may be helpful for population-based treatment and prevention, but it is of little help to the medical provider who treats the individual by seeking to optimize healing through reducing pain and inflammation, increasing strength and flexibility, and immobilizing the affected area when appropriate. Therefore, health care providers treat MSD with antiinflammatory medication, specific therapeutic exercises, splinting, injections, and, when appropriate, surgery. Most health care providers do not have time to go to their patients' work site to examine the workstation or make suggestions regarding the workplace.

Both points of view are correct. A combined view gives the best opportunity for understanding and for formulating solutions. The bucket analogy can be used to demonstrate how this combined approach can blend the ergonomist's and the health care provider's viewpoints into the study of occupational biomechanical ergonomics. The goal of occupational biomechanical ergonomics should be to study the human abilities and characteristics that can affect the design of equipment, systems, and jobs while at the same time provide for the well-being of the individual worker and improved production for the employer.

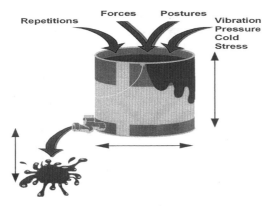

FIG. 2. Individual's response to activities.

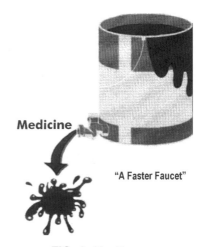

FIG. 4. Health care.

THE BUCKET ANALOGY: A COMBINED VIEW

Occupation-related musculoskeletal pain can occur when the wear and tear of movements exceed the body's ability to heal. Our bodies hold the stresses associated with the activities of daily living, jobs, and hobbies the same way that a bucket holds paint. The amount of paint is proportional to the amount of physical stress (Fig. 2).

Imagine that the buckets come equipped with faucets, allowing stress collected from the day to be drained away during rest and recovery. For most people, the stress collected and drained off daily are about equal. The height of the paint in our bucket moves up and down like the tides of the ocean but stays in a safe range. For some people, however, the amount of stress collected is greater than the amount drained off, and every day the height of the paint rises slightly. When the paint overflows the edges of the bucket, the clinical

symptoms of MSD, such as pain, numbness, and swelling, are felt.

The faucets are controlled by our individual risk factors, including age, gender, inherited genetic makeup, physical fitness, and psychosocial issues. The paint is controlled by the physical stressors that come from activities both at work and leisure and include repetition, force, posture, vibration, temperature, contact stress, and unaccustomed work activities. If we are to decrease MSD from the workplace successfully, we need to address the amount of paint flowing into our buckets (physical stressors = ergonomics = Fig. 3) and the rate of flow out of our buckets from the faucets (individual healing = medicine = Fig. 4). In other words, the ideal solution is to combine the approach of the ergonomist with that of the health care provider.

DEFINING TERMS

The purpose of this chapter is to review the biomechanics and ergonomics of the upper extremities and how they relate to the development of MSDs and CTDs. The goal of a biomechanics and ergonomics program is to establish an ongoing mechanism for systematically identifying affected workers and jobs, for implementation of medical and work interventions, and for evaluating the ef-

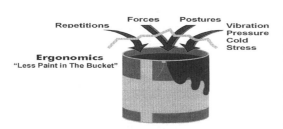

FIG. 3. Ergonomics.

fectiveness of those interventions. Again, the debate regarding causation is discussed in other chapters of this book. Moving beyond the causation debate, a number of sources of information, ranging from biomechanics, epidemiology, and clinical case series, have identified and suggest an association between MSD and activities (1,23,36,37). These activity factors or physical stressors can occur in the workplace or with leisure activities and include repetition, force, posture, vibration, temperature, contact stress, unaccustomed work activities, and psychosocial stress. Each of these physical stressors has specific attributes or characteristics that can affect or alter the effect on each individual as outlined in Table 1 (physical stressors, attributes, and assessment methods).

Ergonomics

Ergonomics is defined as the study of the relationship of humans to machines, based on information from the fields of engineering, biomechanics, physiology, anthropology, and psychology (38). *Ergonomic* is an adjective and *ergonomics* is a noun (39). When trying to decide which is which, use the following rule. If the word can be replaced with the terms *productive* or *user friendly*, it is *ergonomic*. If it can be replaced with the terms *productivity* or *user friendliness*, the term is *ergonomics*. For example, the correct phrase is not "consult an ergonomic expert." Rather, it is "consult an ergonomics expert" (unless the person happens to be quite productive or user friendly). The distinction is difficult because often the grammatically correct usage does not sound right. Incidentally, someone who specializes in ergonormics is called an *ergonomist* (40).

Occupational Biomechanics

Occupational biomechanics can be defined as a science concerned with the mechanical behavior of the musculoskeletal system and component tissues when physical work is performed (22). As such, it seeks to provide an understanding of the physics of manual activities in industry and complements other sciences of the workplace. Similarly, psychologists over the last 50 years have provided the behavioral knowledge necessary to define a human factors discipline useful in the evaluation and design of information displays and controls. Likewise, exercise physiologists have provided the basic concepts necessary to define a work physiology discipline that predicts the metabolic, respiratory, and cardiovascular effects of prolonged, strenuous activities in industry.

Human Factors and Ergonomics

These two terms are synonymous, although in the past within the United States there has been a tendency to refer to cognitive design issues (how does the control panel appear = brain) as *human factors* (often in the department of psychology at a university) and physical design issues (how does the control panel work = body) as *ergonomics* (often in the department of engineering). This field of science developed in World War II to help in aircraft cockpit design. In Europe, the term *human factors* is generally not used, and *ergonomics* traditionally has been defined to include cognitive and physical issues. In the United States, considerable debate about this terminology has taken place within the profession. Sometimes making a firm distinction between the two branches is useful, but in general the two terms should be synonymous. To think otherwise is to split the human being into a traditional "mind" versus body" dichotomy, which has definite disadvantages. From a design standpoint, both cognitive and body cognitive issues must be taken into account (40).

Human and Machine Interface

Studying the human and machine interface is the essence of ergonomic redesign. Er-

TABLE 1. *Physical stressors, attributes, and assessment methods*

Stressor	Attributes	Work factors	Assessment methods
Repetition	Exertion frequency Recovery time Percent recovery Cycle time Velocity and acceleration Force Posture	Production standard Pacing Incentives Work quantities/unit time Methods/materials Work incentives Worker rotation Manufacturing process Mechanical aids Quality control Machines	Observation Time studies Work sampling Interviews Rankings/ratings Force measurements Goniometers Accerlerometers Keystroke counts EMG
Force	Amplitude probability distribution Peak Average Static vs. Dynamic Smooth vs. Jerky	Friction Weight of work objects Balance Reaction forces/torques Drag forces Mechanical aids Gloves/handles Quality control Machines	Observation Interviews Rankings Ratings Force transducers EMG
Posture	Range of motion Average Time position	Work location Work orientation Work object shape Methods/materials Machine Environment	Observation Interviews Rankings Ratings Force measurements Work equipment specifications
Vibration	Frequency Displacement Velocity Acceleration Duration	Abrasive Tool drive train Bit condition Isolation/dampening Gloves	Observation Interviews Rankings/ratings Work equipment specifications
Temperature	Low temperature Conductivity Duration	Temperature of air Work object temperature Air exhaust Gloves Protective clothing	Observation Interviews Rankings/ratings Thermometers
Contact stress	Force Area Location Duration	Force factors Area of contact Location of contact Gloves	Observation Interviews Rankings/ratings Force measurements Work equipment specifications
Unaccustomed activities	Duration Hours Days Percent time	Work schedules Work standards Incentives Methods/environment	Interviews Time cards Production records

EMG, electromyography.

gonomic designs are an applied science that coordinate the physical features, devices, and working conditions within a selective job, along with the capacities of the people working within that environment. A systems approach to the study of the human–machine interaction has as its purpose to enhance productivity, quality, usability, safety, health, comfort, well-being, rehabilitation. Productivity typically is measured by machine output. Frequently, to change productivity, workers adjust their output to the machine. With ergonomic design, the human and machine interface is a balance that is not machine driven.

Anthropometry

Anthropometry is the gathering and interpretation of data on the shapes and sizes of humans and can include height, weight, and other dimensional measurements. This data then are analyzed statistically for variance from the average. Anthropometry is uscd as a basis for designing tools, equipment, workplaces, and accommodating living spaces to the people who occupy them (12) (Fig. 5).

Individual Risk Factors

Individual risk factors include the individual's age, gender, inherited characteristics, nonwork activities, psychosocial issues and

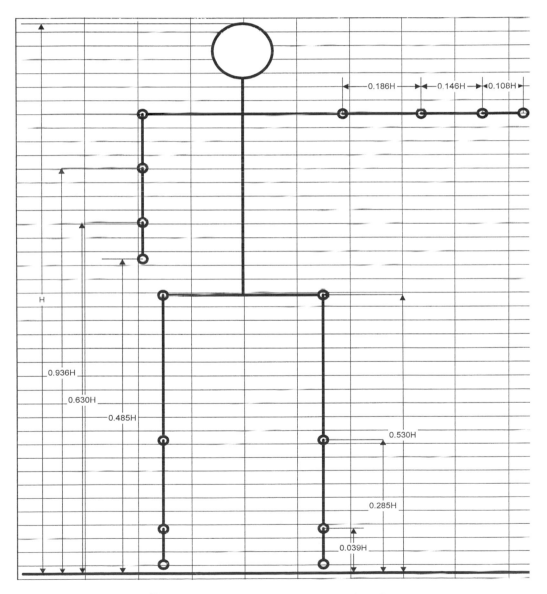

FIG. 5. Anthropometry body segment lengths.

factors, economic concerns, and return-to-work issues. Individual risk factors are commonly cited as one of the reasons why not every person who does a job will develop musculoskeletal symptoms. These factors are based on the medical model (41).

Workplace Risk Factors

Workplace risk factors include any part of the production process (the manufacturing of a product). The production process usually includes *input* (raw materials), production (methods, materials, machines, environment, physical stressors), and the output (the finished product) (42).

Repetition

Repetition is defined as the act or process of repeating or performing the same acts or motions over and over again (5). Repetition refers to the temporal aspect of work. Health care providers tend to think of repetitiveness in terms of joint motions whereas ergonomists look at the task cycle or standard task completion time. Some investigators have characterized repetition in terms of the number of exertions per unit time or frequency. An *exertion* is defined as the contraction of a muscle to produce force or movement. Other investigators have characterized repetition as the number of parts produced per unit time or cycle time. A *cycle* is defined as a sequence of exertions and can be obtained from production records and interviews with workers and supervisors. Repetition is an index of the frequency of movement or exertions, the speed of the motion, and the recovery time. At one extreme, the hands are idle with almost continuous recovery time. At the other extreme, the hands are moving as rapidly as imaginable with no recovery time. An *exertion* can be defined, therefore, as the effort to overcome weight, resistance, or inertia of the body or of a work object (6).

Acceptable dose relationships and tolerance thresholds have not been established. Suggested threshold characteristics have been defined as more than 1,000 per hour or a work cycle of less than 30 seconds (using the same muscle group), exposure duration exceeding 4 hours per day, more than 2,000 repetitions per hour for all muscle groups, and lift and carries of more than 30 per hour. Attributes that can modify how the individual experiences repetition can include frequency, recovery time, cycle time, velocity, acceleration, force, and posture (12).

Force

Force is defined as the capacity to do work or to cause physical change (5). Force is an index of the effort exerted to get, hold, or use a work object or to support the weight of the body. Both average and peak forces should be assessed. Repeated and sustained static exertions defined as maintaining the same position throughout the work cycle or for prolonged periods may require a reduction to 15% of maximum force to avoid exhaustion. As the time decreases, the percentage of maximum force increases. Both average and peak forces should be evaluated when establishing recommendations. Force can be assessed from observations of the worker and from consideration of task factors (6).

Acceptable dose relationships and tolerance thresholds have not been established. Suggested threshold characteristics have been defined as unsupported tool weight of greater than 1.8 kg, mechanical compression to the palm, base or other area of the hand resulting from tool use or job task requirements, or force or torque levels exceeding 4 to 6 kg (12). In the workplace, force can be reduced by (a) adding a better gripping surface such as rubber slips to tool handles; (b) reducing the weight held by workers through the use of fixtures, jigs, or balancers, keeping hand forces to 225 N maximum (6); (c) keeping pinches to 45 N maximum or 30 N for repetitive work; (d) aligning the object's center of gravity; (e) reducing rotating motions caused by either the tool or work design; and (f) reducing power tool speeds and torque (43). Attributes that can modify how the individual experiences force can include static versus dynamic, smooth controlled exertions versus jerky motions, frequency, weight, resistance, reaction forces, size, and shape of the object (12).

Posture

Posture is defined as a position or attitude of the body or of a body part (5). Some positions require more effort than others or result in compression or stretching of tissues in or around the joints. Consideration for both the position and the length of time in the position is critical. Posture includes the concept of movement or bending of the joints.

In general, upper-extremity postural requirements should include keeping the elbows close to the body, keeping the work within arm's length, shoulder abduction angles below 20 to 30 degrees, forward arm flexion below 25 to 30 degrees, wrist at neutral, and hand pinch grips minimized. Inside-grip diameter is suggested at 1.5 to 2.2 inches (6). The study of posture has been enhanced by stick-figure, template manipulations, and computer-aided drafting systems. These systems provide the ability to create engineering drawings and models. Unfortunately, there is no single best location, orientation, or tool for any one job (6).

Vibration

Vibration is defined as the act of vibrating (5). Vibration results from contact with something that shakes or jerks and is a vector quantity with periodicity and properties of frequency, displacement, velocity, and acceleration. *Velocity* is displacement/time; however, the velocity is not constant over the displacement. The time rate of change of velocity is acceleration (distance/time/time). The *periodicity*, or *frequency*, of the vibration is the time it takes to complete one cycle measured in cycles per second (Hz) (44). Quantitative vibration measurements require triaxial accelerometers, amplifiers, and frequency analyzers. As a practical matter, such measurements are not feasible, and vibration may be indicated categorically as "yes" or "no" or as hours of exposure.

In 1986, the International Organization for Standardization (ISO) published ISO 5349 (45) for vibration white finger (VWF). A dose-response relationship was established with the prevalence of VWF blanching directly proportional to the square of the vibration magnitude, the square of the lifetime exposure, and the daily vibration exposure. The prevalence is inversely proportional to the square of the vibration frequency above 16 Hz, meaning that if the acceleration is halved, daily exposure can be increased by a factor of 4 and lifetime exposure by a factor of 2. If the frequency is halved, the daily exposure must be decreased by a factor of 4 or the lifetime exposure by a factor of 2 (46). Unfortunately, even with these complex dose-relationships, there is concern regarding the validity of this relationship and its application in the workplace (44,46).

Temperature

Temperature is defined as the degree of hotness or coldness of a body or environment (5). Favorable working temperatures are from 68 to 78° F with 20% to 60% humidity (47). Cold environments are defined as 52 to 55° F. Skin temperatures below 70° F adversely affected sensitivity and dexterity (47). Skin temperature is related to the air temperature, the temperature and conductivity of work objects, and clothing. It is not known whether low temperature affects tissue tolerance to mechanical stressors, but it does affect sensory and motor performance. Temperature-exposure measurements are assessed from the temperature of ambient air and from the temperature of work objects. The measurements may be influenced by the insulative value of clothing, thermal conductivity of work objects, and air exhaust from hand tools (12).

Contact Stress

Contact stress is defined as force divided by the area of contact or as a pressure (48). In some cases, contact stress can be calculated from force and area measurements. Contact stress is the force per unit area acting between the body and an external object. Although it can be expressed as pounds per square inch or Newtons per square meter, it is necessary to assess the force and area of contact. In a recent laboratory study (49), pain-pressure thresholds of all areas of the hand were calculated using force measurements and knowledge of the area of contact and compared with self-reported physical exposure. Lundborg and colleagues (50) investigated the relationship between pressure on the palmar side of the wrist and intracarpal canal pressure. Pressure was measured inside the wrist by using a catheter and pressure transducer; pressure on the base of the palm was measured simply as the force applied to a known area. Once the relationship between palmar wrist pressure and intracarpal canal pressure was determined, force was applied to the base of the palm to study the effect of intracarpal pressures on median nerve function. Quantitative contact stress measurements are seldom possible in most held settings. Contact stress is usually characterized as a "yes" or "no" categoric variable. In some cases, it is characterized in terms of worker-comfort patterns. Workers are asked to point to areas of discomfort on their hands or to shade areas of discomfort on a drawing of a hand.

Unaccustomed Activities

Unaccustomed activities are defined as changes from the usual activity level. There is an increasing body of knowledge that suggests that safe levels of work can be established by using psychophysical and psychoscaling tools to assess the worker's perception of exertion (51). To assess work capacity and the potential for musculoskeletal injury, investigators (52) rely on one of two approaches: If the work is heavy but intermittent, biomechanical measures of strength may serve as indicators of work capacity. If the work is light but continuous, physiologic measures of endurance may be needed. Ulti-

mately, what work a person is willing to do each day depends on the level of fatigue he or she experiences. When discomfort from muscle fatigue exceeds a personal threshold, the worker seeks ways in which to reduce the aversive state. Attempts at evaluating the effects of fatigue on worker behavior have been largely impeded by the lack of adequate methods of measurement. Work fatigue can be regarded as a perceptual issue, an experienced self-evaluation, integrating psychological (motivational) and sensory (physical) information. *Psychophysics* is concerned with the quantitative relationship between physical changes in stimulation and the subject's awareness of that stimulation. Interest in psychophysical techniques emanates from industry demands for guidelines or limits designed to prevent MSD, combined with the difficulties inherent in assessing upper-extremity work using more objective approaches. Currently, additional evidence is needed to demonstrate that designing work in accordance with psychophysically derived limits will eliminate or reduce the rate of musculoskeletal injury associated with manual work.

Work Requirements

Work requirements include production or work standards, work processes, workplace layout, tools, equipment, and materials. Individual factors include the worker's abilities, skills, size, and fitness. *Environmental factors* include vibration and ambient air temperatures. Work requirements may include the quantity and quality of work to be performed in a given period. They also specify the method, tools, and workstation to be used to attain the standard. Consequently, the standard is an important determinant of how many exertions a worker will perform in a given amount of time, how much recovery time will be available, how much force a worker will have to exert to hold and use work objects, where a worker will have to reach, and how long a worker will hold a vibrating object. The posture also may be affected by worker size. A short worker will have to reach higher than a tall worker for a work object at a fixed location; however, if the work object is held in one hand while it is worked on with the other hand, posture will not be affected. Employers can exercise some control over posture by making work locations adjustable and providing workers with adjustable seating.

Physical stressors can be increased or decreased in some cases by worker behavior. Worker skill affects how many exertions are required to complete some jobs and also may influence the force of exertion and posture. Skills training may help to reduce exposure to these stressors in certain tasks, such as typing. Methods such as biofeedback may be helpful in some aspects of worker training. Workers can be taught how to arrange their work and adjust their workstation to minimize posture stresses and needless exertion of force. They also can be trained in how to select the best tools and how to use them most efficiently.

Psychosocial Factors

Psychosocial factors in the workplace are increasingly indicated as being involved in the etiology of work-related MSD (53). The International Labor Office (ILO) has defined workplace psychosocial factors in broad terms, synonymous with conditions that give rise to job stress (54). In this definition, *psychosocial factors* is used to refer to the attributes of both the job and the individual worker, including the worker's nonwork environment, that contribute to job stress. The expression *work organization* is used broadly in reference to any work-related risk factor for job stress and includes individual factors that interact with working conditions in the development of stress. It is currently believed that (a) psychosocial demands and job stress may produce increased muscle tension and exacerbate task-related biomechanical strain, (b) psychosocial demands may affect awareness and reporting of musculoskeletal symptoms or perceptions of their cause, or (c) a causal or correlated relationship exists between psychosocial and physical workload demands (7). Therefore, the development of symptoms is not a direct or predetermined response to some internal physical event as a result of an activity; rather, it is a highly interpretive process subject to influences from contextual factors. These contextual factors include social and cultural factors (55), legal issues, workers' compensation systems (56), and workplace industrial relations (24).

Modeling

Based on the presumed relationship between activity and potential MSDs, it has been proposed that external stressors produce a series of internal biomechanical and physiologic disturbances. Biomechanical models, in this context, have been used to describe the motions of, and forces acting on, the limb segments, including joint motion during function using rigid body models. For example, through the use of external forces and limb accelerations, moments of force at the elbow during pitching can be predicted. In addition, through the incorporation of the biologic materials properties, the response of the tissue to load can be grossly predicted (26,27,57). The models available to study activity-related MSDs are in the preliminary stages of development. Therefore, specific models for the mechanisms of injury are not available. Modeling is also lacking a good animal model to help in understanding the delicate balance of physical strain and restorative responses that can occur in MSD. Additionally, models are only as good as their parameters. Current modeling research is developing a better database of quantitative anatomy (shapes of joint surfaces, sizes of muscles, geometry of the carpal canal) as well as properties of the various tissues. By comparing a model's behavior with the actual behavior of the system, further insights into how components of the system function and how to build a better are gained.

Biomechanical models of the upper limb can provide the link between the physical activities that people do and the disorders they acquire. Because the upper limb is a multilink chain with a large number of degrees of freedom, it becomes difficult to relate a description of the activity to MSDs without a conceptual model to provide guidance. For example, in the depiction of manual material handling tasks, to elucidate the link between work and low back pain, one could describe the load lifted by a person and the distance away from the body of this mass. It is more useful to compute the joint movement (the product of the force and the distance), based on a biomechanical model that demonstrates that tissue loads are better reflected by movement than by either load or posture separately. Unfortunately, these data frequently are collected in the laboratory under conditions that are not representative of sports or work (e.g., low strain rate, acute [minutes or hours] exposures). The biofidelity of these models, therefore, remains to be shown for the study of work- related MSDs.

Although modeling is not the only method by which the relationships between activity and MSDs can be studied, it appears to possess a number of strengths. Models help us to understand the many simultaneous and interacting physical stressors that act on the upper limb during activity. If based on sound anatomy and solid pathophysiology, such models may form a bridge between the performance of work and sport and the cellular or other descriptions of the degenerative or inflammatory processes involved in activity-related MSDs.

Return to Work after Injury

Employees are an employer's greatest asset. In companies of all sizes and types, employees are expected to give 100% effort every day. With an increased incidence of injury comes a focus on accident prevention. Despite the focus on prevention, injuries still occur. Injured employees represent a significant business expense but one that can be controlled. Workers' compensation laws in all states require the employer to bear the cost (payment of income as well as medical expenses) of an employee injury or illness resulting from work done for the employer. Most employers, therefore, can gain much from a program that keeps workers at work in a productive capacity (58).

Return-to-work programs make it possible for employees to return to the workplace as soon as possible after an occupational injury or illness. The ideal situation is for the worker to return to his or her regular job. Two types of disabilities occur with injuries: *temporary* and *permanent*. Most injuries cause a temporary disability, in which case the worker cannot return to the previous job until healing is complete. Programs can be designed to return these workers to the workplace earlier, albeit in a different, temporary capacity, to the benefit of the employee, the employee's family and co-workers, and the employer and insurance carrier. Return-to-work programs create a winning solution for all interested parties. In the event of a permanent disabling injury, the worker may need an altogether new job (41,59).

Suggestions from the ergonomist and occupational health care provider regarding return to work should include (a) worker rotation, (b) frequent breaks, (c) gradual orientation to job and demands, (d) appropriate temperature, (e) appropriate job placement (current skill matches essential functions of the job), and (f) education and or training for new or different tools and job requirements (9).

Regulatory Issues: Occupational Safety and Health Administration (OSHA)

In section 5.(a)(1), the "general duty clause" states that each employer (1) shall furnish to each employee a place of employment free of recognized hazards that are causing or are likely to cause death or serious physical harm to employees (60); section 8.(c)(2) on record keeping states that "each employer shall make, keep and preserve, and make available to the Secretary...such records regarding his activities relating to this Act." Section 8.(c)(1) states, "The Secretary...shall prescribe regulations requiring employers to maintain accurate records of, and to make periodic reports on, work-related deaths, injuries and illnesses other than minor injuries requiring only first aid treatment and which do not involve medical treatment, loss of consciousness, restriction of work or motion, or transfer to another job." Section 8.(c)(2) OSHA-200 states that "Cumulative trauma disorders are classified as illnesses (7f. disorders associated with repeated trauma, e.g., synovitis, tenosynovitis and bursitis)." Because work-related carpal tunnel syndrome cases almost always result from repetitious movement, they should be classified as *occupational illnesses*. Recording an injury or illness under the Occupational Safety and Health Administration (OSHA) system does not necessarily imply that management was at fault, that the worker was at fault, that a violation of an OSHA standard has occurred, or that the injury or illness is compensable under workers' compensation or other systems.

Workplace Assessment

Numerous observation schemes, checklists, numeric methods, and instrumental methods have been proposed for observing and characterizing the risk of work-related MSDs of the upper limb (22,61,62). Often these systems are more sensitive to one factor than to another and consequently will be found to work better in one situation than in another, which probably explains why each investigator has a favorite system. It is important that users understand the factors present in each situation before conducting a detailed analysis. Often these factors can be assessed through evaluation of work factors, such as production standards and tool and equipment attributes. They also may be assessed through observation of the job. Observations may be performed on site or from videotapes. In either case, it is recommended that the analysis include a thorough documentation of what the worker under study does. Videotapes of selected jobs should be saved as benchmarks for each attribute. Jobs can be rated periodically by a team of two to five people, who will discuss and agree on the what affects each factor. Workplace assessment should include an understanding of manual materials handling, which has four parts: (a) worker characteristics, (b) material and container characteristics, (c) task and workplace characteristics, and (d) work practices characteristics:

Worker Characteristics

Physical characteristics include general worker measures, such as age, sex, anthropometry, and postures. *Sensory measures* of a worker's sensory processing capabilities include visual, auditory, tactual, kinesthetic, vestibular, and proprioceptive factors. *Motor measures* include the worker's motor capabilities, such as strength, endurance, range of movement, kinematic characteristics, and muscle-training state. *Psychomotor measures* of worker capabilities include interfacing mental and motor processes, such as information processing, reaction and response times, and coordination. *Personality* measures of a worker's values and job satisfaction includes attitude profiles, attribution, risk acceptance, and perceived economic need. *Training and experience* include measures of the worker's educational level in terms of formal training or instruction in manual material handling skills, informal training, and work experience. A worker's *health status* includes measures from the worker's general health appraisal, such as previous medical complaints, diagnosed medical status, emotional status, regular drug use, pregnancy, diurnal variations, and deconditioning. *Leisure-time activities* include measures of the person who chooses to be involved in physical activities during leisure hours, such as holding a second job or regular participation in sports.

Material and Container Characteristics

Load is the measure of force, weight, pushing and pulling force requirements, and mass moment of inertia. *Dimensions* include measures of the size of unit workload, such as height, width, and breadth when indicating the form as rectangular, cylindrical, spherical, or other shape. *Distribution of load* is the measure of the location of the unit load center of gravity with respect to the worker for one- or two- handed carrying. *Couplings* are measures of simple devices used to aid in grasping and manually manipulating the unit load, such as texture and handle size, shape, and location. *Stability of load* includes measures of the location of the load's center of motion and its consistency as a concern in handling liquids and bulk materials.

Task and Workplace Characteristics

Workplace geometry includes measures of the spatial properties of the task, such as movement distance, direction and extent of path, obstacles, and nature of destination. *Frequency/duration/pace*: measures of the time dimensions of the handling task, including frequency, duration, and required dynamics of activity over the short and long term. *Complexity* includes measures of combined or compounding demands of the load, such as manipulation requirements of movement, objective of activity, precision of motion tolerance, and number of kinetic components. *Environment* includes measures of added deteriorative environmental factors, such as temperature, humidity, lighting, noise, vibration, foot traction, and seasonal toxic agents.

Work-practices Characteristics

Individual characteristics include measures of operating practices under the control of the individual worker, such as speed and accuracy in moving objects and postures (i.e., lifting techniques) used in moving objects. *Organizational* characteristics include measures of work organization, such as the size of the physical plant and staffing of medical, hygiene, engineering, and safety functions and utilization of teamwork. *Administrative* characteristics include measures of the administration of operating practices, such as work and safety incentive system, compensation scheme, safety training and control, hygiene and safety surveys, medical aid and rescue, long work shifts, rotation, and personal protective devices.

DEVELOPING ERGONOMIC PROGRAMS

The development and implementation of a ergonomics program reduce the number and severity of work-related MSDs. In addition to lower costs resulting from fewer MSDs, benefits include decreased absenteeism, reduced workers' compensation premiums, increased productivity, and higher product quality (63–68). Relying on information published from the General Accounting Office and the National Institute for Occupational Safety and Health (NIOSH), the following section outlines six critical elements found in successful ergonomic programs (23,68).

Element 1: Management Commitment

Occupational safety and health literature stresses management commitment as a key, and perhaps controlling, factor in determining whether any work-site hazard control effort will be successful (68,69). This commitment can be expressed in several ways.

1. Establishing policy statements that:
    a. Treat ergonomic efforts as furthering the company's goals of maintaining and preserving a safe and healthful work environment for all employees
    b. Expect full cooperation of the workforce in working together toward realizing ergonomic improvements
    c. Give ergonomic efforts priority with other cost-reduction, productivity, and quality assurance activities
    d. Have the support of the local union or other worker representative(s)
2. Assigning staff to be specifically responsible for the program and providing the resources, time, and authority to operate the program on a daily basis

3. Conducting meetings between employees and supervisors that allow full discussion of the policy and plans for implementation

4. Establishing goals and objectives with target-completion dates and accountability mechanisms

5. Securing the financial resources for training and implementing controls

6. Ensuring that middle management support is sustained

Element 2: Employee Involvement

Promoting worker involvement in efforts to improve workplace conditions increases employee motivation and job satisfaction and also increases the chances for accepting change (70). Worker input is critical to identify problem jobs, processes, or equipment and is an excellent resource for obtaining suggestions about ways to control suspected hazards. Contributions can come from direct individual input or through a joint labor management safety and health committee.

Element 3: Identifying Problem Jobs

Once a decision has been made to initiate an ergonomics program, a necessary step is to gather information to determine the scope and characteristics of the potential problem(s). This can be done by examining the health and medical indicators or identifying risk factors in jobs.

Health and Medical Indicators

1. Worker reports: Encouraging employees to report, as early as possible, symptoms of physical stress is a key component of any ergonomics program. Early reporting allows corrective measures to be implemented before the effects of a job problem worsen. Incentive programs that discourage workers from reporting symptoms will probably lead to more severe problems eventually as a result of the delay in seeking medical attention.

2. Reviewing OSHA 200 logs and other existing records: Inspecting the logs of injuries and illnesses as required by OSHA and plant medical records can yield information about the nature of work-related MSDs, as can workers' compensation claims, insurance claims, absentee records, and job-transfer applications. Finding workers in certain departments, operations, or jobs presenting with more MSDs than others would suggest some immediate areas for study.

3. Other instruments: If worker reports or existing records have not yielded identified higher risks departments, jobs, or processes, consideration should be given to conducting symptom surveys or periodic medical examinations.

Identifying Risk Factors in Jobs

Efforts to identify jobs or tasks that have risk factors for MSD can provide the groundwork for changes aimed at risk reduction. Even without clear medical evidence, screening jobs for physical risk factors can offer a basis for early interventions. Tools in the form of worksite checklists can be used to identify physical stressors such as high repetition, high force, extreme postures, vibration, and static posture (Tables 2A through F). These checklists have been used widely and successfully in many ergonomics programs; however, they have not been scientifically validated. Combining checklist observations with symptoms data offers a means of overcoming uncertainly.

Element 4: Analyzing and Developing Controls for Problem Jobs

Once problem jobs or tasks are identified, ergonomic job analysis can be performed. Job analysis breaks a job into its various elements or actions, describes them, measures and quantifies risk factors inherent in the elements, and identifies conditions contributing to the risk (71). Job analyses usually are done by persons who have considerable experience and training in these areas and will not be described more fully here. A three-tier hierarchy

TABLE 2A. *General ergonomic risk analysis checklist*

Fill in the "O" if your answer is "yes" to the question. A "yes" response indicates that an
  ergonomic risk factor may be present that requires further analysis.

Manual material handling
  O   Is there lifting of loads, tools, or parts?
  O   Is there lowering of tools, loads, or pans?
  O   Is there overhead reaching for tools, loads, or pans?
  O   Is there bending at the waist to handle tools, loads, or pans?
  O   Is there twisting at the waist to handle tools, loads, or pans?
      For further analysis, refer to Table 2E.
Physical energy demands
  O   Do tools and pans weigh more than 10 lb?
  O   Is reaching greater than 20 in.?
  O   Is bending, stooping, or squatting a primary task activity?
  O   Is lifting or lowering loads a primary task activity?
  O   Is walking or carrying loads a primary task activity?
  O   Is stair or ladder climbing with loads a primary task activity?
  O   Is pushing or pulling loads a primary task activity?
  O   Is reaching overhead a primary task activity?
  O   Do any of the above tasks require five or more complete work cycles to be done within a minute?
  O   Do workers complain that rest breaks and fatigue allowances are insufficient?
      For further analysis, refer to Table 2E.
Other musculoskeletal demands
  O   Do manual jobs require frequent, repetitive motions?
  O   Do work postures require frequent bending of the neck, shoulder, elbow, wrist, or finger joints?
  O   For sealed work, do reaches for tool and materials exceed 15 in. from the worker's position?
  O   Is the worker unable to change his or her position often?
  O   Does the work involve forceful, quick, or sudden motions?
  O   Does the work involve shock or rapid buildup of forces?
  O   Is finger-pinch gripping used?
  O   Do job postures involve sustained muscle contraction of any limb?
      For further analysis, refer to Table 2B, 2C, 2D.
Computer workstation
  O   Do operators use computer workstations for more than 4 hours a day?
  O   Are there complaints of discomfort from those working at these stations?
  O   Is the chair or desk nonadjustable?
  O   Is the display monitor, keyboard, or document holder nonadjustable?
  O   Does lighting cause glare or make the monitor screen hard to read?
  O   Is the room temperature too hot or too cold?
  O   Is there imitating vibration or noise?
      For further analysis, refer to Table 2F.

of controls is widely accepted as an intervention strategy for controlling ergonomic hazards: engineering controls, administrative controls, and personal protective equipment.

Engineering Controls

The preferred approach to prevent and control work-related MSD is to design the job to take into account the capabilities and limitations of the workforce. *Engineering controls* eliminate or reduce the physical stresses identified in the checklists, which can be accomplished through automation, mechanical-assist devices, power-tool devices, height-adjustable bins, changing workstation layout, redesigning tools (particularly the position of hand grips), and changing the way materials, parts, and products are transported. Engineering controls frequently take a significant amount of time and money to develop and implement. Until these changes can be made, administrative controls are useful interventions.

Administrative Controls

Administrative controls are management-dictated work practices and policies to reduce or prevent ergonomic risk factors. Examples of administrative controls include reducing

TABLE 2A. Continued.

Environment
- O   Is the temperature too hot or too cold?
- O   Are the worker's hands exposed to temperatures less than 70 degrees Fahrenheit?
- O   Is the workplace poorly lit?
- O   Is there glare?
- O   Is there excessive noise that is annoying, distracting, or producing hearing loss?
- O   Is there upper extremity or whole body vibration?
- O   Is air circulation too high or too low?

General workplace
- O   Are walkways uneven, slippery, or obstructed?
- O   Is housekeeping poor?
- O   Is there inadequate clearance or accessibility for performing tasks?
- O   Are stairs cluttered or lacking railings?
- O   Is proper footwear worn?

Tools
- O   Is the handle too small or too large?
- O   Does the handle shape cause the operator to bend the wrist in order to use the tool?
- O   Is the tool hard to access?
- O   Does the tool weigh more than 9 lb?
- O   Does the tool vibrate excessively?
- O   Does the tool cause excessive kickback to the operator?
- O   Does the tool become too hot or too cold?
      For further analysis, refer to Table 2D.

Gloves
- O   Do the gloves require the worker to use more force when performing job tasks?
- O   Do the gloves provide inadequate protection?
- O   Do the gloves present a hazard of catch points on the tool or in the workplace?

Administration
- O   Is there little worker control over the work process?
- O   Is the task highly repetitive and monotonous?
- O   Does the job involve critical tasks with high accountability and little or no tolerance for error?
- O   Are work hours and breaks poorly organized?

Adapted from The University of Utah Research Foundation "Checklist for General Ergonomic Risk Analysis," available from the ERGOWEB Internet site (http://ergoweb.com/).

TABLE 2B. *Workstation checklist*

Fill in the "0" if your answer is "no" to the question. A "no" response indicates that an ergonomic risk factor may be present that requires further analysis.

- O   Does the work space allow for full range of movement?
- O   Are mechanical aids and equipment available?
- O   Is the height of the work surface adjustable?
- O   Can the work surface be tilted or angled?
      Is the workstation designed to reduce or eliminate
  - O   Bending or twisting in the wrist?
  - O   Reaching above the shoulder?
  - O   Static muscle loading?
  - O   Full extension of the arms?
  - O   Raised elbows?
- O   Are the workers able to vary posture?
- O   Are the hands and arms free from sharp edges on work surfaces?
- O   Is an armrest provided where needed?
- O   Is a foot rest provided where needed?
- O   Is the floor surface free of obstacles and flat?
- O   Are cushioned floor mats provided for employees required to stand for long periods?
- O   Are chairs or stools easily adjustable and suited to the task?
- O   Are all task elements visible from comfortable positions?
- O   Is there a preventive maintenance program for mechanical aids, tools, and other equipment?

TABLE 2C. *Task analysis checklist*

Fill in the "O" if your answer is "no" to the question. A "no" response indicates that an ergonomic risk factor may be present that requires further analysis.

Does the design of the primary task reduce or eliminate
- O Bending or twisting of the back or trunk?
- O Crouching?
- O Bending or twisting the wrist?
- O Extending the arms?
- O Raised elbows?
- O Static muscle loading?
- O Clothes wringing motions?
- O Finger pinch grip?

O Are mechanical devices used when necessary?
O Can the task be done with other hand?
O Can the task be done using two hands?
O Are pushing or pulling forces kept minimal?
O Are required forces judged acceptable by the workers?

Are the materials
- O Able to be held without slipping?
- O Easy to grasp?
- O Free from sharp edges and corners?

O Do containers have good handholds?
O Are jigs, fixtures, and vises used where needed?
O When needed, do gloves fit properly, and are they made of the proper fabric?
O Does the worker avoid contact with sharp edges when performing the task?
O When needed, are push buttons designed properly?
O Do the job tasks allow for ready use of personal equipment that may be required?

Are high rates of repetitive motion avoided by
- O Job rotation?
- O Self-pacing?
- O Sufficient pauses?
- O Adjusting the job skill level of the worker?

Is the employee trained in
- O Proper work practices?
- O When and how to make adjustments?
- O Recognizing signs and symptoms of potential problems?

TABLE 2D. *Handtool analysis checklist*

Fill in the "O" if your answer is "no" to the question. A "no" response indicates that an ergonomic risk factor may be present that requires further analysis.

Are tools selected to limit or minimize
- O Exposure to excessive vibration?
- O Use of excessive force?
- O Bending or twisting the wrist?
- O Finger pinch grip?
- O Problems associated with trigger finger?

O Are tools powered where necessary and feasible?
O Are tools evenly balanced?
O Are heavy tools suspended or counterbalanced in ways to facilitate use?
O Does the tool allow adequate visibility of the work?
O Does the tool grip/handle prevent slipping during use?
O Are tools equipped with handles of textured, non-conductive material?
O Are different handle sizes available to fit a wide range of hand sizes?
O Is the tool handle designed not to dig into the palm of the hand?
O Can the tool be used safely with gloves?
O Can the tool be used by either hand?
O Is there a preventive maintenance program to keep tools operating as designed?

Have employees been trained
- O In the proper use of tools?
- O When and how to report problems with tools?
- O In proper tool maintenance?

TABLE 2E. *Materials handling checklist*

Fill in the "0" if your answer is "no" to the question. A "no" response indicates that an ergonomic risk factor may be present that requires further analysis.

O   Are the weights of loads to be lifted judged acceptable by the workforce?
O   Are materials moved over minimum distances?
O   Is the distance between the object load and the body minimized?
Are walking surfaces
     O   Level?
     O   Wide enough?
     O   Clean and dry?
Are objects
     O   Easy to grasp?
     O   Stable?
     O   Able to be held without slipping?
O   Are there handholds on these objects?
O   When required, do gloves fit properly?
O   Is the proper footwear worn?
O   Is there enough room to maneuver?
O   Are mechanical aids used whenever possible?
O   Are working surfaces adjustable to the best handling heights?
Does material handling avoid
     O   Movements below knuckle height and above shoulder height?
     O   Static muscle loading?
     O   Sudden movements during handling?
     O   Twisting at the waist?
     O   Extended reaching?
O   Is help available for heavy or awkward lifts?
Are high rates of repetition avoided by
     O   Job rotation?
     O   Self-pacing?
     O   Sufficient pauses?
O   Are pushing or pulling forces reduced or eliminated?
O   Does the employee have an unobstructed view of handling the task?
O   Is there a preventive maintenance program for equipment?
O   Are workers trained in correct handling and lifting procedures?

---

shift length or curtailing overtime, job rotation in which workers rotate through several jobs with different physical demands, scheduling more rest breaks, enlarging the job task, adjusting the work pace to give employees more control over the work process, training employces in the proper work technique, and recognizing ergonomic risk factors.

Personal Equipment

One of the most controversial areas for preventing work-related MSD is whether the use of personal equipment worn or used by the employee (such as wrist splints, back belts, or vibration attenuation gloves) is effective. Some authorities consider these devices to be personal-protection equipment (PPE). In the field of occupational safety and health, PPE generally provides a barrier between the worker and the hazard sources (e.g., respirators, ear plugs, goggles, chemical aprons, safety shoes, hard hats). Whether braces, wrist splints, back belts, and similar devices can be regarded as offering personal protection against biomechanical hazards remains open to question. Although in some situations these devices may reduce the duration, frequency, or intensity of exposure, evidence of their effectiveness in injury reduction is inconclusive (72).

Element 5: Training and Education

Identifying and controlling MSD requires some level of knowledge of ergonomics and skills in remedying biomechanical hazards. Recognizing and filling different training

TABLE 2F. *Computer workstation checklist*

Fill in the "O" if your answer is "no" to the question. A "no" response indicates that an ergonomic risk factor may be present that requires further analysis.

Does the workstation ensure proper worker posture, such as
    O Horizontal thighs?
    O Vertical lower legs?
    O Feet flat on floor or footrest?
    O Neutral wrists?
Does the chair
    O Adjust easily?
    O Have a padded seat with a rounded front?
    O Have an adjustable backrest?
    O Provide lumbar support?
    O Have casters?
O Are the height and tilt of the work surface on which the keyboard is located adjustable?
O Is the keyboard detachable?
O Do keying actions require minimal force?
O Is there an adjustable document holder?
O Are arm rests provided where needed?
O Are glare and reflections avoided?
O Does the monitor have brightness and contrast controls?
O Do the operators judge the distance between eyes and work to be satisfactory for their viewing?
O Is there sufficient space for knees and feet?
O Can the workstation be used for either right- or left-handed activity?
O Are adequate rest breaks provided for task demands?
O Are high stroke rates avoided by
    O Job rotation?
    O Self-pacing?
    O Adjusting the job to the skill of the worker'?
Are employees trained in proper postures?
    O Proper work methods?
    O When and how to adjust their workstations?
    O How to seek assistance for their concerns?

needs is an important step in building an effective program. The different types of training that a facility might offer include the following:

Overall ergonomics awareness training for employees so they can recognize general risk factors, learn the procedures for reporting MSD or symptoms, and become familiar with the process the facility is using to identify and control problem jobs. Targeted training for specific groups of employees is done because of the jobs they hold, the risks they face, or their roles in the program. For example, it is important for line supervisors and managers to recognize the early signs and symptoms of MSD; for engineers to prevent and correct ergonomic hazards through equipment design, purchase, or maintenance; and for members of an ergonomics team to perform job analysis and develop controls.

Element 6: Health Care Management

In general, health care management emphasizes the prevention of impairment and disability rather than the prevention of MSD. It does this through early detection (discussed earlier), prompt treatment, and timely recovery. Early diagnosis of MSD can alert management to the need for job analysis of that employee's job or the need for further analysis if the job already has been evaluated. The responsibility of health care providers in this setting is to evaluate the symptomatic employee, seek information, review materials regarding the employee's job activities, and be familiar with the management of MSD cases or refer to a practitioner who is familiar with such management.

As the practitioner evaluates the employee, the following items should be addressed:

A medical history (occupational and nonoccupational)

A description of work activities as reported by the employee and the employer

A physical examination appropriate to the presenting symptoms and history

An initial assessment or diagnosis, and an appropriate treatment plan

An opinion about whether occupational risk factors did, or did not, contribute to or exacerbate the condition

Determine time frames for expected improvement and resolution of the condition

The practitioner should conduct follow-up for symptomatic employees to document symptom improvement or resolution. Employees who have not improved should be reevaluated. Inquiry regarding compliance with the use of light or restricted duty jobs and other aspects of the treatment plan should be undertaken. If the employer has been following the work restrictions and the employee has been following the treatment plan but the symptoms persist beyond the expected time frames, consideration should be given to referring the worker to another practitioner who has specialty training.

APPLICATION OF ERGONOMICS

Task Analysis

Ergonomics task analysis means many things to many people. To a physical therapist, an ergonomist, or an OSHA inspector, the job may be to perform an ergonomics task analysis, but the methods and the results are likely to be quite different. The physical therapist will tend to document the specific number, types, and duration of activities performed. The ergonomist will tend to list options for improving the problems associated with the task. The OSHA inspector will tend to compare the task demands to relevant threshold limits to determine whether a problem exists. All these methods of ergonomics task analysis have value, depending on the reason for and the goals of the analysis. Regardless of the method used, ergonomics task analysis is a key element in any comprehensive ergonomics program. Benefits from ergonomics task analysis include the following:

Improved productivity
Elimination of human error
Improvement in employee satisfaction
Prevention of MSDs and CTD
Making return-to-work decisions
Optimization of job rotations
Conducting before and after studies

Method

Two types of task analysis exist: documenting job requirements and development improvements (40). Which method is selected depends on the information needed. A good task analysis can be quite simple and yet provide good insight into issues and potential improvements. The key is to be systematic and have a good understanding of ergonomic principles. There is no one best way to do a task analysis that is equally valid in all workplaces. Task analysis is a means to an end, not a goal in itself. The technique and approach used must fit the needs and goals of the specific workplace. The first step is to determine why the analysis is to be done. The critical question that must be asked before ergonomics task analysis is performed is, What will be done with the task analysis when it is complete? The answer to this question will be invaluable in leading to the right task analysis method for the goal. Subsequently, the task analysis method that is chosen will dictate the instruments and equipment that will be needed to perform the analysis. If the goal is to document job requirements, precision in conducting the analysis is vital. If the goal is to find improvements, the analysis part can be much simpler, with the focus shifting to evaluating options for improvements. This distinction is important, because if the goal is to correct problems, then time spent documenting job requirements can be a distraction, especially in the early stages of an ergonomics program.

Pitfalls of Using the Wrong Method

The most common mistakes of ergonomics practitioners is to use the wrong method for conducting ergonomics task analysis. If the goal is to develop improvements that reduce the risk of employees for developing a MSD, spending time documenting job requirements can be counterproductive. For example, often an ergonomics committee will waste time debating the definition of repetition or what constitutes a high, moderate, or low number of repetitions. This debate is not productive in the day-to-day application for workplace improvement, because in many cases the problem jobs and what part of the job is at higher risk are already apparent. The focus should be on addressing the known, or likely, problem aspects of the job. Although less common, the inverse situation also wastes valuable resources. That is, if the goal is detailed documentation of the job risk factors, the qualitative approach to task analysis will not provide the needed data.

Tools

Task analysis requires tools. Over the years, a multitude of ergonomics task analysis formats and methods have been developed. Given the variety of tools available for task analysis, a discussion of each is beyond the scope of this chapter but several examples are listed for review (23,71,73,74):

Employee symptom surveys
Heat stress analysis
Job severity index (JSI)
Methods-time-measurement system (MTM)
NIOSH lifting equations
Ovako Work Analysis System (OWAS)
Psychometric lifting, pushing, pulling, carrying tables
Risk factor analysis (various)
University of Michigan Three-dimensional Static Strength Prediction Model (3DSSPM)
Work/recovery cycles analysis
RULA (rapid upper limb assessment): a survey method for the investigation of work-related upper limb disorders

Task Analysis Instruments

Task analysis requires instruments for measurements. Table 3 is a brief list of the instruments typically used to conduct ergonomics task analysis for various risk factors.

Videotaping for Ergonomics Analysis

Videotape can play a valuable role in the problem-solving process. Although not essential, video can provide the following advantages:

Ability to replay task
Ability to review in slow motion
Ability to isolate individual aspects of task
Eliminate distractions of plant floor during analysis (e.g., noise, other personnel)

To take full advantage of these benefits, some specific techniques in recording the tape are necessary.

Before Videotaping. To ensure that the video has value for persons who did not participate in the taping or at some later date, the following information should be recorded on tape:

Name and location of facility
Name of person shooting the video
The name of the job being taped
The date and time of taping

TABLE 3. *Risk factor instruments*

Risk factor	Instruments
Repetition	Stopwatch
	Videotape
Force	Pinch gauge
	Hand dynamometer
	Electromyography
	Force sensing resistors
	Force gauge
	Biomechanical models (software)
Posture	Visual checklist
	Videotape
	Computer posture analysis
	Goinometer
	Electric goinometer
	Inclinometers
Vibration	Accelerometers
Cold	Wet bulb globe temperature

This information can be recorded in a number of ways:

By writing the information neatly on a sheet of paper and then, after zooming in on the page, recording the sign for about 10 seconds (a large, dark marker usually works best)

By stating the information aloud at the start of the taping (some facilities with high noise content make this option difficult)

By keying in and displaying information at the beginning of taping in camcorders equipped with character-generating capabilities

Any combination of the above.

The last step before actually taping is to ensure that the settings on the camcorder are correct for the conditions in which the job is to be taped. Although most camcorders adjust well for most conditions, the following should be checked:

Time orientation: useful in performing quantitative task analysis. A working stopwatch or clock is important.

Battery power: a back-up battery should be brought.

Light level settings: if the camcorder has a high-speed shutter, it should be turned off. More light is required than most industrial settings can supply. When taping a worker wearing dark clothing against a bright background, the back light switch of the camcorder should be activated.

Videotaping. Videotaping should start with a wide shot of the task to allow the viewer to gain a sense of perspective on the whole task, the equipment used, and the general layout of the area. In general, at least three cycles should be captured. If the task has a long cycle, this may not be possible. (Tip: When taping, it often seems as though recording has lasted much longer than it actually has (especially if this type of taping has not been done before). It is a good idea to use a watch and count the task cycles.

After taping the big picture, the activity of a particular body part of interest can be fo-

cused on (e.g., the hands, wrists, arms) by choosing an angle and a zoom that best shows the body part's activities and postures of interest. This body part should be taped without movement, if possible, for about ten cycles of the task. (Tip: The camcorder can be held still while shooting. Tripods are helpful, but if one is not available, the right elbow can be placed firmly against the side and the left hand placed under the camcorder to give it additional support. Simultaneously, the eye should be pressed firmly to the view-finder cup. It is important not to walk while taping unless absolutely necessary. Moving or panning the camcorder should be done slowly and smoothly while recording.

All body parts should be taped by using various angles and zooms, and taping is stopped before resetting for the next shot. If possible, taping is done from both the left and right sides, from the front, the back, and overhead. For thorough analysis, these steps can be repeated using another worker from another shift. Tip: If videotaping is new to the facility, someone should explain and gain approval from the subject before taping. This activity represents an opportunity to spread the word about ergonomics.

After Videotaping. To allow total quality management (TQM) in application of the ergonomics intervention program, the following steps are helpful:

Identification information is entered onto the tape and on associated documents.

The appropriate ergonomics task assessment method is chosen.

Data are compiled and assessment forms completed.

Data are analyzed for patterns.

Conclusions about relationships are formed.

Intervention plans are developed and implemented.

The benefits of an intervention plan are assessed.

Task Analysis: Training Requirements

The training required for workers to participate in ergonomics task analysis is minimal, but it is advantageous for all participants to have basic knowledge about what CTDs are and how they occur. The "bucket analogy" is helpful for communication with and understanding by the worker. In particular, special emphasis should be placed on the MSD risk factors associated with physical activity. Finally, the four fundamental steps of ergonomics task analysis for generating options for improvement should be reviewed: (a) description of a task in terms of its MSD risk factors, (b) association of the risk factors with requirements of the task, (c) creation of options for reducing the requirements, and (d) implementation of the best option.

Application of Task Analysis by Developing Improvements

Most industrial ergonomists use the ergonomics intervention method of developing improvements. The process of developing improvements is completed by qualitative risk factor analysis (75). If the goal is to make improvements, often the step of determining the problem is fairly simple. The ergonomic issues might be fairly obvious, and there is no particular need to stop to quantify or evaluate the problem further. On some occasions, detailed job analysis may be used to document the problem, but the study may become so complex that the analysis becomes easily distracted from the real goal of lower risk and improving jobs. Further study and additional detail may lend no additional insights to the problem and often cause a loss of focus. Therefore, the focus should remain on identifying the problem and finding solutions. Four steps are involved in this method: (a) description of a task in terms of its MSD risk factors, (b) association of the risk factors with requirements of the task, (c) creation of options for reducing the requirements, and (d) implementation of the best option (75).

The analysis needs to list the risk factors and provide for the relative impact of each risk factor. Risk factors and their relative impact can be better understood using the heart disease model. Table 4 demonstrates two risk fac-

TABLE 4. *Medical—MSD risk factors*

Heart disease risk factors	MSD risk factors
Smoking	Repetition
Fatty diet	Force
Sedentary lifestyle	Awkward postures
High blood cholesterol	Direct pressure
Family history of heart disease	Vibration
Obesity	Temperature extremes
Stressful conditions	Stressful conditions

MSD, musculoskeletal disorders.

tor models. In both models, the more risk factors present, the higher the risk of developing a disorder; but some risk factors have a greater impact and are therefore more likely to cause the worker to develop a disorder. This risk factor modeling logically leads to the steps required to generate options for improvement.

Screwdriver Example

Congratulations! You have just inherited a futon-making business. The business works as follows. You receive prefabricated futon parts from a wholesaler. Your business assembles the futon parts using a screwdriver, adds custom cushions that are also provided by the wholesaler, and sells them for a profit. Thus, your primary assembly process is repetitive use of a standard screwdriver. The ergonomics improvement steps are the following:

Step 1: Description of the task in terms of its MSD risk factors. The risk factors associated with using a screwdriver in the manner described here are observation of the risk factors; repetitions to turn the screwdriver; force to hold the screwdriver, turn the screwdriver, and push the screwdriver to keep it from stripping the screw; awkward postures to maneuver the screwdriver into tight locations and around obstacles; direct pressure from contact with the screwdriver; and possibly stress, if production demands are high and cold if production occurs in the winter in an unheated environment.

Step 2: Association of the risk factors with the source. Although several risk factors are listed in step 1, this discussion is limited to repetitions associated with using the screwdriver. The goal here is to associate the risk factor observed with its source at the job. Thus, the question is, What is the source of repetitions when using a screwdriver? This is a difficult question and requires some reflection to answer: risk factor, work task repetitions, choice of fastener, and choice of tools.

Step 3: Creation of options for changing the source that reduces the risk factor. Now that the risk factor (workplace stressors = repetitions in this example) have been identified, the work task can be reviewed and a choice made. The following is a list of possible options for each source: work task options for improvement; fasteners, glue, bolts, screws with fewer threads, nails (screws with no threads); change handle, shape, handle angle; use power tool; use ratchet driver.

Step 4: Implementation of the best option. Although many of the options for improvement may be beneficial, a quick review of the commercially available vendor products indicates that a power screwdriver with an adjustable handle is available at modest cost. This option was implemented and resulted in drastically less repetition with a simultaneous increase in productivity.

This solution may have been obvious without going through the intermediate steps, but this example was used to drive home the principles involved. In most cases, especially when commercially available vendor solutions do not exist, the intermediate steps are critical to developing a solution. This is the exciting part of ergonomics. Developing ergonomics solutions usually requires thinking beyond normal paradigms and often requires creating unique methods of completing tasks that may have been performed in a certain manner for many years. This requirement of thinking outside the box, however, often will create drastically improved methods that positively impact safety considerations but also improve quality and productivity.

Application of Task Analysis by Documenting Job Requirements

There are many important instances when documenting precise job tasks is a requirement. A partial listing would include the following:

Conducting epidemiologic studies to compare job conditions with effects on health (i.e., *NIOSH Lifting Guide)*

Matching jobs to employee restrictions to determine the tasks for which a worker with restrictions is suited

Evaluating the appropriateness of job rotations in preventing MSD

Proving whether MSD risks are present, either to management or in reference to legal or regulatory issues

Conducting before-and-after studies to evaluate the effectiveness of job improvements

Improving a problem when common sense and simple evaluations are not sufficient

The specific methods, instruments, and equipment required for ergonomics task analysis by documenting job requirements will vary based on what is to be done with the information. For example, the following is a generic description of documenting task requirements for the purpose of counting repetitions.

Measuring Repetitions

In many instances, the number of repetitions per unit of time is needed. This may be for lifts, carries, bends, or other steps that occur during a 1-hour period. Two techniques used to make these calculations would be the product flow or the timed measurement method (76).

Measuring Repetitions by the Product Flow Method. The *product flow method* is the preferred technique and may be used when the rate of work is controlled by machine output, moving conveyors, or known quantity of daily output. To calculate the motions per hour using the product flow method, the following steps should be taken:

1. Counting the number of motions per piece
2. Determining the maximum product flow out of the machine (or down the conveyor) in terms of pieces per hour
3. Multiplying the number of motions per piece by the product flow rate to calculate the overall motions per hour
4. Determining the number of workers performing the job
5. Dividing the overall motions per hour by the number of workers performing the job to calculate the number of motions per hour done by each worker
6. Checking the motions per hour per person on the job requirements form in the appropriate category

This same technique can be expressed in math form:

$$\frac{\text{Motions/Hour}}{\text{Person}} = \left[\frac{(\text{Motions/Piece}) \times (\text{Pieces/Hour})}{\text{Number of Workers}} \right]$$

Example: Calculate motions/hour when packaging widgets into a box for shipment.

1. Sixteen wrist motions are required in the right hand to package the widgets (including grabbing the box, packing six widgets, and sealing the box).
2. The maximum output is 2,500 packaged boxes per hour.
3. 16 x 2,500 = 40,000 motions per hour.
4. Twenty-four people perform this job.
5. 40,000/24 = 1,667 motions per hour per person.
6. Select the 1,250–2,500 per hour (20–40/min) category for dominant-hand repetitions on the job requirements form.

Measuring Repetitions by Timed Measurement Method. If the work flow varies over time and is dependent on the employee (self-paced), motions per hour can be calculated using the timed measurement method. This approach is not as accurate as the product flow method because a single snapshot of a task may not take into account variations occurring throughout the day. Therefore, whenever possible, the product flow method should be used to calculate repetitions. Additionally, taking several measurements at random times of the day and averaging the findings will help reduce possible estimation errors.

Example: For a 1-minute period:

1. Count the number of motions which occur.
2. Multiply the motions per minute by 60. This will give you the number of motions per hour done by each worker.
3. Note: For jobs having cycle times greater than 15 seconds (four or less per minute), use a 5-minute timing period and multiply by 12. It is important to capture several complete cycles per sample.

Conclusion for Application of Ergonomics: Task Analysis

In general, performing ergonomics task analysis means at least two distinctly different methods: documenting task requirements or creating options for improvement. For maximum effectiveness, the ergonomist must have both approaches in the ergonomics "tool box."

THE FUTURE OF BIOMECHANICS AND ERGONOMICS OF THE UPPER EXTREMITY

Foundation

From a public health perspective of prevention, enough evidence has been found to begin to reduce risks for MSD in the workplace by engineering, administrative controls, and individual risk identification. Further research is needed to develop standard methods of quantifying exposure that can be applied in a wide variety of industries and occupations (36). In addition, further research is needed to develop standardized and validated methods to define specific MSDs (77). Additional biomechanical and epidemiologic studies are necessary to establish a dose-response relationship between the physical stressors and medical outcomes that can be used to specify acceptable workplace standards.

Prevention by individual risk assessment currently provides the best opportunity while additional data are obtained from current research (78). Any attempt at prevention of MSD in the workplace will need employee and employer support to ensure success. Giving the workforce some lead time before implementing any new program is critical to the prevention program's success. An ergonomic improvement without an education and orientation period for employees is of limited value. For proof of the need for education, many of us need to look no farther than where we sit. Many offices have adjustable chairs that cost 200 to 300 dollars, but the average person will report never having adjusted his or her chair. Therefore, the ergonomic benefit is lost. On paper, purchasing all these chairs looks like a successful initiative, but in reality it is of no benefit. On paper, this company has a successful ergonomics program, but the reality is that the only goal that has been accomplished is the purchase of new chairs.

Gaining Support

Successful reduction of work-related MSDs requires a team approach: the employer, the employee, the ergonomist, and the health care provider. Before implementing this process, it is important to address concerns. The first step is to elicit support from management. Management must realize that ignoring MSDs is not the best approach and does not save money. This requires management placing a price tag on the "do nothing" option.

Management often has a fear that providing education to employees about MSD will lead to increased awareness and that to do so is akin to opening "Pandora's Box." It is a little naive to believe that the employees for any company operate in a vacuum: The Internet, printed materials, and word-of-mouth information (accurate or inaccurate) are currently available to employees. Employers have been encouraged to do workplace screening by NIOSH and OSHA (1), but employers have been reluctant. A prospective study by author JMM (79) was designed to review the effects

and possible impact of workplace screening for MSD and CTD on the number of OSHA 200 injuries; reporting of MSD was started in 1997. The employer in this study implemented an individual risk screening program, education, and employee awareness for randomly assigned groups of employees in an effort to stimulate their awareness and possible reporting of musculoskeletal pain associated with the workplace. After 11 months, the employer has not experienced an increase in the incidence of work-related musculoskeletal pain or OSHA 200 reportable cases. This study suggests that employers should be encouraged to develop, implement, and use screening programs because they provide the best opportunity for prevention of MSDs and do not appear to increase the incidence of MSD in the workplace. On the other hand, other studies have reported a slight increase in the incidence of CTD, but this increase has been offset by a reduction in the severity of the disorders (80).

As important as management support is to the success of such efforts, the support of the plant supervisors is equally crucial. The supervisors are on the front line and have the ability to correct dangerous postures or actions instantly. The key is training supervisors to recognize what is unsafe and providing them with the knowledge and problem-solving skills to address concerns immediately. If these efforts are successful, it is like having a safety director in every department.

THE AT-RISK EMPLOYEE

Identification

To be both cost-effective and efficient, it makes sense to identify the employees who require intervention and to focus attention on these employees rather than attempting the shotgun approach of training the entire employee population. In addition to being more effective, less disruption occurs in the plant and makes the process easier for management to support. It is also possible that if global changes are made, some of the low-risk employees could become high-risk or sympto-matic employees (i.e., do not "fix" the person who does not need to be fixed) (78,81–83).

Several outcome measure instruments are available to assist the employer in identifying the at-risk employee (84–93). Most of these instruments use an employee questionnaire or physical measures or both that examine age, gender, inherited genetic characteristics, the workplace, the nonwork environment, and psychosocial issues. The at-risk worker then can receive appropriate risk management. Successful prevention of MSD is not about ignoring everything that is known about ergonomics and focusing on decreasing personal risk, nor is it about ignoring an employee's medical history and focusing solely on ergonomics.

Intervention

Numerous benefits are derived from employee education. One benefit of educating employees about MSD is that they will report their symptoms early. Although this might increase the OSHA 200 reportables, it can decrease the lost workday case incident rate, lost time case incident rate, and the lost time day severity rate. In a 2-year study by author JMM (currently under review for publication), a risk reduction intervention program was initiated for new hires with only a 3% increase in recordable case incidence rate by OSHA 200 log but a 16% decline in total workers' compensation costs the first year and 24% the second year, despite a 56% increase in total man hours for the same period. The employer estimated direct savings of $1.3 million dollars with a cost-to-benefit ratio of 271% over 2 years.

Therefore, having employees report symptoms is crucial. Conservative medical treatment is most effective in the early stages of the inflammatory process. If an employee continues to take part in all the activities that are causing the discomfort without any intervention, he or she will reach a point at which day-to-day activities cause pain and inflammation. As a general rule, workers should not

be experiencing symptoms from the previous day's work at the beginning of their workshift. Persistence of such symptoms indicates that something may be more seriously wrong than fatigue from an "honest day's work." Early modification in these day-to-day activities is key. The longer the employee waits to report or the employer to respond, the less likely the symptoms will respond to a few days of light or restricted work.

An additional benefit of employee education is that it gives the employer the opportunity to invite employees to share with management the responsibility for injury prevention. Safety is an area where management and employees can find common ground. Employee education also provides the employer with the opportunity to teach employees to work in a biomechanically sound way, which is not as complicated as it sounds. A few basic principles can make a big difference. Working with the wrists in neutral, shoulders relaxed, and the elbows at about 90 degrees can make a significant impact not only on employee comfort but can increase production and quality as well. A comfortable employee is more efficient and makes fewer mistakes. These principles are most effectively taught in small groups, and the employer should start with those employees identified as high risk or with the employees who are in the most demanding jobs (94).

SUMMARY

Exposure to physical stressors, such as repetitive and forceful exertions, posture stresses, contact stresses, vibration, and low temperature, probably are related to the development of work-related MSDs. Many of these physical stressors are present in the workplace; therefore, in some employees, work can be a contributing factor to their development. Physical work requirements of a job include work rate, methods, equipment, and work objects, and thus they specify what workers do and how they do it. In specifying these aspects of a worker's job, physical work requirements in part determine the level at which the worker is exposed to stressors.

Although methods for quantifying exposure to physical stressors have not been standardized, many useful methods have been adapted from existing methods of job analysis and physiologic measurement. Observation, direct measurement, calculation, electromyography, goniometry, and psychophysics are all used to quantify exposure to the various stressors. The choice of which method to apply in a given situation depends on the particular characteristics of the workplace and job under consideration, the available resources, and the level of precision required.

Further research is needed to develop standard methods of quantifying exposure that can be applied in a wide variety of industries and occupations. Although the physical stressors appear to be related to the pathogenesis of these disorders, more biomechanical and epidemiologic studies are necessary to establish a dose-response relationship between the physical stressors and medical outcomes that can be used to specify acceptable work designs. Until this information is available, prevention by individual risk assessment remains the best treatment for MSDs (i.e., CTDs) in the workplace.

ACKNOWLEDGMENT

Reference support was by Wanda K. Roehl, CSP, of Raytheon Aircraft Company, Workers' Compensation Manager.

REFERENCES

1. U.S.Department of Health and Human Services. *Musculoskeletal disorders and workplace factors: a critical review of epidemiologic evidence for work-related musculoskeletal disorders of the neck, upper extremity, and low back.* Cincinnati: NIOSH, 1997, pp. 1–14.
2. Bureau of Labor Statistics. *Survey of occupational injuries and illnesses, 1996.* Washington, DC: U.S. Government Printing Office, 1998, pp. 1–16.
3. Bureau of Labor Statistics. BLS issues 1996 Lost-work-time injuries and illnesses survey. *American College of Occupational and Environmental Medicine (ACOEM) Report* 1998:6–7.
4. Brady W, Bass J, Royce M, Anstadt G, Loeppke R, Leopold R. Defining total corporate health and safety costs—significance and impact. *J Occup Med* 1997;39: 224–231.
5. Mish FC, Gilman EW. *Webster's ninth new collegiate dictionary.* Springfield: Merriam-Webster Inc., 1991, pp. 87–88.
6. Armstrong TJ. Ergonomics and cumulative trauma disorders, In: Kasdan ML, ed. *Occupational injuries.* Philadelphia: WB Saunders, 1994:553–567.
7. Frazier LM, Stenberg CR, Finc LJ. Is it time to integrate psychosocial prevention with ergonomics for cumulative trauma disorders?, In: Moon SD, Sauter SL, eds. *Beyond biomechanics: Psychosocial aspects of musculoskeletal disorders in office work.* London: Taylor & Francis, 1998, pp. 1–24.
8. Melhorn JM. Epidemiology of musculoskeletal disorders in the workplace. In: Zeppieri JP, Spengler DM, eds. *Workers' compensation case management: a multidisciplinary perspective.* Rosemont, IL: American Academy of Orthopaedic Surgeons, 1998:45–55.
9. Melhorn JM. Physician support and employer options for reducing risk of CTD. In: Spengler DM, Zippieri JP, eds. *Workers' compensation case management: a multidisciplinary perspective.* Rosemont, IL: American Academy of Orthopaedic Surgeons, 1997:21–34.
10. Chaplin ER. Chronic pain and the injured worker: a sociobiological problem, In: Kasdan ML, ed. *Occupational hand and upper extremity injuries and diseases.* Philadelphia: Hanley & Belfus, 1991:13–46.
11. Stutts JT, Kasdan ML. Disability: a new psychosocial perspective. *J Occup Med* 1993;35:825–827.
12. Falkenburg SA, Schultz DJ. Ergonomics for the upper extremity, In: Kasdan ML, ed. *Occupational diseases of the hand.* Philadelphia: WB Saunders, 1993:263–271.
13. Kasdan ML, Weiland AJ. Repetitive strain injuries and cumulative trauma disorders [Letters]. *J Hand Surg* 1997;22A:168–169.
14. Louis DS, Kasdan ML. Lifestyle and money, not job, drive CTS. *AAOS Academy News* 1998;2:11–12.
15. Johnson RK. Psychologic asessment of patients with industrial hand injuries, In: Kasdan ML, ed. *Occupational diseases of the hand.* Philadelphia: WB Saunders, 1993: 221–229.
16. Kasdan ML, Louis DS. Repetitive strain injuries and cumulative trauma disorders [Letter]. *J Hand Surg* 1997;22A:165–166.
17. Vender MI, Kasdan ML, Truppa KL. Upper extremity disorders: a literature review to determine work-relatedness. *J Hand Surg* 1995;20A:534–541.
18. Stark RH. Repetitive strain injuries and cumulative trauma disorders [Letter]. *J Hand Surg* 1997;22A: 166–167.
19. Hadler NM. Clinical perspective. Repetitive upper-extremity motions in the workplace are not hazardous. *J Hand Surg* 1997;22A:19–27.
20. Mackinnon SE, Novak CB. Repetitive strain in the workplace. *J Hand Surg* 1997;22A:2–15.
21. Murphy PL, Sorock GS, Courtney TK, Webster BS, Leamon TB. Injury and illness in the American workplace: A comparison of data sources. *Am J Public Health* 1996;30:130–141.
22. Chaffin DB, Andersson GBJ. *Occupational biomechanics.* New York: John Wiley & Sons Inc., 1991, pp. 1–35.
23. Cohen AL, Gjessing CC, Fine LJ. *Elements of ergonomics programs: a primer based on workplace evaluations of musculoskeletal disorders.* Cincinnati: U.S. Department

of Health and Human Services, Public Health Services, Centers for Disease Control, National Institute for Occupational Safety and Health, DHHS (NIOSH), 1997.

24. Bureau of National Affairs. *Cumulative trauma disorders in the workplace: costs, prevention, and progress.* Washington, D.C.: Bureau of National Affairs, 1991.

25. U.S. Department of Health and Human Services. Cumulative trama disorders in the home and in the work place. OSHA Publication no. 1-250.

26. Sjogaard G, Sogaard K. Muscle injury in repetitive motion disorders. *Clin Orthop* 1998;351:21–31.

27. Allan DA. Structure and physiology of joints and their relationship to repetitve strain injuries. *Clin Orthop* 1998;351:32–38.

28. Feuerstein M, Miller VL, Burrell LM, Berger R. Occupational upper extremity disorders in the federal workforce. *J Occup Environ Med* 1998;40:546–555.

29. Baker EL, Melius JM, Millar JD. Surveillance of occupational illness and injury in the United States: current perspectives and future directions. *Journal of Public Health Policy* 1988;9:198–221.

30. Silverstein BA, Stetson DS, Keyserling WM, Fine LJ. Work-related musculoskeletal disorders: comparison of data sources for surveillance. *Am J Ind Med* 1997;31:600–608.

31. Henderson AK, Payne MM, Ossiander E, Evans CG, Kaufman T. Surveillance of occupational diseases in the United States. *J Occup Environ Med* 1998;70:714–719.

32. Hadler NM. Cumulative trauma, carpal tunnel syndrome in the workplace—epidemiological and legal aspects, In: Gelberman RH, ed. *Operative nerve repair and reconstruction.* Philadelphia: JB Lippincott, 1991:949–956.

33. Hadler NM. Coping with arm pain in the workplace. *Clin Orthop* 1998;351:57–62.

34. Louis DS. Presidential address are we there yet? *J Hand Surg* 1998;23A:191–195.

35. Hadler NM. Arm pain in the workplace: a small area analysis. *J Occup Environ Med* 1992;34:113–119.

36. American Academy of Orthopaedic Surgeons. *Repetitive motion disorders of the upper extremity.* Rosemont, IL: American Academy of Orthopaedic Surgeons, 1995

37. Blume RS, Sandler HM. *Final report: evaluation of the OSHA approach and cited literature critique draft proposed ergonomics protection standard.* Health Effects Document, Causal Association Section. Sandler Occupational Medicine Associates, Washington, D.C., 1996, pp. 1–45.

38. Gassett RS, Hearne B, Keelan B. Ergonomics and body mechanics in the work place. *Orthop Clinic North Am* 1996;27:861–879.

39. Scheer SJ, Mital A. Ergonomics. *Arch Phys Med Rehabil* 1997;78:S36–S45

40. MacLeod D. *The ergonomics edge.* New York: Van Nostrand Reinhold, 1995, pp. 1–22.

41. Melhorn JM, Wilkinson LK. *CTD solutions for the 90's: a comprehensive guide to managing CTD in the workplace.* Wichita: Via Christi, 1996, pp. 1–19.

42. Melhorn JM. Management of work related upper extremity musculoskeletal disorders, In: *Kansas Case Managers Annual Meeting.* Wichita, KS: Wesley Rehabilitation Hospital, 1998;16–25.

43. Roberts SL, Falkenburg SA. *Biomechanics--problem solving for functional activity.* St. Louis, MO: Mosby-Year Book, 1992, pp. 36–47.

44. Halder NM. Vibration white finger revisited. *J Occup Environ Med* 1998;40:772–779.

45. International Organization for Standardization. *Mechanical vibration guidelines for the measurement and the assessment of human exposure to hand transmitted vibration.* [International Standard ISO 5349]. Geneva: International Organization for Standardization, 1986, pp. 17–22.

46. Pecora LJ, Udel M, Christman RP. Survey of current status of Raynaud's phenomenon of occupational origin. *Ind Hyg J* 1998;2140:80–83.

47. Pheasant S. *Ergonomics, work and health.* Baltimore, MD: Aspen Publishers, 1991.

48. Armstrong TJ, Fine LJ, Goldstein SA, Lifshitz YR, Silverstein BA. Ergonomic considerations in hand and wrist tendinitis. *J Hand Surg* 1987;12A:830–837.

49. Fransson-Hall C, Bystrom S, Kibom A. Self-reported physical exposure and musculoskeletal symptoms of the forearm-hand among automobile assembly-line workers. *J Occup Environ Med* 1995;37:1136–1144.

50. Lundborg G, Myers R, Powell H. Nerve compression injury and increased endoneurial fluid pressure: a "miniature compartment syndrome." *J Neurol Neurosurg Psychiatry* 1983;46:1119–1124.

51. Putz-Anderson V, Grant KA. Perceived exertion as a function of physical effort, In: *Repetitive motion disorders of the upper extremity.* Rosemont: American Academy of Orthopaedic Surgeons, 1995:49–64.

52. Viikari-Juntura E. Risk factors for upper limb disorders. *Clin Orthop* 1998;351:39–43.

53. Sauter SL, Swanson NG. The relationship between workplace psychosocial factors and musculoskeletal disorders in office work: suggested mechanisms and evidence. In: *Repetitive motion disorders of the upper extremity.* Rosemont: American Academy of Orthopaedic Surgeons, 1995;65–76.

54. The Joint ILO/WHO on Occupational Health. *Psychosocial factors at work: Recognition and control.* Geneva, Switzerland: International Labour Office, 1986, pp. 101–124.

55. Bonzani PJ, Millender LH, Keelan B, Mangieri MG. Factors prolonging disability in work-related cumulative trauma disorders. *J Hand Surg* 1997;22A:30–34.

56. Bednar JM, Baesher-Griffith P, Osterman AL. Workers compensation effect of state law on treatment cost and work status. *Clin Orthop* 1998;351:74–77.

57. Novak CB, Mackinnon SE. Nerve injury in repetitive motion disorders. *Clin Orthop* 1998;351:10–20.

58. Roehl WK. Return to work—clearing the liability and productivity hurdles that trip up even the most savvy employers. Workers' Compensatin Update: Walnut Creek, CA: Council on Education in Management, 1998;13–30.

59. Melhorn JM. CTD injuries: an outcome study for work survivability. *Journal of Workers' Compensation* 1996;5:18–30.

60. U.S. Congress. *Occupational Safety and Health Act of 1970,* 29 USC 651. Washington, D.C.: U.S. Government Printing Office, 1970, pp. 1–350.

61. McAtamney L, Corlett EN. RULA: a survey method for the investigation of work-related upper limb disorders. *Applied Ergonomics* 1993;24:91–99.

62. Hales TR, Bertsche PK. Management of upper extremity cumulative trauma disorders. *American Association*

Occupational Health Nursing Journal (AAOHN J) 1992;40:118–129.

63. OTA (Office of Technology Assessment). *Preventing illness and injury in the workplace.* Washington, DC: Office of Technology Assessement, 1995, pp. 1–37.

64. McKenzie F, Storment J, VanHoom P. A program for control of repetitive trauma disorders in a telecommunications manufacturing facility. *Am Ind Hyg Assoc J* 1985;46:674–678.

65. Lapore BA, Olson CN, Tomer GM. The dollars and cents of occupational back injury prevention training. *Clinical Management* 1984;4:38–40.

66. LaBar G. Safety at Saturn: a team effort. *Occupatioinal Hazards* 1994;56:41–44.

67. LaBar G. Employee involvement yields improved safety record. *Occupational Hazards* 1989;51:101–104.

68. GAO. *Worker protection: private sector egronomics programs yield positive results.* Washington, D.C.: U.S. General Accounting Office, Report to Congressional Requesters. GAO/HEHS 97-163, 1997.

69. Hoffman DA, Jacbos R, Landy F. High reliability process industries: individual, micro, and macroorganizational influences on safety performance. *J Safety Res* 1995;26:131–149.

70. Noro K, Imada AS. *Participatory ergonomics.* Bristol, PA: Taylor & Francis, 1991, pp. 1–21.

71. Keyserling WM, Stetson DS, Silverstein BA, Brouwer ML. A checklist for evaluating ergonomic risk factors associated with upper extremity cumulative trauma disorders. *Ergonomics* 1993;36:807–831.

72. National Institute for Occupational Safety and Health (NIOSH). *Workplace use of back belts: review and recommendations.* Cincinnati, OH: U.S. Dept of Health and Human Services, Public Health Service, Center for Disease Control, National Institute for Occupational Safety and Health, DHHS, 1994.

73. Wilson JR. Devolving ergonomics: the key to ergonomics management programmes. *Ergonomics* 1994;37: 579–594.

74. Feuerstein M, Hickey PF. Ergonomic approaches in the clinical assessment of occupational musculoskeletal disorders, In: Turk DC, Melzack R, eds. *Handbook of pain assessment.* New York: Guilford Press, 1992; 71–79.

75. Liker JK, Joseph BS, Armstrong TJ. From ergonomic theory to practice: Organizational factors affecting the utilization of ergonomic knowledge, In: Henrick J, Brown JA, eds. *Human factors in organizational design and management.* New York: John Wiley and Sons, 1984;1–256.

76. Grandjean E. *Fitting the task to the man: an ergonomic approach.* London: Taylor and Francis, 1980, pp. 1–29.

77. Rempel DM, Evanoff BA, Amadio PC, et al. Consensus criteria for the classification of carpal tunnel syndrome in epidemiologic studies. *Am J Public Health* 1998;88: 1447–1451.

78. Melhorn JM. Cumulative trauma disorders and repetitive strain injuries: the future. *Clin Orthop* 1998;351: 107–126.

79. Melhorn JM. The impact of workplace screening on the occurrence of cumulative trauma disorders and workers' compensation claims. *J Occup Environ Med* 1999; 41:84–92.

80. Moore JS, Garg A. A job analysis method for predicting risk of upper extremity disorders at work: preliminary results. *Advances in Industrial Ergonomics and Safety* 1987;1:1–252.

81. Nakaseko M, Tokunage R, Hosokawa M. History of occupational cervicobrachial disorders in Japan and remaining problems. *J Hum Ergol (Tokyo)* 1982;11:7–16.

82. Melhorn JM. Prevention of CTD in the Workplace, In: *Workers' comp update 1998.* Walnut Creek, CA: Council on Education in Management, 1998;101–124.

83. Melhorn JM. Upper-extremity cumulative trauma disorders on workers in aircraft manufacturing [Letter, Response] Upper extremities cumulative trauma disorders. *J Occup Environ Med* 1998;40:103–104.

84. Melhorn JM. Cumulative trauma disorders: how to assess the risks. *Journal of Workers' Compensation* 1996; 5:19–33.

85. Jette DU, Jette AM. Health status assessment in the occupational health setting. *Orthop Clinic North Am* 1996; 27.891–902.

86. American Academy of Orthopaedic Surgeons. *Upper limb—DASH outcomes data collection questionnaire.* Des Plaines, IA: Musculoskeletal Outcomes Data Evaluation and Management System, 1998, pp. 1–17.

87. Stewart AL, Hays RD, Ware JE, Jr. The MOS short-form general health survey. Reliability and validity in a patient population. *Med Care* 1988;7:724–735

88. Chung KC, Pillsbury MS, Hayward RA. Reliability and validity testing of the Michigan hand outcomes questionnaire, In: *American Society for Surgery of the Hand Annual Meeting.* Denver: American Society for Surgery of the Hand, 1997:52–53.

89. Chung KC, Pillsbury MS, Walters MR, Hayward RA. Reliability and validity testing of the Michigan hand outcomes questionnaire. *J Hand Surg* 1998;23A:575–587.

90. Laing MH, Fossel AH, Larson MG. Comparisons of five health status instruments for orthopedic evaluation. *Med Care* 1990;28:632–642.

91. Martin DP, Engelberg R, Agel J, Swiontkowski MF. Comparison of the musculoskeletal function assessment questionnaire with the short form-36, the Western Ontario and McMaster universities osteoarthritis index, and the sickness impact profile health-status measures. *J Bone Joint Surg Am* 1997;79A:1323–1335.

92. Levine DW, Simmons BP, Koris MJ, et al. A self-administered questionnaire for the assessment of severity of symptoms and functional status in carpal tunnel syndrome. *J Bone Joint Surg Am* 1993;75A:1585–1592.

93. L'insalata JC, Warren RF, Cohen SB, Altchek DW, Peterson MGE. A self-administered questionnaire for assessment of symptoms and function of the shoulder. *J Bone Joint Surg Am* 1997;79A:738–748.

94. Melhorn JM. A prospective study for upper-extremity cumulative trauma disorders of workers in aircraft manufacturing. *J Occup Environ Med* 1996;38:1264–1271.

Occupational Musculoskeletal Disorders
edited by T. G. Mayer, R. J. Gatchel, and P. B. Polatin.
Lippincott Williams & Wilkins, Philadelphia © 2000.

9

Lower-extremity Occupational Musculoskeletal Disorders

Ankle-complex Inversion Injuries as a Model for Studying a Nontraditionally Considered Work-related Injury

*Takuma Ozaki, †David Lord, and *Mark D. Grabiner

*Department of Biomedical Engineering, Lerner Research Institute, The Cleveland Clinic Foundation, Cleveland, Ohio 44106; †Department of Mechanical Engineering, Case Western Reserve University, Cleveland, Ohio 44106

An *occupational injury* is any injury resulting from a work-related accident or exposure involving a sudden event in the work environment (1). In contrast, an *occupational illness* is an abnormal condition or disorder, excluding those resulting from an occupational injury, caused by exposure to employment-related factors (1). *Cumulative trauma*, or *repetitive motion disorders*, are considered occupational illnesses. The 1994 statistics from the Bureau of Labor Statistics revealed that the number of occupational illnesses was less than 10% of the number of occupational injuries (514,700 versus 6,252,200, respectively).

Most occupational injuries that lead to work loss involve the musculoskeletal system. Published statistics from the Bureau of Labor Statistics for the year 1987 revealed that more than 70% of occupational injuries were associated with three classes. Overexertion, being struck by or against an object, and falling accounted for 32.1%, 23.6%, and 17.0% of occupational injuries, respectively. Of the total number of occupational injuries affecting the musculoskeletal system, sprains and strains accounted for 43%. The term *sprain* is usually applied to ligament injuries, whereas *strain* is used in reference to injuries to muscle-tendon units. Occupational sprain and strain injuries demonstrate a gender effect and generally occur more often in women.

The anatomic site most often affected occupationally by sprains and strains is the trunk. Defined by the Bureau of Labor Statistics to range from the shoulder joints to the hip joints inclusively, sprains and strains to the trunk accounted for about 61% of all occupationally related sprains and strains in 1987. Within the segment broadly referred to as the trunk, approximately 80% of the total sprains and strains occurred to the back. The hip joint accounted for only 1% of the total number of occupation-related sprains and strains.

The incidence of sprains and strains of the trunk was approximately three times that of the lower extremity (below the hip joint). The knee, ankle, and foot accounted for 7.9%, 7.0%, and 1.6% of the total number of occupation-related sprains and strains, respectively. These lower-extremity sprains and strains represent a substantial economic burden considering lost work, reduced productivity, and medical and rehabilitation costs.

With the exception of the epidemiologic aspects of occupation-related injuries, the greatest attention of basic and clinical researchers has been given to injuries affecting the upper extremity and lower back. The lower extremity has been studied less frequently from an occupational medicine vantage. The previously mentioned statistics suggest that this lack of attention does not likely reflect a much lower incidence of occupation-related injuries to the lower extremity but, rather, may reflect the typical placement of many lower-extremity injuries and disorders, including those resulting from repetitive motion, such as stress fractures (actually a repetitive loading disorder), Achilles tendonitis, and some types of patellofemoral syndrome, in a sports medicine context because of their association with participation in athletic and recreational, as opposed to vocational, activities. Nevertheless, recognition that lower-extremity injuries can have a significant impact on the workplace represents the initial step in the formulation of a framework by which preventative efforts and rehabilitation techniques can be designed, studied, and improved. Such a framework should encompass a knowledge of the mechanics of the particular tissues involved in the injury; an understanding of the mechanics of the injury itself, the effects of the injury on the tissues, and the manner in which the tissues heal biologically; and an es-

tablished classification system for the injuries that reflects information garnered from the other elements. These elements can contribute to determining the effect of the injury on motor function and to specifying a rehabilitation program that can address the functional impairments.

The general area of acute and chronic lower-extremity injuries is clearly beyond the scope of a single chapter. Thus, the purpose of this chapter is to serve as a point of departure for the long-term objective of refining the aforementioned framework. To achieve this purpose, we selected ankle-complex inversion injuries in general and chronic ankle-complex instability in particular. Ankle-complex inversion injuries have been selected because they have not only a high incidence in the general population but also a high rate of becoming chronic injuries.

Figure 1 is a general model of disability prevention strategies proposed by Jette (2) in which, for the context of ankle-complex inversion injuries, the term *injury* has replaced *disease*. An ankle-inversion injury creates an ankle-complex impairment, or abnormality, that may be anatomic or physiologic. Such an impairment often is accompanied by pain and may be characterized by reductions in range of motion, muscle strength, and power. Impairment can digress to become functional limitation(s), resulting in an inability to perform specific motor tasks that are considered normal. For example, a lateral ankle-complex instability arising from a ligamentous injury could impair the ability of the individual to move laterally during locomotion. Functional

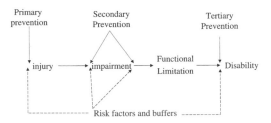

FIG. 1. A model of disability-prevention strategies. (From ref. 2, with permission.)

limitations can degrade further to become physical disabilities that are the functional effects of chronic conditions. Such limitations may impair the ability to participate in societal activities or roles that may be both expected and desired.

Figure 1 also illustrates the various stages in which efforts can be undertaken to prevent the development of physical disabilities. In the context of ankle-complex inversion injuries, primary prevention may be represented by efforts to avoid the initial injury. Preventative efforts may be effective in reducing the number of ankle-complex inversion injuries, for example, reducing the presence of environmental factors that increase the risk of injury. It is arguable, however, as to whether these reductions can have a substantial impact on the estimated 23,000 ankle injuries occurring per day in the United States (3).

Once an injury occurs, secondary preventative efforts can influence the extent to which impairments digress toward functional limitations. Such efforts include early detection of conditions that may give rise to functional limitations and the use of various interventions that can retard or reverse the digression of impairments (2). Clearly, secondary prevention is the key component in efforts directed toward reducing the incidence of ankle-complex inversion injuries resulting in chronic instabilities. Secondary prevention must be considered superior to tertiary prevention efforts that are directed toward restoring functional abilities in persons who have reached the level of disability.

Jette (2) further developed the model of disablement by addressing issues related to factors that modify the likelihood of injuries developing to impairments, limitations, and disabilities. Risk factors present before or after the development of a chronic condition increase the likelihood of disablement. These factors include education, income level, and job satisfaction. Unlike risk factors, buffers serve to reduce the likelihood of disablement. Physical and occupational therapy as well as lifestyle and environmental changes are considered buffers. In this overall model of disablement, physical and occupational therapy are buffers contributing to the pivotal role of secondary prevention.

Ankle-complex inversion injuries account for about 85% of all ankle sprains (3); furthermore, they are the most common injuries to the lower extremity. It has been estimated that there is one ankle sprain per day per 10,000 population members. These injuries most often are limited to soft-tissue damage. The sporting arena is not the only venue, although it is the most common, in which a substantial incidence of ankle sprains occurs. For example, Kaikkonen and colleagues (4) reported that 12% of the ankle injuries reviewed retrospectively were work-related injuries. Clearly, some occupations place workers at higher risk for sustaining ankle sprains. For example, the incidence of ankle injuries in military personnel is, perhaps not surprising, quite high. The injury rate occurring during training jumps for paratroopers has been reported to be about 20 per 1,000 jumps (5). Of these injuries, 36% occurred to the ankle. In special military units in which a technique called *fast-roping* is common, ankle injuries account for up to 30% of all injuries (6). Sprained ankles were the most commonly encountered lower-extremity injury in army recruits and the most prevalent injury sustained by cadets at the U.S. Military Academy (7–9).

Whereas the military, like some types of professional sports, increases the probability of ankle-complex inversion injuries, even workers who find themselves in a relatively safe work environment are not immune to such injuries. The present-day awareness of physical fitness and lifestyle is associated with participation in a spectrum of individual and team sports. Some of these activities may even be sponsored by the employing institution. The net effect of a worker sustaining an ankle injury while at work or during recreational hours is similar: reduced productivity. Turning once again to the military for an example, during a 6-month deployment of a navy aircraft carrier, injuries occurring during recreational activities represented 19% of all injuries and resulted in lost duty time about

50% of the time, whereas work-related injuries resulted in lost duty time only about 33% of the time (10). The point here is that vocationally derived injuries can become significant vocational concerns.

BIOMECHANICS OF LIGAMENTS

The structural (ligament as a whole) and material (standardized ligament sample) properties of human ankle-complex ligaments have not been widely studied (11,12), but an understanding of basic tissue biomechanics is necessary to appreciate issues related to ligament injury and healing. Ligaments are parallel-fibered collagenous tissues that are sparsely populated with cells but possess abundant extracellular matrix, which may represent 80% of the ligament. Furthermore, about 70% of the extracellular matrix is water. The remaining 30% is composed of collagen, ground substance, and elastin.

Collagen fibers, specifically type I collagen, provide strength and stiffness to the ligament. Type I collagen comprises three polypeptide chains (α-chains) that are combined in a right-handed triple helix. Intrachain bonding, or cross-linking, is the result of hydrogen bonds formed by the three main amino acids of type I collagen: glycine, proline, and hydroxyproline. The strength and stiffness of collagen arise from intermolecular cross-links.

Up to 20% of the solid components, the ground substance, of ligaments is composed of proteoglycans. A proteoglycan aggregate, formed by the proteoglycan bonded to a hyaluronic acid chain, is responsible for binding most of the extracellular water. The ground substance serves also to maintain the geometric arrangement of collagenous fibers, thereby contributing to the strength and stiffness of the ligament. Elastin fibers contribute to the reversible extensibility of the ligament; however, elastin is present in only small amounts in ligaments of the extremities compared with elastic ligaments such as the ligamentum flavum.

The structural and material properties of ligaments are influenced by the orientation of the ligament fibers and the properties of the constituent fibers. The present discussion is limited to a brief introduction to some basic biomechanical principles. For excellent reviews of the broader biomechanical principles and issues related to ligament, the reader is referred to Woo and associates (13) and Hawkins (14). Based on their biomechanical role, the meaningful structural and material properties of ligaments are determined by tensile tests.

An introduction to biomechanical testing can begin with a Newtonian spring subjected to the load of an attached mass suspended from one end of the spring. The force f is the product of the mass m and the acceleration of the mass due to gravity g (Fig. 2A). The physics of such a spring tells us that the restoring force F exerted by the spring on the body is proportional to the elongation of the spring ΔL. That is, $F = k\Delta L$. Figure 2B illus-

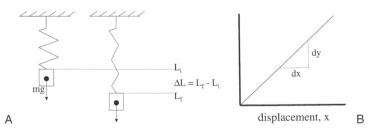

FIG. 2. A: A simple linear, or Newtonian spring, subjected to elongation by an applied force. The stiffness of the spring k can be determined by measuring ΔL the change in length. ΔL is measured knowing the initial length L_i and the final length L_f after applying a load, mg. **B**: Determination of the stiffness k of the spring depicted in panel A. $k = dy/dx$ = spring constant.

trates the relationship between the displacement to which a Newtonian spring is subjected and the resulting restorative force at any given displacement. The slope of the line defining the relationship k is the spring constant, or stiffness. The *spring constant* may be considered the magnitude of the restoring force per unit of elongation. By rearranging the simple relationship to $\Delta L = F/k$, it is clear that for a given force, a large stiffness value will be associated with a small elongation.

Figure 3A illustrates a body under uniaxial loading, having an initial length L and a cross-sectional area A ($d \times W$), subjected to a tensile load by the axially applied forces. Under the influence of the applied forces, the body is elongated by a distance ΔL. In a manner similar to that of the Newtonian spring, the structural properties of the body are given by the relationship between elongation of the body (*displacement*) and the applied force illustrated in Fig. 3B. The linear region of the relationship, below the yielding point, is called the *elastic region*. The region of the curve above the yield point is referred to as the *plastic region*. When an axial load whose magnitude is less than the force corresponding to the yielding point F_y is applied to the body, the deformation of the body remains in the elastic region, and the body will return to its original length after the load is removed. If the applied load is greater than F_y but less than the load corresponding to failure F_f, the body will elongate into the plastic region and will not return to its original

length after the load is removed but rather to an elongated length (d"). In this case, the elongation has caused permanent structural damage. Ultimately, any load equaling or exceeding the magnitude of F_f will cause the material to rupture completely. The slope of the force-displacement curve in the elastic region is the structural stiffness of the body; however, the structural stiffness of the body measured in this way is dependent on a number of factors: the geometry of the body, that is, the original length (L) and cross-sectional area (A) of the body, and the value E, which is referred to as the *modulus*.

The important structural variables related to the strength of the body that may be determined from the relationship illustrated in Figure 3B are (a) the maximum load that the body can sustain prior to failure, (b) the maximum elongation that the body can sustain prior to failure, and (c) the stiffness of the body.

To determine the material properties of the body, its geometrical influences must be eliminated. This is accomplished by dividing the applied force by the cross sectional area of the body (A) and by dividing the elongation (ΔL) by the original length of the body L. When the geometry of the specimen is controlled, the previously discussed force-displacement relationship becomes a stress-strain relationship (Fig. 3C). Stress (σ) is the description of the intensity of internal force. Strain (ε) is the description of the intensity of elongation. The

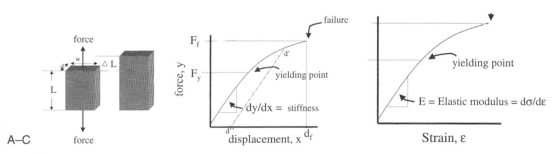

FIG. 3. A: A rigid body subjected to uniaxial loading. The change in the length of the body δL is reliant on the applied forces and the geometry of the body, specifically its cross-sectional area ($d \times w$).
B: Determination of the structural properties of the rigid body subjected to uniaxial loading (see text).
C: Determination of the material properties of the rigid body subjected to uniaxial loading (see text).

slope of the stress-strain curve in the elastic region, computed so as to be independent of the geometry of the structure, is the modulus of elasticity, or modulus, or Young's modulus. It is a measure of the material, as opposed to structural, stiffness.

Ligaments do not behave as simple linear springs. Indeed, ligaments possess viscoelastic properties that arise due to interaction between the collagen and ground substance. Viscoelastic properties of ligaments are demonstrated by strain-rate sensitivity, stress relaxation, creep, and hysteresis. For human knee ligaments tested in isolation and subjected to high strain rates, the specimens required greater forces to cause total tissue failures and underwent larger elongations (15). *Stress relaxation* is a phenomenon observed when ligaments are stretched and maintained at a constant length. Over time, the internal ligament force diminishes, resulting in decreased stress. *Creep*, on the other hand, occurs when a ligament is subjected to a constant force and, over time, the ligament stretches. *Hysteresis* occurs during cyclic loading of a ligament and is the difference in the areas of the force-displacement curves for loading and subsequent unloading. The reader is referred to Woo et al. (13) and Hawkins (14) for reviews of the time dependence and history dependence of ligament properties as well as other factors influencing these properties including age, exercise, disuse, and injury.

As previously mentioned, the structural and material properties of human ankle-complex ligaments have not been well described. Compared with other lower-extremity ligaments, such as the anterior cruciate ligament and the medial collateral ligament, little is known about the ankle-complex ligaments.

ANATOMY OF ANKLE-COMPLEX INVERSION INJURIES

The position and motion of the foot relative to the tibia can be described as occurring about three orthogonal axes that are convenient for analysis but may not accurately reflect motion of the foot about its anatomic axes. The position and motion of the foot are a complex interaction between the geometry of the articulating bones, muscles, tendons, ligaments, and internal and external forces. Normally, these factors contribute to stabilization of the foot and thereby prevent injury resulting from undesirable kinematics. The foot may become unstable, however, about its rotational axes as a result of intrinsic (*motor control*) or extrinsic (*environmental*) factors. In the presence of instability, even typically encountered reaction forces can result in excessive joint motion that exceeds the mechanical strength of the restraining tissues, giving rise to tissue damage.

Bony Architecture

The articulating bones producing foot movements include the tibia, fibula, talus, and calcaneus. The architecture of these bones, depicted in Fig. 4, dictate the orientation of the foot relative to the tibia and the range of foot motion about its axes. The expansion of the distal fibula forms the lateral malleolus. The medial aspect of the lateral malleolus serves as the facet in which the lateral talus rotates. Similarly, the distal expansion of the tibia creates the medial malleolus. The tibiofibular articulation completes the mortise in which the proximal talus (*trochlea*) articulates. Distal to the talus and extending beyond the tibiofibular mortise both posteriorly and anteriorly is the calcaneus, the largest bone in the foot that serves to transmit body weight to the ground.

Movements of the foot, relative to the tibia, can be approximated by assuming two fixed axes. Articulation of the talus with the tibia and fibula occurs about the talocrural axis, which passes through the medial and lateral malleoli. Articulation of the calcaneus with the talus occurs about the subtalar axis, which passes through the distal posterior calcaneus and the proximal anterior navicular bone. By virtue of their positions and orientations, rotations about the talocrural and subtalar axes are combinations of rotations about the three previously de-

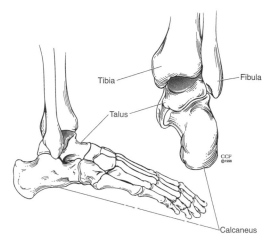

FIG. 4. Schematic diagram of the bones contributing to the articulation of the foot relative to the shank from the lateral and posterior views.

scribed axes. To simplify the nomenclature associated with describing movements about the three orthogonal axes, rotation about the talocrual axis is commonly referred to as *plantarflexion* or *dorsiflexion* and that about the subtalar axis as *inversion* or *eversion*.

When viewed from above in the transverse plane, the trochlea possesses a wedgelike shape that is wider anteriorly than posteriorly. This irregular shape provides stability to the ankle complex when the foot is in dorsiflexion. In this position, the wider anterior talus fits snugly within the tibiofibular mortise. In plan-

tarflexion, the more narrow posterior portion of the talus rotates in the mortise, and a small gap is created between the medial talus and the facet of the medial malleolus. This small gap enables the talus to rotate internally or externally, depending on the direction(s) and magnitude(s) of the ground reaction forces.

Ligaments

Of all ligamentous injuries to the ankle complex, 85% involve sprain to the lateral ligaments (16). These ligaments are shown in Fig. 5

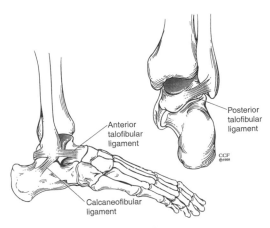

FIG 5. Schematic diagram of the ankle joint complex showing the attachments and orientations of the lateral collateral ligaments that protect the complex against extreme plantarflexion and/or inversion.

and include the anterior talofibular ligament, calcaneofibular ligament, and posterior talofibular ligament. The contribution to the stability of the ankle complex by each ligament is highly dependent on the position of the foot.

Anterior Talofibular Ligament

The anterior talofibular ligament is the most frequently injured ligament in the human body (17) because of its location and inability to resist high forces. This ligament is a thickening of the anterior ankle-complex capsule. It serves to restrict the motion of the foot anteriorly with respect to the tibia and runs nearly horizontally from its origin on the anterior aspect of the lateral malleolus to its insertion on the talus, anterior to its lateral articular facet. This anatomy allows the anterior talofibular ligament to resist plantarflexion and inversion. The anterior talofibular ligament is about 18 mm long with a cross-sectional area of 13 mm^2 (17,18). This ligament is the shortest of the lateral ligaments and requires the least amount of force to rupture.

Calcaneofibular ligament

The calcaneofibular ligament, which resists medially directed motion of the calcaneus away from the fibula, runs posteriorly and inferiorly from its origin at the apex of the fibular malleolus to its insertion on the lateral aspect of the calcaneus. This ligament is somewhat integrated with the tendon sheaths of the peroneus longus and brevis muscles and stabilizes the inverted or dorsiflexed foot. The calcaneofibular ligament, the longest of the lateral ligaments, crosses both the talocrual and subtalar joint. It is about 2.5 times stronger than the anterior talofibular ligament and measures an average 28 mm long with a cross-sectional area of 10 mm^2.

Posterior Talofibular Ligament

The posterior talofibular ligament, which resists medially directed motion of the talus away from the fibula, runs mostly horizontally from its origin on the posterior aspect of the lateral malleolus to its attachment on the posterior surface of the talus. It serves as a weak restraint against posterior displacement of the talus within the ankle mortise. The posterior talofibular ligament usually is injured only in the case of severe ankle trauma (19). This ligament is the strongest of the lateral ligament complex and requires the highest force to be ruptured. It measures 21 mm long and has a cross-sectional area of 22 mm^2.

Musculature

Lower-extremity skeletal muscles can generate large contraction forces that contribute to the dynamic stability of the ankle complex. Passive forces generated by stretching muscles are a function of the structural properties of the tissue. Active force is generated by the contractile machinery, that is, the interaction between actin and myosin. The maximum active force that a muscle can generate is a function of a number of architectural characteristics but also is influenced by the length of the muscle and the velocity of muscle contraction. For an in-depth review of skeletal muscle properties, the reader is referred to Lieber (20).

The muscles of the lower leg that influence the ankle complex may be categorized as the anterior crural muscles, the posterior crural muscles, and the lateral crural muscles. The *anterior crural muscles* include the tibialis anterior (causes dorsiflexion and supination), extensor hallucis longus (causes dorsiflexion and supination), the extensor digitorum longus (causes dorsiflexion and pronation), and peroneus tertius (causes dorsiflexion and pronation). The muscles of the *posterior crural group* are subdivided into a *superficial* group and a *deep* group. The superficial group consists of the gastrocnemius (causes plantarflexion), the soleus (causes plantarflexion), and the plantaris (causes plantarflexion). The deep group consists of the politeus (no ankle-complex action), the flexor hallucis longus (causes plantar flexion and supination), the flexor digitorum longus (causes plantar flexion and supination), and the tibialis posterior (causes plantar flexion and supination). Lastly, the *lateral crural group* includes the peroneus longus (causes plantarflexion and pronation) and the peroneus brevis (causes plantarflexion and pronation).

MECHANISMS OF ANKLE-COMPLEX INVERSION INJURY

The lateral ligament complex is injured most often when the foot is subjected to simultaneous plantarflexion and inversion and is common when descending stairs and curbs, encountering uneven or unstable surfaces, or during the landing phases of running and jumping. The orientation of a plantarflexed and inverted foot is illustrated in Fig. 6. As the an-

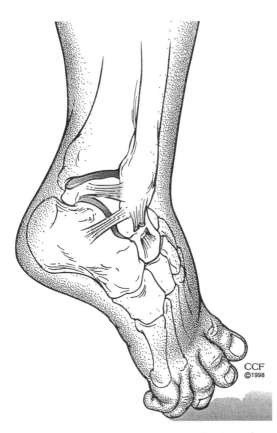

FIG. 6. Schematic illustration of the plantarflexed and inverted foot. With its attachments, the anterior talofibular ligament is more likely to be strained to rupture followed by the calcaneofibular ligament. The more narrowed posterior talus is within the tibiofibular mortise; as such, the ankle complex is most unstable with this foot orientation.

kle complex is plantarflexed, the anterior talofibular ligament experiences increased strain. The calcaneofibular ligament acts in a synergistic manner to the anterior talofibular ligament to control lateral ankle-complex stability; that is, the calcaneofibular ligament experiences increased strain as the ankle complex is dorsiflexed. In the presence of inversion, however, both the anterior talofibular ligament and the calcaneofibular ligament experience strain. Temporally, injury of the anterior talofibular ligament precedes that of the calcaneofibular ligament. Isolated injuries of the calcaneofibular ligament are not common. Broström (21,22) reported that 66% of inversion injuries are isolated anterior talofibular ligament injuries and that 20% of inversion injuries were combined anterior talofibular and calcaneofibular ligament injuries. Continued inversion will subsequently subject the posterior talofibular ligament to strain.

CLASSIFICATION OF ANKLE-COMPLEX INVERSION INJURIES

The manner in which an ankle-complex inversion injury is treated, and of course the prognosis, is linked to the extent of the damage caused to the ligaments. A *grade I* (*mild*) sprain is one in which some of the fibers within the ligament have experienced strain injury but no macroscopic tearing; that is, ligament elongation has exceeded that of the elastic region. The ligament is intact, however, and there is no evidence of ankle complex laxity. This type of injury is associated with little swelling or pain, and there is no functional impairment. A *grade II* (*moderate*) sprain is one in which there is a partial tear in the fibers of the anterior talofibular ligament or the anterior talofibular ligament and calcaneofibular ligament. This sprain is associated with some ankle-complex laxity, swelling, and pain that give rise to some functional impairments. Both grade I and grade II sprains recover relatively quickly and are well managed with conservative treatment. Conservative treatment consists of *r*est, application of *i*ce to the injury, *c*ompression, and *e*levation

(RICE), immediately following the injury and then a brief period of immobilization and protection of the ankle complex, generally provided by taping or bracing (23–28). Finally, conservative treatment ends with progressive exercises to increase joint range of motion and to improve neuromuscular control (29).

A *grade III* (*severe*) sprain is a complete rupture of the ligament(s). This injury is associated with substantial swelling and pain, hemorrhage, and the presence of ankle-complex laxity. There is a significant functional impairment. Kannus and Renström (3) reviewed 12 prospective studies that had been conducted to characterize the treatment of choice for grade III sprains. The result of this review led the authors to conclude that the treatment of choice is not surgical but rather the same type of conservative treatment that is used for grade I and grade II sprains.

LIGAMENT HEALING

The temporal aspects and the mechanical and biological details of ligament healing probably demonstrate reasonable ligament and animal model specificity (30). Variables such as age, nutritional status, various systemic pathologies, and local factors such as blood supply, synovial environment, mechanical and biological stress can influence the physiology of ligament healing.

Ligament healing may be considered to have three clinical phases (30). Within the initial 72 hours following the injury, there is a period of acute inflammation and reaction marked by swelling, redness, warmth, and pain (*phase 1*). The inflammation phase comprises vascular, cellular, and biochemical events that are crucial to the healing and repair process. These events serve to remove damaged tissue and promote tissue regeneration that underlies the return of normal tissue function. Histologically[1], the early inflamma-

tion phase, within a few hours of injury, is characterized by the arrival of erythrocytes, polymorphonuclear leukocytes, and lymphocytes to the injury site. Within 24 hours of the injury, monocytes and macrophages initiate the process of phagocytosis, in which necrotic tissue and cellular debris are removed from the injury site. Late in the inflammation stage, fibroblasts engage in production of a scar tissue matrix.

During *phase 2*, repair and regeneration, the inflammation subsides and healing is initiated. This phase may last from 48 to 72 hours postinjury to 6 weeks after the injury. The early part of this phase is characterized by the beginning of cellular and matrix proliferation. The latter part of this phase is marked by a cellular scar tissue and the emergence of vascular endothelial capillary buds. The extracellular matrix becomes less cellular and better organized with healing. The concentration of ligament matrix collagen increases during this phase but is still less than that found in an uninjured ligament. Finally, during this phase, the collagen matrix will become more aligned with the functional axis of the ligament, the diameter of the collagen fibrils increases, and the fibrils themselves become more densely situated.

The last phase, *phase 3*, may require a year or longer. This phase, during which remodeling and maturation occur, is marked by contraction of the healing ligament and increases in the tensile strength of the ligament. The scar tissue matures and, albeit still hypercellular and disorganized, has histologic qualities resembling the uninjured tissue.

INSUFFICIENCY OF REHABILITATION: CHRONIC ANKLE COMPLEX INSTABILITY

The prognosis for most sprains of the ankle-complex ligaments treated conservatively is good to excellent, although up to 40% of patients with these injuries develop chronic symptoms. Typically, chronic symptoms include pain, the feeling of giving way, swelling, and muscle weakness (3,19,31).

---

[1]The physiological aspects of the clinical phases of ligament healing reflect those processes that are associated with a complete in-substance rupture of the rabbit medical collateral ligament.

Surgery is an option for some patients who experience chronic ankle-complex instability that is nonresponsive to conservative treatment and whose symptoms can be traced specifically to a surgically addressable problem; this may account for up to 20% of patients with acute ligament ruptures (19). Even accounting for this percentage of potential surgical candidates, however, a large group of patients have persistent symptoms of chronic ankle complex instability.

Various explanations for chronic ankle-complex instability have been offered in the literature. The information that underpins proprioception arises from the skin, muscle spindles, tendon organs, and joint receptors ligaments and from the motor commands generated by the central nervous system (32). *Proprioception*, or *kinesthesia*, refers to the ability to recognize the position and motion of body segments relative to one another, effort and heaviness, and the perceived timing of motion-related events. Diminished ankle-complex proprioception often is associated with chronic ankle-complex instability. Indeed, Freeman and associates (33) first suggested that ankle-complex functional instability could result from ligament trauma affecting the reflex stabilization of the foot during locomotion. Injury to the ligament was proposed to interrupt the normal sensory information arising from the mechanoreceptors located in said ligament. In that original study, Freeman and colleagues (33) measured proprioception as the ability to maintain balance on one leg. In addition to the ability to balance on a single leg, other studies of proprioception test the hypothesis that disruption of this sense is a contributor to chronic ankle complex instability and, thus, should be a focus of the rehabilitation process (34–39).

Peroneal muscle strength is a second factor to which chronic ankle complex instability is attributed. The importance of the strength and/or power of the peroneal muscles for the stabilization of the ankle complex against inversion is found in its primary functional role as an ankle complex evertor. A dogma of rehabilitation from ankle complex inversion in-

juries has been to direct efforts at increasing the strength of the peroneal muscles (3,8,19,40). Strengthening the peroneal muscles poses considerable obstacles to rehabilitation efforts, however (41). For example, simulation of the dynamic conditions during which the ankle complex experiences inversion injuries and during which the peroneal muscles have been proposed to offer dynamic stabilization of the ankle complex cannot practically be conducted clinically. In addition, the short functional range of ankle complex motion associated with normal peroneal muscle contraction and the complex multiaxial motion of inversion precludes accurate and meaningful clinical measures of peroneal strength. Thus, the difficulty of specifically training peroneus longus and measuring performance of this muscle is underscored.

Therefore, although the underlying rationale seems reasonable, the quantitative support for the contentions related to peroneal strength and ankle-complex proprioception are not considered compelling. We propose a conceptual model by which the mechanisms of chronic ankle-complex instability can be investigated further. In part, the basis for the model is a set of established criteria that may be used to establish causal relationships between various factors (42). These criteria are the following:

- *Temporal ordering*: The cause is present before the effect
- *Temporal contiguity*: The effect closely follows the cause
- *Covariance*: In the absence of cause there is no effect
- *Congruity*: The size of the cause is related to the size of the effect
- Absence of other plausible explanations for the observed effects

Generally, the literature related to proprioception, strength, and chronic ankle-complex instability reflects well-designed and executed studies; however, the proposed relationships have not been subjected to rigorous, systematic prospective investigation, which tends to diminish the level of certainty associated with the findings. These criteria may be broadly applied to test the external validity of the relationships proposed in the literature.

Is diminished proprioception (and strength) of patients evident before the development of chronic ankle-joint instability? The answer to this question is not known because of the absence of any published longitudinal studies. Cross-sectional studies, however, suggest that patients with chronic ankle instability have a diminished ability to balance on a single limb. Cross-sectional studies also suggest that patients with chronic ankle instability have diminished eversion strength.

Does ankle complex instability develop in concert with diminished proprioception (and strength)? Again, the answer is not known because of the absence of any published longitudinal studies.

Can diminished proprioception (and strength) be present in the absence of chronic ankle complex instability? The gerontologic literature is replete with reports of diminished strength and diminished ability to maintain balance on one leg; however, the subjects did not have chronic ankle-complex instability.

Is the extent to which proprioception (and strength) diminished directly related to the extent of the instability? This type of analysis in which the magnitudes of the instability is correlated with the size of the functional impairment has not been reported in the literature. Further, an argument similar to older adults can be made here.

The final criterion against which a cause-and-effect argument may be held is *whether any alternative explanations exist for the reported relationships between diminished proprioception, diminished eversion strength, and chronic ankle-complex instability.* The findings of the published studies are not in dispute; however, the extrapolation that seems to have been accepted, that is, that diminished proprioception and diminished eversion strength are the causes of chronic ankle complex instability, may be challenged because the contention seems to be supported only by cross-sectional studies. In the absence of support for a cause-and-effect relationship that can be derived by prospective studies, the published findings of diminished proprioception and strength in patients with ankle injuries and functional instability arguably can be explained as the influence of detraining or disuse. Indeed, Pintsaar and colleagues (39) reported that subjects with functional instabilities improved performance on a postural task following 8 weeks of ankle-disk training. The authors did not report whether this outcome was associated with an improvement in the extent of the functional instability.

Based on the preceding discussion, it can be concluded that determination of the physiologic basis of chronic ankle-complex instability may require further systematic study, including prospective designs. Figure 7 illustrates a conceptual model on which such study may be based. The figure presents a relationship between injury to the lateral ankle-complex ligaments and the development of chronic-ankle complex instability. The injury, which occurs at the time indicated by the arrow, results in immediate physical effects, such as pain, swelling, hemorrhage, and, of course, physical damage to the ligament tissue. Two such effects, pain and damage to the ligament tissue, are marked by the dotted and dashed lines, respectively. The intent is to demonstrate that the resolution of pain, which may arise from numerous anatomic locations, likely follows a different time course than that required for the various stages of ligament healing.

Concurrent with these physical effects are functional effects, such as diminished range of motion, pain-related inhibition of skeletal muscle activation, loss of coordination, the inability to bear weight, and joint instability. Inhibition of skeletal muscle activation and inability to bear weight generally contributes to secondary effects such as the loss of muscle mass (*atrophy*) and the loss of muscle strength and power. The collective effects are marked by the solid line. Generally, conservative treatment tends to alleviate these physical effects until pain, swelling, and hemorrhage are reduced to baseline or near-baseline levels. The return to baseline levels of function do not follow the same time course, however.

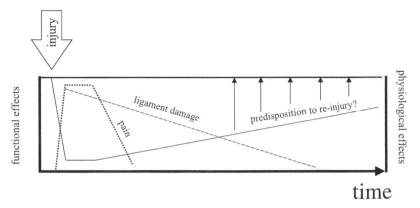

FIG. 7. A conceptual model by which the physiologic basis of chronic ankle-complex instability may be subjected to systematic study that includes prospective designs (see text). The predisposition to further injury may be a function of the extent to which function (*solid line*) remains displaced from the original uninjured state. In this model, an impairment can remain, the cause of which may be unidentified, even though the physiologic effects such as pain, swelling, and ligament damage have been resolved (*dashed line*).

The ultimate use of the conceptual model presented in Fig. 7 is to serve as a means by which patients suffering ankle-complex ligament injuries can be rehabilitated in the most expedient manner and with the best clinical and functional result. A second use is to provide an accurate clinical picture of the likelihood of a particular patient developing chronic ankle complex instability. Presently, however, the use of the model is to provide a framework by which basic and clinical research may continue systematically toward answering questions related to what variables are most meaningful to collect, the most appropriate time to measure these variables, and to what benchmark the derived variables can be compared? In addition, with respect to the influence of clinical interventions on the measures deemed most appropriate, it is important to address issues such as the extent to which preinjury functional status can be achieved and the length of time required by rehabilitation efforts to achieve that level.

REFERENCES

1. Praemer A, Furner S, Rice DP. *Musculoskeletal conditions in the United States*. Park Ridge, IL: American Academy of Orthopaedic Surgery, 1992, p. 98.
2. Jette AM. Musculoskeletal impairments and associated physical disability in the elderly: insights from epidemiological research. In, *Musculoskeletal soft-tissue aging:* impact on mobility. Rosemont, IL: American Academy of Orthopaedic Surgeons, 1993:7–22.
3. Kannus P, Renstrom P. Treatment for acute tears of the lateral ligaments of the ankle: operation, cast, or early controlled mobilization. *J Bone Joint Surg Am* 1991;73:305–312.
4. Kaikkonen A, Hyppänen E, Kannus P, Järvinen. Long-term functional outcome after primary repair of the lateral ligaments of the ankle. *Am J Sports Med* 1997;25:150–155.
5. Ekeland A. Injuries in military parachuting: a prospective study of 4499 jumps. *Injury* 1997;3:219–222.
6. Kragh JF. Fast-roping injuries among Army Rangers: a retrospective survey of an elite airborne battalion. *Mil Med* 1995;160:277–279.
7. Jackson DW, Ashley RL, Powell JW. Ankle sprains in young athletes. *Clin Orthop* 1974;101:201–215.
8. Balduini FC, Vegso JJ, Torg JS, Torg E. Management and rehabilitation of ligamentous injuries to the ankle. *Am J Sports Med* 1987;4:365–380.
9. Hopkinson WJ, St.Pierre P, Ryan JB, Wheeler JH. Syndesmosis sprains of the ankle. *Foot Ankle Int* 1990;10:325–330.
10. Krentz MJ, Li G, Baker SP. At work and play in a hazardous environment: injuries abourd a deployed US Navy aircraft carrier. *Aviat Space Environ Med* 1997;68:51–55.
11. Colville MR, Marder RA, Boyle JJ, et al. Strain measurement in lateral ankle ligaments. *Am J Sports Med* 1990;18:196–200.
12. Nigg BM, Skarvan G, Frank CB, Yeadon MR. Elongation and forces of ankle ligaments in a physiological range of motion. *Foot Ankle Int* 1990;11:30–40.
13. Woo S L-Y, An K-N, Arnoczky SP, Wayne JS, Fitian DC, Myers BS. Anatomy, biology, and biomechanics of tendon, ligament, and meniscus. In: Simon SR, ed. *Orthopaedic basic science*. American Academy of Orthopaedic Surgeons. Park Ridge: IL, 1994:45–88.

14. Hawkins D. Ligament biomechanics. In: Grabiner MD, ed. *Current issues in biomechanics.* Champaign, IL: Human Kinetics Publishers, 1993:123–150.

15. Kennedy JC, Hawkins RJ, Willis RB, Danylchuk KD. Tension studies of human knee ligaments: yield point, ultimate failure, and disruption of the cruciate and tibila collateral ligaments. *J Bone Joint Surg* 1976;58:350–5.

16. Cawley PW, France EP. Biomechanics of the lateral ligaments of the ankle: an evaluation of the effects of axial load and single plane motions on ligament strain patterns. *Foot Ankle Int* 1991;12:92–99.

17. Lutter LD, Mizel MS, Pfeffer GB. *Foot and Ankle:* Orthopaedic Knowledge Update. American Academy of Orthopaedic Surgeons, Rosemont: IL 1994, pp. 241–253.

18. Burks RT, Morgan J. Anatomy of the lateral ankle ligaments. *Am J Sports Med* 1994;22:72–77.

19. Peters JW, Trevino SG, Renstrom PA. Chronic lateral ankle instability. *Foot Ankle* 1994;12:182–191.

20. Lieber RL. *Skeletal muscle structure and function:* implications for rehabilitation and sports medicine. Baltimore: Williams & Wilkins, 1992, pp. 54–63.

21. Brostrom L. Sprained ankles. VI. Surgical treatment of "chronic" ligament ruptures. *Acta Chir Scand* 1966;132: 551–565.

22. Brostrom L. Sprained ankles. I. Anatomic lesions in recent sprains. *Acta Chir Scand* 1964;128:483–495.

23. Cetti R. Conservative treatment of injury to the fibular ligaments of the ankle. *Br J Sports Med* 1982;16:47–52.

24. Vaes P, De BH, Handelberg F, et al. Comparative radiologic study of the influence of ankle joint bandages on ankle stability. *Am J Sports Med* 1985;13:46–50.

25. Kay DB. The sprained ankle: current therapy. *Foot Ankle Int* 1985;6:22–28.

26. Zwipp H, Schievink B. Primary orthotic treatment of ruptured ankle ligaments: a recommended procedure. *Prosthet Orthot Int* 1992;16:49–56.

27. Shapiro MS, Kabo JM, Mitchell PW, et al. Ankle sprain prophylaxis: an analysis of the stabilizing effects of braces and tape. *Am J Sports Med* 1994;22:78–82.

28. Anderson DL, Sanderson DJ, Hennig EM. The role of external nonrigid ankle bracing in limiting ankle inversion. *Clin J Sport Med* 1995;5:18–24.

29. Seto JL, Brewster CE. Treatment approaches following foot and ankle injury. *Clin Sports Med* 1994;13:695–718.

30. Andriacchi T, Sabiston P, DeHaven K, et al. Ligament: injury and repair. In: Woo SLY, Buckwalter JA, eds. *Injury and repair of musculoskeletal soft tissues.* Park Ridge, IL: American Academy of Orthopaedic Surgeons, 1987:103–128.

31. Yeung MS, Chan KM, So CH, et al. An epidemiological survey on ankle sprain. *Br J Sports Med* 1994;28: 112–116.

32. Enoka RM. *Neuromechanical basis of kinesiology.* Champaign, IL: Human Kinetics Publishers, 1988, pp. 134–143.

33. Freeman MAR, Dean MRE, Hanham IMF. The etiology and prevention of functional instability of the foot. *J Bone Joint Surg Br* 1965;47B:678–685.

34. Tropp H, Odenrick P, Gillquist J. Stabilometry recordings in functional and mechanical instability of the ankle joint. *Int J Sports Med* 1985;6:180–182.

35. Tropp H, Ekstrand J, Gillquist J. Factors affecting stabilometry recordings of single limb stance. *Am J Sports Med* 1984;12:185–188.

36. Tropp H, Ekstrand J, Gillquist J. Stabilometry in functional instability of the ankle and its value in predicting injury. *Med Sci Sports Exer* 1984;16:64–66.

37. Fridén T, Zätterström R, Lindstrand A, Moritz U. A stabilometric technique for evaluation of lower limb instabilities. *Am J Sports Med* 1989;17:118–122.

38. Golie PA, Evans EM, Bach TM. Postural control following inversion injuries in the ankle. *Arch Phys Med Rehabil* 1994;75:969–975.

39. Pintsaar A, Brynhildsen J, Tropp H. Postural corrections after standardized perturbations of single limb stance: effect of training and orthotic devices in patients with ankle instabiltiy. *Br J Sports Med* 1996;30:151–155.

40. Boruta PM, Bishop JO, Braly WG, Tullos HS. Acute lateral ankle ligament injuries: a literature review. *Foot Ankle Int* 1990;11:107–113.

41. Ozaki T, Mizuno K, Grabiner MD. Peroneus longus cannot be fully activated during ankle complex exercises by uninjured subjects. To be published in *The Kobe Journal of Medical Sciences*, Vol. 45, no. 3, 1999.

42. National Research Council, Steering Committee for the Workshop on Work-related Musculoskeletal Injuries. *Work-Related Musculoskeletal Disorders.* Committee on Human Factors, National Academy Press, Washington, D.C., 1998, pp. 9–11.

Occupational Musculoskeletal Disorders
edited by T. G. Mayer, R. J. Gatchel, and P. B. Polatin.
Lippincott Williams & Wilkins, Philadelphia © 2000.

10

Relevance of Biomechanics in Occupational Musculoskeletal Disorders

A. Kim Burton and *Chris J. Main

Spinal Research Unit, University of Huddersfield, Queensgate, Huddersfield HD1 3DH, United Kingdom; *Department of Behavioural Medicine, Hope Hospital, Scott Lane, Salford M6 8HD, United Kingdom

The term *occupational musculoskeletal disorder* (OMD) covers a wide spectrum, from trivial aches and pains related in some way to work, to significant injury (and possibly irreparable damage). No doubt, OMDs (in the broad sense) are extremely common in the workforce of industrialized nations, but so too are identical syndromes among nonworkers. This situation presents a challenge for both epidemiology and clinical or workplace management. It is exceedingly difficult to substantiate relationships with work in complaints that are highly prevalent among the population at large, and it is similarly difficult to relate them to specific aspects of work. The results of epidemiologic surveys, which have tended to form the basis of our understanding of OMDs, are dictated by the various definitions of what is being studied, which has led to some measure of obfuscation and inappropriate patterns of response both by scientists and society.

It is axiomatic that OMDs are an increasing problem for industrialized societies, and serious concern has been expressed about the fact that the problem shows no sign of diminishing, despite the substantial efforts of a considerable body of scientists (1–6). It is a commonly held tenet that physically demanding work must, in some way, be at the root of most OMDs and that control can be achieved through minimization of the physical forces (whether they be dynamic or static) that are inherent in work. This tenet, attractive as it may be, seemingly is in the process of being contradicted; despite a couple of decades in which workloads have been decreased, there is little sign of the problem lessening.

This chapter does not set out to offer a systematic review; rather, it takes as its starting point the stand that "somewhere along the line we must have got it wrong" and examines a selection of the literature to test the injury concept and seek alternative mechanisms to explain the phenomenon of OMDs. Much of what is presented relates to the low back, the area for which there is most evidence, but it is becoming apparent that other OMDs have much in common with low back trouble (7,8).

EPIDEMIOLOGIC INCONSISTENCIES

A recent National Institute of Occupational Safety and Health (NIOSH) publication (9) that reviewed the evidence on musculoskeletal disorders and physical workplace factors concluded that strong evidence exists for increased risk of work-related musculoskeletal disorders for some body parts (back, neck, upper limbs); but the fact remains that most workers do not succumb. It was also pointed out that all these disorders can be caused by nonwork exposures. The focus was largely on the relationship between the work exposures and the presence of the disorders; the issue of disability and workloss was not the purpose of the review. The corollary of the findings is that prevention and control can be achieved by reducing physical exposures at the workplace.

Is there a rationale for reducing mechanical stress on the musculoskeletal system, or is mechanical stress both necessary and beneficial? This question is stimulated by the discrepancy that has emerged between the differing approaches advocated by clinicians and nonclinicians. On the one hand, ergonomists, biomechanists, and legislators strive to reduce exposure to physical stress at the workplace, whereas clinicians incorporate physical challenges to the musculoskeletal system in their rehabilitation programs (10,11).

There is a simple history of how this dichotomy developed. The concept of work being detrimental to the musculoskeletal system became established around the middle of the nineteenth century when the social movement in Europe pressed for policies to provide monetary compensation for injured workers. Although originally focused on obvious maiming injuries, the concept of compensation for those who developed musculoskeletal problems gradually developed; but to receieve compensation, the worker had to have a disorder that was due to an "injury." It would seem that laymen and the medical profession inadvertently colluded to promote a simple injury model. This model, suggesting that exposure to physical stress can result in tissue damage and that further exposure will lead to further damage and eventually result in disability, is intuitively reasonable. Consequently, elements in society have striven to reduce the physical stress of work, and clinicians initially were encouraged to cooperate by prescribing rest and avoidance as the treatment of choice for these purported injuries. As the failure of this strategy became apparent, clinical research turned to strenuous active rehabilitation strategies, for which there is evidence of benefit (12,13). To understand the relevance of biomechanics in OMDs requires a critical exploration of evidence from a variety of perspectives.

The literature contains numerous inconsistencies about the nature of OMDs, their risk factors, pathology, and management. It is known that low back pain in adolescents has a prevalence approximating 50% by age 16, which is not much different from that found in working-age adults; but few adults, on questioning, will admit a history of low back trouble before the age of 18 years (14). Presumably, the adolescent experience is not sufficiently intrusive to become memorable, perhaps because back pain in children is rarely accompanied by disability (15). The lifetime prevalence of adult back pain (based on clinically reported cases) is about 59%, with a 1-month prevalence of the order of 40%; there is little obvious relationship to occupational physical stressors, but there is a slightly higher prevalence with advancing age (16). A 1996 random population survey in the United Kingdom found an annual prevalence of 40% for back pain lasting more than a day, with no difference between genders; the point prevalence was 15%. The symptoms started before the 12-month period for 80% of people, and 16% said they had had symptoms for the whole year. Care seeking during the previous 12 months was reported by 46%, with female patients more likely to seek care (17), a feature mirrored in the clinical survey (16).

There is no scarcity of industrial epidemiologic studies finding a relationship between work that stresses the spine and the prevalence of back symptoms (9), but this is not a universal finding (18,19). Similarly, occupations that place stress on the upper limbs have been shown to be related to high levels of self-reported upper-limb symptoms (20), but other jobs that involve substantial upper-limb use do not show the presupposed high levels of upper-limb disorders (8). A study of construction workers did find a dose-response relationship between severe low back pain and stooping and kneeling, but back pain in general was associated more with a range of psychosocial parameters (21). It would appear that some jobs entailing low spinal stress (such as clerical work) can have similar prevalence rates for low back pain as found in blue-collar work (22). The neck is not subjected to the same loading patterns as the low back, but the prevalence of cervical symptoms is similar to that of lumbar symptoms (23).

Further inconsistency is found when looking at physical spinal stress from whole-body vibration (WBV). The high-vibration environment of racing cars has been linked specifically with back symptoms (24), and a study of police officers in the United Kingdom found long-term driving to be a hazard for back pain (25), but this finding was not confirmed in a study of Canadian police officers (26). Neck pain, as well as back pain, has been related to urban transit driving, but the higher prevalence among female drivers could not be explained by ergonomic factors. A combination of WBV and heavy or frequent lifting by occupational drivers carries a higher risk for back pain than either factor alone (27), but higher risk from combinations of risk factors is not always reported (25).

When looking at work loss, about 5% of workers took absence for back pain in the 4 weeks prior to a national survey, whereas for all respondents, downtime in the preceding 4 weeks was reported by 8%; both absence and downtime were for only a few days for about three quarters of people (17). Heavy jobs are associated with increased work loss resulting from low back pain (28), although that increase may be due to longer spells rather than to more spells (29). The association between heavy work and absence rates is not, however, a consistent finding (30). Where WBV has been seen to be related to symptoms, work loss was related to psychosocial factors (i.e., distress and work stress) rather than physical aspects of the work (25,27). This finding gains some support from a study of office workers that showed absence resulting from back pain was inversely related to employment grade (reflecting psychological job stress) (22).

A recent national survey of the UK labor force looked at self-reported work-related disorders (31) and revealed that musculoskeletal disorders far outweighed any other category. Lower back symptoms dominated (55% of those reporting musculoskeletal symptoms), followed closely by neck and upper limb symptoms (44%); interestingly, the next highest category was stress, depression, or anxiety.

ATTRIBUTION OF CAUSE

Nearly 80% of those in the UK survey with musculoskeletal symptoms identified a work task (or set of tasks) as leading to their complaint (31). For low back pain, the most commonly perceived causes were manual handling (66%) and posture (33%), whereas for upper limbs and neck, it was repetitive work (38%) and manual handling (37%). Workload or pace and lack of support were implicated as causative in the stress category. Surprisingly, attribution to work did not decline substantially for symptoms starting after ceasing to work (except for stress), a finding noted previously in Swedish shipyard workers (32). In the UK population survey (which was not confined to workers), men were more likely than women to attribute back pain to their job (30% versus 18%) (17); it is uncertain whether this finding reflects differing perceptions on attribution or whether the women had less strenuous jobs. Low back pain attributed to work has been reported to be more common in female nurses than in female teachers, but nonoccupationally attributed back pain had the same prevalence in both groups (33). Worker ratings of job-required physical abilities may be correlated with back injury rates (34); but, because both parameters are subject to possible reporting bias, the relationship may, in part, represent subjective attribution. Confounding of physical workload with psychosocial workload has been shown among various branches of agricultural work with differing prevalence rates, rendering clear identification of risk factors difficult (35).

Although workers frequently relate their symptoms and disorders to characteristics of their work, the question presented is, Are they physically connected with work (and, if so, how)? Should the symptoms result in disability? Or are symptoms largely a consequence of being a human in modern times?

WORK AND DAMAGE

It can be expected that a high proportion of workers will believe that their work has, in some way, damaged them, a belief fostered by society in various ways (36); but are workers likely to sustain substantial damage from typical work systems?

The structure presumed at greatest risk for damage from heavy work (including WBV) is the intervertebral disc, which has been the subject of major investigation. Whereas it has been indicated that heavy work is associated with lumbar disc degeneration (37,38), much may depend on the measurement methods, imaging techniques, and population studied. Recent investigation involving multivariable statistical techniques confirmed that disc degeneration, as measured by magnetic resonance imaging (MRI), is influenced only modestly by work history; the greatest proportion of the explained variance in degeneration scores can be accounted for by genetic influences, but age does exert some influence (39).

Disc herniations (as opposed to generalized degenerative changes) theoretically can be associated with work activities involving flexion and torsion (40), but this hypothesis remains to be confirmed epidemiologically in occupational settings. Of some interest is that similar movements by fast bowlers in cricket are associated with disc disruption (41). The clinical presence of disc herniations, however, is poorly correlated both with symptoms and physical stress. Disc herniations were found in 76% of an asymptomatic control group (matched for age, sex, and work-related factors), compared with 96% in a symptomatic group. The presence of symptoms was related to neural compromise and psychosocial aspects of work but not to exposure to physical stressors (42).

Primary mechanical overload damage to the discs and vertebral bodies (as opposed to disc herniations or degenerative changes) are

to be expected from *in vitro* studies (43), assuming the normal biologic repair processes do not obscure the evidence (44). The predicted irreparable overload damage has now been confirmed *in vivo* but only for extreme physical tasks of the sort that rarely are found in modern workplaces (45). This radiologic study, which compared cohorts exposed to strenuous physical work with a normative database, demonstrated that heavy manual labor and WBV do not result in damage to vertebral bodies (except two cohorts exposed to work in flexed postures). Overload damage to discs was associated with two types of work exposure that involved handling heavy objects, especially in confined spaces, or driving vehicles with totally unsprung seats. Cohorts doing work that was broadly covered by existing manual handling guidelines did not display signs of overload damage. The study could not specifically address symptomatology, but fortuitous data concerning two of the cohorts studied suggest that there is no simple relation between overload damage and symptoms. Indeed, severe trauma leading to vertebral body fractures, such as can happen in ejection from military aircraft, may present few, if any, symptoms; even when symptoms do ensue, recovery can be relatively swift, with no lasting disability or reduced effectiveness (46).

Of course, structures other than vertebrae and discs (i.e., muscles and ligaments) may be injured (40), but for the most part we do not have objective means for detecting such damage. We might expect, from fields such as sports medicine, that muscle and ligament injuries (in the absence of complete rupture) generally resolve in 4 to 8 weeks. Perhaps 85% of those taking time off from work because of back trouble will have returned to work during that time (47), but a sizeable number remains for whom an obvious physiological explanation for persisting disability is lacking. Current knowledge is insufficient, in the vast majority of cases, for accurate identification of the structure or structures that are "injured" or the extent to which they might be injured. New modeling techniques suggest that spine stability is closely related to muscle activity, such that deficient intrinsic spine muscles or a lack of motor control may reduce the mechanical stability of the spine and increase the risk of straining muscles or ligaments (48). On balance, the evidence shows that the back certainly can be injured in various ways (whether at work or leisure), but the injury model lacks explanatory power where prolonged disability is concerned.

WORK SYMPTOMS—DISABILITY

The biomechanical approach to the identification of occupational risk factors for low back trouble (LBT) has shifted from static models of spinal loading to dynamic models that use accelerations and velocity to estimate forces acting on the spine (49), whereas other models incorporate muscle synergy and co-contraction patterns (50). Evidence for a link between dynamic lifting and LBT has been available for some time (51), and more recently this parameter has been linked to epidemiologic findings with quantitative biomechanical findings in a large working population (52). A multiple logistic regression model revealed that a combination of five trunk motion and workplace factors distinguished between high and low risk; the factors were lifting frequency, load moment, trunk lateral velocity, trunk-twisting velocity, and trunk sagittal angle. The outcome variable (i.e., risk of LBT) was derived from medical and injury records, which admittedly suffer from confounding effects of reporting bias and inadequate information about previous trouble. When looking at worker-rated job demands (including ratings of dynamic components) and back injury rates, it is apparent that high-risk jobs can have quite diverse demands (i.e., not all jobs with high injury rates require the same physical abilities) (49). A study of nurses in Belgium and The Netherlands, using a quasiobjective rating system for task demands, showed a significantly lower prevalence of OMDs in the Dutch nurses, despite the fact that their average workload was substantially greater than their Belgian counter-

parts. Overall, symptoms and work loss in the previous 12 months were not related to workload, nor was attribution that work was causative. What was significant was that the Dutch nurses differed from the Belgian nurses on a range of psychosocial variables; they were significantly more positive about pain, work, and activity and reported less depressive symptoms (53).

It is known that a previous history of back pain is highly predictive of future episodes (18,54,55); therefore, it might be more illuminating to investigate the relationship between occupational physical stressors and first-time back injury rather than to use prevalence rates. Videman and colleagues (56) studied nursing aides and trained nurses and found that young nursing aides (with high workloads but low likelihood of previous LBT history) had a higher prevalence than the trained nurses, suggesting that skill and training may be important; it also was noted that the aides tended to have children at an earlier age. Thus, domestic spinal loading was possibly a confounding influence. Although the annual incidence rate of LBT in nurses is higher than in teachers, the annual prevalence and point prevalence rates were the same (57). Experienced industrial workers show a reduced risk for LBT compared with inexperienced workers, but this difference is not necessarily because they experience reduced spinal loads; rather, their smoother motions may be related to muscular coordination aiding spinal stability (58).

PSYCHOSOCIAL INFLUENCES

A large general population study (59) found that new episodes of LBT are more likely for those who are psychologically distressed, a relationship that held true even for first onsets. In the large prospective study at the Boeing plant (55), reported first injuries were not related specifically to job demands but rather to psychosocial factors; the workers, however, worked in an environment in which job tasks were not particularly stressful on the back. Some clarification of the issue could emerge from the study of first onsets in workers exposed to the same substantial physical stressors over long periods. Police officers in Northern Ireland compulsorily wear body armor (weighing >8 kg) for up to 12 hours per day; they do so irrespective of rank and return to the same work on recovery from back trouble. This police force was compared with an English police force that did not wear armor. The physical stress of wearing body armor reduced survival time to first onset, and over time the hazard increased slightly. The proportion of officers with persistent (chronic) back complaints did not depend on the length of exposure (to the same stressors) following first onset; rather, chronicity was associated with psychosocial factors (such as distress and blaming work) (25).

A study that examined musculoskeletal symptoms among supermarket cashiers used a multivariable model to seek factors related to symptom reports. Factors related to work equipment and work tasks had little relationship with symptom prevalence compared with age and distress and, particularly, dissatisfaction with the work. The dissatisfaction was not targeted to physical matters such as work equipment; rather, dissatisfaction with anything at work had the same association. Reported severity and disability had the same strong association with distress and dissatisfaction but not with the physical parameters (8).

An enhanced instrument, the Psychosocial Aspects of Work questionnaire, has been described. This questionnaire separately evaluates job satisfaction, social support, and mental stress (60). It has been possible to show that workers with current low back pain have a lower score for job satisfaction and social support, but absenteeism (60) and physical demands of the work (53) were not related to these parameters. Although attitudes about work itself may not influence absenteeism, other attitudes and beliefs seem relevant. Psychosocial factors, such as negative beliefs about the inevitable consequences of LBT (measured by the Back Beliefs Questionnaire) (60), inadequate pain-control strategies (60),

fear-avoidance beliefs (61), and belief that work was causative (25) have been found to relate to absenteeism. The relationship between attribution of cause, job satisfaction, and pain perception is complex and, in part, related to job level; matters related to attribution in particular are believed to be important influences on compliance with intervention strategies (62). Educational intervention that steers workers away from inappropriate attribution can be effective in reducing absenteeism. Workplace broadcasting of a simple educational pamphlet (stressing the benign nature of LBT, the importance of activity, and the desirability of early work return) has been shown to be capable of creating a positive shift in beliefs with a concomitant reduction in extended sickness absence (63).

RETURN TO WORK

The question of when and how to return workers with LBT to their job is an important consideration. A popular belief states that too early a return to the same task would risk recurrence of symptoms (or do further damage). Indeed, back-injured workers may perceive their back problem as lifelong trouble and believe that their back injury has made them more vulnerable to reinjury and disability (64). There is accumulating evidence that such beliefs are probably erroneous. A large prospective study of employees in various industries found that recurrence of symptoms was common; a figure of 44% in the first year dropped to 31% in the second year. It was suggested that recurrence rates may be more a feature of the natural history of the disorder than a reflection of continued exposure to the work environment (65). Support for this notion has come from other studies involving multivariable analyses, which have found little relationship between recurrence and work demands (18,54,55). Bearing in mind the role of psychosocial factors (including inappropriate attribution), it has been suggested that the concept of reinjury may be a misconception (55).

A recent review concluded that returning workers to modified work is a successful strategy (in terms of actual return and reduction of lost workdays). If workers believe work has been the cause of their problem (or that they are vulnerable), it is understandable that modified work programs can have success, but a real need for modified work can be questioned. The use of work restrictions does not necessarily correlate with reduced symptoms following return to work. A 3-year follow-up of reported occupational musculoskeletal injuries (including LBT) found that those for whom workloads had been reduced did not report fewer problems (66). In fact, a successful rehabilitation program for patients with subchronic back pain has advocated early return to unrestricted duties as part of a combined graded activity/behavioral therapy approach (67). Prospective study of even the most severe chronic disabling spinal disorder workers' compensation patients who completed a functional restoration program and returned to work found that they were at relatively low risk for recurrence (68). The study of working police officers revealed that change of duties after developing LBT was rare, and persistence of symptoms was unrelated to the length of exposure (to the same physical stressors at work) following first onset (25).

Even when there is known damage to lumbar structures, activity restriction seems not to be an absolute necessity. A prospective study of patients operated for lumbar disc herniation who were urged to return to full activity as soon as possible showed that the mean return to work time was 1.7 weeks with 25% returning within 1 to 2 days. Almost all patients returned to their previous jobs and had returned to full work by 8 weeks; no patient changed job because of symptoms, and only 6% had a recurrence during follow-up averaging some 4 years (69). Clinical studies in workers' compensation back pain patients found that delayed functional recovery was associated with psychosocial factors more than with perceived task demand (70) and that longer spells away from work were associated with a poor outcome (71).

The impact of ergonomics in primary prevention is limited (72) and largely anecdotal

(73). Where secondary prevention is concerned, the importance of personnel issues (as opposed to ergonomics intervention) are being recognized (74). A large industrial study found that ergonomic solutions failed to reduce lost workdays and that reliance on case monitoring and wellness orientation actually increased work loss. Diligent safety programs and an emphasis on systematic return-to-work programs did reduce lost workdays (75). Similarly, a comparison of a personnel program (designed to increase communication between claimants and their employer, their doctor, and the Workers' Compensation Board) with a back program (designed to reduce back injuries through intensive feedback training) found that it was the personnel program that was by far the most effective (76). The subject is complex, and it remains to be determined whether the obstacles to return to work are predominantly at the individual level or whether organizational issues are more relevant.

OBSTACLES TO RECOVERY

Sufficient evidence now exists to challenge seriously the power of a simple injury/damage model to explain the current phenomenon of occupational back trouble; the same is probably true for other OMDs. Biomechanics may help to explain some initial injury mechanisms but contributes little to our understanding of recurrence or persisting trouble. Epidemiology can link certain working practices to reported symptoms but rarely to objective injury, and it would seem that it is only extremely strenuous work that can result in irreparable overload damage (at least insofar as the spine is concerned). Thus, one might reasonably expect virtually all OMDs, by virtue of known physiological processes, to resolve within a reasonably short time without leading to marked disability. The fact that many workers do not recover rapidly probably has little to do with the nature of the purported injury.

The reluctance to confront normal physical challenges seen in back-disabled workers has been termed *activity intolerance*, which is variously linked to the individual response to pain, the belief that a specific injury must be the cause of the pain, and behavioral roles such as suffering. This led to the proposal that treatment and financial benefits should not, in general, be pain contingent but rather time-contingent such that there is a clear incentive to return to work within an allotted time (77). Such a proposal may seem rather draconian and may well be suboptimal without first addressing other issues that can act as obstacles to recovery or return to work. It has been advocated that workplaces should be comfortable when we are well and accommodating when we are ill (78), but the words *comfort* and *accommodating* should be taken to encompass the milieu of psychosocial influences (both individual and occupational).

SUMMARY

This chapter attempted to illustrate, albeit briefly, that our dismal record for understanding and managing OMDs may, in large part, be due to adherence to an incomplete and partially false conceptualization of the phenomenon. We suggest that medical concepts of prevention and cure are inappropriate (and unrealistic); attention should shift to an acceptance that people will hurt no matter what we do. Our honest response should be to invoke a paradigm shift and concentrate on the removal of obstacles to recovery.

These obstacles seem to fall into three basic categories: medical, ergonomic, and psychosocial (7). Accumulating evidence indicates that the first two categories exert a modest influence compared with the third, but it is apparent that these psychosocial variables constitute a heterogeneous category. Certain clinical psychosocial *yellow flags* (79) can alert the clinician to a risk for chronicity (80). These essentially psychological parameters, such as distress, depression, coping strategies, and beliefs, will operate alongside a number of work-related obstacles that might be termed *blue flags*. These include individual worker-specific factors such as attribution of blame, beliefs about the work/injury relationship, and psychosocial aspects of work, in addition to work-specific issues such as managerial attitudes, return-to-work policies, work organization, and perceived work demands. The need to consider such factors in designing effective secondary intervention programs has been recognized (7), but the immediate challenge is to discover precisely how the yellow flags and blue flags interact to present obstacles to recovery; only when these interactions are understood can optimal interventions be formulated.

REFERENCES

1. Nachemson AL. Low back pain in the industrial world. In: Aspden RM, eds. *Lumbar spine disorders.* Chesterfield, UK: Arthritis & Rheumatism Council for Research, 1996:1–5.
2. Waddell G. Nordin M, Vischer TL, eds. Biopsychosocial analysis of low back pain. *Common low back pain: prevention of chronicity.* London: *Baillieres Clin Rheumatol* 1992;6:523–557.
3. Bigos SJ, Battié MC, Weinstein JN, Wiesel SW, eds. Industrial low back pain: risk factors. In: *The lumbar spine.* Philadelphia: WB Saunders, 1990:846–859.
4. Winkel J, Westgaard RH. Editorial: a model for solving work related musculoskeletal problems in a profitable way. *Applied Ergonomics* 1996;27:71–78.
5. Burton AK. Back injury and work loss: biomechanical and psychosocial influences. *Spine* 1997;22: 2575–2580.
6. Hadler NM. Arm pain in the workplace: a small area analysis. *J Occup Med* 1992;34:113–119.
7. Feuerstein M, Huang GD. Preventing disability in patients with occupational musculoskeletal disorders. *American Pain Society Bulletin* 1998;8:9–11.
8. Mackay C, Burton K, Boocock M, et al. *Musculoskeletal disorders in supermarket cashiers.* London: HSE Books, 1998.
9. Bernard BP, ed. *Musculoskeletal disorders and workplce factors:* a critical review of epidemiologic evidence for work-related musculoskeletal disorders of the neck, upper-extremity, and low back. Cincinnati: NIOSH, 1997:1-1.
10. Mayer T, Gatchel R. *Functional restoration for spinal disorders:* the sports medicine approach. Philadelphia: Lea & Febiger, 1988.
11. Lindstrom I, Ohlund C, Eek C, et al. The effect of graded activity on patients with subacute low back pain: a randomized prospective clinical study with an operant-conditioning behavioural approach. *Phys Ther* 1992;72:279–290.
12. Kohles S, Barnes D, Gatchel RJ, Mayer TG. Improved physical performance outcomes after functional restoration treatment in patients with chronic low-back pain: early versus recent training results. *Spine* 1990;15: 1321–1324.
13. Bendix AF, Bendix T, Ostenfeld S, Bush E, Andersen A.

Active treatment programs for patients with chronic low back pain: a prospective, randomized, observer-blinded study. *Eur Spine J* 1995;4:148–152.

14. Burton AK, Clarke RD, McClune TD, Tillotson KM. The natural history of low-back pain in adolescents. *Spine* 1996;21:2323–2328.

15. Burton AK. *Patterns of lumbar sagittal mobility and their predictive value in the natural history of back and sciatic pain* [Doctoral Thesis]. Huddersfield Polytechnic/CNAA, 1987.

16. Papageorgiou AC, Croft PR, Ferry S, Jayson MIV, Silman AJ. Estimating the prevalence of low back pain in the general population: evidence from the South Manchester Back Pain Survey. *Spine* 1995;20:1889–1894.

17. Dodd T. *The prevalence of back pain in Great Britain in 1996*. London: The Stationery Office, 1997.

18. Burton AK, Tillotson KM, Troup JDG. Prediction of low-back trouble frequency in a working population. *Spine* 1989;14:939–946.

19. Spengler DM, Bigos SJ, Martin NA, Zeh J, Fisher L, Nachemson A. Back injuries in industry: a retrospective study. I. Overview and cost analysis. *Spine* 1986;11: 241–245.

20. Williams NR, Dickinson CE. Musculoskeletal complaints in lock assemblers, testers and inspectors. *Occup Environ Med* 1997;47:479–484.

21. Holmstrom EB, Lindell J, Mortiza U. Low back and neck/shoulder pain in construction workers: occupational workload and psychosocial risk factors. Part 2: Relationship to neck and shoulder pain. *Spine* 1992;17:672–667.

22. Hemingway H, Shipley MJ, Stansfield S, Marmot M. Sickness absence from back pain, psychosocial work characteristics and employment grade among office workers. *Scand J Work Environ Health* 1997;23: 121–129.

23. Cote P, Cassidy JD, Carroll L. The Saskatchewan Health and Back Pain Survey: the prevalence of neck pain and related disability in Saskatchewan adults. *Spine* 1998; 23:1689–1698.

24. Burton AK, Sandover J. Back pain in Grand Prix drivers: a 'found' experiment. *Applied Ergonomics* 1987; 18:3–8.

25. Burton AK, Tillotson KM, Symonds TL, Burke C, Mathewson T. Occupational risk factors for the first-onset of low back trouble: a study of serving police officers. *Spine* 1996;21:2612–2620.

26. Brown JJ, Wells GA, Trottier AJ, Bonneau J, Ferris B. Back pain in a large Canadian police force. *Spine* 1998; 23:821–827.

27. Magnusson ML, Pope MH, Wilder DG, Areskoug B. Are occupational drivers at an increased risk for developing musculoskeletal disorders? *Spine* 1996;21:710–717.

28. Riihimaki H, Tola S, Videman T, Hanninen K. Low-back pain and occupation. A cross-sectional questionnaire study of men in machine operating, dynamic physical work, and sedentary work. *Spine* 1989;14: 204–209.

29. Andersson GBJ, Svensson H, Oden A. The intensity of work recovery in low back pain. *Spine* 1983;8:880–804.

30. Lindstrom I, Ohlund C, Nachemson A. Validity of patient reporting and predictive value of industrial physical work demands. *Spine* 1994;19:888–893.

31. Jones JR; Hodgson JT; Clegg TA, et al. *Self-reported work-related illness in 1995:* results from a household survey. London: HSE Books, 1998.

32. Berg M, Sanden A, Torell G, Jarvholm B. Persistence of muscuoloskeletal symptoms: a longitudinal study. *Ergonomics* 1988;31:1281–1285.

33. Cust G, Pearson JCG, Mair A. The prevalence of low back pain in nurses. *Int Nurs Rev* 1972;19:169–79.

34. Skovron ML, Nordin M, Halpern M, et al. Do worker ratings of job-required physical abilities correlate with back injury rates? Heidelberg: ISSLS, 1991.

35. Hildebrandt VH. Musculoskeletal symptoms and workload in 12 branches of Dutch agriculture. *Ergonomics* 1995;18:2576–2587.

36. Hadler NM. Workers with disabling back pain. *N Engl J Med* 1997;337:341–343.

37. Kellgren JH. Osteoarthrosis in patients and populations. *BMJ* 1961;July:1–6.

38. Riihimaki H, Mattison T, Zitting A, Wickstrom G, Hanninen K, Waris P. Radiologically detectable changes of the lumbar spine among concrete reinforcement workers and house painters. *Spine* 1990;15: 114–123.

39. Battié MC, Videman T, Gibbons L, Fisher L, Manninen H, Gill K. Determinants of lumbar disc degeneration: a study relating lifetime exposures and MRI findings in identical twins. *Spine* 1995;20:2601–2612.

40. Adams MA, Dolan P. Recent advances in lumbar spinal mechanics and their clinical significance. *Clin Biomech* 1995;10:3–19.

41. Elliott BC, Davis JW, Khangure MS, Hardcastle P, Foster D. Disc degeneration and the young fast bowler in cricket. *Clin Biomech* 1993;8:227–234.

42. Boos N, Reider V, Schade K, Spratt N, Semmer M, Aebi M. The diagnostic accuracy of magnetic resonance imaging, work perception, and psychosocial factors in identifying symptomatic disc herniations. *Spine* 1995; 20:2613–2625.

43. Brinckmann P, Biggemann M, Hilweg D. Fatigue fracture of human lumbar vertebrae. *Clin Biomech* 1988; 3(Suppl 1):S1–S23

44. Brinckmann P. Pathology of the vertebral column. *Ergonomics* 1985;28:77–80.

45. Brinckmann P, Frobin W, Biggemann M, Tillotson M, Burton K. Quantification of overload injuries to thoracolumbar vertebrae and discs in persons exposed to heavy physical exertions or vibration at the work-place. Part II. Occurrence and magnitude of overload injury in exposed cohorts. *Clin Biomech* 1998;13(Suppl 2): S(2)1–S(2)36.

46. Laurell L, Nachemson A. Some factors influencing spinal injuries in seat ejected pilots. *Aerospace Medicine* 1963;7:726–729.

47. Clinical Standards Advisory Group. *Epidemiology review:* the epidemiology and cost of back pain. London: HMSO, 1994.

48. Cholewicki J, McGill SM. Mechanical stability of the *in vivo* lumbar spine: implications for injury and chronic low back pain. *Clin Biomech* 1996;11:1–15.

49. Halpern M, Nordin M, Vischer TL, eds. *Common low back pain:* prevention of chronicity. London: Bailliere Tindall, vol 9, *Prevention of low back pain:* basic ergonomics in the workplace and clinic, 1992:705–730.

50. Cholewicki J, McGill SM, Norman RW. Comparison of muscle forces and joint load from an optimization and EMG assisted lumbar spine model: towards development of a hybrid approach. *J Biomech* 1995;28:321–332.

51. Bigos SJ, Spengler DM, Martin NA, et al. Back injuries

in industry: a retrospective study. II. Injury factors. *Spine* 1986;11:246–251.

52. Marras WS, Lavender SA, Leurgens SE, et al. The role of dynamic three-dimensional trunk motion in occupationally-related low back disorders: the effects of workplace factors trunk position and trunk motion characteristics on risk of injury. *Spine* 1993;18:6117–6128.

53. Burton AK, Symonds TL, Zinzen E, et al. Is ergonomics intervention alone sufficient to limit musculoskeletal problems in nurses? *Occup Environ Med* 1997;47:25–32.

54. Troup JDG, Foreman TK, Baxter CE, Brown D. The perception of back pain and the role of psychophysical tests of lifting capacity. *Spine* 1987;12:645–657.

55. Bigos SJ, Battié MC, Spengler DM, et al. A prospective study of work perceptions and psychosocial factors affecting the report of back injury. *Spine* 1991;16:1–6.

56. Videman T, Numinen T, Tola S, et al. Low back pain in nurses and some loading factors of work. *Spine* 1984;9: 400–404.

57. Leighton DJ, Reilly T. Epidemiological aspects of back pain: the incidence and prevalemce of back pain in nurses compared to the general population. *Occup Environ Med* 1995;45:263–267.

58. Granata KP, Marras WS, Kirking B. 20th Annual Meeting. Georgia Tech, Atlanta, USA: American Society of Biomechanics; 1996; *Influence of experience on lifting kinematics and spinal loading.*

59. Croft PR, Papageorgiou AC, Ferry S, Thomas E, Jayson MIV, Silman AJ. Psychologic distress and low back pain: evidence from a prospective study in the general population. *Spine* 1995;20:2731–2737.

60. Symonds TL, Burton AK, Tillotson KM, Main CJ. Do attitudes and beliefs influence work loss due to low back trouble ? *Occup Environ Med* 1996;46:25–32.

61. Waddell G, Newton M, Henderson I, Somerville D, Main CJ. A fear avoidance belief questionnaire (FABQ) and the role of fear—avoidance beliefs in chronic low back pain and disability. *Pain* 1993;52:157–168.

62. Linton SJ, Warg L. Attributions (beliefs) and job satisfaction associated with back pain in an industrial setting. *Percept Mot Skills* 1993;76:51–62.

63. Symonds TL, Burton AK, Tillotson KM, Main CJ. Absence resulting from low back trouble can be reduced by psychosocial intervention at the work place. *Spine* 1995;20:2738–2345.

64. Tarasuk V, Eakin JM. Back problems are for life: perceived vulnerability and its implications fro chronic disability. *J of Occup Rehab* 1994;4:55–64.

65. Troup JDG, Martin JW, Lloyd DCEF. Back pain in industry—a prospective survey. *Spine* 1981;6:61–69.

66. Kemmlert K, Orelium-Dallner M, Kilbom A, Gamberale F. A three-year follow-up of 195 reported occupational over-exertion injuries. *Scand J Rehabil Med* 1993;25:16–24.

67. Lindstrom I, Ohlund C, Eek C, Wallin L, Peterson L, Nachemson A. Mobility strength and fitness after a graded activity program for patients with subacute low back pain: a randomized prospective clinical study with a behavioral therapy approach. *Spine* 1992;17:641–652.

68. Garcy P, Mayer T, Gatchel RJ. Recurrent or new injury outcomes after return to work in chronic disabling spinal disorders: tertiary preventation efficacy of functional restoration treatment. *Spine* 1996;21:952–959.

69. Carragee EJ, Helms E, O'Sullivan GS. Are postoperative activity restrictions necessary after posterior lumbar discectomy? A prospective study of outcomes in 50 consecutive cases. *Spine* 1996;21:11893–11897.

70. Hadler NM, Carey TS, Garrett J. The influence of indemnification by works' compensation insurance on recovery from acute backache. *Spine* 1995;20:2710–2715.

71. Lancourt J, Kettelhut M. Predicting return to work for lower back pain patients receiving workers compensation. *Spine* 1992;17:629–640.

72. Frank JW, Kerr MS, Brooker AS, et al. Shannon HS, Norman RW, Sullivan TJ, Wells RP. Disability resulting from occupational low back pain: Part I: what do we know about primary prevention? a review of the scientific evidence on prevention before disability begins. *Spine* 1996;21:2908–2917.

73. Smedley J, Coggon D. Will the manual handling regulations reduce the incidence of back disorders? *Occup Environ Med* 1994;44:63–65.

74. Frank JW, Brooker AS, DeMaio SE, et al. Disability resulting from occupational low back pain: Part II: what do we know about secondary prevention? a review of the scientific evidence on prevention after disability begins. *Spine* 1996;21:2918–2929.

75. Hunt A, Habeck R. The Michigan Disabilty Prevention Study. Kalamazoo, Michigan: Upjohn Institute for Employment Research, 1993.

76. Wood DJ. Design and evaluation of a back injury prevention program within a geriatric hospital. *Spine* 1987; 12:77–82.

77. Fordyce WE, ed. *Back pain in the workplace:* management of disability in nonspecific conditions. Seattle: IASP Press, 1995.

78. Hadler NM. Back pain in the workplace. What you lift or how you lift matters far less than whether you lift or when. *Spine* 1997;22:935–940.

79. Kendall NAS, Linton SJ, Main CJ. *Guide to assessing psychological yellow flags in acute low back pain:* risk factors for long-term disability and work loss. Wellington, NZ: Accident Rehabilitation & Compensation Insurance Corporation of New Zealand and the National Health Committee, 1997.

80. Burton AK, Tillotson KM, Main CJ, Hollis S. Psychosocial predictors of outcome in acute and subchronic low back trouble. *Spine* 1995;20:722–728.

PART **III**

Prevention

Occupational Musculoskeletal Disorders
edited by T. G. Mayer, R. J. Gatchel, and P. B. Polatin.
Lippincott Williams & Wilkins, Philadelphia © 2000.

11

Preemployment and Preplacement Screening

William S. Shaw, *Glenn S. Pransky, and †Sharona Hoffman

*Integrated Health Management, Denver, Colorado 80210; *Department of Family and Community
Health, University of Massachusetts Medical School, Worcester, Massachusetts 01655; and
†Case Western Reserve University School of Law, Cleveland, Ohio, 44106-7148*

Evaluating the fitness or risk of employees at the beginning of their employment creates one of the greatest challenges faced by the clinician. Although these evaluations may be the most common types performed by occupational physicians, there is limited scientific support for the efficacy or validity of this practice (1–3). An individual's skills, past experience, attitude, job requirements, and related standards are much more important determinant for the vast majority of hiring decisions. The process of entering or reentering employment is predominantly a nonmedical one. Instances in which physician input is critical to the decision-making process are rare. When these situations occur, physician input may be important to ensure that considerations of personal freedom, work ability, and protection of health and safety are addressed appropriately. In this context, the physician becomes an adjunct to the human resource department. The role of the clinician in the preplacement setting is becoming more complex as a result of scientific and legal developments. The American College of Occupational and Environmental Medicine's Section of Work Fitness and Disability Evaluation summarized some of these challenges in its introduction to the section's function and objectives as follows: "Multiple considerations must be weighed in reaching a conclusion regarding a worker's fitness for duty. We must take into account worker capacity, a job's requirements, medical diagnosis, direct threat implications and ADA [Americans with Disabilities Act] to name just a few. Yet no task is more integral to our practice of occupational medicine than this determination" (4). The physician's role in worker fitness and risk evaluation has been comprehensively reviewed (5).

Often, however, the role of the physician in this context is unclear. Expectations of the various parties (e.g., worker, employer, society) may differ. Under most circumstances, potential conflicts in the preplacement setting occur. The applicant desires the job and has the expectation that he or she can perform the essential functions of the job safely and satisfactorily. The employer needs an employee to perform these functions and has reasons independent of this applicant's health to hire the applicant but seeks to minimize the costs of hiring workers who cannot do the job. If physical problems arise in the course of employment, the financial repercussions may include workers' compensation and group health budgets as well as disruption of productivity. These considerations may motivate employers to avoid any potential risks of future injury to a new hire or to coworkers. Society benefits from full employment of all potential workers. The preplacement examination often becomes the focal point for the tensions inherent in this process.

This chapter attempts to outline some of the considerations clinicians should keep in mind as they perform this routine but important determination; presents a brief history of preemployment medical evaluations; distinguishes between *preemployment* and *preplacement* evaluations; gives an overview of the ADA and its critical impact on this process; and focuses on the preventive goals of this process and explores the techniques used to reach these goals; comments on the scientific support (or lack of it) for specific measures and tests, including efforts used to estimate functional capacity; and explores the practical aspects of and provides recommendations for various approaches. Finally, this chapter comments on the appropriate use and dissemination of information by the clinician.

SCOPE OF PREEMPLOYMENT AND PREPLACEMENT EVALUATIONS

Preemployment and preplacement examinations can be defined as medical evaluations conducted to determine the fitness or risk of a worker in relation to a specific job (6). Preemployment examinations usually are conducted after a job offer has been made. They are intended to determine, through medical evaluation, whether an individual is fit (i.e., capable of performing the task required by the job) and whether the worker poses a risk of injury to self or to others or poses risk of other adverse outcomes. The term *preplacement* is often used instead of *preemployment* to emphasize the timing of the evaluation, that is, after a job offer has been made. These evaluations also may be intended to establish baseline levels of biologic measures, for later comparison, to determine whether significant work-related changes have occurred. They can serve as an opportunity for wellness interventions related to general preventive health issues.

Most evaluations are conducted on workers who are new hires, although many are performed on those who have been out of work because of injury or illness to determine the ability to return to work safely. In these contexts, the examinee is evaluated in relation to a specific job or classification of jobs. Similar evaluations occur in the context of disability evaluations, in which medical evaluators are asked to determine whether impairments exist that lead to inability to perform a range of jobs, or any work at all. In this context, there may not be a specific job under consideration.

These evaluations are common, arguably the most common evaluations in the scope of occupational medicine practice. It is estimated that almost half of the 2.2 million U.S. workers hired each year are subjected to a preplacement medical evaluation (7). More than two million U.S. workers lose a day or more of work due to work-related injuries (8). Their physicians usually are required to make a decision about the appropriate length of work absence, risks involved in returning to work, and need for accommodations. More than half a million formal evaluations of impairment and ability to work are conducted each year within the workers' compensation system (9), and more than a half million medical evaluations of impairment are conducted on applicants for disability payments each year within the U.S. Social Security system alone (10).

HISTORY OF MEDICAL EVALUATIONS OF FITNESS AND RISK

Before the 1900s, medical evaluations of fitness or risk for work were rare, and few citations are found in the medical literature for any reasons to involve medical professionals. Employers simply relied on personal and professional references, past work history, and observations of work performance to determine whether an employee was fit or safe.

During World War I, significant concerns about the spread of contagious disease led to a new program of preinduction medical examinations of new recruits. This program disclosed a number of significant reasons for rejection (e.g., active tuberculosis, limb deformity, chronic illness) as well as reasons that were of more dubious relationship to ability to serve in the armed forces (e.g., flat feet).

The Metropolitan Life Insurance Company began the practice of medical evaluations before issuing policies in the 1920s, with apparent success in identifying those with high risk for early mortality. Most insurers today continue to use similar methods as a routine part of their underwriting process. These programs reinforced the perception that medical evaluators to determine risk accurately. The development and deployment of industrial medical departments throughout all major U.S. corporations in the first quarter of this century provided a milieu for administering physician examinations to many persons applying for work. In 1984, the American Medical Association summarized the objectives for preplacement examinations as follows (11).

To evaluate the medical fitness of individuals to perform their duties without hazard to themselves or fellow workers

To assist employees in the maintenance or improvement of their health

To detect the effects of harmful working conditions and advise corrective measures

To establish a record of the medical condition of the employee at the time of each examination

Questions about the rationale and effectiveness of these evaluations appeared in the medical literature in the early 1970s. Several authors concluded that nonphysicians could perform these evaluations equally effectively. Others suggested that many employers and employees do not benefit from preemployment medical evaluation programs at all (12). The medical community failed to produce a definitive study demonstrating the apparent levels of success and risk avoidance that stimulated interest in these examinations a half century earlier.

In the 1980s, a community of persons with a range of disabilities began to organize, asserting their rights to equal access to all benefits from full participation in society, including work. Advocates perceived the industrial medical clinic and the practice of medical evaluation for fitness to work as "...yet another barrier that disabled individuals face in attempting to secure employment." This sentiment was an important consideration in for-

mulating the proposed ADA in the late 1980s and was clearly reflected in the congressional debate before its passage (13).

The Americans with Disabilities Act (ADA)

The ADA represents a significant legislative attempt to change the scope and nature of preemployment evaluations, although it builds on preexisting federal law. The Rehabilitation Act of 1973 prohibited unreasonable exclusion of disabled persons from governmental employment for more than 15 years before passage of the ADA (14). Title I of the ADA specifically addresses the timing, nature, scope, and use of results of these evaluations and limits the ability of employers to require medical evaluations of those who are already employed. It prohibits disability-based discrimination in all aspects of employment and mandates that medical examinations be conducted only after an offer of employment is made to an applicant. It prohibits employers from rejecting candidates because of concerns about insignificant or uncertain future risks or inability to perform nonessential job functions. Employers are required to maintain the confidentiality of medical information and to provide reasonable accommodations for qualified applicants who have disabilities.

Although the ADA applies to all aspects of employment, many cases brought under the ADA have concerned preemployment medical evaluations. The primary contention has been that the employer wrongly regarded an applicant as disabled and incapable of performing the job or erroneously considered the candidate to be high risk for future injury. In the past, physicians have been inclined to recommend to employers that they not hire applicants based on speculative risks of injury or the costs of accommodation. Under the ADA, incorrect medical advice can result in significant and costly litigation.

The ADA protects a broad range of persons with disabilities. A person with a disability is one with a "physical or mental impairment that substantially limits one or more...major life activities" (15). These are "functions such as caring for oneself, performing manual tasks, walking, seeing, hearing, speaking, breathing, learning, and working" (16). Even if the only life function affected by a disability is the capacity to work, a person is disabled if the employee is significantly restricted in the ability to perform an entire class or range of jobs (17). If an individual's restrictions apply only to a single, specific job, however, he or she may not be disabled with respect to the ability to work. The ADA also covers those who are not actually disabled, but an employer wrongly regarded them as disabled (18). These definitions have been further explored and refined by recent court cases, some of which are discussed herein. Individuals with covered disabilities are protected from discrimination in regard to hiring, advancement, or discharge from employment, compensation, job training, and other terms, conditions, and privileges of employment (19).

Employers may require an applicant to undergo a physical examination before beginning employment, but only after a job has been offered. The reasons for conducting such an evaluation may include medical determination of the ability to meet job performance requirements or medical standards, legal requirements for an examination, identifying risk of employment, establishment of a baseline for subsequent medical surveillance testing, and identification of opportunities to improve the general health of workers (20). The ADA clearly specifies that a medical examination can be conducted only after a *bona fide* offer of employment has been made (21).

The ADA allows an employer to reject a person with a disability if stringent criteria are met. An applicant may be rejected who poses a direct threat to himself, herself, or others in the workplace (22), a disability prevents performance of essential job functions, or where accommodations cannot be made without undue hardship (23). In determining whether an accommodation would impose an undue hardship on an employer, courts consider the

nature and cost of the accommodation, the financial resources and size of the employer, the specific facility involved, and the nature of the employer's operations (24). Physicians should recognize that some accommodations, such as scheduling changes, additional breaks, equipment adjustments, and the purchase of special tools or devices to facilitate job performance, are relatively inexpensive and thus should be provided by employers.

The ADA allows employers to decline hiring a candidate if employment in a particular job would "pose a direct threat to the health or safety of other individuals in the workplace" or to his or her own physical welfare (25). The "direct threat defense" requires a high threshold of proof. Relevant Equal Employment Opportunity Commission (EEOC) regulations provide that in determining whether an individual would pose a direct threat, the factors to be considered include (a) the duration of the risk, (b) the nature and severity of the potential harm, (c) the likelihood that the potential harm will occur, and (d) the imminence of the potential harm (26). A speculative, remote, or purely hypothetical risk is not sufficient to support the existence of a direct threat (27). The courts have that an employer is not justified in rejecting for employment a person whose disability does not constitute a direct threat, regardless of the advice received from an examining physician.

In an important case, a physician advised an airport van line not to hire an obese bus driver because she might not be able to move around swiftly in case of an accident. The conclusion was based on a cursory medical examination and the physician's assessment that the examinee walked slowly and "waddled" as she moved from the waiting room to the examining room, but no test of mobility or agility was performed. The court held that there was no basis to conclude that the employee would constitute a direct threat and that discrimination based on perception of impairment had occurred (28). The involvement of a doctor in the decision-making process did not shield the employer from liability.

In another case, an employer excluded all applicants with asymptomatic abnormalities on low back radiographs because it believed that a substantial risk of significant harm existed. The case was settled with the company agreeing to cease the practice of subjecting all job applicants to low back radiographs, except when specific indications were present. The presence of abnormalities would no longer imply automatic exclusion from a job involving lifting (29).

Other Recent Court Cases Reflecting the ADA

The case cited here, although it defines the law at the time of publication, may not reflect future decisions, especially those from the Supreme Court, which would preempt any appeals court findings. Therefore, the citations given here should be regarded in that context and are not to be relied on as definitive but rather as examples that reflect areas of present discussion and debate. The cases most relevant to the readers of this chapter address definitions of disability, record of an impairment, regarded as having an impairment, and otherwise qualified for the position at issue.

As noted earlier, courts have had difficulty determining whether a condition actually constitutes a disability. This problem becomes manifest as courts struggle to decide whether impaired function relates to one specific job or to work in general. A clear pattern has yet to emerge.

With regard to carpal tunnel syndrome (CTS), several cases are relevant. In *Wooten v Farmland Foods* (30), a meat cutter with CTS was deemed as not disabled because her condition prevented her from pursuing only a narrow range of jobs, but she was still capable of performing many other jobs.

In *McKay v Toyota Motor Manufacturing, U.S.A., Inc.* (31), the court held that CTS was not a disability as a matter of law. In *EEOC v Joslyn Manufacturing Co.* (32), however, the court held that there was still a triable issue after an applicant was denied employment as a punch-press operator because of previous bilateral CTS surgery. Future considerations at trial were to include whether the perceived impairment substantially limited the applicant's ability to work while taking into account access to the job market of low and semiskilled manual labor, given his educational and employment background. Many factors considered in the *Joslyn* case obviously take employment decision-making were obviously beyond the arena of the examining clinician.

Other cases tend to support a narrower definition of disability. In *Ray v Glidden Co.* (33), discharge because of inability to continuously lift 44- to 56-pound containers secondary to multiple musculoskeletal disorders (avascular necrosis and bilateral shoulder replacements) was determined not to be grounds for an ADA claim, because limitations applied to a narrow range of jobs. Similarly, in *Hughes v Bedsole* (34), tennis elbow was not deemed a disability.

In the arena of "record of" or "regarded as having" an impairment, several cases are relevant. In *Flasza v TNT Holland Motor Express, Inc.* (35), it was determined that an applicant who had a history of filing five previous workers' compensation claims against a former employer does not have a record of an impairment or should be regarded as having an impairment, because the impairment from which he suffered did not limit any of life's major activities.

Issues of whether an individual is otherwise qualified to perform the job and thus protected under ADA have been frequently addressed. Although most of these cases have addressed persons who are already employed, there are possible implications for the applicant in the preplacement setting as well. One relevant case is *Cannon v Principal Health Care of Louisiana* (36). Here, termination after a work-related back injury precluded continuation on the job, but did not constitute discrimination because the employee was not otherwise qualified for the job, he could not perform an essential job function. Similarly, in *Lawrence v IBP, Inc.* (37), a meat cutter with carpal tunnel syndrome was determined to be not otherwise qualified as she could not do the essential functions of the job.

A recent case that reached the Supreme Court and is relevant to the definition of disability is *Abbott v Bragdon*, a case of a dentist who refused to treat a patient positive for human immunodeficiency virus (HIV), instead saying that he needed to perform the procedure (filling a cavity) in the hospital for adequate infection control. The Supreme Court said that asymptomatic HIV was indeed a disability, if a person who desired to reproduce was substantially limited in her ability to do so by this illness. This finding might lead to a reversal of some of the district cases that limited the scope of coverage, but such a result has yet to occur.

PREEMPLOYMENT VERSUS POST-HIRE PREPLACEMENT EVALUATIONS

A distinction is made between pre-offer and post-offer preplacement evaluations. Before an offer of employment is made, certain evaluations can be performed, including drug and skill testing. The employer may describe the job and ask the applicant whether he or she can perform the essential functions. The employer may ask whether the individual needs reasonable accommodations to perform the essential functions. Agility tests, including measures of physical and functional capacity, are allowed if they are consistently applied and job-related.

Medical evaluations are permitted only in the post-offer setting. These evaluations are acceptable after a conditional offer of employment has been tendered and if all applicants to that job are required to undergo such an evaluation. Although some states may limit testing to job-related abilities, the ADA does not impose such restrictions. Essentially, any appropriate medical evaluation is allowed. Initial evaluations should be identical for all applying to the same job category; however, the subsequent content of the evaluation may be modified and adjusted according to the individual's circumstances and medical condi-

tion. If medical records are provided, the employer must abide by confidentially requirements outlined under the law. Physicians would do well to remind employers in writing of this requirement when providing information of a medical nature to employers. An applicant may be rejected by the employer based on inability to do the job's essential functions, failure to satisfy a regulatory medical standard, and direct threat.

Prevention

As noted earlier in this chapter, the prevention aspects of preplacement evaluations often were designed to reduce risk and expense for the employer. When first instituted, the goal of these evaluations was to eliminate costly future expenditures on injured and disabled workers. This goal often was couched in the context of protecting the prospective worker from injury and disability. Unfortunately, as noted, the methods used for screening were often arbitrary and were not supported by data demonstrating their ability to predict risk for the individual applicant. They were almost always exclusionary. If applicants could not do the work as it has always been done, then there was no place for them in that workplace.

With the advent of the ADA, prevention has assumed a new perspective. Part of the preventive responsibility assumed by the clinician must be protection from liability under the ADA. As such, it is critical for all clinicians who perform preplacement evaluations to become familiar with the details of this law. Since the Act is undergoing continual definition through case law, regular updates are obligatory.

In the context of the ADA, prevention is achieved most effectively through reasonable accommodation. The interests of multiple parties must be considered and include the individual applicant, co-workers, and the employer. Safety and productivity of all parties are the goals of a successful preplacement process. This goal is consistent with the ideals of primary prevention. There may be collateral preventive benefits of providing an opportunity for a general health screening examination and interaction between a physician and persons who may have rarely visited a physician for preventive health care in the past. Some companies also involve the medical staff in safety training, respirator fitting and clearance, and other preventive functions.

Determining Functional Capacity and Work Fitness

Multiple factors must be considered to understand more fully the differing perspectives of the involved parties. From the applicant's perspective, there may have been previous health problems. Concerns about functionality and general ability to work safely may be present. Fears of specific injury or reinjury may be consciously or unconsciously present. On occasion, a conscious effort may be made to deny or mislead. Rarely, there may be intent to defraud.

From the employer's perspective, increased workers' compensation and group health costs, and lost productivity may be interpreted as concerns associated with the placement of new employees. Fears of fraudulent intent on the part of applicants are not uncommon in the employer community. The impact of injury, particularly musculoskeletal, is well appreciated.

Part of the tension inherent in this process lies in the distinction among the capacity of a worker, factors that determine employability, and economic factors that drive prospective employees and employers. Final decisions bring into play multiple related interests and measures. Determinants of employability differ markedly from determination of worker fitness or functional capacity. Determinations of employability relate primarily to what jobs are available to a worker at the time and what an employer values in a prospective employee. A worker's fitness depends upon that worker's functional capacity, job demands, and employer expectations. Functional capacity is a complex combination of physical strength, dexterity, mental abilities,

psychosocial factors, and motivation (38–40).

The determination of functional capacity and work fitness may be quite different in the pre-placement setting than it is in the return to work setting following an injury or illness. There is a process of choice each individual makes based on his or her own personal estimation of the overall benefit versus the risk of a particular action in relation to all possible actions. Psychosocial factors play an important, though often immeasurable role in an individual's choice regarding employment. Most models used to determine fitness for work ignore the psychosocial factors in favor of the biological influences. Variables that affect human output include more than the method of the task, the conditions in which the task is performed, and the technical skill of the worker. Voluntary efforts will be the limiting factor in many real situations. Fitness and function may be not so much determined by capacity as volition.

Functional Capacity Evaluations

One popular technique presently in use is the functional capacity evaluation (FCE), which is generally described as a standardized set of tests intended to provide an accurate prediction of an individual's general work capacity. It is based on the observation of that individual's actual performance of stereotypic activities, which usually incorporate aspects of static and dynamic lift and carry, posture, and body movements. Observations for the maintenance of proper body mechanics, an estimate of the sincerity of effort assessed by a coefficient of variation, and simple measurements of physiologic response to exercise are included.

Efforts have been made to demonstrate the validity of such evaluations (41–45). Whereas variants of an FCE are widely used, caution must be employed before relying on data produced from them. To understand the weakness of these tests, an understanding of the foundation on which they are based is necessary. Most FCEs are based on an engineering stress/strain model in which the physical demands of a job are compared with the measured physical capacity of the person being tested and then a comparison is made between that which is expected and actual performance.

One standard approach to worker fitness and risk evaluation is based on a combination of: (a) the *Dictionary of Occupational Titles* (DOT), a compendium of occupations that was devised as a vocational counseling tool incorporating broad categories of the physical strength required for each generic occupational title and (b) the National Institute for Occupational Safety and Health (NIOSH) lifting guide, which is a model for predicting the risk of injury in certain types of manual materials handling tasks. Definitions of the frequency of an activity are delineated in Table 1, and definitions of lifting categories are outlined in Table 2.

The DOT was created as a vocational counseling aid and compendium of occupations. Estimates incorporated in the DOT are crude and inexact. No attempt was made to analyze the method and mechanism of lifting and associated postures as was done in the NIOSH lifting guides. NIOSH guides point out the import of posture and mechanics of lifting over the specific weight lifted. The intent of the DOT was to categorize the physical requirements for each generic occupational title and provide a standard method to analyze and classify jobs. It was never intended to analyze people and their performance.

The *NIOSH Work Practices Guide for Manual Lifting* represents a simplified model focusing on forces generated at the lumbosacral disc. The entire second chapter of this guide is

TABLE 2. *Definition of job categories by lifting requirement (in pounds)*

Job category	Frequent lifting	Maximum occasional lifting
Sedentary		<10
Light	10	20
Medium	20	50
Heavy	50	100
Very heavy	100	>100

DOT, *Dictionary of Occupational Titles.*

devoted to the shortcomings of the model. Inconsistencies were clearly understood (46). It is also not intended as guidelines for worker fitness and risk evaluations. This guide provides an appropriate model to evaluate specific job tasks and design work in a less risky fashion. It is not a mechanism to evaluate individual physical capacity. It is recognized that a most occupational injuries do not involve the low back, and only about one-third of low back injuries are associated with a specific episode of lifting or bending to which the guidelines could be applied (47).

Stereotypic functional measures ignore the impact of training and experience and other factors that influence safety. They are also based on the assumption that a job will be performed without the benefit of individualization and accommodation. Most of the comparative standards used were obtained from measurements made of healthy people under ideal settings. There is little data to compare how these standards may apply to injured or disabled people in less than ideal real-life work settings. Futhermore, the impact of the ADA, with its legal directives to accommodate has not been determined. Other problems exist with FCEs. With only a single measure, they represent a "snapshot" in time. It is sometimes difficult to know whether the measurements obtained represent a minimum level at which the individual almost certainly can function or if they represent a true maximum above which he or she cannot reasonably go (48). Measurement of various functions and activities in isolation does not necessarily allow reconstruction of the parts into a whole. Some have a more accurate and

TABLE 1. *Definitions of frequency used in the DOT*

Description	Range of activity performed (%)
Occasional	1–33
Frequent	34–66
Constant	67–100

DOT, *Dictionary of Occupational Titles.*

predictive method of determining functional capacity (50); however, this technique is not widely applied to a broad scope of different job duties. While reports are often impressive with tables and charts, it is critical for the clinician to understand the multiple suppositions on which the report is built. Otherwise, the FCE represents nothing more than subjectivity wrapped in a cloak of objectivity. The validity of the coefficient of variation as a predictor of sincerity of effort is open to question and sometimes difficult to confirm (49).

One study that uses computerized measures (an ERGOS machine) and has showed good correlation between test performance with simple tasks such as push/pull and lift/carry and the actual ability to work. However, correlation began to break down with more complex activities. Work ability was consistently underestimated and predictive ability was unknown. Finally, the test is rapid but expensive (52). A particularly innovative concept of preplacement evaluations has been described that considers employer, societal, and applicant interests (51). Although it is creative and thought provoking, this decision analysis model has yet to find applicability for individual practitioners performing examinations.

Some published reports have indicated that in evaluating patients after an injury, clinical and mechanical methods of evaluation are comparable in terms of the information they can yield about a subject's performance in relation to his or her capacity (53,54).

Back Radiographs

The general consensus in the medical literature has been that preemployment radiographs of the low back are ineffective and costly when used to predict future injury risk. They can reveal significant lumbar disc degenerative changes, spondylolysis, or spondylolisthesis in more than 10% of asymptomatic patients (55). One study found that those with "low-risk" radiographs actually had a higher risk of injury compared with those who had abnormalities (56). A carefully controlled, ret-

rospective study found that the introduction of a radiographic screening program in a steel plant, where most of the workers were performing heavy work, did not significantly influence the subsequent incidence of low back pain (57). The incidence of spondylolysis in the general population is about 5%, but the rate of significant, disabling back pain in these persons is only 0.5% (58). Gibson concluded that if anyone with a degenerative change would be rejected, at best the incidence of significant back pain would be reduced by 3% to 5% at the expense of rejecting at least 25% of all applicants. He further calculated that for spondylolysis or spondylolisthesis, 5% of the screened population would be rejected, with probably no measurable effect on the number of back pain episodes (59).

A recent case in the Eastern District of Texas was settled after the employer agreed to eliminate the practice of subjecting all successful applicants to having radiographs of the back. Specifically, the employer agreed to implement the following policy:

> [The employer] will require back x-rays only in those instances where they are medically indicated, in the physician's discretion, on account of the individual's past or ongoing medical history of significant back problems, or abnormal physical or clinical findings made during the physical examination or objective functional testing, such as surgical scars on the back, severe scoliosis, abnormal range of motion or flexibility, or abnormal neurological findings. The condition that necessitates the taking of the back x-ray shall be documented in detail in the applicant's file. [The company] . . . will utilize a doctor who, in its judgment, is sufficiently skilled to be able to determine, based on valid medical findings, which candidates require back x-rays and which do not" (60).

Physicians and employers alike would be wise to adopt similar policies. Requirement of routine preemployment back radiographs can no longer be supported scientifically or legally. Other preemployment evaluations have been disappointing in detecting and preventing low back disability as well (61–63).

Practical Aspects and Recommendations

Physicians conducting preemployment examinations would be well advised to take several steps to reduce the likelihood of violation of the ADA. This will protect both the employer and the physician. Employers who are found liable for discrimination under the law may have grounds, in turn, to take legal recourse against the examining physician.

Examining physicians should obtain from employers detailed and accurate job descriptions for each job for which they are examining applicants. The physician should discuss the job descriptions with the employer to ensure that they are fully updated and do not exaggerate the physical requirements of the work. Discussion with the applicant regarding expectations of job requirements is also appropriate. Physicians should be aware that worker reports of job requirements may be inaccurate (64). When possible, physicians should visit the job site to observe employees engaged in the tasks related to each job. If the physician cannot personally observe workplace tasks, videotapes of persons performing their various job duties can be helpful. Familiarity with the physical requirements of each position is essential for purposes of evaluating whether particular individuals are medically qualified to perform the essential functions of the job (65).

In addition, doctors conducting preemployment examinations should endeavor to understand the relevant provisions of other applicable regulations. Most commonly, these will include Department of Transportation regulations on medical qualifications of drivers and state antidiscrimination regulations. Examining physicians must recognize that a physical condition that limits an applicant's ability to perform particular job duties does not automatically make the individual disqualified. Rather, if the applicant is a qualified individual with a disability, the employer must explore whether the disability can be reasonably accommodated without undue hardship. The doctor may serve as a facilitator by suggesting possible accommodations, such as the adjustment of equipment or realistic lifting restrictions.

Examining physicians must understand the stringent scope of the "direct threat" defense. A doctor cannot declare an individual unfit to work if there is only a minimal chance of injury to the the worker himself or herself or to others or if the condition is a degenerative one and no harm is likely to occur for many years. Tension may exist between the ADA standard and the doctor's inclination to take every precaution with each patient to minimize, if not eliminate, the risk of harm. Although the doctor may in good faith believe that even a small risk of injury justifies the disqualification of a particular applicant, under federal law, persons with disabilities cannot be deprived of the opportunity to work unless serious and specific hazards are imminent.

The examining physician should discuss any problematic medical findings with the applicant before making any hiring recommendation. A history of prior symptoms, past work history, and the frequency of other physical activities will be critical to making an educated recommendation. Additional past records may be necessary before any conclusions are reached. An individual's previous history of performing heavy physical labor is often a better predictor of job capacity than the existence of certain physical abnormalities (66,67).

Appropriate communication among the physician, employer and the applicant is valuable to each party. The applicant should be informed of the doctor's medical assessment in order to seek further treatment and to make appropriate decisions concerning his or her future activities. After learning of the diagnosis and the physician's concerns, some candidates may decide to seek other employment that would not similarly jeopardize their health or to obtain second opinions from their own specialists. A candid and detailed discussion with the employer may reduce the risk of potential litigation.

A letter documenting the content and outcome of the discussion should follow verbal contact with the employer. Copies of all relevant information should be retained in the patient's file. It is insufficient for the physician to send the employer a standardized form that lacks specificity. Evidence of individualized assessment of each applicant's health and ability to work is needed.

The doctor should discuss the accuracy and predictive value of the testing done with each individual who may receive a negative hiring recommendation and the potential employer. Many physicians, including specialists, who conduct preemployment examinations are unfamiliar with the paucity of scientific bases for most medical determinations of direct threat and limited predictive value of many tests. If the physician is not confident in his or her ability to predict the risk of future injury with respect to a particular applicant, this cer tainty should be disclosed uncertainty to the employer.

Limited Versus Comprehensive Approach

Employers, ideally in consultation with physicians, must decide the extent to which preplacement evaluations will be performed. Choices range from doing nothing to performing comprehensive evaluations. Individual circumstances should determine the course to be taken.

If no evaluation is performed, risks under Title 1 of the ADA are essentially eliminated, and initial medical costs are lowered. With little evidence of the efficacy of these screenings, justification for this minimalist approach can be argued. On the other hand, many managers are skeptical of this approach because of safety and productivity concerns.

A conservative approach may be taken. Preemployment evaluations, such as drug screening, may discourage certain applicants and provide a modicum of the protection management expects. Agility tests may be customized to assist both applicants and employers in recognizing whether a job is a reasonable fit for the employee. Administration of a simple medical questionnaire is less costly than a full

medical evaluation. This approach is supported in recent respiratory certification regulations.

A limited physical examination is less costly than a full post-hire, preplacement medical evaluation. Follow-up to questionnaires will be required frequently enough that delays in hiring may offset savings accrued. Safety issues are still only partially resolved. Incomplete data may expose employers and employees alike to some increased future risks.

A comprehensive physical examination approach provides the greatest opportunity for implementing preventive strategies. Individualized assessment provides reasonable compatibility with the ADA. Physician involvement in the process allows correlation of clinical conditions to workplace requirements. Opportunity for contact with a physician and the perceived value of medical examinations provides unknown but widely embraced benefits. Initial costs of this approach are higher than other alternatives.

Regardless of the approach taken, it must be applied consistently to all applicants. In general, efforts should be made to make evaluations as simple, inexpensive, and noninvasive as possible. This need should be balanced against a valid, reliable, and specifically targeted determination that is appropriate to the task anticipated. Examiners, applicants, and employers all must understand that these evaluations are not definitive and will not replace an ongoing relationship between a patient and provider.

When designing specific tests for applicants, care must be taken to ensure that the function tested is actually important to job performance and is not based on a theoretic possibility. Particularly when performing agility or strength tests, it is important to consider whether *present* employees are capable of performing at the level required of applicants.

In certain circumstances, baseline range of motion may be useful for apportionment of future determinations of impairment; however, this technique can be costly and requires a certain level of expertise. Sensitivity, stability of results over time, and cost effectiveness of this approach have not yet been documented. The agility test most likely to provide valid information on work capacity is a simulation of actual work activities.

Clinician's Role

The role of the clinician has changed dramatically with the advent of the ADA. In times past, the clinician would often make a determination regarding employability. Multiple examples exist of physicians asserting that an applicant was not physically fit for a job. In essence, these decisions were determinants in the context of employment. In the post-ADA era, the clinician should refrain from absolute pronouncements about whether the applicant can do a particular job. If there are still boxes to be checked on examination forms that state "not qualified," they should be eliminated. Instead, the clinician's role is to define medical conditions and to estimate their impact on function and risk.

In general, medical determinations might include findings, opinions, and conclusions. An example of one format for this report is shown in Fig. 1. Note that the findings are described as possibilities, and the impact is further delineated. Conclusions are stated in terminology consistent with the ADA. When appropriate, further medical information is requested and medical recommendations are deferred. Additional clarification of the individual's condition (including additional medical history) and discussion regarding job requirements may be appropriate. Final conclusions are always individualized. Standardized or boilerplate responses should be avoided.

The most important fact for the clinician to keep in mind is that the responsibility for determination regarding employability resides with the employer. It is not the job of the clinician to make this decision. The clinician's role is solely that of an advisor and consultant.

Clinicians should supply objective information about an applicant's job-related functional abilities and limitations. Comparison of the measured abilities and the job description is important and appropriate. Comparisons also may be made with an employer's health and safety standard. Employers should provide the clinician with current job descriptions and functional requirements of the job as well as any relevant information relating to job performance, including the requirements for shift work, productivity standards, and other such factors. Distinction between essential and marginal job functions should be provided. Exclusion from a job may occur only if essential job functions cannot be performed after reasonable accommodation. Marginal job functions such as escaping a burning building or lifting a heavy item once a year are not generally relevant in making a determination of fitness for duty. It may be appropriate to contact employer representatives (often in the Human Resource Department) to discuss findings and explore possible accommodations. The ability to accommodate and determine what is reasonable is a management decision, however. Final discussions regarding accommodations most appropriately take place between the employer and the applicant using medical information as but one component of the total information employers need to resolve these questions. Accommodations are appropriate when requested by the applicant and after an individualized interactive problem-solving process.

ACKNOWLEDGMENTS

This work was supported in part by Grant 525495 from the National Institute of Occupational Safety and Health. Special thanks to Pamela M. Harris, Esq., of Minneapolis, Minnesota, who compiled and succinctly summarized most of the ADA cases quoted. This article does not represent the opinion or official position of the EEOC.

REPORT OF POST-HIRE / PRE-PLACEMENT MEDICAL EVALUATION

<u>by</u>

CORPORATE MEDICAL CONSULTANT

Name	SSN
Company	Job Title

FINDINGS AND OPINIONS:

Based on all the information available to me, it is my medically probable opinion that the above named individual has:

A: _____ No abnormal medical conditions

B: _____ Has a medical condition(s) that:
Is unlikely to interfere with the regular performance of normal job duties.
Explain: _____
_____
_____

C: __ Has a medical condition(s) that:
May endanger him/herself or others in the regular performance of normal job duties.
May be aggravated in the regular performance of normal job duties.
May interfere with the regular performance of normal job duties.
Explain: _____
_____

Requires the following additional information:
1. _____
2. _____
3. _____
4. _____

CONCLUSIONS AND RECOMMENDATIONS:

Based on all the information available to me, including my findings and opinions, I recommend that:

No restrictions or accommodations appear necessary. This individual has the physical capacity to perform the essential functions of the job without direct threat to self or others. **(Findings A or B)**

Decision regarding placement be deferred. In order to determine if reasonable accommodation is appropriate, further consideration is necessary to delineate this individual's condition. Additional information may be required. **(Finding C)**.

Examiner:

_____   _____   _____
Print Name   Signature   Date

FIG. 1. Sample medical report. (From Integrated Health Management, Denver, Colorado.)

REFERENCES

1. *National Occupational Hazard Survey I*, Vol III: Survey analysis and supplemental tables. National Institute for Occupational Safety and Health, DHEW (NIOSH) publication 78-114, 1978.
2. Loeser JD. Sullivan M. Doctors, diagnosis, and disability: a disastrous diversion. *Clin Orthop* 1997;336:61–66.
3. Elder AG, Symington IS, Symington EH. Do occupational physicians agree about ill-health retirement? A study of simulated retirement assessments. *Occup Med* 1994;44:231–235.
4. ACOEM Section on Work Fitness and Disability Evaluation.
5. Himmelstein JS, Pransky GS, eds. Worker fitness and risk evaluations. *Occupational Medicine State of the Art Reviews* 1988;3:179–191.
6. Himmelstien JS. Worker Fitness and Risk Evaluations in context. *Occup Med* 1988;3:169–178.
7. *National Occupational Hazard Survey I*, Vol III: Survey Analysis and Supplemental Tables. National Institute for Occupational Safety and Health, DHEW (NIOSH) publication 78-114, 1978.
8. Berkowitz M, Burton JF. *Permanent disability benefits in workers' compensation*. Kalamazoo, MI: Upjohn Institute, 1987.
9. National Council on Compensation Insurance, Countrywide Workers' compensation experience including certain competitive state funds, First Report Basis, NCCI: Boca Raton, 1982.
10. Social Security Administration. Statistical Summary. Social Security Bulletin, v52, 1989:3–91.
11. *Guiding principles for medical examinations in industry*. Chicago: American Medical Association, 1984:1.
12. Hainer BL. Pre-placement evaluations [Review] *Primary Care Clinics in Office Practice* 1994;21:237–247.
13. Congressional record for the ADA.
14. Rothstein MA. Legal considerations in worker fitness evaluation. *Occup Med* 1988;3:209–218.
15. 42 U.S.C. § 12102(2)(A).
16. 29 C.F.R. § 1630.2(h)(2)(I).
17. 29 C.F.R. § 1630.2(j)(3)(I).
18. 42 U.S.C. § 12102(2)(C).
19. 42 U.S.C. § 12112(a).
20. Cowell JWF. Guidelines for fitness-to-work examination. *Can Med Assoc J* 1986;135:985–988.
21. 42 U.S.C. §12112(d)(4).
22. 42 U.S.C. § 12113(b), 29 C.F.R. 1630 app. § 1630.2(r).
23. 42 U.S.C. §§ 12112(b)(5)(A), 12113(a).
24. 42 U.S.C. § 12111(10).
25, 42 U.S.C. § 12113(b), 29 C.F.R. 1630 app. § 1630.2(r).
26. 29 C.F.R. 1630 app. §1630.2(r).
27. *EEOC v Texas Bus Lines*, 923 F.Supp. 965, 980 (S.D. Tex 1996).
28. 923 F.Supp. 965 (S.D. Tex. 1996).
29. The case was filed in the Eastern District of Texas, Beaumont Division, Civil Action No. 1:96CV0367 (1996). This language appears in the consent decree by which the case was resolved. The name of the employer is being withheld pursuant to a confidentiality agreement.
30. 58 F.3d 382 (8th Cir. June 28, 1995).
31. 878 F. Supp. 1012 (E.D. Ky. 1005).
32. 5AD Cases 122 (N.D. Ill. 1996).
33. 5AD Cases 991 (5th Cir. 1996).
34. 48 F.3d 1376 (4th Cir. 1995).
35. 159 F.R.D. 672, 4 AD Cases 11 (N.D. Ill. 1994).
36. 4 AD Cases 873, 1995 WL 131099 (E.D. La. 1995).
37. 4 AD Cases 632, 1995 WL 261144 (D. Kan. 1995).
38. Menard MR, and Hoens, AM. Objective evaluation of functional capacity: medical, occupational, and legal settings. *J Orthop Sports Phys Ther* 1994;19:249–260.
39. Reisine S, McQuillan J, Fifield J. Predictors of work disability in rheumatoid arthritis patients: a five-year followup. *Arthritis Rheum* 1995;38:1630–1637.
40. Mazanec DJ. The injured worker: assessing "return-to-work" status. *Cleve Clin J Med* 1996;63:166–171.
41. Lechner DE, Jackson JR, Roth DL, Straaton KV. Reliability and validity of a newly developed test of physical work performance. *J Occup Med* 1994;36:997–1004.
42. Reimer MS, Halbrook BD, Dreyfuss PH, Tibiletti C. A novel approach to preemployment worker fitness evaluations in a material-handling industry. *Spine* 1994;19:2026–2032.
43. Fishbain DA, Abdel-Moty E, Cutler R, Khalil TM, Sadak S, Rosomoff RS, and Rosomoff HL. Measuring residual functional capacity in chronic low back pain patients based on the *Dictionary of Occupational Titles*. *Spine* 1994;19:872–880.
44. Velozo CA. Work evaluations: critique of the state of the art of functional assessment of work [Review]. *Am J Occup Ther* 1993;47:203–209.
45. Kraus J. The independent medical examination and the functional capacity evaluation. *Occup Environ Med* 1997;12:525–56.
46. *NIOSH work practices guide for manual lifting*. NIOSH technical report 81-122, 1981:34.
47. Waters TR, et al. Revised NIOSH equation for the design and evaluation of manual lifting tasks. *Ergonomics* 1993;36:749–776.
48. Leavitt F. The physical exertion factor in compensable work injuries: a hidden flaw in previous research. *Spine* 1992;17:307–310.
49. Hendriks EJ, Brandsma JW, Heerkens YF, Oostendorp RA, Nelson RM. Intraobserver and interobserver reliability of assessments of impairments and disabilities. *Phys Ther* 1997;77:1097–1106.
50. Jackson AS. Pre-employment physical evaluation. *Exerc Sport Sci Rev* 1992;22:53–90.
51. Harber P, Hsu P, Fedoruk MJ. Personal risk assessment under the Americans with Disabilities Act: a decision analysis approach. *J Occup Environ Med* 1993;35:1000–1010.
52. Dusik LA, Menard MR, Cooke C, Fairborn SM, Beach GN. Concurrent validity of the ERGOS work simulator versus conventional functional capacity evaluation techniques in a workers' compensation population. *J Occup Environ Med* 1993;35:759–767.
53. Menard MR, Cooke C, Locke SR, Beach GN, and Butler TB. Pattern of performance in workers with low back pain during a comprehensive motor performance evaluation. *Spine* 1994;19:1359–1366.
54. Abdel-Moty E, Fishbain DA, Khalil TM, et al. Functional capacity and residual functional capacity and their utility in measuring work capacity [Review]. *Clin J Pain* 1993;9:168–173.
55. Lawrence JS. Disc degeneration: its frequency and rela-

tionship to symptoms. *Ann Rheum Dis* 1969;28: 121–127.

56. Redfield JT. The low back x-ray as a pre-employment screening tool in the forest products industry. *J Occup Environ Med* 1971;13:219–226.

57. Gibson ES, Martin RH, Terry CW. Incidence of low back pain and pre-placement x-ray screening. *J Occup Environ Med* 1980;22:515–519.

58. Bailey W. Observation on the etiology and frequency of spondylolisthesis and its precursors. *Radiology* 1947; 48:107–112.

59. Gibson ES. The value of pre-placement screening radiography of the low back. *Occ Med* 1988;3:91–107.

60. Eastern District of Texas, Beaumont Division, Civil Action No. 1:96CV0367 (1996). This language appears in the consent decree by which the case was resolved. The name of the employer is being withheld pursuant to a confidentiality agreement.

61. Cohen JE, Goel V, Frank JW, Gibson ES. Predicting risk of back injuries, work absenteeism, and chronic disability: the shortcomings of preplacement screening. *J Occup Environ Med* 1994;36:1093–1099.

62. Frymoyer WB. Predicting disability from low back pain. *Clin Orthop* 1992;279:101–109.

63. Lancourt J, Kettelhut M. Predicting return to work for lower back pain patients receiving worker's compensation. *Spine* 1992;17:629–640.

64. Linstrom I, Ohlund C, Nachemson A. Validity of patient reporting and predictive value of industrial physical work demands. *Spine* 1994;19:888–893.

65. Hoffman S, Pransky G. Pre-employment examinations and the Americans with Disability Act: how best to avoid liabilities under federal law. *J Occup Rehabil* (*in press*).

66. Texas Workers' Compensation Research Center. Factors Affecting Return to Work for Injured Workers with Permanent Impairments. *Research Review* 1995.

67. Mihous RL, Haugh LD, Frymoyer JW, et al. Determinants of vocational disability in patients with low back pain. *Arch Phys Med Rehabil* 1989;70:589–593.

Occupational Musculoskeletal Disorders
edited by T. G. Mayer, R. J. Gatchel, and P. B. Polatin.
Lippincott Williams & Wilkins, Philadelphia © 2000.

12

Workplace Fitness Programs and Other Preventive Approaches

Mohamad Parnianpour

Department of Industrial, Welding & Systems Engineering, Ohio State University, Columbus, Ohio 43210

The significant human suffering and economic cost due to work-related musculoskeletal disorders (WMSDs) have motivated many to work in an interdisciplinary fashion to develop and implement prevention programs. This chapter begins with defining some essential terminology and concepts to guide readers in evaluation of the efficacy of workplace fitness programs in the prevention of WMSDs. The theoretical bases for worksite fitness programs have been developed, and some exemplary programs have been reviewed. However, it has been argued that any single intervention strategy may be less effective than multiple intervention strategies that address the multifactorial causal model of WMSDs. A systematic approach to prevention and management of WMSDs must identify the causes of these disorders and eliminate or substantially reduce workers' exposure to these risk factors. A prevention program must consider all elements of the work system and must start by securing management commitment and employee involvement, leading to empowering the workers to address the ergonomic hazards in their workplace and participate in the problem-solving process. Total quality management requires regular program review and evaluation. An effective occupational and safety program to implement the prevention strategy must have these elements:

- Worksite analysis,
- Hazard prevention and control,
- Medical management,
- Training and education.

The above guidelines have been suggested by the Occupational Safety and Health Administration (OSHA) (1) for management of cumulative trauma disorders (CTDs) in meatpacking plants and can be the minimum basis of a successful strategy.

DEFINITION AND CONCEPTS

The literature on the etiology and epidemiology of WMSDs can be labeled as an "unhelpful polemic," in part because terminology use is consistent and clarity is lacking regarding *a priori* distinctions of competing conceptual frameworks (2). Any critical reconstruction of this literature requires recognition of the sources of bias and inherent limitations of the diverse methodologies employed. For example, "low back pain" (LBP), "low back injury," and "low back disorders" are often used interchangeably without regard to their ontologic and epistemologic distinctions. The problem may be not only lack of precision in the quantification of causal factors (using job titles for determination of the occupational load) but also detection of the manifestation of the effects (i.e., there is no objective method of detection of LBP). The lack of correspondence between structural impairment, functional deficit, and pain behavior due to LBP poses another methodologic obstacle.

The distinctions among impairment, disability, and handicap have been provided elsewhere (3). The implications of these distinctions in design and implementation of prevention programs cannot be overemphasized. For example, prevention of LBP may be an unattainable goal, while management of LBP to prevent (chronic low back) disability has been recognized to be more effective in reducing the associated human suffering and economic costs. Battie (4) summarized the literature by enumerating factors that affect the onset and persistence of low back disability: job demands, symptom severity, cultural norms, socioeconomic conditions, opportunities for compensation, emotional distress, job satisfaction, and the physical and social work environment. It is clear that any prevention strategy must be designed and implemented to address these multifactorial dynamics.

A WMSD is defined by Kuorinka and Forcier (5) as a descriptor for disorders and diseases of the musculoskeletal system having a proven or hypothetical work-related causal component. The natural history of a WMSD relates the response of the system to environmental and other pathophysiologic factors triggering the pathologic condition, which could lead to observable measures in terms of signs and symptoms, defect and disability, or death. In response to stimuli, tissues could adapt positively with an enhanced capacity to sustain subsequent exposure or negatively by diminishing their capacity (5). Armstrong et al. (6) proposed a conceptual model for the development of WMSDs that related the functional state of the system in terms of the four cascading and interacting variables of exposure, dose, capacity, and response. Internal dose is defined as a set of mechanical, physiologic, or psychologic factors that are caused by external factors determined by work requirements called exposure. The response to the dose, which is a function of capacity, can act as a dose for a secondary response. Little is known about the stress-induced modeling or remodeling in various tissues (i.e., bone, ligament, tendon, and muscle). How various stressors interact and

augment the capacity of the system is also poorly understood. Hence, the most fundamental issue of how much of a stressor (risk factor) or a combination of risk factors is too much remains illusive. This weakness is confounded by the fact that real-world stressors are time-varying, and many may coexist at the same time (7). The failure of the mechanistic approach to the study of WMSDs often stems from the inability of such paradigms to capture the complexity of the intricately interconnected subsystems. Often, with the reduction of the dimensionality of the problem to only a limited sphere (i.e., biomechanics, psychosocial, etc.) the separability of distinctive patterns of behaviors is reduced.

The following topologic example may provide insight into this problem. Let us imagine a particle that spirals up on the surface of a cylinder. The trajectory of this particle in the three-dimensional space determines the precise location of the particle as a function of time. Observer A, who is only provided a top view of this physical system, will accurately describe the motion of the particle as a limit cycle—the particle is going around in a circle repeatedly. The loss of one dimension (depth) causes observer A to conclude that the particle is occupying the same space at different points in time. However, observer A's description is considered false by observer B, who has access to the three-dimensional view (data)—since the particle will never occupy its old location during its spiraling ascent. Of course, observer B is in position to verify that the radius of cylinder is the same as the radius of the circle measured by observer A, despite his or her false description of the particle's path. Here lies a fundamental difficulty in our understanding of the etiology and prevention of WMSDs: We are not sure whether we are observing the phenomenon in its appropriate "space." Are we considering all the relevant dimensions that specify the behavior of this complex system? Are we measuring all dimensions as accurately? Are the dimensions that we are measuring independent of each other? The purpose of this chapter is not to exhaust all these methodologic concepts. The natural history of the disease or disorder is akin to the trajectory of the particle in this example. We must realize that the observable states of a system may vary as a function of time, and a multidimensional (multifactorial) assessment is needed to study the evolution of the trajectory. Efficient prevention strategies cannot be realized without a better delineation of the risk factors.

The deleterious effects of immobilization on biologic tissues indicate that too little activity is harmful, while too much loading can accelerate degeneration and the risk of tissue failure. Battie and Videman (8) considered the important distinctions between risk indicators and risk factors. They argued that it is crucial to the design of an optimal prevention strategy to investigate whether the intervention is changing a risk factor or risk indicator. They cited Leino's (9) work that suggested that those engaged with higher levels of exercise activity had fewer reports of low back symptoms. Could exercise participation be a marker for a set of other factors affecting the reporting of low back troubles (e.g., lifestyle behavior, lower occupational physical demand, or higher job satisfactions)? Other studies have also associated some type of exercise with higher spinal pathologies (10). Hence, it is not clear whether exercise is a positive or negative risk factor, or is solely an indicator. More important, it is unclear where the prescription of exercise *per se* could be a beneficial intervention strategy. What determinants of exercise must be studied to investigate the threshold of its effectiveness? How do time and content of exercise affect the outcome of the intervention on different populations at different stages of development of WMSDs?

Biomechanical injury models consist of two mechanisms: acute (overload) and cumulative trauma. The former occurs with single application of load above the threshold of tissue tolerance (its ultimate strength), while the latter requires repetitive application of submaximal load. The gradual onset of most back symptoms without a specific precipitating accident or an unusual activity further complicates the

identification of risk factors (11). A given factor may also play different roles in different circumstances. Whether heavy loads cause low back disorders is still unclear (11), but it is rational to assume that they tremendously affect the coping mechanism of workers afflicted with back symptoms. Hence, heavy loads may be a causal risk factor or a modifying factor (catalyst). The complex interaction can be only detected by appropriately designed studies that attempt to accurately quantify the risk factors in prospective studies.

Two typical but rather comprehensive conceptual frameworks are presented in Figs. 1 and 2 (12). The lack of organizational factors is evident in Fig. 2, while a more detailed delineation of the short- and long-term responses is provided (13). It is clear on the basis of this framework that it will be ideal to reduce the stressors and/or increase worker personal attributes such as strength or fitness to affect the short- and long-term responses to a condition. Fundamentally, the conceptual basis for the prevention programs assumes that there is an underlying process that determines the evolution of a WMSD in a well defined, sequential manner. If one reduces the strength of negative inputs while augmenting the strength of positive inputs, then the output of the process could be changed in the desired direction. Unfortunately, the detailed mapping of many of these processes is unknown. It is postulated that future advances in the understanding of cell biomechanics could determine the responses of tissues to different mechanical environments (14).

The next logical question is whether the existing literature permits determining the strength of causal relationships between controllable parameters of a task and the risk of WMSDs. Once these relationships are estimated, one could optimize the task in light of the existing tradeoffs to reduce the risk due to satisfaction of system's constraints (satisfactory performance of the task while not overtaxing the system's available resources or violating its tolerance limits). For example, controllable parameters in a manual material-handling task from an assembly line could be

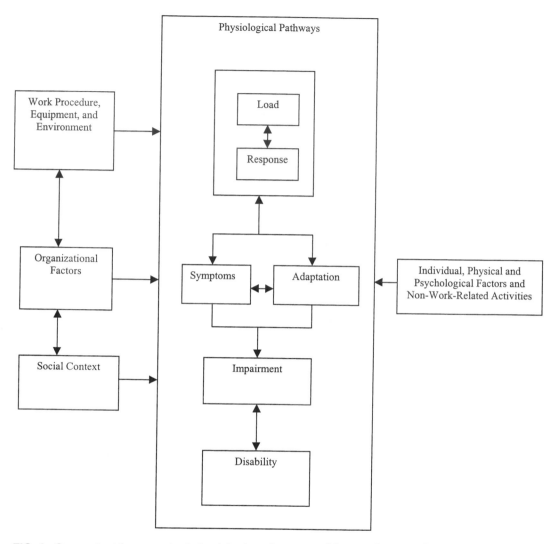

FIG. 1. Conceptual framework of physiologic pathways and factors that contribute to musculoskeletal disorders. (From ref. 12, with permission.)

the pace and height of the assembly line and the weight and size of object to be lifted. These parameters could be adjusted to minimize the risk of low back WMSD. In this context, ergonomics can be defined as the study of humans at work for the purpose of fitting tasks to the capability of humans to enhance safety, health, comfort, efficiency, ease of use, and productivity. The concept of fitness from human performance or exercise physiology may be based on the relation of one's score to normative values obtained experimentally and stratified based on sex and age. However, the concept of "fitness" in ergonomics is enlarged by consideration of both the task demands and individuals' functional capacity. Training to enhance functional capacity along its various dimensions, such as strength, coordination, endurance, speed, mobility, steadiness, and so on, can only be considered one of the many strategies for fitting the task to the person. Administrative and engineering controls could be introduced to accommodate an individual's capacity while satisfying the es-

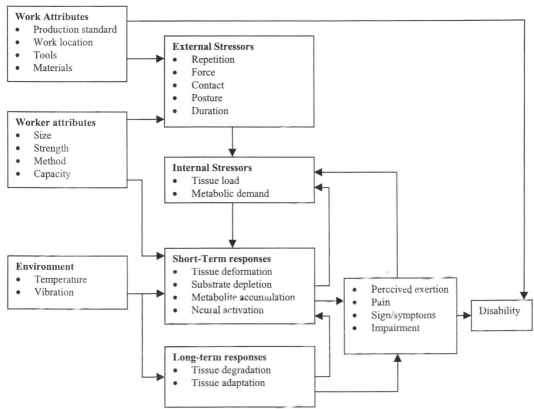

FIG. 2. Worker impairment and disability as related to worker and work attributes and environmental factors. (From ref. 13, with permission.)

sential functions of the task. The latter strategies are often more effective, as they change the work instead of the worker (15,16).

It is clear that the earlier signs of WMSDs in their asymptomatic stages should guide the continuous control of the risk management. This points to the need for having a workforce trained in fundamentals of ergonomics and the presence of active and passive surveillance systems (5). Prompt attention to early symptoms by engineering, and clinical management of both symptoms and causes, can lead to more effective prevention strategies.

PREVENTION PROGRAMS

Prevention programs can be divided into three main categories: primary, secondary, and tertiary (17). There is a considerable de-

gree of overlap among these programs. *Primary* prevention strategies aim at preventing the clinical manifestation of WMSDs, while *secondary* prevention considers measures to avoid the symptomatic stages of WMSDs and *tertiary* prevention takes measures to minimize the consequences of WMSDs once their symptomatic manifestations become evident. Pope and Andersson (17) cited the following as examples of primary prevention strategies for lower back disorders:

• Preemployment/preplacement,
• Worker training in safe techniques for performance of tasks,
• Ergonomic job design,
• Job modification,
• Back school education,
• Use of lifting belts,
• Employee fitness programs.

Reduction of identified risk factors is the goal of primary prevention. Secondary prevention programs consist of treatment, education, ergonomic counseling, and job modification. Tertiary prevention programs include treatment and functional restoration programs to reduce the duration of chronicity and disability, with the goal of returning patients to work. The above examples clearly show how much overlap exists among these programs. However, in the design and implementation of a prevention program, the program goals must become clear to all stakeholders, and their rights and responsibilities in the process must be well defined and transparent (1).

Based on the above description, it must be clear why the system approach to prevention of WMSDs has been recommended, given the complex interactions of various subsystems describing the time-varying responses of an individual to the exchanges of energy and information with his or her environment. Lastly, to detect the risk factors, one must select the appropriate observable parameters at various levels of understanding of the process. Tissue responses to external and internal loading are characterized by the mechanical and material properties (poroviscoelasticity) of the tissue (i.e., its creep or stress relaxation). At this level of analysis, the determination of safe levels of stressors is mostly determined by cell or tissue biomechanics (14,18), while investigation for the determinants of the filing of an industrial claim, the development of disability or chronicity, or return to work will understandably require macroergonomic analysis (consideration of the whole work system [19], as shown in Figs. 1 and 3). Hence, much energy is wasted in an attempt to gauge the global importance of biomechanical versus psychosocial determinants of WMSDs, while the system approach affords to each determinant its relative importance at various stages of an WMSD's evolution in time.

More and more companies in industrialized countries are implementing fitness or wellness programs to promote the value of a healthier workforce. Advocates of such programs point to benefits in health care cost reduction, de-

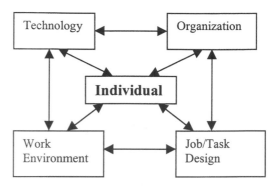

FIG. 3. A work system requires a balance among technology, organization, environment, job, and individuals. Work-related musculoskeletal disorders indicate a work-system imbalance. Any changes in the factors will cause adaptations in other parts of the system that may increase or decrease risk factors. (From ref. 19, with permission.)

creased employee absenteeism, increased productivity, stress reduction, improved job satisfaction, and improved employee–employer relationship (20). Companies can provide fitness programs in three ways: company-reimbursed, -sponsored, or -operated programs.

Operated programs in the worksite have the disadvantage of requiring the financial commitment of startup and operational expenses, while they have the advantage of increasing employee participation and allowing greater employer control over the program, including the chance of modifying the content based on research outcomes (20). Is there a rationale for promoting workplace fitness programs for prevention of WMSDs? How successful have such programs been? Is there an inherent problem in approaching prevention in such a narrowly defined manner? On the basis of recent models of human performance, a task can be defined in terms of the amount of resource that it requires across the dimensions of performance such as strength, mobility, speed, endurance, steadiness, and so on. Using resource economics, utilization ratios can be estimated, based on the ratio of demand to the maximum available resource for each dimension of performance (21,22). The system is constrained by its maximum available resource, and overload occurs if demand exceeds the available resource. Hence, theoretically, having a higher magnitude of available resources increases the margin of safety with regard to overload for a given level of demand. Therefore, intuitively, if one can increase performance capability by various training and exercise programs in or outside the workplace, one can expect to enhance the margin of safety against overloading the system. It should be noted that higher initial reserves for a prolonged low level of activity, or repetitive application of low loads, provide less protection if the number of repetitions and/or duration of activity are very large. In short, higher muscular strength or endurance may not be as effective a deterrent to CTDs as it is to acute soft tissue injuries (overload injuries). For CTDs affecting the tendons, tendon sheaths, and nerves, few data are available as how to increase the tolerance limits of these tissues to frictional work, hydrostatic pressure, or contact, compressive, or shear forces. In this context, alterations of work techniques or tasks are needed to allow more rest periods and/or prescribed physical activities; for example, pauses with stretching serve to supply nutrition to tissues and allow recovery (23–25).

Justification for the implementation of fitness programs can be sought in the epidemiologic literature. Battie and Videman (8) compiled an extensive literature from prospective studies that provided mixed results in terms of the significance of strength, endurance, flexibility, and cardiovascular fitness as risk indicators of low back symptoms on health surveys and back complaints in the workplace. Trunk muscles provide torque-generation capability while stabilizing the spine (26). Both functions are important in protecting the passive tissues of the spine during work-related or leisure physical activities. Trunk muscle strength, endurance, and coordination have been significant areas of research in both healthy and LBP patients. Hence, review of this literature could provide a rationale for suggesting programs that enhance trunk muscle strength, endurance, and coordination, as well as overall cardiovascular fitness.

Strength and Low Back Pain

Several authors have published data showing that symptom-free subjects have stronger trunk muscles than subjects complaining of LBP (27). It seems not only that the muscles are weaker but also that there are modifications in the extensor-to-flexor strength ratio. In healthy subjects, trunk extension strength is greater than flexion strength. In LBP subjects, there is a significant loss of both flexor and extensor strength, but the main loss seems to be in extensor muscles (27). Other investigators, using isoinertial techniques, reported that subjects with LBP tend to have slower movements than normal individuals (28) and that velocity in extension shows the main reduction (29). Muscle-strengthening therapies have been prescribed to remedy the altered strength balance. Addison and Schultz (30) reported that inpatients with severe back disorders have less back strength than matched symptom-free individuals, but outpatients with low back disorders were as strong as normal individuals. Nicolaisen and Jorgensen (31), studying a group of postal workers, did not demonstrate any differences in isometric strength among subjects who experienced back troubles to the extent that work was impossible, those who experienced back pain to a lesser degree, and those without any history of back troubles. Newton et al. (32), using an isokinetic device, found that LBP patients are indeed weaker than healthy controls, but they did not find any changes in the extension–flexion ratio. Despite these conflicting results, there seems to be agreement that patients with LBP have weaker trunk muscles than symptom-free subjects in control groups.

Chronicity may be an additional factor contributing to the deconditioning of trunk muscles. Nachemson and Lindh (33) found that isometric strength is significantly reduced in chronic versus acute LBP patients. Hultman et al. (34) found a reduction in the isokinetic strength of back muscles in subjects with chronic back pain compared with intermittent sufferers, but Suzuki and Endo (35) found no differences in isokinetic strength between chronic and nonchronic patients.

Biering-Sorensen (36) demonstrated that in a general population without acute back pain, isometric trunk muscle strength was reduced in subjects who experienced recurrence of low back troubles in the follow-up year, compared with those without recurrence. However, trunk strength in subjects who experienced first-time low back troubles in the follow-up year did not differ from that of subjects without low back troubles. Battie et al. (37) conducted a prospective study to determine the physical risk factors associated with back pain report among 3,020 aircraft manufacturing employees. They found that isometric lifting-strength measurements were not predictive of back pain incidence. This was probably due to their using standard isometric lifting tests that were not specific for the job. It seems that the injury-predictive capability of isometric strength testing is limited to jobs requiring workers to use a high percentage of their strength potential (38). Mostardi et al. (39), studying a group of 174 nurses with an isokinetic device, failed to show any predictive value of strength measures. In this study, lifting strength was measured, which takes into account more factors than just trunk strength.

Troup et al. (40) showed that psychophysical lifting tests were not good predictors of first-time LBP incidence during the follow-up year; however, lifting capability was significantly lower in subjects with chronic LBP. These results tend to invalidate the theory that lack of strength is the cause of LBP and may indicate instead that loss of strength is a process resulting from recurrent LBP (27). However, the number of confounding variables associated with psychophysical testing must also be taken into account. In a small sample of 66 symptom-free subjects followed for an average of 30 months, Newton et al. (32) found no difference in initial isometric or psychophysical lifting simulation between subjects in whom LBP did and did not appear. However, testing in this study was not job-specific. Despite certain contradictory results, it seems that lifting-strength measurements

have some predictive value if they are made highly task-specific (27).

Trunk Muscle Endurance and Low Back Pain

It is conceivable that when individuals with low trunk muscle endurance are exposed to postural stress, they will fatigue more quickly and may recruit muscles less optimally and/or allow the passive tissue to carry more load because of muscle insufficiency. This impaired coordination and additional loading may result in subsequent back troubles. Indeed, it is classically assumed that local muscular fatigue predisposes to injury (41) . Many reports have been published to indicate that a worker's skill is affected by fatigue (42). Chaffin (41) demonstrated that reduction of precise motor control accompanies muscular fatigue.

Parnianpour et al. (43) studied the effect of fatiguing isoinertial flexion and extension trunk movements on the movement pattern (angular position and velocity profile) and the motor output (torque) of the trunk. They showed that with fatigue there is a reduction of the functional capacity in the main sagittal plane. There is also a loss of motor control, leading to greater range of motion in the transverse and coronal planes while the primary sagittal task is being performed. Association of sagittal with coronal and transverse movements is considered more likely to induce back injuries; thus, the effect of fatigue and reduction of motor control and coordination may be an important risk factor leading to injury-prone working postures. The endurance limit is a more useful predictor of the incidence and recurrence of low back disorders than the absolute strength values (43).

Few studies have investigated trunk muscle endurance and low back disorders. Biering-Sorensen (36) demonstrated that isometric back endurance was significant for prediction of first-time occurrence of low back troubles among men in the follow-up year. However, women showed a nonsignificant trend in the opposite direction. Trunk muscle endurance does differ between healthy subjects and those reporting LBP. During isometric endurance testing, trunk flexors develop fatigue faster than extensors in symptom-free subjects (35). Flexor fatigability appeared significantly higher in patients with LBP than in controls, but no difference in extensor endurance was demonstrated.

Hultman et al. (34) showed reduced abdominal isometric endurance in intermittent LBP sufferers compared to healthy individuals. Chronic LBP patients showed reduced abdominal as well as back muscle endurance relative to healthy controls, and lower back muscle endurance than those in the intermittent LBP group. Holmstrom et al. (44) demonstrated a similar loss of extensor endurance relative to LBP severity. Finally, Nicolaisen and Jorgensen (31) found that individuals with a history of debilitating LBP demonstrated less isometric trunk extensor endurance than either normal individuals or patients with a history of lesser LBP.

Fitness and Low Back Pain

The most widely cited work in favor of fitness programs is a study of firefighters (45). The composite score of physical fitness based on strength, aerobic capacity, and flexibility measures was related to back injury report over a 3-year period in 1,652 firefighters. Those with the highest fitness levels had the fewest back problems. In their Boeing prospective study of 3,020 employees, Battie et al. (46) found that after controlling for sex and age, cardiovascular fitness as measured by maximum oxygen uptake was not predictive of future back injury reports. Several studies have investigated physical fitness relative to the incidence of injury in the military (47–49). These studies are interesting because they may also give us some indication of the determinants of exercises that may cause injury during new recruits' intense physical training (50). In a retrospective review of soldiers' medical records for the 6-month period before the fitness testing of a cohort of 298 male soldiers, the association of age and physical fitness with injuries was investigated

(47). Slower two-mile run times and fewer situps were associated with a higher incidence of musculoskeletal injuries, indicating that a low physical fitness level may be a risk factor for injuries. Two other, prospective studies also associated lower physical fitness with a higher risk of injuries (48,49).

Exercise and Risk of Training-related Injuries

The design parameters of exercise programs that allow aerobic fitness training effects are intensity, duration, and frequency. It is interesting that these are also the determinants of injuries due to training (50). The total amount of exercise is the product of the three parameters that have been most consistently associated with exercise-related injuries. At some level, an increased amount of exercise may not only cause more fitness but also result in greater risk of injury.

Multivariate models of training-related injuries in military recruits have identified older age, cigarette smoking, sedentary jobs and lifestyle, high and low flexibility, high arches of the feet, low past running mileage, and unit training as risk factors. Better knowledge of the effects of the parameters of training and other factors on the risks of exercise-related injuries is necessary to design exercise content to achieve the benefits of exercise while preventing injuries.

Neuromuscular adaptation during heavy-resistance strength training has shown that the initial gains during the first weeks are due to neural factors, with gradually more contribution from muscular hypertrophy as training continues (51). Adaptation in facilitatory and/or inhibitory neural pathways allows more efficient recruitment and higher outcome. Increase in muscle fiber size accompanies higher strength. The overload principle indicates that to increase strength, the loading intensity must exceed muscles' daily activities. Hence, worksite exercises to promote strength must be not only set appropriately to cause the desired gain but also pursued frequently so that the strength can be maintained. There are different types of strength, and because muscle training is specific, job-specific training programs may have more preventive potential. Often, the intensity and duration of exercises are not specified, and that makes interpretation of results of ergonomic interventions difficult. The effects of age and sex on strength training should be considered for industrial programs, given the aging workforce. Short strengthening programs without proper maintenance strategy may not have a lasting effect (52).

ERGONOMIC INTERVENTIONS

Frank et al. (16) reviewed primary prevention studies after summarizing three types of low back WMSD risk factors: individual, biomechanical, and psychosocial. The likelihood of success for work-changing interventions is higher than that for worker-changing interventions. Several studies have reviewed cost-effective ergonomic intervention programs (53–55). Saunders et al. (56) suggested that an injury-prevention strategy must include four elements:

• Management practices (organizational, medical, and claims management),
• Ergonomics,
• Fitness for work,
• Education and training.

Goldenhar and Schulte (15) reviewed occupational health and safety intervention studies published between 1988 and 1993. They concluded that these studies, in general, often lacked a theoretical basis, used small samples, and tested interventions lacking the intensity to cause the desired changes. They criticized the belief that a single causal relationship can be modified by intervention (given the complex multistep causal processes with a wide range of outcomes that may extend over time). They described the control-implementation hierarchy recommended by the National Institute for Occupational Safety and Health (NIOSH): Engineering control is the preferred intervention strategy, followed by administrative controls and lastly behavioral

controls. Many experts believe that interventions targeting multiple levels will be more effective. Clearly, it is hard to modify an individual's behavior without changing the culture of the organization in which the individual works. This concept was reinforced by Wood (57), who quoted Katz and Kahan's (58) description of psychologic fallacy: Attempts to change organizations by changing individuals has a long history of failure because concentration on individuals without regard to the situational factors that shape their behavior is a great oversimplification.

Lahad et al. (59) summarized the results of four interventions to prevent low back injuries in asymptomatic individuals: back and aerobic exercises, education, mechanical support (corsets), and risk-factor modification. They concluded that there is some limited evidence based on randomized trials and epidemiologic studies that increasing strength and overall fitness can reduce the incidence and duration of LBP episodes. Despite the identified methodologic difficulties, the randomized trials that were reviewed all showed fewer episodes or shorter duration of LBP episode for the exercise group. Seven of the epidemiologic studies reviewed indicated a significant association of increased strength and fitness with LBP, while four found no protective effects. The evidence in support of education is minimal, while insufficient evidence exists for the use of corsets. These results must be considered with caution for two reasons: (a) By design, the authors considered primarily studies conducted in the workplace rather than the clinical setting, and (b) they assumed that the response to exercises by asymptomatic individuals with and without a history of LBP would be the same. Linton et al. (60) studied early active intervention for acute musculoskeletal pain in first-time sufferers and patients with a previous history of musculoskeletal pain. Early intervention reduced the likelihood of chronicity in first-time sufferers by a factor of eight, compared to usual treatments. The content and timing of treatment significantly affected the outcome. Patients in early intervention received a median of one physician appointment and three meetings with a physical therapist. When evaluating prevention studies in the literature in general, and particularly those using exercise programs, one must consider the target population (healthy, acute, subacute, or chronic patients) and the content, intensity, frequency, and duration of the programs. Generic approaches seem to be less effective, and appropriately matching the intervention to the needs of each category of patients seems to be more effective.

Faas (61) reviewed recent trials investigating the efficacy of exercise for LBP patients. He concluded that exercise therapy is ineffective for acute back pain, but exercises with a graded activity program deserve attention in subacute back pain and intensive exercise deserves attention in chronic back pain. It is important to note that in one study of acute LBP, patients in an exercise group fared worse than those who were instructed to do their ordinary activities within the limits of pain (62). Among patients with acute LBP, continuing ordinary activities within the limits permitted by the pain was more effective than either bed rest or back-mobilizing exercises. Lindstrom et al.'s (63) study of subacute LPB patients showed positive results for a graded activity program with a behavioral therapy approach. This program significantly increased patients' mobility, strength, and fitness and caused higher rates of return to work.

In a recent critical review of 92 studies, Westgaard and Winkel (64) categorized the ergonomic intervention studies aimed to improve musculoskeletal health into three classes:

- Mechanical-exposure interventions (reducing the level, duration, or repetition of external forces),
- Production-system interventions (arrangement of material, premises, equipment, and workforce required to make the product),
- Modifier interventions (putting workers in a better position to deal with existing demands [i.e., exercise programs], without any change in external demands.

Sixteen studies passed their inclusion criteria and used exercise as their sole intervention. These studies varied greatly in terms of intensity and duration of the exercises, including light pause gymnastics, strength training, and aerobics. The lack of random selection to treatment and control groups confounds the results of many of these studies. The exercise intervention must reach a certain intensity level to improve musculoskeletal health. More studies are needed to specify the optimal content and intensity of worksite exercises that can achieve prevention objectives. Melnik (65) distinguished among exercise, warmup, and stretching activities. Exercise aims to increase maximum performance capacity in terms of strength, endurance, or flexibility. A warmup is for preparing muscles to do work, while a stretching program restores circulation and oxygen after sustained periods of activity. Due to the viscoelastic nature of muscle, flexibility exercises can be performed holding the muscle for 20 seconds in a lengthened position. However, stretching requires a much shorter duration in the lengthened position. The precise characteristics of exercise or fitness programs must be better described in the literature to address the dose–response relationship that is crucial for optimum design of these programs (66).

Westgaard and Winkel (64) concluded that the best chance of success belonged to intervention strategies that identified risk factors and utilized multiple interventions to reduce the risk factors relevant for individuals at risk. High commitment of stakeholders also seems to be important in changing the organizational culture. They also identified that modifier interventions that addressed the medical management of workers at risk, physical training, active training in work techniques, or a combination of these approaches were more successful. Many studies recommend a process-oriented approach to prevention of WMSDs, given their multifactorial nature.

Examples of Studies Using Exercise to Prevent WMSDs

Kellet et al. (67) conducted a prospective randomized clinical trial to evaluate the effect of physical exercise (performed 1 hour per week for a 1.5-year period) on LBP-related sick leave in a major kitchen unit producer. Participants were workers with short (less than 50 days) episodes of LPB in the prior 1.5 years. They were instructed to increase the intensity of exercise until they felt warm and sweaty. The exercise program (detailed in the paper) consisted of warmup, gentle stretching, strengthening, and cardiovascular fitness. Subjects in the exercise group had significantly (50%) fewer episodes of back pain and sick-leave days attributable to back pain, while no change in cardiovascular fitness was detected.

Donchin et al. (68) reported on secondary-prevention study of LBP in 142 hospital employees. A 45-minute at-work calisthenics program with a biweekly session of flexion exercises showed significantly better results in the number of painful months in the follow-up year than the control or back school groups. There was a significant relationship between the rate of participation in the exercise program and the gain in trunk forward flexion. At 6 months postintervention, the trunk forward flexion decreased, while between-group differences remained significant; however, there was no difference in abdominal strength between the groups.

Gundewall et al. (69) performed a prospective, randomized study at a geriatric hospital using 20 minutes of exercise at work as a primary-intervention strategy. The exercises were intended to increase dynamic endurance, isometric strength, and functional coordination using very modest tools. It is important to consider that 100 hours of physiotherapist time were spent answering questions regarding the low back trouble in the exercise group. The 13-month intervention increased the back muscle strength by 20% and lowered the incidence of back pain, back pain intensity, and work absence. Each exercise participant had on average 3.8 fewer absence days, compared with the control group. The authors attributed the positive results to two factors: (a) increased back muscle strength and (b) psychosocial effects.

Linton et al. (70) used a combination of exercise and back-education treatment as secondary prevention for nurses with LBP. The intervention was successful in improving participants' pain intensity, anxiety, sleep quality, fatigue ratings, observed pain behavior, activities, mood, and helplessness. These differences were generally maintained at 6-month follow-up. It is, however, not possible to partition the contribution of each element of the interventions.

Hilyer et al. (71) reported that a flexibility training program reduced the severity and lost-time costs of joint injuries in 469 municipal firefighters, although incident rates were not significantly different from those in the control group. Thirty minutes of flexibility exercises were performed each day on every shift in the experimental group.

Guo et al. (52) examined the effects of four job-simulated flexibility and strength–flexibility training protocols on the dynamic strength, endurance, and flexibility of 24 maintenance employees engaged in a manual material-handling task. The training program consisted of 30 minutes of exercises 5 days per week for 4 weeks. Significant increases in physical capacity measures were found, but these temporary gains were not maintained during follow-up periods, in which training was performed only twice per week. This study proved that indeed the strength and endurance of industrial workers can be enhanced but the protective effects of these increases must be explored.

Harma et al. (72) showed that a 4-month physical training program for 75 nurses and nurses' aides working irregular shifts had reduced their work-dependent fatigue and musculoskeletal symptoms while increasing their physical fitness. The physical training program activated both the circulatory and musculoskeletal systems, based on age, submaximal ergometer performance, and sport habits.

Silverstein et al. (24) found no reduction in localized postural discomfort in 178 participants after 1 year of an on-the-job exercise program to control musculoskeletal symptoms in the neck and upper limb. However, the exercises made 67% of respondents feel better. Workers were involved in repetitive assembly operations, and the exercises lasted 7 minutes and were performed twice per shift along with accompanying music in the manufacturing area. The details of the exercise program are not described, but the authors provided two examples that promoted stretching of the shoulder girdle area and blood flow through and strengthening of the hand. It is highly doubtful that any strengthening could be gained by gripping a soft cloth.

Lutz and Hansford (23) reported on the results of an ergonomics program to control CTDs at Ethicon, Inc. After a 3-month exercise program for 33 workers in microswagging departments, work-related CTD visits to the medical department were reduced from 76 to 28 per month. The unspecified exercise program was performed for 7 minutes twice a day.

Takala et al. (73) used dynamic gymnastic neck exercises for 45 minutes once a week for 10 weeks in a randomized, crossover design matched by age, work task, and frequency of symptoms. No significant effect in terms of the neck pain was detected in the gymnastic group, despite the presence of a seasonal variation in neck symptoms among these 44 women in a printing company. The authors suggested that the results may be due to the light level of exercises used.

Genaidy et al. (74) investigated the effect in an administrative-control intervention of active microbreaks on the discomfort perceived by 28 employees in a meatpacking plant. Employees were given control over work and rest periods and could use an active break of up to 2 minutes at a time to perform the stretching exercises for the parts of the body experiencing discomfort on the job. The total duration of active microbreaks was not allowed to exceed 24 minutes (5% of an 8-hour workday). The study was conducted over a 4-week period, and the rate of perceived discomfort (RPD) was assessed during the second and third weeks. The average total of microbreaks and frequency were 48 seconds and 2.1 (the units of the frequency are missing in the text). Upper extremity RPD was significantly lower with microbreaks. Although the results are intriguing, methodologic problems cast doubt on the generalizability of these results.

Kuorinka et al. (75) randomly assigned a group of 315 workers from three manufacturing companies into two interventions and a control group to prevent the neck–shoulder WMSDs. The intervention group consisted of (a) dynamic training and relaxation program of neck and shoulder muscles and (b) ergonomics improvement in the workplace. At 1-year follow-up of a 10-week training program (completed by 50% of the subjects) and various changes made in one-third of workplaces of the second group, the results indicated a preventive effect of training in terms of new cases of neck–shoulder disorders. The ergonomics program, despite workers' subjective feelings, did not show any preventive effect over the control group. The authors indicated that because some major changes were made by companies in both intervention and control groups, the validity of the results may have been affected. The following study illustrates the difficulty in interpreting some ergonomic field studies, since conditions in a company cannot be kept under control.

Ergonomics Standards

OSHA's circulation of the draft ergonomic standard in 1995 faced considerable resistance from industry, which claimed that the scientific literature does not support a causal relationship between workplace risk factors and WMSDs. In addition, industry indicated that identifying and reducing ergonomics hazards required an unreasonable effort. In response to these criticisms, NIOSH conducted a very substantial review of the epidemiologic and biomechanical literature to partially fill this void (76). The summary results of this undertaking are presented in Table 1. Second, OSHA has been conducting a number of national meetings to further inform all stakeholders with regard to its programs. Third, in a report to Senator Edward Kennedy (Massachusetts) and Senator Major R. Owens, the results of the successful implementation of five ergonomics programs by the private sector were reported (77). These case studies included the core elements and varied according to need in some specific areas. To be

TABLE 1. *Summary results of a critical review of epidemiologic evidence for work-related musculoskeletal disorders performed by the National Institute for Occupational Safety and Health*

Risk factor	Strong evidence	Evidence	Insufficient evidence
Neck and neck/shoulder			
Repetition		*	
Force		*	
Posture	*		
Vibration			*
Shoulder			
Repetition		*	
Force			*
Posture		*	
Vibration			*
Elbow			
Repetition			*
Force		*	
Posture			*
Combination	*		
Hand/wrist			
Carpal tunnel syndrome			
Repetition		*	
Force		*	
Posture			*
Vibration		*	
Combination	*		
Tendinitis			
Repetition		*	
Force		*	
Posture		*	
Combination	*		
Hand–arm vibration syndrome			
Vibration	*		
Back			
Lifting/forceful movement	*		
Awkward posture		*	
Heavy physical work		*	
Whole-body vibration	*		
Static work posture			*

From ref. 76, with permission.

effective, the following essential elements should be present in an ergonomics program:

- Management commitment,
- Employee involvement,
- Identification of problem jobs,
- Development of controls for problem jobs,
- Training and education for employees,
- Appropriate medical management.

These are in keeping with OSHA's *Ergonomics Program Management Guidelines for Meatpacking Plants* (1).

Recently, the National Academy of Sciences and National Research Council released a report reviewing the evidence on WMSDs (12), partly in response to questions posed by Representative Robert Livingston (Louisiana). Many scientists from various disciplines represented the fields of orthopedic surgery, occupational medicine, public health, epidemiology, risk analysis, decision making, ergonomics, and human factors. The report concluded that "there is a strong biological plausibility to the relationship between the incidence of musculoskeletal disorders and the causative exposure factors in high-exposure occupational settings." But, more important in the context of this communication, it pointed out that

Research clearly demonstrates that specific interventions can reduce the reported rate of musculoskeletal disorders for workers who perform high-risk tasks. No known single intervention is universally effective. Successful interventions require attention to individual, organizational, and job characteristics, tailoring the corrective actions to those characteristics.

Although much research remains to be done, using the above guideline, a multilevel intervention strategy for prevention should be implemented. The likelihood of the success of such a program is higher than with single-intervention strategies, such as worksite fitness programs. Which specific additional programs should be included to optimize the performance of these strategies remain to be explored on an individual, case-by-case basis. These issues remain an active area of multidisciplinary research.

REFERENCES

1. Occupational Safety and Health Administration. *Ergonomics program management guidelines for meatpacking plants.* Washington, DC: US Government Pringing Office, 1993. OSHA publication 3123.
2. Frank JW, Pulcins IR, Kerr MS, Shannon HS, Stansfeld SA. Occupational back pain—an unhelpful polemic. *Scand J Work Environ Health* 1995;21:3–14.
3. Parnianpour M, Engin AE. A more quantitative approach to classification of impairments, disabilities, and handicaps. *J Rheumatol Med Rehabil* 1994;5:52–64.
4. Battie MC. Minimizing the impact of back pain: workplace strategies. *Semin Spine Surg* 1992;4:20–28.
5. Kuorinka I, Forcier L, eds. *Work-related musculoskeletal disorders: a reference book for prevention.* London: Taylor and Francis, 1995.
6. Armstrong TJ, Buckle P, Fine LJ, et al. A conceptual model for work-related neck and upper-limb musculoskeletal disorders. *Scand J Work Environ Health* 1993; 19:73–84.
7. Fathallah FA, Marras WS, Parnianpour M. The role of complex, simultaneous trunk motions in the risk of occupation-related low back disorders. *Spine* 1998;23: 1035–1042.
8. Battie MC, Videman KT. Epidemiology of the back. In: Nordin M, Andersson GJ, Pope MH, eds. *Work-related musculoskeletal disorders in the workplace:* principles and practices. St. Louis, MO: Mosby–Year Book, 1997: 253–268.
9. Leino PI. Does leisure time physical activity prevent low back disorders? A prospective study of metal industry employees. *Spine* 1993;18:863–871.
10. Sward L, Hellstrom M, Jacobsson B, Nyman R, Peterson L. Disc degeneration and associated abnormalities of the spine in elite gymnasts: a magnetic resonance imaging study. *Spine* 1991;16:437–443.
11. Volinn E. The epidemiology of low back pain in the rest of the world: a review of surveys in low- and middle-income countries. *Spine* 1997;22:1747–1754.
12. The Research Base, Committee on Human Factors, National Research Council. *Work-related musculoskeletal disorders:* a review of the evidence steering committee for the workshop on work-related musculoskeletal injuries. National Academy Press, Washington, D.C., 1998.
13. Armstrong TJ, Martin BJ. Adverse effects of repetitive loading and segmental vibration. In: Nordin M, Andersson GJ, Pope MH, eds. *Work-related musculoskeletal disorders in the workplace:* principles and practices. St. Louis, MO: Mosby–Year Book, 1997:134–151.
14. Lotz JC, Colliou OK, Chin JR, Duncan NA, Liebenberg E. Compression-induced degeneration of the intervertebral disc: an *in vivo* mouse model and finite-element study. *Spine* 1998;23:2493–2506.
15. Goldenhar LM, Schulte PA. Intervention research in occupational health and safety. *J Occup Med* 1994;36: 763–775.
16. Frank JW, Kerr MS, Brooker AS, et al. Disability resulting from occupational low back pain. Part I: what do we know about primary prevention? A review of the scientific evidence on prevention before disability begins. *Spine* 1996;21:2908–2917.
17. Pope MH, Andersson GJB. Prevention. In: Nordin M, Andersson GJ, Pope MH, eds. *Work-related musculoskeletal disorders in the workplace:* principles and practices. St. Louis, MO: Mosby–Year Book, 1997: 244–252.
18. Wang JL, Parnianpour M, Shirazi-Adl A, Engin AE. The simulation of viscoelastic behaviors under experimental controlled loading and the failure criterion of collagen fiber. *J Theoret Appl Fracture Mech* 1997;27:1–12.
19. Smith MJ, Sainfort PC. A balance theory of job design for stress reduction. *Int J Ind Ergon* 1989;4:67–79.
20. Voleki RV. Employee fitness programs. In: Key GI, ed. *Industrial therapy.* St. Louis, MO: Mosby–Year Book, 1995:181–193.
21. Khalaf KA, Parnianpour M, Sparto PJ, Simon SR. Modeling of functional trunk muscle performance: interfacing ergonomics and spine rehabilitation in response to the ADA. *J Rehabil Res Dev* 1997;34:459–469.
22. Kondraske GV. Quantitative measurement and assessment of performance. In: Smith RV, Leslie JH, eds. *Rehabilitation engineering.* Boca Raton, FL: CRC Press, 1990:101–120.
23. Lutz G, Hansford T. Cumulative trauma disorder controls: the ergonomics program at Ethicon, Inc. *J Hand Surg [Am]* 1987;12:863–866.
24. Silverstein BA, Armstrong TJ, Longmate A, Woody D. Can in-plant exercise control musculoskeletal symptoms? *J Occup Med* 1988;30:922–927.
25. Putz-Andersson V, ed. *Cumulative truama disorders:* a manual for musculoskeletal diseases of the upper limbs. Philadelphia: Taylor and Francis, 1988.
26. Quint U, Wilke HJ, Shirazi-Adl A, Parnianpour M, Loer F, Claes LE. Importance of the intersegmental trunk muscles for the stability of the lumbar spine: a biomechanical study *in vitro. Spine* 1998;23:1937–1945.
27. Szpalski M, Parnianpour M. Trunk performance, strength and endurance: measurement techniques and application. In: Weisel S, Weinstein J, eds. *The lumbar spine,* 2nd ed. Philadelphia: WB Saunders, 1996:1074–1105.
28. Hirsch G, Beach G, Cooke C, et al. Relationship be-

tween performance on lumbar dynamometry and Waddell score in a population with lowback pain. *Spine* 1991;16:1039–1043.

29. Carlier P, Szpalski M, Vanderbecken F, Hayez JP. Isoinertial functional assessment of lowback disorders in paediatric nurses: ergonomic and rehabilitation guidelines. *J Occup Rehabil* 1992;2:131–139.

30. Addison R, Schultz A. Trunk strength in patients seeking hospitalization for chronic low back disorders. *Spine* 1980;5:539–544.

31. Nicolaisen T, Jorgensen K. Trunk strength, back muscles endurance and low back trouble. *Scand J Rehabil Med* 1985;17:121–129.

32. Newton M, Morag T, Somerville D, et al. Trunk strength testing with iso-machines, part 2: experimental evaluation of the Cybex II back testing system in normal subjects and patients with chronic low back pain. *Spine* 1993;18:812–824.

33. Nachemson A, Lindh M. Measurement of abdominal and back muscle strength with and without low back pain. *Scand J Rehabil Med* 1969;1:60–63.

34. Hultman G, Nordin M, Saraste H, et al. Body composition, endurance, cross-sectional area, and density of MM erector spinae in men with and without low back pain. *J Spinal Disord* 1993;6:114–123.

35. Suzuki N, Endo S. A quantitative study of trunk muscle strength and fatigability in the low back pain syndrome. *Spine* 1983;8:69–74.

36. Biering-Sorensen F. Physical measurements as risk indicators for low back trouble over one-year period. *Spine* 1984;9:106–119.

37. Battie MC, Bigos SJ, Fisher LD, et al. Isometric lifting as a predictor of industrial back pain. *Spine* 1989;14:851–856.

38. Chaffin DB, Herrin GD, Keyserling WM. Preemployement strength testing: an updated position. *J Occup Med* 1978;20:403–408.

39. Mostardi RA, Noe DA, Kovacik MW, et al. Isokinetic lifting strength and occupational injury: a prospective study. *Spine* 1992;17:189–193.

40. Troup JDG, Martin JW, Lloyd DC. Back pain in industry: a prospective study. *Spine* 1981;6:61–69.

41. Chaffin DB. Localized muscle fatigue-definition and measurement. *J Occup Med* 1973;15:346–354.

42. Holding DH. *Stress and fatigue in human performance.* New York: John Wiley and Sons, 1983:145-165.

43. Parnianpour M, Nordin M, Kahanovitz N, Frankel VH. The triaxial coupling of torque generation of trunk muscles during isometric exertions and the effect of fatiguing isoinertial movements on the motor output and movement patterns. *Spine* 1988;13:982–992.

44. Holmstrom EB, Andersson M, Moritz U. Trunk muscle strength and back muscle endurance in construction workers with and without low back disorders. *Scand J Rehabil Med* 1992;24:3–11.

45. Cady LD, Bischoff DP, O'Connel ER, et al. Strength and fitness and subsequent back injuries in firefighters. *J Occup Med* 1979;21:269–272.

46. Battie MC, Bigos SJ, Fisher LD, et al. A prospective study of the role of cardiovascular risk factors and fitness in industrial back pain complaints. *Spine* 1989;14:141–147.

47. Knapik J, Ang P, Reynolds K, Jones B. Physical fitness, age and injury incidence in infantry soldiers. *J Occup Med* 1993;35:598–603.

48. Jones BH, Bovee MW, Harris JM III, Cowan DN. Intrinsic risk factors for exercise-related injuries among male and female army trainees. *Am J Sports Med* 1993;21:705–710.

49. Jones BH, Cowan DN, Tomlinson JP, Robinson JR, Polly DW, Frykman PN. Epidemiology of injuries associated with physical training among young men in the army. *Med Sci Sports Exerc* 1993;25:197–203.

50. Jones BH, Cowan DN, Knapik JJ. Exercise, training and injuries. *Sports Med* 1994;18:202–214.

51. Hakkinen K. Neuromuscular adaptation during strength training, aging, detraining, and immobilization. *Critical Reviews Physical Rehabil Med* 1994;6:161–198.

52. Guo L, Genaidy A, Warm J, Karwowski W, Hidalgo J. Effects of job-simulated flexibility and strength-flexibility training protocols on maintenance employees engaged in manual handling operations. *Ergonomics* 1992;35:1103–1117.

53. Shi L. A cost-benefit analysis of a California county's back injury prevention program. *Public Health Rep* 1993;108:204–211.

54. Aaras A. The impact of ergonomic intervention on individual health and corporate prosperity in a telecommunications environment. *Ergonomics* 1994;37:1679–1696.

55. Garg A, Owen B. Reducing back stress to nursing personnel: an ergonomic intervention in a nursing home. *Ergonomics* 1992;35:1353–1375.

56. Saunders HD, Stultz MR, Saunders R, Anderson MA. Back injury prevention. In: Key GI, ed. *Industrial therapy.* St. Louis, MO: Mosby–Year Book, 1995:123–148.

57. Wood DJ. Design and evaluation of a back injury prevention program within a geriatric hospital. *Spine* 1987;12:77–82.

58. Katz D, Kahan RL. *The social psychology of organizations,* 2nd ed. New York: John Wiley and Sons, 1978.

59. Lahad A, Malter AD, Berg AO, Deyo RA. The effectiveness of four interventions for the prevention of low back pain. *JAMA* 1994;272:1286–1291.

60. Linton SJ, Hellsing AL, Andersson D. A controlled study of effects of an early intervention on acute musculoskeletal pain problems. *Pain* 1993;36:197–207.

61. Faas A. Exercises: which ones are worth trying, for which patients, and when? *Spine* 1996;21:2874–2878.

62. Malmivaara A, Hakkinen U, Aro T, et al. The treatment of acute low back pain—bed rest, exercises, or ordinary activity? *N Engl J Med* 1995;332:351–355.

63. Lindstrom I, Ohlun C, Eek C, et al. Mobility, strength, and fitness after a graded activity program for patients with subacute low back pain. *Spine* 1992;17:641–652.

64. Westgaard RH, Winkel J. Ergonomic intervention research for improved musculoskeletal health: a critical review. *Int J Ind Ergon* 1997;20:463–500.

65. Melnik MS. Upper extremity injury prevention. In: Key GI, ed. *Industrial therapy.* St. Louis, MO: Mosby–Year Book, 1995:148–180.

66. McGill SM. Low back exercises: evidence for improving exercise regimens. *Phys Ther* 1998;78:754–765.

67. Kellet KM, Kellett DA, Nordham LA. Effects of an exercise program on sick leave due to back pain. *Phys Ther* 1991;71:283–293.

68. Donchin M, Woolf O, Kaplan L, Florman Y. Secondary prevention of low back pain: a clinical trial. *Spine* 1990;15:1317–1320.

69. Gundewall B, Liljeqvist M, Hansson T. Primary preven-

tion of back symptoms and absence from work. *Spine* 1993;18:587–594.

70. Linton SJ, Bradley LA, Jensen I, Spangfort E, Sundell L. The secondary prevention of low back pain: a controlled study with follow-up. *Pain* 1989;36:197–207.

71. Hilyer JC, Brown KC, Sirles AT, et al. A flexibility intervention to reduce the incidence and severity of joint injuries among municipal firefighters. *J Occup Med* 1990;32:631–637.

72. Harma MI, Ilmarinen J, Knauth P, Rutenfranz J, Hanninen O. Physical training intervention in female shift workers: I. The effects of intervention on fitness, fatigue, sleep, and psychosomatic symptoms. *Ergonomics* 1988;31:39–50.

73. Takala EP, Viikari-Juntura E, Tynkkynen EM. Does group gymnastics at the workplace help in neck pain? *Scand J Rehabil Med* 1994;26:17–20.

74. Genaidy AM, Delgado E, Bustos T. Active microbreak effects on musculoskeletal comfort ratings in meatpacking plants. *Ergonomics* 1995;38:326–336.

75. Kuorinka I, Alaranta H, Erich I. Prevention of musculoskeletal disorders at work: validation and reliability in a multicenter intervention study. *Int J Ind Ergon* 1995; 15:437–446.

76. Bernard BP, ed. *Musculoskeletal disorders and workplace factors:* a critical review of epidemiological evidences for work-related musculoskeletal disorders of the neck, *upper extremity, and low back.* Washington, DC: Department of Health and Human Services. NIOSH publication 97-141.

77. *Private sector ergonomics programs.* Washington DC: Government Accounting Office/Health, Education, and Human Service Division 97-163, 1997.

Occupational Musculoskeletal Disorders
edited by T. G. Mayer, R. J. Gatchel, and P. B. Polatin.
Lippincott Williams & Wilkins, Philadelphia © 2000.

13

Employer Experiences, Outcomes, and Challenges in Implementing Effective Ergonomics Programs[1]

Lori Rectanus

*U.S. General Accounting Office, Heath, Education, and Human Services Division,
Washington, D.C. 20548*

Employers spend billions of dollars annually on workers' compensation claims associated with musculoskeletal disorders (MSDs), a wide range of illnesses and injuries resulting from repetitive stress or sustained exertion on the body (1–5). Although controversy surrounds which specific workplace conditions may cause MSDs and what actions are necessary to eliminate MSDs, more and more employers realize that they must do something to address their increasing workers' compensation costs. Many employers who have taken action to reduce MSDs in the workplace report lowered costs, as well as improvements in employee productivity and morale. It is a challenge, however, for employers to find out how well a program is really working, given the reality of business and differences in local conditions (6). This chapter highlights what are commonly believed to be the necessary components of an effective program to prevent MSDs—often referred to as an "ergonomics" program. Based on the experiences of facilities at five companies, this chapter explores how these components may be successfully implemented, what challenges must be overcome, and the outcomes that result from this process.

BASIC COMPONENTS OF EFFECTIVE PROGRAMS

An ergonomics program designed to prevent the occurrence of MSDs must include several basic components to ensure that workplace conditions that contribute to or cause MSDs are identified and addressed (7,8). Necessary components of such a program include management commitment, employee involvement, employee training and education, reduction of workplace hazards, and active medical treatment and prevention (3,6,8–11). A wide variety of alternatives have been suggested to carry out these components that call for varying degrees of effort on the part of employers and employees.

Management Commitment and Employee Involvement

Employers must demonstrate a commitment to a safe and healthy work environment for all employees and can do so in a number of ways. Designated staff can be assigned responsibility for a safety program and be provided time during the workday to address ergonomic concerns. Impoved equipment and workplace designs confirm an employer's interest in employment safety, as does demonstrating positive outcomes from an effective ergonomics program (3,6,8,10–13). Involv-

---

[1]This chapter is based on and summarized from ref. 6.

ing employees in key decisions about workplace safety increases the likelihood that they will accept changes in their job or work methods. One of the simpler ways to achieve such involvement is to establish a simple, well-understood procedure that encourages employees to promptly report symptoms of MSDs. Employers may also solicit employee reports of potential hazards and suggestions for improving job operations, or administer periodic surveys to obtain employee reactions to workplace conditions. Committees or teams of employees might be established to receive information on problem areas, analyze these problems, and make recommendations for corrective action.

Employee Training and Education

Training and education for employees is critical because identifying and controlling MSDs require some knowledge of ergonomics and skills in remedying hazards. General ergonomics awareness training can be provided to all employees so that they can recognize general risks, know the procedures for reporting MSDs, and become familiar with the process of identifying hazards and problem jobs. Training can also be more targeted to specific groups of employees because of the jobs they hold, the risks they face, or their roles in the program (3,8,9,14).

Hazard Identification

The identification of hazards contributing to MSDs is at the heart of any ergonomics program. One way to identify hazards or problem jobs is to use existing data, such as Occupational Safety and Health Administration (OSHA) Form 200 logs, workers' compensation records, or reports by employees to health care providers of symptoms or discomfort, to see where injuries or symptoms are occurring. This "incidence-basis" is the easiest as it focuses on problems that are already documented. Employers can also interview workers or administer surveys to find what symptoms employees are experiencing, even

if they have not yet reported them. The most resource-intensive approach often called "risk-based" is to review all jobs or operations for particular risk factors such as awkward postures, forceful exertions, repetitive motion, or vibration. In this manner, employers can determine which jobs have the potential for MSDs, whether or not any symptoms have yet been reported (3,8–11,14–17).

Hazard Reduction: Developing Solutions for Problem Jobs

A wide range of alternatives have been suggested for how hazards can be addressed. They can be as simple as watching a worker perform a job or a particular task for a short time to determine where the likely hazard is and then, with that information, brainstorming possible solutions (controls) to rectify the particular problem. Taking measurements of employees' workstations (e.g., work-surface heights or required reach distances) helps determine whether the physical layout requires changes. Such an approach would address a particular hazard but would not necessarily change an entire job or operation. A more expensive and complex way to identify all risk factors in a particular job would be to videotape the entire job or activity, take still photos, and make biomechanical calculations (e.g., how much muscle force is required to accomplish a task) or break down the job into individual tasks. Controls would then be developed that would seek to change the entire job or operation (3,8–11,14–17).

The types of solutions (e.g., controls) that can be put in place vary in complexity and expense. "Engineering" controls that reduce or eliminate employees' exposure to hazards through the job process include changing the way materials, parts, and products are transported, or changing the workstation layout or tool design to better accommodate employees. "Administrative" controls are work practices and policies that reduce employee exposure to hazards and include such measures as scheduled rest breaks, rotation of workers through hazardous jobs, and implementation of work practices that ease workloads (3, 8–11,14,15).

Medical Treatment and Prevention

Any good medical management program for employees should emphasize the prevention of impairment and disability through early detection of injuries, prompt treatment, and timely recovery. It is essential to ensure that whatever medical management program already exists is integrated with an employer's efforts to reduce MSDs. Suggested ways to implement this integration include the following:

- Encouragement of employees to report symptoms of MSDs early, without fear of reprisal or discrimination;
- Prompt evaluation by health care providers of any MSD reports;
- Education of health care providers to individual job requirements so that employees with diagnosed MSDs are given appropriate restrictions or transitional duty assignments until effective controls are installed on the problem job;
- Follow-up monitoring to ensure that recovering employees continue to be protected from exposure to hazards (3,8–11,14).

VARIETY AND SIMPLICITY: KEYS TO SUCCESSFUL PROGRAM IMPLEMENTATION

Based on experiences in five facilities, variety in implementation of program components appears to be essential in accounting for differences in industrial or production operations, corporate culture, and experiences during program evolution. Moreover, simplicity in execution—characterized by implementation of the relatively easiest of the suggested alternatives in terms of cost or operation—was often necessitated by business conditions and made the most sense when the program was just beginning. This simplicity was especially evident in activities to identify and control problem jobs: Facilities included in this study generally identified problem jobs on an incidence basis, undertook simple methods to identify controls, and implemented "low-tech" controls—those that did not significantly change the job and were generally fairly inexpensive (6).

Facilities Selected for Review

The five facilities selected for review represent different industries, geographic locations, and numbers of employees. They include manufacturing, health care, and financial services, industries either known for a high incidence of MSDs (e.g., manufacturing and health care) or associated with problems involving computer use (e.g., financial services). The facilities are located in five states (Maine, Minnesota, Ohio, Pennsylvania, and Texas) and range in size from 300 to more than 5,000 employees. Only one facility has a unionized workforce. Each facility had a "fully implemented" ergonomics program in place at the time of this review. The oldest program had been implemented in 1992 and the newest in 1994.

1. *American Express Financial Advisors, Inc.* (AEFA), headquartered in Minneapolis, Minnesota, is the largest of the facilities studied; it has a nonunion workforce of about 5,300, providing financial planning services. AEFA's efforts to implement an ergonomics program began in 1986 as a commitment to improving employee comfort and satisfaction and as a result of a major staff reorganization required a physical relocation of the staff and the purchase of new furniture. However, the program was not fully implemented until 1993, when a full-time ergonomist was hired to lead the program. Most of AEFA's employees work in an office environment using computers.

2. *AMP, Inc.*, located in Tower City, Pennsylvania, manufactures electrical and electronic connection devices. It is the smallest facility studied, with a nonunion workforce of about 300. Employees operate mechanical presses to form the electronic terminals and connectors. The majority of workers are die machinists and mechanics. Its ergonomics

program has largely focused on these manufacturing operations and has been evolving since the late 1980s. At that time, the safety department began to offer ergonomics training courses, corporate productivity initiatives were being launched, and different units of employees across AMP formed teams to identify production problems. The program was fully implemented in 1993, when the facility formed an ergonomics team that is now the heart of the program.

3. *Navistar International*, in Springfield, Ohio, assembles heavy- and medium-duty trucks, although it was originally designed to produce pickup trucks. The majority of the facility's 4,000 employees are represented by the United Auto Workers, and the union's 1984 collective bargaining agreement was a major influence in Navistar's pilot ergonomics program. In 1991, the facility hired its first ergonomist, but the current program was fully implemented in 1994 with the hiring of the current ergonomist. She was placed in the safety, rather than the engineering, department. Although there are office-related occupations at the facility, most of the program's efforts have focused on the production workers on the floor who assemble the trucks.

4. *Sisters of Charity Health System's* (SOCHS) Lewiston, Maine, nursing home and acute/behavioral medical care facility employs about 800 nonunion workers. SOCHS officials said their major concerns were the certified nursing assistants (CNAs) responsible for patient handling and employees working in the laboratory, medical records, registration, and other computer- and phone-intensive operations. This program became fully implemented in 1994 after SOCHS received an invitation from OSHA to participate in the "Maine 200" program, which targeted employers with high numbers of lost workdays to help them reduce workplace injuries and illnesses.

5. *Texas Instruments'* (TI) Lewisville, Texas, facility manufactures electronics for "smart" weaponry. Ergonomic efforts have been ongoing there since the 1980s, but the ergonomics program was fully implemented in 1992, the

year after the facility's workers' compensation costs for MSDs exceeded $2 million. About 3,000 nonunionzed employees work at the facility—about two-thirds engineers and others representing electrical assemblers, machinists, manufacturing aides, and equipment technicians. The program has focused both on manufacturing and office-related operations. In 1997, the facility was purchased by Raytheon Systems.

Variety in Program-component Implementation

All the programs of the facilities included in this review contain all the previously mentioned program components, but there is significant variety in how these components are structured. For example, all the facilities assign staff to be responsible for the program along with the resources, time, and authority to operate the program on a daily basis, thereby demonstrating management commitment. The AEFA facility employs an ergonomist to lead the program, while the AMP and TI facilities rely on leadership provided by teams of line employees because their organizations' culture uses employee teams for most projects. At the Navistar facility, management decided to use an ergonomist and a union representative to lead the program because early experience with employee teams had not proved successful. Other employees are brought in on an *ad hoc* basis to address specific problems. All facilities also emphasize employee involvement by establishing processes whereby employees may request action based on real or potential MSDs. At the Navistar facility, employees fill out a one-page "Request for Ergonomic Study" form and submit it to the ergonomist or the union representative. At the AEFA facility, employees request evaluations of their workstation through a phone call, electronic message, or scheduling them themselves on an electronic calendar designed for such purposes. In some cases, facilities administer different kinds of campaigns to obtain employee involvement. The AEFA facility uses "discomfort" surveys to help the ergonomics staff identify areas of concern for employees and the type of discomfort employees are feeling in various body parts. The TI facility sponsors "wing-by-wing" measurement campaigns, in which all employees are measured and their workstations adjusted, even for employees who have not requested services but might be at risk.

All the facilities provide training for employees, which varies depending on corporate culture, occupation held, and industry standards. Not every facility offers general awareness training to all employees. When it is offered, it is generally required by the industry or is a part of larger training efforts. For example, at the SOCHS facility, employees must participate in a yearly 90-minute safety training session that includes instruction on patient handling and the use of video display terminals. At the TI facility, all employees are required to take 1 hour of general ergonomics awareness training every 3 years. More commonly at these facilities, training is targeted to specific groups of workers. For example, because most employees in AEFA's ergonomics program work on computers, weekly training is offered on how to identify and address computer-related hazards, and employees are required to take this training before their workstations will be adjusted. The TI facility emphasizes instruction for production teams within their own work areas. Team members work together to develop controls for problem jobs.

At each facility, the ergonomics program is strongly linked to the existing medical management program, but the type of linkage varies. In all cases, report of a MSD automatically triggers an evaluation of the job or workstation. For facilities with on-site health care providers, the providers themselves can request evaluations of particular activities based on reported symptoms of MSDs, participate in developing controls for problem jobs, or serve on ergonomics teams. At the Navistar facility, an on-site physical therapist walks the floor with the union representative to watch employees performing jobs and to identify potential problems. At the SOCHS facility, the on-site health care provider evaluates employees prior to placement, as well as prior to job transfers, so the facility knows how employees should or should not be used. The health care provider also evaluates designs for new construction or office layouts to ensure that they are ergonomically sound. Where health care providers are not on-site, facilities have a list of several local health care providers who are familiar with MSDs, are conservative in their treatment approach, and have knowledge of the facilities' jobs. These providers are encouraged to visit the facility to understand the jobs that these workers perform, or are provided physical descriptions of the facility's jobs. All the facilities emphasize a return-to-work policy that gives employees with diagnosed MSDs the opportunity to work on restricted- or light-duty assignments during their recovery period, but procedures used to identify and monitor such work varies. The TI facility developed a database of available jobs for workers on restriction and created a special account that covers the payroll costs of employees on transitional duty so that the costs are not charged to the budget of the home work area. The AEFA facility returns injured employees to their original jobs but modifies the work requirements, when necessary, so that employees do not perform any activity to further aggravate their injury. The SOCHS facility establishes particular jobs that employees on restriction can perform and charges their activity to that unit as an incentive to return employees to full duty as soon as possible. Each facility also monitors employees after they have been given a restriction or have returned to work. AEFA allows a 12-week return-to-work policy before employees are required to return to their original work schedule. Navistar allows employees 30 days of light duty before they lose any union seniority or job classification rights.

Simplicity in Program-component Implementation

In many cases, facilities implement the less complex of suggested alternatives. Problem jobs or activities are typically identified on an incidence basis through reports of MSDs or employee discomfort, employee requests for assistance, OSHA 200 logs, or workers' compensation data. For example, the TI facility identifies problem jobs based on the high numbers of injuries and illnesses recorded in its workers' compensation database. Because every job has some inherent risk factors, using a more proactive, risk-based approach requires that every job be scrutinized, an expensive and time-consuming process. Beginning the program where the problems have already been identified provides the best return.

Only after problem jobs identified on an incidence-basis are dealt with do these facilities focus their efforts on proactive methods for identifying workplace hazards. At this point, they typically do not screen jobs for risk factors but instead use key work-related factors. For example, the Navistar facility began to identify problem jobs as those with high employee turnover or low union seniority, on the premise that if employees with seniority consistently declined a particular job, then there were likely problems associated with that job. Because the TI facility had already addressed many of the hazards at the manufacturing workstations, it recognized that the facility needed to shift its focus to identify potential hazards at administrative workstations and started conducting an administrative workstation adjustment campaign.

All the facilities use a simple, fairly informal procedure to analyze problem jobs, and often their efforts focus only on a particular job element thought to be the problem (e.g., drilling or lifting). For example, as the basis for its evaluations, the AMP facility uses a one-page "Ergonomic Evaluation" form that is tailored to the specific job and asks simple "yes/no" questions about the employee's ease and comfort when performing certain job tasks. After reviewing this form, a member of the ergonomics team will interview the employee and observe him or her performing the job. Program officials at AEFA and TI facilities take workstation and personal measurements (e.g., height of work surface, appropri-

ate height of chair when the employee is seated properly), in addition to collecting information through interviews. When in some cases the problem job is particularly complex, hazardous, or labor-intensive, a detailed job analysis may be performed; however, this is rarely required.

The process of developing hazard controls is also informal, relying heavily on brainstorming, in-house engineering, and available medical resources. At the Navistar facility, the *ad hoc* committee of employees informally develop prospective solutions, brainstorm options, and look at other operations within the facility with similar job elements to get ideas for controls. At TI, in addition to its own employees and line supervisors, its production engineering department and the team of employees assigned to the job are also resources for developing controls on more complex or technical jobs.

Although facilities use a mix of the controls described in the literature in their attempts to eliminate or reduce ergonomic hazards for problem jobs, they generally implement "low-tech" engineering controls—those that do not drastically change a job's requirements and do not require significant capital investments. In many cases, the types of controls implemented depend on the facility layout, jobs, or product line. For example, because the Navistar facility's layout constrains an overhaul of many jobs, engineering controls are used to reduce some of the problem activities in particular jobs. These include hoists to lift heavy fuel tanks, mechanical articulating arms to transport carburetors, and replacing impact guns used to drill in bolts with nutrunner guns, which expose employees to lower levels of vibration. Because most AEFA employees work on computers, the facility found that the most effective controls involve adjusting employee workstations (e.g., repositioning monitors, designing corner work surfaces, providing equipment to support forearm use) and introducing ergonomic chairs. Because transporting patients was identified at the SOCHS facility as a major cause of employee back injuries, the facil-

EMPLOYERS AND EFFECTIVE ERGONOMICS PROGRAMS

ity purchased numerous automatic lifts, doing away with manual lifting. Facilities also use administrative controls, particularly for problem jobs in which they are unable to eliminate the ergonomic hazards through engineering controls. Where production of a particular product is being phased out, it does not make sense to invest resources in an engineering control. For example, in one job at the AMP facility, employees were rotated every 2 hours so that they were not performing the same hand motion over long periods of time. At the Navistar facility, for one job in which it would be too costly to implement engineering controls, employees were provided padded gloves and elbow supports to help minimize exposure to hazards.

REDUCED MSD WORKERS' COMPENSATION COSTS AND INCREASED PRODUCTIVITY

One sign of a successful ergonomics program is reduced workers' compensation costs associated with MSDs. In addition to reductions in MSD costs, however, these facilities also saw general improvements in facility-wide indicators, such as number of lost and restricted workdays. Facility officials also reported improved worker morale, productivity, and product quality, although evidence of these improvements was primarily anecdotal.

Before implementation of these programs, the cost of MSD claims at these facilities accounted for at least 50% of each facility's total annual workers' compensation costs; as a result, high MSD claims' costs were a major influence on the initiation of these programs. Several years after fully implementing their programs, these facilities experienced often dramatic declines in workers' compensation costs for MSDs. Comparing the year prior to full implementation to 1996 or 1997 (depending on which data were available), facilities' workers' compensation costs for MSDs declined 37% to 91% (Fig. 1). At the TI facility, where the ergonomics program had been in place for the longest time, workers' compensation costs for MSDs dropped from millions

of dollars in 1991 to hundreds of thousands of dollars in 1996.

For four of the facilities, the average cost of MSD claims also dropped 49% to 77% during this same time (see Fig. 1) as a result of early identification and treatment. However, at the SOCHS facility, the average cost for MSD-related claims did not decline since full implementation of the program because the number of claims declined faster than the cost of those claims. Facility officials said that treatment for several back injury claims was expensive and has kept costs from declining more quickly.

Along these lines, if an important part of a medical management program is getting injured employees back to work as soon as possible, then reducing the number of lost or restricted workdays should also be a program goal. In fact, officials at several facilities said one of their first activities when implementing their ergonomics programs was to assist employees in returning to work during this period. Not surprisingly then, during this time, the facilities generally experienced declines in the number of lost workdays (according to their OSHA 200 log records) for all employees at the facilities. As shown in Fig. 2, the four facilities required to keep OSHA 200 logs found that they had reduced the number of lost workdays per 100 employees by 20 to 122 days.

One would expect to see a reduction in restricted days if a facility is in fact returning an employee to full work as soon as possible. As shown in Fig. 2, three of the four facilities required to keep an OSHA 200 log decreased the number of restricted workdays per 100 employees by 15 to 80 days. On the other hand, officials at the AMP facility, which actually experienced an increase in the number of restricted days, said that this increase reflects their policy of bringing workers back to work as soon as possible, although these workers have not yet been taken off restricted duty.

Facility officials report improved employee morale since implementation of their programs, although evidence of this outcome is primarily anecdotal. Some facility officials

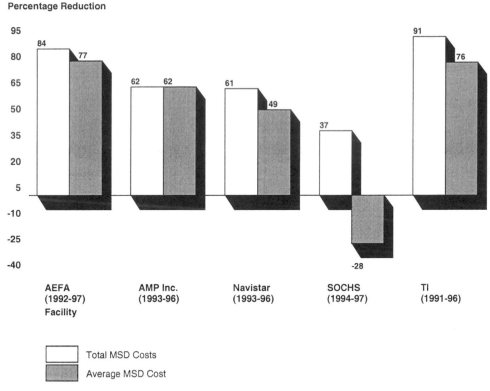

FIG. 1. Percentage reduction in total and average cost of musculoskeletal disorder (MSD) claims for the facilities reviewed in this chapter. Note: Data are not adjusted for inflation. Years presented generally represent the year prior to full implementation at each of the facilities compared to 1996, with several exceptions. Neither AMP, Inc., nor the Sisters of Charity Health System (SOCHS) had data available for the year prior to their program's full implementation. In addition, American Express Financial Advisors, Inc. (AEFA) and SOCHS were able to provide data through 1997. (Adapted from ref. 6, with permission.)

say that as a consequence of their programs, employees are now more likely to exercise control over their jobs and be more actively involved with line supervisors in how jobs are performed. Officials from the SOCHS facility believe that turnover and absenteeism have been reduced. They are able to hire better qualified employees as a result of their efforts, even though there was initial employee resistance to some of the changes proposed, such as automatic lifts to move patients. Results from AEFA's annual discomfort survey show that about 75% of employees surveyed in 1993 experienced headaches and discomfort in the neck and back, but only about a

one-third of employees surveyed reported such discomfort in 1997.

The facilities provided primarily anecdotal evidence of improvements in productivity and quality of work associated with implementation of ergonomic controls. Several facilities found that these hazards had often contributed to production bottlenecks or problems, so that by addressing ergonomic-related problems, they made productivity gains as well. By minimizing employees' stressful hand exertions during a windshield installation process, the Navistar facility was able to increase the quality of the installation, reducing a previously high rate of warranty claims.

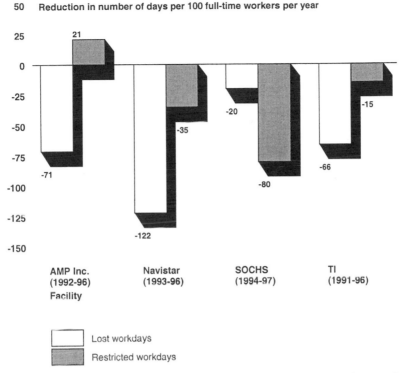

FIG. 2. Change in lost and restricted workdays for the facilities reviewed in this chapter. See note in Fig. 1 legend. In addition, as a financial institution, American Express Financial Advisors, Inc., is not required to maintain an OSHA Form 200 log, from which these data are obtained. As a result, it is not included in this figure. (Adapted from ref. 6, with permission.)

CHALLENGES IN DEMONSTRATING OVERALL PROGRAM PERFORMANCE

Although officials at all the facilities are adamant that their programs are effective—pointing to reductions in MSD workers' compensation costs, lost and restricted workdays, and improved employee morale and productivity—they admit that a number of confounding factors make it impossible to determine whether a program is as effective as it should or could be. These factors include the following:

- Uncertainties in determining what types of injuries should be included as MSDs,
- Difficulties in analyzing changes in these injuries as a result of ergonomic program implementation because management and

business conditions are changing at the same time,
- Accepting the idea that these programs are in a constant state of evolution and therefore will change in effectiveness over time.

Identifying the Types of Injuries to Track

A major influence on the initiation of the program at these facilities was a concern about increased workers' compensation costs due to MSDs. However, in the early stages of implementing the ergonomics program, some facilities reported uncertainties about which injuries and illnesses should be categorized as MSDs. AEFA officials said the lack of agreement about MSDs made it difficult to know what to track when trying to isolate MSDs from other kinds of injuries and illnesses. SOCHS officials said that incident reports had to be reviewed to identify whether an in-jury was caused by a lack of ergonomic con-ditions or other factors. In another facility, differences of opinion existed between the er-gonomist and corporate managers as to what categories should or should not be included as MSDs. Workers' compensation databases of-ten include different categories or types of in-juries. There continues to be a lack of consen-sus on which types of injuries or illnesses should be counted as MSDs. For example, while all the facilities include injuries or ill-nesses that result from obviously repetitive activity, some also include those that are the result of a one-time occurrence.

Using cost data, such as workers' compen-sation expenditures, to identify problem areas or jobs can also be difficult, depending on the facility's medical practices or local workers' compensation insurance policies. For exam-ple, if a state does not cover certain MSDs as compensable injuries under workers' compen-sation, then these data would not provide a good basis for such analysis. For adequate data analysis, a facility must have complete infor-mation on its actual workers' compensation costs. Four of these facilities operate on a self-insured basis. Because they pay out of pocket for claims, they are probably aware of true costs. Other companies, may not have a true sense of actual workers' compensation costs.

OSHA 200 logs, another source of injury and illness data available to most facilities, were found not to be very helpful. The logs, which should record any injury or illness re-quiring more than first aid, provide limited in-formation about the circumstances of inci-dents, so that the cause cannot be determined in some cases. This is especially the case for injuries or illnesses that may have occurred over a long time. Logs are often completed by nonmedical personnel, who do not diagnose the injury and do not record the proper term (e.g., recording a wrist injury rather than carpal tunnel syndrome). There is some ambi-guity about what types of injuries and ill-nesses should be reported on the OSHA Form 200. This form is used by OSHA to assess a facility's safety and health performance, and

therefore there may be some administrative bias in its utilization. Industrial facilities do not like to be identified as hazardous to their workers. For all of these reasons, health care providers serving several of these facilities did not know for sure whether the OSHA 200 log accurately reflected all MSDs occurring at the facilities.

As a result, facilities use information ob-tained from OSHA 200 logs along with other work-related data in which they have more confidence. For example, the number of in-juries recorded in the OSHA 200 log for a particular job classification might be com-pared with the number of personnel com-plaints received about that job, the number of employees working on it, or the number of employees performing it who have been seen by a health care provider. Other facilities also balance the above information against the number of requests that they have received from employees to investigate hazards on a particular job.

Several facilities found that they lacked the capability to track any changes in these in-juries or costs, so that program effectiveness could not be accurately monitored. To facili-tate the tracking of their programs' progress, these companies, either on their own or through their workers' compensation insurer or a third-party administrator, often had to set up a system or method for tracking MSD-re-lated injuries and associated costs. In some cases, these systems were actually separate databases, run by the safety department or by the officials leading the ergonomics program.

Analyzing Changes in Injury and Cost Experience

Although the goal of any ergonomics pro-gram is to see reductions in MSDs and asso-ciated costs, facility officials warn that it takes several years to see results, and often re-sults can be affected by business conditions.

An overriding problem faced by these facil-ities was that none of them had a cost-account-ing system that determined how much they spent on ergonomic investments alone. As a result, regardless of how great a reduction they experienced in workers' compensation and associated costs, these facilities could not conduct a reliable cost–benefit analysis to determine whether the program was saving more money than it was costing. Facility officials point out that any facility will always be making financial expenditures to improve productivity, and it will be difficult to differentiate benefits as a result of investments made to reduce ergonomic hazards from other productivity and quality investments.

After full implementation of an ergonomics program, there might actually be an initial increase in recorded costs, claims, complaints, and other identified "problems." This means that employees are more freely reporting problems and that established systems to obtain this information are working. In fact, at each of these facilities, there was an increase in the total cost of MSD claims in the first year after the program was fully implemented.

If the facility is trying to bring employees back to work, there may actually be an increase in the number of restricted days, as occurred with the AMP facility. This may be a necessary interim cost for the facility. Bringing employees back to work as soon as possible may also require a greater number of light-duty positions than are currently available. If these positions are not available, then a facility may continue to experience high lost-workday rates. At the Navistar facility, light-duty positions for returning employees must be allocated according to the seniority provisions of the collective bargaining agreement. If an injured employee does not have sufficient seniority, there may not be any light-duty jobs available, or the jobs available, such as cleanup duty, are often not appealing to employees who desire productive work. How does a facility ensure that workers are productive when they are working under restriction? SOCHS facility officials reported some cases in which the employees were so restricted that the cost of keeping them on light duty exceeded their productivity.

Even after a program has been in place for a few years and passed the initial hurdles,

there will always be other confounding factors that will affect injury and cost experience. Health care costs in general continue to rise, so a facility may not see a decrease in MSD-associated costs. In some cases, maintenance of a certain level of expenditure reflects actual cost containment. Often, there is a lag of several years between the time when an injury occurs and the date when a worker's compensation claim is finally closed; or, as with the AEFA facility, new management may emphasize closing cases, which can skew any particular year's costs, reflecting indemnification rather than new injuries.

Changes in injury and claim experience are also affected by the number and type of employees. Significant hiring could contribute to increased claims and costs, since new employees are more likely to get hurt than experienced ones. If no new workers are hired and the workforce is aging, this may also contribute to injuries, as older workers may be more likely to experience injury, especially if they have already suffered injury in the past. Workers' compensation claims tend to increase prior to an announcement of a layoff or a shutdown, and then decline again when employees are recalled to work or the shutdown is averted.

Management and business changes can affect the availability of data or results. In 1996, the TI facility was purchased by Raytheon Systems. Since then, the existing ergonomics program has undergone changes, as a result of which data for 1997 will not be comparable to those of earlier years. The SOCHS facility recently instituted a behavioral medicine clinic that provides outpatient services to children and adults. Because this clinic's employee injuries resulting from combative patients are now included in the facility's ergonomics program, officials cautioned that current data may not be truly comparable to those of earlier years. Other business-related factors may be relevant but are hard to address through an ergonomics program, such as the results of employee stress and perceived lack of control over work. Furthermore, if resource limitations extend the amount of time it takes to put a control in place, then injury reduction may not result as quickly. Navistar's willingness to provide customized trucks as orders dictate causes frequent production and schedule changes that may affect newly implemented ergonomics controls. It will therefore be difficult to know what long-term impact these controls have on injury and claim experience.

The staff of an ergonomics program must continually review changes that have been made to ensure that controls are working. At the AMP facility, the ergonomics team administers a post-"Ergonomics Evaluation" form, the same form administered when the job is first analyzed, to determine whether or not the controls are working.

As an interim measure, progress in program implementation can be assessed. Some corporate-wide audits include ergonomics; these audits look for the existence of particular program components such as an established team, ergonomics training, or analyses of problem jobs. The Navistar facility recently instituted a 5-year strategic plan that includes process-oriented goals for the program, such as a certain number of work operations to be redesigned ergonomically. Both the TI and AEFA facilities have developed databases that contain the results of workstation evaluations and employee preferences. At both of these facilities, because employees are relocated frequently, the information in the databases is used to ensure that upon relocation an employee's new workstation will be properly set up. Other facilities are tracking the number of people trained or the number of requests for assistance received from employees.

Accepting Continual Program Evolution and Change

A good ergonomics program is a moving target. Its structure and operations should continually be modified to keep up with changes in corporate goals and culture. To obtain and sustain the commitment of management is a challenge, even after initial cost reductions have been achieved.

These ergonomic programs, as they existed during this review, represent a culmination of years of effort and experimentation. This gradual evolution makes it difficult for facilities to identify at what point a program actually "began." This is why the term *fully implemented* (when all of the components are in place and implemented in a manner that works for the facility) is used. It also makes it difficult to determine when to start expecting results. Taking the time to learn how to properly adapt program components for a local facility is essential to success, as is learning from mistakes made during a program's early years. It is difficult, however, to change program structure in midstream without appearing to lose previously documented progress.

All of the facilities achieved various cost reductions and are pleased with their progress. However, they also realize that as programs evolve, goals need to change as well. Programs need to move from goals of reducing workers' compensation costs to increasing productivity and quality. Developing measures of productivity and quality presents new challenges. Officials at the TI facility stress that they are now moving toward using productivity and other quality measures as indicators of their program's success. AEFA is starting to include anecdotal measures of productivity in employee discomfort surveys.

CONCLUSION

While effective ergonomics programs must include a core set of components to ensure that hazards are identified and controlled, experience suggests that there must be variety and simplicity in how the components are actually implemented at the local level for a program to be effective. The best way to initially identify problem jobs or hazards is an incidence basis, with movement toward a more proactive approach as the program matures. Decisions appear to be based more on business-related factors than theoretical "risk factors."

Reductions in MSD-related workers' compensation costs and overall injury and illness rates and increases in productivity and morale are attainable by using a simple, informal, site-specific approach. While officials at the facilities reviewed in this chapter agree that their programs are effective, they emphasize that data limitations and the confounding effects of local conditions are factors limiting their ability to prove quantitatively that their programs were cost-beneficial or optimally effective. The facilities address some of these limitations by establishing process measures to review the implementation of program components.

ACKNOWLEDGMENTS

I wish to thank Charles Jeszeck, Assistant Director, and Jacquelyn B. Werth, Senior Evaluator, at the U.S. General Accounting Office for their work supporting this chapter. I also wish to thank officials at the respective facilities, especially Christine Meier, PhD, CPE, and Kelly Byrkit from American Express Financial Advisors, Inc.; Robin S. Baver, MD, MPH, from Navistar International; and Judy Caron, Don Estabrook, Jennifer Heutz, and Jonathan K. Torres, MD, MPH, from Sisters of Charity Health System, for providing updated information about their respective programs. The conclusions expressed in this chapter are solely mine.

REFERENCES

1. *Preventing repetitive stress injuries.* Washington, DC: U.S. Department of Labor, Dec 10, 1996. [Press release.]
2. Occupational Safety and Health Administration. *Ergonomics: the study of work.* Washington, DC: U.S. Department of Labor, 1991.
3. Occupational Safety and Health Administration. *Ergonomics program management guidelines for meatpacking plants.* Washington, DC: U.S. Department of Labor, 1993.
4. National Institute for Occupational Safety and Health. *Cumulative trauma disorders in the workplace: bibliography.* Cincinnati, OH: U.S. Department of Health and Human Services, 1995.
5. National Institute for Occupational Safety and Health. *Musculoskeletal disorders and workplace factors: a critical review of epidemiologic evidence for work-related musculoskeletal disorders of the neck, upper extremity, and low back.* Cincinnati, OH: U.S. Department of Health and Human Services, 1997.
6. *Worker protection: private sector ergonomics programs yield positive results.* Washington, DC: U.S. General Accounting Office, 1997. GAO/HEHS publication 97-163.
7. Occupational Safety and Health Administration. *Draft safety and health program management standard.* Washington, DC: U.S. Department of Labor, 1997.
8. National Institute for Occupational Safety and Health. *Elements of ergonomics programs.* Cincinnati, OH: U.S. Department of Health and Human Services, 1997.
9. Occupational Safety and Health Administration. OSHA draft proposed ergonomic protection standard: summaries, explanations, regulatory text. *Occup Safety Health Rep* 1995;24(42, suppl).
10. *Ergonomics and the newspaper industry.* Reston, VA: Newspaper Association of America, 1996.
11. *Office ergonomics management program.* Rosslyn, VA: Center for Office Technology, 1993.
12. *Occupational safety and health: options for improving safety and health in the workplace.* Washington, DC: U.S. General Accounting Office, 1990. GAO/HRD publication 90-66BR.
13. National Institute for Occupational Safety and Health. *Participatory ergonomic interventions in meatpacking plants.* Cincinnati, OH: U.S. Department of Health and Human Services.
14. Moore JS. *Best practices for office ergonomics programs: a descriptive study of North American corporations.* Tyler, TX: University of Texas Press, 1995.
15. Gauf M. *Ergonomics that work: case studies of companies cutting costs through ergonomics.* Haverford, PA: CTD News, 1996.
16. National Institute for Occupational Safety and Health. *Ergonomic interventions for the soft drink beverage delivery industry.* Cincinnati, OH: U.S. Department of Health and Human Services, 1996.
17. Bettendorf RF. *Office ergonomics solutions: six case studies.* Rosslyn, VA: Center for Office Technology, 1994.

Occupational Musculoskeletal Disorders
edited by T. G. Mayer, R. J. Gatchel, and P. B. Polatin.
Lippincott Williams & Wilkins, Philadelphia © 2000.

14

Factors Affecting the Transition from Acute to Chronic Back Pain

Malcolm I.V. Jayson

Rheumatic Diseases Centre, University of Manchester, Salford M6 8HD, United Kingdom

Back pain is remarkably common. Many surveys have indicated a population prevalence between 30% and 40% and a lifetime prevalence up to 80%. In a survey conducted by our institution in a primary care setting in South Manchester, the question was asked, "Thinking over the past month, have you had any ache or pain that lasted for 1 day or longer?"(1). The estimated 1-month prevalence rate was 35% for men and 37% for women. The overall prevalence rate for ever having back pain was about 60%.

Back problems are clearly one of the most common causes of morbidity.

PREDICTION OF BACK PAIN

Factors predicting the initial development of episodes of back pain clearly are directly relevant to the risk of persistent problems. Most epidemiologic data relate to the initial development of low back problems. Studies principally have been cross-sectional, comparing back pain patients with controls, but there is a limited number of prospective studies examining pain-free populations.

In an extensive study of a large population of pain-free individuals followed over the subsequent 12 months, the consulting rate for new episodes of back pain was 3% in men and 5% in women, and for episodes of back pain not resulting in a medical consultation, it was 31% in men and 32% in women (2). Those with a history of previous low back pain

(LBP) had double the rate of new episodes for both consulting and nonconsulting back pain episodes, compared to those with no LBP in the past. Neck pain or pain in other musculoskeletal sites at baseline also doubled the risk of a subsequent new episode of LBP. These observations confirm that not only previous back problems but also musculoskeletal pains in general are important risk factors for the future development of back pain.

The Rheumatic Diseases Centre recently completed an analysis of factors predicting the development of persistent, disabling LBP (3). Three premorbid factors were identified as predictive of outcome—female sex, history of LBP, and job dissatisfaction—as well as three episode-specific factors: widespread pain, radiating leg pain, and restriction in spinal and other movements (Table 1). When combined in a multivariate model, these factors correctly predicted outcome in 74% of subjects, with a negative predictive value of 77% and a positive predictive value of 60% (Table 2).

In a prospective workplace study in the Boeing Aircraft factory in Seattle, Washington, Bigos et al. (4) found that work dissatisfaction and poor relations with a supervising officer were important predictors of future back problems. The Centre's study in South Manchester showed that symptoms of psychologic distress in individuals without back pain provide an important predictor of subsequent onset of new episodes of back pain (5).

TABLE 1. *Predictors of the presence of persistent disabling low back pain*

Predictive factor	Odds ratio	95% Confidence interval
Gender		
Male	Reference	
Female	2.26	1.0–5.1
First episode of low back pain		
Yes	Reference	
No	2.76	0.8–9.9
Satisfied with employment situation		
Yes	Reference	
No	2.62	1.2–5.8
Radiating leg pain		
No	Reference	
Yes	1.89	0.8–4.4
Widespread pain		
No	Reference	
Yes	3.44	1.3–9.3
Spinal restrictions		
None or 1	Reference	
2–5	3.08	1.3–7.3

From ref. 3, in press, with permission.

It was calculated that the proportion of episodes of new back pain attributable to such psychologic factors in the general population is 16%. More specifically, my fellow investigators and I sought associations among LBP, work dissatisfaction, perceived inadequacy of income, and lower social class (6). All these factors were associated with significant increases in risk for back problems. The increased risk with work dissatisfaction and perceived inadequacy of income was not explained by general psychologic distress or social status.

Once an episode of back pain has developed, psychologic factors play an important part in predicting outcome. In a study of 252 back pain patients in a primary care osteopathic setting, patients showing significant

psychologic distress at presentation had a much worse outcome than those without psychologic distress (7).

Physical factors also likely play some role. There appears to be an increased incidence of back pain in workers in heavy manual industries. It is commonly difficult to distinguish an increased risk for back pain and an increased disability as a result of heavy manual work with inability to cope with heavier work with the same amount of back problems.

In a prospective study of back pain–free individuals, we found that occupational factors such as working with heavy weights or standing or walking for long periods were associated with the future development of back pain (8). This was greater in magnitude and was statistically significant in women, whereas it

TABLE 2. *Presence of persistent disabling low back pain*

Factors present (no.)[a]	Subjects	Subjects with persistent symptoms	Observed proportion with persistent symptoms
5 or 6	30	21	0.7
4	43	15	0.35
3	45	12	0.27
0–2	49	3	0.06

[a]Factors predicting persistence include female sex, dissatisfaction with employment situation, history of low back pain, radiating leg pain, widespread pain, or two or more restrictions in spinal movement.
From ref. 3, in press, with permission.

appeared less important in men. Analysis of cumulative exposure to long-standing and heavy lifting failed to demonstrate any increase in risk with prolonged exposure. Indeed, in men the excess risk decreased with increasing duration of exposure, and in women the excess risk was less in those exposed for the longest time.

This analysis is complicated by possible selection problems. If a worker has a back complaint, he or she may not be able to spend prolonged periods standing or undertake heavy work. As a result, an association with heavy work may not be demonstrated. The relationships between the demands of work and the development of back problems therefore appear uncertain.

Excess physical stresses on the spine may also be a result of obesity, with increased mechanical demands leading to premature degenerative change. An extensive review about to be published found little evidence of a causal link, with inconsistent results. Positive associations between obesity and back pain principally related to demands for health care rather than actual back pain itself.

An increased risk for back problems has been identified as being associated with having children. The physical stresses associated with pregnancy—the accompanying laxity of spinal ligaments, epidural injections, and the process of parturition—have all been identified as risk factors. However, recent evidence has identified child-rearing rather childbearing as the significant factor (9). The increased risk, if anything, is greater in men than women. There is increasing risk with increasing numbers of children. It appears that the physical demands of pregnancy are less important than the general increase in lifting, carrying, and other mechanical activities with increased numbers of children. Increased psychologic distress and greater potential for adverse events may also play important parts.

PROGNOSIS OF ACUTE BACK PAIN

It is commonly stated that most episodes of acute back pain will resolve rapidly, and Wad-

dell (10) estimated that in 90% of episodes recovery will occur within 6 weeks. Recent surveys, however, indicate that this is a grossly overoptimistic view. Once a patient has suffered an episode of back pain, he or she is at greatly increased risk of either current or recurrent back problems.

In a prospective cohort study of patients seen in primary care, Cherkin et al. (11) found good outcomes in only 67% of patients after 7 weeks, and 1 year later only 71% were satisfied with their condition. In an extension of our study, only 21% had recovered completely at 3 months, and at 1 year only 25% had done so (12). In contrast, however, most patients ceased to consult after the initial episode of LBP. These results suggest that 90% of patients with LBP in primary care stop seeing their doctor but most will continue to experience LBP and related disability.

In a prospective study, 1,213 adults with back pain were assessed 1 month after first consultation for back problems in a primary care setting and were followed at annual intervals thereafter (13). Out of 100 factors initially documented, psychosocial factors such as degree of somatization, depression, functional limitation, and pain were the strongest predictors of the 2-year outcome. Physical factors also played a role initially. We undertook an analysis of the perpetuation of back symptoms in 3 and 12 months (14). Among 4,501 adults who initially were pain-free, back pain developed in 246 and was followed up at 3 (n=217) and 12 (n=102) months later. Significant associations with a persistence of symptoms were related to low levels of physical activity, longer duration between onset and consultation, and the presence of concurrent leg pain, widespread pain, and restriction of lateral flexion.

MECHANISMS OF CHRONICITY OF BACK PROBLEMS

Much effort is expended attempting to provide a pathologic basis for the chronicity of back symptoms. A wide variety of degenerative pathologies may be demonstrated, but their correlations with the presence of symptoms are poor. For example, in a careful study comparing magnetic resonance imaging in back pain sufferers and controls, Jensen et al. (15) found that the prevalence of degenerative changes in intervertebral discs was more frequent in back pain sufferers but similar appearances could be found in symptom-free individuals. It is only the presence of a sequestrated disc that seemed specifically associated with back symptoms. Annular tears, spinal stenosis, and spondylolisthesis are also commonly sought but only show modest associations with the presence of back symptoms.

Increasing evidence indicates that vascular damage plays a fundamental role in the pathogenesis of mechanical back pain problems. Degenerative disc disease is associated with atherosclerosis and spinal artery stenosis, and the various degrees of disc degeneration and obliteration are associated with increased vascularity in the annulus fibrosus (16). Correlations between back pain and cardiovascular disease and smoking are in keeping with a possible role for arterial disease. Disc degeneration and protrusion are associated with pressure on the epidural venous plexus, leading to venous dilatation, nerve root edema, intra- and perineural fibrosis, and neuronal atrophy (17). Venous compression may be present at two or more levels in the spine, leading to isolated segments of poor perfusion (18).

An inflammatory response is often observed secondary to mechanical spine damage (19). Pathologic studies show that the local tissue reaction to herniated nuclear material seems to be due to endothelial proliferation, vascular activation, and collagen proliferation (20,21). Nociceptive fibers may be identified within this proliferating vascular tissue, extending into the outer layers of the degenerative disc and toward its center (22). These changes are not easily recognized in life; nevertheless, they clearly provide the potential for pain production and relate to the epidemiologic associations with vascular disorders.

Some patients have back and lower limb pain associated with hyperesthesia, hyperpathia, allodynia, vasomotor changes, and sensitivity to cold. Clinically, the appearances are suggestive of a sympathetic dystrophy otherwise known as the complex regional pain syndrome (CRPS).

Sympathetic chains run down along the sides of the vertebral column, but are anastomosing sympathetic fibers around and within the spine and the intervertebral discs. There are several case reports of the association of disc herniation with a sympathetic dystrophy (23,24). Indeed, a careful physiologic study by Maigne et al. (25) showed physiologic vasomotor changes typical of sympathetic dystrophy occurring in the majority of cases with root symptoms due to a herniated disc.

The characteristics of patients with well established CRPS consist of pain in the lower limb referred from the spine; it is described as continuous and burning with hyperpathia and/or allodynia, cold sensitivity, and vasomotor and pseudomotor changes. Symptom relief by a sympathetic block helps with the diagnosis. Although sympathectomy provides short-term relief, the long-term results have proved disappointing and the syndrome frequently recurs. It appears that some mechanism for establishing sympathetic hyperactivity reestablishes itself. More recent research has suggested that sympathetic pain may be centrally mediated through hypersensitized cells in the dorsal region of the spinal cord and is a feature of central nervous system sensitization.

Recognition of CRPS is relatively easy when the problem is unilateral. Comparison with the contralateral normal limb facilitates recognition of cold sensitivity, allodynia, hypopathia, and reduced skin temperature. Thermography can be very helpful. However, if the problem is bilateral, it would be extremely difficult to recognize. We see many patients with pain radiating to both lower limbs in whom the underlying pathology is uncertain. I believe that many of these are cases of CRPS and this syndrome is fundamental in causing many back problems to become chronic.

The concept that increased nervous system excitability may follow some peripheral injury has been known for many years. Indeed, Sturge (26) first proposed that many of the symptoms associated with angina may arise on this basis.

Afferent impulses are translated through complex synapses in the dorsal horn of the spinal cord before being relayed up the spine into the brain. Experimental studies have shown that after nociceptive stimulation there is increased dorsal horn activity, with prolonged periods of discharge lasting long after the actual nociceptive stimulus has stopped (27–30). This means that back pain patients may continue to feel pain long after the physical cause of the problem has been removed. The dorsal horn cells have increased sensitivity to afferent impulses. As a result, patients may experience disproportionate pain compared with the evidence of tissue damage and peripheral nociception. This gives rise to the phenomena of hyperpathia and allodynia. There may be expansion of the dorsal horn receptor fields so that the pain is experienced over a much wider area than the nociceptive damage would predict. This means that patients will experience widespread pain. Coderre et al. (31) provided an extensive review of this whole mechanism.

Hypersensitivity of the dorsal horn is believed to underlie CRPS. As a result, the mechanisms within the dorsal horn that can lead to persistence and chronicity of back and referred pain are just beginning to be understood. As a consequence of an increased sensitivity to minor stimulation, minor stresses on the back may be sufficient to provoke a severe painful response. The severity and widespread nature of the pain may become grossly disproportionate to the objective evidence of tissue damage.

The mechanisms for integrating the physical problems of back and nerve root damage with psychologic influences are now beginning to be understood. Descending impulses from the brain have the potential to stimulate these sensitized cells so that as a result of psychologic distress, patients experience much more severe symptoms.

Investigation is now moving into the area of examining the processing of pain perception within the brain. In chronic pain, the pain processing system is abnormal (32). Application of this approach to the study of back pain problems is currently in progress.

CONCLUSION

Overall hypotheses for the mechanisms of chronicity of back problems are beginning to be developed. Clearly, physical factors may initially precipitate the development of back pain, and such physical damage in itself contributes toward the perpetuation of symptoms. However, more detailed analysis indicates that psychosocial factors are important in predicting the development of back pain and its perpetuation. These are likely to have an organic basis, and how the physical and psychologic factors integrate is beginning to be understood. Purely mechanical factors such as disc degeneration and herniation are inadequate to explain the perpetuation of symptoms in the majority of cases. Of fundamental importance appear to be secondary vascular, neurologic, and fibrotic changes in and around the neural structures and the complex secondary changes within the central nervous system itself that lead to perpetuation and amplification of the pain-producing process. Understanding these mechanisms should help in the future to prevent the development and improve the treatment of chronic back pain.

REFERENCES

1. Papageorgiou AC, Croft PR, Ferry S, Jayson MIV, Silman AJ. Estimating the prevalence of low back pain in the general population. *Spine* 1995;20:1889-1894.
2. Papageorgiou AC, Croft PR, Thomas E, Ferry S, Jayson MIV, Silman AJ. Influence of previous pain experience on the episode incidence of low back pain: results from the South Manchester Back Pain Study. *Pain* 1996;66: 181–185.
3. Thomas E, Silman AJ, Papageorgiou AC, Macfarlane GJ, Croft PR, Jayson MIV. Predicting who develops chronic low back pain in primary care: a prospective study. *BMJ.*
4. Bigos SJ, Battie M, Spengler DM, et al. A prospective study of work perceptions and psychosocial factors affecting the report of back injury. *Spine* 1991;16:1–6.
5. Croft PR, Papageorgiou AC, Ferry S, Thomas E, Jayson MIV, Silman AJ. Psychological distress and low back pain: evidence from a prospective study in the general population. *Spine* 1996;20:2731–2737.

6. Papageorgiou AC, MacFarlane GJ, Thomas E, Croft PR, Jayson MIV, Silman AJ. Psychosocial factors in the workplace: do they predict new episodes of low back pain? *Spine* 1997;22:1137–1142.

7. Burton AK, Tillotson KF, Main CJ, Hollis S. Psychosocial predictors of outcome in acute and subchronic low back trouble. *Spine* 1995;20:722–728.

8. MacFarlane GJ, Thomas E, Papageorgiou AC, Croft PR, Jayson MIV, Silman AJ. Employment and physical activities as predictors of future low back pain. *Spine* 1997;22:1143–1149.

9. Silman AJ, Ferry S, Papageorgiou AC, Jayson MIV, Croft PR. Number of children as a risk factor for low back pain in men and women. *Arthritis Rheum* 1995; 38:1232–1235.

10. Waddell GC. A new clinical model for the treatment of low-back pain. *Spine* 1987;12:632–644.

11. Cherkin DC, Deyo RA, Street JH, Barlow W. Predicting poor outcomes of back pain seen in primary care using patients' own criteria *Spine* 1996;21:2900–2907.

12. Croft PR, MacFarlane GJ, Papageorgiou AC, Thomas E, Silman AJ. Outcome of low back pain in general practice: a prospective study. *BMJ* 1998;316: 1356–1359.

13. Dionne CE, Koepsall TD, von Korff M, Deyo RA, Barlow WE, Checkoway H. Predicting long-term functional limitations among back pain patients in a primary care setting. *J Clin Epidemiol* 1997;50:31–43.

14. Jayson MIV, Thomas E, Papageorgiou AC, MacFarlane GJ, Silman AJ. Factors predicting the persistence of disabling low back pain. *Spine* 1995;20:722–1142.

15. Jensen MC, Brant-Zowadzki MN, Obuchowski N, Modic MT, Malkasian D, Ross JS. Magnetic resonance imaging of people without back pain. *N Engl J Med* 1994;331:69–71.

16. Kauppila L. Igrowth of blood vessels in disc degeneration. *J Bone Joint Surg [Am]* 1995;77:26–31.

17. Hoyland JA, Freemont AJ, Jayson MIV. Intervertebral foramen venous obstruction: a cause of periradicular fibrosis? *Spine* 1989;14:558–568.

18. Olmarker K, Holm S, Rydevik B. Single versus double level root compression. *Clin Orthop* 1992;279:35–39.

19. Saal J. The role of inflammation in lumbar pain. *Spine* 1995;16:1821–1827.

20. Cooper RG, Freemont AJ, Hoyland AJ, et al. Herniated intervertebral disc-associated periradicular fibrosis and vascular abnormalities occur without inflammatory cell infiltration. *Spine* 1995;20:591–598.

21. Gronblad M, Virri J, Ronkko S, et al. A controlled biochemical and immunohistochemical study of human synovial type (group II) phospholipase A2 and inflammatory cells in macroscopically normal, degenerated and herniated lumbar disc tissue. *Spine* 1996;21:2531–2538.

22. Freemont AJ, Peacock TE, Goupille P, Hoyland JA, O'Brien J, Jayson MIV. Nerve ingrowth into diseased intervertebral disc in chronic back pain. *Lancet* 1997; 350:178–181.

23. Bernini PM, Simeone FA. Reflex sympathetic dystrophy associated with low lumbar disc herniation. *Spine* 1981; 6:180–184.

24. Chodoroff B, Ball RD. Lumbosacral radiculopathy, reflex sympathetic dystrophy and carpal tunnel syndrome: an unusual presentation. *Arch Phys Med Rehabil* 1985;66: 185–187.

25. Maigne J-Y, Treuil C, Chatellier G. Altered lower limb perfusion in patients with sciatica secondary to disc herniation. *Spine* 1996;21:1657–1660.

26. Sturge WA. The phenomena of angina pectoris and their bearing on the theory of counter irritation. *Brain Res* 1883;5:492–510.

27. Cervero F, Handworker HO, Laird JMA. Prolonged noxious stimulation of the rat's tail: response and encoding properties of dorsal horn neurones. *J Physiol* 1988;404: 419–436.

28. Devor M, Wall PD. Reorganisation of spinal and senory map after peripheral nerve injury. *Nature* 1978;267: 75–76.

29. Mendell LM. Physiological properties of unmyelinated fibre rejection to the spinal cord. *Exp Neurol* 1966;16: 316–332.

30. Schoenberg J, Dickenson A. The effects of a distant noxious stimulation on A and C fibre-evoked flexion reflexes and neuronal activity in the dorsal horn of the cat. *Brain Res* 1985;328:23–32.

31. Coderre TJ, Katz JL, Vaccarino AL, Melzak RR. Contribution of central neuroplasticity to pathological pain: review of clinical and experimental evidence. *Pain* 1993; 52:259–283.

32. Derbyshire SWG, Jones AKP, Devani P, et al. Cerebral responses to pain in patients with atypical facial pain measured by positron emission tomography. *J Neurol Neurosurg Psychiatry* 1995;57:1166–1172.

PART IV

Acute Occupational
Musculoskeletal Disorders

Occupational Musculoskeletal Disorders
edited by T. G. Mayer, R. J. Gatchel, and P. B. Polatin.
Lippincott Williams & Wilkins, Philadelphia © 2000.

15

Epidemiology of Musculoskeletal Disorders and Workplace Factors

J. Mark Melhorn

Section of Orthopaedics, Department of Surgery, University of Kansas School of Medicine—Wichita, Kansas 67208

This chapter on the epidemiology of musculoskeletal disorders (MSDs) and workplace factors is designed to provide quick access and a summary of references for epidemiology, epidemiologic evidence of work-related MSDs, and the financial costs of MSDs in the workplace. It is divided into five sections: summary, introduction and definition of terms related to work-related MSDs, risk factor analysis by body part, the scope of occupational MSDs, and the cost of work-related MSDs. The first section—summary and outline—provides information about the conclusions of studies and assists the reader in exploring the epidemiology of MSDs by using the outline. The second section introduces epidemiology and defines terms as they relate to the epidemiologic evidence of work-related MSDs. The third section focuses on epidemiologic evidence by body part, with each body part's risk evaluated for the effect of repetition, force, posture, and vibration. To facilitate the use of this chapter as a reference source, the conclusion of the evidence for each body part is presented first, followed by the specific details and the two best reference articles. This format allows the reader to assess the key information with additional details, if needed. The fourth section provides the numbers of current occupational injuries and illnesses. The fifth section contains cost information on work-related injuries.

SUMMARY

The term *musculoskeletal disorder* refers to a condition that involves the nerves, tendons, muscles, and supporting structures of the body. The only routinely collected national source of information about the occupational injuries and illnesses of workers in the United States is the annual survey of occupational injuries and illnesses conducted by the Bureau of Labor Statistics (BLS) of the U.S. Department of Labor. The most current available issue, published in 1997, contains 1994 information (1). This survey, which the BLS has conducted for the past 25 years, is a random sample of about 250,000 private-sector establishments and provides estimates of workplace injuries and illnesses on the basis of information provided by employers from their Occupational Safety and Health Administration (OSHA) Form 200 log of recordable injuries and illnesses. The OSHA Form 200 log column 7, line F, headed "Disorders Associated with Repeated Trauma" has been criticized as misleading and resulting in overreporting of occupational injuries and illnesses (2). In response to these and many other concerns, OSHA is embarking on a campaign to introduce additional regulations and newer reporting forms (OSHA Form 300) with more stringent requirements and penalties (3).

Even with these limitations and concerns, this survey is still the most comprehensive database available for review. In 1994, the BLS reported that approximately 52% of the total 705,800 cases of occupational injuries and illnesses were the result of overexertion or repetitive motion. Specifically, 367,424 injuries were due to overexertion in lifting, of which 65% affected the back; 93,325 injuries were due to overexertion in pushing or pulling objects, of which 52% affected the back; and 68,992 injuries were due to overexertion in holding, carrying, or turning objects, of which 58% affected the back. Across these three categories, there were 47,861 disorders affecting the shoulder. An additional 83,483 injuries or illnesses were categorized as other or unspecified overexertion events. There were 92,576 injuries or illnesses due to repetitive motion, including typing or key entry, repetitive use of tools, and repetitive placing, grasping, or moving of objects other than tools. Of these injuries or illnesses, 55% affected the wrist, 7% the shoulder, and 6% the back.

Carpal Tunnel Syndrome

The incidence of overexertion (in lifting) was 41.1 per 10,000 workers and of repetitive motion disorders 10.1 per 10,000 workers (1). A 1998 study by Stevens et al. (4) reported 11 cases of carpal tunnel syndrome (CTS) per 10,000 person-years in the community surrounding Rochester, Minnesota, for the years 1960 to 1980. Unfortunately, their study did not address the work-related component of these cases. A survey of health care providers in the San Francisco area suggested that approximately 47% of all CTS cases were work-related (5). Data from the Washington State workers' compensation program showed the overall incidence of work-related CTS for the 5-year 1984 through 1988 was 17.4 cases per 10,000 full-time workers (6). In 1974, Allander (7) reported incidences of 2 per 100 people aged 42 to 46 per year for painful shoulder and 1 per 100 people per year for tennis elbow in Stockholm, Sweden, in 1965 to 1968. Unfortunately, this study also did not address the cases considered to be work-related. The author reported that the average cost to employers

(workers' compensation) for care for an employee with bilateral CTS that required surgery was $74,000 (8). This cost included direct expenses for medical care, indemnity, legal matters, and job or work rehabilitation. It did not include the indirect costs of lost production, training of new personnel, or increased workers' compensation insurance cost.

Upper Extremity Musculoskeletal Disorders

The prevalence of upper extremity MSDs depends on the occupation studied, the risk factors present, and the specific body part studied. In 1988, the National Health Interview Survey found that 8% of the 127 million active workers reported prolonged hand discomfort (20 days or more in the past year, or 7 or more consecutive days in the past month). Approximately 0.5% (635,000 current workers) reported both prolonged hand discomfort and "medically called" CTS; 356,000 (56%) of these respondents reported that the medical person said that the CTS was work-related (9). Hagberg et al. (10) reviewed the literature on work-related CTS, finding a widely ranging prevalence (0.6% to 61%), depending on the occupational group studied. Allander (7) reported a prevalence of painful shoulder ranging from less than 10% to more than 20%, depending on the age group studied; the prevalence of epicondylitis also depended on the age group studied, ranging from less than 1% to more than 5%. The mean cost per case of upper extremity cumulative trauma disorder (CTD) was $8,070, compared to only $824 for other workers' compensation cases in 1992. With more than 5 million U.S. workers affected by upper extremity CTDs, the cost was more than $4.04 billion (11,12). In 1996, the direct health care costs were more than $418 billion, and lower-range estimates for indirect costs were more than $837 billion for a total cost of $1.256 trillion (13).

Back Disorders

Low back pain (LBP) is a common ailment. Most studies report a lifetime prevalence of

60% to 80% and a yearly prevalence of 6% to 20%. Fortunately, most episodes of LBP are relatively mild and self-limited (5). Approximately 90% of those affected spontaneously recover and regain activity tolerance within a month (14,15). Approximately 20% of individuals with back pain seek health care. Only about 10% of workers with work-related back pain seek compensation (16). The incidence of compensation for back injury ranges from 0.3 to 3.3 cases per 100 workers per year (17,18). Spengler et al. (19) found that a small proportion of cases become chronic and these accounted for a higher proportion of compensation costs. The direct workers' compensation cost for low back disorders (LBDs) in 1989 was estimated to be $11.4 billion (20). This figure does not include the indirect costs, which are considered to be two to three times the direct costs (10). Including indirect costs with the direct compensation costs results in an estimate of $30 billion per year for the total costs of compensable work-related LBDs (21). Adding the cost of uncompensated LBP to that figure (using the 10% as work-related), the total cost to society is estimated to be between $50 billion and $100 billion (16,22).

Physical, Psychologic, and Work-related Causation Factors

Because the relationship between exposure to physical work factors and the development and prognosis of a particular disorder may be modified by psychosocial factors, the literature about psychosocial factors and the presence of musculoskeletal symptoms or MSDs will also be reviewed. Understanding these associations and relating them to the cause of disease is critical for identifying exposures amenable to preventive and therapeutic interventions. In July 1997, the U.S. Department of Health and Human Services, sections of the Public Health Service, the Centers for Disease Control and Prevention (CDC), and the National Institute for Occupational Safety and Health (NIOSH) completed the most comprehensive compilation of the epidemiologic research on the relation between selected MSDs and exposure to physical work factors (23). On the basis of its review of the literature, NIOSH concluded that a large body of credible epidemiologic research exists, showing a consistent relationship between MSDs and certain physical factors. This relationship was considered to be stronger at higher levels of exposure and with combination exposures to more of the physical factor. This document is currently available for review at the CDC's web site (www.cdc.gov/niosh/ergosci1.html) or for purchase at 800-356-4674. Current NIOSH data (see ref. 23) are also available (www.cdc.gov/niosh/homepage.html). This document is not without its critics. In 1996, Blume and Sandler (24) stated that OSHA's approach in reviewing the literature to support a causal relationship between the workplace and MSDs was flawed because such an approach to finding a causal association did not yield the scientific certainty engendered by critical analysis of the medical literature. Also, they believed that there was a bias in the articles selected for review. Additionally, three editorials published in the *Journal of Hand Surgery* in 1995, 1996, and 1998 expressed concern about the lack of carefully designed prospective studies, suggested delaying additional regulations until better scientific data are available, and recommended avoiding the terms *CTD* and *repetitive strain* as diagnostic terms (2,25,26). In 1995, Vender et al. (27) reviewed the medical literature to establish whether there was a causal relationship between upper extremity disorders and work activities. Based on their article selection, only 14 of 52 articles reviewed were felt to encompass medical criteria, and many of these contained major validity flaws in research design. This article also had its critics. In a letter to the editor, Silverstein et al. (28) outlined their concerns with Vender and Kasdan's medical literature review.

Despite the continuing debate on causation, the NIOSH study is the largest accumulated review of the medical literature (23). Its goal was to identify factors associated (positively or negatively) with the development or recurrence of adverse medical conditions. The evaluation and summary of the epidemiologic evidence focused chiefly on MSDs affecting the neck and upper extremities, including tension neck syndrome, shoulder tendinitis, epicondylitis, CTS, and hand–arm vibration syndrome (HAVS). Additional studies reviewed dealt with work-related back pain and the way in which work organizational and psychosocial factors influence the relationship between exposure to physical factors and work-related MSDs. A search of bibliographic databases identified more than 2,000 studies. Because the focus was on the epidemiology literature, laboratory-based or -focused studies, clinical treatment studies, and nonepidemiologically oriented studies were eliminated from the NIOSH review. This arbitrary selection may have injected a bias in the outcome data. The remaining 600 studies that were included underwent a detailed review process, with specific attention given to analysis of the weight of the evidence for the strength of the association between these MSDs and work factors.

Epidemiologic Risk-factor Classification

In the NIOSH study, the epidemiologic strength of the associations in each individual study was analyzed for specific risk factors and compared to body parts. In general, the largest increases in risk were generally observed in studies with a wide range of exposure conditions and careful observation or measurement of exposures. The risk factors included repetition, force, posture, vibration, and combination. The body parts included the neck and neck/shoulder, shoulder, elbow, hand/wrist for CTS, hand/wrist for tendinitis, HAVS, and back. Using this framework, the epidemiologic evidence for a relationship between a workplace factor and the development of a MSD was classified into one of four categories:

- **Strong epidemiologic evidence (+++):** Consistently positive findings from a large number of cross-sectional studies, strengthened by the limited number of prospective studies, provided strong evidence for increased risk of work-related MSDs for

some body parts. This was based on the strength of associations, lack of ambiguity in or consistency of the results, and adequate control or adjustment for likely confounders in cross-sectional studies and for temporal relationships in prospective studies, with reasonable confidence levels in at least several of those studies.

- **Epidemiologic evidence (++):** Some convincing epidemiologic evidence showed a causal relationship when the epidemiologic criteria of causality for intense or long-duration exposure to the specific risk factor(s) are used. In this category of evidence, a positive relationship was observed between exposure to a specific risk factor and a MSD in studies in which chance, bias, and confounding factors were not the likely explanation.

- **Insufficient epidemiologic evidence (+/0):** Available studies were of insufficient number, quality, consistency, or statistical power to permit a conclusion regarding the presence or absence of a causal association. Some studies suggested a relationship to specific risk factors, but chance, bias, or confounding may explain the association. Either there was an insufficient number of studies from which to draw conclusions, or the overall conclusions from studies were equivocal. The absence of existing epidemiologic evidence should not be interpreted to mean that there is no association between work factors and MSDs.

- **No epidemiologic evidence (–):** Adequate studies were not found that consistently showed that specific workplace risk factors were not related to the development of MSDs.

Categorization of the epidemiologic evidence suggestive of a relationship between physical work factors and MSDs is summarized in Table 1.

Methods for Analyzing Studies

The epidemiologic studies reviewed for this chapter had a participation rate of 70%, health outcomes were defined by symptoms

TABLE 1. *Epidemiologic evidence suggestive of a relationship between physical work factors and musculoskeletal disorders*

Risk factor	Strong evidence (+++)	Evidence (++)	Insufficient evidence (+/−)	Evidence of no effect (−)
Neck and neck/shoulder				
Repetition		*		
Force	*			
Posture	*			
Vibration			*	
Shoulder				
Repetition		*		
Force			*	
Posture		*		
Vibration			*	
Elbow				
Repetition			*	
Force		*		
Posture			*	
Combination	*			
Hand/wrist				
Carpal tunnel syndrome				
Repetition		*		
Force		*		
Posture			*	
Vibration		*		
Combination	*			
Tendinitis				
Repetition		*		
Force		*		
Posture		*		
Combination	*			
Hand–arm vibration syndrome				
Vibration	*			
Back				
Lifting/forceful movement	*			
Awkward posture		*		
Heavy physical work		*		
Whole-body vibration	*			
Static work posture			*	

and physical examination, the investigators were blinded to health or exposure status when assessing health or exposure status, and the body area under discussion was subjected to an independent exposure assessment. The second step of the analytic process was to divide the studies into those with statistically significant associations between exposures and health outcomes and those without statistically significant associations. The third step of the analytic process was to review and summarize studies with regard to strength of association, consistency in association, temporal association, and exposure–response relationship. Each of these factors is discussed in greater detail in the next section.

Criteria for Causality

No single epidemiologic study will fulfill all criteria for causality. However, the results of many epidemiologic studies can contribute to evidence of causality in the relationship between workplace risk factors and MSDs. Greenberg et al. (29) defined a cause as "an event, condition, or characteristic that plays an essential role in producing an occurrence of the disease." Causality has been further modified by Hill (30,31) and by Susser (32).

Strength of Association

Odds ratios (ORs) and prevalence rate ratios (PRRs) from the reviewed studies were used to examine the strength of the association between exposure to workplace risk factors and MSDs, with the higher values indicating a stronger association. The greater the magnitude of the relative risk (RR) or the OR, the less likely will the association be spurious (33–35). Weaker associations are more likely to be explained by undetected biases. Debate is ongoing in the epidemiologic literature about studies with small sample sizes that find increased ORs or PRRs but have confidence intervals (CIs) that include 1.0. The question is whether such studies simply show no significant association or can be seen as useful estimates of associated risk. Nonetheless, it is useful to identify trends across such studies and consider whether they have valuable information after other epidemiologic principles are taken into account. If the studies with and without significant findings both have similarly elevated ORs or PRRs, this information is useful in estimating the overall level of risk associated with exposure.

Consistency

Consistency refers to the repeated observation of an association in independent studies. Multiple studies yielding similar associations support the plausibility of a causal interpretation. Finding the same association with different and valid ways of measuring exposure and disease may show that the association is not dependent on measurement tools. Similar studies that yield diverse results weaken a causal interpretation.

Specificity of Effect or Association

This criterion refers to the association of a single risk factor with a specific health effect. This criterion has not been emphasized because of the different views of its utility in determining causality. If it is interpreted to mean that a single stressor can be related to a specific outcome (e.g., forceful exertion alone can be related to hand/wrist tendinitis), it becomes an important criterion for MSD. However, this criterion can be interpreted and applied too simplistically. Schlesselman (36) noted that the concept of specificity is generally too simplistic and that multiple causes and effects are more often the rule than the exception. Rothman (37) referred to specificity of effect as "useless and misleading" as a criterion for causality.

Temporality

Temporality refers to documentation that the cause precedes the effect in time. Prospectively designed studies ensure that this criterion is strictly adhered to. However, cross-sectional studies are not designed to allow strict adherence to this criterion because both exposure information and adverse health outcome are obtained at the same time. Even though the cross-sectional study design precludes strict establishment of cause and effect, additional information can be used to make reasonable assumptions that exposure preceded the health effect—particularly when the relationship between physical exposures is measured by observation or direct measurement and by MSD-related health outcomes. If the exposure was directly measured or observed, it is also unlikely that the measurement was influenced by the presence or absence of the MSD in the employee. Rothman (37) stated that it is important to realize that cause and effect in an epidemiologic study or epidemiologic data cannot be evaluated without making some assumptions (explicit or implicit) about the timing between exposure and disease. For example, from a cross-sectional study of hand/wrist tendinitis and highly forceful, repetitive jobs, a researcher can determine when exposure began from recorded work histories or from interviews. The researcher can also reasonably determine the time of tendinitis onset by interviews. Kleinbaum et al. (38) said that in cross-sectional studies, risk factors and prognostic factors cannot be distinguished empirically without additional information. With additional information (e.g., laboratory experiments or biomechanical findings), an investigator can deduce that the adverse health outcome followed exposure. For example, with other confounders taken into account, it is unreasonable to deduce that persons with hand/wrist tendinitis are likely to seek employment in jobs that require highly forceful, repetitive exertion of the hand/wrist area.

Exposure–Response Relationship

This relationship relates disease occurrence with the intensity, frequency, or duration of an exposure (or a combination of these factors). For example, if long-duration, forceful, repetitive work using the hands and wrists is associated with an increased prevalence of hand/wrist tendinitis, this association would tend to support a causal interpretation. Some have challenged the importance of physical factors as causal agents, but prospective studies have shown that reduced exposures result in a decreased incidence of disease (39). In occupational health, important and effective preventive actions have been initiated without prospective demonstration that reduced exposure decreases the incidence of disease.

Coherence of Evidence

Coherence of evidence means that an association is consistent with the natural history and biology of a disease. For example, an observed association between repetitive wrist motion and CTS (defined by nerve conduction criteria) must be supported by biologic plausibility: Repeated wrist movement can cause swelling of tissue in the carpal tunnel, resulting in injury to nerves. It is important to remember, however, that epidemiologic studies can identify new associations for further study.

Individual Risk Identification and Prevention

These epidemiologic categories are useful in MSD research but offer little insight into medical care for treating physicians seeing individual workers. The benefit of this information is the opportunity that it provides to develop preventive measures in the workplace (40). In general, there is limited detailed quantitative information about exposure–disorder relationships between risk factors and MSDs. The risk of each exposure depends on a variety of factors, such as the frequency, duration, and intensity of physical workplace exposures. Most of the specific exposures associated with strong epidemiologic evidence involved exposure to the factors under investigation for 8 hours per day. Individual factors may also influence the degree of risk from specific exposures. There is evidence that individual risk factors influence the occurrence of MSDs. Examples include elevated body mass index, sex, and inherited systemic diseases for CTS or a history of past back pain for current episodes of LBP. There is evidence that these individual factors (age, sex, and genetics) interact synergistically with physical factors (workplace and nonwork environment) and are modified by linked factors (social, cultural, and economic) (41). Additionally, all of these disorders can also be caused by nonwork exposures. The majority of epidemiologic studies involve health outcomes that range in severity from mild (workers reporting these disorders continue to perform their routine duties) to more severe disorders (workers are absent from the workplace for varying periods of time). The milder disorders are more common. A limited number of studies investigated the natural history of MSDs and attempted to determine whether continued exposure to physical factors alters their prognosis. Individuals who remain at work in a modified or alternate work pattern were more likely to remain employable at 2 years and did not show any increased likelihood of recurrence (42). Prevention will remain the cornerstone for reduction of work-related MSDs, and identification of individuals at risk for MSDs provides the best opportunity for effective prevention (40,43-47).

INTRODUCTION AND DEFINITION OF TERMS FOR WORK-RELATED MUSCULOSKELETAL DISORDERS

MSDS are disorders involving the soft tissues (nerves, tendons, muscles, and supporting structures) not caused by an acute event (23). Examples of acute events include injuries from lacerations, cuts, fractures, sprains, strains, slips, or falls. The magnitude of MSDs is reflected in the BLS's annual survey of occupational injuries (1).

For epidemiologic evaluation, MSDs can be clinically grouped as follows:

- Well defined disorders, such as tendinitis, CTDs, or HAVS;
- Less well defined disorders, such as tension neck syndrome;
- Nondefined or nonspecific disorders, such as CTSs (Carpal Tunnel Syndrome), repetitive strain injury, overuse syndrome, or cervicobrachial disorders.

When this information is lumped together and nonspecific subjective musculoskeletal pain is incorrectly labeled with a specific pathoanatomic diagnosis, confusion can occur. Many of the current myths regarding musculoskeletal pain in the workplace can be attributed to this inappropriate grouping (46,48–50). This misunderstanding has been compounded by widespread public awareness of these disorders and enhanced by frequent reports in the public media (51–56). Health care providers can easily relate to clinically defined disorders for which the criteria for epidemiologic case definition are similar to physicians' diagnostic criteria. However, when the emphasis shifts from diagnostic criteria to the more inclusive surveillance case definitions used by epidemiologists to identify risk factors and to institute preventive measures, confusion does occur. For example, Vender et al. (27) reviewed the medical literature for articles that encompassed medical criteria to validate a causal relationship between upper extremity MSDs and work activities. Their conclusions were that the medical literature currently fails to incorporate sound medical diagnostic criteria in defining and identifying MSDs and does not establish a causal relationship between distinct medical disorders and work activities.

This confusion over terminology and case definitions has had a dramatic impact on the recognition, reporting, surveillance, and individual diagnoses of MSDs (57–59). It is somewhat ironic that the orthopedic literature seems to have originated the terms *overuse syndrome* to describe athletic injuries (60) and *repetitive strain injury* to describe injuries in long-distance runners (61). In these cases, the terms were used to describe specific medical conditions that demonstrated a direct dose–response relationship without apparent secondary gains. As an epidemiologist, Riihimaki (62) also recognized the weakness of using epidemiologic research based on the lack of specific criteria to establish causation of MSDs by work activities.

MSDs are considered to be work-related, using a legal definition, when the work environment and the performance of work contribute significantly to their development (63). Based on this legal definition, epidemiologic studies have identified several workplace risk factors associated with the development of MSDs in workers. Work-related MSDs are therefore distinguishable from occupational diseases in that occupational diseases have a direct cause–effect relationship between a single hazard and a specific disease (e.g., asbestos and asbestosis or silica and silicosis), whereas MSDs do not have such a relationship.

In the 1980s, to improve reporting and research, the U.S. government defined the term *CTD* as any musculoskeletal pain that an individual believes is associated with activities performed at work (50). Musculoskeletal pain is defined as any pain that may involve the muscles, nerves, tendons, ligaments, bones, or joints. This pain can be defined as real or imagined. For the pain to be considered work-related, state governments legislated a variety of work-contribution requirements. These state requirements range from a scale of no actual contribution (0%) to full work contribution (100%). Additionally, some states provided specific legislation to exclude specific conditions, such as CTS. Workers' compensation was created to provide benefits for work-related pain that meets specific legislative requirements (64). This system resulted in a shift from "medical diagnostic criteria," to "epidemiologic case definition," to government-defined "musculoskeletal pain" that becomes state-defined as "compensable pain in the workplace" (50). As I (45) pointed out, although it would be desirable to find an exact diagnosis for every worker with workplace pain, in most cases this diagnosis will be impossible, and therefore it would be desirable to intervene in the workplace before explicit signs of disease develop.

Epidemiology

Before the evidence is dealt with, the following section lays the foundation for health professionals without epidemiologic training to interpret the results of MSD epidemiologic studies. It has been stated that the objective of any science is the accumulation of systematized verifiable knowledge and that this is to be achieved through observation, experiment, and thought (31). Clinicians are concerned primarily with individual patients, while epidemiologists study the occurrence of disease or other health-related conditions or events in defined populations. Epidemiologic research is based on the systematic collection of observations related to the phenomenon of interest in a defined population. These data then are subjected to quantification including measurement of random variables, estimation of population parameters, and statistical testing of hypotheses (65). Epidemiology is the biomedical discipline focused on the distribution and determinants of disease in groups of individuals who happen to have some characteristics, exposures, or diseases in common. Viewed as the study of the distribution and societal determinants of the health status of populations, epidemiology is the basic science foundation of public health. With the changing profile of health care delivery systems, clinicians must go beyond individual patients and consider their practices in terms of their effects on the lives entrusted to them. Clinicians should recognize the increasing responsibility for understanding the field of population medicine.

Definition of Epidemiology

Epidemiology is a basic medical science that focuses on the distribution and determinants of disease frequency in human populations and the application of this study to disease control (29,66). It is important to note that this definition recognizes the epidemiologists' role in describing both the distribution (i.e., person, place, and time) and determinants (i.e., risk factors) of disease and linking these findings to prevention programs. Studies in epidemiology seek to find associations between exposure and disease (cause and effect). The need to identify and interpret associations is greatest for conditions accounting for a large share of society's health problems. Given the magnitude of work-related MSD problems in the United States, MSDs fulfill this criterion.

Epidemiologic Observations

It has been stated that any work that stands to elucidate the cause of disease, the mechanism of disease, the cure of disease, or the prevention of disease must begin and end with observations of humans, whatever the intermediate steps may be (67). Observations and measurements form the fundamental units of data. The quality of data is commonly described using four terms:

- *Accuracy*: the degree to which a measurement represents the true value of the attribute being measured;
- *Precision*: the quality of being sharply defined through exact detail;
- *Reliability*: a measure of how dependably an observation is exactly the same when it repeated; it refers to the measuring procedure rather than to the attribute being measured. (Reliability is not synonymous with repeatability or reproducibility; rather, it is a broader term that includes the concept of

consistency, which refers to how closely findings in different samples or populations conform to one another under different conditions or at different times);

- *Validity*: the ability to measure what the work purports to measure (29).

Bias is defined as any trend in the collection, analysis, interpretation, publication, or review of data that can lead to conclusions that are systematically different from the truth (66).

Confounding is a distortion in an effect measure (e.g., RR) that results from an effect of another variable (the confounder) associated with the disease and exposure being studied. Confounding can lead to an overestimate or an underestimate of the true association between a disease and an exposure, and can even change the direction of the observed effect. For a factor to be a confounder, it must in and of itself be a risk factor for the disease in the unexposed population, and it must be associated with the exposure variable in the population from which the cases were derived.

An *effect modifier* is a factor that changes the magnitude of an effect measure (e.g., RR or OR). Effect modification differs from confounding in that the latter is a bias that the investigator tries to prevent or remove from the data, whereas the former is a constant of nature.

Selection bias refers to a distortion in the estimation of an effect due to systematic differences in characteristics between subjects who are selected for a study and those who are not.

Information or *observation bias* refers to a distortion in the estimation of an effect that results from error in the measurement of either an exposure or a disease or from the misclassification of subjects with regard to at least one variable (65).

Epidemiologic Study Design Issues

Epidemiologic studies seek to identify factors associated, positively or negatively, with the development of adverse health outcomes. These individual factors can be demographic (age and sex), genetic (inherited characteristics), environmental (workplace or occupational), nonwork environmental (lifestyle and hobbies), or linked elements (behavioral, social, and economic). To measure these factors, several study designs are used. Each study design has strengths and weakness for evaluations of each of the individual factors. These studies can be group into two basic types: descriptive and analytic. Descriptive studies can be case reports or case series. Analytic studies are case–control, cohort (prospective or retrospective) or cross-sectional studies. A brief review of the study types used in occupational MSDs follows.

Case Reports and Case Series

Case reports and case series are reports of disorders identified during the clinical evaluation of individual employees or several members of a workforce. Authors typically describe some interesting or intriguing observations among the employees. Case reports and case series typically generate hypotheses that can then be investigated in analytic epidemiologic studies, such as cross-sectional, case–control, and cohort studies. These reports or series should not be viewed as providing evidence for causal association between a particular exposure and a MSD. In addition, because case reports and case series do not involve hypothesis testing or have comparison groups, many epidemiologists do not consider them to be epidemiologic studies.

Case–Control Studies

Subjects in case–control studies are selected based on their disease status. Differences in exposures are compared between employees who are MSD cases and those who are noncases (controls). A ratio is generated between the proportion of cases exposed to the risk factor versus the proportion of noncases exposed. This ratio is known as the OR. The OR informs the reader regarding the strength of the association between an exposure and a work-related MSD. An OR of 3 for a particular exposure factor, for example, suggests that it will increase the risk of getting the disease threefold. Two statistical measures are used to ensure that associations are not attributable to chance. They are the p value and the CI (68). By convention, scientists often use a p value less than 0.05 to conclude that the results observed were unlikely to have arisen by chance (in 95 times out of 100, the results would not be attributable to chance). The CI indicates the probable range in which the OR actually falls. Again, by convention, scientists typically use a 95% CI (66). If the CI includes 1, the association between the exposure and a MSD may have occurred by chance alone; therefore, the OR is not considered statistically significant. Case–control studies are good for evaluating rarely occurring conditions or those that include a small number of cases. The main limitation of these studies is the inability to determine the temporal relationship between exposure and disease condition. Another important consideration for case–control studies is how the control population was selected and whether it represents an appropriate comparison group.

Cohort Studies

Cohort studies involve the identification of an exposed worker population (cohort), follow-up over time, and a determination of disease frequency in relation to the exposure type and level. If a MSD has not yet occurred when the exposure status is being ascertained, the study is considered a prospective cohort study. If a MSD has already occurred when the exposure status is being ascertained, the study is considered a retrospective cohort study. The incidence (defined subsequently) of MSD cases among the exposed employees is compared with the incidence of MSDs among the nonexposed employees. This comparison establishes a RR, which assesses the relationship between exposures and MSDs. A RR greater than 1 implies that the incidence of a MSD was greater in the exposed than the nonexposed group, thereby suggesting an association between that exposure factor and the MSD. A CI is used to indicate the probable range in which the RR actually falls.

Cross-sectional Studies

The most common study design used in investigating work-related MSDs is the cross-sectional study. Employees are usually selected for study based on their exposure to a particular factor in their employment within a particular industry, occupation, plant, or department. Exposure is usually stratified into at least two categories, and MSD prevalences (defined subsequently) are determined among exposed and nonexposed workers. The prevalences of MSDs among the exposed and the nonexposed are usually evaluated by a PPR; an OR can also be derived. Interpretation of the OR, CI, and p value were discussed earlier. It is important to note that both the MSD and exposure status are determined at approximately the same time. This inability to establish a temporal relationship or to track exposure status over time is a major limitation of cross-sectional studies. An employee who acquires a work-related shoulder tendinitis attributable to factors from one job may be assigned to another job, for example. This situation both would obscure the association of shoulder tendinitis with the original job and may erroneously associate the tendinitis with the second job.

Epidemiologic Causality

Causation is an empiric definition that requires the fulfillment of the following criteria:

- The characteristic referred to as the "cause" is associated with the disease (effect); that is, it occurs in the same individual as the disease more often than expected by chance alone;
- The cause has been shown to precede the effect; that is, the cause acts at a time before the disease has developed;
- Altering only the cause has been shown to alter the probability of the disease (effect) (66).

Additional criteria have been developed for the interpretation of epidemiologic data (29,65,69–71). The criteria relevant to the study of work-related MSDs are strength of the association, dose–response relationship, consistency of the association, coherence, reversibility, statistical significance, specificity, temporal relationship, incidence, prevalence, bias, and statistics. A brief review of how these criteria are used in occupational MSDs follows:

The *strength of association* is measured by the size of the RR or the OR. In general, strong associations (RR or OR >3) are unlikely to be attributable to chance or unidentified confounding associations and therefore support a potential causal association (65). If the risk of disease increases as exposure to a risk factor increases, a dose–response relationship is said to exist.

A *dose–response relationship* is relatively strong evidence for a causal association, but its absence does not rule out a causal association because of a potential threshold effect or inability to adequately quantify the exposure.

Consistency refers to whether the association has been reported in other studies. Diverse study designs conducted by a variety of researchers in several countries that yield similar associations support a causal association. Review of the literature in a more formal approach, known as metaanalysis, can synthesize data from many studies and derive a single best estimate of the strength of association.

Coherence implies that the cause–effect interpretation for an association does not conflict with the known natural history and biology of the disease. In other words, it is the biologic plausibility or believability of the potential association.

Reversibility refers to whether the disease risk is lower with the elimination or reduction of the exposure to the risk factor. Obviously, this criterion is only applicable to intervention studies. Given the inability to control many of the potentially confounding factors for MSDs, intervention studies are difficult to perform and therefore uncommon.

Statistical significance refers to the process by which an association is estimated to be attributable to chance. Too often, statistical significance has been equated with clinical or public health significance. Taken out of context, the *p* value or CI has little meaning (68).

Specificity assumes that a cause leads to a single effect, not multiple effects. Given the multifactorial nature of most criteria, specificity may not always be appropriate for interpreting MSD epidemiologic studies.

Temporal relationship refers to the condition required for causal associations; therefore, the exposure precedes the disease.

The *incidence* is defined as the number of new cases of a disease in a population within a certain period of time. The basic characteristic of incidence data is that time is part of the units (i.e., cases per population per time). Incidence rates are usually measured in experimental and cohort studies.

Prevalence measures the number of cases present at or during a specified time. The prevalence equals the incidence multiplied by the average duration of the disease. The two types of prevalence used by investigators are point prevalence and period prevalence. Point prevalence refers to the number of cases present at a specified moment. Period prevalence refers to the number of cases present during any part of a specified time (e.g., 1 year). Prevalences are usually measured in cross-sectional studies.

Bias is the alteration of data by including or excluding population that influences a disease's being measured.

Statistics is derived from the Latin *status*, meaning state or condition, denoting that statistics should be used to describe how things are. Inferential statistics is the process of estimation and hypothesis testing that allows going beyond describing characteristics about a group that has been measured to making statements or inferences about much larger groups or populations. Statistical inference is founded in logic and philosophy, rather than existing as a body of coherent technical knowledge (72).

The following work-related definitions are from the U.S. Department of Health and Human Services, Office of Workers' Compensation Programs (73):

- *Accleration*: a documented physiologic mechanism or process by which an occupational act, exposure, or occurrence can be shown to have increased the expected speed of progression in a preexisting condition documented to be progressive in nature (e.g., asbestosis).

- *Aggravation*: a documented physiologic mechanism or process by which an occupational act, exposure, or occurrence can be shown to have made worse, intensified, or increased the severity of a physical or mental problem known to preexist that exposure or occurrence. With *temporary* aggravation, the preexisting condition is worsened or made more severe for a time, with no residual alteration of the underlying condition and without leaving any continuing impairment beyond that time. With *permanent* aggravation, there is a continuing and irreversible change in the underlying condition, thus adversely altering the course of the condition or disease process.

- *Causal relationship*: To a physician, "cause" may refer only to a direct or principal cause, but for workers' compensation, a variety of contributing causes must be considered. Under the Federal Employees Compensation Act, any disease or disability is compensable when it is proximately caused or materially aggravated by employment-related injury or condition(s) of employment. Proximate cause is that which, in a natural and continuous sequence, produces the disability. However, natural progression of a disease while a person is working does not constitute cause or aggravation. For conditions of employment to bring about aggravation of an underlying disease, the employment factors must be capable of aggravating or accelerating the disease.

NIOSH STUDY OF EPIDEMIOLOGIC CAUSALITY CRITERIA

Four evaluation criteria were used to analyze each study in this chapter. These four evaluation criteria are essential for considering the validity of epidemiologic studies and their results. Ideally, each article should meet all four criteria. At the end of each section for the body parts are included those articles that meet the following four evaluation criteria:

- Participation rate of 70%: This criterion limits the degree of selection bias in a study;
- Defining health outcome by symptoms and physical examination: This criterion reflects the preference of most reviewers to have health outcomes that are defined by objective criteria;
- Blinding of investigators to health or exposure status when assessing health or exposure status: This criterion limits observer bias in classifying exposure or disease;
- Subjecting the joint under discussion to an independent exposure assessment, with characterization of the independent variable of interest (e.g., repetition or repetitive work): This criterion indicates whether the exposure assessment was conducted on the joint of interest and involved the type of exposure being examined (e.g., repetitive work, forceful exertion, extreme posture, or vibration) or whether the exposure was measured independently or in combination with other types of exposures.
- Exposure was also characterized by the method used to measure the level of exposure. Studies that used either direct observation or actual measurements of exposure were considered to have a more accurate exposure classification scheme, whereas studies that exclusively used job titles, interviews, or questionnaire information were assumed to have less accurate exposure information.

Neck and Neck/Shoulder

Summary: Neck and Neck/Shoulder

Interpreting association for individual workplace factors is difficult, as most epidemiologic studies of MSDs selected populations because of multiple factors (e.g., forceful exertion and repetitive tasks). Unlike in laboratory experiments, one cannot isolate exposure factors or alter some factors while keeping others constant to ensure accuracy in examining, recording, and interpreting results. However, one can examine the body of epidemiologic evidence and infer relationships as in Table 1.

More than 40 epidemiologic studies focused on work factors and their relationship to neck and neck/shoulder MSDs. Many studies identified individuals in heavier industrial occupations and compared them to workers in light industry or office environments. Other studies identified a symptomatic group of workers or those with symptoms and physical examination abnormalities and compared them to asymptomatic workers at the same worksite or to population referents, looking for differences in exposure. These approaches, although quite different, have largely chosen to focus on similar workplace risk factors. These factors include repetition, forceful exertions, and constrained or static postures, usually found in combination. Some of these studies meet rigorous epidemiologic criteria and appropriately address important issues so that causal inferences can be made. The majority of studies involved working groups with a combination of interacting work factors, but certain studies assessed specific work factors. Each study (with negative, positive, or equivocal findings) contributed to the overall pool of data used in assessing the strength of work-relatedness using causal inference (23).

Evidence is strong that working groups with high levels of static contraction, prolonged static loads, or extreme working postures involving the neck/shoulder muscles are at increased risk for neck/shoulder MSDs. Consistently high ORs were found (12 statistically significant studies with ORs >3.0), providing evidence linking tension neck syndrome with static postures or static loads.

Evidence exists for a causal relationship between highly repetitive work and neck and neck/shoulder MSDs. Most of the epidemiologic studies reviewed defined "repetitive work" for the neck as work activities that involve continuous arm or hand movements that affect the neck/shoulder musculature and generate loads on the neck/shoulder area. Fewer studies examined relationships based on actual repetitive neck movements. The two studies that measured repetitive neck movements by measuring head position (using frequency and duration of movements) fulfilled the most stringent epidemiologic criteria, showing strong associations with neck/shoulder MSDs. Among studies that defined repetitive work involving continuous arm or hand movements affecting the neck/shoulder, nine were statistically significant and had ORs greater than 3.0.; eight studies fulfilled all the epidemiologic criteria, except the exposure criteria, and measured repetition for the hand/wrist and not for the neck. Of these nine studies, only three were statistically significant and had ORs greater than 3, while five studies had nonsignificant ORs.

There is reasonable evidence for a relationship between forceful exertion and the occurrence of neck MSDs in the epidemiologic literature. Most of the epidemiologic studies reviewed defined "forceful work" for the neck/shoulder as work activities involving forceful arm or hand movements that generate loads to the neck/shoulder area. No study examined a relationship based on actual forceful neck movements. Of the 16 studies addressing force as one of the exposure factors, five studies found statistically significant associations but did not derive ORs; two studies found ORs greater than 3.0, seven studies found ORs ranging from 1.0 to 3.0, and two studies had ORs less than 1.0. Many of the studies relating measured force (e.g., workload, etc.) to MSDs are in the biomechanical and ergonomic literature.

Reasonable evidence exists demonstrating a causal relationship between highly repetitive work and neck and neck/shoulder MSDs. Most of the epidemiologic studies reviewed defined "repetitive work" for the neck as work activities that involve continuous arm or hand movements that affect the neck/shoulder musculature and generate loads to the neck/shoulder area. Fewer studies examined relationships based on actual repetitive neck movements. The two studies that measured repetitive neck movements by head position (using frequency and duration of movements) and fulfilled the four criteria found strong associations with neck/shoulder MSDs. In those studies defining repetitive work as continuous arm or hand movements affecting the neck/shoulder, nine found statistically significant ORs greater than 3.0. Eight studies fulfilled all the criteria, except for objective exposure assessment, and measured repetition for the hand/wrist, not the neck. Of these, three had statistically significant ORs greater than 3.0, and five had nonsignificant ORs, all less than 2.0.

The epidemiologic data were insufficient to provide support for the relationship of vibration to neck disorders. At this time, further studies must be done before a decision regarding causal relationships can be made.

Details: Neck and Neck/Shoulder

Studies from the United States have generally classified neck disorders separately from shoulder disorders when evaluating work-related risk factors. On the other hand, Scandinavian studies examining work-related factors have often combined neck and shoulder MSDs into one health outcome variable, based on the concept that several muscles act on both the shoulder girdle and the upper spine together. Epidemiologic studies have defined neck MSDs in one of two ways: (a) by symptoms occurring in the neck (usually concerning a specific duration, frequency, or intensity) or (b) by using both symptoms and physical examination findings. The prevalence of reported MSDs is generally lower when they are defined using both symptoms and physical examination results rather than symptoms alone. For example, the prevalence rate (PR) of tension neck syndrome among male industrial workers in the United States was reported to be 4.9% from interview data and 1.4% when case definitions included physical examination findings (74). The percentage of work-related MSD cases defined by physical examination findings and those defined solely by symptoms has ranged from approximately 50% (75–78) to approximately

85% (79). Forty-seven studies included physical examination findings in the health outcome assessment criteria.

References: Neck and Neck/Shoulder

The following studies meet all four criteria for neck and neck/shoulder:

- Olsson et al. (80)
- Jonsson et al. (81)

Shoulder

Summary: Shoulder

Workplace factors and their relationship to shoulder MSDs have been examined in more than 20 epidemiologic studies. In general, workers in jobs with higher levels of exposure were compared to workers with lower levels of exposure, following observation or measurement of job characteristics (23).

There is evidence for a positive association between highly repetitive work and shoulder MSDs, with some important limitations. Only three studies specifically addressed the health outcome of shoulder tendinitis, and these studies involved combined exposure to repetition with awkward shoulder postures or static shoulder loads. The other six studies with significant positive associations dealt primarily with symptoms. Evidence reinforces a relationship between shoulder MSDs and repeated or sustained shoulder postures with greater than 60 degrees of flexion or abduction. There is evidence to suggest a link between tendinitis and shoulder pain and their relationship to work. The evidence for specific shoulder postures and their link to work is strongest where there is combined exposure to several physical factors, such as holding a tool while working overhead. The association was positive and consistent in the six studies that used diagnosed cases of shoulder tendinitis or a constellation of symptoms and physical findings consistent with tendinitis as the health outcome. Only one of the 13 studies failed to find a positive association with exposure and symptoms or a specific shoulder disorder (82). These results are consistent with the evidence found in the biomechanical, physiologic, and psychosocial literature.

Evidence is insufficient for positive associations between force and shoulder MSDs and vibration and shoulder MSDs, based on current available epidemiologic studies.

Details: Shoulder

Shoulder MSDs and their relationship to work risk factors have been reviewed by several authors (73,83,84). These authors attributed the majority of shoulder problems occurring in a variety of occupations to workplace exposure. When looking specifically at shoulder tendinitis, they concluded that the epidemiologic literature is "most convincing" regarding work-relatedness, demonstrating an increased risk for overhead and repetitive work. The current review focused on the evidence for a relationship between shoulder tendinitis and workplace exposures to the following: awkward postures, forceful exertions, repetitive exertions, and segmental vibration. Also included were studies relevant to shoulder disorders, as defined by a combination of symptoms and physical examination findings or by symptoms alone but not specifically defined as tendinitis, and studies in which neck and shoulder disorders were combined in the health outcome but where the exposure was likely to have been specific to the shoulder.

References: Shoulder

The following studies meet all four criteria for the shoulder:

- Chiang et al. (85)
- Kilbom et al. (86)
- Ohlsson et al. (87)
- Ohlsson et al. (80)

Elbow

Summary: Elbow

The epidemiologic studies reviewed in this section focused principally on the risk of epicondylitis in workers performing repetitive job tasks requiring forceful movements. More than 20 epidemiologic studies examined physical workplace factors and their relationship to epicondylitis. The majority of studies involved study populations exposed to some combination of work factors, and some of these studies included assessment of specific work factors. Each study examined (with negative, positive, or equivocal findings) contributed to the overall pool of data regarding the strength of work-relatedness.

Most of the relevant occupational studies were cross-sectional and based on current estimates for the level of exposure compared to estimated past exposure. Despite the cross-sectional nature of the studies, it is likely that the exposures predated the onset of disorders in most cases for forceful movements that included but were not limited to repeated dorsiflexion, flexion, pronation, and supination, sometimes with the arm extended. Clinical case series of occupationally related epicondylitis and studies of epicondylitis among athletes suggested that repeated forceful dorsiflexion, flexion, pronation, and supination, especially with the arm extended, increased the risk of epicondylitis. In general, the epidemiologic studies have not quantitatively measured the fraction of forceful hand motions most likely to contribute to epicondylitis; rather, they have used as a surrogate qualitative estimation the presence or absence of these types of hand movements. Studies that based their exposure assessment on quantitative or semiquantitative data showed a solid relationship.

Insufficient evidence exists for the association of repetitive work and epicondylitis. For extreme posture in the workplace, the epidemiologic evidence, thus far, is also insufficient. No studies having repetitive work as the dominant exposure factor met all four epidemiologic criteria. When the sports medicine literature was considered in evaluating the risk of the single factors of repetition and posture, some supportive evidence was suggested.

With regard to the relationship between work factors and epicondylitis, the strongest evidence by far is for a combination of factors, especially at higher levels of exposure. The strong evidence for a combination of factors is consistent with evidence found in the sports medicine and biomechanical literature. Based on the epidemiologic studies reviewed above, especially those with some quantitative evaluation of the risk factors, the evidence is clear that an exposure to a combination of exposures, especially at higher exposure levels (as seen in meatpacking or construction work), increases the risk for epicondylitis. Studies outside the field of epidemiology also suggested that forceful and repetitive contraction of the elbow flexors or extensors (which can be caused by flexion and extension of the wrist) increases the risk of epicondylitis. The one prospective study that had a combination of exposure factors demonstrated a particularly high incidence rate (6.7) and illustrated a temporal relationship between physical exposure factors and epicondylitis. Epidemiologic surveillance data, both nationally and internationally, consistently indicated that the highest incidence of epicondylitis occurs in occupations and job tasks that are manually intensive and require high work demands in dynamic environments. Examples include mechanics, butchers, construction workers, and boilermakers.

Studies that based exposure assessment on quantitative or semiquantitative data tended to show a stronger relationship for epicondylitis and force. Eight studies fulfilling at least one criterion showed statistically significant relationships. Epicondylar tenderness was also found to be associated with a combination of higher levels of forceful exertions, repetition, and extreme postures of the elbow. Some data indicated that a high percentage of individuals with severe elbow pain are not able to do their jobs and they have a higher rate of sick leave than individuals with other upper extremity disorders. Therefore, considering biologic plausibility, the studies with quantitative evaluation of exposure factors and evidence for the occurrence of MSDs when combinations of factors occurred at higher levels of exposure provide evidence for the association between repetitive, forceful work and epicon-

dylitis. There are several important qualifications to this conclusion. Forceful and repetitive work is most likely a surrogate for repetitive, forceful hand motions that cause contractions of the muscles whose tendons insert in the area of the lateral and medial epicondyles of the elbow. While the studies did not identify the number or intensity of forceful contractions leading to the increased risk epicondylitis, the levels were likely to be substantial. The majority of studies were positive for some relationship of elbow MSDs to work. However, one study showed no evidence of increased risk. The association between forceful and repetitive work involving dorsiflexion, flexion, supination, and pronation of the hand is definitely biologically plausible. These motions can cause the contraction of the muscle–tendon units that attach in the area of the medial and lateral epicondyles of the elbow. The evidence for a qualitative exposure–response relationship overall was considerable for the combination of exposures, with studies examining differences in levels of exposure for the elbow with corresponding evidence for greater risk in the highly exposed group.

There is insufficient evidence to draw conclusions about the relationship of postural factors alone and epicondylitis at this time.

Using epidemiologic criteria to examine these studies and with account taken of issues of confounding, bias, and strengths and limitations of the studies, the studies suggest that there is epidemiologic evidence for the relationship between forceful work and epicondylitis. Additionally, there is strong evidence for a relationship between exposure to a combination of risk factors (e.g., force and repetition, force and posture) and epicondylitis. There is also evidence for the association of forceful work and epicondylitis. Future studies should focus on the types of forceful and repetitive hand motions, such as forceful dorsiflexion, pronation, and supination, that result in forceful contractions of the muscle–tendon units that insert in the area of the lateral and medial epicondyles. Common nonoccupational activities, such as sport activities, that cause epicondylitis should be considered. Older workers may be at some increased risk. Finally, even though the epidemiologic literature shows that many affected workers continue to work with definite symptoms and physical findings of epicondylitis, survivor bias should be addressed.

Details: Elbow

Epicondylitis is an uncommon disorder with an overall prevalence in the general population of 1% to 5% (7). Fewer epidemiologic studies have addressed workplace risk factors for elbow MSDs than for other MSDs. Most of these studies compared the prevalence of epicondylitis in workers whose jobs are known to have highly repetitive, forceful tasks (e.g., meat processing) to that in workers in less repetitive, forceful work (e.g., office jobs); the majority of these studies were not designed to identify individual workplace risk factors. There were 19 studies: 18 cross-sectional studies and one cohort study. Studies using symptom and physical examination findings to define epicondylitis used consistent criteria—almost all studies using physical examination for diagnosis identified epicondylitis with palpation of the epicondylar area and pain at the elbow with resisted movement of the wrist. However, studies using a definition based on symptom data alone used various criteria; some were based on frequency and duration of symptoms, while others were based on elbow symptoms preventing work activities. This lack of a case definition may explain why there are no studies that met all four evaluation criteria.

Hand/Wrist

Summary: Hand/Wrist

More than 30 epidemiologic studies examined physical workplace factors and their relationship to CTS. These studies generally compared workers in jobs with higher levels of exposure to workers with lower levels of exposure following observation or measurement of job characteristics. Several studies fulfilled the four epidemiologic criteria used in this review and appropriately addressed important methodologic issues. The studies generally involved populations exposed to a combination of work factors, but a few assessed single work factors, such as repetitive motions of the hand. Each study was reviewed for positive, negative, or equivocal findings to evaluate the strength of work-relatedness using causal inference. Using epidemiologic criteria and with account taken of issues of confounding, bias, and strengths and limitations of the studies, the following observations can be made.

Studies that based exposure assessment on quantitative or semiquantitative data tended to show a stronger relationship for CTS and repetition. The higher estimates of RR were found when highly repetitive jobs were contrasted to low-repetitive jobs and when repetition was combined with high levels of forceful exertion. Individual variability in work methods among workers in similar jobs and the influence of differing anthropometry on posture were among the difficulties noted in measuring postural characteristics of jobs in field studies. Findings from laboratory-based studies of extreme postural factors support a positive association with CTS, and there is evidence of a positive association between work involving hand/wrist vibration and CTS. Ten studies allowed a comparison of the effect of individual versus combined work risk factors (9,55,75,85,88–92). Based on the epidemiologic studies reviewed, especially those with quantitative evaluation of the risk factors, the evidence is clear that exposure to a combination of the job factors studied (repetition, force, posture, etc.) increased the risk for CTS. This conclusion is consistent with the evidence found in the biomechanical, physiologic, and psychosocial literature. Nine of these studies demonstrated higher estimates of RR when exposure involved a combination of risk factors compared to the effect of individual risk factors.

Based on currently available epidemiologic data, positive associations are apparent between force and CTS, between highly repetitive work alone or in combination with other factors and CTS, between forceful work and CTS, and between jobs with exposure to vibration and CTS. Evidence, however, is insufficient for an association between extreme postures and CTS.

Evidence is strong for a positive association between exposure to a combination of risk factors (e.g., force and repetition, force and posture) and CTS. Epidemiologic surveillance data, both nationally and internationally, also consistently indicated that the highest rates of CTS occur in occupations and job tasks with high work demands for intensive manual exertion. Examples include meatpackers, poultry processors, and automobile assembly workers.

Details: Hand/Wrist

In 1988, the estimated population prevalence of CTS was of 53 cases per 10,000 workers (9). Of these, 20% reported absence from work because of CTS. In 1994, the BLS reported that the rate of CTS cases resulting in "days away from work" was 4.8 per 10,000 workers. The BLS also reported that the median number of days away from work for CTS was 30, which is even greater than the median reported for back pain cases (93). In 1993, the incidence rate for CTS workers' compensation cases was 31.7 per 10,000 workers, and only a minority of these cases involved time off from work (6,94). These data suggest that about 5 to 10 workers per 10,000 will miss work each year due to work-related CTS.

In recent years, the literature relating occupational factors to the development of CTS has been extensively reviewed by numerous authors (10,95–99). Most reviews reached a similar conclusion: Work factors are one of the important causes of CTS. One review found the evidence more equivocal but stated that the epidemiologic studies revealed a fairly consistent pattern of observations regarding the spectrum and relative frequency of CTS, among other MSDs, among jobs believed to be hazardous (98).

Researchers relied on a variety of methods to assess exposure to suspected occupational risk factors for CTS. These methods included direct measurement, observation, self-reports, and categorization by job titles. Most investigators agreed that observational or direct-measurement methods increase the quality (both the precision and accuracy) of ergonomic exposure assessments, but these methods also tended to be costly and time-consuming. In general, misclassification errors tended to dilute the observed associations between disease and physical workload (97).

In the literature reviewed, assessment of CTS was based on symptoms alone, a combination of symptoms and physical findings, or symptoms and physical findings supported by electrophysiologic nerve tests. Electrodiagnostic testing—nerve conduction studies (NCS)– has been considered by some to be a requirement for a valid case definition of CTS, as it is similarly used for a clinical diagnosis of individuals with CTS. A few studies that looked at the relationship of occupational factors to CTS used a health outcome based on electrodiagnostic testing alone (55,89, 100). However, some authors discouraged the use of labeling workers as having CTS or median nerve mononeuropathy based on abnormal sensory nerve conduction alone (without symptoms) (101,102). The reason for this view is illustrated in a recent prospective study by Werner et al. (101). On follow-up 6 to 18 months after initial evaluation, they found that asymptomatic active workers with abnormal sensory median nerve function by NCS were no more likely to develop symptoms consistent with CTS than those with normal nerve function. Studies using NCS for epidemiologic field studies employed a variety of evaluation methods and techniques (55,78,103,104). Normal values for NCS also varied from laboratory to laboratory. NCS results were found to vary with electrode placement and temperature, as well as age, height, finger circumference, and wrist ratio (91), suggesting that "normal" values may need to be corrected for these factors.

Several epidemiologic studies used a surveillance case definition of CTS based on symptoms in the median nerve distribution and abnormal physical examination findings using Phalen's maneuver and Tinel's sign, and did not include NCS. As questionnaire-based research evolves, two recent studies looked at CTS diagnosis based on questionnaire and physical examination findings and its association with the "gold standard" of NCS for the ability to diagnose CTS (78, 105). Both studies found statistically significant evidence to support the use of an epidemiologic CTS case definition based on symptoms and physical examination (not requiring NCS) for epidemiologic surveillance studies. Nathan et al. (88) also found a strong relationship between symptoms and prolonged sensory median nerve conduction. (It is important to note that a case definition used for epidemiologic purposes usually differs from one used for medical diagnosis and therapeutic intervention.)

Confounders and CTS

It is clear that CTS has several nonoccupational causes. When the relationship of occupational factors to CTS is examined, it is important to take into account the effects of these individual factors, that is, to control for their confounding or modifying effects. Studies failing to control for the influence of individual factors may either mask or amplify the effects of work-related factors (48). Most epidemiologic studies of CTS that address work factors also take into account potential confounders.

Almost all the studies reviewed controlled for the effects of age in their analysis (85,91, 92,106,107). Likewise, most studies included sex in their analyses either by stratification (85,89), selection of single-sex study groups (108,109), or inclusion of the variable in the logistic regression model (91,106). Through selection of the study population and exclusion of those with metabolic diseases, most researchers were able to eliminate the effects of these conditions. Other studies controlled

for systemic disease (85). Anthropometric factors have also been addressed in several studies (88,91,101).

As more is learned about confounding, more variables tend to be addressed in more recent studies (e.g., smoking, caffeine, alcohol, hobbies). In older studies that may not have controlled for multiple confounders, it is unlikely that they are highly correlated with exposure, especially those with ORs greater than 3.0. When studies that included good exposure assessment, widely contrasting levels of exposure, and control for multiple confounders are examined, the evidence supports a positive association between occupational factors and CTS.

References: CTS

The following studies met all four criteria for CTS:

- Chatterjee (110,111)
- Chiang et al. (85,92)
- Melhorn (112)
- Moore and Garg (113)
- Osorio et al. (104)
- Silverstein et al. (106)

Hand/Wrist Tendinitis

Summary: Hand/Wrist Tendinitis

Eight epidemiologic studies examined physical workplace factors and their relationship to hand/wrist tendinitis. Several studies fulfilled the four epidemiologic criteria used in this review and appropriately addressed important methodologic issues. The studies generally involved populations exposed to a combination of work factors. One study assessed single work factors, such as repetitive motions of the hand. Each study was reviewed for findings that were positive, negative, or equivocal to evaluate the strength of work-relatedness using causal inference.

There is evidence of an association between any single factor (repetition, force, and posture) and hand/wrist tendinitis, based on currently available epidemiologic data. There is strong evidence that job tasks that require a combination of risk factors (e.g., highly repetitious, forceful hand/wrist exertions) increased risk for hand/wrist tendinitis.

Details: Hand/Wrist Tendinitis

Because the hand/wrist area may be affected by more than one MSD, only studies that specifically addressed hand/wrist tendinitis are considered here. Studies with outcomes described as hand/wrist disorders or symptoms in general or those in which hand/wrist tendinitis was combined with epicondylitis were excluded from this section because it was not possible to evaluate evidence for work-related hand/wrist tendinitis from the data. The eight studies provided data specifically addressing hand/wrist tendinitis. In each study, the outcome was determined using physical examination criteria, although the case definitions varied among studies. Prevalence or incidence rates of hand/wrist tendinitis reported in exposed groups ranged from 4% to 56% and in unexposed groups from 0% to 14% (114,115). Such wide ranges of PRs probably reflect the variability in diagnostic criteria as much as they do the range of workplace exposures in these studies. For example, one study used very strict criteria (116). The case definition required observation of swelling along the tendon at the time of the physical examination. The only cases of tendinitis diagnosed were de Quervain's disease; no other cases of tenosynovitis or peritendinitis were diagnosed among 199 automobile assembly line workers. In contrast, the studies with the highest PRs either did not clearly state what diagnostic criteria were used to determine the case definition or also considered recurrences of tendinitis as new cases. Whether case definitions were inclusive or exclusive would not affect the RR as long as they were applied nondifferentially between groups designated as exposed or unexposed.

Although several studies reported ORs, published data were reanalyzed and the results showed PRs of 1.4 to 6.2 (114–117).

This analysis was done to make estimates of RR comparable across studies, because ORs may overestimate RR when PRs are high. In studies that presented ORse original articles, the recalculation of data as PRs resulted in lower estimates of the RR. In the one prospective cohort study, incidence rates and risk ratios were presented (118).

Except for a study reported by Armstrong et al. (114), risk estimates were not reported separately for single risk factors. This study also used a formal quantitative exposure assessment as the basis for determining exposure groups. Other studies grouped together jobs with similar risk factors and compared them to jobs without those risk factors. Typically, the selection of jobs for the exposed and unexposed groups was based on general knowledge of the jobs, previously published literature, or questionnaire data. Repetition, force, and extreme postures were considered in combination to determine which workers were exposed or unexposed. Formal exposure assessment (e.g., videotape analysis for cycle time, repetition, extreme postures, and estimates of force) was usually conducted on a sample of jobs and used as the rationale for grouping jobs into exposed and unexposed categories, rather than creating quantitative measures of risk factors. In some cases, the investigators noted the difficulty in examining risk factors separately because of job rotation (115). Review of tendinitis demonstrated several potential confounders: sex, age, and years on the job.

The association between sex and tendinitis is not uniform. Bystrom et al. (116) reported a higher prevalence of de Quervain's tendinitis in men than in women and proposed the explanation that men in their study group used hand tools more often than women. Ulnar deviation and static muscle loading were likewise more often reported among men. Armstrong et al. (114) reported a higher prevalence of tendinitis among women but found no significant associations with other medical factors or activities outside of work. However, significant differences in posture were observed between men and women.

Differences in postures may be due to differences in height between men and women whose workstations have uniform dimensions. In McCormack et al.'s (90) study of textile workers, three of the four exposed groups were largely female (89% to 95%), limiting the ability to separate the effect of sex from job effect. However, in an analysis that included sex and job as risk factors, they reported that sex was a significant predictor of tendinitis ($p = 0.01$) but not as significant a predictor as job category ($p = 0.001$). The other studies reviewed did not have both male and female subjects.

Several investigators noted that tendinitis appears to be more prevalent in younger age groups. Bystrom et al. (116) reported that most cases of de Quervain's tendinitis occurred in the younger-than-40 age group. McCormack et al. (90) reported that age was not a significant predictor of tendinitis, but years on the job was inversely associated: Prevalence was higher with fewer than 3 years on the job. Armstrong et al. (114) noted that "a significant interaction between sex, age, and years on the job suggested that the risk of hand/wrist tendinitis might actually decrease with an increased number of years on the job, but the effect was too small to merit further discussion." Roto and Kivi (119) noted that "the few cases of tenosynovitis occurred in younger workers." Kuorinka and Koskinen (120) and Luopajarvi et al. (115) found no significant association between age and tendinitis.

McCormack et al. (90) reported that race was not associated with tendinitis. Armstrong et al. (114) found no significant associations with personal factors: birth control pills, hysterectomy, oophorectomy, or recreational activities. No subjects with seropositive rheumatic disease were included in the Kuorinka and Koskinen (120) study. They reported that their earlier unpublished questionnaire found no correlations between illness and extra work, work outside the factory, work at home, or hobbies. Luopajarvi et al. (115) excluded subjects with previous trauma, arthritis, and other pathologies.

References: Hand/Wrist Tendinitis

The following studies met all four criteria for hand/wrist tendinitis:

- Armstrong et al. (114)
- Luopajarvi et al. (115)

Hand–Arm Vibration Syndrome

Summary: Hand–Arm Vibration Syndrome

Hand–arm vibration (HAV) is defined as the transfer of vibration from a tool to a worker's hand and arm. The amount of HAV is characterized by the acceleration level of the tool when grasped by the worker and in use. The vibration is typically measured on the handle of the tool while in use to determine the acceleration levels transferred to the worker (23).

In general, HAV studies show strong evidence for a positive association between high-level exposure to HAV and vascular symptoms of HAVS. These studies involved workers with high levels of exposure such as forestry workers, stone drillers, stone cutters or carvers, shipyard workers, or platers. These workers were typically exposed to HAV acceleration levels of 5 to 36 m/s^2. The studies typically were cross-sectional studies that compared workers with high levels of exposures to HAV with a nonexposed control group. There is substantial evidence that as intensity and duration of exposure to vibrating tools increase, the risk of developing HAVS increases. There also is evidence that an increase in symptom severity is associated with increased exposure. As intensity and duration of exposure are increased, the time from exposure onset and beginning of symptoms is shortened. The relationship of vibration to HAVS was also supported by epidemiologic causality criteria of consistency, coherency, and temporal sequence of exposure and outcome.

Support for the exposure was provided by a few longitudinal studies of workers exposed to HAV. In general, all showed strong evidence that decreasing the acceleration level of a handheld vibrating tool has a positive relationship with the prevalence of HAVS. In a study of Finnish forestry workers using chain saws, Koskimies et al. (121) found that the prevalence of HAVS symptoms declined from a peak of 40% to 5% after the introduction of lightweight, low-vibration chain saws with reduced acceleration from 14 to 2 m/s². Likewise, a study of similar workers in Japan found that the prevalence of vascular symptoms among chain saw operators who began their jobs before the introduction of various engineering and administrative controls peaked at 63%. (Vibration acceleration levels for chain saws used during this period ranged from 111 to 304 m/s².) In contrast, the peak prevalence for chain saw operators who began working after the introduction of antivibration chain saws (acceleration level: 10 to 33 m/s²) and exposure duration limits (2 hours per day) was only 2% (122,123).

NIOSH (124) ranked 23 cross-sectional studies that measured HAV acceleration levels and estimated a PR for vascular symptoms. To test whether a linear relationship existed between the HAV level and the prevalence of vascular symptoms, a correlation coefficient was calculated. The correlation analysis found a statistically significant linear relationship between HAV acceleration level and the prevalence of vascular symptoms (PR 0.67, $p<0.01$), indicating that the prevalence of vascular symptoms tends to increase as the HAV acceleration level increases. However, the absorption of vibration energy by the hand is influenced by the vibration intensity, as well as by frequency, transmission direction, grip and feed forces, hand–arm postures, and anthropometric factors (125). Several studies found relationships between the prevalence of HAVS and the duration of vibration-exposed work (126–129). One cross-sectional study with a very poor response rate found no association with duration of exposure (130). Justification for a relationship between dose and HAVS prevalence and symptom severity was provided by Bovenzi et al. (131) and Mirbod et al (132). In a study of stone-cutters using rock drills and chisel hammers, Bovenzi et al. (131) found that HAVS prevalence increased linearly with the total number of working hours from about 18% for persons with 6,000 hours of exposure to more than 50% among persons with more than 26,000 hours of exposure. Likewise, in a study of 447 workers using chain saws, Mirbod et al. (132) found that the prevalence of HAVS increased from 2.5% among workers with less than 14 years of exposure to 11.7% among workers with 20 to 24 years' exposure.

Details: Hand–Arm Vibration Syndrome

The 20 epidemiologic studies in this review were chosen according to the four main selection criteria. Additional criteria included adequate participation rate, definition of health outcome by both symptoms and medical examination criteria, blinding of investigators to exposure or outcome status, and independent or objective measure of exposure. When bias factors were removed, the criteria of strength of association, temporal relationship, consistency of association, coherence of association, and exposure–response relationships supported a strong evidence for a relationship between vibration and HAVS. Confounding factors for HAVS include age and metabolic diseases.

References: Hand–Arm Vibration Syndrome

The following study met all four criteria for HAVS: Bovenzi et al. (127).

Back

Summary: Back

More than 40 recent articles provided evidence regarding the relationship between low back disorders (LBDs) and the five physical workplace factors that were considered in this review: heavy physical work, lifting and forceful movements, bending and twisting (awkward postures), whole-body vibration

(WBV), and static work postures. Many studies addressed multiple work-related factors. All articles that addressed a particular workplace factor contributed to the information used to draw conclusions about that risk factor regardless of whether results were positive or negative.

The review provided evidence for a positive relationship between back disorders and heavy physical work, although risk estimates were more moderate regarding lifting or forceful movements, awkward postures, and WBV. These findings were perhaps due to subjective and imprecise characterization of exposures. Evidence for a dose–response relationship was equivocal for this risk factor.

There is strong evidence that LBDs are associated with work-related lifting and forceful movements. Of 18 epidemiologic studies reviewed, 13 were consistent in demonstrating positive relationships. Those using subjective measures of exposure showed a range of risk estimates from 1.2 to 5.2, and those using more objective assessments had ORs ranging from 2.2 to 11. Studies using objective measures to examine specific lifting activities generally demonstrated risk estimates greater than 3 and found dose–response relationships between exposures and outcomes. For the most part, higher ORs were observed in high-exposure populations (e.g., one high-risk group averaged 226 lifts per hour with a mean load weight of 88 newtons). Most of the investigations reviewed adjusted for potential covariates in analyses; nevertheless, some of the relatively high ORs observed were unlikely to be caused by confounding or other effects of lifestyle covariates. The review provided evidence that work-related awkward postures are associated with LBDs. Results were consistent in showing positive associations, with several risk estimates greater than 3. Exposure–response relationships were demonstrated. Many studies adjusted for potential covariates and a few examined the simultaneous effects of other work-related physical factors. Several studies suggested that both lifting and awkward postures were important contributors to the risk of LBD. The observed relationships were consistent with biomechanical and other laboratory evidence regarding the effects of lifting and dynamic motion on back tissues.

There is strong evidence of an association between exposure to WBV and LBDs. Of 19 studies reviewed, 15 were consistent in demonstrating positive associations, with risk estimates ranging from 1.2 to 5.7 for those using subjective exposure measures and from 1.4 to 39.5 for those using objective assessment methods. Most studies that examined relationships in high-exposure groups using detailed quantitative exposure measures found strong positive associations and exposure–response relationships between WBV and LBDs. These relationships were observed after adjusting for covariates.

Both experimental and epidemiologic evidence suggest that WBV may act in combination with other work-related factors, such as prolonged sitting, lifting, and awkward postures, to cause an increased risk of back disorder. It is possible that effects of WBV may depend on the source of exposure (type of vehicle).

With regard to static work postures and LBDs, results from the studies reviewed provided insufficient evidence that a relationship exists. Few investigations examined the effects of static work postures, and exposure characterizations were limited.

Details: Back

Low back pain (LBP) is common in the general population. Lifetime prevalence has been estimated at nearly 70% for industrialized countries, and sciatic conditions may occur in 5% of those experiencing back problems (133). Studies of workers' compensation data suggest that LBP represents a significant portion of morbidity in working populations. Data from a national insurer indicate that back claims account for 16% of all workers' compensation claims and 33% of total claims' costs (20,134). Studies demonstrate that back disorder rates vary substantially by industry, occupation, and job within given industries or facilities (14,82,135,136).

Back disorder is multifactorial in origin and may be associated with both occupational and nonwork-related factors and characteristics. The latter may include age, sex, cigarette smoking status, physical fitness level, anthropometric measures, lumbar mobility and strength, medical history, and structural abnormalities (137). Psychosocial factors, both work- and nonwork-related, have been associated with back disorders.

The relationship of LBDs with employment can be complex. Individuals may experience impairment or disability at work because of LBDs whether or not the latter were directly caused by job-related factors. The degree to which ability to work is impaired often depends on the physical demands of a job. Furthermore, when an individual experiences a LBD at work, it may be a new occurrence or an exacerbation of an existing condition. Originally, the LBD may have been directly caused by work or by nonwork-related factors. Those suffering back pain may modify their work activities in an effort to prevent or lessen pain. Thus, the relationship between work exposure and MSDs may be direct in some cases, but in other cases there is no direct relationship.

In the consideration of causal factors for LBDs, it is important to distinguish among the various outcome measures, such as LBP, impairment, and disability. LBP can be defined as chronic or acute pain of the lumbosacral, buttock, or upper leg region. Sciatic pain refers to pain symptoms that radiate from the back region down one or both legs. Lumbago refers to an acute episode of LBP. In many cases of LBP, specific clinical signs are absent. Low back impairment is generally regarded as a loss of ability to perform physical activities. Low back disability is defined as necessitating restricted duty or time away from the job. Although it is not clear which outcome measure is best suited for determining the causal relationship between LBD and work-related risk factors, it is important to consider severity when the literature is evaluated.

In addition to the level of severity, outcomes may be defined in several other ways ranging from subjective to objective. Information on symptoms can be collected by interview or questionnaire self-report. Back "incidents" or "reports" include conditions reported to medical authorities or in injury/illness logs. These conditions may be symptoms or signs that an individual has determined a need for medical or other attention. The need may be due to acute symptoms, chronic pain, or injury related to a particular incident, and it may be subjectively or objectively determined. Whether an incident is reported depends on the individual's situation and inclinations. Other back disorders can be diagnosed using objective criteria, for example, various types of lumbar disc pathology.

Many conditions in the low back may cause back pain, including muscular or ligamentous strain, facet joint arthritis, or disc pressure on the annulus fibrosus, vertebral endplate, or nerve roots. In most patients, the anatomic cause of LBP, regardless of its relationship to work exposures, cannot be determined with any degree of clinical certainty. Muscle strain is probably the most common type of work or nonwork back pain. While there is sometimes a relationship between pain and findings on magnetic resonance imaging of disc abnormalities (e.g., a herniated disc and clinical findings of nerve compression), the most common form of back disorder, unfortunately, involves nonspecific symptoms that often cannot be diagnosed. It is important to include subjectively defined health outcomes in any consideration of work-related back disorders because they compose such a large subset of the total. It may be too restrictive to define cases of back disorder using "objective" medical criteria. Therefore, in contrast to chapters for MSDs or other anatomic regions, this literature review on the back included slightly different evaluation criteria. For consideration of back disorders, use of a subjective health outcome was not necessarily considered a study limitation. Furthermore, because back disorders were rarely defined by medical examination criteria, the evaluation criterion related to blinding of assessors (to health or exposure status) was also less relevant to a discussion of this literature.

In this review, epidemiologic studies of all forms of back disorder were included. The term *back disorder* is used to encompass all health outcomes related to the back. It should be pointed out that in some studies disorders of the low back were not distinguished from total back disorders. Therefore, articles for LBP and total back disorders were grouped together for the review.

The 42 epidemiologic studies reviewed were chosen according to the epidemiologic selection criteria. Thirty studies used a cross-sectional design; five were prospective cohort studies, four case–control studies, and two retrospective cohort studies. One study combined both cross-sectional and cohort analyses. Twenty-four investigations defined the health outcome only by report of symptoms on questionnaires or in interviews (e.g., total back pain, LBP, and sciatica); 10 studies used symptoms plus medical examination (back pain, low back syndrome, sciatica, back insufficiency, lumbago, herniated lumbar disc, and lumbar disc pathology), six used injury or illness reports, and two used sick leaves and medical disability retirements. Injury or illness reports included outcomes defined as "low back complaints," "injuries caused specifically by lifting or mechanical energy", and "acute industrial back injury." The 42 studies used outcome definitions that corresponded to several regions of the back and included disorders that may have been acute or chronic and were based on subjective and objective findings.

Back disorders are multifactorial in origin and may be associated with both occupational and nonwork-related factors. Confounders may include demographics, leisure-time activities, history of back disorder, and structural characteristics of the back (137). The relative contributions of these covariates may be specific to particular anatomic areas and disorders. For example, a recent study of identical twins demonstrated that occupational and leisure-time physical loading contributed more to disc degeneration of the upper than the lower lumbar region (138). For both anatomic areas, age and twin effects (ge-

netic influences and early shared environment) were the strongest identifiable predictors for this particular health outcome.

Psychosocial factors, both work- and nonwork-related, have been associated with back disorders. In the studies reviewed, sex and age effects were addressed in most (86% and 74%, respectively). Approximately 40% of the studies addressed work-related psychosocial factors.

References: Back

The following studies met all four criteria for the back:

- Burdorf (139)
- Marras et al. (140, 141)

Psychosocial

Summary: Psychosocial

Not only are the etiologic mechanisms of psychosocial factors poorly understood, but there is increasing evidence that psychosocial factors related to the job and work environment play a role in the development of work-related MSDs of the upper extremity and back. Although the findings of the studies reviewed were not entirely consistent, they suggested that perceptions of intensified workload, monotonous work, limited job control, low job clarity, and low social support are associated with various work-related MSDs.

The purpose of this discussion is to summarize research evidence linking work-related psychosocial factors, as described above, to MSDs of the neck, shoulder, elbow, hand/wrist, and back. It should be recognized at the outset, however, that the linkages between work-related psychosocial factors and health outcomes of all varieties are often complex and influenced by a multitude of conditions. In particular, both personal and situational characteristics may lead to differences in the way individuals exposed to the same job and work environment perceive and/or react to the situation (40,45,142). Recent theoretical models of the relationship between psychosocial factors and MSDs clearly reflect the complexity and multifactorial nature of the problem (143,144).

In general, four plausible types of explanations have been suggested to account for associations between work-related psychosocial factors and MSDs (45,78,143,145–148):

- Psychosocial demands may produce increased muscle tension and exacerbate task-related biomechanical strain.
- Psychosocial demands may affect awareness and reporting of musculoskeletal symptoms and/or perceptions of their cause. Included within this second explanation is "perverse incentive" view, in which societies may provide workers with systems (e.g., workers' compensation) that may lead to overreporting of MSD symptoms (59).
- Initial episodes of pain based on a physical insult may trigger a chronic nervous system dysfunction, physiologic as well as psychologic, that perpetuates a chronic pain process.
- In some work situations, changes in psychosocial demands may be associated with changes in physical demands and biomechanical stresses, and thus associations between psychosocial demands and MSDs occur through either a causal or effect-modifying relationship.

As some of these factors are seemingly unrelated to physical demands and several studies found associations even after adjusting for physical demands, the effects of these factors on MSDs may be partly or entirely independent of physical factors. It is also evident that these associations are not limited to particular types of jobs (e.g., video display terminal [VDT] work) or work environments (e.g., offices) but rather seem to be found in a variety of work situations. These findings suggest that psychosocial factors represent generalized risk factors for work-related MSDs.

At present, two difficulties in determining the relative importance of physical and psychosocial factors are (a) that psychosocial factors are usually measured at the individual level, while physical factors are more often measured at the group (e.g., job or task) level and often by methods with limited precision or accuracy; and (b) that "objective measures" of aspects of the psychosocial work environment are difficult to develop and are rarely used, while objective methods to measure the physical environment are more readily available. Until most workplace and individual variables can be measured with more comparable techniques, it will be hard to determine precisely their relative importance.

For most clinicians, the term *psychosocial factor* is ill-defined and difficult to grasp. As a result, considerable confusion and misunderstanding exist regarding the contribution of psychosocial factors or stressors to MSDs. Workplace psychosocial factors can be placed into three broad categories (68):

- Job or task demands,
- Organizational structure,
- Physical work environment.

In addition, individual characteristics (e.g., personality traits, coping ability, attitude toward one's health) and factors outside the work can be independent contributors, moderators, or buffers. Examples of individual factors include personality traits, psychologic dysfunction (depression), coping ability, job dissatisfaction, attitude toward life, overall poor health, lower socioeconomic status, and lower intelligence. Nonwork factors include marital problems, living alone, financial problems, child-rearing problems, and interpersonal conflicts. These latter factors may influence why individuals' perceptions or reactions to the same workplace situation differ (142).

Three mechanisms have been suggested to account for associations between psychosocial factors and MSDs (78,147–150):

- Psychosocial demands may overwhelm an individual's coping mechanism and produce a stress response, which may increase muscle tension or static loading of muscles (151,152).
- Psychosocial demands may affect MSD awareness and reporting or increase its attribution to the work environment.

• Psychosocial demands in some work situations may be highly correlated with increased physical demands (68).

Details: Psychosocial

Considerable confusion exists regarding the contribution of psychosocial factors to musculoskeletal illness and injury. Because of the complexity of this issue, it is examined in this separate section. Unlike the more finite (and generally more familiar) range of physical factors (e.g., force, repetition, and posture), psychosocial factors include a vast array of conditions. Indeed, the term *psychosocial* is commonly used in the occupational health arena as a catchall term to describe a very large number of factors that fall within three separate domains: (a) factors associated with the job and work environment, (b) factors associated with the extrawork environment, and (c) characteristics of the individual worker. Interactions among factors within each of these domains constitute what is referred to as a *stress process,* the results of which are thought to affect both health status and job performance (144,149,153,154).

Included in the domain of job and work environment is a host of conditions, sometimes referred to as "work organizational factors." These include the following:

• Aspects of job content (e.g., workload, repetitiveness, job control, mental demands, job clarity, etc.),
• Organizational characteristics (e.g., tall versus flat organizational structures, communications issues),
• Interpersonal relationships at work (e.g., supervisor–employee relationships, social support),
• Temporal aspects of the work and task (e.g., cycle time and shift work),
• Financial and economic aspects (e.g., pay, benefit, and equity issues),
• Community aspects (e.g., occupational prestige and status).

These work and job environmental factors are often thought of as demands, or "risk factors," that may pose a threat to health (142).

Extrawork environment parameters typically include factors associated with demands arising from roles outside work, such as responsibilities associated with a parent, spouse, or children. Finally, individual worker factors are generally of three types (8,112,155,156):

• Genetic factors (e.g., sex and intelligence),
• Acquired aspects (e.g., social class, culture, educational status),
• Dispositional factors (e.g., personality traits, characteristics and attitudes such as life and job satisfaction).

The research evidence reviewed in the following discussion is organized into two separate sections. The first section includes studies of disorders of the neck, shoulder, elbow, hand, and wrist, discussed under the rubric of upper extremity disorders. This convention was adopted because many studies utilized measures that combine symptoms associated with several upper extremity body areas (e.g., neck and shoulder). In the review of these studies, it was not possible to isolate the effects of psychosocial variables under consideration on more specific areas. The second section examines studies of back disorders. Associations reported in this review are statistically significant in nearly all cases (at the $p<0.05$ level and frequently also at the $p<0.01$ level). Where possible, ORs are also reported.

It is necessary to be aware in the interpretation of the studies reviewed that in general researchers have not used standardized methods for assessing psychosocial factors in relationship to MSDs. Thus, individual psychosocial factors assessed by investigators vary from study to study. Moreover, even when work-related psychosocial factors (e.g., workload, job control, social support, job satisfaction, etc.) included by various investigators are the same or similar, they may be measured by different methods and different kinds of scales that can vary in psychometric quality. These methodologic limitations complicate the process of drawing definitive conclusions regarding the literature as a whole; when comparing results between studies, one must take these differences into account.

Upper Extremities: Psychosocial Factors

Overall, the epidemiologic studies suggest that certain psychosocial factors, including intensified workload, monotonous work, and low levels of social support, have a positive association with MSDs involving the upper extremities. Lack of control over job and job dissatisfaction also appears to be associated with upper extremity MSDs, although the data are not as supportive.

Evidence for the relationship between psychosocial factors and upper extremity MSDs appears to be stronger for neck/shoulder disorders or musculoskeletal symptoms in general than for hand/wrist disorders. This stronger association for neck/shoulder disorders may be due to the following: (a) the large number of studies performed in the Nordic countries have focused more on neck/shoulder MSD health outcomes than on hand/wrist MSD outcomes; (b) many neck/shoulder studies included numerous psychosocial variables in their models, whereas studies of hand/wrist MSDs did not as a rule include as extensive psychosocial variable testing (therefore the variables are absent from the risk factor models); and (c) most studies with extensive psychosocial scales were in office settings, where physical factors may be less important than psychosocial factors in their relationship with MSDs. This finding can be contrasted with studies in heavy industrial settings, where higher exposure to physical factors may have played a greater role than psychosocial factors in the development of MSDs. In addition, pathophysiologic processes resulting from adverse psychosocial and work organizational factors may exert a greater effect on the neck/shoulder musculature than on the hand/wrist region in producing increased muscle tension and strain.

Individual and Extrawork Environmental Factors. Various psychosocial factors associated with both individual workers and the extrawork environment have been linked to upper extremity MSDs (143,147,157). These factors included conditions such as depression and anxiety (158), symptoms of psychologic distress (159), and "home problems" (160). However, the connection between factors of this nature and the job and work environment is unclear. While affective problems (e.g., anxiety and depression) and symptoms of distress may certainly be a consequence of the work situation, they may also be causally related to nonwork circumstances only. Likewise, while extrawork environmental conditions (e.g., home problems) may be exacerbated by the work situation (e.g., shift work), their work-relatedness remains unclear. Because of the uncertainty regarding the work-relatedness of these individual and extrawork environmental factors only the individual psychosocial factor of job dissatisfaction is examined here.

Job Dissatisfaction. Several studies suggested associations between low levels of satisfaction with work and upper extremity musculoskeletal symptoms and MSDs. For example, in a study of 1,174 machine operators, 1,054 carpenters, and 1,013 office workers, Tola et al. (161) found an association (OR 1.2) between job dissatisfaction and neck/shoulder physical findings or symptoms after adjusting for confounders. Hopkins (162) reported a positive association between job dissatisfaction and musculoskeletal symptoms. Low job satisfaction, however, was not found to predict neck/shoulder problems 1 year later in a study of 154 Finnish workers (163). Similarly, in a study of 273 nursing aides employed in a geriatric hospital, job satisfaction was found to be unrelated to reports of ever having cervical pain (164).

Intensified Workload. One factor most consistently associated with upper extremity MSDs has been the perception of an intensified workload, as measured by indices of perceived time pressure, workload, work pressure, and workload variability. For example, in a cross-sectional study of 222 VDT operators, Pot et al. (165) found high levels of perceived time pressure associated with the reporting of upper extremity musculoskeletal complaints. Bongers et al. (149) found perceived time pressure to be associated with upper extremity complaints (in the preceding 12 months) among 158 male bus drivers. Likewise, in a longitudinal study of 351 female bank cashiers, Takala and Viikari-Juntura (166) reported a positive association between perceived time pressure and symptoms of the neck and shoulder after adjusting for postural load. However, Theorell et al. (167) found that perceived time pressure was not significantly correlated with neck or shoulder symptoms in a sample of 206 workers from six occupations.

Positive associations with upper extremity MSDs have also been found in studies using measures of perceived work pressure and workload. High levels of perceived workload, for example, were found to be positively associated with musculoskeletal symptoms by Pot et al. (165) and Theorell et al. (167) (whose studies adjusted for physical demands such as lifting and awkward postures). In a case–control study of 112 cases and 112 age- and sex-matched controls from an engineering firm, Kvarnstrom and Halden (168) found sick leave due to fatigue or shoulder muscle soreness to be positively associated with a high perceived workload. Karasek et al. (160) found perceived workload to be positively associated with musculoskeletal aches, as measured by a combination of several questions (OR 1.1 for men and 1.2 for women), in 8,700 full-time members of the Swedish white collar labor union federation. Likewise, in a study of 248 VDT users, Sauter et al. (144) found perceived workload and demands for attention to be associated with neck, back, and shoulder discomfort after adjusting for a wide variety of variables denoting physical demands. Bernard et al. (78) found perceived increased workload demands (increased time working under deadline and increased job pressure) among 1,050 newspaper employees to be positively associated with neck, shoulder, and hand/wrist symptoms. Similarly, in a study of 553 telecommunications workers, Hales et al. (76) found increased work pressure to be associated with neck (OR 1.2) and upper extremity MSDs (OR 1.1), as defined

by physical examination and questionnaire. Ryan and Bampton (169), using a total sample of 143 data processors, compared 41 individuals reporting a number of neck symptoms to 28 reporting very few neck symptoms (middle group left out) and found a positive association between symptom reports and reports of having to increase production (OR 3.9). Ekberg et al. (170) compared 109 workers who consulted a physician for new neck/shoulder MSDs with 637 controls and found a positive association (OR 3.5) with a rushed work pace. In a representative sample of 5,865 workers in the Netherlands, Houtman et al. (171) found a high work pace associated with muscle or joint symptoms (OR 1.3) after adjusting for physical stressors and modifying personal characteristics. However, Dehlin and Berg (164) found no relationship between reports of high perceived physical and psychologic demands and reports of ever having pain in the cervical region.

Variability in workload (surges in workload) has also been linked to upper extremity MSDs. Studies by Hales et al. (76) of 553 telecommunication workers and Hoekstra et al. (172) of 108 teleservice representatives found perceived workload variability to be associated with elbow (OR 1.2) and neck (OR 1.2) MSDs, but not with shoulder or hand disorders.

Monotonous Work. Monotonous work has been positively linked to the prevalence of upper extremity symptoms. In their study of 143 data processors, Ryan and Bamptom (169) found that self-reports of "being bored most of the time" were highly associated with neck symptoms (OR 7.7). Similarly, in a study of approximately 22,200 Swedish workers undergoing a screening examination by the occupational health care service, Linton (173) found that monotonous work was positively associated with neck/shoulder pain (OR 2.3). Ekberg et al. (170) found an association between "low quality work' (lacking stimulation and variation) and neck/shoulder problems (OR 2.6). Similarly, Kvarnstrom and Halden (168) found monotonous work to be associated with sick leave due to fatigue or tenderness in the shoulder muscles. Finally, Hopkins

(162) found high levels of boredom in around 280 clerical workers to be associated with musculoskeletal symptoms (in any part of the body) during work hours.

Job Control. Many studies reported positive associations between limited job control or autonomy at work and upper extremity problems, including neck symptoms: Ryan and Bamptom (169) (OR 3.9), Hales et al. (76) (OR 1.6), Sauter et al. (144) (neck, back, and shoulder symptoms), Theorell et al. (167), Karasek et al. (160) (musculoskeletal aches), and Hopkins (162) and Houtman et al. (171) (muscle and joint symptoms).

Job Clarity. Several studies, including those of Ryan and Bamptom (169), Karasek et al. (160), and Ekberg et al. (170), showed positive associations between reports of role ambiguity (uncertainty about job expectations) and upper extremity MSDs, particularly neck disorders. Similarly, uncertainty regarding job future was found to be predictive of neck/shoulder discomfort by Sauter et al. (144) and of elbow, neck, and hand/wrist symptoms by Hales et al. (76).

Social Support. Limited social support from supervisors and coworkers has been found to be positively associated with a various upper extremity symptoms. Studies by Pot et al. (165), Hopkins (162), Sauter et al. (144), and Hales et al. (76) all supported a positive association. Linton (173) reported a positive association between neck symptoms and limited support from supervisors. Ryan and Bampton (169) reported an effect of limited support from coworkers (OR 6.7), but not supervisors, on neck symptoms. While Kvarnstrom and Halden (168) reported an effect of limited support from supervisors resulting in more coworkers on sick leave due to shoulder muscle symptoms. Dehlin and Berg (164), however, found no effect of social support on neck/shoulder symptoms; nor did Theorell et al. (167) for neck/shoulder symptoms or symptoms of the other joints (with or without adjustment for physical load). Likewise, Karasek et al. (160) found no significant association between musculoskeletal aches and social support at work.

Back: Psychosocial Factors

In general, the studies reviewed suggested an association between back disorders and perceptions of intensified workload as measured by indices of both perceived time pressure and workload. Despite considerable differences in the types of methods used to assess both independent and dependent variables, four of the five studies that explicitly included measures of intensified workload found significant associations. It is also noteworthy that all four studies attempted to control or adjust for potential covariates. Five of the seven studies that assessed job dissatisfaction also found positive associations with back disorders.

Individual and Extrawork Environmental Factors. As with upper extremity MSDs, back disorders also have a host of psychosocial factors associated with individual workers (e.g., personality, psychologic status) and the extrawork environment (e.g., living alone) linked to back pain and disability (143). As the work-relatedness of these factors is unclear, with the exception of job dissatisfaction, they will not be extensively reviewed (143). In general, these studies showed clear associations between measures of psychologic distress or dysfunction and self-reported back pain. However, the temporal relationship between psychologic factors and musculoskeletal symptoms or MSDs remains unclear. One possibility relating to back disorders is that psychologic distress is simply a consequence of chronic LBP, with no etiologic role in the development of the disorder. Alternatively, it is possible that psychologic factors may have some etiologic role in the transition experienced by employees with a history of back pain to the status of unemployed patients with chronic back pain due to fear of reinjury or other factors that would make it impossible to perform a job (174).

While there are several prospective studies of LBP and individual physical factors, only a few prospective studies appear to incorporate individual and extrawork environmental psychosocial factors. In a 4-year study of 3,020 hourly wage earners at an aircraft manufacturing plant, Bigos et al. (39) defined an outcome as reporting a back pain complaint to the company medical department, filing a back-related incident report, or filing an industrial insurance claim. The psychosocial assessment included personality traits, as measured by the Minnesota Multiphasic Personality Inventory (MMPI), and limited information on family support, health locus of control, and work social support. One question about enjoyment of tasks in the job was also included. Of the 37 variables used to evaluate the role of social support, health locus of control, and personality traits, three were found to be significant in a multivariate analysis. They were scale 3 of the MMPI tendencies toward somatic complaints or denial of emotional distress (RR 1.4), dissatisfaction with work (RR 1.7), and prior back pain (RR 1.7). Although significant, these variables explained only a small fraction of the back pain reports in this population. The number of back pain reports was three times higher in the group with the highest scores on these three variables compared with the group with the lowest scores, although only 9% of the workforce was in the highest risk group. Because this study focused on the reporting of back pain complaints and not the actual development of back pain, it would be a mistake to generalize the results to workers developing back pain. This study suggested that individual premorbid personality traits only explain a small fraction of work-related low back problems.

Job Dissatisfaction. Job dissatisfaction has been associated with back disorders in both longitudinal and cross-sectional investigations. Bergenudd et al. (175), studying 575 residents of Malmo for over 19 years, found job dissatisfaction to be associated with self-reported back pain. As described above, Bigos et al. (39) found a positive association between job dissatisfaction and workers filing compensation claims for back injury. In this study, subjects who stated that they "hardly ever" enjoyed their job tasks were 2.5 times more likely to report a back injury than

those who "almost always" enjoyed their job tasks. However, as Frank (59) pointed out, some reviewers argued that the airplane manufacturing jobs with the highest levels of dissatisfaction were also the most physically demanding. He also noted that, unfortunately, the extent of the interaction is difficult to assess because of the limited measurement of workplace biomechanical exposures in the studies by Bigos and colleagues (39,176, 177).

The cross-sectional study by Dehlin and Berg (164) of nursing aides found an association between dissatisfaction and self-reported back symptoms. However, this study did not adjust for confounders. Likewise, in a mailed survey study of Israeli workers in eight occupational categories, Magora (178) found job satisfaction to be associated with reports of sick leave due to LBP. This study also did not adjust for potential confounders. Svensson and Andersson (179) found an association after adjustment in a cross-sectional study of 1,746 Swedish residents. However, in a cross-sectional study by Astrand (180) of 391 male Swedish paper company workers (clerks and manual workers), no association was found between dissatisfaction and back disorders, as assessed by symptoms and physical examination after confounder adjustment.

Job and Work Environmental Factors. Several studies reported associations between perceptions of intensified workload, as measured by reports of time pressure and high work pace, and self-reports of back pain. In a study of approximately 5,600 Finns, Heliovaara et al. (181) found a composite measure (containing items on perceived time pressure at work, monotony, and fear of mistakes) to be associated with back disorders (OR 2.0, defined by interview and physical examination) after adjusting for potential confounders, including physical load and previous back pain. Lundberg et al. (182) found perceived time pressure to be associated with perceived back load among 20 workers on a Swedish assembly line. In a similar vein, Houtman et al.'s (171) study of 5,865 Dutch workers across all occupations reported above found an association (OR 1.21) between reporting a high work pace and self-reported back pain, defined as back pain for more than three months or at least three times in the study period. Magora (178) found high levels of concentration to be associated with reports of sick leave due to LBP (OR 2.9). However, Astrand (180) found no association between "hustling" and "nerve wracking work" and back pain in male paper company workers.

Monotonous Work. Heliovaara et al. (181) and Houtman et al. (171) reported associations between perceived monotony and reports of back complaints. Similarly, in a study of 940 male residents of Goteborg, Sweden, between the ages of 40 and 47, Svensson and Andersson (183) found monotonous work (rated "absolutely" or "unacceptably" boring) to be associated with back complaints. This relationship remained after adjustment for several physical factors. However, they found no relationship between monotony and back pain complaints among Swedish women in a multivariate analysis that included measures of job and task satisfaction. Similarly, Houtman et al. (171), controlling for a combination of physical stressors (dangerous work, heavy physical load, noise at work, dirty work, and bad smell at work) reduced the magnitude of the relationship; for back complaints, the OR decreased from 3.90 to 3.46. The authors suggested that this relationship may exist because monotonous work is often work that also either is short-cycled or involves a high static (postural) load.

Job Control. After controlling for a number of individual and work-related factors, Hoekstra et al. (172) found perceived job control at work to be inversely associated with back disorders (OR 0.6); that is, the less perceived job control at work, the higher were the odds of back disorders. Likewise, Sauter et al. (144) found that low job control was related to neck, back, and shoulder discomfort.

Social Support. Bigos et al. (177) found a significant univariate relationship between limited social support at work and back trouble.

OCCUPATIONAL INJURY AND ILLNESS COUNTS, RATES, AND CHARACTERISTICS FOR WORK-RELATED MUSCULOSKELETAL DISORDERS

The BLS has long been interested in developing data on safety and health conditions for workers. The only routinely collected national source of information about occupational injuries and illnesses of U.S. workers is the BLS's annual survey; the most current available issue, published in 1997, is for 1994 (1). This survey, conducted for the past 25 years, is a random sample of about 250,000 private-sector establishments and provides estimates of workplace injuries and illnesses on the basis of information provided by employers from their OSHA Form 200 log of recordable injuries and illnesses. The 1994 national survey marks the third year that the BLS has collected additional information, such as the demographic and case characteristics data, that is detailed in the report. This additional data enable analysis for industries, occupations, and worker groups for risks for lost work time (184).[1]

Summary

To correctly understand occupational injury and illness counts, rates, and characteristics, it is necessary to understand what is being counted. The BLS survey seeks to measure the number of work-related illness cases that are recognized, diagnosed, and reported during a year. Some conditions (e.g., long-term latent illnesses caused by exposure to carcinogens) are often difficult to link to the workplace and therefore may not be recognized and reported. The reporting is only from the private sector. Government employees, military employees, and not-for-profit organizations are not included.

---

[1]A supplement with this information is available from the Bureau of Labor Statistics, Office of Safety, Health, and Working Conditions, U.S. Department of Labor, 2 Massachusetts Avenue, NE, Room 3180, Washington, DC 20212. Phone: (202) 606-6170; URL for web site: http://stats.bls.fov.oshhome.htm.

The BLS defines an *occupational injury* as one that results from a work-related event or from a single instantaneous exposure in the work environment. Injuries are reported if they result in lost work time or require medical treatment (other than first aid), or if the worker experiences loss of consciousness or restriction of work activities or motion or is transferred to another job (1).

The BLS defines an *occupational illness* as any abnormal condition or disorder (other than one resulting from an occupational injury) caused by exposure to a factor or factors associated with employment. Included are acute and chronic illnesses or diseases that may be caused by inhalation, absorption, ingestion, or direct contact (1).

The BLS defines *lost workday* cases as cases that involve days away from work or days in which work activity is restricted, or both (93).

The BLS defines *incidence rates* as the rate representing the number of injuries and/or illnesses per 100 full-time workers, calculated as the number of injuries and/or illnesses divided by the total hours worked by all employees during the calendar year times 200,000 (the base for 100 full-time-equivalent workers working 40 hours per week for 50 weeks per year) (93).

Counts, Rates, and Characteristics for 1994

There were 6.8 million nonfatal injuries and illnesses in private industry workplaces in 1994. These occurred at a rate of 8.4 cases per 100 full-time-equivalent workers. During the last 10 years, the rates of injuries and illnesses have fluctuated within a range of 7.9 to 8.9 cases. Of the 6.8 million total, a majority of cases (about 3.7 million) resulted neither in workdays lost nor in restricted workdays. However 2.4 million cases involved at least 1 day away from work after the day of injury or onset of illness. Information on worker and case characteristics was collected only for cases with days away from work. The balance of the total, about 825,000 injuries and ill-

nesses, resulted in restricted work activity only, such as no heavy lifting. In 1994, 6.25 million lost workdays were attributed to injuries and 500,000 lost workdays were attributed to illnesses.

Injury and illness rates varied from 12.2 per 100 full-time workers in manufacturing to 2.7 per 100 for finance, insurance, and real estate. At 11.8 per 100 full-time workers, the 1994 rate in construction fell below the rate in manufacturing for the first time since 1972. The rate of injuries and illnesses involving days away from work declined for the fourth year in a row to its lowest level, 2.8 per 100 full-time workers. In general, injury rates were higher for midsize establishments (50 to 249 workers) than for small and large establishments. This pattern, however, varies somewhat by industry, with manufacturing dominating the list of industries with the highest injury rates (18.2 per 100 full-time worker) followed by nursing and health care (16.5), trucking (14.8), and trades and services such as hotels and department stores (10.8). Injury rates for an industry producing or delivering similar types of goods and services can vary. For example, household furniture manufacturing rates at 17.4 per 100 full-time workers can be compared to furniture upholstering at 10.7.

Illnesses were reported when they could be directly related to workplace activity. This can result in significant underreporting because each state can define work-relatedness (40). In 1994, nearly two-thirds of reported illnesses were disorders associated with repeated trauma, such as CTS. Manufacturing continues to dominate illnesses reported, accounting for more than 60% of all new illness cases in the 1994 BLS survey. Services industries, such as hospitals, represented another 16% of the illness total. The majority of these cases were repetitive trauma injuries.

Occupational injury and illness counts, rates, and characteristics can be grouped by sex, age, occupation, and length of service:

Sex. Men accounted for 66% of the 2.4 million cases in 1994, a proportion higher than their share (about 55%) of private wage and salary employment. Although working women numbered fewer cases overall, women nevertheless accounted for a larger share of certain injury and illness categories, such as assaults and repetitive motion disorders.

Age. Workers aged 25 to 44 accounted for nearly 60% of the 2.4-million case total; the rest of the cases were about evenly divided between younger and older workers. The risk of injury and illness generally declines with age, although older workers typically miss more workdays than younger workers.

Occupation. Operators, fabricators, and laborers accounted for a larger share (40%) of the survey's case total than any other major occupational grouping. This group's injury and illness share far exceeded its one-sixth share of total private wage and salary employment. Three individual occupations had 100,000 cases each: truck drivers, nonfarm and nonconstruction laborers, and nursing aides or orderlies. All three of these occupations represented injury and illness case numbers that were more than double their shares of total employment. The top five industries with disorders due to repeated trauma were meatpacking at 126 per 1,000 full-time workers, knit underwear manufacturing at 101, motor vehicle manufacturing at 96, poultry processing at 83, and house slippers manufacturing at 73.

Length of service. Most workers had at least 1 year of service with their employer when they sustained their injury or illness. One-fourth had more than 5 years of service, suggesting that many experienced workers also incur lost-work-time injuries.

OCCUPATIONAL COSTS FOR WORK-RELATED MUSCULOSKELETAL DISORDERS

In 1996, direct health care costs were more than $418 billion, and lower-range estimates for indirect costs were more than $837 billion—for a total cost of $1.256 trillion (13). Other studies estimated the national cost of occupational injuries to be between $81 billion in 1989 and $173 billion in 1992 (185–187). This cost estimate would put occupational injuries on par with heart disease and stroke at $110 to $162 billion, cancer at $120 to $170 billion, and acquired immunodeficiency syndrome at $30 billion in 1992 (188).

Efforts to rank occupations based on the costs of job-related injuries and illnesses has only been done in two studies (187,189). In these studies, data from the BLS were combined with the supplementary data system (SDS) of the BLS. The percentage distribution of the SDS data was applied to the annual survey data to arrive at estimated injury and illness costs per job.

Costs can be estimated using either the direct/indirect cost method or the willingness-to-pay (WTP) method. The direct/indirect method, also called the human capital method, is the most widely used method in medical and legal settings, partly because estimates are available and reliable (190) and it is readily understandable to noneconomists. The WTP method attempts to value injuries and illnesses based on prices generated in private market transactions. One example involves the trade-off that consumers have in buying a car: High prices are frequently associated with greater safety. Economists apply econometric techniques and attempt to estimate how much consumers are willing to pay for an additional reduction in risk of injury. The WTP method is more widely used in the economics literature. Many economists believe that it is theoretically more compelling than the direct/indirect method (191). Yet no consistent set of WTP cost estimates is available by workers' compensation severity categories. The following information will use the direct/indirect method, with costs representing actual dollars spent or anticipated to be spent on providing medical care to an injured or ill person as well as on property damage, police and fire services, administrative costs for delivering indemnity benefits, and direct costs to innocent third parties. Medical costs include services of doctors and nurses, hospital charges, drug costs, rehabilitation services, ambulance fees, and payments for medical equipment and supplies. Indemnity-benefit costs do not include the benefits themselves, which are included in the indirect costs (lost wages). Indemnity-benefit costs include administrative costs associated with providing workers' compensation indemnity or Social Security disability payments to injured or sick workers and their families. Property damage includes costs for damage to vehicles, machines, buildings, and so on directly associated with the injuries and illnesses. The largest indirect costs include injured or sick workers' lost earnings, fringe benefits, and home production (192).

Leigh and Miller (187) ranked costs by specific occupations at the national level. Examples of the most expensive include the following: heavy-truck drivers, $365,167,487; laborers, except construction, $330,667,638; machine operators, not specified, $260,453,369; occupations, not classified, $238,922,707; and janitors and cleaners, $226,284,072. Examples of the least expensive include the following: physicians and astronomers, $104; geologists, $98; marine engineers, $93; health and diagnosing practitioners, $92; social scientists, $79; agricultural workers, $2; and atmospheric and space scientists, $2.

They also ranked costs per employee. Examples of the most expensive include the following: timber cutting and logging occupations, $5,733; production helpers, $3,679; laborers, except construction, $1,777; sawing machine operators, $1,691; and millwrights, $1,670 (187). Examples at the lower end include the following: general office clerks, $317; electronic repairers, communications, $314; painters and construction and maintenance workers, $311; and stock and inventory clerks, $310 (187). This type of study demonstrates that the public is frequently misinformed about job hazards, that many occupations are in the lowest status categories, that the most hazardous jobs enjoy the least pay, and that jobs high on both lists should be candidates for greater attention from occupational safety and health researchers for prevention in the workplace.

ACKNOWLEDGMENTS

I wish to express my appreciation for review of this paper by Peggy Gardner, PhD, Executive Director, Research, Via Christi Health System, Kansas, for reference support provided by the Via Christi Medical Libraries, and for funding by The Hand Center.

REFERENCES

1. U.S. Bureau of Labor Statistics. *Occupational injuries and illnesses: counts, rates, and characteristics, 1994.* Washington, DC: U.S. Department of Labor, U.S. Government Printing Office, 1997.
2. Louis DS. Presidential address: are we there yet? *J Hand Surg [Am]* 1998;23:191–195.
3. National Institute for Occupational Safety and Health. *NIOSH public homepage for National Institute for Occupational Safety and Health.* Washington, DC: Centers for Disease Control and Prevention, 1998.
4. Stevens JC, Sun S, Beard CM. Carpal tunnel syndrome in Rochester, Minnesota, 1961 to 1980. *Neurology* 1988;38:134–138.
5. Cummings K, Maizlish N, Rudolph L. Occupational disease surveillance: carpal tunnel syndrome. *MMWR* 1991;38:485–489.
6. Adams ML, Franklin GM, Barnhart S. Outcome of carpal tunnel surgery in Washington state workers' compensation. *Am J Ind Med* 1994;25:527–536.
7. Allander E. Prevalence, incidence, and remission rates of some common rheumatic diseases or syndromes. *Scand J Rheumatol* 1974;3:145–153.
8. Melhorn JM, Wilkinson LK. *Carpal tunnel disease solutions for the 90's: a comprehensive guide to managing CTD in the workplace.* Wichita, KS: Via Christi, 1996.
9. Tanaka S, Wild DK, Seligman PJ, et al. Prevalence and work-relatedness of self-reported carpal tunnel syndrome among U.S. workers: analysis of the occupational health supplement data of 1988 National Health Interview Survey. *Am J Ind Med* 1995;27:451–470.
10. Hagberg M, Morgenstern H, Kelsh M. Impact of occupations and job tasks on the prevalence of carpal tunnel syndrome. *Scand J Work Environ Health* 1992; 18:337–345.
11. The 1990 national executive poll on health care costs and benefits. *Bus Health* 1990;8:25–38.
12. Wright JG. Clincal research now more complex: needs outcomes, clinical trials, cost-effectiveness analyses. *AAOS Bulletin* 1993;Oct:24–26.
13. Brady W, Bass J, Royce M, et al. Defining total corporate health and safety costs—significance and impact. *J Occup Med* 1997;39:224–231.
14. Bigos SJ, Spengler DM, Martin NA, et al. Back injuries in industry: a retrospective study. II. Injury factors. *Spine* 1986;11:246–251.
15. Dixon SJ. Progress and problems in back pain research. *Rheumatol Rehabil* 1973;12:165–167.
16. Chaffin DB. Manual materials handling—the cause of overexertion injury and illness in industry. *J Environ Pathol Toxicol* 1979;2:67–73.
17. Burry HC, Gravis V. Compensated back injury in New Zealand. *N Z Med J* 1988;101:542–544.
18. Klein BP, Jensen RC, Sanderson LM. Assessment of workers' compensation claims for back strains/sprains. *J Occup Med* 1984;26:443–448.

19. Spengler DM, Bigos SJ, Martin NA, et al. Back injuries in industry: a retrospective study. I. Overview and cost analysis. *Spine* 1986;11:241–245.

20. Webster BS, Snook SH. The cost of 1989 workers' compensation low back pain claims. *Spine* 1994;19: 1111–1116.

21. Pope MH, Andersson GBJ, Frymoyer JW. *Occupational low back pain: assessement, treatment, and prevention.* St. Louis, MO: Mosby–Year Book, 1991.

22. Frymoyer JW, Cats-Baril WL. An overview of the incidence and costs of low back pain. *Orthop Clin North Am* 1991;22:262–271.

23. National Institute for Occupational Safety and Health. *Musculoskeletal disorders and workplace factors: a critical review of epidemiologic evidence for work-related musculoskeletal disorders of the neck, upper extremity, and low back.* Cincinnati, OH: U.S. Department of Health and Human Services, 1997.

24. Blume RS, Sandler HM. *Final report: evaluation of the OSHA approach and cited literature critique draft proposed ergonomics protection standard. Health Effects Document, Causal Association Section.* Sandler Occupational Medicine Associates, Washington, D.C., 1996.

25. Lister GD. Ergonomic disorders. *J Hand Surg [Am]* 1995;20:353–353.

26. Weiland AJ. Repetitive strain injuries and cumulative trauma disorders. *J Hand Surg [Am]* 1996;21:337–338.

27. Vender MI, Kasdan ML, Truppa KL. Upper extremity disorders: a literature review to determine work relatedness. *J Hand Surg [Am]* 1995;20:534–541.

28. Silverstein BA, Armstrong TJ, Buckle P, et al. Can some upper extremity disorders be defined as work-related? [Letter]. *J Hand Surg [Am]* 1996;21:727–729.

29. Greenberg RS, Daniels SR, Flanders D, Eley JW, Boring JR. *Medical epidemiology.* Norwalk, CT: Appleton & Lange, 1993.

30. Hill AB. The environment and disease: association or causation? *Proc R Soc Med* 1965;58:295–300.

31. Hill AB. Observation and experiment. *N Engl J Med* 1953;248:995–1001.

32. Susser M. What is a cause and how do we know one? A grammar for pragmatic epidemiology. *Am J Epidemiol* 1991;133:635–648.

33. Cornfield J, Haenszel WHEC, Lilienfeld AM, Shimkin MB, Wynder EL. Smoking and lung cancer: recent evidence and a discussion of some questions. *J Natl Cancer Inst* 1959;22:173–203.

34. Bross JD. Spurious effects from an extraneous variable. *J Chronic Dis* 1966;19:736–747.

35. Schlesselman J. Assessing the effects of confounding variables. *Am J Epidemiol* 1978;108:3–8.

36. Schlesselman J. Case-control studies: design, conduct, analysis. In: *Monographs in epidemiology and biostatistics.* New York: Oxford University Press, 1982:2–57.

37. Rothman KJ. *Modern epidemiology.* Boston: Little, Brown and Company, 1986.

38. Kleinbaum DG, Kupper LL, Morgenstern H. *Epidemiologic research: principles and quantitative methods.* London: Lifetime Learning Publications, 1982.

39. Bigos SJ, Battie MC, Spengler DM, Fisher LD. A prospective study of work perceptions and psychosocial factors affecting the report of back injury. *Spine* 1991;16:1–6.

40. Melhorn JM. Physician support and employer options for reducing risk of CTD. In: Spengler DM, Zippieri JP, eds. *Workers' compensation case management: a multidisciplinary perspective.* Rosemont, IL: American Academy of Orthopaedic Surgeons, 1997:21–34.

41. Melhorn JM. CTD's: risk assessment applications in the workplace. In: *Science symposium.* McPherson: McPherson College, Kansas, 1985:1–12.

42. Melhorn JM. CTD injuries: an outcome study for work survivability. In: Amadio PC, Hentz VR, eds. *Yearbook of hand surgery 1997.* St. Louis, MO: Mosby–Year Book, 1997:261–262.

43. Melhorn JM. CTD in the workplace: treatment outcomes. In: *Seventeenth annual workers' compensation and occupational medicine seminar.* Boston: Speak, 1997:168–178.

44. Melhorn JM. CTD solutions for the 90's: prevention. In: *Seventeenth annual workers' compensation and occupational medicine seminar.* Boston: Speak, 1997: 234–245.

45. Melhorn JM. Identification of individuals at risk for developing CTD. In: Spengler DM, Zippieri JP, eds. *Workers' compensation case management: a multidisciplinary perspective.* Rosemont, IL: American Academy of Orthopaedic Surgeons, 1997:41–51.

46. Melhorn JM. Upper-extremity cumulative trauma disorders in workers in aircraft manufacturing [Letter, response]. *J Occup Environ Med* 1998;40:103–104.

47. Vannier FP, Rose JF. Etiologies and prevalence of occupational injuries to the upper extremity. In: Kasdan ML, ed. *Occupational hand and upper extremity injuries and and diseases.* Philadelphia: Hanley and Belfus, 1991:53–60.

48. Melhorn JM. CTD: carpal tunnel syndrome, the facts and myths. *Kans Med* 1994;95:189–192.

49. Melhorn JM. Occupational injuries: the need for preventive strategies. *Kans Med* 1994;95:248–251.

50. Melhorn JM. CTD RSI and their relationship to work injury. In: Spengler DM, Zippieri JP, eds. *Workers' compensation case management: a multidisciplinary perspective.* Rosemont, IL: American Academy of Orthopaedic Surgeons, 1997:1–25.

51. Silverstein BA, Fine LJ, Stetson DS. Hand-wrist disorders among investment casting plant workers. *J Hand Surg [Am]* 1987;12:838–844.

52. Nathan PA, Keniston RC, Myers LD, Meadows KD. Obesity as a risk factor for slowing of sensory conduction of the median nerve in industry: a cross-sectional and longitudinal study involving 429 workers. *J Occup Med* 1992;34:379–383.

53. Nathan PA, Meadows KD, Doyle LS. Relationship of age and sex to sensory conduction of the median nerve at the carpal tunnel and associations of slowed conduction with symptoms. *Muscle Nerve* 1988;11: 1149–1150.

54. Nathan PA, Doyle LS, Meadows KD. Comparison of sensory latencies of the median nerve at the carpal tunnel among juveniles and adults. *Bull Hosp Jt Dis Orthop Inst* 1975;49:85–85.

55. Nathan PA, Meadows KD, Doyle LS. Occupations as a risk factor for impaired sensory conductions of the median nerve at the carpal tunnel. *J Hand Surg [Br]* 1988;13:167–170.

56. Melhorn JM. CTD injuries: an outcome study for work survivability. *J Workers' Compensation* 1996;5: 18–30.

57. Gerr F, Letz R, Landrigan PJ. Upper extremity mus-

culoskeletal disorders of occupational origin. *Annu Rev Public Health* 1991;12:543–566.

58. Hadler NM. Arm pain in the workplace: a small area analysis. *J Occup Med* 1992;34:113–119.

59. Frank JW. Occupational back pain—an unhelpful polemic. *Scand J Work Environ Health* 1995;21:3–14.

60. Slocum D. Overuse syndromes of the lower leg and foot in athletes, In: *Instructional course lectures.* Chicago: American Academy of Orthopaedic Surgeons, 1960:359–367.

61. McBryde A. Running injuries. In: *Instructional course lectures.* Chicago: American Academy of Orthopaedic Surgeons, 1984:253–282.

62. Riihimaki H. Hands up or back to work—future challenges in epidemiologic research on musculoskeletal diseases. *Scand J Work Environ Health* 1995;21: 402–403.

63. World Health Organization. *Identification and control of work-related diseases.* Geneva: World Health Organization, 1985. Technical report series no. 714.

64. U.S. Bureau of Labor Statistics. *Survey of occupational injuries and illnesses in 1994.* Washington, DC: U.S. Department of Labor, U.S. Government Printing Office, 1996.

65. Szabo RM. Current concepts review. Principles of epidemiology for the orthopaedic surgeon. *J Bone Joint Surg Am* 1998;80:111–120.

66. Riegelman RK, Hirsch RP. *Studying a study and testing a test.* Boston: Little, Brown and Company, 1989.

67. Pickering GW. Opportunity and the universities. *Lancet* 1952;2:895–898.

68. Hales TR, Bernard BP. Epidemiology of work-related musculoskeletal disorders. *Orthop Clin North Am* 1996;27:679–709.

69. Clinical epidemiology. In: Kasser JR, ed. *Orthopaedic knowledge update 5.* Rosemont, IL: American Academy of Orthopaedic Surgeons, 1996:71–80.

70. Fraumeni JF, Hoover RN. Epidemiology: principles and methods. *Federal Register Part II* 1985;58–64.

71. Kellgren L. Epidemiology. *J Clin Epidemiol* 1992;45: 373–376.

72. Szabo RM. Statistical analysis as related to hand surgery. *J Hand Surg [Am]* 1997;22:376–385.

73. U.S. Department of Health and Human Services. *Accepted definitions for work injuries.* Washington, DC: U.S. Government Printing Office, 1998.

74. Hagberg M, Wegman DH. Prevalence rates and odds ratios of shoulder-neck diseases in different occupational groups. *Br J Ind Med* 1987;44:602–610.

75. Silverstein BA, Fine LJ, Armstrong TJ. Occupational factors in carpal tunnel syndrome. *Am J Ind Med* 1987; 11:343–358.

76. Hales TR, Sauter SL, Peterson MR. Musculoskeletal disorders among visual display terminal users in a telecommunications company. *Ergonomics* 1994;37: 1603–1621.

77. Blader S, Harck-Holst U, Danielsson S, et al. Neck and shoulder complaints among sewing-machine operators: a study concerning frequency, symptomatology and dysfunction. *Appl Ergon* 1991;22:251–257.

78. Bernard BP, Sauter SI, Fine LJ. *Hazard evaluation and technical assistance report:* Los Angeles Times, *Los Angeles, CA.* Washington, DC: National Institute for Occupational Safety and Health, 1993. Report HHE 90-013-2277.

79. Andersen JH, Gaardboe O. Prevalence of persistent neck and upper limb pain in a historical cohort of sewing machine operators. *Am J Ind Med* 1993;24: 677–687.

80. Ohlsson K, Attewell R, Paisson B, et al. Repetitive industrial work and neck and upper limb disorders in females. *Am J Ind Med* 1995;27:731–747.

81. Jonsson BG, Persson J, Kelbom A. Disorders of the cervicobrachial region among female workers in the electronics industry: a two year follow-up. *Int J Ind Ergon* 1988;3:1–12.

82. Schibye B, Skov T, Ekner D, Christiansen J, Sjogaard G. Musculoskeletal symptoms among sewing machine operators. *Scand J Work Environ Health* 1995;21: 427–434.

83. Sommerich CM, McGlothin JD, Marras WS. Occupational risk factors associated with soft tissue disorders of the shoulder: a review of recent investigations in the literature. *Ergonomics* 1993;36:697–717.

84. Winkel J, Westgaard RH. Occupational and individual risk factors for shoulder-neck complaints. Part II. The scientific basis (literature review) for the guide. *Int J Ind Ergon* 1992;10:85–104.

85. Chiang H, Ko Y, Chen S, et al. Prevalence of shoulder and upper-limb disorders among workers in the fish-processing industry. *Scand J Work Environ Health* 1993;19:126–131.

86. Kilbom A, Horst D, Kemfert K, Richter A. Observation methods for reduction of load and strain on the human body: a review. *Abetarskyddsstyrelsen Publikation Service* 1986;171(84):92–110. Gig Tr Prof Zabol 1990; 1990:51–54.

87. Ohlsson K, Hansson GA, Balogh I, et al. Disorders of the neck and upper limbs in women in the fish processing industry. *Occup Environ Med* 1994;51: 826–830.

88. Nathan PA, Keniston RC, Myers LD. Longitudinal study of median nerve sensory conduction in industry: relationship to age, gender, hand dominance, occupational hand use, and clinical diagnosis. *J Hand Surg [Am]* 1992;17:850–851.

89. Schottland JR, Kirschberg GJ, Fillingim R. Median nerve latencies in poultry processing workers: an approach to resolving the role of industrial "cumulative trauma" in the development of carpal tunnel syndrome. *J Occup Med* 1991;33:627–630.

90. McCormack RR, Inman RD, Wells A, Berntsen C, Imbus HR. Prevalence of tendinitis and related disorders of the upper extremity in a manufacturing workforce. *J Rheumatol* 1990;17:958–964.

91. Stetson DS, Silverstein BA, Keyserling WM, Wolfe RA, Albers JW. Median sensory distal amplitude and latency: comparisons between nonexposed managerial/professional employees and industrial workers. *Am J Ind Med* 1993;24:175–189.

92. Chiang H, Chen S, Yu H, Ko Y. The occurrence of carpal tunnel syndrome in frozen-food factory employees. *J Med Sci* 1990;6:73–80.

93. Bureau of Labor Statistics. *Survey of occupational injuries and illnesses, 1995.* Washington, DC: U.S. Government Printing Office, 1997.

94. Washington State Department of Labor and Industries. *Work-related musculoskeletal disorders.* Olympia, WA: Washington State Department of Labor and Industries, Consultation and Compliance Services Division, 1996.

95. Stock SR. Workplace ergonomic factors and the development of musculoskeletal disorders of the neck and upper limbs: a meta-analysis. *Am J Ind Med* 1991; 19:87–107.

96. Armstrong TJ, Buckle P, Fine LJ, et al. A conceptual model for work-related neck and upper-limb musculoskeletal disorders. *Scand J Work Environ Health* 1993;19:73–84.

97. Viikari-Juntura E. The role of physical stressors in the development of hand/wrist and elbow disoders. In: Gordon SL, Blair SJ, Fine LJ, eds. *Repetitive motion disorders of the upper extremity*. Rosemont, IL: American Academy of Orthopaedic Surgeons, 1994: 7–28.

98. Moore JS. Carpal tunnel syndrome. *Occup Med* 1992; 7:741–763.

99. Kuorinka IA, Forcier L. *Work-related musculoskeletal disorders: a reference book for prevention*. London: Taylor and Francis, 1995.

100. Radecki P. Variability in the median and ulnar nerve latencies: implications for diagnosing entrapment. *J Occup Med* 1995;37:1293–1299.

101. Werner RA, Franzblau A, Albers JW, Buchele H, Armstrong TJ. Use of screening nerve conduction studies for predicting future carpal tunnel syndrome. *Occup Environ Med* 1997;54:96–100.

102. Nilsson T, Hagberg M, Burstrom L, Lundstrom R. A five-year follow-up study of nerve conduction across the carpal tunnel among workers at a heavy engineering production plant. In: *International conference on the prevention of musculoskeletal disorders (PREMUS)*. Montreal, Quebec: International Committee on Occupational Safety and Health, 1995:81–83.

103. Nathan PA, Takigawa K, Keniston RC, Meadows KD, Lockwood RS. Slowing of sensory conduction of the median nerve and carpal tunnel syndrome in Japanese and American industrial workers. *J Hand Surg [Br]* 1994;19:30–34.

104. Osorio AM, Ames RG, Jones JA, et al. Carpal tunnel syndrome among grocery store workers. *Am J Ind Med* 1994;25:229–245.

105. Atterbury MR, Limke JC, Lemasters GK, et al. Nested case-control study of hand and wrist work-related musculoskeletal disorders in carpenters. *Am J Ind Med* 1996;30:695–701.

106. Silverstein BA, Fine LJ, Armstrong TJ. Hand-wrist cumulative trauma disorders in industry. *Br J Ind Med* 1986;43:779–784.

107. Wieslander G, Norback D, Gothe CJ, Juhlin L. Carpal tunnel syndrome (CTS) and exposure to vibration, repetitive wrist movements, and heavy manual work: a case-referent study. *Br J Ind Med* 1989;46:43–47.

108. Morgenstern H, Kelsh M, Kraus J, Margolis W. A cross-sectional study of hand/wrist symptoms in female grocery checkers. *Am J Ind Med* 1991;20: 209–218.

109. Punnett L, Robins JM, Wegman DH, Keyserling WM. Soft-tissue disorders in the upper limbs of female assembly workers: impact of length of employment, work pace, and selection. *Scand J Work Environ Health* 1985;11:417–425.

110. Chatterjee DS. Exploratory electromyography in the study of vibration-induced white finger in rock drillers. *Br J Ind Med* 1982;39:89–97.

111. Chatterjee DS. Workplace upper limb disorders: a prospective study with intervention. *J Occup Med* 1992;42:129–136.

112. Melhorn JM. A prospective study for upper-extremity cumulative trauma disorders of workers in aircraft manufacturing. *J Occup Environ Med* 1996;38: 1264–1271.

113. Moore JS, Garg A. A job analysis method for predicting risk of upper extremity disorders at work: preliminary results. *Adv Ind Ergon Safety* 1987;1:1–252.

114. Armstrong TJ, Fine LJ, Goldstein SA, Lifshitz YR, Silverstein BA. Ergonomic considerations in hand and wrist tendinitis. *J Hand Surg [Am]* 1987;12:830–837.

115. Luopajarvi T, Juorinka I, Virolainen M, Holmberg M. Prevalence of tenosynovitis and other injuries of the upper extremities in repetitive work. *Scand J Work Environ Health* 1979;5:48–55.

116. Bystrom S, Hall C, Welander T, Kilbom A. Clinical disorders and pressure-pain threshold of the forearm and hand among automobile assembly line workers. *J Hand Surg [Br]* 1995;20:782–790.

117. Amano M, Gensyo U, Nakajima H, Yatsuki K. Characteristics of work actions of shoe manufacturing assembly line workers and a cross-sectional factor-control study on occupational cervicobrachial disorders. *Jpn J Ind Health* 1988;30:3–12.

118. Kurppa K, Viikari-Juntura E, Kuosma E, Huuskonen M, Kivi P. Incidence of tenosynovitis or peritendinitis and epicondylitis in a meat-processing factory. *Scand J Work Environ Health* 1991;17:32–37.

119. Roto P, Kivi P. Prevalence of epicondylitis and tenosynovitis among meatcutters. *Scand J Work Environ Health* 1984;10:203–205.

120. Kuorinka IA, Koskinen P. Occupational rheumatic diseases and upper limb strain in manual jobs in a light mechanical industry. *Scand J Work Environ Health* 1979;5:39–47.

121. Koskimies K, Pyykko I, Starck J, Inaba R. Vibration syndrome among Finnish forest workers between 1972 and 1990. *Arch Occup Environ Health* 1992;64: 251–256.

122. Futatsuka M, Uneno T. Vibration exposure and vibration-induced white finger due to chain saw operation. *J Occup Med* 1985;27:257–264.

123. Futatsuka M, Uneno T. A follow-up study of vibration-induced white finger due to chain saw operation. *Scand J Work Environ Health* 1986;12:304–306.

124. National Institute for Occupational Safety and Health. *NIOSH criteria for a recommended standard: occupational exposure to hand-arm vibration*. Cincinnati: U.S. Department of Health and Human Services, 1989.

125. Gemne G, Lundstrom R, Hansson J. Disorders induced by work with hand-held vibrating tools: a review of current knowledge for criteria documentation. *Arbete Halsa* 1993;6:1–83.

126. Bovenzi M. Italian study group on physical hazards in the stone industry: hand-arm vibration syndrome and dose-response relation for vibration-induced white finger among quarry drillers and stonecarvers. *Occup Environ Med* 1994;51:779–784.

127. Bovenzi M, Franzinelli A, Mancini R, et al. Dose-response relation for vascular disorders induced by vibration in the fingers of forestry workers. *Occup Environ Med* 1995;52:722–730.

128. Letz R, Cherniak MG, Gerr F, Hershman D, Pace P. A cross-sectional epidemiological survey of shipyard

workers exposed to hand-arm vibration. *Br J Ind Med* 1992;49:53–62.

129. Nilsson T, Burstrom L, Hagberg M. Risk assessment of vibration exposure and white fingers among platers. *Int Arch Occup Environ Health* 1989;61:473–481.

130. Musson Y, Burdorf A, van Drimmelen D. Exposure to shock and vibration and symptoms in workers using impact power tools. *Ann Occup Hyg* 1989;33:85–96.

131. Bovenzi M, Franzinelli A, Strambi F. Prevalence of vibration-induced white finger and assessment of vibration exposure among travertine workers in Italy. *Int Arch Occup Environ Health* 1988;61:25–34.

132. Mirbod SM, Yoshida H, Nagata C, et al. Hand-arm vibration syndrome and its prevalence in the present status of private forestry enterprises in Japan. *Int Arch Occup Environ Health* 1992;64:93–99.

133. Andersson GBJ. Epidemiologic aspects of low back pain in industry. *Spine* 1981;6:53–60.

134. Snook SH. Low back pain in industry. In: *American Academy of Orthopaedic Surgeons symposium on idiopathic low back pain*. St. Louis, MO: Mosby–Year Book, 1998:23–38.

135. Riihimaki H, Tola S, Videman T, Hanninen K. Low-back pain and occupation: a cross-section questionnaire study of men in machine-operating, dynamic physical work, and sedentary work. *Spine* 1989;14:204–209.

136. Skovron ML, Szpalski M, Nordin M, Melot C, Cukier D. Sociocultural factors and back pain: a population-based study in Belgian adults. *Spine* 1994;19:129–137.

137. Garg A, Moore SJ. Epidemiology of low-back pain in industry. *Occup Med State Art Rev* 1992;7:593–608.

138. Battie MC, Videman T, Gibbons LE, et al. Determinants of lumbar disc degeneration: study relating lifetime exposures and magnetic resonance imaging findings in identical twins. *Spine* 1995;20:2601–2612.

139. Burdorf A. Exposure assessment of risk factors for disorders of the back in occupational epidemiology. *Scand J Work Environ Health* 1998;18:1–9.

140. Marras WS, Lavender SA, Ferguson SA, Allread WG. Biomechanical risk factors for occupationally-related low back pain disorders. *Ergonomics* 1995;38:377–410.

141. Marras WS, Lavender SA, Leurgans SE, et al. The role of dynamic three-dimensional trunk motion in occupationally-related low back disorders: the effects of workplace factors, trunk position, and trunk motion characteristics on risk of injury. *Spine* 1993;18:617–628.

142. Hurrell JJ, Murphy LR. Psychological job stress. In: Rom WN, ed. *Environment and occupational medicine*. New York: Little, Brown and Company, 1992:675–684.

143. Principles of tendon transfers to the hand. In: *Principles of tendon transfers to the hand*. Rosemont, IL: American Academy of Orthopaedic Surgeons, 1997:1–25.

144. Sauter SL, Gottlieb MS, Jones KC. Job and health implications of VDT use: initial results of the Wisconsin-NIOSH study. *Communication Assoc Comput Mach* 1983;26:284–294.

145. Bergqvist UO. Video display terminals and health. *Scand J Work Environ Health* 1984;10:68–77.

146. Ewartk CK, Taylor CV, Reese LB. Effects of early postmyocardial infraction exercise testing on self-perception and subsequent physical activity. *Am J Cardiol* 1983;20:1076–1080.

147. Sauter SL, Swanson NG. Psychological aspects of musculoskeletal disorders in office work. In: Moon S, Sauter SL, eds. *Psychosocial factors and musculoskeletal disorders*. London: Taylor and Francis, 1998:225–256.

148. Ursin H, Edresen IM, Ursin G. Psychological factors and self-reports of muscle pain. *Eur J Appl Physiol* 1988;57:282–290.

149. Bongers PM, de Winter CR, Kompier MAJ, Hildebrandt VH. Psychosocial factors at work and musculoskeletal disease. *Scand J Work Environ Health* 1993;19:297–312.

150. Bernard BP, Sauter SL, Fine LJ, Petersen MR, Hales TR. Psychosocial and work organization risk factors for cumulative trauma disorders in the hands and wrists of newspaper employees. *Scand J Work Environ Health* 1992;18:119–120.

151. Waersted M, Bjorklund R, Westgaard RH. Generation of muscle tension related to a demand of continuing attention. In: Knave BG, Wideback PG, eds. *Work with display units*. New York: Elsevier Science North-Holland, 1986:288–293.

152. Westgaard RH, Bjorklund R. Generation of muscle tension additional to postural muscle load. *Ergonomics* 1987;30:911–923.

153. International Labor Organization. *Psychosocial factors at work: recognition and control*. Geveva: International Labour Organization, 1986.

154. World Health Organization. Work with visual display terminals: psychosocial aspects of health. *J Occup Med* 1989;31:957–968.

155. Payne R. Individual differences in the study of occupational stress. In: Cooper CL, Payne R, eds. *Causes, coping, and consequences of stress at work*. Chichester, UK: John Wiley and Sons, 1988:209–232.

156. Melhorn JM. Cumulative trauma disorders: how to assess the risks. *J Workers' Compensation* 1996;5:19–33.

157. Bongers PM, de Winter CR. *Psychosocial factors and musculoskeletal disease: a report of the literature*. The Netherlands: Institute of Preventive Health Care, 1998.

158. Helliwell PS, Mumford DB, Smeathers JE, Wright V. Work-related upper limb disorder: the relationship between pain, cumulative load, disability, and psychological factors. *Ann Rheum Dis* 1992;51:1325–1329.

159. Leino P. Symptoms of stress predict musculoskeletal disorders. *J Epidemiol Community Health* 1989;43:293–300.

160. Karasek RA, Gardell B, Lindel J. Work and non-work correlates of illness and behavior in male and female Swedish white collar workers. *J Occup Behav* 1987;8:187–207.

161. Tola S, Riihimaki H, Videman T, Viikari-Juntura E, Hanninen K. Neck and shoulder symptoms among men in machine-operating, dynamic physical work and sedentary work. *Scand J Work Environ Health* 1988;14:299–305.

162. Hopkins A. Stress, the quality of work, and repetition strain injury in Australia. *Work Stress* 1990;4:129–138.

163. Viikari-Juntura E, Vuori J, Silverstein BA, et al. A lifelong prospective study on the role of psychosocial factors in neck-shoulder and low back pain. *Spine* 1991;16:1056–1061.

164. Dehlin O, Berg S. Back symptoms and psychological perception of work: a study among nursing aides in a geriatric hospital. *Scand J Rehabil Med* 1977;9:61–65.

165. Pot F, Padmos P, Brouswers A. Determinants of the VDU operator's well being. In: Knave BG, Wideback PG, eds. *Work with display units.* New York: Elsevier Science North-Holland, 1986:16–25.

166. Takala EP, Viikari-Juntura E. *Muscle force endurance and neck-shoulder symptoms of sedentary workers: an experimental study on bank cashiers with and without symptoms.* The Netherlands: Elsevier Science, 1991.

167. Theorell T, Harms-Ringdahl K, Ahlberg-Hulten G, Westin B. Psychosocial job factors and symptoms from the locomotor system: a multicausal analysis. *Scand J Rehabil Med* 1991;23:165–173.

168. Kvarnstrom S, Halden M. Occupational cervico-brachial disorders in an engineering company. *Scand J Rehabil Med* 1983;8:1–14.

169. Ryan GA, Bampton M. Comparison of data process operators with and without upper limb symptoms. *Community Health Studies* 1988;12:63–68.

170. Ekberg K, Bjorkqvist B, Malm P, et al. Case-control study of risk factors for disease in the neck and shoulder area. *Occup Environ Med* 1994;51:262–266.

171. Houtman ILD, Bongers PM, Smulders PGW, Kompier MAJ. Psychosocial stressors at work and musculo-skeletal problems. *Scand J Work Environ Health* 1994; 20:139–145.

172. Hoekstra EJ, Hurrell JJ, Swanson NG. *Hazard evaluation and technical assistance report: Social Security Administration Teleservice Centers, Boston, MA; Fort Lauderdale, FL; Cincinati, OH.* Cincinnati: U.S. Department of Health and Human Services, 1994.

173. Linton SJ. Risk factors for neck and back pain in a working population in Sweden. *Work Stress* 1998;4: 41–49.

174. Feyer A, Williamson A, Mandryk J, de Silva I, Healy S. Role of psychosocial risk factors in work-related low back pain. *J Work Environ Health* 1992;18: 368–375.

175. Bergenudd H, Lindgren B, Nilsson BY, Petersson C. Shoulder pain in middle age: a study of prevalence and relation to occupational work load and psychosocial factors. *Clin Orthop* 1988;23:234–238.

176. Battie MC, Bigos SJ, Fisher LD, et al. A prospective study of the role of cardiovascular risk factors and fitness in industrial back pain complaints. *Spine* 1989; 14:141–147.

177. Bigos SJ, Spengler DM, Martin NA, et al. Back injuries in industry: a retrospective study. III. Employee-related factors. *Spine* 1986;11:252–256.

178. Magora A. Investigation of the relation between low back pain and occupation. *Scand J Rehabil Med* 1973; 5:191–196.

179. Svensson H, Andersson GBJ. The relationship of low-back pain, work history and work environment, and stress: a retrospective cross-sectional study of 38- to 64-year old women. *Spine* 1989;14:517–522.

180. Astrand NE. Medical, psychological, and social factors associated with back abnormalities and self-reported back pain: a cross-sectional study of male employees in a Swedish pulp and paper industry. *Br J Ind Med* 1987;44:327–336.

181. Heliovaara M, Makela M, Knekt P. Determinants of sciatica and low back pain. *Spine* 1991;16:608–614.

182. Lundberg U, Granqvist M, Hansson T, Magnusson M, Wallin L. Psychological and physiological stress responses during repetitive work at an assembly line. *Work Stress* 1989;3:143–153.

183. Svensson H, Andersson GBJ. Low-back pain in 40 to 47-year old men: work history and work environment factors. *Spine* 1983;8:272–276.

184. Bureau of Labor Statistics. Lost-worktime injuries: characteristics and resulting time away from work, 1995. *News 1997.* U.S Department of Labor publication, 1997, 97-1888:1–19

185. Hoskin AF, Brand S. *Accident facts.* Itasca, IL: National Safety Council, 1993.

186. Miller TR, Galbraith M. Estimating the costs of occupational injury in the United States. *Accid Anal Prev* 1995;27:741–747.

187. Leigh JP, Miller TR. Ranking occupations based upon the costs of job-related injuries and diseases. *J Occup Med* 1997;39:1170–1182.

188. Leigh JP, Markowitz SB, Fahs MC, Shin C, Landrigan PJ. Occupational injury and illness: estimates of costs, mortality and morbidity. *Arch Intern Med* 1997;157: 1557–1568.

189. Dieterly DL. Industrial injury cost analysis by occupation in an electric utility. *Hum Factors* 1995;37: 591–595.

190. Rice DP, Hodgson TA, Kopstein, AN. The economic costs of illness: a replication and update. *Health Care Finance Rev* 1985;7:61–80.

191. Viscusi WK. *Fatal tradeoffs: public and private responsibility for risk.* New York: Oxford University Press, 1992.

192. Leigh JP, Markowitz SB, Fahs MC, Shin C, Landrigan PJ. *Costs of occupational injuries and illnesses.* Cincinnati, OH: Centers for Disease Control and Prevention, 1995.

Occupational Musculoskeletal Disorders
edited by T. G. Mayer, R. J. Gatchel, and P. B. Polatin.
Lippincott Williams & Wilkins, Philadelphia © 2000.

16

Cumulative Trauma Disorders and Repetitive Strain Injuries and Their Relationship to Work Injury

J. Mark Melhorn and †David W. Florence

Section of Orthopaedics, Department of Surgery, University of Kansas School of Medicine—Wichita, Wichita, Kansas 67208-4510; †Department of Occupational Medicine, Marshfield Clinic, Marshfield, Wisconsin 54449

This chapter is divided into two sections. The first section addresses the concept of cumulative trauma disorders (CTDs) of the upper extremity, and the second section addresses the lower extremities and back. This separation is consistent with the studies and manuscripts that have been published on these topics.

Cumulative trauma disorders is a term that has been used by many organizations and by the federal government to describe any musculoskeletal pain or symptoms that a person believes is associated with activities performed at work (1). *Musculoskeletal pain* is defined as any pain that may involve the muscles, nerves, tendons, ligaments, bones, or joints. This pain or symptom can be real or imagined. For the pain or symptom to be considered work related, state governments have legislated a variety of work contribution requirements. These state government requirements range on a scale of no actual contribution (0%) to full work contribution (100%). Additionally, some states have provided legislation to exclude specific conditions such as carpal tunnel syndrome (CTS) (2). Workers' Compensation was created to provide benefits for work-related injuries that meet the specific legislative requirements (3). Work-related symptoms without a specific trauma injury or event were recent additions to the Workers' Compensation system (4).

Cumulative trauma disorder is not a medical diagnosis but a label for pain perception or symptoms (5). CTD is not a new concept. Symptoms or pains associated with the workplace were discussed indirectly in Greek and Roman times but was first described in a manuscript in 1473 (6). CTD has also been called *repetitive strain injury* (RSI) and *repetitive motion disorder* (RMD). These terms are misleading, however, because in some instances the absence of motion (e.g., static contractions) may be more predictive of CTD. For example, data entry tasks involve prolonged static loading of muscles in the neck and shoulder area that stabilize the arm so that precise repetitive motions can be performed. CTDs then represent a continuum from CTS that has both relatively clear diagnostic criteria and pathophysiology to tension neck syndrome, which is defined primarily by the specific location of pain and has a pathophysiology that is less clearly defined (7).

To help avoid confusion and to separate the emotional link to terms like repetitive strain injury, repetitive motion disorder, cervicobrachial disease, and CTDs, a new term is being suggested. *Musculoskeletal disorder* (MSD) is the newest term to describe these conditions and refers to any condition that involves the nerves, tendons, muscles, and supporting structures of the body (8). MSD is further defined by what activities are being performed at the time of symptoms. This expanded definition allows for the terms *occupational MSD* and *nonoccupational MSD*. This separation is arbitrary and does not represent a medical diagnosis but simply provides an additional modifier to the term MSD. Therefore, CTD and MSD can be considered as being both similar and different. Both terms describe symptoms of the musculoskeletal system, but MSD, unlike CTD, is supposed to have a physiological etiology for the pain. Many studies of MSD indicate, however, that the musculoskeletal pain associated with the workplace (occupational MSD) cannot be separated from and are influenced by psychosocial factors (1,9–11). Therefore, the terms CTD and MSD are more similar than different and can be used interchangeably to describe musculoskeletal pain associated with the workplace; this pain is experienced differently by the individual based on a unique set of risk factors that include: age, gender, genetics (inherited characteristics), nonwork environment, and how these elements are linked by psychosocial factors (12,13).

This conclusion is supported by the fact that CTD and MSD can be clinically grouped as: (a) well-defined disorders such as tendinitis, CTS, and hand-arm vibration syndrome, (b) less well-defined disorders such as tension neck syndrome, and (c) poorly defined or nonspecific disorders such as CTD, RSI, overuse syndrome, or cervicobrachial disorders). Confusion over terminology (CTD or MSD) and case definitions (epidemiological criteria required to consider inclusion compared to medical diagnosis criteria) has had a dramatic impact on the understanding, reporting, and treatment of CTD and occupational MSD. Physicians can easily relate to the clinically well-defined disorders in which the criteria for the epidemiologist's case definition are similar to the physician's diagnostic criteria. Confusion

occurs for the physician when emphasis is shifted from medical diagnostic criteria to the more inclusive surveillance case definitions used by epidemiologists to identify risk factors and to institute preventive measures. In a review of the medical literature, Vender et al. (14) tried to encompass medical criteria to validate a causal relationship between upper-extremity disorders and work activities. Their conclusions were that the medical literature currently fails to incorporate sound medical diagnostic criteria in defining and identifying MSD and does not establish a causal relationship between distinct medical disorders and work activities.

This conclusion also implies that research may be unable to establish a specific dose relationship for each activity and workplace pain, a causational relationship to specific jobs and workplace pain, or a pathoanatomical etiology for every pain that occurs in the workplace. Current epidemiological research has established associations between certain work activities and the development of CTD/MSD. These epidemiological categories are useful in research of MSD but offer little insight into the medical care for the treating physician seeing the individual worker. The benefit of this information lies in the opportunity to develop preventive measures in the workplace (15). Regardless of the preferred descriptive term (CTD or MSD) and the epidemiologists' case surveillance definitions, the cornerstone for treatment will remain identification of risk factors and the institution of prevention rather than diagnosis and treatment of individual patients (15–20).

CUMULATIVE TRAUMA DISORDERS/ REPETITIVE STRAIN INJURY AND COMPENSATION

With the recognition of workplace injury came the concept of compensation. Compensation for injury has a long and complicated history. A brief calendar below highlights key events:

2050 BC	Samaria	Compensation for injury of body part (21)
600 AD	Europe	Compensation without justification (22)
1880	Germany	First comprehensive workers' compensation system (23)
1906	Great Britain	Workman's Compensation Act of 1906 (24)
1920	United States	Workman's Compensation by states (25)
1970	United States	Occupational Safety and Health Administration (OSHA) Public Law 91-596 Safe Work Place (26)
1986	United States	National Institute for Occupational Safety and Health (NIOSH) National Safety and Prevention Plan (27)
1990	United States	Americans with Disability Act signed July 26, 1990 (28)

The roots of the concept that a worker should be compensated for loss date back to about 2050 BC. As detailed in the Nippur Tablet No. 3191 (21) dealing with the law of Ur-Nammu, King of Ur in Samaria, compensation was given for the injury of body parts, such as fractures of the hand, foot, and nose. Monetary relief for the loss was given, and, at times, rewards were given for lost wages and doctors' fees. Sand (22) reported that in 600 AD the Lombards had a system of compensation in which the injured workers did not have to prove blame.

As society became more complex and industrialized, so did the laws regarding workers' compensation. Germany developed the first comprehensive workers' compensation system in the late 1880s. This system replaced the earlier system in which an injured worker had to prove that the employer was at fault. Most workers were not financially able to pursue such a path through the legal system; the advent of the workers' compensation laws and reforms changed this situation. Coincidental with the development of laws regarding workers' compensation was an observed change in the attitude of workers. McKendrick (24) noted that after the Workman's Compensation Act of 1906 in Great Britain, workers applied for benefits for even the most trivial problems that would have been tolerated without medical attention before the enactment of the legislation. Sir John Collie (29) was so upset with this alteration in behavior that he wrote a book, *Malingering and Feigned Sickness*, in 1913. McKendrick (24) also devoted a book to the subject in which he classified malingerers as real, partial, or unconscious according to his appreciation of the worker's intent.

In 1934, Hammer (30) described a condition in workers that was characterized by pain and swelling and was accompanied by burning and numbness in the fingers. He was aware of deQuervain's earlier work and recognized part of the symptom complex for what it was; however, he did not further pursue identification of the symptoms that were no doubt CTS. He observed:

> The advent of the Workmen's Compensation Act has placed upon the surgeon the added responsibility of making careful inquiry into the subject of tenosynovitis in so far as that condition relates to the continued use of certain sets of muscles in daily occupation...It should not then be surprising to find that certain industrial pursuits require the continuous use of special groups of muscles constituting "high speed hand operations" and that such often repeated manipulations predispose to the development of tenosynovitis.

In 1931 Conn (25) commented on the Ohio State Workers' Compensation Act of 1929. Primary tenosynovitis, characterized by a passive effusion or crepitus into the tendon sheath of the flexor or extensor muscles of the hand due to frequent repetitive motions or vibration, was considered compensable. The new code abandoned the need for an etiologic diagnosis and recognized repetitive motion and vibration by themselves as causative factors.

Arthur (31), in discussing Conn's paper, noted the high incidence of tenosynovitis in newly hired employees and those who had returned from vacation. In 1947, in an extensive review of the problems of median nerve compression, Brain et al. (32) concluded that occupation was a causal factor. Each of his six patients had a history of recent or chronic repetitive hand use.

In recent decades, the concept that work could be the cause of symptoms or disease has been the subject of heated debates in the literature relating to two basic issues: (a) whether an activity can cause "symptoms" or "disease" and (b) the extent that emotional or psychological problems may amplify and prolong physical symptoms (5). A review of the history of CTD/RSI can provide some insight into this debate.

CUMULATIVE TRAUMA DISORDERS/ REPETITIVE STRAIN INJURY AND THE WORKPLACE

A World Perspective

Below is a brief calendar of historical events related to awareness of CTD/RSI in the workplace:

BC	Greece	Pain in workplace (33)
1473	Ellenbon	Pain with work of goldsmiths (34)
1567	Paracelsus	Pain with work of miners (34)
1700	Ramazzini	Pain with work of potters (35)
1830	United Kingdom	Writer's cramp (36)
1882	United Kingdom	Telegraphist's cramp (37)
1960	Japan	Cervicobrachial disease (38)
1960	Sweden	Tension headache (39)
1960	Finland	Occupational headache (40)
1962	Switzerland	Tension headache (41)
1979	Scandinavia	Occupational cervicobrachial disease (42)
1980	Australia	RSI (43)
1980	New Zealand	RSI (44)
1985	West Germany	Occupational complaint number 2101 (45)
1988	Hong Kong	Occupational cervicobrachial disease (38)
1990	United Kingdom	RSI (46)
1990	United States	CTD (7)
1995	United States	Occupational MSD (7)

Although we have become increasingly aware of the problems of workers and their pain symptoms associated with the workplace, these conditions have been noted throughout history. Rosen cited early works by Ellenbon in 1473 devoted to goldsmiths and by Paracelsus in 1567 relating to diseases of miners as perhaps some of the first CTD manuscripts (34). In 1700 Ramazzini (35) stood alone as the first to present a comprehensive overview of the general problem. Almost 300 years ago, his observations were as follows:

> Various and manifold is the harvest of diseases reaped by certain workers from the craft and trades they pursue. All the profit that they get is fatal injury to their health, mostly from two causes. The first and most potent is the harmful character of the materials they handle. The second I ascribe to certain violent and irregu-

lar motions and unnatural postures of the body, by reason of which, the natural structure of the vital machine is so impaired that serious disease gradually develops therefrom.

In 1830, Sir Charles Bell described writers' cramp as a condition occurring in persons who consider their job to be primarily one of writing (36). Writers' cramp differs from RSI only in the higher incidence of hand spasm. With continued observation, he noted that writer's cramp sufferers frequently are of distinctively nervous temperament, irritable, sensitive, bearing overwork and anxiety badly, and that this disease is easily imagined by those who have witnessed the disorder. He observed that 50% of writer's cramp occurred bilaterally and finally concluded that it is an occupational neurosis (47). Goodman suggested that the increased incidence of writers' cramp was accompanied by a change from the feather quill to the more productive steel nib (48).

Gowers observed similar occupational neuroses of the time labeled as piano forte player's cramp, violin player's cramp, seamstress cramp, and telegraphist's cramp (49). In 1882, Robinson reviewed the similarity of telegraphist's cramp to writer's cramp (37). In 1908, telegraphist's cramp was added to the schedule of diseases covered by the British Workman's Compensation Act; its incidence steadily increased to affect 60% of operators. In 1910, The Great Britain and Ireland Post Office Departmental Committee of Inquiry removed telegraphist's cramp from the list after concluding that telegraphist's cramp was a nervous breakdown resulting from nervous instability and repeated fatigue (47). Interestingly, telegraphist's cramp developed about the time of introduction of the Morse key.

Another occupational condition, Miner's nystagmus, which bears no relationship to the upper limb, affected up to 34% of British underground coal miners at a time when battery-operated helmet lamps and mechanized coal extraction were introduced early in this century. These two innovations increased coal productivity enormously (50). After several years of increase, the condition disappeared when it was determined that the condition was

not physical and the condition would no longer be considered work-related for compensation (47).

The term *occupational cervicobrachial disorder* (OCD) was first established by the Japan Association of Industrial Health in 1972 (38). In the years between 1960 and 1980, an epidemic of OCDs was reported in Japan (38,51,52). The initial reports of cervicobrachial problems were noted among punch card perforators in 1958, but, subsequently, the disorder was found to affect typists, telephone operators, office keyboard operators, calculator operators, cash-register operators, those in packing-machine jobs, assembly-line workers, and process workers. The frequency varied, with 81% reporting shoulder stiffness, 49% only right shoulder pain, 31% neck pain, 13% wrist symptoms, 19% hand, 13% fingers, 82% general fatigue, 59% headaches, 27% insomnia, and 42% low back pain (53). The term OCD was used to describe a somewhat vague syndrome of pain about the shoulder, posterior neck, and parascapular musculature, the glenohumeral musculotendinous structure, and pain radiating in the upper arm. In other words, it was not a pathologic or clinical diagnosis but a symptom-based diagnosis. In 1964 the problem had become so widespread that the Japanese Ministry of Labor set ergonomic guidelines for keyboard operators, limiting their workday to 5 hours and ordering 10-minute rest breaks each hour (38). Unfortunately, these rigid guides did not decrease the number of new cases reported.

Cervicobrachial disorders have been discussed in Scandinavia (42), Switzerland, and Sweden as *tension neck* (41), in Finland as *occupational disorder* (40), in West Germany as *occupational complaint number 2101*, and in France as *occupational neck pain* (45). Some investigators suggest that high levels of stress and subsequent muscle tension predispose persons to OCD (54,55). Nakaseko et al. (38) concluded that OCD symptoms were associated with light physical work but not with heavy physical work. This conclusion was supported by a cross-sectional study performed in Sweden in which a negative correlation was found between heavy work and neck and shoulder problems (39). This findings should not be taken as an indication that heavy lifting prevents neck and shoulder problems, but it does support the fact that OCD is more prevalent among sedentary and light-assembly workers. The study also found that people who complain about pain from the neck and shoulder area had more sick leave for illnesses of all types than job-matched controls. In a study of various staff members at the University of Hong Kong, back and neck problems were more prevalent in persons aged 31 to 40 years and to have an increased incidence in women (56).

In the 1980s, the United Kingdom experienced its epidemic of upper-limb pain. The pain was often nonspecific and did not conform to the pattern of various well-recognized rheumatologic entities. The syndrome was known by a number of terms, some of which imply an etiologic link to workplace activities unsubstantiated by hard evidence. The syndrome was considered largely psychosocial and analogous to the chronic fatigue syndrome (46). Studies based on a random sample of more than 1,000 working-age people in the north of England revealed that, at any time, 9% of men and 12% of women had an arm or neck pain sufficiently severe enough to cause them to consult their physician (42). Other studies have drawn attention to the prevalence of neck and arm pain experienced by the patient during normal activities of daily living (57,58). The Australian RSI experience differs only in its epidemic spread and high incidence compared with OCD (43,59–61). The epidemic of RSI spread to involve a wide spectrum of occupations, including data processors, process workers, typists, clerks, cashiers, bank tellers, musicians, packers, and textile-industry machinists whose manual tasks and productivity had not changed significantly for decades. It then spread to workers who were not engaged in repetitive movements, such as retail sales assistants. In Australia in 1985, 34% of the national telephone company's operators complained of this phenomenon (59). Repetitious use was suggested as the cause for RSI, but medical studies could not demonstrate a common denominator for motion of the upper limb and RSI. In one Australian study of Telecom (the government-run national telephone company), the highest incidence of RSI occurred in the following groups: 34% in telephonists who had the lowest keystroke rate, followed by 28% in clerks and 3.4% in keyboard operators, who had the most repetitious tasks and highest keystroke rate (59). Other studies showed the frequency of occurrence to be different for RSI, with keypunch operators at 16% to 28%, cash register operators at 11% to 16%, typists at 13%, calculator operators at 10%, and light-assembly workers at 16%. A 1981 Australian survey of 122 data-processing workers showed that 78% had symptoms of RSI. Most symptoms, however, were mild, and only 26% of the group had obtained medical treatment. No specific work-related explanation was found (61–64). Suggestions for why RSI developed in Australia in the early 1980s vary. It was a time of relative prosperity in a country with as many physicians and pharmacists per capita as any industrialized nation and one in which more patented medicines were consumed per capita than in the United States. The inability to work because of a physical ailment became more socially acceptable. Perhaps most importantly, the epidemic occurred at a time of technologic change: computerization of clerical tasks. This change increased a worker's productivity but threatened those less adaptable to change who then had to compete with younger, computer-educated applicants. Some believe the increased reporting of RSI was similar to the changes that occurred with other technologic advances. Others suggested that RSI was encouraged by ergonomists and their costly ergonomic redesign of the workplace, work furniture, and equipment and by the trade union movement that fostered demands for 15-minute work breaks for every hour of work and that work health and safety officers be stationed in workplaces for early recognition of RSI. In addition, a publication entitled *The*

Sufferer's Hand Book (45) was issued to most members of the Public Service, which employs—through federal, state, and local governments—one in three Australians (65).

Members of the medical profession (the so-called industrial rehabilitation specialists and their clinics proved to be a rapid growth area in the 1980s in the health industry) were required to provide periodic certification requirements of continuing unfitness for work. Members of the legal community saw an increase in the case for employer negligence litigation and publicly solicited their specialty as RSI negligence claims (65). Many sections of the paramedical industry, including physiotherapy, occupational therapy, and the fringe providers saw an increase in services for ergonomic furniture designs and equipment. The RSI subculture also included such occupations as tactile therapists and management consultants, who regularly advertised cures for RSI in the computer sections of the print media. RSI was used by the antifluoridation lobby in their claims that fluoridated water supply was causative. The print and electronic media industries, which thrive on controversy, were responsible for disseminating misinformation. RSI became a costly sociopolitical phenomenon in Australia and RSI concerns diverted huge government resources to research committees, inquiries, social workers, and other rehabilitators, all of whom depended on the continuity of RSI (66).

The estimated cost of lost work from July 1984 to June 1985 in the Australian Commonwealth Public Service (excluding state public servants and private enterprise employees) was $24.13 million. In June 1985, 26% of Commonwealth Public Service employees in the Australian Capital Territory suffered from RSI, and most of them were certified as being unfit for work in the year 1984 to 1985. From December 1983 until November 1984, the Commonwealth Banking Corporation saw a 275% increase in the incidence of RSI (65).

The Australian Medical Community Official statement was that although the term *repetition strain injury* was conceived in good faith, the term was inappropriate, misleading, and unscientific, as it commonly affects young to middle-aged, predominantly female employees engaged in low-paying, monotonous, low-prestige occupations. Many but not all RSI patients had symptoms that failed to respond to any form of physical treatment, including rest, splinting, symptomatic physical therapy, and antiinflammatory medications. Frequently, such treatment was often accompanied by a deterioration in the individual's condition. RSI was not associated exclusively with repetitious tasks. It affected data processors, video display unit (VDU) operators, process workers, typists, clerks, cashiers, bank tellers, musicians, packers, machinists, and textile workers, occupations where the manual tasks and work practices had not changed substantially for a decade before or during the epidemic. These occupations required different tasks, used different joints and muscles at different rates, and were performed with different degrees of difficulty. It was also seen in workers not engaged in repetitive movement, such as retail sales assistants, implying that repetitious use and motion of the upper limb was not the common denominator (66). Miller and Topliss (67) completed a systematic cross-sectional study on Australian patients with chronic upper-limb pain syndrome (i.e., RSI). The results demonstrated that 29 of 229 patients had been inappropriately grouped as RSI patients. When this group was treated appropriately, they improved and responded to treatment as would be expected. In a similar study, Littlejohn (68) found evidence that most of the Australian workers with work-related complaints did not have classic conditions associated with repetitive muscle tendon unit activities or postural strains but had clinical characteristics of chronic pain syndromes. These studies suggest that work-related symptoms are multifactorial.

Just as RSI was not new, its meteoric rise and less precipitous decline were predictable based on the historical precedent of writer's cramp, telegraphist's wrist, and miner's nystagmus. This change was based on the acceptance by general medical practitioners and the public of the following: (a) a change in the editorial perspective of the *Australian Medical Journal* in 1986 which allowed publication of articles emphasizing the nonphysical origin of RSI, including a resolution from the 1985 Annual General Meeting of the Australian Hand Surgery Society that RSI is an occupational neurosis is not associated with localized pathology, is reversible with normal use, and leaves no residual or permanent disability (61,64); (b) a coordinated and well-orchestrated education campaign by the Australian Hand Surgery Society with nominated delegates in each state to communicate with both the media and the Colleges of General Practitioners (43); and (c) the judicial decision by the Supreme Court of Australia in the cases *Zabaneh v Commonwealth of Australia* in 1985 and *Cooper v the Commonwealth* in 1987, which found the employer not guilty of negligence and that the plaintiff had not suffered an injury and awarded all costs against the plaintiff. Subsequently, many suits pending by RSI sufferers against their employers were withdrawn (66).

When Australian physicians reflected on their RSI patients, they concluded that few were malingerers. The patients genuinely experienced the pain of which they complained. RSI had become a multimillion dollar business that targeted a specific cohort, employees engaged in low-paying, boring, repetitious, low-prestige jobs, who genuinely believed, through no fault of their own, that their work caused the injury. Once the "secondary gain" of the vested interests in the RSI business was removed, the patients were dumped and soon disappeared. Even as the Australian epidemic came to an end, the debate regarding etiology continued. Two groups remained: one that supported the opinion that most patients and their treating physicians were simply pawns to the many opportunists who gained financially from the unproven notion that repetitive tasks cause injurious tissue strain and that the effect of soft-tissue trauma is cumulative and represents a disorder (43,66,69); and a second group who believed that many patients did not receive adequate evaluation and were inappropriately grouped as RSI and therefore did not respond to treatments (67,68).

The United States Experience

In the United States, CTD experience has been similar to that in other countries except for the descriptive name of the musculoskeletal pain that is associated with the workplace. As pointed out earlier, CTD is a term that has been used by the federal government to describe any musculoskeletal pain that an individual believes is associated with activities performed at work (70), and it implies a presumptive etiology. To the clinician treating a patient with a painful upper extremity, this etiologic inference is only of minor relevance. Activity-related MSDs have complex multifactorial etiology, including not only the physical aspects of activity that people perform but also the psychosocial factors. These disorders may involve muscular, tendinous, ligamentous, and nervous tissues, and onset may be either acute (*overexertion*) or chronic (*overuse*) (1).

With a need to understand the pathophysiology of CTD and a desire to develop effective treatment protocols, the American Academy of Orthopaedic Surgeons held a workshop symposium on CTD in Bethesda, Maryland on June 20–22, 1994. This symposium was supported by the National Institute of Arthritis and Musculoskeletal and Skin Diseases, the National Institute for Occupational Safety and Health, the National Center for Medical Rehabilitation Research, the National Institute of Child Health and Human Development, Orthopaedic Research and Education Foundation, The Center for Vocational Development Training and Health Research, and the Public Health Services Advisory Committee on Employment of Persons with Disabilities. A textbook was edited by Gordon et al. and was titled *Repetitive Motion Disorders of the Upper Extremity* (7). The preface stated the following:

> There is overwhelming evidence that the number of reported cases of repetitive motion is rapidly growing. These disorders have become

an extremely costly public health issue. In many cases, more is unknown than known about an issue. There are many research opportunities in this field. Most epidemiologic studies of CTD have considered almost exclusively the physical attributes of work, such as the number of wrist movements per hour; however, psychosocial factors are increasingly recognized as important factors to be investigated as well. From a public health perspective of prevention, there is enough information to begin to reduce these risk factors with engineering and administrative controls while the research continues.

In May 1996, the *Journal of Hand* presented an editorial on "Repetitive Strain Injuries and Cumulative Trauma Disorders" as follows:

Over the past year, members of the American Society for Surgery of the Hand's Industrial Injuries and Prevention Committee have expressed concern about the use of the terms CTD and RSI. The following statement written to express these concerns has been adopted by the Council of the American Society for Surgery of the Hand, Andrew J. Weiland, MD, President: "The American Society for Surgery of the Hand is concerned that patients with upper extremity pain are being assigned specific diagnoses on the basis of subjective complaints without objective physical findings. There is also a tendency to assign a causal relationship to work for this pain when there is a lack of epidemiological evidence. As part of our normal process of providing the best care for our patients, it is important that the diagnosis be accurate and the assignment of causation be correct. The Society feels that the diagnoses of cumulative trauma disorder (CTD) and repetitive strain injury (RSI) are not appropriate and may actually lead the patient to believe that he or she has a condition that is something more than the ordinary aches and pains of life. Tendinitis is a term that clearly indicates inflammation of tendons or tendon–muscle attachments, while tenosynovitis indicates inflammation of a tendon sheath. These terms are examples of clearly definable and diagnosable entities with a known histologic appearance. In the absence of edema, erythema, or crepitation, it is inappropriate to assign the provisional diagnosis of conditions such as tendinitis or tenosynovitis to patients with upper extremity pain. If patients are told they have one of these conditions, the oppressive power of these words may lead them to believe they are severely injured. A treating physician would do better to explain to their patients

that they have pain or fatigue that may or may not be related to their occupation, but there is no definable diagnosis.

In January 1997, the *Journal of Hand Surgery* published the editorial on "Repetitive Strain: Putting it in Perspective" by Manske (71):

Alternative points of view, contrary opinions, and full-blown controversies have always surrounded hand surgery. For example: reattachment of amputated digits by anastomosis of minute blood vessels using high-powered magnification was at one time championed by a few and considered a radical idea by many; similarly, primary repair of flexor tendons was not only challenged as an inappropriate practice, a paper at the ASSH Annual Meeting advocating its use instigated an investigation to determine whether the results had been reported honestly (they had); more recently, release of the carpal tunnel using an endoscope and a miniature blade has been considered trivial, dangerous, and an expensive form of medical gadgetry by some, while others regard it as a state-of-the-art, cutting edge, way-of-the-future technology. The opposing views in each of these issues were ardently debated with intense emotional fervor— concepts were scorned, egos bruised, and clever terms competed with innovative thoughts for validity. Nevertheless the exchange of ideas was valuable to hand surgery. The diversity of expressed opinions and the richness of the discussions contributed in time to a deeper understanding of the issues and the subsequent advancement of our specialty. Traditional concepts were reevaluated, unproven and fanciful opinions were set aside, and new ideas were sharpened and focused. We became better educated. A current 'hot topic' is the controversy regarding repetitive activities in the workplace as a causative factor of upper extremity disorders. The responses to an American Society for Surgery of the Hand Industry Injuries and Prevention Committee position statement 21A:357, 1996 in Letters to the Editor attest to the heightened level of interest. Although the current issue is disease causation rather than treatment application, the opposing positions are held with the same intensity and passion.

The Individual and Cumulative Trauma Disorders/Repetitive Strain Injury

Human behavior is determined in part by influences beyond control. One's actions are partially programmed by one's genetic heritage. One cannot escape this control system. It is implanted permanently. Although behavior may be modified, humans' ancestors are always looking over their shoulders, influencing and sometimes dictating their actions; however, humans are not robots. Alhough genes influence the individual, much leeway exists for decision-making. Most members of the healing arts believe a patient's desire to improve influences the "getting well" process, but we have given more lip service than study to the concept (72). Just how important motivation is in functional outcome was demonstrated in a study of 183 surgeons who had lost parts of a hand: Only three claimed significant professional disability (73).

Physicians recognize that a hand injury does not occur in a psychological vacuum. Assessment of the psychosocial factors that either complicate recovery or aid in rehabilitation adds valuable diagnostic and therapeutic information about a patient. Although it has been recommended that all patients with financially compensable injuries should be assessed for the possibility of malingering, and although others believe that roughly one-half of injured workers have preexisting psychologic conditions that complicate their recovery, it is critical that the physician realize that patients do suffer intensely and that the common psychologic symptoms of anxiety, depression, and anger are often results of their injuries and not the cause of their current suffering (74,75).

The question of what pain is has been difficult to answer. People have tried to define pain for centuries. Aristotle considered pain an emotion, the opposite of pleasantness, and a quality of the soul (76,77). Modern Western medicine has regarded the body in mechanical terms and has held pain to be a problem of sensory input. The International Association of Pain Study defines pain and pain-related syndromes as follows: Pain is an unpleasant sensory and emotional experience associated with actual or potential tissue damage, or described in terms of tissue damage. Pain is always subjective. Each individual learns the application of the word through experience related to injury. This definition emphasizes that pain is an experience and therefore subjective. It also separates pain from tissue damage. Pain in general, and chronic pain in particular, is a multidimensional experience (78).

Ergonomics

As an approach to the prevention of CTD, ergonomics has gained recognition in recent years. Ergonomics, however, is much more. The term, coined during World War II, was applied to efforts to improve the design of aircraft cockpits. Since then, ergonomics has had a major role in the aerospace and defense industries, in design projects ranging from space capsules to software (33). The concepts of ergonomics now are entering much of the rest of industry, not only to prevent CTD but also as an effective tool for promoting innovation, improving quality and productivity, and increasing job satisfaction.

Currently, ergonomics is a broad field that covers issues such as biomechanics, work physiology, anthropometry, and man–machine interface; from a CTD perspective, it is the lack of ergonomic considerations that increase risk of discomfort or injury. A deficiency in ergonomic design or work organization may lead to the presence of risk factors. Industrial ergonomics has as its major focus the identification, quantification, evaluation and elimination or control of occupational risk factors which may contribute to or aggravate musculoskeletal disorders (CTD). Determining whether ergonomic efforts are worthwhile and effective is difficult and, therefore, ergonomic issues often go unaddressed. Examples of how the lack of good ergonomics can interfere with production are evident when: people working in awkward and uncomfortable positions may not be able to do their jobs properly, fatigue results in errors and inconsistent work, and poor layout and design result in unnecessary work, mistakes, and inefficiency. Studies have shown that ergonomically designed work stations have improved productivity not by making anyone work harder or faster but by better enabling employees to do the best job of which they are capable without hindrances.

Epidemiology is the study of distribution of determinants of disease in human populations (79). A precise epidemiology model for CTD is lacking. However, there is a consensus that the development of CTD involves multifactorial causes rather than a single stimulus. *Epidemiology* allows for analysis of the population risk factors, whereas screening allows for the analysis of the individual's risk factors for the development of CTD.

The sciences of epidemiology and biostatistics are necessary for an analysis of the association of CTD to the workplace. The validity of clinical research relies on a number of factors. The hypothesis must be formulated specifically enough to be testable. The appropriate study subjects should be eligible, and there should not be differential participation. The information collected should be appropriate to the hypothesis and accurate. The study design and information sources should avoid potential information biases. Potential confounders should be eliminated in the study design or controlled in the statistical analysis. At the time the study is designed, clinically significant hypothesized results should be defined, the plan of statistical analysis determined, and the necessary number of study subjects defined. Study management should avoid the introduction of differential loss to follow-up, unblinding, and other potential problems. The statistical analysis should be appropriate to the structure of the data and to the hypothesis. Finally, although the discussion should place the study in the content of other work and what is already known about the question, the specific conclusions should not go beyond what is actually tested in the study (80).

The Debate Continues

The answer to the debate of whether CTD/RSI is or is not caused by work depends on the definition of *causation*. When the medical definition of causation is asked, the an-

swer is "no," but for the epidemiologic definition the answer is "possibly," and for the legal definition, the answer is "yes." A review of the literature provides insight into why the same question can have several answers.

That CTD/RSI is caused by work is supported by the acknowledgment that acute injuries can occur in sports, in dance, and at work. Similarly, most authorities would agree that sports can cause disorders of gradual onset related to repetitive motion (such as lateral and medial epicondylitis and rotator cuff tendinitis). The terms *overuse syndrome* or *chronic overuse injuries* have been used in the orthopedic literature to describe injuries recognized in the athlete, dancer, or musician, and efforts have been directed toward treatment of these chronic disorders; yet confusion arises when this term is applied to work-related injuries. It is possible that the worker may assume similar repetitive movements and static postures. For the worker, however, we are asked to prove that these disorders exist, to determine causality, and establish blame (81). The case for CTD being caused by work is limited by flaws in study design. The case for CTD being work related can be compelling. There is evidence to show that tissue damage can occur in a cumulative and additive fashion (82–94). In theory, tissue damage requires exposure to physical stressors. The amount of damage depends on the duration of exposure, repetition, force, posture, and vibration. An investigation into hand–arm vibration syndrome and dose–response relation for vibration induced white finger among quarry drillers and stone carvers has demonstrated a relationship for a vasospastic phenomenon and ultimately a disease. Unfortunately, many epidemiologic studies that have no clear diagnostic criteria and that lack standardization in data collection result in more confusion and controversy than answers. At the basic science level, it can be concluded that physical factors of force, duration, repetition, and posture have a deleterious effect on muscles, tendons, ligaments, and nerves; however, the point of damage on the continuum of the physical factors and the degree to which this injury occurs have yet to be established. Physical stressors are not the only factors contributing to the development of neuromusculoskeletal disorders. Physical, individual, and psychological factors are jointly associated in this population. Individual factors such as age, gender, physical fitness, and weight also have been linked to the development of these disorders. Although age has been associated with osteoarthritis, studies associating CTS with age are mixed in their conclusions. Repetition and force can eventually result in neuromusculoskeletal disorders. Physiologic evidence shows that the rate and degree of tissue damage depends on the amount of force and repetition and the duration of exposure. With high repetition and high load, tissue changes may occur more quickly, and the association between occupation and injury is more easily discernible. The difficulty comes in determining at what point repetition and strain are sufficient to account for the disorders and apportioning weight to the multiple factors that influence development of neuromusculoskeletal disorders. Also, these factors differ with the individual. Psychological factors, both occupational and nonoccupational, cannot be overlooked. Occupational stressors, including job control, job demands, job security, and type of supervision or supervisor, may influence an individual's response to the onset of symptoms. Nonoccupational stressors, including financial status, family, and social support, also should be considered in patient management, particularly in patients with chronic illness. Chronic neuromusculoskeletal disorders are painful; thus, an awareness of the medical definition of pain is important for the hand surgeon treating these patients (95).

Examples that CTD/RSI *is* caused by work include (a) a study designed to address the question of why some people develop CTS whereas others do not? Two matching female populations, one with a known history of CTS and one without a known history of CTS, were selected, and differences in hand size and work methods were studied. Both populations were employed in the same production sewing jobs. Although differences in hand size were not found, the use of forceful exer-

tions and of deviated wrists, grip and pinch, hand positions, particularly during forceful exertions, were associated with CTS (96). (b) A workplace study was conducted to review repetitiveness, force, awkward posture, and vibrating and nonvibrating hand tools as risk factors for the development of CTD. Repetitiveness appeared to be more important than force as a risk factor for CTS. The prevalence of CTD in women was twice that of men, but no significant association was found between gender and CTS, exposure, and health history or recreational activities. CTD increased with age and years on the job, but this association was not statistically significant (97–100). See Table 1 for CTD RSI Study tables for a detailed list of additional studies (7).

That CTD/RSI is *not* caused by work is supported by the concept of regional arm pain that occurs in response to particular patterns of use. Regional arm pain is described as some local tenderness, but in the physician's opinion, there is no obvious explanation for the pain (101). The clinical categorization of regional arm pain represents a challenge for current Western medicine. A diagnosis of "your arm hurts here" flies in the face of 250 years of the desire of medicine to objectify the experience of illness. However challenging, the term CTD is not a medical diagnosis and is not available for International Classification of Diseases (ICD)-9 coding. The term "pain in limb" 729.5 is an ICD-9 code (102).

In 1986 the National Institute for Occupational Safety and Health (NIOSH) defined CTD and proposed national strategies for the prevention of CTD in the workplace with the following concept: "When job demands...repeatedly exceed the biomechanical capacity of the worker, the activities become trauma-inducing. Hence, traumatogens are workplace sources of biomechanical strain that contribute to the onset of symptoms affecting the musculoskeletal system" (27).

In 1986 the strongest arguments against the CTD hypothesis were the telling experiences in other countries, notably Australia, and the fact that the studies offered in support were flawed (43,103). The hypothesis suggests that

TABLE 1A. *Studies of cumulative trauma disorders and repetitive strain injuries:carpal tunnel syndrome (CTS)*

Study	Design	Exposure ascertainment	Disease ascertainment	Risk factor	OR/RR
Cannon LJ. Personal and occupational factors associated with carpal tunnel syndrome. J Occup Environ Med 1981;23:255–258.	Case referent	Job category	Clinical assessment	Vibration Repetition	7.0[a] 2.1
Punnett et al. Soft-tissue disorders in the upper limbs of female assembly workers: impact of length of employment, work pace, and selection. Scand J Work Environ Health 1985;11:417–425.	Cross sectional	Questionnaire and videotape	Questionnaire	Repetition	3.0[a]
Silverstein BA, Fine LJ, Armstrong TJ. Occupational factors and the carpal tunnel syndrome. Am J Ind Med 1987;11:343–358.	Cross sectional	Electromyelograph and videotape	Questionnaire & physical exam	Lowforce-lowrep Highforce-lowrep Lowforce-hirep Highforce-hirep	1.0 1.8 1.9 15.5[a]
Weislander G, et al. Capral tunnel syndrome (CTS) and exposure to vibration, repetitive wrist movements, and heavy manual work: a case-referent study Br J Ind Med 1989;46:43–47.	Case referent	Questionnaire	Clinical assessment and NCT	Vibration Repetition Force Obesity	6.1[a] 4.5[a] 2.7[a] 3.4[a]
DeKrom MC, et al. Risk factors for carpal tunnel syndrome. Am J Epidemiol 1990;132:1102–1110	Case referent	Questionnaire	Clinical assessment and NCT	Flexed wrist Extended wrist	8.7[a] 5.4[a]
Chiang H, et al. The occurrence of carpal tunnel syndrome in frozen food factory employees. Tsay-Chih 1990;6:73–80.	Cross sectional	Observation	Clinical assessment and NCT	Lowrep, notcold Highrep, notcold High rep, verycold	1.0 2.2 9.4[a]
Barnhart S, et al. Carpal tunnel syndrome among ski manufacturing workers. Scan J Work Environ Health 1991;17:46–52.	Cross sectional	Observation	Physical exam and NCT	Repetition	1.9[a]
Schottland JR, et al. Median nerve latencies in poultry processing workers: an approach to resolving the role of industrial "cumulative trauma" in the development of carpal tunnel syndrome. J Occup Environ Med 1991;33:627–631.	Cross sectional	Current vs preemployment	NCT	2/16 measures of median nerve conduction different between groups	
Nathan PA, Meadows KD, Doyle LS.Occupation as a risk factor for impaired sensory conduction of the median nerve at the carpal tunnel. J Hand Surg 1988;13B:167–170.	Cross sectional	Observation	NCT	Very lightforce-lowrep Lightforce-Modrep Modforce-Himodrep Heavyforce-hirep Very heavyforce Vhirep	1.0 1.0 1.7[a] 1.4 2.2[a]
Bjelle A, Hagberg M, Michaelson F. Clinical and ergonomic factors in prolonged shoulder pain among industrial workers. Scand J Work Environ Health 1979;5:205–210.	Case referent	Interview and observation	Clinical evaluation	Posture (work above shoulders)	11
Nathan PA, et al. Obesity as a risk factor for slowing of sensory conduction of the median nerve in industry: a cross-sectional and longitudinal study involving 429 workers. J Occup Environ Med 1992;34:379–383.	Prospective cohort	Observation	NCT	Body mass index Age Wrist dimension Hand dominance Exercise level Weight	0.6%[a] 3.3%[a] 2.1%[a] 1.0%[a] 0.6%[a] 0.4%[a]

TABLE 1A. Continued.

Study	Design	Exposure ascertainment	Disease ascertainment	Risk factor	OR/RR
Herberts P, et al. Shoulder pain in industry: an epidemiological study on welders. *Acta Orthop Scand* 1981;52:299–306.	Cross sectional	Observation and electromyelograph	Clinical evaluation	Posture (work above shoulders)	13[a]
Herberts P, et al. Shoulder pain and heavy manual labor. *Clin Orthop* 1984;191:166–178.	Cross sectional	Observation	Clinical evaluation	Posture and force	9[a]
Wells JA, et al. Musculoskeletal disorders among letter carriers. *J Occup Environ Med* 1983;25:814–820.	Cross sectional	Weight	Questionnaire	Load (force)	4[a]
Hagberg M, Wegman DH. Prevalence rates and odds ratios of shoulder-neck diseases in different occupational groups. *Br J Ind Med* 1987;44:602–610.	Cross sectional	Observation	Questionnaire and physical exam	Posture (work above shoulders)	11[a]
National Institute for Occupational Safety and Health (NIOSH) evaluation and technical assistance report: Shoprite & Co, NJ. NIOSH report no. HETA 88-344-2092. Cincinnati: USDHHS, CDC, 1992.	Cross sectional	Observation and videotape	Questionnaire and physical exam	Lack of sufficient rest	4[a]
Elbow					
Roto P, Kivi P. Prevalence of epicondylitis and tenosynovitis among meatcutters. *Scan J Work Environ Health* 1984;10:203–205.	Cross sectional	Observation	Clinical evaluation	HighForce and posture	7
Kurppa K, et al. Incidence to tenosynovitis or peritendinitis and epicondylitis in a meat processing factory. *Scand J Work Environ Health* 1991;17:32–37.	Cohort	Observation	Clinical evaluation	High force	6
Viikari-Juntura E, et al. Prevalence of epicondylitis and elbow pain in the meat-processing industry *Scand J Work Environ Health* 1991;17:38–45.	Cross sectional	Observation	Clinical evaluation	High force	1
Hand-Wrist					
Kuorinka I, Koskinen P. Occupational rheumatic diseases and upper limb strain in manual jobs in a light mechanical industry. *Scand J Work Environ Health* 1979;5(Suppl 3):39–47.	Cross sectional	Job analysis	Clinical evaluation	Repetition and posture	1
Luopajarvi T, et al. Prevalence of tenosynovitis and other injuries of the upper extremities in repetitive work. *Scand J Work Environ Health* 1979;5(Suppl 3):48–55.	Cross sectional	Questionnaire and videotape	Clinical evaluation	Repetition and posture	8*
Armstrong TJ, et al. Ergonomic considerations in hand and wrist tendinitis. *J Hand Surg* 1987;12A:830–837.	Cross sectional	Electromyelograph and videotape	Questionnaire and physical examination	LowForce-LowRep / HiForce-LowRep / LowForce-HiRep / HiForce-HiRep	1.0 / 2.0 / 2.0 / 29.0[a]
McCormack RR Jr, et al. Prevalence of tendinitis and related disorders of the upper extremity in a manufacturing workforce. *J Rheumatol* 1990;17:958–964.	Cross sectional	Job category	Clinical evaluation	Repetition	4[a]
Moore JS. Function, structure, and response of components of the muscle-tendon unit. In: Moore JS, Garg A, eds. *Occupational medicine, state of the art reviews.*Philadelphia: Handley & Belfus, 1992:713–740.	Cohort	Observation	Clinical evaluation	Force	24[a]

From ref. 7, with permission.
[a]Statistically significant at $p < 0.05$.
OR, odds ratio; RR, relative risk; NCT, nerve conduction test; MOD,moderate; Rep, repetitions.

TABLE 1B. *Studies of cumulative trauma disorders and repetitive strain injuries: tenosynovitis or peritendinitis studies*

Study	Task	Independent variable(s)	Dependent variable(s)	Psychophysical method(s)	Results/ recommendations
Snook SH. Maximum frequency of lift acceptable to male industrial workers. *Am Ind Hyg Assoc J* 1968;29, 531–536 and Psychophysical studies of physiological fatigue criteria. Hum Factors, 1969;11: 291–300.	Lifting boxes using arms	Box weight, lift height	MAF of lift Heart rate	MAF adjustment over 1 h	MAF decreased with height and weight of lift. No difference in heart rate between conditions
Garg A. Maximum frequency acceptable to female workers for one handed lifts in the horizontal plane *Ergonomics* 1982; 25:839–853	One-handed horizontal lifting	Load, reach distance	MAF of lift Heart rate FPE	MAF adjustment over 40-minute Borg RPE scale	Increasing the load weight and lifting distance reduced MAF
Hammarskjöld E. Shoulder-arm muscular activity and reproducibility in carpenters' work. *Clin Biomech* 1990;5:81–87.	Sawing, nailing, screwing	Task type, day, time of day	FPE EMG Force Motion Work time	Borg RPE scale	Screwing consistently rated as hard or very hard, sawing as somewhat hard, and nailing as fairly light
Armstrong TJ. Subjective worker assessments of hand tools used in automobile assembly *Am Ind Hyg Assoc J* 1989;50:639–645	Powered hand tool use (assembly work)	Tool and handle diameter. Vertical and horizontal work distance, gender, stature, hand size	Rating of weight, handle size, grip force, and comfort of tools used	Attribute rated using a continuous scale (0–10), anchored at 0, 5, and 10	Weight and grip force assessments correlated with tool mass Perceived handle size related to handle circumference. Discomfort increased with horizontal and verticalwork distance
Garg A. One-handed dynamic pulling strength with special reference to speed, handle height and angles of pulling. *Int J Industr Ergonomics* 1990;6:231–240.	One-handed handle pulling	Speed of pull; vertical height of handle, angle of pull	RPE—elbow, shoulder, back, comfort, pull strength	Borg RPE scale	RPE and strength decreased, comfort increased with increased pulling speed. Pull height and angle had little effect of RPE
Genaidy AM. Physiological and psychophysical responses to static, dynamic and combined arm tasks. *Appl Ergonomics* 1990;2:63–67	Holding wt. moving the lower arm about the elbow	Task type (static, dynamic, and combination) Weight lift frequency	RPE heart rate. blood pressure, time until exhaustion	Borg RPE scale	RPE increased, endurance time decreased with weight. Static task associated with greatest RPE and blood pressure, shortest endurance time. Lift frequency had no effect.

TABLE 1B. Continued.

Study	Task	Independent variable(s)	Dependent variable(s)	Psychophysical method(s)	Results/recommendations
Park D. Knife replacement studies at an automobile manufacturing plant. Proceedings of the Human Factors Society 35th Annual Meeting, San Francisco, CA, 1991.	Carpet trimming (3 studies)	Carpet type and direction of cut Knife temperature Blade angle	RPE, EMG Wrist position Grip force Length of cut	Borg CR-10 scale	RPE affected by carpet type and blade angle (straight blade associated with lowest RPE)
Snook SH. Psychophysical studies of repetitive wrist motion: Part I: Two day per week exposure. Ergonomics, (in press) and Part II. Five day per week exposure. Ergonomics (in press).	Wrist motion against resistance (2 studies)	Wrist motion and grip type Repetition rate Days of exposure (2 vs 5 days/wk)	MAT wrist strength isometric Tactile sensitivity force time	MAT ave record each minute for 7 h Discomfort recorded on series of graded scales (0–3)	MAT decreased with repetition and hour of day; greater for wrist flexion than extension. No MAT difference between days. Increase in weekly workload (day 2–5) produced 36.3% decrease in MAT
Examination of the effect of tool mass and work postures on perceived exertion for a screw driving task. Int J Indust Ergonomics 1993;12:105; Perceived exertion and discomfort associated with driving screws at various work locations and at different work frequencies. Ergonomics 1993;36:833–846; Preferred tool shapes for various horizontal & vertical work locations.Appl Occup Environ Hyg 1992;7:327–337; Effect of tool shape & work location on. Am Ind Hyg Assoc J 1993;54:383–391.	Driving screws (4 studies)	Vertical and horizontal work location; tool type; tool mass work rate	RPE discomfort rating	Borg CR-10 scale Body part discomfort survey	RPE increased with tool mass, vertical and horizontal work distance, and work pace
Marley RJ. Psychophysical frequency and sustained exertion at varying wrist posture for a drilling task. Ergonomics 1995;38:303–325; Kim Psychophysical frequency for a drilling task. Int J Indust Ergonomics 1993;12:209–218; Dahalan psychophysical frequency for a gripping task. Int J Indust Ergonomics 1993;12: 219–230.	1. Drilling sheet metal 2. Wire crimping simulated	1. Force, wrist flexion 2. Grip force as a % of MVC, grip duration	MAF RPE, BP EMG. No discomfort measure	MAF adjustment over a 20-min period. RPE-Borg scale	MAF decreased, RPE increased with increasing force, duration, and wrist flexion, RPE and MAF (−) correlated. RPE, HR, EMG, and blood pressure (+) correlated

Reference	Task	Variables	Measures	Results
Krawczyk S. Psychophysical determination of work design guidelines for repetitive upper extremity transfer tasks over an eight hour workday. Ann Arbor, MI, University of Michigan, 1993, Unpublished dissertation	3 studies:Moving plastic bottles and containers (combination task)	Bottle wt. freq. & distance & time. % time spent on each task.	1. RPE, discomfort 2. PW, RPE, discomfort 3. RPE, discomfort	RPE—10 cm visual analog scale (anchored at ends) Discomfort of 11 body parts determined over 8-hour period	RPE increased with weight and frequency but not distance of transfer. For combination task, RPE and discomfort were minimized when time was evenly split between tasks. PW decreased with increased frequency and distance of movement RPE and PW stable during workday; discomfort increased
Putz-Anderson V. Psychophysically determined work duration for limiting shoulder girdle fatigue from elevated manual work. Int J Indust Ergonomics 1993;36:833–846.	Lifting and lowering a tool handle (4 studies)	Discomfort level, force as a % of MVC & rate/force Repetition rate, tool weight & reach height	Work duration (time until onset of a specified level of fatigue)	Borg CR-10 scale used to designate fatigue/ discomfort criterion	Work duration increased with fatigue criterion; decreased with increased force, tool weight, reach, and repetition. Increases in force or repetition attenuated the other's effect. No change in average work time through workday. Limiting fatigue maintained rest effectiveness
Harber P. Subject-based rating of hand-wrist stressors. J Med 1994;36:84–89.	Repetitive grasping motions	Wrist position Force Repetition rate	RPE comfort (overall and wrist)	Brog CR-10 scale RPE Discomfort scale (1–8)	RPE and discomfort affected by grip type, force, wrist position, and rapid repetition
Grant KA. Psychophysical and EMG Correlates of force exertion in manual work. Int J Indust Ergonomics 1994;13:31–39.	Grasping and moving tool handles (3 studies)	Handle shape/ diameter Tool weight	RPE grip force forearm EMG	RPE measured using Borg CR-10 scale	RPE increased with weight, not affected by handle shape or diameter. RPE correlated with grip force, EMG

RPE, rating of perceived exertion; EMG, electromyography; MAF, max. acceptable frequency; MAT, max. acceptable torque; PW, preferred container weight; MVC, max. voluntary contracture; HR, heart rate; BP, blood pressure.
From ref. 7, with permission.

a particular exposure and some repetitive upper-extremity use lead to a particular health effect, commonly termed an *injury*. To test the hypothesis, *exposure* and *health effects* must be defined and some systematic way must be devised to determine the likelihood that the exposures and health effects are cause and effect in some way that minimizes biases. Examples cited to support that CTD/RSI is *not* caused by work include the following: (a) the incidence of Dupuytren's contracture appears to be greatest in Northern Europe and in emigrants of Celtic origin but is rare in Africa and Asia. At this time, the consensus favors the view that heavy manual labor in itself cannot cause Dupuytren's contracture but that a mild form of the disease can be aggravated by traumatizing an early nodule. (b) Beyond the poorly understood familial predisposition to primary generalized osteoarthritis that is manifest most prominently in women, considerable population differences are seen in the prevalence of osteoarthritis carpal metacarpal joint of thumb. The major factors accounting for these differences in the upper extremity appear to be both environmental and heritable in nature. Postmortem chimpanzee material has failed to demonstrate any evidence of severe osteoarthritis disease, suggesting that the configuration of modern man's trapeziometacarpal joint represents an evolutionary design compromise and a lack of anatomic evolution sufficient to keep pace with the changing functional demands of humans (104). (c) CTS and fitness studies showed deconditioned workers to be vulnerable to the risks of physical disuse. The incidence of CTS is two to three times greater in women than in men and peaks in premenopausal women (a possible relationship to retention of fluids and general swelling). Females employed outside the home have a lower incidence rate than female homemakers (59,105–108). Several other studies support the lower incidence rate among employed women, with keyboard users (including clerical workers and managers) having the lowest incidence of CTD and CTS (82,109,110). The incidence rate in workers covered by workers' compensation is strongly dependent on the method of reporting and legislative considerations. Legislative considerations were exemplified in the state of Oregon, where in 1988 passage of a law making CTD compensable resulted in a 52% increase in disabling claims for CTS the year after the law was enacted. This increase was followed by a steady decline in claims rate as loopholes were closed and criteria for causation were defined more sharply (82) (these are, of course, legal and political effects and indicators of a change CTD). (d) CTS studies of risk factors showed the strongest relationship to increased weight and body mass index (suggesting the effects of deconditioning on increasing the risk of the individual's musculoskeletal symptoms with increasing activities), followed by diabetes, thyroid disease, connective tissue disorders, amyloidosis, acromegalia, age, gender, oral contraceptive use, oophorectomy, and wrist dimension (111–118). (e) CTS is found in adults of all ages and often "runs" in families. Many times, these persons are not performing any unusually repetitive or forceful activities. CTS is also found in all occupations studied, regardless of the level of occupational hand use. Within a given group or occupation, persons with CTS are on average older, more overweight, less physically active, and have deeper, squarer wrists than those without CTS. Studies have identified 20-year veteran workers without CTS and novice workers who report CTS symptoms almost as soon as they begin work, in all occupations surveyed (again suggesting the effects of deconditioning) (111,114,118–121). Workers who report engaging in frequent avocational aerobic exercise were much less likely to report symptoms than workers who describe a sedentary lifestyle (113, 114,118). Work factors in 1984 made only a minimal contribution to predicting CTS in 1995, and most of that effect was to predict less, not more, CTS. Neither vibrations nor repetitions made an independent contribution, and hours of keyboard use was not associated with increased NCS (Nerve Conductor Study) values or CTS. These studies did not find median neuropathy and CTS to be specific to or characteristic of any occupation, but personal characteristics and lifestyle factors, including age, body mass index, wrist dimensions, and lack of aerobic exercise were more predictive of median-nerve slowing and CTS. Work factors such as duration of employment, keyboard time, keyboard rate, and sitting time (diagnosis by symptoms not clinical examination) were not independent predictors of median-nerve slowing or CTS. Their conclusions were that if multiple-factor causation is considered, CTS is not typically aggravated by work activities (119,122–124).

Therefore, the debate of causation for CTD/RSI and its relationship to work is likely to continue. How causation is defined is the key to how to answer the question; however, there are sufficient epidemiologic data to support a relationship to work activities. Because two factors make humans unique among living creatures, their psyche and their hands, the answer to the question will have many qualifiers. Current understanding suggests that activity related musculoskeletal pain (CTD, RSI, or MSD) has a complex multifactorial etiology, including not only the physical aspects of activity but also the psychosocial factors. Musculoskeletal disorders may involve muscle, tendons, ligaments, bones, joints, skin, and nerves. Their onset may be either acute (overexertion) or chronic (overuse). *Intrinsic* risk factors include age, gender, genetic, and linked elements. *Extrinsic* risk factors include activities in the workplace and nonwork environment. All activities have extrinsic risk factors associated with forcefulness, adverse posture, repetition or continuous activity, duration of exposure, temperature, vibration, and use of gloves. Most current models for musculoskeletal or neuromusculoskeletal injury are incomplete and frequently are based on tissue loads. They fail to compare tissue tolerance or failure data to the body's ability to repair. Although these models may help document the exposure of people to physical stressors during work, leisure, sports, and the activities of daily living, they will be difficult to develop and implement. Therefore, the solution lies in development of prevention while research continues for a better understanding of musculoskeletal pain, called CTD or RSI, in the workplace.

The Future

Work-related musculoskeletal symptoms or pain can be real, perceived, or fabricated. As important as the diagnosis and the treatment are for the restoration of the injured worker to the workplace, they cannot—except administratively—address the cause of CTD. Health professionals and employers alike must direct their attention to prevention of CTD, RSI, and MSD. Traditional approaches to injury reduction in the workplace have focused heavily on ergonomics and the methods of effecting change through manipulation of the physical environment. Beyond ergonomics and education, medical consultation broadens the scope of intervention to include active surveillance of the worker population by means of health screens, clinical examinations, and, when indicated, early referral for conservative management. A physician knowledgeable about CTD and familiar with the risks within the workplace is able to treat and rehabilitate work-related injuries optimally for the worker and the employer.

CUMULATIVE TRAUMA DISORDERS/REPETITIVE STRAIN INJURY OF THE BACK AND LOWER EXTREMITIES

Although causation of CTD/RSI in the upper extremity (work related versus non-work related) is still in dispute, the literature is resplendent with references for CTD/RSI of the back and lower extremities and their work-related relationship. Temporarily setting aside CTD/RSI of the upper extremity, this chapter now reviews CTD/RSI of the lower extremities.

For those who evaluate and treat great numbers of back strains and injuries, a system or algorithm should be set up based on whether he or she functions in a primary care or specialty capacity. The experienced examiner can determine readily real impairment from fabrication. Being deconditioned is a frequent cause of low back problems, but solid prevention programs, ongoing education, and practically applied ergonomics create a solid barrier against low back strains. The occasional frank disc herniation seems to defy all rules and predictions and may or may not be of repetitive or overuse origin. The literature gives some definitive insight about certain activities (work-related or recreational) and their relationship to spine pathology.

For example, a report from the University of Tokushima, Japan (125), states that children and adolescents who are actively involved in sports can demonstrate lesions of the posterior lumbar endplates, manifesting clinically in low back pain. The lesions, diagnosed by magnetic resonance (MR) imaging, were seen at the posterior inferior rim of the body of L-4 and at the superior rim of the sacrum. The posterior endplate lesions were considered to be nonarticular osteochondrosis. The University of Kumamoto, School of Medicine, in Japan (126), reported on acquired coccygeal nodules in long-distance bicycle riders with radiographic evidence of anterior bending or dislocation of the coccyx. The repetitive irritation of the bicycle saddle was believed to be the repeated stress etiology. Repetitive stress pain and injuries to the back and lower extremities in soccer referees in Denmark (127) were alleviated by shock-absorbing heel inserts, which proved to be both therapeutic and preventative. In a prospective study of 395 male infantry recruits in Israel (128), overexertional back pain was found in 18% during the 14 weeks of basic training. Increased lumbar lordosis was a risk factor for overexertional thoracic pain. Of the recruits with overexertional back pain, 65% were asymptomatic by the end of basic training, demonstrating the therapeutic effect of conditioning. Human tolerance of physical stresses and strains does have a limit, however, exemplified in the report by Volpin (129), from Haifa, relative to three military recruits who, during rigorous elite basic train-

ing (similar to U.S. Army Special Forces) sustained stress fractures of the sacrum following strenuous training. These recruits were in excellent physical condition before beginning the rigorous elite basic training; so deconditioning was not a factor, but rather human endurance was the key.

The University of Western Australia (130) gave a report on lumbar spine injuries from "fast bowling" in the game of cricket. The study, limited to persons aged 16 to 18 years, demonstrated a high incidence of back pain, always associated with radiologic abnormalities, especially pars interarticularis defects (seen in 54% of the cases) and intervertebral disc degeneration (seen in 63% of the cases). Actions involving "counterrotations" in the game were associated with a higher incidence of both injuries.

Some researchers consider ballet to be a sport, and others consider it a type of employment. In either case, the American Ballet Theater, of New York, was the focus of a study by Marshall (131) on overuse injuries in an occupation that rivals any other when looking at the extremes of kinesiology. The reduction of predisposing factors was considered to be of utmost importance in the successful management of overuse injuries to the spine and lower extremity, especially the foot. In fact, prevention was believed to require greater skill and attention than treatment of a primary lesion. The most common anatomic site of pain, stress lesions, and disability in ballet dancers is the forefoot (132). Schon (133), of the Department of Orthopedics, Union Memorial Hospital, Baltimore, published an article entitled "Foot and Ankle Problems in Dancers," which described the importance of both static and dynamic biomechanical evaluation of the leg, foot, and ankle conditions in dancers. He stated that the contributing factors may be of paramount importance and must be corrected by changes in techniques or training if the area of complaint is to be resolved.

The importance of stretching and strengthening exercises in the prevention of overuse running injuries is stressed by Ballas et al. (134) in *The American Family Physician.*

Overuse due to training errors is critical [too far, too fast, too soon]. He admonishes: "never run through pain."

Other articles of interest relative to overuse factors of the lower extremities are as follows: "Lower Limb Morphology and Risk of Overuse Injury among Male Infantry Trainees," by Cowan et al. (135), from Walter Reed Hospital, who describes the effect of anatomic variation on the risk of overuse injuries. He reported that the relative risk of overuse injury was significantly higher among participants with the most valgus knees, especially a Q-angle of more than 15 degrees, resulting in a significantly increased risk for stress fractures.

"A Prospective Study of the Effect of the Appropriateness of Foot-Shoe Fit and Training Shoe Type on the Incidence of Overuse Injuries Among Infantry Recruits" is a study by Finestone et al. (136), of the Israeli Defense Forces, who found that three shoe widths were required for each shoe length size to prevent overuse injuries in recruits. Recruits who trained in basketball shoes had a lower incidence of overuse injuries than those who trained in infantry boots. "Achilles Tendon Overuse Injuries," a study by Galloway et al. (137), of Yale, stressed the importance of stretching exercises to prevent injury and admonished the use of steroid injections into the Achilles tendon for tendonitis.

"Epidemiology of Podiatric Injuries in US Marine Recruits Undergoing Basic Training" is a study by Linenger and Shwayhat (138), of the University of California, San Diego, who analyzed 233,946 recruit days at risk among U.S. Marine recruits in basic training. They found that stress fractures of the foot were the most prevalent injury, followed by ankle sprains and Achilles tendonitis. "Patellofemoral Pain Caused by Overactivity, a Prospective Study of Risk Factors in Infantry Recruits" is a study by Milgrom et al. (139), who found that of 390 infantry recruits, the medial tibial intercondylar distance and isometric strength of the quadriceps (tested at 85 degrees knee flexion) had a statistically significant correlation with the incidence of patellofemoral pain caused by overactivity.

"The Accident-prone and Overuse-prone Profiles of the Young Athlete" is a report by Lysens et al. (140), of Belgium, who stated that the overuse-prone profile is based mainly on physical traits: a combination of muscle weakness, ligamentous laxity, muscle tightness, large body weight, long body length, a high explosive strength, and a malalignment of the lower limbs.

"Orthopedic History and Examination in the Etiology of Overuse Injuries," a contribution by Montgomery et al. (141), of the Department of Military Medicine, Uniformed Services University of Health Sciences, in Bethesda, Maryland, reported on pretraining factors that predispose to overuse injuries. Of 505 trainees entering an intense military training school, those whose running history exceeded 25 miles per week had a significantly lower incidence of stress fractures compared to those running 4 or fewer miles per week in the previous year.

Alignment and Anatomic Factors

Lower-extremity alignment and anatomic factors have been reported as major issues in overuse injuries of the lower extremities. Such reports are as follows:

"Lower Extremity Alignment and Risk of Overuse Injuries in Runners" is a report by Wen et al. (142), of the University of California—Los Angeles (UCLA) in which a group of 304 runners enrolled in a marathon training program was studied. The following relationships were reported: mileage with hamstring injuries, interval training with shin injuries, hard surfaces with back and thigh injuries, shoe-use patterns with foot and overall injuries, and body mass index with heel injuries. This group concluded that the lower-extremity alignment was not a major risk factor and admitted that prospective studies were needed to clarify this point.

"Anatomical Factors Associated with Overuse Sports Injuries" by Krivickas (143), of Harvard, gave a different opinion, stating that anatomic factors such as bony alignment, flexibility deficits, and ligamentous laxity do predispose athletes to develop overuse injuries. He described malalignment of the lower extremity as excess femoral anteversion, increased Q-angle, lateral tibial torsion, tibia vara, genu varum or valgum, subtalar varus, and excessive foot pronation. He also discussed the role of muscle inflexibility as a predisposition to overuse injuries. The importance of prehabilitation conditioning to decrease the risk of overuse injury was emphasized. Krivickas stated that overuse injuries develop when repetitive stress to bone and musculotendinous structures occurs at a greater rate than that at which the body can repair itself.

"Combined Effect of Foot Arch Structure and an Orthotic Device on Stress Fractures" is a paper by Simkin et al. (144), in Israel. Femoral and tibial stress fractures were more prevalent in the presence of feet with high arches, whereas the incidence of metatarsal fractures was higher in feet with low arches.

Biomechanical Factors

Rzonca and Baylis (145) describe in *Clinics in Podiatric Medicine and Surgery* that the common preventable causes of overuse injuries include training errors and biomechanical factors. They reported that biomechanical treatment would decrease the vast majority of lower-limb injuries.

Gresegor and Wheeler (146), of the Department of Physiology, UCLA, described how an alteration of bike-pedal design showed evidence of reducing the high injury overuse rate in cyclists by altering the shoe–pedal interface. This biomechanical change significantly alters the stresses on the lower extremity.

Perhaps many of the risk factors to overuse symptoms and injuries to the back and lower extremities can be lessened or minimized by such biomechanical means. Recent development and experimental use of antivibratory materials are another example of biomechanical alterations. The potential for improvement in this area is unlimited.

SUMMARY FOR CUMULATIVE TRAUMA DISORDERS/REPETITIVE STRAIN INJURY AND THEIR RELATIONSHIP TO WORK INJURY

Although theories and references have been presented in abundance, the treating physician or provider must deal with the patient on a one-to-one basis, looking at the individual issues pertinent to that case rather than a generic theory or philosophy. Although identification of risk factors and institution of prevention and ergonomics are touted as the keys to resolving the CTD dilemma, such activities or policies would have occurred long before the patient comes face-to-face with the provider. At the point of treatment, the various theories, philosophies, opinions, and biases are of no value to the provider who is required to analyze the complaint, formulate the diagnosis, and develop an appropriate treatment plan, which should including early return to work, if possible. The patient's musculoskeletal symptoms may be real, perceived, or fabricated. It is the physician's task ultimately to sort out which is which and to develop algorithms to treat the complaints and physical findings or lack thereof. Preexisting conditions, if they exist, must be considered. An absolute or definitive diagnosis of tissue damage is not necessary and may not be possible before reasonable treatment is implemented. Physicians tend to believe that every presenting problem must be categorized as some form of pathology and given a diagnostic code. Is that of reimbursement necessity or a matter of habit? Perhaps treating cumulative symptoms (even though such have a vague or disputed acronym) is more appropriate and cost effective by facilitating an early return to work. Frequently, patients' anxiety, depression, and anger are the results of a prolonged workers' compensation process (or lack thereof). Such emotional states preclude recovery and early return to work. The provider should intervene in such situations and function as a facilitator or a minicase manager. Early return to work results in a better self-image (147), an improved ability to cope (148), greater work survivability (149), an an enhanced ability to be self-sufficient; therefore, it is in the patient's (i.e., the employee) best interests (150–154).

Unfortunately, some authors have become so preoccupied with the debate of whether CTD/RSI is work related that the goal of prevention and early return to work is lost. Because a condition or diagnosis is overused or abused, the etiology is not necessarily altered. Because CTD/RSI are terms for symptoms or musculoskeletal pain, reasonable healthcare providers can conclude that these symptoms can and do occur with workplace activities and during regular living activities. In contrast to many stated calculations, most awake time (i.e., during the work week) of many people is spent in the workplace or on the job, particularly in recent years. Therefore, it can be reasonably concluded that at least some of the CTD/RSI can be linked to aggravation with work activities. It is the system's responsibility to determine whether the CTD/RSI symptoms are work related or not. This determination should be based on individual issues, the opinion of physicians, and the specific requirements of each state's workers' compensation program. If a dispute develops, the legal system must make a determination based on the facts. It is the physician's task to determine whether the complaints are diagnostic or not and to treat the symptoms and condition in accordance with the diagnosis. This responsibility may include appropriate management of the patient or referral to another facility, assisting with the bureaucratic determination of work relationships; if all other mechanisms have failed, the suggestion may be made for the patient to talk with an attorney.

So where does the answer lie? Not only are risk factors, prevention, and ergonomics required; but there must be a commitment from employers and employees to work together. This mutual involvement also requires the appropriate support from the legal community and government. The keys are identification of worksite risks; analyzing risk factors; train-

ing workers to deal with risks appropriately; developing management and worker cooperation; providing familiarity with respective worksites; employee input; and surveys, education, work conditioning, worksite research, and redesigning when needed.

The need for conditioning of a worker for a job or job task is often overlooked in our current workers' compensation system. Although Oriental cultures have known of this necessity and pursued it for decades, our culture and system rarely "condition" a worker for repetitive motions, positions, or tasks, even though athletes have appreciated and practiced the necessity in all major physical sports for years. Risk-reduction programs that include individual risk assessment in the posthire preplacement and use of conditioning or break-in periods have been quite successful in reducing occurrences of CTD, reducing costs, and improving work performance (13,155,156).

Research relative to forces, postures, motions, vibrations, temperature, magnitudes, repetitions, durations, and other conditions can go on forever, but no absolute solution will be found, because each factor varies with the individual worker. The confounders are endless. Some practical working solutions have been offered by the American College of Occupational and Environmental Medicine (ACOEM) in the articles "Ergonomic Tips to Prevent CTD" in *Business & Health* (157), "1997 Labor Day Checklist: Ergonomic Tips to Prevent Cumulative Trauma" in *ACOEM* (158), and "ACOEM's Eight Best Ideas for Workers' Compensation Reform" in *ACOEM Conference* (159). These reports offer concrete and reasonable immediate steps for prevention and for improvement of the workers' compensation system.

When considering the information in this text, it becomes apparent that the etiology of MSD/CTD is multifactorial for the individual and dependent on the individual's environment. Even with similar environments, each person has a highly variable presentation. When these individual presentations are combined with the unlimited individual confounders, the likelihood of establishing an absolute *objective paradigm* for etiology, diagnosis, and treatment becomes impossible. Additionally, science will have a hard time convincing the American public that workers should not be compensated if the workplace is a substantial factor in precipitating the pathology, even though the same condition would not have occurred in another person with a different physical makeup. For these and other reasons, it is our firm belief that the present issue of MSDs (CTDs or RSI) *ultimately* will be resolved at the political and administrative levels rather than on a scientific basis. Although physicians rely on science to produce answers, politics and industry actually dictate the application of such scientific knowledge. Therefore, scientific knowledge may be logically and reasonably applied to the workplace, or it may not. Fortunately for the individual worker, prevention based on individual risk factors offers the best opportunity to decrease the likelihood of MSD.

ACKNOWLEDGMENTS

Peggy Gardner, Ph.D., Executive Director, Research, Via Christi Health System reviewed this chapter. Reference support was by the Via Christi Medical Libraries, Kansas, and funding by The Hand Center.

REFERENCES

1. U.S. Bureau of Labor Statistics. *Survey of occupational injuries and illnesses, 1995.* Washington, DC: U.S. Government Printing Office, 1997.
2. Carrico HL. Virginia declares carpal tunnel not a job injury. *Occupational Health Management* 1996; July:79–80.
3. U.S. Bureau of Labor Statistics. *Survey of occupational injuries and illnesses in 1994.* Washington, DC: U.S. Department of Labor, U.S. Government Printing Office, 1996.
4. Luck JRJV, Florence DW. A brief history and comparative analysis of disability systems and impairment rating guides. *Orthop Clinic North Am* 1988;19: 839–844.
5. Melhorn JM. CTD RSI and their relationship to work injury, In: Spengler DM, Zeppieri JP, eds. *Workers' compensation case management: a multidisciplinary perspective.* Rosemont, IL: American Academy of Orthopaedic Surgeons, 1997:1–25.
6. Kaplan SJ, Glickel SZ, Eaton RG. Predictive factors in the non-surgical treatment of carpal tunnel syndrome. *J Hand Surg* 1990;15B:106–108.
7. American Academy of Orthopaedic Surgeons. *Repetitive motion disorders of the upper extremity.* Rosemont, IL: American Academy of Orthopaedic Surgeons, 1995.
8. U.S. Bureau of Labor Statistics. *Occupational injuries and illnesses: counts, rates, and characteristics, 1994.* Washington, DC: U.S. Department of Labor, U.S. Government Printing Office, 1997, pp. 1–185.
9. Bernard BP, Sauter SL, Fine LJ, Petersen MR, Hales TR. Psychosocial and work organization risk factors for cumulative trauma disorders in the hands and wrists of newspaper employees. *Scand J Work Environ Health* 1992;18:119–120.
10. Hales TR, Sauter SL, Peterson MR. Musculoskeletal disorders among visual display terminal users in a telecommunications company. *Ergonomics* 1994;37: 1603–1621.
11. BLS. *Survey of occupational injuries and illnesses, 1996.* Washington, DC: U.S. Government Printing Office, 1998.
12. Melhorn JM. CTD: Carpal tunnel syndrome, the facts and myths. *Kans Med* 1994;95:189–192.
13. Melhorn JM. Occupational injuries: the need for preventive strategies. *Kans Med* 1994;95:248–251.
14. Vender MI, Kasdan ML, Truppa KL. Upper extremity disorders: a literature review to determine work-relatedness. *J Hand Surg* 1995;20A:534–541.
15. Melhorn JM. Physician support and employer options for reducing risk of CTD, In: Spengler DM, Zippieri JP, eds. *Workers' compensation case management: a multidisciplinary perspective.* Rosemont, IL: American Academy of Orthopaedic Surgeons, 1997:21–34.
16. Melhorn JM. CTD in the workplace treatment outcomes, In: *Seventeenth Annual Workers' Compensation and Occupational Medicine Seminar.* Boston: Speak, 1997:168–178.
17. Melhorn JM. CTD solutions for the 90's: prevention. In: *Seventeenth Annual Workers' Compensation and Occupational Medicine Seminar.* Boston: Speak, 1997:234–245.
18. Melhorn JM. Identification of individuals at risk for developing CTD, In: Spengler DM, Zippieri JP, eds. *Workers' compensation case management: a multidisciplinary perspective.* Rosemont, IL: American Academy of Orthopaedic Surgeons, 1997:41–51.
19. Melhorn JM. Upper-extremity cumulative trauma disorders on workers in aircraft manufacturing [Letter, Response] upper extremities cumulative trauma disorders. *J Occup Environ Med* 1998;40:103–104.
20. Vannier FP, Rose JF. Etiologies and prevalence of occupational injuries to the upper extremity, In: Kasdan ML, ed. *Occupational hand and upper extremity injuries and diseases.* Philadelphia: Hanley & Belfus, 1991:53–60.
21. Geerts A, Kornblith B, Urmson J. *Compensation for bodily harm.* Brussels: Editions Labor, 1977.
22. Sand R. *Vers La Medecine Sociale.* University of Paris, Paris: 1948.
23. Louis DS. A historical perspective of workers and the work place, In: Millender LH, Louis DS, Simmons BP, eds. *Occupational disorders of the upper extremity.* New York: Churchill Livingstone, 1992:15–18.

24. McKendrick A. *Malingering and its detection.* Edinburgh: E & S Livingstone, 1912, pp. 1–45.

25. Conn HR. Tenosynovitis. *Ohio State Med J* 1931;9: 713–714.

26. U.S. Congress. *Occupational Safety and Health Act of 1970, 29 USC 651.* Washington: U.S. Government Printing Office, 1970.

27. Viegas SF. Extension block pinning for proximal interphalangeal joint fracture dislocations: preliminary report of a new technique. *J Hand Surg* 1992;17A: 896–901.

28. Equal Employment Opportunity Commission. *ADA enforcement guidance: preemployment disability-related questions and medical examinations.* Washington, D.C.: U.S. Printing Agency, 1998, pp. 1–26.

29. Collie J. *Malingering and feigned sickness.* London: Edward Arnold, 1913.

30. Hammer AW. Tenosynovitis. *Med Rec* 1934;140: 353–354.

31. Arthur WC. Discussion of paper by Conn. *Ohio State Med J* 1931;9:715–716.

32. Brain WR, Wright AD, Wilkerson M. Spontaneous compression of both median nerves in the carpal tunnel: six cases treated surgically. *Lancet* 1947;1: 277–282.

33. Melhorn JM. Management of work related upper extremity musculoskeletal disorders. In: *Kansas case managers annual meeting.* Wichita: Wesley Rehabilitation Hospital, 1998:16–25.

34. Rosen G. *The worker's hand.* Summit, New Jersey: CIBA Symposium, 1942.

35. Ramazzini B. *DeMorbis artificum diatriba: diseases of workers.* Chicago: University of Chicago Press, 1940, pp. 1–11.

36. Bell C. Partial paralysis of the muscles of the extremities, In: *The nervous system of the human body.* London: Taylor and Francis, 1833:57–88.

37. Robinson E. Case of telegraphist's cramp. *BMJ* 1882; 42:880–881.

38. Nakaseko M, Tokunage R, Hosokawa M. History of occupational cervicobrachial disorders in Japan and remaining problems. *J Hum Ergol (Tokyo)* 1982;11: 7–16.

39. Westerling D, Jonsson BG. Pain from the neck-shoulder region and sick leave. *Scand J Soc Med* 1980: 131–136.

40. Luopajarvi T, Juorinka I, Virolainen M, Holmberg M. Prevalence of tenosynovitis and other injuries of the upper extremities in repetitive work. *Scand J Work Environ Health* 1979;5:48–55.

41. Hosman J. *Adaptation to muscular effort.* Stockholm: University of Stockholm, 1967.

42. Hult L. A field investigation of a non-selected material of 1200 workers in different occupations with special references to disc degeneration and so-called muscular rheumatism. *Acta Orthop Scand* 1954;17:7–102.

43. Ireland DCR. Repetition strain injury: the Australian experience-1992 update. *J Hand Surg* 1995;20A: S53–S56.

44. Browne CD, Nolan BM, Faithfull DK. Occupational repetition strain injuries guidlines for diagnosis and managment. *Med J Aust* 1984;140:329–332.

45. Australian Public Service Association. *Sufferer's handbook: repetition strain.* Melbourne: Union Media Services, 1984.

46. Reilly PA. Repetitive strain injury: from Australia to the UK. *J Psychosomat Res* 1995, Aug:783–788.

47. Great Britain and Ireland post office. Telegraphists' cramp report. *Her Majesty's Marationery Office,* 1911, pp. 1–12.

48. Goodman RC. An aggressive return-to-work program in surgical treatment of carpal tunnel syndrome: A comparison of costs. *Plast Reconstr Surg* 1989;89: 715–717.

49. Gowers WR. *A manual for diseases of the nervous system.* Philadelphia: Blakiston, 1888.

50. Silvain PB. Psychological injury evidence in workers' compensation cases: the manipulation of symptoms, In: *Annual Workers' Compensation and Occupational Medicine Seminar.* Boston: Speak, 1997:335–360.

51. Maeda K, Horiguchi S, Hosokawa M. History of the studies of occupational cervicobrachial disorders in Japan and remaining problems. *J Hum Ergol (Tokyo)* 1982;11:17–29.

52. Ohara H, Aoyama H, Itani T. Health hazard among cash register operators and the effects of improved working conditions. *J Hum Ergol (Tokyo)* 1976:31–40.

53. Muto T, Sakurai H. Relation between exercise and absenteeism due to illness and injury in manufacturing companies in Japan. *J Occup Med* 1994;35:995–999.

54. Hagberg L, Slevik G. Tendon excursion and dehiscence during early controlled mobilization after flexor tendon repair in zone II an x-ray stereophotogrammetric analysis. *J Hand Surg* 1991;16:669–680.

55. Langlais F, Thomazeau H, Bourgin T, Derennes A, Allard G. Social and professional status of 184 manual workers treated in a microsurgical emergency unit. *Ann Chir Main Memb Super* 1990;9:252–260.

56. Chan KK, Ling LC. Back and neck problems in a teaching institution. *J R Soc Health* 1988;108:182–184.

57. Melhorn JM. CTD's: risk assessment applications in the workplace, In: *Science symposium.* McPherson, Kansas: McPherson College, 1985:1–12.

58. Lucire Y. Neurosis in the workplace. *Med J Aust* 1986; 145:323–327.

59. Hocking B. Epidemiological aspects of repetition strain injury in telecom Australia. *Med J Aust* 1987;147: 218–222.

60. Task Force. *Repetition strain injury in the Australian public service.* Canberra: Australian Government Publishing Service, 1985.

61. McDermott FT. Repetition strain injury and review of current understanding. *Med J Aust* 1986;144:196–200.

62. Ryan GA, Mullerworth J, Pimble J. The prevalence of repetition injury in data process operators. In: Adams AS, Stevenson MG, eds. *Ergonomics and technological changes.* Sydney, Australia: Ergonomics Society, 1984:279–288.

63. Stone WE. Repetitive strain injuries. *Med J Aust* 1983; 2:616–618.

64. Taylor RS, Pitcher M. Medical and ergonomic aspects of an industrial dispute concerning occupational-related conditoins in data process operators. *Community Health Studies* 1984;8:172–180.

65. Macmillan J. What you must know about repetition strain injury. *Law Institute Journal* 1984;11: 1305–1309.

66. Ireland DCR. A review of the Australian RSI/CTD experience. *ASSH* (American Society for Surgery of the Hand) 1995;2:1–9.

67. Miller MH, Topliss DJ. Chronic upper limb pain syndrome (repetitive strain injury) in the Australian workforce: a systematic cross sectional rheumatological study of 229 patients. *J Rheumatol* 1988;15: 1705–1712.

68. Littlejohn GO. Repetitive strain syndrome: an Australian experience. *J Rheumatol* 1986;13:1004–1006.

69. Morgan RG. RSI. *Med J Aust* 1986;144:56–59.

70. Center for Disease Control. *Cumulative trauma disorders in the workplace. Bibliography.* Cincinnati: US Dept. Health & Human Services, 1995.

71. Manske PR. Repetitive strain: putting it in perspective. *J Hand Surg* 1997;22A:1–2.

72. Kasdan ML. *Occupational hand and upper extremity injuries and diseases.* St. Louis: Mosby--Year Book, 1991.

73. Brown PW. Less than ten—surgeons with amputated fingers. *J Hand Surg* 1982;7:31–37.

74. Adams D. Workers' compensation: psychology's role in treatment and risk management. *Psychotherapy Bulletin* 1992;27:17.

75. Orlandi MA. Health promotion technology transfer: organizational perspectives. *Can J Public Health* 1996;87:S28–33.

76. Bonica JJ. *The management of pain.* Philadelphia: Lea & Febiger, 1990.

77. Dallenback KM. History and present status. *Am J Psychol* 1931;52:331–333.

78. Merskey H. Classification of chronic pain. *Pain* 1986; 3:215–216.

79. MacMahon B, Pugh TF. *Epidemiology: principles and methods.* Boston: Little, Brown and Company, 1970.

80. Wright TW, Glowxzewskie F, Wheller D, Miller G, Cowin D. Excursion and strain of the median nerve. *J Hand Surg* 1996;78A:1897–1903.

81. Kasdan ML, Vender MI, Lewis K, Stallings SP, Melhorn JM. Carpal tunnel syndrome: effects of litigation on utilization of health care and physician workload. *J Ky Med Assoc* 1996;94:287–290.

82. Franklin GM, Haug J, Heyer N. Occupational carpal tunnel syndrome in Washington State, 1984–1988. *American Journal of Public Health* 1991;81:741–745.

83. Armstrong TJ, Fine LJ, Goldstein SA, Lifshitz YR, Silverstein BA. Ergonomic considerations in hand and wrist tendinitis. *J Hand Surg* 1987;12A:830–837.

84. Nilsson T, Hagberg M, Burstrom L, Kihlberg S. Impaired nerve conduction in the carpal tunnel of platers and truck assemblers exposed to hand-arm vibration. *Scand J Work Environ Health* 1994;20:189–199.

85. Meenan RF, Anderson JJ, Kazis LE, et al. Outcome assessment in clinical trails: Evidence for the sensitivity of a health status measure. *Arthritis Rheum* 1984;27: 1344–1352.

86. Silverstein BA, Fine LJ, Armstrong TJ. Hand wrist cumulative trauma disorders in industry. *Br J Ind Med* 1986;43:779–784.

87. Craig EV. *The shoulder.* New York: Raven, 1995.

88. Goldstein SA, Armstrong TJ, Chaffin DB, Matthews LS. Analysis of cumulative strain in tendons. *J Biomechem* 1987;20:1–6.

89. Bovenzi M, Zadinin A, Franzinelli A, Borgogni F. Occupational musculoskeletal disorders in the neck and upper limbs of forestry workers exposed to hand-arm vibration. *Ergonomics* 1991:547–562.

90. Mckenna KM, McGrann S, Blann AD. An investigation into the acute vascular effects of riveting. *Br J Ind Med* 1993:160–166.

91. Bovenzi M. Italian study group on physical hazards in the stone industry: hand-arm vibration syndrome and dose-response relation for vibration induced white finger among quarry drillers and stonecarvers. *Occup Environ Med* 1994:779–784.

92. Weislander G, Norback D, Gothe CJ, Juhlin L. Carpal tunnel syndrome and exposure vibration, repetitive wrist movements, and heavy manual work: a case-referent study. *Br J Ind Med* 1989:43–47.

93. Goodman HV, Gilliatt RW. The effect of treatment on median nerve conduction in patients with the carpal tunnel syndrome. *Ann Phys Med* 1961;6:137–155.

94. Mesgarzadeh M, Schneck CD, Bonakdarpour A, Mitra A, Conaway D. Carpal tunnel: MR imaging. Part II. Carpal tunnel syndrome. *Radiology* 1989;171:749–754.

95. Mackinnon SE, Novak CB. Clinical perspective repetitive strain in the workplace. *J Hand Surg* 1997;22A: 2–15.

96. Armstrong TJ, Chaffin DB. Carpal tunnel syndrome and selected personal attributes. *J Occup Environ Med* 1979;21:481–486.

97. Silverstein BA, Fine LJ, Armstrong TJ. Occupational factors in carpal tunnel syndrome. *Am J Ind Med* 1987; 11:343–358.

98. Armstrong TJ, Silverstein BA. Upper-extremity pain in the workplace-role of usage in causality. In: *Clinical concepts in regulating musculoskeletal illness*, 1987: 333.

99. Fitzpatrick R, Zeibland S, Jenkinson C, Mowat A. A comparison of the sensitivity to change of several health status instrustments in rheumatoid arthritis. *J Rheumatol* 1993;20:429–436.

100. Warwick R, Williams PL. *Gray's anatomy.* Philadelphia: WB Saunders, 1973.

101. Hadler NM. Arm pain in the workplace: a small area analysis. *J Occup Environ Med* 1992;34:113–119.

102. American Academy of Orthopaedic Surgeons. *Orthopaedic ICD-9-CM expanded.* Park Ridge, IL: American Academy of Orthopaedic Surgeons, 1996.

103. Reid J, Ewan C, Lowy E. Pilgrimage of pain: the illness experiences of woman with repetition strain injury and the search for credibility. *Soc Sci Med* 1991; 32:601–612.

104. Kellgren, Lawrence. Epidemiology. *J Clin Epidemiol* 1992;45:373–376.

105. Phalen GS. The carpal tunnel syndrome: clinical evaluation of 598 hands. *Clin Orthop* 1972;83:29–40.

106. Stevens JC, Beard CM, O'Fallon WM. Conditions associated with carpal tunnel syndrome. *Mayo Clin Proc* 1992;67:541–543.

107. Evans RB. A study of the zone 1 flexor tendon injury and implications for treatment. *J Hand Ther* 1990;3: 133–148.

108. Stockbridge H. *Attending doctor's handbook.* Olympia: State of Washington Dept of Labor, 1996.

109. Klasson SC, Adams BD. Biomechanical evaluation of chronic boutonniere reconstructions. *J Hand Surg* 1992;17A:868–874.

110. Nathan PA, Takigawa K, Keniston RC, Meadows KD, Lockwood RS. Slowing of sensory conduction of the median nerve and carpal tunnel syndrome in Japanese and American industrial workers. *J Hand Surg* 1994; 19B:30–34.

111. Nathan PA, Keniston RC, Myers LD. Longitudinal study of median nerve sensory conduction in industry: relationship to age, gender, hand dominance, occupational hand use, and clinical diagnosis. *J Hand Surg* 1992;17A:850–851.

112. Nathan PA, Keniston RC, Meadows KD, Lockwood RS. Predictive value of nerve conduction measurements at the carpal tunnel. *Muscle Nerve* 1993;16:1377–1382.

113. Rockwood CA Jr, Green DP, Bucholz RW, Heckman JD. *Fractures in adults.* Philadelphia: Lippincott-Raven, 1996.

114. Nathan PA, Keniston RC, Meadows KD, Lockwood RS. The relationship between body mass index and the diagnosis of carpal tunnel syndrome. *Muscle Nerve* 1994;17:1491–1493.

115. Werner RA, Albers JW, Franzblau A, Armstrong TJ. The relationship between body mass index and the diagnosis of carpal tunnel syndrome. *Muscle Nerve* 1994;17:632–636.

116. Stallings SP, Kasdan ML, Soergel TM, Corwin HM. A case–control study of obesity as a risk factor for carpal tunnel syndrome in a population of 600 patients presenting for independent medical examination. *J Hand Surg* 1997;22 A:211–215.

117. Radecki P. The familial occurrence of carpal tunnel syndrome. *Muscle Nerve* 1994;17:325–330.

118. Nathan PA, Keniston RC, Meadows KD, Lockwood RS. Nerve conduction studies and carpal tunnel syndrome. *Am J Ind Med* 1995;27:311–312.

119. Nathan PA, Keniston RC, Myers LD, Meadows KD. Obesity as a risk factor for slowing of sensory conduction of the median nerve in industry. a cross-sectional and longitudinal study involving 429 workers. *J Occup Environ Med* 1992;34:379–383.

120. Nathan PA, Meadows KD, Doyle LS. Occupations as a risk factor for impaired sensory conductions of the median nerve at the carpal tunnel. *J Hand Surg* 1988; 13B:167–170.

121. Chen LE, Seaber AV, Urbaniak JR. The influence of magnitude and duration of crush load on functional recovery of the peripheral nerve. *J Reconstr Microsurg* 1993;9:299–307.

122. Nathan PA, Keniston RC. Carpal tunnel syndrome and its relation to general physical condition. *Hand Clin* 1993;9:253–261.

123. Nathan PA, Meadows KD, Doyle LS. Relationship of age and sex to sensory conduction of the median nerve at the carpal tunnel and associations of slowed conduction with symptoms. *Muscle Nerve* 1988;11: 1149–1150.

124. Nathan PA, Doyle LS, Meadows KD. Comparison of sensory latencies of the median nerve at the carpal tunnel among juveniles and adults. *Bull Hosp Jt Dis* 1975; 49:85.

125. Ikata T, Morita T, Katoh S, Tachibana K, Maoka. Lesions of the lumbar posterior end plate in children and adolescents. *J Bone Joint Surg Br* 1995;77B:951–955.

126. Nakamura A, Inoue Y, Ishihara T, Matsunaga W, Ono T. Acquired coccygeal nodule due to repeated stimulation by bicycle saddle. *J Dermatol* 1995;22:365–369.

127. Fauno P, Kalund S, Andreasen I, Jorgensen U. Soreness in lower extremities and back is reduced by use of shock absorbing heel inserts. *Int J Sports Med* 1993; 14:288–290.

128. Milgrom C, Finestone A, Lev B, Wiener M, Floman Y. Overexertional lumbar and thoracic back pain among recruits: A prospective study of risk factors and treatment regimes. *J Spinal Disord* 1993;6:187–193.

129. Volpin G, Milgrom C, Goldsher D, Stein H. Stress fractures of the sacrum. following strenuous activity. *Clin Orthop* 1989;243:184–188.

130. Hardcastle P, Annear P, Foster DH, et al. Spinal abnormalities in young fast bowlers. *J Bone Joint Surg Br* 1992;74B:421–425.

131. Marshall P. Rehabilitation of overuse foot injuries in athletes and dancers. *Clin Sports Med* 1988;7:175–191.

132. Van de Meulebroucke B, Dereymaeker G. Stress lesions of the forefoot in ballet dancers. *Acta Orthop Belg* 1994;60(Suppl 1):47–49.

133. Schon LC. Foot and ankle problems in dancers. *Md Med J* 1993;42:267–269.

134. Ballas MT, Tytko J, Cookson D. Common overuse running injuries: diagnosis and management. *Am Fam Physician* 1997;55:2473–2484.

135. Cowan DN, Jones BH, Frykman PN, et al. Lower limb morphology and risk of overuse injury among male infantry trainees. *Med Sci Sports Exerc* 1996; 28:945–952.

136. Finestone A, Shlamkovitch N, Elvad A, Karp A, Milgrom C. Prospective study of the effect of the appropriateness of foot-shoe fit and training shoe type on the incidence of overuse injuries among infantry recruits. *Mil Med* 1992;157:489–490.

137. Galloway MT, Jokl P, Dayton OW. Achilles tendon overuse injuries. *Clin Sports Med* 1992;11:771–782.

138. Linenger JM, Shwayhat AF. Epidemiology of podiatric injuries in US marine recruits undergoing basic training. *J Am Podiatr Med Assoc* 1992;82:269–271.

139. Milgrom C, Finestone A, Eldad A, Shlamkovitch N. Patellofemoral pain caused by overactivity: a prospective study of the risk factors in infantry recruits. *J Bone Joint Surg Am* 1991;73A:1041–1043.

140. Lysens RJ, Ostyn MS, Vande Auweele Y, Lefevre J, Vuylsteke M, Renson L. The accident-prone and overuse-prone profile of the young athlete. *Am J Sports Med* 1989;17:612–619.

141. Montgomery LC, Nelson FR, Norton JP, Deuster PA. Orthopedic history and examination in the etiology of overuse injuries. *Med Sci Sports Exerc* 1989;21: 237–243.

142. Wen DY, Puffer JC, Schmalzried TP. Lower extremity alignment and risk of overuse injuries in runners. *Med Sci Sports Exerc* 1997;29:1291–1298.

143. Krivickas LS. Anatomical factors associated with overuse sports injuries. *Sports Med* 1997;24:132–146.

144. Simkin A, Leichter I, Giladi M, Stein M, Milgrom C. Combined effect of foot arch structure and an orthotic device on stress fractures. *Foot Ankle* 1989;10:25–29.

145. Rzonca EC, Baylis WJ. Common sports injuries to the foot and leg. *Clin Podiatr Med Surg* 1988;5:591–612.

146. Gregor RJ, Wheeler JB. Biomechanical factors associated with shoe/pedal interfaces, implications for injury. *Sports Med* 1994;17:117–131.

147. Bernacki EJ, Tsai SP. Managed care for workers' compensation: three years of experience in an "employee choice" state. *J Occup Environ Med* 1996;38: 1091–1097.

148. Bigos SJ, Spengler DM, Martin NA, et al. Back injuries in industry: A retrospective study. III. Employee related factors. *Spine* 1986;11:252–256.

149. Melhorn JM. CTD injuries: an outcome study for work survivability. *Journal of Workers' Compensation* 1996; 5:18–30.

150. Burke SA, Harms-Constas CK, Aden PS. Return to work/work retention outcomes of a functional restoration program: a multi-center, prospective study with a comparison group. *Spine* 1994;19:1880–1885.

151. Devlin M, O'Neill P, MacBride R. Position paper in support of timely return to work programs and the role of the primary care physician. *Ontario Medical Association* 1994;61:1–45.

152. Bruce WC, Bruce RS. Return-to-work programs in the unionized company. *Journal of Workers' Compensation* 1996;5:9–17.

153. Dworkin RH, Handlin DS, Richlin DM, Rrand L, Vannucci C. Unraveling the effects of compensation, litigation, and employment on treatment response in chronic pain. *Pain* 1985;23:49–59.

154. Hall H, McIntosh G, Melles T, Holowachuk B, Wai E. Effect of discharge recommendations on outcome. *Spine* 1994;19:2033–2037.

155. Melhorn JM. A prospective study for upper-extremity cumulative trauma disorders of workers in aircraft manufacturing. *J Occup Environ Med* 1996;38:1264–1271.

156. Melhorn JM. Prevention of CTD in the workplace, In: *Workers' Comp Update 1998*. Walnut Creek, CA: Council on Education in Management, 1998:101–124.

157. Ergonomic tips to prevent CTD. *Business & Health* 1998;16:45–47.

158. American College of Occupational and Environment Medicine. 1997 labor day checklist: ergonomic tips to prevent cumulative trauma. *ACOEM Conference* 1997; 9:1–2.

159. American College of Occupational and Environment Medicine. ACOEM's eight best ideas for workers' compensation reform. *ACOEM Conference* 1997;4:4.

Occupational Musculoskeletal Disorders
edited by T. G. Mayer, R. J. Gatchel, and P. B. Polatin.
Lippincott Williams & Wilkins, Philadelphia © 2000.

17

Problems of the Aging Worker

David F. Fardon

Knoxville Orthopaedic Clinic, Southeastern Orthopaedics, Knoxville, Tennessee 37909

The term *aging* poses several difficulties as it relates to work. Aging is inseparable from life. Biologically, aging can be considered to begin with maturity, or even before, and to extend throughout life. Indeed, the work life of some professionals (gymnasts, tennis players, perhaps some theoretical mathematicians) may start to decline at ages not far from biological maturity and long before many careers (judges, executive officers) begin. Posner, whose text explores the nuances of meaning of the terms *aging* and *old age*, defines aging in three general contexts: *bodily decline*, including such functions as reaction time and running speed as well as susceptibility to disease; *cognitive change*, including the normal decline in memory and a shift toward concrete knowledge relative to imagination; and *proximity to death*, with all the related legal, personal, and social implications (1).

Drawing conclusions from the medical literature about the aging worker is confounded by an absence of consistent definition of the group. Many studies of the aging worker address changes that occur between the fourth and sixth decades of life (2,3). Another problem is confounding by selective turnover in employment, which may result in constant complaint rates despite declining health and capacity (4). Most studies of work-related injuries either cut the groupings off at age 64 years or include everyone aged over 64 in one group. Depending on job and individual strengths, many people think of themselves as

being at the top of their work careers at ages well beyond 60.

This chapter considers the problems of the aging worker in the context of the "aged worker" as opposed to the much less specific "aging working." In general, and more because of social than physiologic reasons, persons over age 65 are the subjects of this discussion.

Acute problems the older worker may face in the workplace differ little from those encountered by younger workers; however, the context onto which those problems are imposed may be quite unique and complex. Not only specific medical problems, but also what it means to be "aged" and how concepts and particular circumstances of "work" relate to aging are important factors.

Aging is normal. Normal aging is not the result of accumulated effects of accidents and disease. Aging, quite apart from injury and illness, results from changes that may cause problems for the worker.

Although everyone ages, they do so at different rates. Besides the disparate starting capabilities from which the variable changes of aging occur, time increases the likelihood that illness or injury will superimpose specific medical complications on the normal decline of aging. Normal decline in aerobic and muscular capacities reduces capabilities for certain job tasks, requiring, for some workers, adjustment in the physical workload (5). As effects of accidents and illness accumulate, they affect the older worker more because the disturbed homeostasis of aging reduces the ability to adapt and because comorbidities potentiate the effects of one another. Because normal aging and the diseases that accrue to the aged involve multiple systems and the ability to adapt to a challenge to one system depends on the health of others, it is not possible to isolate the musculoskeletal system in the context of a discussion of their aging worker. As Buckwalter et al. stated, in their excellent review of the effects of aging on the biology of soft tissues, musculoskeletal impairments are among the most prevalent functional impairments of older people (6). Fear of loss of function may be greater among older people than fear of dying and may be the paramount health concern of the elderly (7). Physical disability is a major adverse factor in the health of older adults (8).

Medical and social advances have not only increased longevity but have, for the many who have benefited from modern care of fractures, arthritis, cataracts, vascular disease, and other conditions, improved function during the extended years of life. Health-preserving personal strategies, such as exercise, tobacco avoidance, and weight control, can help to reduce disability late in life (9). The result is a heterogeneous population of older people. What "working" means is less clear for older people. Retirement from a workforce defined by hours employed in exchange for taxable wages may be driven by legal and economic considerations for many who continue to work in other ways. Retirement at an older age correlates with health (10); however, most current data are influenced heavily by arbitrary retirement ages that have relatively little to do with health and function. Work outside the usual parameters, such as volunteer work, household production, and part-time or non-public work, is worth billions of dollars to the national economy and is provided in large part by older, "retired" persons. Medical concerns about the health of the aged have increased in response to the gerontification of developed countries. Eighty editors of major medical journals chose aging as the most important topic for their second (1997) global theme issue (reemerging microbial trends was the first (11). In 1995, the American Academy of Orthopaedic Surgeons launched an initiative to address issues related to the aging orthopedic patient (12). Those efforts and the preponderance of contemporary geriatric medical literature do not directly address problems of the older worker, a topic that has been understudied, perhaps because of the dizzying array of variables that face those who try to define aging, working, and how the two relate.

Although medical reports often are grouped by chronological age, the World Health Organization, since 1959, has recommended that health is best measured by function rather than by age or pathology (13). Besides familiar examples of people like Verdi, Picasso, and Shaw, who created great works in their 80s and 90s, millions of "ordinary" people in their 60s and 70s function as though they are middle-aged and, in fact, think of themselves as middle-aged. John Glenn, at age 77, decided to defer another term in the United States Senate in favor of resuming his career as an astronaut, partly in support of the increasing interest in research for problems of aging (14). An 87-year-old tennis player, asked to define the common denominator driving competitors of tournaments sponsored by the United States Tennis Association for those over 85, said, "The common denominator is that we are still alive" (15).

DEMOGRAPHICS

In 1851, 3% of the U.S. population was over age 65 and 0.37% over age 80; in the year 2000, 12.8% will be over 65 and 3.3% over 80: by 2020, there will likely be 17.5% over age 65 and 3.9% over age 80 (16). At present, an American woman aged 65 can expect to live 19 more years, and those surviving to age 85 can expect to live 10 more years (7). Age-matched gender comparisons indicate that, although at a given age men are closer to death, they are no less healthy and functional than women of the same age (17).

The effects of such numbers on the demand for health care are obvious. Not only do people live longer, but they stay healthier and expect to stay functional into their advanced ages, creating demands on health providers to maintain them. Of Americans over age 65, about 85% have at least one chronic illness; of those over age 85, about 60% have two or more chronic illnesses (18). Whereas more people live with disability, health benefits that have produced longevity also have reduced disabilities, as demonstrated by one study that concluded that there were 1.4 million fewer disabled elders in 1994 than there would have been had the 1982 rate of disability persisted (19). About two-thirds of medical care for the elderly is paid by government programs sponsored for that purpose, and about 11% is paid as private expenditures (20).

Thirteen percent of licensed drivers are over age 65 (21). Although accident rates per mile driven are higher among older than middle-aged (although not compared to young) drivers, older people drive fewer miles and at lower speeds; so the number of accidents and the harm inflicted per accident are less for older drivers (22). Crime is uncommon among the elderly. Arrests of persons over 60, which is approximately 20% of the population, consitute a meager 1.4% of all arrests (23).

Older people, as a whole, in American society are materially well off and influential. Between 1970 and 1984, the median incomes of Americans over 65 rose by 35% (24). The elderly have strong voting records and share many interests on political issues. Among the most powerful forces in American culture, its judiciary is composed of its oldest workforce (1).

Paradoxically, some data show that the retirement age in the United States has been shifting toward earlier retirement (25). The numbers of people who retired at age 65 increased abruptly with passage of the Social Security Act of 1935, but retirement percentages at that age and younger have increased steadily since then. Such figures may be deceiving; if the dramatic increase in the numbers of women in the workforce and postretirement employment are factored into this situation, the total labor force of older people is actually growing (1,26). Partial retirement is common (27), and approximately 25% take other jobs after retirement (28). Many private pension funds specify benefits to be paid out on retirement from the career employer; so it is not uncommon for workers to seek different jobs after "retiring" (29). Regardless of trends, the American geriatric workforce is considerable: In the decade from 1983 to 1992, there were 31,520,176 person-years of public work by those over 65, representing 2.8% of the American workforce (30). Work productivity correlates with age-related health (31). Strength, physical activity, and lean body mass have been shown to be correlated with a wide range of benefits in older people (32). Successful aging is facilitated by nutrition, exercise, autonomy, and being active and productive (33–35). For many, that means work.

CAUSES OF NORMAL AGING WORK-RELATED PROBLEMS

Normal aging may result from preprogrammed genetic cellular mutations and death and may result from exogenous effects on cells, such as the deleterious effects of free radicals (7). Despite those as yet unavoidable generators of the aging process, if one excludes the effects of injury, disease, avoidable abuse, and deconditioning, the population of people well beyond what is generally considered retirement age is remarkably healthy (7). Whether productivity and job fitness are diminished significantly by the effects of normal aging depends, in part, on how close to capacity the job pushed a person before the changes of aging (hence retirement considerations by 20-something world-class tennis players). Careers may be considered according to how early the peak is reached and how long performance can remain close enough to peak. Career profiles must be matched to talent, drive, opportunity, health, and fortune as well as to the effects of normal aging.

Biological effects of the aging process inexorably change the spine and other musculoskeletal tissues (16,36). Such changes predispose to stiffness, weakness, and diminished reaction time, although, as discussed later, loss of function may be countered by exercise. Besides the effects on the musculoskeletal system, cognitive and behavioral changes are linked to the aging process that importantly affect employment choices and opportunities.

As discussed at length by Posner, the thought processes of older people rely more on memory, experience, crystallized knowledge base, and retrospective analysis, whereas the thoughts of the young are based on more fluid, imaginative, forwardly oriented analysis and problem solving. Short-term memory and learning ability are superior in younger persons, whereas judgment may be better for older persons. Given such qualities, it is not suprising that many theoretical physicists are young and many appellate court justices are old. Matching cognitive abilities across the rest of the job market may be less obvious, but it is clear that appropriate matching should be the goal rather than arbitrary exclusion by age group. Older workers may be less impulsive and more careful and therefore safer in some situations and less effective in others. Older workers, being less forward looking, may be more loyal, with reduced absenteeism and turnover (1,37). The recovery of injured workers may depend in part on the type of discouragement or encouragement they receive from coworkers (38), which may be well served by the presence of loyal and less reactive older employees. Burnout from stress may be less common among older workers (39). Such considerations support Butler's thesis that employers need to rediscover the value of older people in the workforce (40).

For the older person, the decision to retire or resume working depends on weighing the cons of potential danger, fatigue, pain, tedium, time, and transportation difficulties against possible benefits of prestige, physical and intellectual stimulation, socialization, and support of estate and personal legacy. Whether certain jobs "age" the worker disproportionately is a topic disputed in many forums. Certainly, heavy, dangerous, strenous jobs become impossible for the aging worker, and it may be difficult to distinguish cause

from effect. Analysis of existing data on nonspecific low back pain, for example, does not reveal a tenable model for the effect of specific work on low back pain (41). Among the problems with approaching nonspecific disorders, such as low back pain, for such analysis are the confounding variables introduced by factors such as work satisfaction and perceptions of fair treatment (42). Relationships of job stresses to site-specific injuries are discussed later in this chapter.

PREVENTION STRATEGIES FOR THE AGING WORKER

This section considers *primary prevention*, that is, prevention before the problem occurs. *Secondary prevention*, from early recognition and correction, and *tertiary prevention*, minimizing the consequences, are discussed under specific disorders. Key to prevention of injury is the match of the worker's capabilities to the demands of the job—the so-called *job severity index* (43). The assessment may be particularly demanding for older workers because many have disabilities, some of which vary with time. Preemployment assessment may need to be uniform for all ages, but certain age-related concerns, such hypertension, diabetes, and breast, prostate, and colorectal cancer are of particular concern. Primary medical prevention strategies such as pneumonia and influenza vaccines may be more applicable to older workers (44). Driving and the physical ability to perform task-specific skills safely are reasonable inclusions for preemployment evaluation, if they are administered regardless of age or disability. As for driving, simple tests of cognition, vision, and physical ability can select those who need more extensive testing (45). If there is concern that the job and the worker are not safely matched, alternatives include strategies to improve the fitness of the worker, modification of the tasks, or change in the equipment needed to perform the tasks.

Musculoskeletal symptoms associated with aging, such as weakness, stiffness, and pain after exertion, diminish with regular, appropriately done exercise (46). Fears that vigorous weight-bearing exercises cause arthritis in normal joints and result in musculoskeletal disabilities are irrational and are not supported by evidence (46,47). Aerobic (walking) and resistive exercises are beneficial to older people with symptomatic knee arthritis (48). High-intensity resistive exercise can improve the strength of nonagenarians (49). Balance training and low-intensity posturing through Tai Chi and related programs may be especially helpful to elderly persons (50). Although everyone must accept a small risk that injury may occur with exercise (51), the benefits for those who remain in the window between too little and too much are well worth the effort.

Falls are the most common type of accident among elderly persons (52). Each year 20% to 30% of people over age 65 fall, about half fall more than once, and 10% to 15% of falls produce serious injury (53,54). In the workplace, falls by all ages cause 13% of work-related deaths and 17% of work-related injuries, with steady increases in the numbers by age group (55).

Elderly persons are more susceptible to falling because of problems with vision, balance, and proprioception and an age-related decrease in response time that reduces the ability to recover from a slip or trip. A seven-center study of persons aged 75 to 85 showed that exercises to improve endurance, flexibility, balance, and strength reduced the incidence of falls (56). Attention to surface irregularities, inclination of walking surface, friction and slip resistance, visual obstructions, and cleanliness can reduce the risk of tripping and slipping. Heights of steps may be particularly important in assessing the risk of stair climbing for older people.

Biomechanics of the workplace require attention for the older worker as they would for the younger except that the older worker is more likely to have adaptations confounded by multiple problems. For example, squat lifting, whether better for the back or not, may not be a reasonable alternative for the worker with arthritic knees. Analysis of ergonomic principles as applied in general to aging workers is appropriate (57), but problems more often require individual attention. Adaptations of tool friction, sharpness, and mechanical advantage to accommodate those with subnormal muscle power may assist the older worker.

LEGAL INTERESTS OF THE AGING WORKER

Federal laws pertinent to older workers include the Age Discrimination in Employment Act and amendments, the Americans with Disabilities Act (ADA), and the Employers Retirement Income Security Act. The last regulates employer controls over pension funds and has little direct effect on medical concerns of the aging worker.

Many states have laws that forbid age discrimination in employment. The U.S. Age Discrimination in Employment Act as passed in 1967 forbade discrimination by employers on the basis of age over 40 but permitted mandatory retirement at 65. In 1978, amendments raised the permissible mandatory retirement age to 70, and in 1986 provisions permitting mandatory retirement were removed altogether. There are some exceptions, such as allowing mandatory retirement of airline pilots at age 60. Whereas these laws create a milieu that may be an advantage to the older worker by discouraging discrimination in employment based on age, critics of the laws reason that some reactions actually may work to the disadvantage of older workers (1). Reliable, valid tests that distinguish who should be encouraged to retire and who should continue to work without being unfairly discriminatory on the basis of gender or the presence of unrelated disabilities present a difficult challenge (58). Only a small minority of the suits filed under these laws are by workers over the age of 65 (1). The ADA was enacted in 1990, and some employment provisions were not effective until 1994; so the judicial history is rather brief, and how it relates to age discrimination laws may not have been fully explored. Because older workers have more disabilities, there are obvious overlaps. Among important provisions of the ADA are that employers may not ask job applicants about the existence or the nature of a disability; questions about the ability to function must be job-specific; physical examinations, including job-specific functional capacity, may be required but only after the job is actually offered and only if the same examinations are required of all potential hires; applicants may be required to demonstrate their abilities to perform tasks but only if those tasks are included in detailed written job descriptions available to the applicant before testing; and the employer is obliged to make reasonable accommodations so that qualified applicants with disabilities can perform their jobs. Accommodations may include job restructuring, provision of accessible facilities, change in time requirements, and modifications of equipment (59). Detailed job analyses may be necessary for the employer to comply with requirements about job descriptions and accommodations. The Job Accommodation Network (JAN) provides information on this subject to businesses, disabled workers, and rehabilitation providers at no cost (60,61). One analysis of a large employer's experience with the ADA concluded that adjustment to the ADA is an evolutionary process, that the law provides a useful framework for employers and employees, and that conforming to its provisions has not been unduly expensive to the employer (60). The most common suits brought under the ADA have involved low back disorders (62).

GENERAL HEALTH PROBLEMS OF THE AGING WORKER

Impaired vision and hearing and the array of hormonal, cardiovascular, gastrointestinal, and genitourinary disorders that have increasing incidences with advancing age are well known to medical providers and, indeed, nowadays, to the general public. Because of their more direct relationship to musculoskeletal disorders, this section considers the problems of polypharmacy and of neuropsychiatric disorders. Because older people are more likely to have mul-

tisystem disabilities, they are more likely to be taking more than one medicine. Further, they may metabolize medication less well than younger people, may be affected by vicissitudes in intestinal absorption, cardiac output, protein binding, and alterations in the ratio of body fat to water (63). Side effects may manifest earlier because of preexisting marginal compensation, as, for example, subclinical renal dysfunction. Sedative effects of some drugs, such as benzodiazapines, may increase the risk of falls (64).

Normal aging is attended by some cognitive decline in short-term memory and the ability to process information quickly, which may at times be hard to distinguish from pathologic early dementia (65). Dementia occurs in about 3.9% of persons aged 65 to 74, in 16.4% of those aged 75 to 84, and in 47.6% of those aged over 85; if mild and moderate cognitive impairment is excluded, however, these figures decrease to 0.3%, 5.6%, and 19.6% for those three age groups (65).

Alzheimer's disease, the most common form of pathologic dementia, is diagnosed by using guidelines provided by the American Association for Geriatric Psychiatry, the Alzheimer's Association, and the American Geriatric Society (66). Early symptoms of Alzheimer's and other forms of chronic dementia, such as Parkinson's disease, Pick's disease, Huntington's chorea, and cerebrovascular insufficiency, include abnormal memory loss, confusion, loss of recognition skills, emotional lability, irritability, deterioration of language skills, and loss of attention to grooming and hygiene (67). It is important to distinguish progression of chronic cognitive dysfunction from causes of acute delirium such as from drugs, emotional disorders, nutritional abnormalities, brain tumors, infections, and hormonal and other general medical disorders (67).

Depression is a common accompaniment of age and coexisting medical disorders. Besides depressive reactions to illness, diability, or other loss, some studies suggest that depression may predispose to physical decline (68). Brief mood and energy swings are normal, but depressed mood and anhedonia of more than 2 weeks, loss of weight and appetite, sleep disturbance, agitation, fatigue, feelings of guilt and uselessness, lapses of memory and concentration, and preoccupation with death are all symptoms of depression (69,70). Depression often can be treated successfully without loss of work time, although the tricyclic medications often used as the first-line treatment may have sedative and cardiovascular side effects that become problems for the aging worker (69). Serotonin uptake inhibitors may be better for the older worker with symptoms of depression.

MUSCULOSKELETAL PROBLEMS OF THE AGING WORKER

General

The older worker, having lived longer, is more likely to have accumulated residuals of musculoskeletal injuries; to have contracted common age-related musculoskeletal problems such as osteoporosis, osteoarthritis, and various inflammatory diseases; and to suffer the ordinary indignities of normal aging. The older worker is therefore more likely to have effects of one musculoskeletal impairment compounding those of another. Painful, stiff, dysfunctional hips or knees may make coexisting degenerative lumbar disease intolerable and *vice versa.*

It is estimated that 66% of musculoskeletal problems of women and 51% of those of men are due to various forms of arthritis, and about 11% are due to osteoporosis (71). Clinically manifest osteoarthritis occurs in about 40% of women and 20% of men over the age of 60 years (71,72). Although osteoarthritis is the most common affliction of the joints of aging workers (73), it is far from the only one. Rheumatoid arthritis may have a geriatric onset, often a fulminant one involving the hips and shoulders more than the smaller joints and striking men more often than women. The incidence of polymyalgia rheumatica peaks at around age 70 and is far from uncommon, with a prevalence of about 600 of 100,000

people over the age of 50. Gout may produce increasing deformities with age, although acute crystal arthritis in elderly persons is more likely to be pseudogout (74,75). Septic arthritis is more common in elderly people, usually striking joints impaired by preexisting arthropathies (76,77). Paget's disease of bone occurs in 3% to 4% of people over age 50 and as many as 10% to 15% in those over 80, but it is often minimally symptomatic (78). For the elderly, Paget's disease, which may cause back pain, joint pain, and long bone deformity, is second to osteoporosis as the most common disease of bone (79).

Osteoporosis

Osteoporosis is commonly classified as type 1, postmenopausal; type 2, senile, usually meaning after age 70; and secondary, a variety of bone-wasting diseases and behaviors. Whereas type 1 is a disorder of women, the senile type also occurs more commonly in women but only by a factor of 2 or 3. Many excellent reviews of the musculoskeletal effects of osteoporosis have been done (80,81). Aside from various long-bone fractures from falls, the unique problem osteoporosis presents to the aging worker is the threat of compression fracture of the spine.

Whereas some evidence exists that the morphology of the vertebral bodies correlates with compression fracture (82), most studies focus on the relationship of bone mineral density (BMD) to the load that the spine will support before compression fracture. BMD of lumbar vertebral bodies decreases with age so that forces of 8,000 N could be tolerated without failure in compression at age 25, deteriorating to around 2,000 N at age 75. A normal BMD of around 1 g/cm^2 can tolerate most ordinary stresses, whereas a BMD of 0.5 g/cm^2 places one at risk from lifting 15 kg and 0.3g/cm^2 may predispose to fracture from tying one's shoes or standing from sitting (83).

Clinically, BMD can be measured by radiography, radiographic absorptiometry, single- or dual-energy radiographic absorptiometry, computed tomography, or ultrasound. Since its introduction in 1987, dual-energy radiographic absorptiometry has become the most widely used tool, especially for the hips and spine (84), although some pitfalls are introduced by deformity or by not accounting for volume (85). Using the criterion of a BMD of less than two standard deviations below the mean of normal, young people, about 30% of postmenopausal white American women have osteoporosis. The disease is somewhat selective in that 16% exceed the limits for the spine and 16% exceed the limits for the hip (86). Lifetime risk of clinically evident osteoporotic fracture for white Americans is 16% in women and 5% in men (86).

Those with osteoporotic spines are somewhat compensated in that osteoporosis may be related inversely to spondylosis (87,88) and therefore to hypertrophic forms of spinal stenosis and in that disc displacement in the osteoporotic spine may be more likely to occur through the endplates into the vertebral bodies than into the canal and foramina, where they could compress neural tissues (89). Prevention of fractures from osteoporosis involves injury-prevention strategy to decrease the risk of falls and the risk of excessive compressive loads to the spine. Alhough weight-bearing exercise is the standard prescription to stimulate bone strengthening (90), some data show that resistive strength training also may be important (91).

Calcium supplementation is recommended for all who are not secure in adequate dietary calcium intake of 1,200 to 1,500 mg daily (92). Hormone replacement therapy (estrogens) to preserve the antiresortive effect of estrogens after the menopausal decline in endogenous estrogens is the hallmark of pharmacologic prevention. Second-generation biphosphonates, such as alendronate, may quite effectively counteract the excessive bone resorption of osteoporosis. Calcitonin, by injection or nasal spray, also may be an effective antiresorptive, especially for the spine (93).

Pharmacologic stimulation of osteoblastic activity has not been approved by the U.S. Food and Drug Administration, although fluorides have shown some qualified promise

and remain under investigation (93), and parathormone in certain regimens may stimulate bone formation (94).

Neck

Range of motion of the neck diminishes in the mid and lower cervical spine with age (95). Nonspecific work-related neck and shoulder pains increase in frequency with age (96,97).

Cervical spondylosis describes degenerative changes in the cervical spine, such as disc-space narrowing, formation of osteophytes around the vertebral bodies, hypertrophy of the facets, and ligamentous changes resulting in either stiffness or instability. Normal aging contributes to such changes and may be difficult to distinguish from superimposed effects of trauma or disease (98,99). Cervical spondylosis occurs with normal aging, being present in 95% of men and in 70% of women in a study of asymptomatic subjects (100). Herniation of nuclear material in the cervical spine, so-called soft disc herniation, peaks in incidence in the fourth decade of life (101). Age-related spondylosis of the cervical spine results in a decreased incidence of soft-disc herniation and acute radiculopathy in older persons, but it increases the risks of chronic, intermittent radiculopathy from foraminal root compression and myelopathy from central canal stenosis.

The uncovertebral joint forms the anteromedial wall of the neuroforamen, and the facet joint forms the posterolateral wall, both common sites for formation of osteophytes and hence jeopardy to the exiting nerve root. Symptoms in the distribution of the specific nerve root may result, usually manifesting by proximal pain and distal paresthesias. Compared with acute soft disc herniation, radiculopathy from spondylosis is more likely to have an insidious onset and less likely to be relieved by abduction of the arm (102).

Spinal cord dysfunction from cervical spondylotic myelopathy occurs most often in people over age 55 (103). Symptoms are usually of insidious onset, although myelopathy may have an abrupt onset after a person with spondylosis suffers a relatively minor injury, such as a fall (104), often in the absence of any obvious radiographic evidence of bone injury (105).

Cervical cord dysfunction, whether from direct compression caused by spondylosis, related vascular impairment, or some combination of the two mechanisms, can produce diverse, often enigmatic symptoms, sometimes confused with degenerative or demyelinating diseases of the central nervous system or with peripheral radiculopathies and neuropathies. Most patients fall into one of five commonly cited manifestations of myelopathy: transverse lesion syndrome, motor syndrome, central cord syndrome, unilateral cord syndrome, and brachialgia with cord dysfunction (106). Symptoms vary accordingly, but common symptoms include gait disturbance, deep aching pain with burning sensations, loss of hand dexterity, diffuse weakness, spasticity, loss of position and vibratory sense, and bladder dysfunction (103). Many have electric shocklike sensations with neck movement (L'Hermitte's phenomenon) (104). Signs and symptoms may run an episodic course with long periods of stasis (107–109). Careful assessment of the duration, degree, and progression of neurologic dysfunction along with analysis of imaging findings and correlation with the other features of the individual's health are necessary to make the decision of whether to treat the problem surgically. Whether a posterior or an anterior surgical approach is best is a source of ongoing argument, although most spine surgeons would agree that neither is preferable to the complete exclusion of the other and that each case must be analyzed to decide on the approach (110,111). Older workers, particularly with those known to have spondylosis, best avoid frequent hyperextension of the neck as from working overhead and avoid activities with higher than usual risk of hyperextension injury. Symptoms of neck pain with accompanying headache and shoulder pain may be reduced by ergonomic changes in the work environment.

Dorsal Spine

Abnormal degrees of dorsal kyphosis correlate with age, osteoporosis, bone mineral density, and fractures but not necessarily with overall health status or back-related disability (112). Slow walking, slow step climbing, and difficulty doing heavy housework have been documented for kyphotic older women (113).

Lumbar Spine

Statistical correlations of age- and work-related low back pain vary: some positive (114, 115), some negative (116,117), and at least one showing increased incidence with age in workers for recurrent low back pain but a decrease for first occurrences (116). Such variations are not surprising given the heterogeneity of the aging population, variations in work demands, and the large number of conditions that may cause low back pain. Psychosocial links with low back pain may further confound conclusions from reports of job-related low back pain because factors such as work satisfaction (118), perceived health (119), and various perceptions of the job and its rewards (120–123) are highly predictive of work-related low back complaints.

Information is further limited by the fact that many large studies that seek correlations between low back pain with age, sex, job, and other demographic factors do not examine the over-65 working group. One study showed a peak incidence for blue-collar workers in the 25- to 44-year-old age group and decreasing occurrences of back pain in the 54 to 64 group, except among executives (124). Study of the entire population shows a peak incidence of low back pain at age 55 to 64, with a decrease after age 65 and peak incidence of sciatica in the 45 to 54 age group, with diminishing numbers with age beyond 50 (125). Normal range of motion of the lumbar spine decreases with advancing age in healthy people (126). Deconditioning that may accompany aging and its comorbidities leads to decreased reaction times and postural control, which may contribute to lumbar pain (127). Chaffin and Ashton-Miller reviewed 92 biomechanics papers related to risk factors for manual labor as related to age, concluding that certain work conditions do pose special risk to the lumbar spines of older workers (128). Burton's analysis, however, concluded that the effects of specific work on low back pain were uncertain (41). The incidence of degenerative changes in lumbar discs increases from near zero at age 20 to 90% at age 70 (116). Subtle changes in disc size, vascularity, water content, and proteoglycan organization that may be harbingers of the degenerative process begin even before skeletal maturity (129). Back pain occurs more frequently in people aged 18 to 55 years who have radiographic signs of traction spurs and disc space narrowing at L4–5, but correlation of other symptoms, other ages, and other radiographic changes with pain or with occupation is tenuous (130).

Workers' compensation claims for relatively minor acute low back injuries, such as sprains and strains, are less common among workers over 65 than among younger workers (117). Conservative care and job modification strategies for acute nonspecific low back pain, sprains, and strains are not unique for the geriatric worker. Similar to their younger colleagues, older people can benefit from exercise in improvements of strength, decreased symptoms, and improved function (131,132).

Lumbar disc herniation decreases in incidence after age 65 (71,133). Disc herniation occurs with proportionally less frequency at L5–S1 relative to L4–5 and more craniad discs with advancing age (133). Disc herniation also is a somewhat different pathologic entity among older people with more endplate avulsion and separation of anular fibers compared with the predominantly nuclear tissue displacement of younger patients (134).

Whereas sprains, strains, disc herniation, and nonspecific low back pain may have peak incidences in middle age, the two most common underlying causes of lumbar spinal stenosis (i.e., degenerative spondylolisthesis and lumbar spondylosis) occur with increasing frequency and severity with age.

Stenosis may result in the progressive loss of standing tolerance and walking ability to the point of interference with job performance, depending on the job and the existence of comorbidities. The symptoms may be those of back pain, unilateral or bilateral radiculopathy, or the central stenosis syndrome of intermittent cauda equina compression manifesting by bilateral paresthesias, pain, or weakness brought on by standing and relieved by sitting. The severity of the stenosis correlates in general with severity of walking impairment, although individual variations may be great (135). Some patients have night and other rest pain as well as standing intolerance.

Denerative spondylolisthesis, usually at L4–5, occurs five to six times as often in women as in men (136,137). The common denominators are arthritic, often sagittally oriented, facet joints, with ligamentous laxity. Initial treatment always should be conservative, including modification of tasks to avoid prolonged standing. For those with sufficiently severe compromise despite conservative care and job modification, about 76% get good to excellent results from decompression and fusion (138–140). Decompression alone may yield satisfactory results in the short-term, especially for those with limited activities, but people active enough to be working are better served by fusion even though postoperative care may require a longer period of limited activity (141).

Spinal stenosis may accrue from spondylotic changes of aging without spondylolisthesis or segmental instability. Narrowing of the disc space from desiccation, bulging of discs, settling of facet joints, synovial cysts, osteophytes and hypertrophic thickening of laminae, facets, and vertebral body endplates, and infolding of the ligamentum flavum all compromise the space available to the neurologic tissues. Such changes may become symptomatic at an early age and with less severe pathology if superimposed on a congenitally small canal. The midlumbar spine is most often affected, with L5–S1 and L1–2 relatively spared (142). The average of patients requiring surgical treatment of central spinal stenosis is 65 years (143). Many people with lumbar spinal stenosis do not have progressive loss of function and pain and do not require surgery (144). Improvement in symptoms, however, is more likely with surgical than with conservative care; consequently, stenosis has become the most common diagnosis for back surgery in people over age 65 (145). Maximum benefits from surgical decompression of the stenotic spine usually are achieved at about 3 months. Improvement may deteriorate with time; for example, one study showed that 18% required reoperation within 5 years (140).

Fractures of the lumbosacral spine differ for the geriatric population because of osteoporosis. Preaxial forces, as from lifting, may exceed the limited capacity of the osteoporotic vertebral body to resist compression fracture, as described. Stress fractures of the sacrum are not uncommon for people with osteoporosis and can cause severe pain and standing intolerance (146,147).

Shoulder

Shoulder strength decreases with age (148). Changes of aging predispose to tendinitis of the rotator cuff (149–151). Rotator cuff tendon tears may occur from one or more predisposing factors such as impaired circulation or bony impingement (152,153).

Older patients who suffer a traumatic anterior dislocation of the shoulder, although they are less likely to redislocate (154), often tear their rotator cuffs (155,156). The biceps tendon is functionally a component of the shoulder cuff complex and may rupture along with tears of the rotator cuff (157). Most rotator cuff tears in older people are tears of attrition and can be treated conservatively, but full-thickness tears with loss of motion and persisting pain may be treated surgically with reasonable expectations of good result if there are adequate tissues to allow good repair (158). Rupture of the biceps tendon does not, in itself, produce significant loss of strength and rarely is disabling for elderly people (159). Rotator cuff tendinitis, impingement syndromes, and acromioclavicular arthritis usually can be treated without surgery.

All may limit the ability to perform work with the shoulder at or above 90 degrees of flexion and abduction.

Rheumatoid arthritis is more likely to involve the shoulder in the geriatric population, often symmetrically and with substantial pain and constitutional symptoms (160).

Fractures of the proximal humerus are common injuries in older people, because of osteoporosis. Comminuted or substantially displaced fractures may require complex treatment (161). Minimally displaced fractures are best treated by early mobilization to maintain function (162).

Wrist and Hand

Carpal tunnel syndrome has been related to various work-related stresses and has become a commonly reported work injury (163). Although the age of onset of carpal tunnel syndrome in the general population peaks in the 50- to 60-year-old group (164), the incidence in the industrial population peaks in persons in their 30s (165). Osteoarthritis, the effects of which progress with age, commonly afflicts the hand with painful and motion-limiting nodules adjacent to the distal interphalangeal (Heberden's nodes) or proximal interphalangeal (Bouchard's nodes) joints and by painful degeneration of the carpometacarpal joint of the thumb (74). Depending on the job and the particular manifestations of the disease, osteoarthritis of the hand can be a substantial problem in industry (166,167). Medication and hand therapy may improve the capability of the worker, and modifications of tools and other ergonomic measures may preserve the worker's abilities to perform work tasks. Exercise may counteract the loss of grip strength, which occurs with aging, particularly for women (168).

Hip

Arthritis of the hip has several etiologies, but in the older age group, it most commonly results from osteoarthritis. In 1990 approximately 80,000 total hip arthroplasties were performed for persons over 65 years old in the United States. If trends continue, by 2010 the number will reach 100,000. Nearly half of those procedures are for people aged over 75 (12).

Hip fractures are even more common, with at least 280,000 treated in 1990 and 390,000 predicted by 2010 (12). Falls and osteoporosis are the major determinants; so the trend could be altered by strategies to control those factors.

Guidelines for return to work after successful hip-fracture repair or total-hip arthroplasty for the geriatric age group are not well supported by data because overall figures are skewed by a preponderance of those otherwise not fit for work, and numbers of those actually working at the time of injury are small. In a recent study of 759 community dwelling people over 65 with hip fractures, only 30 were employed at the time the fracture occurred (169). Generally, people can return to sedentary work at 1 to 2 months and some lifting and bending at 3 to 4 months after total-hip arthoplasty or stable repair of a hip fracture.

Knee

Osteoarthritis is a major source of pain and disability for elderly people (170). The synergy of knee and or hip osteoarthritis with other age-related conditions may be more than additive (73). The incidence of osteoarthritis of the knee increases from 2.3% of 45-year-olds to 18% at age 74 (171). Some studies indicate that the risk of osteoarthritis of the knee in older people is higher for those with physically demanding jobs or for those who engage in activities that are stressful to the knee (171–174), although the association is not as strong as it is with obesity (175,176). A task force of the International League of Associations for Rheumatology and the Osteoarthritis Research Society concluded in 1997 that there was not enough information to correlate occupation with knee osteoarthritis (177). In 1990, 109,000 total knee arthroplasties were performed for people over 65, including 43,000 for those over 75 (12).

Workplace and job performance for the older worker with arthritic or postreplacement knees requires limitation of squatting and particular attention to climbing, stair-stepping, and inclined surfaces. Risk of falling is increased for those with stiff, weak, or painful knees. Quadricep-strengthening programs have obvious preventive advantages.

Foot and Ankle

Foot problems exist in 75% of the geriatric population (178). Hallux valgus and bunion deformities increase in severity with age, as do osteoarthritis and hallux rigidus of the metatarsophalangeal joint of the great toe. Calluses, untreated, will increase in severity with repeated stress. The safety footwear recommended in certain industrial settings may aggravate existing foot conditions (179). Because of osteoporosis, stress fractures of the foot are common in the geriatric population (178). Diabetes, vascular disease, edema, venous insufficiency, gout, and other arthridites all produce foot problems that increase in severity with age. Onychauxis (thick nails) and onychomycosis are also common, annoying, sometimes disabling age-related toe problems. Hygiene, careful fitting and prescription of shoes, pads, and orthotics, and early attention to even seemingly minor injuries become increasingly important for the active older person.

RESEARCH AND PLANNING

Understanding the aging process and the diseases and injuries related to the changes that come with aging will continue to accumulate at increasing rates because society's interest has turned to the support of the needed biological and clinical research. Society also must respond in three ways, as suggested by Chan and Koh: (a) by stimulating individuals to prevent avoidable decline in physical capacity and adaptibility; (b) by adjusting work demands to conform to functional capacity; and (c) by educating employers and fellow workers about the benefits of the experience, judgment, and motivation of the aging worker (180).

REFERENCES

1. Posner RA. *Aging and old age.* Chicago: University of Chicago Press, 1995, pp. 18–19.
2. Nygard CH, Huuhtanen P, Tuomi K, Martikainen R. Perceived work changes between 1981 and 1992 among aging workers in Finland. *Scand J Work Environ Health* 1997;23,Suppl 1:12–19.
3. Tuomi K, Ilmarinen J, Martikainen R, Aalto L, Klockars M. Aging, work, life-style and work ability among Finnish municipal workers in 1991–1992. *Scand J Work Environ Health* 1997;23(Suppl 1): 58–65.
4. Broersen JP, deZwart BC, van Dijk FJ, Meijman TF, van Veldhoven M. Health complaints and working conditions experienced in relation to work and age. *Occup Environ Med* 1996;53:51–57.
5. de Zwart BC, Frings-Dresen MH, van Dijk. Physical workload and the aging worker: a review of the literature. *Int Arch Occup Environ Health* 1995;68:1–12.
6. Buckwalter JA, Woo SL-Y, Goldberg VM, et al. Soft-tissue aging and musculoskeletal function. *J Bone Joint Surg Am* 1993;75:1533–1547.
7. Perron VD, Robinson BE. The aging process and functional assessment. *Archives of the American Academy of Orthopedic Surgeons* 1998;2:1–8.
8. Fried LP, Guralnik JM. Disability in older adults: evidence regarding significance, etiology, and risk. *J Am Geriatr Soc* 1997;45:92–1000.
9. Vita AJ, Terry RB, Hubert HB, Fries JF. Aging, health risks, and cummulative disability. *N Engl J Med* 1998; 338:1035–1041.
10. Parnes HS, Sommers DG. Shunning retirement: work experience of men in their seventies and early eighties. *J Gerontol* 1994;49:S117–S124.
11. Winker MA, Glass RM. The aging global population. *JAMA* 1996;276:1758.
12. Canale ST, Buckwalter JA. *Orthopaedic aspects of aging: agenda and background materials.* Rosemont, IL: American Academy of Orthopaedic Surgeons, 1995, pp. 1–102.
13. World Health Organization. *The public health aspects of the aging population.* Copenhagen: World Health Organization, 1959.
14. Butler RN, Luddington AV. Aging research: John Glenn's new mission. *Geriatrics* 1998;53:42–48.
15. Shaughnessy D. Seniors serve as inspiration. *Boston Globe* Sept 7, 1994:57–59.
16. United Nations, Department of International Economic and Social Affairs. *The sex and age distribution of population: the 1990 revision of the United States global population estimate and projections.* Population Study 122, 1991.
17. Penning MJ, Strain LA. Gender differences in disability, assistance, and subjective well-being in later life. *J Gerontol* 1994;49:S202–S208.
18. United States Bureau of Census. *Current population reports, special studies—sixty-five plus in America.* Washington DC: United States Government Printing Office, 1992.
19. Manton KG, Corder L, Stallard E. Chronic disability trends in elderly United States populations 1982–1994. *Proc Natl Acad Sci USA* 1997;94: 2593–2598.
20. United States Senate Special Committee on Aging. *Aging in America:* Trends and projections. Washington DC, United States Government Printing Office, 1991, p. 133.
21. Fitten LJ, Perryman KM, Wilkinson CJ. Alzheimer and vascular dementias and driving. *JAMA* 1995;273: 1360–1365.
22. Evans L. Older driver involvement in fatal and severe traffic crashes. *J Gerontol* 1988;43:S186–S193.
23. United States Department of Justice, Federal Bureau of Investigation. *Uniform crime reports:* crime in the United States 1992; Washington DC: United States Government Printing Office, 1993, p. 228.
24. Auerbach AJ, Kotlikoff LJ. The impact of the demographic transitions on capital formation. In: Rappaport AM, Schieber J, eds. *Demography and retirement: the twenty-first century.* Westport, CT: Praeger, 1993, pp. 163–174.
25. Streib GF. Discussion. In: Ricardo-Campbell R, Lazear EP, eds. *Issues in contemporary retirement.* Stanford CA: Hoover Institute Press, 1988, p. 27.
26. Bennett A. More and more women are staying on the job later in life than men. *Wall Street Journal.* New York:Dow Jones. Sept 1, 1994;B:1.
27. Ruhm CJ. Bridge jobs and partial retirement. *Journal of Labor-Economics* 1990;8:490–493.
28. Myers DA. Work after cessation of a career job. *J Gerontol* 1991;46:S93–S100.
29. Kaufman RL, Spilerman S. The age structure of occupations and jobs. *American Journal of Sociology* 1982; 87:827–839.
30. Bailer AJ, Stayner LT, Stout NA, Reed LD, Gilbert SJ. Trends in rates of occupational fatal injuries in the United States (1983–1992). *Occup Environ Med* 1998; 55:485–489.
31. Robertson A, Tracy CS. *Scand J Work Environ Health* 1998;14:85–97.
32. Davis JW, Ross PD, Preston SD, Nevitt MN, Wasnick RD. Strength, physical activity, and body mass index: relationship to performance based measures and activities of daily living among older Japanese women in Hawaii. *J Am Geriatr Soc* 1998;46:274–279.
33. Clark F, Azen SP, Zemke R, et al. Occupational therapy for independent-living older adults. *JAMA* 1997; 278:1321–1326.
34. Berkman LF, Seeman TE, Albert M, et al. High, unusual, and impaired functioning in community swelling older men and women. *J Clin Epidemiol* 1993;46:1129–1140.
35. Fisher BJ. Successful aging, life satisfaction and generativity in later life. *Int J Aging Hum Dev* 1995;41: 239–250.
36. Gruber HE, Hanley EN. Analysis of aging and degeneration of the human intervertebral disc. *Spine* 1998; 23:751–757.
37. Campanelli L. The aging workforce: implications for organizations. *Occup Med* 1990;5:817–826.
38. Weiser S. Psychological aspects of occupational musculoskeletal disorders. In: Nordin M, Andersson GBJ, Pope MH, eds. *Musculoskeletal disorders in the workplace: principles and practice.* St Louis: Mosby-Year Book, 1997, pp. 52–61.

39. Cordes CL, Dougerty TM. A review and an integration of research on job burnout. *Academy of Management Review* 1993;18:621–633.

40. Butler RN. Living longer, contributing longer. *JAMA* 1997;278:1372–1373.

41. Burton AK. Back injury and work loss: biomechanical and psychosocial influences. *Spine* 1997;22:2575–2580.

42. Papageorgiou AC, Macfarlane GJ, Thomas E, Croft PR, Jayson MIV, Silman AJ. Psychosocial factors in the workplace—do they predict new episodes of low back pain? *Spine* 1997;22:1137–1142.

43. Kumar S, Konz S. Workplace adaptation of the low back region. In: Nordin M, Andersson GBJ, Pope MH, eds. *Musculoskeletal disorders in the workplace: principles and practice.* St. Louis: Mosby-Year Book, 1997, pp. 316–326.

44. Reed R. Preventive interventions. In: Yoshikawa TT, Cobbs EL, Brummel-Smith K, eds. *Practical ambulatory geriatrics.* St. Louis: Mosby Year Book, 1998, pp. 173–183.

45. Marottoli RA, Richardson ED, Stowe MH, et al. Development of a test battery to identify older drivers at risk for self-reported adverse driving events. *J Am Geriatr Soc* 1998;46:562–568.

46. Buckwalter JA, Mooney V, Buckwalter KC. Loss of conditioning and mobility. *Archives of the American Academy of Orthopedic Surgeons* 1998;2:97–102.

47. Fries JF, Gurkirpal S, Morfeld D, O'Driscoll P, Hubert H. Relationship of running to musculoskeletal pain with age. *Arthritis Rheum* 1996;39:64–72.

48. Ettinger WH, Burns R, Messier SP, et al. A randomized trial comparing aerobic exercise and resistance exercise with a health education program in older adults with knee osteoarthritis. *JAMA* 1997;277:25–31.

49. Fiatrone MA, Marks ED, Ryan ND, et al. High intensity strength training in nonagenerians. *JAMA* 1990;263:3029–3034.

50. Wolf SL, Barnhart HX, Kutner NG, McNeely E, Coogler C, Xu T. Reducing frailty and falls in older persons: an investigation of tai chi and computerized balance training. *J Am Geriatr Soc* 1996;44:489–497.

51. United States Dept of Health and Human Services. *Physical activity and health: a report of the surgeon general.* Atlanta GA: US Dept of Health and Human Services, Center for Disease Control and Prevention, 1996.

52. Weindruch R, Hadley EC, Ory MG. *Reducing frailty and falls in older persons.* Springfield IL: Charles C Thomas, 1991, pp. 5–11.

53. Prudham D, Evans JG. Factors associated with falls in the elderly: a community study. *Age Aging* 1981;10:141–146.

54. Blake AJ, Morgan K, Bendall MJ, et al. Falls by elderly people at home: prevalence and associated factors. *Age Aging* 1988;17:365–372.

55. National Safety Council. *Accident facts.* Chicago: National Safety Council, 1991.

56. Province MA, Hadley ED, Hornbrook MC, et al. The effects of exercise in elderly patients: a preplanned meta-analysis of the FICSIT trials. *JAMA* 1995;273:1341–1347.

57. Garg A. Ergonomics and the older worker: an overview. *Exp Aging Res* 1991;17:143–155.

58. Shephard J. Human rights and the older worker: changes in work capacity with age. *Med Sci Sports Exerc* 1987:168–173.

59. Leger D, Kemp JD. The Americans with Disabilities Act. In: Nordin M, Andersson GBJ, Pope MH, eds. *Musculoskeletal disorders in the workplace:* principles and practice. St. Louis: Mosby-Year Book, 1997, pp. 634–639.

60. Blanck PD. Implementing the Americans With Disabilities Act: 1996 follow-up report on Sears, Roebuck and Co. *Spine* 1996;21:1602–1608.

61. President's Committee on Employment of People with Disabilities. *Job Accommodation Network (JAN) reports.* Washington, D.C.: United States Government Printing Office, 1994.

62. Blanck PD. Recent developments in ADA case law and implications for spine professionals. *Spine* 1995;20:116–119.

63. Brummel-Smith K. Polypharmacy and the elderly patient. *Archives of the American Academy of Orthopedic Surgeons* 1998;2:39–44.

64. Herrings RMC, Stricker BH, deBoer A, Bakker A, Sturmans F. Benzodiazapines and the risk of falling leading to femur fractures. *Arch Intern Med* 1995;155:1801–1807.

65. Jutagir R. Psychological aspects of aging: when does memory loss signal dementia? *Geriatrics* 1994;49:45–53.

66. Small GW, Rabins PV, Barry PP, et al. Diagnosis and treatment of Alzheimer's disease and related disorders: consensus statement of the American Association for Geriatric Psychiatry, the Alzheimer's Association, and the American Geriatric Society. *JAMA* 1997;278:1363–1371.

67. Buckwalter KC, Buckwalter JA. Chronic cognitive dysfunction (dementia). *Archives of the American Academy of Orthopedic Surgeons* 1998;2:20–32.

68. Penninx BWJH, Guralnik JM, Ferrucci L, Simonsick EM, Deeg DJH, Wallace RB. Depressive symptoms and physical decline in community-dwelling older persons. *JAMA* 1998;279:1720–1726.

69. Robinson BE. Depression. *Archives of the American Academy of Orthopedic Surgeons* 1998;2:33–38.

70. American Psychiatric Association. *Diagnostic and statistical manual of mental disorders,* 4th ed. Washington, D.C.: American Psychiatric Association, 1994.

71. Praemer A, Furner S, Rice DP. *Musculoskeletal conditions in the United States.* Park Ridge, IL: American Academy of Orthopaedic Surgeons, 1992.

72. Lawrence RC, Hochberg MC, Kelsey JL, et al. Estimates of the prevalence of selected arthritis and musculoskeletal diseases in the United States. *J Rheumatol* 1989;16:427–441.

73. Ling SM, Bathon JM. Osteoarthritis in older adults. *J Am Geriatr Soc* 1998;46:216–225.

74. Levy RN, Sethi PM. Joint pain in the elderly patient. *Archives of the American Academy of Orthopedic Surgeons* 1998;2:66–73.

75. Michet CJ Jr, Evans JM, Fleming KC, O'Duffy JC, Jurrison ML, Hunder GC. Common rheumatologic diseases in eldery patients. *Mayo Clin Proc* 1995;70:1205–1214.

76. Gilbert RS, Strauss E, Gilbert MS. Infection in the aged: septic arthritis. *Archives of the American Academy of Orthopedic Surgeons* 1998;2:74–80.

77. McGuire NM, Kauffman CA. Septic arthritis in the elderly. *J Am Geriatr Soc* 1985;33:170–175.

78. Kaplan FS, Singer FR. Paget's disease of bone: pathophysiology, diagnosis, and management. *J Am Acad of Ortho Surg* 1995;3:336–344.

79. Ankromma MA, Shapiro JR. Pagets Disease of bone (osteitis deformans). *J Am Geriatr Soc* 1998;46:1025–1033.

80. Lane JM, Riley EA, Wirgonowiccz PZ. Osteoporosis: diagnosis and treatment. *J Bone Joint Surg Am* 1996; 78:618–633.

81. Lucas TS, Einhorn TA. Osteoporosis: the role of the orthopaedist. *J Am Acad of Ortho Surg* 1993;1:48–56.

82. Oda K, Shibayama Y, Abe M, Onomura T. Morphogenesis of vertebral deformities in involutional osteoporosis. *Spine* 1998;23:1050–1056.

83. Myers ER, Wilson SE. Biomechanics of osteoporosis and vertebral fracture. *Spine* 1997;22:25S–31S.

84. Seeger LL. Bone density determination. *Spine* 1997; 22:49S–57S.

85. Antonacci MD, Hanson DS, Heggeness MH. Pitfalls in the measurement of bone mineral density by dual energy x-ray absorptiometry. *Spine* 1996;21:87–91.

86. Melton LJ III. Epidemiology of osteoporosis. *Spine* 1997;22:2S–11S.

87. Nutti R, Righi G, Martini G, Turchetti V, Lepore C, Doretti V. Diagnostic approach to osteoporosis and spondyloarthrosis in post-menopausal women by total body dual-photon absorptiometry. *Clin Exp Rheuma tol* 1988;6:47–51.

88. Verstraeten A, Ermen HV, Haghebaert G, Nijs J, Geusens P, Dequeker J. Osteoarthritis retards the development of osteoporosis: observation of the coexistence of osteoarthrosis and osteoporosis. *Clin Orthop* 1991;264:169–177.

89. Harada A, Okuizumi H, Miyagi N, Genda E. Correlation between bone mineral density and intervertebral density and intervertebral disc degeneration. *Spine* 1998;23:857–862.

90. Kelley G. Aerobic exercise and lumbar spine bone mineral density in postmenopausal women: a meta-analysis. *J Am Geriatr Soc* 1998;46:143–152.

91. Swezey RL. Exercise for osteoporosis—is walking enough? The case for site specificity and resistive exercise. *Spine* 1996;21:2809–2813.

92. Dawson-Hughes B. Calcium supplementation and bone loss: a review of controlled clinical trials. *Am J Clin Nutr* 1991;54:274S–280S.

93. Lane JM. Osteoporosis: medical prevention and treatment. *Spine* 1997;22:32S–37S.

94. Finkelstein JS, Klibanski A, Arnold AL, Toth TL, Hornstein MD, Neer RM. Prevention of estrogen deficiency-related bone loss with human parathyroid hormone-(1–34). *JAMA* 1998;280:1067–1073.

95. Dvorak J, Antinnes JA, Panjabi M, Loustalot D, Bonaro M. Age and gender-related normal motion of the cervical spine. *Spine* 1992;17:S393–S398.

96. Westerling D, Jonsson BG. Pain from the neck and shoulder region and sick leave. *Scand J Soc Med* 1980; 8:131–136.

97. Holmstrom EB, Lindell J, Moritz U. Low back pain and neck-shoulder pain in construction workers; occupational workload and psychosocial risk factors. Part 2: relationship to neck and shoulder pain. *Spine* 1992; 17:672–677.

98. Connell MD, Wiesel SW. Natural history and pathogenesis of cervical disk disease. *Orthop Clin North Am* 1992;23:369–380.

99. Lestini WF, Wiesel SW. The pathogenesis of cervical spondylosis. *Clin Orthop* 1989;239:69–93.

100. Gore DR, Sepic SB, Gardner GM. Roentgenographic findings of the cervical spine in asymptomatic people. *Spine* 1986;11:521–524.

101. Kelsey JL, Githens PB, Walter SD, et al. An epidemiologic study of acute prolapsed cervical intervertebral disc. *J Bone Joint Surg Am* 1984;66:907–914.

102. Beatty RM, Fowler FD, Handson EJ. The abducted arm as a sign of ruptured cervical disc. *Neurosurgery* 1988;21:731–732.

103. Clark CR. Cervical spondylotic myelopathy. History and physical findings. *Spine* 1988;13:847–849.

104. Foo D. Spinal cord injury in forty-four patients with cervical spondylosis. *Paraplegia* 1986;24:301–306.

105. Regenbogen VS, Rogers LF, Atlas SW, Kim KS. Cervical spinal cord injuries in patients with cervical spondylosis. *Am J Radiol* 1986;146:277–284.

106. Crandall PH, Batzdorf U. Cervical spondylytic myelopathy. *J Neurosurg* 1966;25:57–66.

107. Clark E, Robinson PK. Cervical myelopathy: A complication of cervical spondylosis. *Brain* 1956;79:483–510.

108. Epstein JA, Janin Y, Carras R, Levine LS. A comparative study of the treatment of cervical spondylotic myeloradiculopathy: experience with 50 cases treated by means of extensive laminectomy, foraminotomy, and excision of osteophytes during the past 10 years. *Acta Neurochir (Wien)* 1982;61:89–104.

109. Lees F, Turner JWA. Natural history and prognosis of cervical spondylosis. *BMJ* 1963;2:1607–1610.

110. Whitecloud TS, Werner JG. Cervical spondylosis and disc herniation: the anterior approach. In: Frymoyer JW, ed. *The adult spine.* Philadelphia: Lippincott-Raven, 1997:1357–1379.

111. Ducker TB, Zeidman SM. Cervical radiculopathies and myelopathies: posterior approaches. In: Frymoyer JW, ed. *The adult spine.* Philadelphia: Lippincott-Raven, 1997:1381–1400.

112. Ensrud KE, Black DM, Harris H, Ettinger B, Cummings SR. Correlates of kyphosis in older women. *Am J Geriatr Soc* 1997;45:682–687.

113. Ryan SD, Fried LP. The impact of kyphosis on daily functioning. *J Am Geriatr Soc* 1997;45:1479–1486.

114. Gyntelberg F. One year incidence of low back pain among male residents of Copenhagen aged 40–59. *Dan Med Bull* 1974;21:30–36.

115. Troup JDG, Foreman TK, Baxter CE, Brown D. The perception of back pain and the role of psychophysical tests of lifting capacity. *Spine* 1987;12:645–657.

116. Miller JAA, Schmatz C, Shultz AB. Lumbar disc degeneration: correlation with age, sex, and spine level in 600 autopsy specimens. *Spine* 1988;13:173–178.

117. Klein BP, Jensen RC, Sanderson LM. Assessment of workers' compensation claims for back strains/sprains. *J Occup Environ Med* 1984;26:443–448.

118. Bigos S, Battie M, Spengler D. A prospective study of work perceptions and psychological factors affecting the report of back injury. *Spine* 1991;16:1–6.

119. Linton ST. Psychological factors related to health, back pain, and dysfunction. *J Occup Rehabil* 1994;4: 3–10.

120. Burton AD, Tillotson KM, Troup JDG. Prediction of low-back trouble fequency in a working population. *Spine* 1989;14:517–522.

121. Magora A. Investigation of the relation betweeen low

back pain and occupation. V. Psychological aspects. *Scand J Rehabil Med* 1973;5:191–196.

122. Ryden LA, Molgaard CA, Bobitt S, Cohn J. Occupational low-back injury in a hospital employee population: an epidemiologic analysis of multiple risk factors of a high-risk occupational group. *Spine* 1989;14:315–320.

123. Svensson HO, Andersson GBJ. The relationship of low-back pain, work history, work environment, and stress. *Spine* 1989;14:939–946.

124. Gluck JV, Oleinick A. Claim rates of compensable back injuries by age, gender, occupation, and industry. *Spine* 1998;23:1572–1587.

125. Deyo RA, Tsui-Wu YJ. Descriptive epidemiology of low-back pain and its related medical care in the United States. *Spine* 1987;12:264–268.

126. Sullivan MS, Dickinson CE, Troup JDG. The influence of age and gender on lumbar spine sagittal plane range of motion. *Spine* 1994;19:682–686.

127. Luoto S, Taimela S, Hurri H, Aalto H, Pyykko I, Alaranta H. Psychomotor speed and postural control in chronic low back pain patients. *Spine* 1996;21:2621–2627.

128. Chaffin DB, Ashton-Miller JA. Biomechanical aspects of low-back pain in the older worker. *Exp Aging Res* 1991;17:177–187.

129. Buckwalter JA. Aging and degeneration of the human intervertebral disc. *Spine* 1995;20:1307–1314.

130. Frymoyer JW, Newberg A, Pope MH, Wilder DG, Clements J, MacPherson B. Spine radiographs in patients with low-back pain. An epidemiologic study in men. *J Bone Joint Surg Am* 1984;66:1048–1055.

131. Holmes B, Leggett S, Mooney V, Nichols J, Negri S, Hoeyberghs A. Comparison of female geriatric lumbar-extension strength: asymptomatic versus chronic low back pain patients and their response to active rehabilitation. *Spine* 1996;9:17–22.

132. Frontiera WR, Meredith CN, O'Reilly KP, Knuttger HG, Evans WJ. Strength conditioning in older men: skeletal muscle hypertrophy and improved function. *J Appl Physiol* 1988;64:1038–1044.

133. Spangfort EV. The lumbar disc herniation. *Acta Orthop Scand Suppl* 1972;142:1–95.

134. Tanaka M, Nakahara S, Inoue H. A pathologic study of discs in the elderly. *Spine* 1993;18:1456–1462.

135. Jonsson B, Annertz M, Sjoberg C, Stromqvist B. A prospective and consecutive study of surgically treated lumbar spinal stenosis. Part I. Clinical features related to radiographic findings. *Spine* 1997;22:2932–2937.

136. Herkowitz H. Degenerative spondylolisthesis. *Spine* 1995;20:1084–1090.

137. Rosenberg NJ. Degenerative spondylolisthesis. *J Bone Joint Surg Am* 1975;57:467–474.

138. Fischgrund JS, Mackay M, Herkowitz HN, Brower R, Montgomery DM, Kurz LT. Degenerative lumbar spondylolisthesis with spinal stenosis: a prospective, randomized study comparing decompressive laminectomy and arthrodesis with and without spinal instrumentation. *Spine* 1997;22:2807–2812.

139. Katz JN, Lipson SJ, Lew RA, et al. Lumbar laminectomy alone or with instrumented or noninstrumted arthrodesis in degenerative lumbar spinal stenosis. *Spine* 1997;22:1123–1131.

140. Jonsson B, Annertz M, Sjoberg C, Stromqvist B. A prospective and consecutive study of surgically treated

lumbar spinal stenosis. Part II. Five year follow-up by an independent observer. *Spine* 1997;22:2938–2944.

141. Herkowitz HN, Kurz LT. Degenerative lumbar spondylolisthesis with spinal stenosis. A prospective study comparing decompression with decompression and intertransverse progressive arthrodesis. *J Bone Joint Surg Am* 1991;73:802–808.

142. Lange M, Hamburger C, Waldhauser E, Beck OJ. Surgical treatment and results in patients suffering from lumbar spinal stenoses. *Neurosurg Rev* 1993;16:27–33.

143. Jonsson B, Stromquist B. Symptoms and signs in degeneration of the lumbar spine: a prospective, consecutive study of 300 operated patients. *J Bone Joint Surg Br* 1993;75:381–385.

144. Johnsson KE, Rosen I, Uden A. The natural course of lumbar spinal stenosis. *Clin Orthop* 1992;279:82–86.

145. Atlas SJ, Deyo RA, Keller RB, Chapin AM, Patrick DL, Long JM, Singer DE. The Maine lumbar spine study, part III: 1-year outcomes of surgical and nonsurgical management of lumbar spinal stenosis. *Spine* 1996;21:1787–1795.

146. Lourie H. Spontaneous osteoporotic fracture of the sacrum. An unrecognized syndrome of the elderly. *JAMA* 1982;248:715–716.

147. Newhouse KE, El-Khoury GY, Buckwalter JA. Occult sacral fractures in osteopenic patients. *J Bone Joint Surg Am* 1992;74:1472–1477.

148. Murray MP. Shoulder motion and muscle strength of normal men and women in two age groups. *Clin Orthop* 1985;192:268–273.

149. Brewer BJ. Aging of the Rotator Cuff. *Am J Sports Med* 1979;7:102–110.

150. Olsson O. Degenerative changes of the shoulder joint and their connection with shoulder pain: a morphological and clinical investigation with special attention to the cuff and biceps tendon. *Acta Chic Scand Suppl* 1953;181:5–130.

151. Daigneault J, Cooney LM. Shoulder pain in older people. *J Am Geriatr Soc* 1998;46:1144–1151.

152. Moseley HF, Goldie I. The arterial pattern of the rotator cuff of the shoulder. *J Bone Joint Surg Br* 1963;45:780–789.

153. Neer CS. Anterior acromioplasty for the chronic impingement syndrome in the shoulder. *J Bone Joint Surg Am* 1972;54:41–50.

154. Rowe CR, Sakellarides HT. Factors related to recurrences of anterior dislocation of the shoulder. *Clin Orthop* 1961;20:40–47.

155. Neviaser RJ, Neviaser TJ, Neviaser JS. Concurrent rupture of rotator cuff and anterior dislocation of the shoulder in the older patient. *J Bone Joint Surg Am* 1988;70:1308–1311.

156. Hawkins RJ, Bell RH, Hawkins RH, Koppert GJ. Anterior dislocation of the shoulder in the older patient. *Clin Orthop* 1986;206:192–195.

157. Slatis P, Aalto K. Medial dislocation of the tendon of the long head of the biceps brachii. *Acta Orthop Scand* 1979;50:73–77.

158. Iannotti JP. Full-thickness rotator cuff tears: factors affecting surgical outcome. *Journal of the American Academy of Orthopedic Surgeons* 1994;2:87–95.

159. Warren RF. Lesions of the long head of the biceps tendon. *American Academy of Orthopedic Surgeons Institute Course Lectures* 1985;34:204–209.

160. Deal CL, Meenan RF, Goldenberg DL, et al. The clnical features of elderly-onset rheumatoid arthritis. *Arthritis Rheum* 1985;28:987–974.

161. Schlegel TF, Hawkins RJ. Displaced proximal humeral fractures: evaluation and treatment. *Journal of the American Academy of Orthopedic Surgeons* 1994;2:54–66.

162. Kristiansen B, Augermann P, Larsen TK. Functional results following fractures of the proximal humerus: a controlled clinical study comparing two periods of immobilization. *Arch Orthop Trauma Surg* 1989;108: 339–341.

163. Stock SR. Workplace ergonomic factors and the development of musculoskeletal disorders of the neck and upper limbs: a meta-analysis. *Am J Ind Med* 1991; 19:87–107.

164. Stevens JC, Sun S, Beard CM, O'Fallon WM, Kurland LT. Carpal tunnel syndrome in Rochester, Minnesota 1961–1980. *Neurology* 1988;38:134–138.

165. Franklin GM, Haug J, Heyer N, Checkoway H, Peck N. Occupational carpal tunnel syndrome in Washington State, 1984–1988. *Am J Public Health* 1991;81: 741–746.

166. Hadler NM, Gillings DB, Imbus HR, et al. Hand structure and function in an industrial setting. *Arthritis Rheum* 1978;21:210–220.

167. Williams WV, Cope R, Gaunt WD, et al. Metacarpophalangeal arthropathy associated with manual labor. *Arthritis Rheum* 1987;30:1362–1371.

168. Pantanen T, Era P, Heikkinen E. Physical activity and the changes in maximal isometric strength in men and women from the age of 75 to 80 years. *J Am Geriatr Soc* 1997;45:1439–1445.

169. Brainsky A, Glick H, Lydick E, et al. The economic cost of hip fractures in community-dwelling older adults: a prospective study. *Am J Geriatr Soc* 1997; 45:281–287.

170. Davis MA, Ettinger WH, Neuhaus JM, Mallon KP. Knee osteoarthritis and physical conditioning: evidence from the NHANES I epidemiologic follow up study. *J Rheumatol* 1991;18:591–598.

171. Andersson JJ, Felson DT. Factors associated with osteoarthritis of the knee in the first national Health and Nurtrition Examination Survey (HANES I). Evidence for an association with overweight, race, and physical demands of work. *Am J Epidemiol* 1988;128: 179–189.

172. Felson DT, Hannan MT, Naimark A, et al. Occupational physical demands, knee bending, and knee osteoarthritis: results from the Framingham Study. *J Rheumatol* 1991;18:1587–1592.

173. Lindberg H, Montgomery F. Heavy labor and the occurence of gonarthrosis. *Clin Orthop* 1987,214: 235–236.

174. Buckwalter JA. Osteoarthritis and articular cartilage use, disuse, and abuse: experimental studies. *J Rheumatol* 1995;22:13–15.

175. Kohatsu N, Schurman D. Risk factors for the development of osteoarthritis of the knee. *Clin Orthop* 1990;261:242–246.

176. Hult L. The Monkfors investigation. *Acta Orthop Scand* 1954;16(Suppl):1–76.

177. Dieppe P, Altman R, Lequesne M, Menkes J, Pelletier JP, Lartel-Pelletier J. Osteoarthritis of the knee: report of the task force of the International League of Associations for Rheumatology and the Osteoarthritis Research Society. *Am J Geriatr Soc* 1997;45:850–852.

178. Karpman R. Foot problems in the geriatric patient. *Clin Orthop* 1995;316:59–62.

179. Marr SJ, Quine S. Shoe concerns and foot problems of wearers of safety footwear. *Occup Med* 1993;43: 73–77.

180. Chan GC, Koh DS. The ageing worker. *Ann Acad Med Singapore* 1997;26:781–786.

Occupational Musculoskeletal Disorders
edited by T. G. Mayer, R. J. Gatchel, and P. B. Polatin.
Lippincott Williams & Wilkins, Philadelphia © 2000.

18

Misuse of Diagnostic Imaging Tests in Low Back Pain

Michael E. Goldsmith and Sam W. Wiesel

Department of Orthopaedics, Georgetown University Medical Center, Washington, D.C. 20007

Low back pain will affect 80% of people at some point in their lifetime. The effect of low back pain on the U.S. workforce is devastating: Each year, 2% of the workforce will be afflicted by industrially related back injuries (1). The financial impact of compensation for low back pain is estimated to surpass 25 billion dollars in annual expenditures by the end of the 1990s, not including the cost to the economy for lost work (2). Interestingly, a small percentage of patients who receive disability payments account for a disproportionate amount of the total costs associated with back pain. Fewer than 10% of back pain cases account for nearly 75% of lost days, medical costs, and indemnity payments (3).

In light of these staggering statistics, industry has turned to medicine for an answer to the problem of the rising costs of industrial back pain. To achieve these goals, an organized approach to the evaluation, diagnosis, and treatment of low back pain needs to be instituted. This process begins with the proper diagnosis of back pain and the sensible use of diagnostic tests. The goal of the treating physician should be first and foremost to make the appropriate diagnosis. The diagnosis is arrived at through a combination of taking a thorough history, performing a proper physical examination, and using appropriate diagnostic tests. Diagnostic tests cannot be used in isolation because of the proven high rates of false positives, but instead must be viewed in the individual context of each patient. The purpose of this chapter is to discuss the proper use of diagnostic tests in the evaluation of industrial low back pain to prevent the misuse of diagnostic tests.

PREEMPLOYMENT SCREENING

Medicine's first response to the problem of industrial low back pain was the idea of preemployment screening, which, in 1929, moved toward preemployment roentgenographic screening (4). It has taken almost 70 years to break employers and doctors of this habit, as multiple studies have demonstrated that standard lumbosacral radiographs are not predictive of future back problems (5,6). Rowe demonstrated that predicting people at risk for low back pain was not possible using x-rays. He reported that the prevalence of leg length differences, increased lumbosacral angle, spondylolisthesis, transitional lumbosacral vertebrae, and spina bifida occulta among low back pain patients was not significantly different from that in a control group (7). In addition, no correlation was noted with back pain and transitional vertebrae, Schmorl's nodes, or the disc vacuum sign. The finding of traction spurs or disc-space narrowing between L4–5, however, was correlated with a slightly increased incidence of severe low back pain (8). Currently, the American Association of Occupational and Environmental

Medicine recommends that the lumbar spine roentgenographic examination should not be used as a routine screening procedure for back problems. Instead, radiographs of the lumbosacral region should be reserved as a diagnostic tool in the appropriate clinical circumstance (9).

UNDERSTANDING PREDICTIVE VALUE OF A STUDY

Diagnostic tests should be used to confirm the core of information gathered from a thorough history and physical examination. Used in isolation, imaging modalities become dangerous tools, because they are overly sensitive and relatively nonselective. When these same imaging studies are teamed with clinically relevant information obtained from a thorough history and physical examination, the power of these studies to diagnose true pathology increases exponentially. The use of imaging modalities as screening tools is neither cost effective nor clinically efficacious. Many iatrogenic catastrophes in the management of patients with low back pain can be directly attributed to excessive reliance on diagnostic studies without clinical correlation.

To understand the power of a diagnostic modality, the clinician must be able to evaluate the sensitivity and specificity of each test. *Sensitivity* is the ability of a test to detect disease when it is present and is a reflection of the false negatives. If a test is highly sensitive, almost everyone with the disease will be detected, although it does not specifically determine whether a person actually has the disease.

Specificity is the ability of a test to remain negative in the absence of disease and is a reflection of the false positives. If a test is highly specific when it is positive, the specific disease process in question is almost certainly the diagnosis, but it makes no statement about the test's failing to detect the diagnosis.

In addition, the idea of prevalence rate must be noted. The *prevalence rate* refers to the percentage of people in an asymptomatic population who will have a specific finding. For example, a certain number of people, say 25 of 100 asymptomatic patients or 25%, will have disc space narrowing.

The physician's challenge is to select an appropriate diagnostic test that is cost effective, incurs little morbidity, and adds information that will alter treatment depending on its result.

PLAIN RADIOGRAPHS

The importance of rigid discipline in the diagnostic workup of a patient with low back pain cannot be overemphasized. To maximize patient outcome, the core of information derived from a thorough history and physical examination must be the basis for all subsequent decision making. To prevent treatment problems, diagnostic tests should be *confirmatory* of a clinical impression but should not be used as screening tests, because most tests are overly sensitive and highly nonselective. Not surprisingly, most of the iatrogenic problems in the management of low back pain can be directly attributed to overreliance on radiographic findings, which may have no positive clinical correlation. Boden et al. expressed concern that a dangerous thought process begins with the habit of approaching diagnosis by stating, "Let's get a magnetic resonance image (MRI) to see if there is anything wrong with the spine." A recurring theme with diagnostic tests is that pathology visualized on any imaging study is not necessarily painful and may not be the cause of a particular patient's pain. This statement becomes more appropriate as the resolution of both computed tomography (CT) and MR imaging improve with advancing technology.

The cause of most industrial low back pain is probably muscle strain or disc herniation. The diagnosis of both of these entities can be made on the basis of a good history and physical examination. The natural history for most patients with these diagnoses is benign, with resolution of most signs and symptoms within 2 to 4 weeks. The addition of any diagnostic test in this period not only adds unnecessary cost to the management of these patients, but it may cloud the picture by adding information that may appear pathologic on the x-ray (or other study) but has no true correlation to the clinical entity currently being entertained (Fig. 1). In addition, the search for organic pathology justifies continued physician patient interactions in the attempt to find the occult cause of back pain when no mechanical cause exists. The continued use of diagnostic tests in the search for pathology when none exists may convince the patient that some-

thing is wrong and that a search must go on until that entity is found (10).

In the presentation of low back pain, plain radiographs of the spine rarely add any information. They may be unnecessary for at least 6 weeks in most cases of acute low back strain (11). Exceptions exist to this rule, and in the case of any "red flags," radiographs should be obtained. Red flags (Table 1) include patients younger than 20 years of age or older than 50 years of age; a history of trauma, cancer, or generalized systemic disease; constitutional symptoms; rest or night pain; or a history of recent infection or immune suppression. In addition, immediate diagnostic evaluation

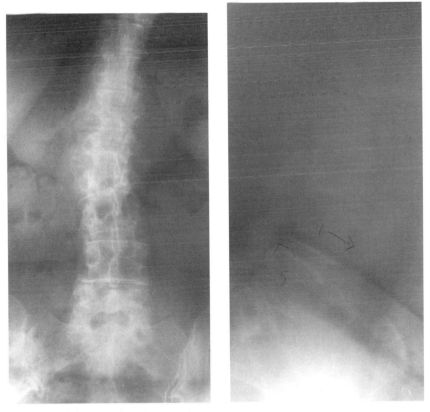

A B

FIG. 1. Anteroposterior (**A**) and lateral (**B**) radiographs of a 65-year-old woman with acute onset of low back pain (without radiculopathy) after bending down to pick up a box. She has had no prior history of back pain. The patient was treated with activity modification and nonsteroidal antiinflammatory drugs; symptoms resolved in 2 weeks. At 4 years, the patient continues to be symptom free. The findings of spondylolisthesis at L4–5 and degenerative scoliosis do not correlate to any clinical findings.

TABLE 1. *Red flags: indications for immediate imaging study on first presentation of a patient with low back pain*

Age <20 or >50 yr
Trauma
Cancer
Night Pain
Fevers
Weight loss
Pain at rest
Immune suppression
Neurologic deficit
Diabetes

should be obtained for any patient with saddle anesthesia, sphincter dysfunction, or a lower-extremity neurologic deficit (12). A medical evaluation should be initiated in patients with constitutional signs and symptoms, because many serious medical conditions present with back pain.

A patient who does not fit any of the red flag criteria should be started on conservative measures, including warm compresses to the back, nonsteroidal antiinflammatories (NSAIDS), a short course of muscle relaxants (carisoprodol or cyclobenzaprine) if indicated, and activity modification (13). At this stage, the specific diagnosis is not important to the therapy, because the entire population is treated in a similar fashion. A few patients eventually may need an invasive procedure, but at this point, there is no way to predict who will respond to conservative therapy and who will not. If the back pain is not resolving with appropriate conservative management by 4 to 6 weeks, plain radiographs are indicated and usually include standing films anteroposterior (AP), lateral, and spot lateral views of the lumbosacral junction and may help to make the diagnosis of congenital spinal stenosis, spondylolisthesis, segmental instability, spondyloarthopathy, or occult fractures and infections. When the diagnosis of spondylolysis is being entertained, additional views can be added although they usually add little information. If after interpreting the three basic views a question exists of a pars interarticularis defect, oblique views can be obtained.

Radiographs may demonstrate spondylolysis with or without spondylolisthesis, which affects 5% of the population (14). Most patients, however, will be able to perform the activities of daily living with little to no discomfort. If symptoms do exist, conservative measures usually are sufficient for the patient to return to full activity. In a small percentage of patients, all conservative measures fail, and a fusion is required (15).

Plain radiographs can be especially helpful in defining instability. Lateral weight-bearing flexion and extension bending films may demonstrate instability at a spinal motion segment. More than 3 mm of sagittal translation is abnormal in the lumbar spine, and angular rotation can be quantified as well (16). Although plain radiographs after 4 to 6 weeks of conservative treatment may be more beneficial than at the outset of the process of low back pain, these radiographs still may be misleading. Degenerative changes such as disc-space narrowing, traction osteophytes, vacuum disc phenomenon, and endplate sclerosis are prevalent in older patients and show a poor correlation with clinical symptoms (17).

Although occupational back pain may present after a significant traumatic incident, numerous microscopic injuries occur daily with normal wear and tear and permit a certain amount of leakage and desiccation of the nuclear material from the disc space. Because this process is gradual, the loss of nucleus usually is asymptomatic. Therefore, as a person ages, the disc spaces will narrow and usually remain symptom free until a superimposed injury occurs. Thus, the narrowing and radiographic changes are usually not relevant to the clinical picture unless rationally correlated with the patient's symptoms and signs (18).

MYELOGRAPHY AND COMPUTED AXIAL TOMOGRAPHY (CT)

Myelography has been the time-honored gold standard against which other tests, such as CT and MRI, have been measured. Myelography has proven efficacy in the diagnosis of lumbar herniated discs and has shown usefulness in the preoperative evaluation of stenosis as well as the evaluation of the patient with the failed back syndrome (19). For most diagnoses, including lumbar disc herniation, however, CT and MRI exceeded the accuracy of myelography while causing less morbidity and radiation exposure to the patient. In addition to its limited utility, myelography, like other studies, has a significant false-positive rate in asymptomatic persons. Hitselberger and Witten reported a 24% false-positive rate in asymptomatic patients undergoing myelography for acoustic neuromas (20). For these reasons, myelography is indicated only when specific criteria are met, such as in cauda equina syndrome (CES), as a preoperative study, and in the postoperative spine patient with pain to diagnose entities such as arachnoiditis or residual stenosis (Fig. 2).

Computed tomography can directly visualize the neural elements and their potential compressing structures. In this respect, it differs from myelography, in which neural compression is inferred through changes in the contrast-filled structures. Unlike MRI and myelography, CT usually is performed only on the vertebra requested, usually the lower three, and therefore can miss unsuspected pathology in other segments. The accuracy of CT can be enhanced by routinely imaging the spine after introduction of water-soluble contrast agents (post-myelography CT). These

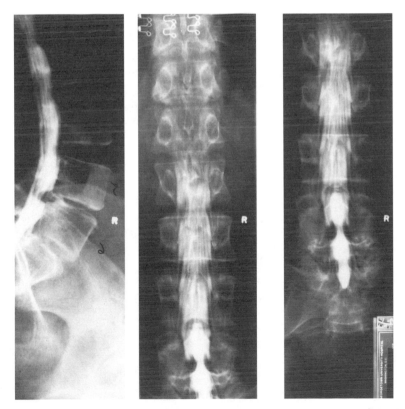

FIG. 2. Myelogram of a 58-year-old woman with back and left leg pain that has failed 3 months of conservative therapy. Plain radiographs were unremarkable. Myelogram demonstrates central and lateral recess stenosis at L4–5 and below. The patient underwent decompression and fusion with resolution of symptoms.

tests are indicated as a preoperative study for herniated disc and stenosis to define clearly the area requiring surgical attention.

At present, CT scans still show bony detail better than MRI; however, their use, much like that of radiography and MRI, should be used only in the appropriate settings. Strict guidelines for ordering CT scans are essential to avoid the pitfalls of such a highly sensitive test. Wiesel et al. reported a 36% incidence of CT abnormalities in a group of asymptomatic volunteers, and these abnormalities increased with age (21). As with other imaging techniques, the clinical significance of the findings on CT can be determined only by correlation with symptoms and objective physical findings.

MAGNETIC RESONANCE IMAGING

Magnetic resonance imaging is the newest diagnostic imaging modality and is widely used in the workup of low back pain and back disorders. The quality of MRI makes it the modality of choice for imaging infection, tumor, and soft-tissue trauma in the spine. In fact, MRI has been shown to be more accurate than discography or the previous gold standard, myelography, in the detection of degenerative disc disease (22,23). Compared with CT scanning, MRI is at least as accurate for diagnosing spinal stenosis and lumbar disc herniations (24). If it is not used properly, however, MRI can be as dangerous as it is useful.

Most studies that have defined the accuracy of MRI in diagnosing pathology in the spine were based on correlation with intraoperative findings and have lacked long-term clinical follow-up documenting the resolution of symptoms. Therefore, these studies are not able to demonstrate that the pathoanatomy visualized on MRI and found at surgery is actually correlated to the patient's complaint.

Although the sensitivity is high for MRI, the false-positive rate, a reflection of the specificity, in asymptomatic persons has been shown to be significant. In the lumbar spine, 22% of asymptomatic subjects younger than

60 years and 57% of those older than 60 years had significantly abnormal MR images that included spinal stenosis and disc herniations. In addition, increasing age has been correlated to decreasing specificity in respect to disc degeneration as diagnosed on MRI. Abnormal images demonstrating changes consistent with disc degeneration on T2-weighted images increased from 34% in asymptomatic 20- to 39-year-old patients to 93% in patients older than 60 (25). Obviously, if MRI was the sole determinant in a preoperative assessment, much unnecessary surgery would be performed (Fig. 3).

The first goal of the physician seeing a patient with low back pain should be to identify any conditions that would require emergent diagnosis and immediate treatment. In a patient presenting with low back pain, CES is the major entity that would demand emergent attention by the treating physician. This setting is one of only a few in which the use of a diagnostic modality should be ordered on first visit. Immediate MRI or myelography should be obtained, and if the suspicion of CES is confirmed, immediate surgical decompression is indicated. Other settings for urgent imaging include infection and pathologic fractures.

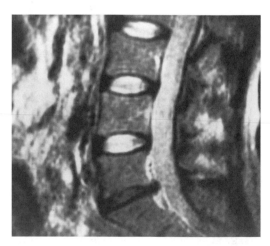

FIG. 3. Sagittal magnetic resonance images of an asymptomatic 45-year-old woman with a disc herniation at L5–S1.

If the patient does not respond, other pathologic processes must be suspected, and a more sophisticated diagnostic test is indicated, such as a bone scan or an MRI. If radiographs are unremarkable and further treatment such as trigger-point injections are not helpful, MRI is indicated. In addition, if other pathologic processes are being considered after radiographs (e.g., tumor or infection), an MRI is indicated. MRI is also indicated as a preoperative study in patients with stenosis to clearly define the levels that require surgical decompression.

NUCLEAR STUDIES

Scintigraphy or bone scanning uses radiation emitted from injected chemicals to detect pathology through a disturbance in vascularity or osteogenesis. Although bone scans are highly sensitive, they have a low specificity, and therefore it is vital to use the information in conjunction with a thorough history and physical examination as well as other diagnostic modalities. As with other studies, it is essential to have a diagnosis in mind before obtaining a bone scan. Bone scans can locate an area of suspected pathology, but usually without much ability to differentiate between pathologic entities. In a patient in whom the area of pain is already localized, the benefit of bone scan is low. A useful indication, however, is in a patient with isthmic spondylolisthesis. Bone scan can rule out an acute fracture as the cause by demonstrating a cold lesion, which is diagnostic of a more chronic process.

A bone scan can identify early bone tumors or infections not visible on routine radiographic examinations. In the patient with nonmechanical low back pain, a bone scan can help detect an occult neoplasm or metabolic disorder. In addition, a thorough medical examination can help to detect most of the extraspinal causes of apparent low back pain, which account for about 3% of back pain presenting to orthopaedists (26).

Single-photon emission computed tomography (SPECT) scanning is a newer modality, consisting essentially of tomographic images following radionuclide injection. SPECT scanning has found utility in the assessment of the patient with pain after spinal fusion. In the symptomatic postoperative spine, the sensitivity and specificity of SPECT scanning have been reported to be 78% and 83%, respectively (27).

DISCOGRAPHY

Historically, the three indications for discography have been to define the morphology of the disc, to augment other studies radiographically, and to determine disc disease by pain provocation. The use of discography as an adjuvant to define the morphology of the disc is no longer a useful test because of the availability of CT and MRI. CT discography appears to be a sensitive and accurate indicator of intradiscal architecture and pathology. High accuracy, greater than 90%, can be achieved in the confirmation of foraminal or extraforaminal lumbar disc herniations, which is higher than with other modalities (28).

The use of discography for identification of the pain generator in patients with low back pain is a much debated topic. It has been proposed as a diagnostic tool to identify internal disc disruption, which may cause low back pain. Proponents believe that if pain is reproduced during injection into the disc, in similar character and distribution to that of which the patient typically complains, the area of pathology has been localized and therefore can be surgically addressed. Holt (1968) reported a false-positive rate of 37% in asymptomatic prisoners, and this modality has been highly controversial ever since (29). Walsh et al. discredited Holt's study by demonstrating a zero false-positive rate in normal subjects (30). The Position Statement on Discography offered by the North American Spine Society states the following:

Discography is indicated in the evaluation of a patient if unremitting spinal pain, with or without extremity pain is greater than four months duration and when the pain has been unresponsive to all appropriate methods of conservative therapy. Furthermore, discography should only be used when a decision has been made that the clinical problems may require surgical treatment (31).

The greatest use for discography is in a patient with nonradicular low back pain with questionable MRI findings because of the involvement of multiple levels or equivocal MRI findings at a certain level. MRI findings in which adjuvant discography is useful include dark discs, speckled discs, and bulging (not herniated) discs. In these cases, demonstration of a positive pain response by discography is recommended before proceeding

with surgery (Fig. 4). In low-probability findings on MRI, such as a white or flat disc with no cleft, discography will be of low yield. In single-level abnormalities with a high probability for a positive provocation test, such as a dark or torn disc, discography usually should be avoided because of the high likelihood of superfluous information at a high expense (32).

STANDARDIZED APPROACH

The evaluation and treatment of low back pain still represent leading costs for medical expenditure in the United States. The vast ma-

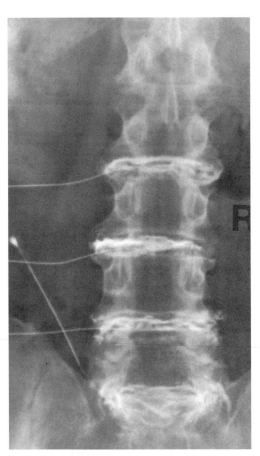 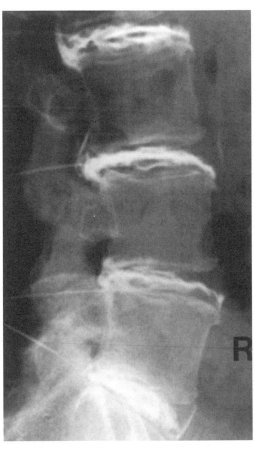

A   B

FIG. 4. Discogram with anteroposterior (**A**) and lateral (**B**) images of a 54-year-old man with low back pain that was unresponsive to 6 months of conservative therapy. Magnetic resonance imaging revealed dark disc disease at L3–4, L4–5, and L5–S1. Discogram reproduced the patient's symptoms at L4–5 only. L4–5 was surgically addressed with an interbody fusion, and the patient's symptoms fully resolved.

jority of industrial low back pain is not serious, however, and most employees can return to work in a short time. Employees return to work sooner and incur lower medical and compensation costs if an organized approach is made in evaluating, diagnosing, and treating the condition (33). Therefore, to maximize resources and efficiently use medical care while treating patients effectively, a standardized approach to the treatment of low back pain must be undertaken.

One of the manners in which to achieve the efficient and precise use of diagnostic studies in the evaluation of low back pain is the use of an algorithmic guideline approach, either standardized or individualized by each physician to fit his or her practice patterns. With the availability of significant technology and imaging modalities, the physician often must resist the impulse to use every modality currently available and to meet the often insistent demands of the patient for the latest study. A proper time and indication exist for each diagnostic study, as discussed in this chapter. In fact, the decision-making process can be made more difficult and less efficient when too much data are made available too early in the treatment process. Once emergent problems have been ruled out, the remainder of a protocol should be directed at the systematic evaluation and treatment of other diagnostic entities, such as a herniated disc, spinal stenosis, or back strain. Again, the goal of the physician is to make the correct diagnosis by using the appropriate studies in the proper time frame.

CONCLUSION

In conclusion, in a medical era in which technology continues to advance at a rapid pace, physicians need to resist the temptation of relying on expensive and nonspecific tests in the low back, in occupational injury or general health. The keys to the diagnosis and treatment of industrial low back pain continue to be based on a thorough history and physical examination. Diagnostic entities including radiography, CT, and MRI have specific indi-

cations, which need to be adhered to for the efficient use of medical resources and delivery of care. Even in a technologically advanced era, our current armamentarium of diagnostic tests is highly sensitive and less specific. Through a sensible approach to the diagnosis of low back pain, physicians can deliver ideal medical care in a precise fashion to benefit both society and the patient.

REFERENCES

1. Boden SD, Wiesel SW, Spengler DM. Workers' compensation as it affects the spine. In: Rothman RH, Simeone FA, eds. W.D. Saunders Company, Philadelphia, PA, 1992, pp. 1909–1921.
2. Snook SH. The costs of back pain in industry. In: Deyo RA, ed. *Occupational medicine:* state of the art reviews, vol 3. Philadelphia: Hanley and Belfus, 1988:1–5.
3. Abenhaim L, Rossignol M, Gobeille D, Bonvalot Y, Fines P, Scott S. The prognostic consequences in the making of the initial medical diagnosis of work-related back injuries. *Spine* 1995;20:791–795.
4. Bigos SJ, Battie MC, et al. A longitudinal, prospective study of industrial back injury reporting. *Clin Orthop* 1992;279:21–34.
5. Bigos SJ, Spengler DM, et al. Back injuries in industry: a retrospective study. *Spine* 1986;11:246–251.
6. Rowe ML. Are routine spine films on workers in industry cost or risk benefit effective: *J Occup Med* 1982;24:41–3.
7. Rowe ML. Low back pain in industry—a position paper. *J Occup Med* 1969;11:161–69.
8. Frymoyer JW, Nauberg A, et al. Spine radiographs in patients with low back pain. *J Bone Joint Surg Am* 1984;66A:1048–55.
9. Boden SD, Wiesel SW, Spengler DM. Worker's compensation as it affects the spine. In: Rothman RH, Simeone FA, eds. *The spine*, 3rd ed. 1992:1909–1920.
10. Loeser JD, Sullivan M. Doctors, diagnosis, and disability. *Clin Orthop* 1997;336:61–66.
11. Boden SD, Wiesel SW. Errors in decision making following radiographic investigations of the spine. *Seminars in Spine Surgery* 1993;5:90–100.
12. Hanley EN. Lumbar degenerative disease. In: *Orthopaedic Knowledge Update 5*. AAOS, Rosemont, IL, 1996:609–623.
13. Boden SD, Wiesel SW, Spengler DM. Lumbar spine algorithm. In: Wiesel SW, ed. *The lumbar spine*, ed. Philadelphia: WB Saunders, 1996:447–458.
14. Wiesel SW, Feffer HL, Rothman RH. Low back pain: development and five-year prospective application of a computerized quality-based diagnostic and treatment protocol. *J Spinal Dis* 1988;1:50–58.
15. Wiesel SW, Boden SD, Feffer HL. A quality-based protocol for the management of musculoskeletal injuries: a ten year prospective outcome study. *Clin Orthop* 1994;301:164–76.
16. Boden SD, Wiesel SW. Lumbosacral segmental motion in normal individuals: have we been measuring instability properly? *Spine* 1990;15:571–576.

17. Torgenson WR, Dotter WE. Comparative roentgeno-graphic study of the asymptomatic and symptomatic lumbar spine. *J Bone Joint Surg Am* 1976;58:850–853.

18. Cailliet R. Assessment and relative importance of physical findings and diagnostic procedures. In: Wiesel SW, Feffer HL, Rothman RH. *Industrial low back pain*. The Michie Company, Charlottesville, VA, 1985:489–491.

19. Haughton V, Eldevik O, et al. A prospective comparison of computed tomography and myelography in the diagnosis of herniated lumbar discs. *Radiology* 1982;142:103–110.

20. Hitselberger W, Witten R. Abnormal myelograms in asymptomatic patients. *J Neurosurg* 1968;28:204–206.

21. Wiesel SW, Tsourmas N, et al. A study of computer-assisted tomography: the incidence of positive CAT scans in an asymptomatic group of patients. *Spine* 1984;9:549–551.

22. Gibson MJ, Buckley J, et al. MRI and discography in the diagnosis of disc degeneration. *J Bone Joint Surg Br* 1986;68:369–373.

23. Weisz GM, Lamond TS, Kitchener PN. Spinal imaging: will MRI replace myelography: *Spine* 1988;13:65–68.

24. Modic MT, Masaryk T, et al. Lumbar herniated disk disease and canal stenosis: prospective evaluation by surface coil MR, CT, and myelography. *Am J Neuroradiol* 1986;7:709–717.

25. Boden SD, Davis DO, et al. Abnormal magnetic resonance scans of the lumbar spine in asymptomatic subjects: a prospective investigation. *J Bone Joint Surg Am* 1990;72:403–408.

26. Wiesel SW, Boden SD. Musculoskeletal injuries in the workplace: defining quality care. *J Am Acad Orthop Surg* 1994;2:231–238.

27. Slizofski WJ, Collier BD, et al. Painful pseudarthrosis following lumbar spinal fusion: detection by SPECT. *Skeletal Radiol* 1987;16:136–141.

28. Jackson R, Cain J, et al. The neuroradiographic diagnosis of lumbar HNP. *Spine* 1989;14:1362–1367.

29. Holt E. The question of lumbar discography. *J Bone Joint Surg Am* 1068;720–726.

30. Walsh T, Weinstein J, et al. Lumbar discography in normal subjects: a controlled prospective study. *J Bone Joint Surg Am* 1990;72:1081–88.

31. Mooney V. Position statement on discography. *Spine* 1988;13:1343.

32. Horton W, Daftari T. Which disc as visualized by MRI is actually a source of pain. A correlation between MRI and discography. *Spine* 1992;17:s164–s171.

33. Wiesel SW, Feffer HL, Rothman RH. Industrial low-back pain—a prospective evaluation of a standardized diagnostic and treatment protocol. *Spine* 1984;9:199–203.

Occupational Musculoskeletal Disorders
edited by T. G. Mayer, R. J. Gatchel, and P. B. Polatin.
Lippincott Williams & Wilkins, Philadelphia © 2000.

19

Primary and Secondary Therapy for the Acute Musculoskeletal Disorder

Susan J. Isernhagen

Isernhagen and Associates, Duluth, Minnesota 55802

COMPLEX CONCEPTS

Specific concepts are interrelated in the development and provision of therapy for musculoskeletal disorders in an occupational setting. Primary and secondary therapy do not stand alone as interventions or processes provided by one profession. Competence and intervention move beyond hands-on treatment and beyond a clinical setting. To be truly occupational, the therapy must be worksite related. Because occupational medicine is multifaceted and includes employer and payer relationships, therapy in an occupational setting also must have these characteristics.

A FOCUSED SPECIALTY

Occupational rehabilitation is a focused specialty. There is some similarity to sports medicine concepts. The focus of occupational rehabilitation is to create and maintain a healthy, productive worker. The playing field is the worksite; the game is the specific job tasks or occupational group that a worker performs. The goals are to prevent work injury, to return the patient to work as soon as injuries can be accommodated, to enhance healing, to rehabilitate the patient to the fullest potential, and to prevent reinjury. The outcome after injury is return to full duty or return to productive duty, and the proof of effectiveness is functional outcome: Specifically, can the worker perform the demands of the job?

DEFINING ACUTE DISORDERS

In delivering therapy for acute disorders, the therapist is faced with the need to put the disorder in context with work and health history. There are three categories that characterize acute in an occupational health setting. Distinctions are made because of perceived differences in motivation between athletes and workers. Although there is basis for this observation, it merely adds challenges to the therapist and other practitioners because the focus must remain worker related and outcomes are expected. Greater attention to confounding aspects is necessary. The therapist involved in primary and secondary care will use concepts and methods beyond the scope of traditional treatment. With successful and work-related interventions in primary and secondary therapy, motivation issues can be directed toward positive goals and prevent chronicity and disability.

1. A perceived sprain, strain, pain or dysfunction that is at an early stage does not create the need for medical treatment and can be treated with "first aid."
2. An acute musculoskeletal sprain, strain, injury, or exacerbated illness requires evaluation and treatment for a cumulative or sudden onset of symptoms.
3. A reinjury or recurrence of a previous similar musculoskeletal disorder may be categorized as acute even though it may

be the second, third, fourth, or other report of a similar condition in a chain of events. Thorough history taking and record keeping will allow this acute episode to be identified accurately as part of a sequence, thus creating a need for more comprehensive evaluation, functional restoration, and case management.

The therapist evaluating and treating acute injuries should classify them correctly. The failure to identify the types of injuries listed in number 3 (i.e., reinjuries or recurrences) can lead to increased severity of the problem, increased lost time and medical expenses, and ongoing mismatch of the worker's capabilities to the job. Eighty-two percent of back patients with non-recent onset and 69% of those with recent onset had back pain within the last month (1). Back pain is a recurrent condition (2). Upper-extremity cumulative traumas, by nature, are also potentially recurrent. If mismatch of a worker's physical capability and the work demands can be a cause of reported injury (as well as an outcome), then failure to identify a work mismatch in relationship to recurrent injuries will facilitate ongoing reports of "acute" musculoskeletal disorders.

OCCUPATIONALLY FOCUSED TREATMENT

Treatment of occupational musculoskeletal disorders differs from that of traditional treatment in a nonoccupational setting. One primary difference is the goal: return to full productive work. The following are the goals of traditional musculoskeletal treatment:

- Pain relief
- Restoration of function of a part that has impairment (internal outcome)
- Patient satisfaction

The following are the goals of occupation-based treatment:

- No loss of the "worker" perception or role
- Return to work as soon as safe and possible in either full or modified duty, (external outcome)

- Worker recognition of the mechanism of illness, exacerbation, or injury with subsequent prevention of reinjury
- Worker self-responsibility for treatment, ergonomic changes, functional restoration, and safe work habits
- Pain relief
- Restoration of function of a part that has impairment (internal outcome)
- Patient satisfaction
- Worker satisfaction
- Employer satisfaction

If the worker is treated in a traditional sense and therapists focus on pain and impairment, then the goal of medical treatment will be perceived by the worker as reduction of pain. If the work function context is maintained and the goal is return to safe full work, however, then the worker's perception will be that return to work is expected, desirable, and a way to measure success.

Treatment of acute musculoskeletal and secondary musculoskeletal disorders by therapists and physicians have been explored in the literature (3–14). The focus of this chapter is to define primary and secondary treatment in an occupation-focused manner that adds to the science of traditional treatment.

Primary treatment for acute musculoskeletal disorder refers to initial evaluation and treatment to reduce dysfunction and improve safe workability. This acute treatment is done as immediately as possible, on site or as close to the work site as possible, and in conjunction with return to work. Secondary treatment is treatment that takes place beyond acute care. It infers that acute care has not been completely able to provide the outcome of return to full duty. Secondary treatment has greater components of job-related rehabilitation.

CONCEPTUAL FRAMEWORK FOR OCCUPATIONAL MUSCULOSKELETAL TREATMENT

On Site and Immediate

Therapy rendered at the worksite provides the most efficient application of therapeutic interventions because it facilitates several important concepts in musculoskeletal treatment. First, it allows the worker to retain a worker role. Second, it does not create the need for travel away from the worksite, which may delay treatment or create more lost time than necessary. Onsite therapists, who provide a continuum of care, are fully aware of the types of jobs the workers do and potential modifications of the work or work requirements. After treatment, the therapist can go to the worksite to identify changes in the job or job method that will allow safe work practices to be performed.

The interaction of worker and therapist in identifying safe work practices in the midst of a treatment regimen creates a positive functional focus similar to the sports medicine concept. The worker feels confident that the therapist who encourages function knows the job, has made sure the job is safe, and has given the worker information and methods to provide safety parameters. There is a continuum of care when the therapist and worker are in the same physical location. This continuum of care may be enhanced if a physician and occupational health nurse are part of the team. Improving function is most able to be done in the "real world."

With small and medium-sized companies, it may not be possible to generate enough volume to justify on-site therapy. In these cases, therapists would have their occupational health clinic in an area of relative close proximity to, and ease of access for, the smaller industries. In this way, travel time is minimized. In addition, worksite analysis, ergonomic modification, and return to work planning are possible because the therapist can go to the worksite easily. The same parameters of the worker and therapist functioning together at the worksite hold true. A clinical setting off site should not remove the therapist from the rehabilitative construct of working with the worker at his or her job.

The close proximity of the therapist can be combined with the employer's request for workers to report symptoms, dysfunctions, injuries, or illnesses early. To do so results in early reporting of problems and prevents the first report from being one of a chronic condition. It also allows proper restorative treatment to begin at a stage where loss of work time can be minimized and results are faster and more successful (7,12).

Worker Oriented, not Patient Oriented

When seeking medical help for an illness or injury, the worker is most often interested in immediate symptoms and does not have a "patient" mindset. The problem is viewed as resolvable, and the worker expects to continue as a healthy, productive person.

It is "medicalization" of illnesses and injuries that force the worker into a "patient" role. Workers in traditional treatment are beset with medical terms, medical treatments, and often little discussion about self-responsibility. These factors encourage the worker to become a patient who is dependent, sick, needing medical attention, and suddenly unable to function in the normal realm. This medicalization of musculoskeletal problems is a large contributor to a "sick" role.

If the medical provider, therapist, or physician is part of the decision to remove the worker from productive work, then the "sick" role becomes set even deeper. The occupational health musculoskeletal injury becomes an event that shapes the worker's self-image. A worker with a problem that can be solved thus becomes a patient who is passive in a sickness system.

Pain Behavior Versus Functional Focus

One aspect of chronic behavior that is perceived as negative to medical providers is that of "pain focus." A system to avoid the development of pain behaviors begins in the acute phase and should be analyzed from a preventive as well as a treatment mode. To prevent pain focus, the medical provider must avoid this focus from the first moment. On entry into a therapy or physician office, the worker will be asked about his or her condition. If the primary questions are "where does it hurt," "how much does it hurt," "what type of pain do you have," "make a drawing of your pain," and similar queries, the worker is immediately focused on the fact that the pain is the most important issue. The worker status becomes that of a patient. In the patient status, pain is the number one priority. Whereas therapists and physicians realize that their questions regarding pain have to do with diagnostic work, the worker does not understand that construct of scientific inquiry.

When patients become focused on pain as a mechanism of reporting the seriousness of their injury, they begin to think of their life in terms of how pain relates to it. Thus begins the chronic pain behavior of quantifying the "pain level" (1–10), describing in detail the type of pain (sharp, stabbing,) and identifying each time pain is present ("it hurts when I sit, stand, walk"). Patients have been taught that qualifying and quantifying how they feel (rather than how they function) is important.

The functional focus, which begins in the first intervention, provides a different means of measuring the problem and the process. Ability to concentrate on performing safely, rather than rating pain, allows the worker to maintain a functional role with focus on positive progression.

Attitude and Perception of Disability

Of the total workers' compensation costs, only one-third is provided for medical benefits, whereas two-thirds go to disability benefits. Self-limiting behaviors of workers can play into the physical aspects of injury (15). Preventing disability requires that the provider of primary and secondary therapy create treatment programs that minimize lost time and a self-defeating worker mindset. The Boeing studies (16), retrospective studies of factors linked with reports of back pain, indicated that the relationship between worker and supervisor appears to be the most important. This study did not include physical work variables such as the results of functional testing, matching the worker with the job demands, or heaviness of the work. The fact that the relationship between supervisor and worker is related to "reporting" injuries is of

significant interest. It is important to identify *when* other factors are involved rather than the actual musculoskeletal injury (13,15). Being able to be compensated for injury can have a powerful effect on an injured worker. If a reward system were implemented for returning to work rather than being off work, the effects would be much different (17).

The behavioral aspect of workers in the recovery and rehabilitation process have been described (18). The emphasis on the whole person and eliciting cooperation rather than adversarial relationships is considered pivotal in having the injured worker accept the concept of return to work as a positive goal. Functional testing as part of the recovery process also imprints the worker with different perceptions (19). Workers who went through functional capacity evaluation demonstrated improvement in their perception of ability. Because functional capacity evaluation is not treatment, and a 3-day testing intervention is not likely to produce an actual physical progress, the improvement in perception of those injured people could be related to the process of performing safe functional activities and its meaning to their functional image.

COMPONENTS OF PRIMARY AND SECONDARY THERAPY

Active Therapy Versus Passive Therapy

Successful protocols for treatment can be based on the literature (4). Specific goals are decreased pain, improved active movement through altering fluid dynamics and input into the central nervous system, modifying connective tissue, enhancing neuromuscular performance, and educating the patient about safe biomechanical movement.

Active physical therapy on site is largely responsible for statistics that demonstrate reduced lost time and reduced cost (7,12). Passive therapy should be used only as an adjunct to therapy and never as a stand-alone treatment (11). The active realm of trauma disorders should be similar to "heart disease prevention included in treatment." Exercise, education, and functional activities should be the main components of physical therapy for work-related injuries. Other researchers and research groups (10,13,15) demonstrate that science supports the active approach. Their work demonstrates that passive measures have not been proven effective. The focus of active treatment should be on functional testing and activity (8). Equipment that is not specifically work related has not been demonstrated to improve functional outcomes of the worker returning to a specific job. Testing that does not have a work relationship does not predict whether a worker can return to work and may not predict the difference between a patient and nonpatient (20,21).

Obtaining cooperation for active therapy is linked to the worker retaining the worker role (22). Both the employer and the medical provider should be aware of their effect on the worker; early intervention and an emphasis on active treatment are important. Goal setting regarding the return to work is the hallmark of therapy for the acute musculoskeletal injury (11,22).

Physical therapists can affect both low back pain and the onset of the movement toward disability (23). The role of the therapist would be one of improving motion and function and achieving return to work health. It is stated that early and aggressive rehabilitation should be sought in treatment of work injuries. For occupation-based musculoskeletal injuries, the active approach is scientifically supported but has the additional benefit of natural transference into functional work skills. Focus on movement and self-awareness of safe activity precedes work testing and return to actual job duties. Specific combinations of treatment and return to work options are found in Table 1.

TABLE 1. *Job functioning combined with treatment[a]*

5-Level job modification	Suggested treatment regimen (must be individualized by therapist for client's specific needs)

Original job/original tasks
  Perform task with stressors fewer hours per shift
  Rotate tasks with stressors with nonstressful tasks
	Active treatment to alleviate weakness, tightness
	Functional testing to indicate readiness for full-duty capability

Full work schedule, original job, partial Perform tasks of the original job that do not stress injured part, work full shift	Active treatment to alleviate weaknesses, tightness Functional testing to indicate readiness for full duty capability

Original job category but lighter rotation, full shift
The lighter work portion of the job description
  e.g., Machine that makes lighter parts,
  nurse in pediatric unit rather than
  orthopedic unit
	Active treatment to alleviate weaknesses, tightness
	Functional testing to indicate readiness for full duty capability
	Specific work rehabilitation exercise and work simulation 1–2 h per session

Original job with ergonomic changes
  Basic: headphones, sit-stand work station,
  moving heavier objects to waist level,
  office ergonomics
  Advanced: Do moving of loads with fork truck
  instead of manually, use a vaccuhoist for
  lifting product, new ergonomic office furniture
	Treatment required only if functional improvement has not plateaued
	Ergonomic changes are often the outcome of functional testing with job matching

Different job in the business/industry that worker can perform productively and safely Different productive job Transitional/light duty area	Treatment of the injury/illness is often completed at this point because plateau has been reached Sequential functional testing if return to higher function job is a goal Intensive work rehabilitation if higher function job is a goal

[a]Note: Modifications can be combined: e.g., 1 can be combined with 4; 4 and 5 can be alternated in a shift (4 hour original job, 4 hour transitional work).

Education

As previously described, on-site therapists are able to provide education in a prevention mode when they are involved at the worksite. Effectiveness of back schools at Bath Iron Works have been described (12). In Department 50, the incident rate was lowered from 28 in 1990 to 15.9 in 1998, and 26 fewer lost time injuries occurred, at a cost of $7,071. each. The cost of the back school was $18,232. which afforded a net cost reduction for back injuries in attendees of $165,614.

Education in the entertainment industry from 1992 to 1995 has been impacted by education and exercised programs (24). The exercise program included instruction in exercise technique and instruction about how to use work equipment properly. It resulted in a 50% decrease in the reported sprains and strains injuries and a 66% reduction in workers' compensation costs.

The history of specific education, "back school," includes the use of prevention and the proper spine position (25), emphasizing stabilization of the spine. Exercise, which promotes strength for stabilization, can be used in home, recreational, or work-related activities. Similarly, the educator in on-site therapy clinics would demonstrate to the worker that prevention techniques taught in the clinics would be useful in these three areas (home, recreation, work) as well. It is important for workers to realize that injury prevention takes place 24 hours a day, not just at work (26).

Key elements in injury prevention include risk identification and control; maintenance of wellness, education, an attitude that work-related injuries can be prevented; and a focus on safety and training. Management must support the concepts of injury prevention. This principle is used by the therapist to collaborate with supervisors and management in promoting total safety in the workplace (26).

Being industry specific in the design of injury prevention programs optimizes learning (26–28). The on-site therapist who is able to evaluate work practices and changes is in a prime position to specify not only the general parameters of prevention programs but also how they relate specifically to the individual worker. For example, back education in the railroad industry would be developed differently from from that of preventing back and neck injury in the office.

Yet, even though a specifically industry designed program is used, elements of the individual worker must be included. The tall worker or the male worker, may have different ways of doing the work than a shorter or female worker. Therefore, the individual facets of education need to be customized as well as generalized. The education process integrates with both primary and secondary therapy both before and after reporting the disorder. If the therapist has previously educated the worker, safety concepts are reinforced in treatment. If not, the industry-specific education program is integrated into the restorative process.

Job Analysis and Ergonomics On Site

Analyzing the job objectively is as important as analyzing the function of the worker objectively. Job analysis methods can be specifically used to provide written descriptions of the essential functions of the job (29). Because of the need to adhere to antidiscrimination laws, job descriptions (used for matching workers to jobs) will be stronger if they have been validated by current workers.

Once job analysis has been performed, ergonomic analysis can evaluate factors that make the job unusually heavy, involving stressors that might lead to cumulative trauma disorders (CTDs) or make productivity lower than optimum. *Ergonomics* is the application of scientific principles of how to design work and workplace to match the functions of the worker. Ergonomic principles involve the use of physiologic measures to prevent fatigue; the use of safety measures to provide a workplace free of hazards; the use of kinesiology and engineering principles to design the methods, tools, and workplaces that best suit the greatest number of workers (30–34). The addition of job analysis to active therapy treatment brings the work and worker together in a match that can progress from modified through full return to work. It also has been noted by those providing services on site that many ergonomic changes made for an individual worker provide an opportunity to do similar ergonomic changes for the entire workforce (35,36).

Prework Screening

The therapist working with employees who have had acute musculoskeletal injuries will find that job-specific testing is an excellent finish to the treatment program. The therapist who has worked within the industry already may have been called in to design or perform prework screening (37). If the screening has been developed based on analysis of the job and developed in a validated manner, then prework screening is specifically job related to each job within an industry, allowing it to be used in conjunction with acute therapy, secondary therapy, functional testing, or work rehabilitation. The prework screening identifies the strength and coordination components necessary to do the work. In addition, the data used in developing the prework screen can be used also to develop expanded testing to provide a base for return-to-work functional-capacity evaluation and design of work rehabilitation. The goal is to develop additional strength and endurance in a worker to allow work to be done in either a frequent or continuous category. Moving the worker up the "physiologic ladder" allows more repetition to be done during the day (30). The basic prework screen can be used and additional exercise developed for endurance building, thus assisting primary and secondary therapy by validating work-specific physical parameters.

If the therapist was not involved in the development of job-specific prework screening, the necessity of defining reentry criteria will still exist. Once essential functions are identified and critical physical testing is developed, the therapist will have a base of prework screening if it is desired later.

Functional Testing

The therapist working with acute musculoskeletal problems is cognizant of the need to evaluate the match of worker and work and will employ aspects of functional testing. Treatment of a part will not necessarily improve the ability to function. For example, in low back injury, not only is the reduction in spasm necessary, but the ability to stabilize the spine and safely functionally perform lifts and carries is required to obtain a return to work goal. In the case of epicondylitis, resumption of gripping equipment will be necessary to perform work tasks. Only testing of functional work tasks will provide the work goal and reduce the chance of reinjury by ensuring safety to resume the job.

Reliability of observation for safety in evaluating body mechanics in functional capacity testing has been demonstrated to be reliable (38). Secondary-therapy functional-capacity evaluation and work tolerance testing are used as a more intensive tests of what the person can do in relation to specific jobs or a grouping of jobs available in the plant or to determine the level at which a person can work. Functional-capacity testing is different from physicians' restrictions in that the purpose of the functional testing is to identify a cadre of abilities of the worker, specified as to positional tolerances, weight capacities, and work activities that the worker can perform on a frequent basis during the day. These evaluations generally have the following characteristics:

- Standardized: Because return to work is in question and becomes a medical, vocational, and potentially legal issue, standardized protocols and test measures assist in creating both reliability of testing procedures and validity, which ensures that the capacities identified can be performed in the work setting.
- Objectivity: These evaluations are performed objectively. Even though the therapist may work on site or near the site, the therapist must retain the role of objective evaluator. The therapist does not work for either the employer or the worker groups.

Rather, functional testing is a measure of what a person can do, using objective scoring criteria (39).

In addition, functional capacity testing assists in the decision making about the worker's return to work. It can create worker confidence, and its information is easily used by the team that makes the decision to return the worker to work. Safety is a primary objective of functional testing, and it should transfer into safety in the workplace (40,41). Interactions with the worker to identify the worker's capability, as well as any precautions that must be taken during work activity, are important. The worker should know his or her maximum weight-lifting limit so that it will be clear what jobs can be performed in the workplace and what must be modified. Functional-capacity testing of the kinesiophysical approach also provides interactions for the worker to learn ergonomic postures, stretch breaks, proper body mechanics, and similar information that can be reinforced in the workplace (41–43). If functional testing identifies deficiencies in physical capability, worker movement problems, or lack of endurance, then referral to work conditioning can be directed.

As often as possible, functional testing should be matched with a job or jobs currently available within the industry. If a work-tolerance test is done, the actual job components will be added to functional testing. In both ways, the worker, the employer, the physician, supervisors, and other team members can identify specifically how and why a person is capable of returning to a specific job with or without modifications.

WORK CONDITIONING/ WORK HARDENING

In secondary therapy, the worker has not returned to work in a timely manner, and the physical deficits that are preventing this return to work need further remediation. Methods of working with the worker to improve work capability are divided into three areas:

Work conditioning is focused on restoring work capability by minimizing deficits caused by neuromusckosketetal problems. It has four components:

- Exercise to improve muscular strength and endurance
- Aerobic capacity training to improve aerobic capacity for working a full shift
- Work simulation that provides an opportunity to do job-specific neuromusculoskeletal tasks
- Education that allows specificity, which provides training for the specific job and review of cumulative trauma prevention and back-injury prevention guidelines

Work conditioning is time limited and goal focused, and it treats the worker as the rehabilitator. The therapist is the evaluator, a program progresser, and a medical professional who evaluates any physical difficulties that arise during the work restoration (5,6,44,45). The worker is asked to use work behavior such as being on time for the program, working to maximum, following the work/rehabilitation plan, and using positive worker behaviors. Also, physical restoration can be used before tertiary care (46). Secondary care is focused on neuromusculoskeletal restoration and involves a team of worksite professionals as well as medical professionals.

Work hardening is a more comprehensive form of work rehabilitation that requires a team, because the problems identified are more comprehensive. Work hardening is used for the worker who has vocational and psychosocial problems in addition to neuro-musculoskeletal deficits.

Work hardening requires considerable more team effort, because multiple goals are involved and multiple professionals are working with the employee. It tends to be longer in scope (hours per day), although its duration is similar to work conditioning. Behavioral issues are addressed as an important part of the rehabilitation, and psychological treatment is used to identify problems. Because the worker may have difficult vocational issues, components of vocational rehabilitation employer relations are emphasized in work hardening.

Work conditioning and work hardening are both performed in a clinical setting but also can be blended with the return-to-work process. The current practice is to integrate the worker part-time back into the workplace while the clinical program continues. A typical progression is found in Table 2.

On-site Work Rehabilitation

In many cases of an injured or ill worker, the employer is dedicated to keeping the person in the work environment and fosters relationships between employers and coworkers. The employer will provide policies and procedures within the workplace to allow an injured or ill worker to return to work when the the worker is stable and ready for progression. The therapist accompanies the worker; does an evaluation with job matching on the original job, a modified job, or a different job; develops a rehabilitation plan; and works toward the goal of as high a function as possible. These steps require the therapist to monitor closely for safety and work progression, although the therapist generally does not have

TABLE 2. *Design of modified work by injury severity*

Severity of injury and job significance	Example	Modified work options examples
Minimal Injury of body part is minimal or body part not used significantly at work	Finger sprain Ankle sprain in a sitting job Back strain that requires change of position every 30 min but this does not disrupt work	*Continue original job* Protect the injured finger Tape or splint ankle for protection is eliminated from work activity due to sitting Change worksite to allow sit/stand alternate work tasks
Moderate Area of body is utilized in same work processes. Area cannot be immobilized or rested Work processes and increased dysfunction and symptoms	Lateral epicondylitis in job that requires repeated gripping Hip arthritis exacerbation that limits standing to 5 min Back strain that is exacerbated by lifting and static forward strain	*Same job modified* Perform parts of job that do not require repetitive or forceful pinching/gripping Provide a high stool for up right activities Temporarily eliminate lifting portion of the job that is beyond safe limits Reposition chair, stool or work to reduce forward flexion
Significant A major body area requires immobilization or protection from pathological stresses; the loss of this area affects function of other body parts as well	Severely strained rotator cuff that is in healing phase of 4 wk; job requires two handed overhead work Fracture of fibula casted: job requires walking outdoors L-5 fusion in 6-month healing phase	*Provide different job* Perform job that does not require anti-gravity flexion or repeated shoulder motion Can use elbow, wrist and fingers Perform job that has minimal to moderate walking or standing on level surfaces Perform job that avoids lifting and allows lumbar non-neutral position
Whole body One severe injury or several injuries resulting in loss of full body movement or function	Accident resulting in arm and leg fractures Immediate post surgical L4–5 fusion	*Off work during whole-body healing time* Continually review safe functional ability and design RTW options for first level of safe productive function

to be on the worksite during the entire shift. The worker begins at a safe level of work. The therapist then continually reevaluates, progressing the worker through increasingly difficult work activities. The goal is return to full duty or to as high a safe function as possible. Medical records start with evaluation, use progressive record keeping as in a clinical site, and have clear goals and outcome records when the worker is discharged into full work status. Table 3 provides a model that combines active therapy and work simulation.

The advantages of allowing the therapist to interact with the worker in the workplace are that any flareup or unrecognized need for modification can be noted immediately by the therapist, and the worker who begins to have problems or doubts can be reassured by the therapist (47). In addition, the team who is accepting the worker back sees that there is objective monitoring of the worker and positive proof that the worker is capable of returning to the job. This interaction with the team is important on the worksite because, often, it is team or supervisor attitudes that can be negative toward a returning worker, either for fear that the worker will not try hard or that the worker will be reinjured, which is a detriment to the team. The therapist assures a more positive outcome.

If the therapist who works with the employees and with the company is the same therapist who developed functional job analysis and prework screens, the rehabilitation will be accepted well by employees because they understand that their therapist does know the physical requirements of the job. The trust between the worker and the medical provider

TABLE 3. *Active therapy and work simulation*

Provide multipurpose exercise
Progress aerobic conditioning, (steps, walk, treadmill)
Match body parts from work activities to exercise for rehabilitation
Teach flexibility stretches
Teach rest break stretches
Bring tools/materials to department or go to usual work area for work simulation

is enhanced by the work-related knowledge base of the medical professional.

Employer Involvement

Employers managing work-injury systems struggle with potential issues regarding a worker's motivation to return to work after illness or injury and the potential of defending themselves against false or exaggerated claims. Employers form philosophies that foster either trust or suspicion. Employers who have worked proactively to create positive relationships with workers have been rewarded with decreased workers' compensation costs, claims, and litigation (48,49). An employer's respect of the worker facilitates the therapist's work not only in the rehabilitation plan and optimum medical treatment but also makes it much easier to provide modified work when it becomes necessary. The enlightened employer understands that loyalty, work ethics, and reduced lost time are outcomes of a strong relationship between the employer and the worker.

To facilitate the employer relationship with the injured worker, the therapist has the responsibility of providing clear and objective information with return to work goals. Return to work is most effective when the physical capacity of the worker matches the physical demands of the job, which is clearly stated in writing to the worker, the physician, the supervisor, and other team members. Employer involvement in returning more difficult workers to work involves an understanding of the workers' needs as they return to productivity (9).

Progression of work intensity requires ongoing evaluation and progression of the worker to higher levels. The therapist and employer must interact so that the worker has the benefit of increasing his or her workload only when medically and functionally feasible and when work can be kept to the level that a worker can tolerate safely. Employees are important in the process, and interaction with the employees is critical (50). The employee must feel welcomed in the workplace, able to do the job safely, and supported by both supervisors and team members. The therapist again plays a strong part in solving problems in the physical return-to-work process and should be available if any functional issues arise. The availability of the therapist after return to work cannot be underestimated, because it is rare that a worker's return to work after a more severe injury is not accompanied by unanticipated issues that need to be resolved. The therapist can return to the worksite to look at modifications, exercises, work motions, and other factors.

Transitional Work

In cases of injury that are more severe and the job requirements exceed safety guidelines or physical capacity, other work should be considered to bring the worker back to the worksite. Two primary types have been identified by employers.

1. *Light duty* is work that has minimal productive importance. It generally done in an area where workers can go during their workshift, considered out of the normal mainstream of work. The light-duty area often draws negative reactions because of its nature.

   - It is not truly productive work; therefore, there is less pride of the worker in doing the work and little respect from coworkers for the work that is being done.
   - It is seen as a "sick" area; so those in the area are not considered well or healthy. This attitude impacts both a worker's self-image and the image of coworkers regarding the lack of health and ability in people in this work group.
   - Because light duty is not perceived as "hard work," light-duty workers may be perceived as not wanting to do their full share of work. There is a suspicion in some workplaces that those on light duty are drawing their pay but do not wish to contribute to the actual work; therefore, a bad attitude on the part of light-duty workers may be inferred.

   - If light duty does not have an endpoint, it becomes an endpoint for undesirable work and undesirable workers. Light-duty workers who feel labeled negatively by their former coworkers and supervisor also may fear that returning to the old work group will mean being chastised.
   - Working in a light-duty area where there is no progression to higher work does not provide an opportunity to improve physical progress toward the ability to do the demands of the job. Light duty does provide "healing time," but it does not have a rehabilitative nature.

   Whereas light duty does have aspects that can create problems in industries where transitional work has not been developed, it does at least offer the option to have employees maintain a work identity while rehabilitation or healing is taking place. A redevelopment of the program into more proactive transitional work will be beneficial.

2. *Transitional work* is progressive and functional. It takes the return to work concept of light duty and adds structure, focus, and goal achievement (51–55).

   - It provides work that is productive. It may be the lighter work in the plant, use smaller materials, produce lighter parts, or doing quality inspection of a lighter nature, but the common thread is that the work is valuable to the company.
   - The placement in transitional work is time limited, and workers in the transitional work area are seen in a temporary phase of activity before return to the regular job. It is not an endpoint but rather a transitional mode.
   - Transitional work offers the opportunity to progress workers to higher levels of productive standards either through increasing heaviness of work or increased repetitions as physical ability improves.
   - Transitional work that demonstrates a positive outcome by having workers return to the regular job in a healthy and

productive manner has demonstrated effectiveness (54,55).

Transitional work is accepted by management and labor because it provides business-related benefits as well as respect for the employees.

ON-SITE THERAPY AND COST REDUCTIONS

Onsite therapy is beneficial because the therapists understand the jobs, make themselves available to go the worker's worksite, and can make immediate and appropriate suggestions for full work, modified work, and light duty. In addition, on returning injured workers from lost time, the therapist will be available to monitor the actual physical ability of the worker to perform the job; so the worker does not fail in a return-to-work effort or incur a reinjury. In addition, the therapist plays an intermediary role between supervisor, coworkers, and the worker who has sustained an injury. The legitimacy of an injured worker's return in either a modified or light-duty position will be validated by the fact that a medical professional is there to assist in the process. One of the more important roles is for the therapist to help assure the supervisors and coworkers that the returning worker is capable of doing the job as designated.

Statistics regarding cost savings of on-site therapy services have been described. An onsite program at Frito Lay reduced the frequency of injuries from 39 in 1992 to 7 in 1995 as a result of the therapist being available for prevention components. In addition, the benefit of immediate and thorough acute therapy reduced the average cost of a CTD. Total costs incurred from $238,609 in 1992 to $17,191 in 1995 provided an average cost reduction per CTD of $6,118. The combination of early reporting, prevention, immediate treatment, and an ability to work with the worker as he or she returned to work substantially reduced the effects of CTDs in the workplace (24).

Roofner (24) also describes on-site therapy in the entertainment industry. The average cost per injury after the implementation of on-site physical therapy was studied. The costs were reduced from $1,996 in 1993 to $1,274 in 1994.

Outcomes of on-site physical therapy in a heavy industry show that lost work days per injury began at 31.1 in 1985 and were reduced to 10.9 by the middle of 1987. Total costs of medical indemnity were reduced from $4,128,545 to $935,318 in 1986. In the same period, the lost work days were reduced from $16,929 to $6,838. Yet the total costs for physical therapy services also were reduced from $144,750 to $130,594 (7).

It is indicated that the on-site therapy is successful because it includes aspects of therapy not available off site (7). These aspects are a team approach with others on site, functional outcomes that can be measured by actual work productivity, greater implementation of early intervention, facilitated communication, and the opportunity to provide education within the therapy framework. Working on site and modifying safe work activities while giving the worker support are important (47,56). The opportunity for the therapist to be with the worker during part of the workday gives the worker confidence that he or she is able to do the job, and the therapist can make slight modifications to the work to make it as functional and safe as possible.

DESIGNING PRIMARY AND SECONDARY THERAPY FOR OUTCOMES

Design

Through reviewing the literature and trends in outcome data, the designer of primary and secondary therapy of occupational musculoskeletal disorders will have strong direction (57). In therapy, the focus is activity and exercise. Testing is functional and related to specific work, and communication in planning involves the entire team in the medical and employment realm. The therapist closely interacts with the worker, the work, and the worksite. Return to the highest level of safe function is the goal. Regarding specific design, the optimum place for primary and secondary therapy is at the worksite; however, because many employers cannot provide the space or funding for such departments, the clinic placed close to the worksite and the therapist who is willing to go often to the worksite will be an acceptable alternative.

The physical design of the space will capture the amount of primary or secondary treatment expected and performed. The more the therapist is involved in prevention and education for early reporting, the more the actual therapy assumes the sports medicine model. Early treatment focuses on icing, stretching, resting the injured part, and remedial exercise as soon as feasible. The primary therapy for acute musculoskeletal disorders has only necessary passive modalities to relieve pain, muscle spasm, swelling, and other acute symptoms. Even in the acute phase of injury and the primary type of treatment, exercise, proper positioning, self-modulation of activity, and proper body mechanics become important.

The clinical setting for primary therapy will offer space for both evaluation and treatment of acute injuries, a small area for modalities, and the greater amount of space for active exercise and functional testing. Design for secondary therapy, which is focused on work rehabilitation and progressive functional testing, emphasizes exercise equipment, which is chosen based on the need to strengthen the parts of the body that are most used in the industries that are served. For example, if the work is primarily heavy active work of moving objects, building strength and endurance of the larger muscle groups and aerobic endurance will be important. If the businesses served are primarily offices, emphasis will be on postural muscles and proper positioning. Upper-extremity endurance should be targeted when cumulative trauma is the issue. The secondary therapy that uses the worksite to progress workers will need less exercise space than clinics that do the work

simulation on the clinical site. The therapist evaluating the space will consider how much rehabilitation will be done on site.

In both primary and secondary therapy, education in injury prevention and maintenance of proper body mechanics and proper positioning is included. In department design, space for team meetings should be included. If conference rooms are available in the industry, they may be used. If a clinic site does not have access to meeting space, a conference area will be required for confidential discussions of return-to-work processes that include the medical team and the employer return-to-work team. Communication in the workplace itself takes place, but medical information cannot be shared with others outside the medical team or designated employer representatives. Therefore, the confidentiality of the information discussed in conferences should be protected by closed meeting rooms.

Outcome Measurement

Outcome measurements in the occupational setting are developed through cooperation with the employer, payer, and medical providers. Identifying the components to be analyzed precedes data collection. In this way, return-to-work effectiveness and cost effectiveness can be measured by comparing variables before the implementation of primary and secondary therapy and after it is in place. Table 4 explains variables.

Redesign

Outcome evaluation will identify areas of therapy or related services that need to be altered. The nature of the workforce, the work, and the workplace is constantly in change. In addition, production demands, management–union relationships, and financial stability of a company create outside influences that affect both reporting of injuries and return-to-work activity.

Therapists analyze aspects of treatment for most cost-effectiveness and work outcomes. Constantly evaluating the data and the satis-

TABLE 4. *Outcome variables*

Demographics
  Age
  Gender
  Time at employer
  Time at specific job
  Categorization of physical job heaviness
  Anthropometric measurements
  Previous injuries
Treatment
  Primary
  Secondary
  Diagnostic code
  Diagnostic categorization (severity)
  Treatment duration (weeks, months)
  Treatment time (minutes, hours, per specific
    treatment)
  Time lost from work due to treatment (includes
    travel time)
Outcome
  Return to work
  Full duty
  Modified duty, same job
  Light/transitional job
Reinjury
  Same injury
  Different injury
Financial
  Lost time days and/absenteeism of any type
  Modified work days
  Medical costs of injury
  Disability costs
Affective and perception
  Perceived functional ability
  Perceived discomfort/pain
  Depression
  Worker role
  Team worker role
  Attitude: supervisor to employee, employee to
    supervisor

Both work-related and nonwork-related illnesses/injuries should have primary and secondary therapy available and measurable.

faction of workers and employers is critical in redesigning primary and secondary therapy.

CONCLUSION

Primary and secondary therapy in the occupational setting for acute musculoskeletal injuries traditionally have been available in most socialized industrial countries. Research and outcome data have identified the parameters that create the greatest satisfaction of workers, employers, payers, and the medical team. The successful concepts for optimum primary and secondary therapy are early, active, functional, progressive, and work related. In conjunction with all other aspects of medical care, the use of effective primary and secondary therapy creates an opportunity to diminish the human and financial costs of chronic illnesses. Primary and secondary therapy have the potential to keep workers in a healthier, productive, more functional role and to avoid the negative outcomes of chronic pain focus, dysfunction, and disability.

REFERENCES

1. VinKorff M, Deyo R, Cherkin D, Barlow W. Back pain in primary case: outcomes at 1 year. *Spine* 1993;18:855–862.
2. Skargren EI, Carlsson PG, Oberg BE. One year follow-up comparison of the cost and effectiveness of chiropractic and physiotherapy as primary management for back pain. *Spine* 1998;17:1975–1984.
3. Benz LN. Carpal tunnel syndrome measurement and surveillance management. In: Isernhagen SI, ed. *The comprehensive guide to work injury management.* Gaithersburg, MD: Aspen Publishers, 1995:254, pp. 231–253.
4. DeRosa C, Porterfield JA. The objectives of treatment for mechanical low back pain. In: Isernhagen SJ, ed. *The comprehensive guide to work injury management.* Gaithersburg, MD: Aspen Publishers, 1995:280–302.
5. Darphin L. Work-hardening and work-conditioning perspectives. Isernhagen SJ ed. *The comprehensive guide to work injury management.* Gaithersburg, MD: Aspen Publishers, 1995:443–460.
6. Darphin LE, Smith RL, Green EJ. Work conditioning and work hardening. In: Isernhagen SJ, ed. *Orthopedic physical therapy clinics of North America:* industrial physical therapy. Philadelphia: WB Saunders, 1992:105–124.
7. Dumont DD, Vance S. Industrial physical therapy: a model of on-site intervention. *Work Injury Management* 1992;July/Aug:1–4.
8. Isernhagen DI. The role of equipment in evaluation and treatment of occupational-related injuries. In: Isernhagen SJ, ed. *The comprehensive guide to work injury management.* Gaithersburg, MD: Aspen Publishers, 1995:504–512.
9. Larson BA. Work rehabilitation: the importance of networking with the employer for achieving successful outcomes. In: Isernhagen SJ, ed. *The comprehensive guide to work injury management.* Gaithersburg, MD: Aspen Publishers, 1995:483–494.
10. Quebec Task Force on Spinal Disorders. Scientific approach to the assessment and management of activity-related spinal disorders. *Spine* 1987;12:S1–S59.
11. Saunders R. Physical therapy early intervention. In: Isernhagen SJ, ed. *The comprehensive guide to work in-*

jury management. Gaithersburg, MD: Aspen Publishers, 1995:305–316.

12. Vance SR, Brown AM. On-site medical care and physical therapy impact. In: Isernhagen SJ, ed. *The comprehensive guide to work injury management.* Gaithersburg, MD: Aspen Publishers, 1995:269–276.

13. Waddell G. A new clinical model for the treatment of low back pain. *Spine* 1987;12:632–644.

14. Snook SH, Jensen RC, Pope MH, et al., eds. *Occupational low back pain.* New York: Praeger, 1984:115–121.

15. Waddell G, et al. Nonorganic physical signs in low-back pain. *Spine* 1980;5:117–125.

16. Bigos S, Spengler DM, Martin NA, Zeh J, Fisher L, Nachemson A, Wang MH. Back injuries in industry: a retrospective study II. Injury factors. *Spine* 1986;11: 246–256.

17. Nachemson A. Work for all—for those with low back pain as well. *Clin Orthop* 1983;179:77–85.

18. Green EJ. Behavior modification with the injured worker. In: Isernhagen SJ, ed. *The comprehensive guide to work injury management.* Gaithersburg, MD: Aspen Publishers, 1995:463.

19. Matheson LN. Getting a handle on motivation: self-efficacy in rehabilitation. In: Isernhagen SJ, ed. *The comprehensive guide to work injury management.* Gaithersburg, MD: Aspen Publishers, 1995:514–539.

20. Newton M, Waddell G. Trunk strength testing with iso-machines. Part 1. Review of a decade of scientific evidence. *Spine* 1993;18:801–811.

21. Newton M, et al. Trunk strength testing with iso-machines. Part 2. Experimental evaluations of the Cybex II back testing system in normal subjects and patients with chronic low back pain. *Spine* 1993;18:812–824.

22. Isernhagen SJ. The first minute: the importance of early and proper intervention. *Work (in progress).*

23. Cats-Baril WL, Frymoyer JW. Identifying patients of becoming disabled due to low back pain: the Vermont Rehabilitation Engineering Center Predictive Model. *Spine* 1991;16:605–607.

24. Roofner M. *Cost savings in corporate injury prevention programs.* American Physical Therapy Associates Annual Conference Presentation, 1998.

25. White LA. Back school. In: Isernhagen SJ, ed. *The comprehensive guide to work injury management.* Gaithersburg, MD: Aspen Publishers, 1995:103–112.

26. Baum B. Working with the workers: the "buy in" to maintenance of wellness. In: Isernhagen SJ. ed. *The comprehensive guide to work injury management.* Gaithersburg, MD: Aspen Publishers, 1995:254.

27. Mistal M. Establishing an industrial prevention program. In: Isernhagen SJ, ed. *The comprehensive guide to work injury management.* Gaithersburg, MD: Aspen Publishers, 1995:118–125.

28. Mistal M. Injury prevention education: back injury. In: Isernhagen SJ, ed. *Orthopedic physical therapy clinics of North America:* industrial physical therapy. Philadelphia: WB Saunders, 1992:47–54.

29. Isernhagen SJ. Job analysis. In: Isernhagen SJ, ed. *The comprehensive guide to work injury management.* Gaithersburg, MD: Aspen Publishers, 1995:70–82.

30. Rodgers S. Job evaluation in worker fitness determination. In: Pransky G, Himmelstein J, eds. *Occupational medicine.* Philadelphia: Hanley and Belfus, 1988: 219–240.

31. Rodgers S. A functional job analysis technique. In: Moore JS, Garg A, eds. *Occupational medicine.* Philadelphia: Hanley and Belfus, 1992:679–712.

32. Rodgers S. Matching worker and worksite—ergonomic principles. In: Isernhagen SJ, ed. *Work injury management and prevention.* Gaithersburg, MD: Aspen Publishers, 1988:675–677.

33. Isernhagen SJ. Ergonomic basics. In: Isernhagen SJ, ed. *Orthopedic physical therapy clinics of North America:* industrial physical therapy. Philadelphia: WB Saunders, 1992:23–36.

34. Isernhagen SJ, Hart DL, Matheson LN. Rehabilitation ergonomics perspectives from the field. *Work* 1996;7: 221–223.

35. Isernhagen SJ, Hart DL, Matheson LN. Rehabilitation ergonomists: standards for development. *Work* 1988;10: 199–204.

36. Isernhagen SJ, Hart DL, Matheson LN. Rehabilitation ergonomics: A model for work injury prevention. *Work* 1997;187–189.

37. Miller M. Functional prework screening. In: Isernhagen SJ, ed. *The comprehensive guide to work injury management.* Gaithersburg, MD: Aspen Publishers, 1995:86–96.

38. Smith RL. Therapists' ability to identify safe maximum lifting in low back pain patients during functional capacity evaluation. *J Orthop Sports Phys Ther* 1994;19: 277–281.

39. Isernhagen SJ, Hart DL, Matheson LN. Observation criteria for level of effort, work *(in progress).*

40. APTA Board of Directors. *Occupational health guidelines:* evaluating functional capacity, Appendix D. Alexandria, VA: APTA, 1997.

41. Isernhagen SJ. Contemporary issues in functional capacity evaluation. In: Isernhagen SJ, ed. *The comprehensive guide to work injury management.* Gaithersburg, MD: Aspen Publishers, 1995:410–427.

42. Isernhagen SJ. Functional evaluation and work hardening perspectives. In: *Contemporary conservative care for painful spinal disorders.* Philadelphia. Lea & Febiger, 1991:335.

43. Johnson L. The kinesiophysical approach matches worker and employer needs. In: Isernhagen SJ, ed. *The comprehensive guide to work injury management.* Gaithersburg, MD: Aspen Publishers, 1995:399–408.

44. Smith RS. Integrated work therapy in the small practice. In: Isernhagen SJ, ed. *The comprehensive guide to work injury management.* Gaithersburg, MD: Aspen Publishers, 1995:469–481.

45. Bettencourt CM. Using work simulating to treat adults with back injuries. *Am J Occup Ther* 1986;40:12–18.

46. Mayer TG, Gatchel RJ, Mayer H, Kishino ND, Keeley J, Mooney V. A prospective two-year study of functional restoration in industrial low back injury. *JAMA* 1987; 258:1763–1767.

47. Larson BA. Onsite work rehabilitation: the employer insurer, and provider connection. *Work Programs Special Interest Section Quarterly* 1994;8:1–2.

48. Swanburn NE. Employer point of view. In: Isernhagen SJ, ed. *Work injury:* management and prevention. Gaithersburg, MD: Aspen Publishers, 1988:317–328.

49. Pease DE. An industrial perspective o reducing worker's compensation claims. In: Isernhagen SJ, ed. *The comprehensive guide to work injury management.* Gaithersburg, MD: Aspen Publishers, 1995:689–696.

50. Isernhagen DI. Building occupational health and rehabilitation programs on the consumer's actual needs. In: Isernhagen SJ, ed. *The comprehensive guide to work injury management*. Gaithersburg, MD: Aspen Publishers, 1995:634–652.

51. Daly J. The role of the physical therapist in transitional work programs. In: Shrey DE, Lacerte M, eds. *Principles and practices of disability management in industry*. Boca Raton, FL: GR Press, 1995:107–130.

52. Hofer HO, et al. Ergonomic intervention in the workplace: experiences from 360 patient assessments. In: Fehr K, Kruger H, eds. *Occupational musculoskeletal disorders:* occurrence, *prevention and therapy*. Basel: Eular, 1992:91–106.

53. Lacerte M, Desjardins L. Evaluation of work disability from a worker- work environment perspective. In: Shrey DE, Lacerte M, eds. *Principles and practices of disabil-ity management in industry*. Boca Raton, FL: GR Press, 1995:207–225.

54. Shrey DE. Disability management practice at the worksite: developing, implementing, and evaluating transitional work programs. In: Shrey, DE, Lacerte M. eds. *Principles and practices of disability management in industry*. Boca Raton, FL: GR Press, 1995:55–106.

55. Shrey D, Olsheski J. Disability management and industry based work return transition programs. *Physical Medicine and Rehabilitation:* State of the Art Review 1992;6:303–314.

56. Ellexson MT. Worksite rehabilitation programs: the future for industrial rehabilitation? Work Programs Special Interest Section Quarterly. *American Occupational Therapy Association* 1997;11:1–3.

57. Isernhagen SJ. Challenge for the future. *Orthop Phys Ther Clin North Am* 1992;1:177–180.

Occupational Musculoskeletal Disorders
edited by T. G. Mayer, R. J. Gatchel, and P. B. Polatin.
Lippincott Williams & Wilkins, Philadelphia © 2000.

20

Medical Management in the First Three Months

*Joel S. Saal and †Jeffrey A. Saal

*†SOAR, Physiatry Group, Menlo Park, California 94025

The approach to the low back pain patient within the first 3 months of onset of symptoms should be guided by the integration of our knowledge base of the natural history of each of the clinical and anatomic subsets of low back pain and the known impact of interventions on their clinical outcomes. Rehabilitation of patients with low back pain is a comprehensive process that requires both accurate diagnosis and appropriate early intervention. Although pain may be a patient's initial chief complaint, the primary goal of rehabilitation is to optimize function. Our goal in the first 3 months is to prevent loss of function of the patient as a whole and to integrate a program to improve the function of the spine as a unit to prevent further injury. The rehabilitation process can be divided into three linked phases: diagnosis, pain and inflammation control, and the training phase.

The rehabilitation process should begin as soon as possible after disability onset and should be terminated only at the point when the patient can successfully return to his or her maximal realistic level of active function. Early diagnostic intervention with the establishment of a precise diagnosis is the key to unlocking the rehabilitation plan. An improper or imprecise diagnosis can lead to mistaken paths in the treatment regimen. A careful outlining of the rehabilitation goals before embarking on the program will eliminate the patient's frustration and discouragement. Early intervention will lead to control of the inflammatory processes and speed the recovery of normal articular and soft tissue range of motion (ROM). Adequate control of pain and inflammation plays a critical role in allowing the patient to actively participate in the rehabilitation program.

To facilitate progress and outline its milestones, short- and long-term goals must be set for each individual case. The short-term goals will require continual monitoring and adjustment as the clinical progression is monitored during delivery of the rehabilitation care plan. It is imperative that the patient be integrally involved in the goal-setting process. The patient must fully understand the realistic outcome of his or her clinical condition. Additionally, the patient must understand the time frame required and the methods to be used to achieve this outcome. If the physician and patient are not on the same "wavelength" on all these issues, the outcome will be less than optimal.

The most important task in managing a patient suffering from low back pain is to establish a diagnosis (Tables 1 and 2). Localization of the pain generator is paramount in spinal pain diagnostics. A structure that appears to be most involved on magnetic resonance (MR) imaging scan or other imaging study may not be that which is generating the disabling pain. Therefore, a careful correlation of the history, mechanism of injury, physical examination, and diagnostic studies is imperative to establish the location of the pain generator(s).

TABLE 1. *Differential diagnosis of acute low back pain (musculoskeletal origin)*

Category one: Nonspecific low back pain without radicular referral	Category two: nonspecific low back pain with radicular referral

Primary low back pain syndromes
    Anular tear (i.e., the common "back sprain")
    Contained disc herniation
    Mechanical pain secondary to degenerative
      spinal segment
    Internal disc derangement
    Posterior element pain (facet synovitis,
      spondylolysis)
    Non-specific soft tissue pain
    Sacroiliac joint dysfunction
    Primary psychological disorder
    Osteoporotic stress fracture
	Primary leg pain syndromes
	    Intervertebral disc herniation
	Spinal stenosis
	    Central
	    Lateral
	    Spondylolisthesis causing spinal stenosis
	    Degeneration with spondylolisthesis
	    Anular fissure with noncompressive radiculopathy

TABLE 2. *Primary low back pain syndromes*

Mechanical low back pain of primary posterior element origin
    Facet mediated pain
    Spondylolysis,
    Spondylolisthesis
Primary intervertebral disc disorder
    Degenerative disc disorders (with and without segmental instability)
    Contained herniated nucleus pulposus (HNP)
    Internal disc derangement (chronic anulus tear or fissure)
Back pain of miscellaneous etiologies
    Soft-tissue pain syndromes, ie., fibromyalgia
    Primary psycho-social problems
    Deconditioning syndrome
Early and late postoperative lumbar surgery failure
    Recurrent disc herniation
    Spinal stenosis (missed, secondary)
    Segmental instability
    Infection
    Internal fixation hardware breakage/dislodgement
    Arachnoiditis
    Chronic pain syndrome (associated with emotional/behavioral disorders)
    Spondylolysis aquisita (Iatrogenic pars stress fracture)
    Discogenic pain
    Adjacent spinal segment disease
    Nonspinal pathology (visceral or systemic processes)

DIFFERENTIAL DIAGNOSIS AND DIAGNOSTIC EVALUATION

In the primary screening evaluation, the physician must first look for indicators of neoplasm, infection, systemic disease, or visceral disorders (Table 3). Diagnostic testing after the initial contact will be dictated by the presence or absence of these indicators (Table 4). Additionally, the physician evaluation must screen for gross neurologic deficits and the possible presence of cauda equina syndrome (CES), which typically presents with saddle anesthesia

TABLE 3. *Nonspinal causes of low back pain syndromes: red flags*

Neoplasm: primary spine, metastatic disease retroperitoneal, pelvic, prostate processes

Pelvic disease
Genitourinary disorder
Vascular disease
Systemic arthopathy
Primary neurologic disorder
Paget's disease
Hip and lower limb disorders
Peripheral nerve entrapments

TABLE 4. *Diagnostic evaluation for low back pain disorders value, timing, and level of use*

Evaluation	Timing	Level of use	Value
History	Initial contact	Primary	Important to sort differential diagnosis
Physical examination	Initial contact and serial evaluation	Primary	Important to sort differential diagnosis monitor progress
Radiographic evaluation	>4 wk unless red flags	Primary	Fracture, tumor, deformity, systemic disease
MRI	>4–12 wk unless red flags or neurologic loss	Specialist	Disc disorders, stenosis, tumor, infection, canal compromise
CT	>4–12 wk unless red flags or neurologic loss	Specialist	Less sensitive than MRI for similar disorders, sensitive for osseous evaluation
CT myelography	>4–12 wk unless red flags or neurologic loss	Specialist	Spinal stenosis, preferred in some centers as preoperative evaluation
Bone scan	Red flags only, not routine use	Primary	Fracture, tumor, infection
Lab Studies	Red flags only, not routine use	Primary	Tumor, infection, metabolic systemic disease
Thermography	Never		No proven value
EMG	>4 wk of neurologic loss leg pain referral	Primary or Specialist	Sort out neurologic disorders
SSEP	>4 wk of neurologic loss, leg pain/numbness	Specialist	Spinal stenosis, unusual spinal pathology, spinal cord asessment
Discography	>6 mo	Specialist	Controversial use for discogenic pain
Nerve Blocks	>3–6 mo	Specialist	Preoperative assessment, spinal stenosis, multisegment disease

CT, computed tomography; EMG, electromyogram; MRI, magnetic resonance imaging; SSEP, somatosensory evoked potentials.

and an inability to initiate urination or bowel evacuation. It usually is caused by a large disc herniation at the L4–5 interspace, causing severe compromise of the descending sacral nerve roots in the thecal sac at that level.

PATHOGENESIS OF LOW BACK PAIN

The outer anulus of the intervertebral disc has nociceptive innervation and is therefore of great importance in many back pain syndromes. In the initial approach to the patient with low back pain, one should exclude the disc as the source. Acute or subacute tearing of the anulus through repetitive microtrauma or, less commonly, from a single major stress can result in low back and referred pain into the lower extremities. Repetitive flexion and torsional loads to the lumbar spine have caused anular injury leading to disc degenerative changes. Lifting is a major cause of intervertebral disc injuries especially when twisting or lateral bending is combined with flexion. Attrition of the supporting component of the anulus can result in a degenerative and painful disc that bulges; alternatively, the degenerative process may progress to the development of the herniated disc.

No scientific evidence has been established that muscles themselves cause back pain. Pain referred to the musculature can arise from any source that feeds into and is modulated by the dorsal ramus system. Basic science studies support that ligaments and fascia may be sources of primary pain, but there is no substantiation that they cause pain syndromes that persist longer than 4 to 6 weeks. Thus, soft tissues of the lumbar region must obey the same biologic rules that apply elsewhere in the body. For example, hamstring muscle injuries do not create pain syndromes that persist beyond the normal point of healing.

The lumbar facet joints also may contribute to low back pain (1). Facet joint articular cartilage is exposed to high loading pressures in extension and torsion (1). Bony proliferation will follow cartilage degeneration. These hypertrophic changes, often in combination with vertebral endplate osteophytes, can cause stenosis of either the central or lateral nerve canals resulting in radicular symptoms (2,3). The spinal degenerative process is a continuum. As a given disc degenerates and desiccates, it becomes more susceptible to fissuring, which in turn will lead to poor spinal stability and a risk of disc herniation and discogenic pain syndromes.

Some practitioners believe that the sacroiliac joints are important spinal pain generators; however, the data are inconclusive. It appears that the sacroiliac joints may play a part in some pain syndromes, but they are clearly not a major source of primary low back pain.

CLINICAL SUBSETS

Acute Anulus Tear Syndrome

The acute anulus tear usually occurs as a result of repetitive microtrauma (4); however, it may occur as a result of a single strenuous flexion or torsion, or it may be caused by a seemingly insignificant forward bend. Assessment will reveal that activities and physical examination maneuvers that "load" the disc will increase symptoms. Anular tear pain is classically increased with flexion and is provoked by sitting.

Clinically, the patient presents with guarded motions in all plane, but pain is greatest in flexion. Extension is usually painless or significantly less painful. Back pain usually is generalized across the low back, with varying degrees of lateral intensity, depending on the portion of the disc wall involved. There may be referral of pain to the groin, sacroiliac joint "region" (common), or upper thigh. Physical examination findings include a straight leg raise (SLR) that is negative or that reproduces low back pain only at 70 to 90 degrees of elevation. The neurologic examination is normal, without change in reflexes or muscle strength. Palpation often reveals tenderness to deep pressure over the spinous process at the involved level, typically L-4 or L-5. This syndrome usually resolves spontaneously after 7 to 14 days. Ice, nonsteroidal antiinflammatory drugs (NSAIDs), gentle extension exercises, a day of bed rest if necessary, and limited activity during the painful period are indicated. Education in back care is indicated for these patients in an attempt to prevent further progression of the injury or a recurrence. Repeated episodes of anular tear may lead to a herniated disc.

It is important to note that it is common for a patients suffering from a herniated disc to provide a past history of recurrent episodes of anulus tears, occurring at increasingly frequent intervals. Therefore, a patient with recurrent acute anulus tear episodes should be treated with back school, spine-specific exercise training, and lifestyle modifications. At physician encounter, the recurringly symptomatic patient should also be viewed with a higher index of suspicion of having more serious disc pathology, that is, a disc herniation, or internal disc derangement. Aggressive treatment consisting of an exercise program to improve lumbar dynamic stabilization and fitness and back education may limit the incidence of disc herniation in this recurrent group, which in turn may reduce the severity of the episodes or degree of physical impairment when a disc herniation does occur.

Subacute Low Back Pain Syndromes

A patient who presents with an acute syndrome whose symptoms persist beyond 6 weeks should be suspected of having a more serious disc pathology, that is, a disc herniation, a chronic radial anular fissure, contained herniated nucleus pulposus (HNP), or degenerative segmental disease. On physical examination, this group may have low back pain, which increases with a supine passive SLR test below 60 degrees, coupled with dorsiflexion of the ankle, a finding indicative of dural irritation. A normal neurologic examination is typical and therefore does not exclude a disc herniation. It only excludes patients with a deficit caused by root or canal compression or inflammatory radiculopathy.

In the group of patients who have chronic discogenic pain, that is, anulus tear or HNP, the dural irritation will often respond to ice or corticosteroids (oral or epidural) combined with a specific regimen of therapeutic exercise. The medication will help reduce the inflammation, but it is not effectively used unless to facilitate participation in an exercise program. Exercise improves function and helps to relieve pain. Further, it provides a self-care strategy for the patient to use in preventing and treating future episodes. These patients may not reach clinical stability until 8 to 16 weeks after initial onset. Physiologically, 12 weeks of exercise training is required for the patient to achieve a satisfactory level of fitness to protect his or her spine.

Herniated Nucleus Pulposus

Disc herniations may present with a number of different clinical syndromes. The presentation will vary based on whether the disc is lateral, paracentral, or central in its location in the spinal canal, the spinal level of the lesion, the patient's physical condition, and the size of the patient's spinal canal and available reserve volume.

More than 90% of disc herniations occur at L4–5 or L5–S1 (5). The herniated material extends through a cleft in the anulus. The herniation may be contained by part of the remaining anulus, which is still intact posteriorly (i.e., contained HNP) or openly exposed to the epidural space (i.e., extruded). The extruded disc may be in continuity to the parent disc or separated from it (sequestrated). The prognosis for these patients as a group is good, with appropriate nonoperative treatment. Unless there is progressive neurologic loss (weakness in the extremity that progresses through the treatment course), CES, or an overwhelming social reason, surgery is not indicated unless a comprehensive and appropriately aggressive nonoperative treatment program fails after at least 6 weeks. Usually, a 12-week timeline is necessary to achieve successful results without surgery.

In the only controlled study of surgery versus minimal care for HNP, Weber found little difference in the two groups 4 years after initiation, but a moderate difference was found at 1 year (6). Our cohort study of patients with HNP treated with exercise and epidural cortisone yielded a 93% success rate at 3 months (7). Discectomy for persisting leg pain due to a documented HNP can be expected to yield a 90% chance of relief of leg pain symptoms (8,9), a rate that compares favorably with nonoperative care. Therefore, patients clearly have an option to be treated nonoperatively for HNP. Surgery is indicated only if aggressive nonoperative care fails or if a progressive neurologic deficit occurs. The imaging test findings of an HNP with or without a neurologic loss should not be the sole criterion used to refer patients for operative intervention of their HNP. Nonoperative and natural history studies demonstrate no difference in neurologic recovery whether patients are treated operatively or nonoperatively.

Painful Degenerative Segment with Mechanical and Soft-tissue Pain

A disc need not compress a nerve to cause pain. The pain from a degenerative spinal segment in the absence of a disc herniation or stenosis can occur as the result of a combination of factors: soft-tissue irritation immediately posterior to that spinal level, referral of pain from the osteoarthritic changes within the facet joint, nociceptors within the posterior anulus of the disc, or dural irritation from inflammatory mediators. The degenerative segment may become symptomatic even when subjected to loads within the physiologic range. A degenerative segment is one where degenerative changes have affected the disc and facet joints, thereby altering its biomechanical characteristics.

The clinical presentation of these patients is varied. Patients typically have mechanical pain increased or triggered with movement, with resolution on discontinuation of those particular movements. Historically, the patient may complain of pain with static positions that is, prolonged sitting or standing. The patient may relate that walking or continuous low-level activity permits changes in position to reduce symptoms. The most frequent symptoms in this subgroup include back pain, buttock and thigh pain, and occasionally paresthesias in the foot. It is unusual for these patients to report leg pain as their primary symptom. In that setting, disc herniation, stenosis, or a combination of these features may be suspected.

Physical examination findings may reveal limitations of spine motion in all planes, paraspinal soft-tissue tenderness, and midline deep bony tenderness. SLR may create low back pain, buttock pain, or foot paresthesias at end range. Neurologic examination is typically normal.

These patients respond well to therapeutic exercises. Pain control is achieved through soft-tissue flexibility, application of ice, and NSAIDs, combined with progressive trunk strengthening. Those with persistent pain may be candidates for either an epidural or facet injection with glucocorticoids. In this subgroup, epidural with glucocorticoids is best suited for patients with back or buttock pain, which is increased by forward flexion, and SLR that reproduces back and buttock pain. The patient with low back pain that increases with extension or prolonged standing may be a candidate for a facet injection with glucocorticoids. These injections are best performed under fluoroscopic guidance to ensure accuracy.

Unremitting Low Back Pain

Some patients with unremitting symptoms of low back pain (i.e. for longer than 6 months) will have pain of a primary intervertebral disc origin. This condition is often diagnosed by discography. These patients may not respond to all currently available forms of nonoperative care. Discography will demonstrate the anular fissure and reproduce the patient's symptoms.

Spinal Stenosis and Neurogenic Claudication

Degenerative changes may lead to narrowing of the lumbar nerve canals. This is particularly troublesome in patients with developmentally small diameter spinal canals. The nerve canal stenosis (central, lateral, foraminal, extraforaminal) may create vascular compromise and inflammatory changes resulting in radicular pain referral, which is most commonly exacerbated by walking. MR scanning, coupled with electromyographic studies will readily diagnose this condition. Vascular claudication and peripheral neuropathy (e.g., diabetic, uremic, toxic/metabolic) should be differentiated by appropriate testing. Most spinal stenosis patients will respond to light exercise and NSAIDs and activity modification. Particularly symptomatic patients may benefit from epidural cortisone injection. The natural history of this condition is favorable in most cases, and therefore only limited numbers of patients with spinal stenosis actually require surgical intervention (10). The results of surgery for lumbar spinal stenosis is successful in approximately 65% to 70% of cases (11). Although an individual patient may respond dramatically to decompression surgery, these results are not necessarily generalizable.

TREATMENT

The nonoperative treatment program has many potential tools available to the provider. This program may include the following elements:

- Antiinflammatory medications
- Pain-modulating medications
- Physical modalities for pain control
- Detoxification from addictive and central nervous system (CNS) acting medications
- Therapeutic exercises to
  control pain (flexion range vs. extension range)
  improve flexibility
  improve ROM
  improve muscular strength
  improve muscular endurance
  improve balance
  improve proprioception and coordination
  improve cardiorespiratory aerobic and anaerobic capacity

"work-harden"
train for a particular sport, job, or activity
- Use of braces and orthoses
- Ergonomic evaluation and workplace modification
- Body mechanics instruction
- Psychosocial evaluation and intervention
- Psychiatric intervention (when necessary and appropriate)
- Family counseling
- Vocational counseling
- Nutritional counseling and weight reduction
- Smoking cessation
- Establishing a successful doctor–patient relationship

The decisions for implementation of the specific components of the program include the factors of timing and goal setting, after taking into a account the clinical subtype, the pattern of development of clinical findings, the extent of structural pathology, the patient's age and perceived outcome, as well as activity level, motivation to improve, level of physical conditioning, and psychosocial barriers to recovery.

The treatment of low back pain disorders can be divided into two phases: *pain control* and *education and exercise*. The pain-control phase may include a variety of passive modalities, for example, flexion or extension exercises, lumbar mobilization, traction and selective injection procedures, antiinflammatory analgesic medications, and antidepressant medications. The key element of treatment is the training phase, which emphasizes back school, functional movement training, and specific, dynamic, muscular lumbar stabilization exercises. It cannot be overemphasized that exercise training for the lumbar pain patient is a powerful pain reliever as well as a method for improving their overall function and prevention of further tissue injury.

Pain-control treatment should be instituted as early and efficiently as possible. It is important not to get stuck in the pain-control phase but rather to advance as rapidly as possible to the training phase of treatment. The initial stage of pain control, referred to as *back first-aid*, treats the pain and teaches the patient to control pain and muscle spasm. The treatment includes the application of ice, resting in a position of comfort, and basic instruction in body mechanics to facilitate pain-free movement getting in and out of chairs, cars, bathtubs, and toilet seats. The use of medications then can be kept to a minimum. Depending on the type of injury sustained, anterior structures (the discovertebral joints) or posterior structures (the facet joints and neural arch) determine the position of comfort. During this initial phase, rest is also specifically prescribed. Bed rest is the most abused and overprescribed treatment in lumbar spine care. It should be used to control pain in the early days following the injury. There is absolutely no evidence to support total and absolute bed rest after any injury to the lumbar spine. Excessive bed rest leads to hypomobile lumbar motion segments, tightened soft tissues, loss of muscle strength, blunting of motivation, and loss of mineral matrix from bone. Pain-relieving modalities, such as passive physical therapy modalities and pulsed alternating electric muscle stimulation combined with ice may be useful to reduce the acute pain in certain circumstances when other simple measures (rest, ice, NSAIDs, and activity modification) are not beneficial. Extension exercises are valuable in reducing pain in many discogenic subsets. When extension exercises cause centralization of low back pain without exacerbating or peripheralizing the lower extremity (i.e., radicular pain), they can be used. Peripheralization of the pain (i.e., an increase in radicular referral pain into the buttock or lower extremity) is a contraindication to the use of extension exercises and may indicate the presence of significant stenosis, posterior element pathology, or disc herniation in the subarticular, foraminal or extraforaminal zones. The overuse of extension exercises may lead to facet pain that delays the treatment program.

No one should remain on one particular type of exercise regimen during the entire treatment phase. Flexion exercises are most useful for patients suffering from facet pain or symptomatic neural compromise from a stenotic canal. Flexion has been noted to cause a reduction in articular weight-bearing stress to the facet joints. Flexion exercises have an additional benefit of stretching the dorsolumbar fascia. Flexion must be used cautiously because of the increases in intradiscal pressure that result and the heightened stress it places on the posterior anulus. Flexion exercises in the seated position are the most precarious because of the acute increase in intradiscal pressure that results. In our opinion, this type of William's flexion exercise is contraindicated in most lumbar spine patients. In addition, lumbar flexion exercises performed with the legs fully extended create the greatest degree of flexion on the lower spinal segments and predispose the posterior anulus to the receipt of forces that may disrupt its integrity. Therefore, flexion exercises, if they are to be done, should be done in spine-safe positions. These positions unload the spinal segment while allowing a flexion stretch to occur.

Spinal immobilization with a corset or semirigid brace is rarely necessary but may be useful for patients who are not strong enough to use their own musculature to stabilize the spine, especially senior citizens, and patients with a degenerative spondylolisthesis. Studies of these devices demonstrate the corset's inability to immobilize the lower lumbar spinal segments. Caution must be exercised when prescribing these appliances because their overuse can lead to trunk flexor and extensor muscle weakness. Patients must be instructed to remove the orthotic device at least once daily to exercise the trunk musculature. Patients who have become dependent on the appliance must be weaned slowly while progressively strengthening the supporting musculature to replace the corset. Lumbar bracing may be useful in the treatment of acute spondylolysis to facilitate fracture healing.

The use of mobilization and manipulation techniques may be useful to attain articular as well as soft-tissue ROM. *Mobilization* refers to forceful movement of a joint within physiologic range, manipulation that requires greater force, and moves a joint beyond its physiological range. Stiffened segments should be mobilized and tight soft tissues must be adequately stretched. Ultrasound application is useful only as a deep-heating modality that can facilitate soft-tissue extensibility to allow adequate articular as well as soft-tissue mobilization to occur. Ultrasound treatment as a sole intervention is ineffective and should not be used. Caution must be taken with the use of ultrasound in the presence of an acute radiculopathy. Possible posttreatment exacerbation of radicular symptoms related to neural swelling may occur. Mobilization treatment is appropriate for the thoracolumbar junctional segments, which often become hypomobile and indeed are a pain generator in their own right, often masquerading as a lumbar pain syndrome. Overvigorous mobilization can be harmful in all types of injuries and should be carefully graded and timed during the treatment program. These techniques are most useful for back pain syndromes without significant leg pain of a 14 to 28 days' duration. Manipulation has not been shown to be beneficial in leg pain predominant syndromes or back pain that has persisted longer than 1 month. Manipulation has been shown to be no more effective than transcutaneous electrical nerve stimulation (TENS) or placebo for patients with lumbar pain lasting 6 weeks to 6 months (i.e., subacute).

The use of traction may be useful in obtaining symptomatic relief in the treatment of discogenic injury subtypes; however, the authors rarely find it useful or necessary. There are proponents of gravity inversion, gravity lumbar reduction, auto traction, and pelvic traction. Depending on the size of the patient, the type of equipment available, and the type of disc pathology, all these traction modalities may be useful in providing short-term symptomatic relief. Although many studies report subjective symptom improvement, no scientific evidence has been found to support the contention that any of the traction techniques actually facilitate nuclear migration (12). A force equal to about 26% of the body's weight is required to overcome the surface resistance of the lower half of the body (12). Bed traction, therefore, cannot overcome this enormous resistance, does not facilitate any separation of the vertebral elements, and is therefore not advisable.

One of the most powerful tools in the pain-control phase is the use of selective injections. The list of selective injections include epidural cortisone injections from the translumbar or sacral approach, intraarticular facet injections, and lumbar selective nerve-root blocks. These procedures are indicated when the patient is unable to progress with an active physical rehabilitation program because of excessive pain.

The use of an epidural cortisone injection in the face of a disabling lumbar radiculopathy caused by disc injury or stenosis can provide dramatic relief. The rationale for using corticosteroid antiinflammatory agents is well established. In general, epidural cortisone is most beneficial for patients with more leg pain than back pain and for those who manifest dural tension signs on physical examination. Early aggressive use of epidural cortisone injections in this clinical setting may give tremendous benefit to the successful rehabilitation program. Their use must be considered an adjunct to treatment, however, and not be considered a treatment in themselves. Intraarticular lumbar facet injections under fluoroscopic guidance place corticosteroids into inflamed facet capsules; their role remains limited and controversial. Lumbar selective nerve-root block instills medication around an inflamed nerve root when the major pathology is in the foramen or lateral recesses.

Trigger-point injections with local anesthetic may only be useful to reduce painful muscle spasm associated with persistent trigger zones identified in the offending muscles (13). There is a limited physiologic basis for the addition of corticosteroids in this type of injection. Trigger-point injections followed by soft-tissue stretching and joint mobilization can improve ROM and pain reduction. It is uncommon for the soft-tissue component of pain to act as the principal disabling factor even in the face of a structural diagnosis of discogenic pathology. It has been reported that trigger points are found in predictable locations and correspond to well-established acupuncture points. Dry needling a trigger point is just as effective as injecting the trigger point with lo-

cal anesthetic solution alone, saline alone, or local anesthetics solution plus corticosteroid alone (14,15). Acupuncture may be useful to break a pain cycle, thereby facilitating an active exercise program. It must be kept in mind that acupuncture as well as the other injection procedures are purely facilitators of treatment and should be considered adjunctive therapy only. They are useful in the pain-control phase in a framework and clinical context in which they enhance rehabilitation.

The use of antiinflammatory medication in the early phases of treatment may be appropriate. The recent report of high levels of phospholipase A2 activity in herniated discs supports the contention that inflammation plays a role in symptomatic disc herniation (16). The analgesic effect of the NSAIDs as well as their ability to act as prostaglandin synthetase inhibitors can have a role in treating lumbar pain syndromes. The efficacy of oral corticosteroids has been established in the treatment of acute radiculopathy, although the exact dosage and optimal time frame are questionable. Their use in nonradicular acute back pain syndrome is controversial and limited.

Prescribing so-called muscle relaxants has no physiologic basis. All the currently marketed muscle relaxants are CNS depressants and not peripherally acting muscle relaxants (17). Caution should therefore be exercised against their use on this basis as well as on their potential depressive and addictive nature. The use of opiate analgesics is occasionally necessary in the initial week of treatment of lumbar pain syndromes but rarely is required once the specific treatment program is under way. The proper use of positioning, rest, ice, extension or flexion exercises, and the selective injection procedures normally obviate the need for opiate analgesics.

TRAINING PHASE

Principles of Training Phase

The key element in the phase devoted to exercise training is the accomplishment of adequate dynamic control of lumbar spine forces to eliminate repetitive injury to the intervertebral discs, facet joints, and related structures. This training program is called *stabilization training*. Stabilization exercise routines are to be divided into basic and advanced levels. Before strengthening exercises, the focus of all exercise is soft-tissue flexibility and joint ROM. Flexibility training focuses on the musculotendinous units of the hamstrings, quadriceps, iliopsoas rectus femoris, external and internal hip rotators, and gastrocsoleus. Strict attention is given to the maintenance of neutral spine posture while the stretching exercises are performed. These exercises are performed on a daily basis. Stretching first is performed passively by the exercise trainer and then is included as part of the patient's home program. Continued active assistive stretching is occasionally necessary to overcome soft-tissue contracture resulting from limited mobility and nerve-root irritation.

The patient then is trained in active joint mobilization methods, such as extension exercises in prone and standing positions, as well as alternating midrange flexion and extension while in a four-point stance. Abdominal muscle strengthening begins with simple "curl-ups." Then the patient progresses to dynamic abdominal bracing, an exercise that uses alternate arm and leg movements while lying supine, contracting the abdominal musculature, and holding the spine in neutral position. More advanced exercises include diagonal curl-ups, and diagonal curl-ups performed on an inclined board. Once the patient can carry out three sets of 15 repetitions, more challenging exercises are undertaken. At the end of this stage of the program, lower abdominal muscle strengthening is emphasized using straight leg lowering exercises.

Demonstration of proper form and technique is required for the patient to graduate from the basic level. These same guidelines are applied to the weight-training portion of the program. Aerobic and anaerobic training is incorporated into the total fitness program. Aerobic conditioning is initiated early in the program in the form of walking. Shortly thereafter, the patient rides a stationary bicycle or uses a cross-country ski machine. Swimming is encouraged for interested patients but is not uniformly used with all patients. These activities first are performed under supervision to ensure maintenance of neutral spine posture. Training levels are tailored to the patient's age, medical history, and level of aerobic conditioning according to previously established guidelines of the American College of Sports Medicine (18).

Decisions for advancement to more challenging exercise during the program are be based on functional progress rather than pain level. The program endpoint is determined by maximal functional improvement, which cannot be improved further by exercise training or pain control.

Training Phase of Lumbar Rehabilitation

After successfully passing through the pain-control phase of the rehabilitation program, the treatment program progresses to the training phase. The key element in the training phase is to attain adequate musculoligamentous control of lumbar spine forces to eliminate repetitive injury to the intervertebral discs, facet joints, and related structures. Without progressing beyond the pain-control phase, we would continue to have an individual who is at risk of a repeat injury, further limiting his or her activity. It is crucially important to try to identify why the individual was injured and what risk factors for further injury he or she faces. The patient must be made aware of these factors and trained in specific measures to deal with them to learn preventative measures.

After a lumbar motion segment has been injured, it is at risk of repetitive injury. Numerous studies point out the recidivism rate in low back pain patients (17). Others have demonstrated the benefits of prevention programs in the industrial workplace (19). These prevention techniques can be taught in a back-school setting. Repetitive loading results in fatigue failure of the lumbar intervertebral disc and the progressive development of gradual disc prolapse (4). This supports the biomechanical construct of repetitive injuries to the intervertebral disc, leading to progressive pathology. It also makes us aware of how a simple anular tear can progress to further anular injury to develop into a full-blown disc protrusion or herniation (20). Therefore, the early identification of an anular tear indicates the need for early institution of a back-school program in an attempt to prevent future injury and disability. Our role in spine care delivery must not be simply to provide a "band-aid" symptomatic treatment. Our mandate should be to prevent back pain before it starts. Society can ill afford for the health care profession to ignore prevention and only endeavor to treat pain.

The core of our treatment regimen is an exercise program designed to teach the patient to use dynamic muscle control to maintain stabilization of the spine. This dynamic muscular stabilization program should allow patients to reduce the mechanical stress on their spines and thereby reduce the possibility of symptom production (21). Arguably, the end effect of this training should include not only symptom control but a reduction of the mechanical factors that accelerate the degenerative process. One can conceptualize this exercise training process as creating a muscle fusion to maintain spine stability. The goal, however, is not to make the patient rigid and inflexible (22,23). Quite the contrary, the patient is taught to improve and maintain symmetrical strength, flexibility, balance, proprioception, and trunk control. To apply the muscle fusion, adequate flexibility and spinal range of motion must be attained. Evidence of the diurnal variations and stresses on the lumbar spine note changes in lumbar disc and ligament extensibility as the day progresses (24). These changes are based on the creep of soft-tissue structures, leading to an increased range of motion. Adams et al. noted that bending and lifting activities performed early in the morning, when undertaken by nonextensible ligamentous and anulus fibers, cause fatigue damage to the disc more easily than do similar activities performed later in the day. This finding suggests a need for flexibility of the structures to eliminate this repetitive fatigue stress to the intervertebral joint. We should also think of the muscles that attach to the pelvis as "guidewires" that effectively change the position and symmetry of the pelvis.

Given that the pelvis is the platform upon which the lumbar spine rests, pelvic positioning is a key factor to postural control of the lumbar spine. Therefore, adequate flexibility of hamstring, quadricep, iliopsoas, gastrocsoleus, hip rotators, and iliotibial band muscles is important. There is also a need for flexible neural elements.

Training programs for the rehabilitation of the lumbar spine progress from floor and manual-resistance exercises to the use of resistance equipment. Training for strength and flexibility of the trunk and extremities is integral to the development of adequate postural control and stabilization skills. All patients must demonstrate a baseline level of skill in the floor exercise program before advancing to a gym training program. It is inadequate simply to tell a patient to "go to the gym and work out." Similarly, distributing exercises to patients on handout sheets yields unsatisfactory results (25). A properly structured training program in a gym can minimize the risk of injury through the use of weight-training equipment and maximize the gains from combined and coordinated muscle group activity. That type of training program should conceptually match the program of floor exercises, because both are based on the principles of dynamic muscular stabilization of the spine.

It is important to emphasize that every spine patient does not need to commit to an extensive weight-training program. The overall rehabilitation program should be designed for an individual patient's needs, with realistic and functional goals. Patients who are avid recreational athletes usually require additional strength gains that are attainable only through a weight-training program. This is certainly true of professional and high-level competitive athletes. These same considerations exist for patients involved in manual labor or in activities that require performing repetitive tasks with heavy loads. The training goals of a gymn program are similar to those of a floor exercise program. Development of trunk strength is essential for functionally stabilizing the spine (25). Increasing the strength and endurance of extremity musculature will limit the amount of stress placed on the spine and trunk during the performance of daily activities. Patients should be taught to use resistance equipment with spine-safe techniques and in spine-safe positions.

Extremity strength training techniques are targeted for the muscle groups that stabilize the trunk. These techniques are most commonly used during floor exercises and spine-safe lifting and bending. The benefits of performing extremity strength exercises are more than the targeting and training of specific sites of extremity strength. In addition, patients are instructed in cocontraction techniques that consist of active use of the trunk musculature to stabilize the spine while an extremity is working against resistance. Specific exercises are targeted for the prime trunk stabilizers, including the abdominal obliques, the latissimus dorsi (including all of its segments), the spine extensors, and the interscapular musculature (middle trapezius, serratus anterior, and rhomboids). A specific strengthening program is always tailored to the needs of the individual. The patient's physical capacity for occupational and recreational activities serves as a guide to structuring the program. The weight-training program is not geared solely toward strengthening the truncal musculature. Taken a step further, it becomes a total fitness program. Incorporated in this total fitness program is aerobic and anaerobic training. Teaching an individual to stabilize the spine while riding a stationary bicycle, while running on the treadmill, or while swimming becomes integral stages of the training program. Careful instruction that demonstrates proper spinal positioning while performing each of these activities is required. The injured worker is schooled in body mechanics and transferring the newly found skills to the job site. Ergonomic evaluation and modification of the job site also may be required.

The goal of exercise training is to develop an engram (26) of the motor control to accomplish stabilization. An *engram* is a neuro-physiologic phenomenon that describes the motor information necessary to perform a complex movement. All the individual components of a complex motor act are stored together as a unit forming an engram. These data, which are stored in the motor cortex, are retrievable without the need for conscious control. This phenomenon is identical to the training of athletic skill, such as a golf swing or a tennis stroke. During early training, conscious control is necessary. Later, the movement pattern becomes automatic and no longer requires conscious control. Isolation patterns are difficult to obtain, but the ease of use of the machine and the multiple stations make this type of equipment extremely practical. The use of cammed equipment, such as the Nautilus, has many distinct advantages. This type of equipment is designed with a cam, which varies the resistance offered by a given load to try to match the average torque curves for each of a large number of muscle groups. Theoretically, this eliminates the dead areas noted in certain portions of the ROM when an individual trains with free weights. Another advantage to cammed equipment is the individualized stations, which allow adjustment of foot rests and seat height.

The use of elastic bands is extremely practical, especially for home strengthening programs. Elastic bands can be used not only to supply resistance but also for flexibility programs. Isolation patterns can be accomplished with the use of elastic bands. This type of exercise is extremely practical because the patient is able to travel with the exercise equipment. Maintenance programs using elastic bands can be helpful. Occasionally, the buoyancy produced by water is useful during the initial phase of strengthening programs. An individual can be placed in the pool and with use of a life vest he or she can begin to use water and his or her own body weight as resistance for strengthening. These hydroprograms allow the individual to maintain lower-extremity strength and ROM as well as aerobic endurance.

This program satisfies not only physiological goals but also the psychological goals of the patient. Performing stabilization exercise in water allows some lower-level patients to advance more easily. Additionally, patients should be taught proper swimming techniques to avoid repetitive reinjuries.

Program Prescription

It is important for the physician prescribing the exercise program to communicate certain key information to the physical therapist. At the time of the initial prescription, the medical report must contain detailed pathoanatomic diagnostic information that relates the pain generator and whether a flexion or extension bias is preferred. Most typically, a flexion bias will be most appropriate for the patient with a painful spondylolisthetic condition (27). A similar approach may be indicated for a patient with lumbar spinal stenosis, whereas an extension bias works best in the setting of a herniated disc. Precautions regarding peripheral joint pathology that may interrupt active exercise training (e.g., patellofemoral pain) syndromes must be adequately communicated. Additionally, specialized lower-extremity or upper-extremity rehabilitation programs should be incorporated into the lumbar exercise program. For example, the patient with rotator cuff tendinitis (i.e., an impingement syndrome) and lumbar disc herniation will require a combined program. If the shoulder pathology is not addressed, the lumbar program will falter because of the patient's inability to carry out any exercises that involve the upper extremities.

Time goals must be given to the patient and the physical therapist. If these goals are not met, the program will require modification. For example, in the case of the patient with an acute disc herniation, the physician should inform the physical therapist that leg pain that limits progress in exercise persisting beyond three sessions should prompt return of the patient to the physician for an epidural injection of cortisone or other aggressive approaches to reduce radicular inflammatory response (28).

The decision to discharge the patient from the supervised exercise program and transition to a maintenance program must be a team decision. Because of their athletic background and motivation, some patients can learn the program quickly, that is, in six to eight visits, and thereby complete the supervised portion of the program. The deconditioned nonathletic patient, however, may need 18 sessions of supervised physical therapy to assume a level that will allow the transitional program to begin.

Exercise training is not finished in the physical therapy gymnasium. All patients must be transitioned to home programs. The patients must receive detailed and clear information regarding their precise program at discharge. The program should be updated 4 to 6 weeks after discharge as well. In many circumstances, the exercise program will continue at a neighborhood gym. In this case, the physical therapist or trainer must accompany the patient to the gym to instruct the patient about the program and proper weight-training activities using the specific equipment that is available. In some circumstances, the duration of supervised physical therapy can be shortened by having a trained exercise instructor work with the patient. The exercise trainer can monitor the program progression and act as the patient's coach during the recovery process. The exercise trainer will give feedback in the form of progress reports to the treating physician to allow smooth program progression.

REFERENCES

1. Adams MA, Hutton WC. The mechanical function of the lumbar apophyseal joints. *Spine* 1983;8:327–330.
2. Farfan HF. Muscular mechanism of the lumbar spine and the position of power and efficiency. *Orthop Clin North Am* 1975;6:135–144.
3. Yong-Hing KW, Kirkaldy-Willis. The pathophysiology of degenerative disease of the lumbar spine. *Orthop Clin North Am* 1983;14:491–504.
4. Adams MA, Hutton WC. Gradual disc prolapse. *Spine* 1985;10:524–531.
5. Kelsey JL. An epidemiological study of acute herniated lumbar intervertebral discs. *Rheumatol Rehabil* 1975; 14:144–159.
6. Weber H. Lumbar disc herniation: a controlled prospective study with ten years of observation. *Spine* 1983;8: 131–140.
7. Saal JA, Saal JS. Nonoperative treatment of herniated lumbar intervertebral disc with radiculopathy: an outcome study. *Spine* 1989;14:431–437.
8. Salenius P, Laurent L. Results of operative treatment of

lumbar disc herniation. *Acta Orthop Scand* 1977;48: 630–634.

9. Shannon N, Paul E. L4/5 and L5/S1 disc protrusions: Analysis of 323 cases operated over 12 years. *J Neurol Neurosurg Psychiatry* 1979;42:804–809.

10. Johnsson KE, Rosen I, Uden A. The natural course of lumbar spinal stenosis. *Acta Orthop Scand* 1993;251:67–68.

11. Johnsson K, Uden A, Rosen I. The effect of decompression on the natural course of spinal stenosis. *Spine* 1991;16:6–15.

12. Judovich BD. Lumbar traction therapy-elimination of physical factors that prevent lumbar stretch. *JAMA* 1955;159:159–162.

13. Walters CE, Partridge MJ. EMG study of the differential action of the abdominal muscles exercise. *Am J Phys Med* 1957;36:259–268.

14. Frost FA, Jessen B, Siggard-Andersen J. A control, double-blind comparison of mepivacaine injection versus saline injection for myofascial pain. *Lancet* 1980;1:499–500.

15. Lippitt AB. The facet joint and its role in spine pain: Management with facet joint injections. *Spine* 1984;9: 746–750.

16. Sjolund BH, Eriksson MBE. *Endorphins and analgesia produced by peripheral condition.* 1979, New York: Raven Press, pp. 29–41.

17. Goodman AG, Gilman LS, Gilman A. *The pharmacological basis of therapeutics.* New York: Macmillan, 1980, pp. 686–699.

18. Saal JA. Saal JA. Later stage management of lumbar spine problems. In: Herring SA, ed. *Physical medicine clinics of North America,* vol 2. Philadelphia: WB Saunders, 1991:205–222.

19. Moffett JA, Chase SM, Porteck BS, et al. A controlled prospective study to evaluate the effectiveness of back school in the relief of chronic low back pain. *Spine* 1986;11:120–123.

20. Moore RJ, Osti OL, Vernon-Roberts B, et al. Changes in end plate vascularity after an outer anulus tear in sheep. *Spine* 1992;17:874–878.

21. Saal JA. Dynamic muscular stabilization in the non-operative treatment of lumbar pain syndromes. *Orthop Rev* 1990;19:691–700.

22. Saal JA. Rehabilitation of football players with lumbar spine injury (Part 1). *Phys Sports Med* 1988;16:61–74.

23. Saal JA. Rehabilitation of football players with lumbar spine injury (Part 2). *Phys Sports Med* 1988;16: 117–125.

24. Adams MA, Hutton WC. The relevance of torsion to the mechanical derangement of the lumbar spine. *Spine* 1981;8:241–248.

25. Oldridge NB, Steiner DL. The health belief model: predicting compliance and dropout in cardiac rehabilitation. *Med Sci Sports Exerc* 1990;22:678–683.

26. Harris FA. Facilitation techniques and technological adjuncts in therapeutic exercise. In: Basmajian JV, ed. *Therapeutic exercise.* Baltimore: Williams & Wilkins, 1984;110–178.

27. Sinaki M, Lutness MP, Ilstrup DM, et al. Lumbar spondylolisthesis: retrospective comparison and three year follow up of two conservative treatment programs. *Arch Phys Med Rehabil* 1989;70:594–598.

28. Saal JS, Franson RC, Dobrow R, et al. High levels of inflammatory phospholipase A2 activity in lumbar disc herniations. *Spine* 1990;15:674–678.

Occupational Musculoskeletal Disorders
edited by T. G. Mayer, R. J. Gatchel, and P. B. Polatin.
Lippincott Williams & Wilkins, Philadelphia © 2000.

21

The Future of Musculoskeletal Disorders (Cumulative Trauma Disorders and Repetitive Strain Injuries) in the Workplace

Application of an Intervention Model

J. Mark Melhorn

Section of Orthopaedics, Department of Surgery, University of Kansas School of Medicine— Wichita, Wichita, Kansas 67208-4510

In 1975 the National Center for Health Statistics Interview Survey estimated that 16 million upper-extremity injuries occur yearly and that these injuries result in 16 million days lost from work (1). Recently, the U.S. government predicted that by the year 2000, 50% of the American work force will have occupational injuries annually and that 50 cents of every dollar will be spent on cumulative trauma disorders (CTDs). Currently, occupational illnesses affect 15% to 20% of all Americans; 56% of these occupational illnesses are CTD. These numbers continue despite the 1986 National Institute for Occupational Safety and Health (NIOSH) national strategy for the prevention of work-related diseases and injuries (2). There is little agreement on the three controversial aspects of CTD: (a) appropriate definition of work-related musculoskeletal pain; (b) the best ergonomic and epidemiologic model for CTD; or (c) the specific exposure relationships of the individual as they relate to the activities in the workplace. There is, however, common agreement on the need for reduction of CTD in the workplace. In 1996 direct health care costs exceeded 418 billion dollars, and lower-range estimates for indirect costs exceeded 837 billion dollars, for a total cost of 1.256 trillion dollars (3).

As the costs for CTD have risen, an effort has been made to redefine the term CTD by using the term *musculoskeletal disorders* (MSDs) (4). *Musculoskeletal pain* is defined as any pain that may involve the muscles, nerves, tendons, ligaments, bones or joints. This pain can be defined as real or imagined. MSD pain has been described by the U.S. government and other organizations as any musculoskeletal pain that a person believes is associated with activities performed at work. For the pain to be considered work related, state governments legislated a variety of work-contribution requirements (5).

The need for screening and prevention for MSD and CTD is documented in important publications such as *Repetitive Motion Disorders of the Upper Extremity* (6) and *Musculoskeletal Disorders and Workplace Factors: A Critical Review of Epidemiologic Evidence for Work-Related Musculoskeletal Disorders of the Neck, Upper Extremity, and Low Back* (7). The former publication (6) recommends screening for CTDs and states the following:

... workers with physically demanding jobs should undergo careful screening to disqualify those with unacceptable intrinsic risk factors, and a program of continuing physical condition should be required. In addition, it should be recognized that after 10 to 20 years, a worker should be transferred to a less demanding task. The belief that any worker can do any job until age 65, which is a premise of much workers' compensation policy and labor union rhetoric, is not realistic.

The latter publication (7) recommends prevention and states: "NIOSH concludes that a large body of credible epidemiologic research exists that shows a consistent relationship between MSD and certain physical factors, especially higher exposure levels. NIOSH will continue to address these inherently preventable disorders."

As important as diagnosis and treatment are for the restoration of the worker to the workplace, they cannot, except administratively, address the larger scope of MSD/CTD. To control this increasing workplace problem, health professionals and employers alike must direct their attention to prevention of MSD/CTD. Traditional approaches to injury reduction in the workplace have focused heavily on ergonomics and methods of effecting change through manipulation of the physical environment (8–10). Beyond ergonomics and education, medical consultation broadens the scope of intervention to include active surveillance of the worker population by means of health screens, clinical examinations, and, when indicated, early referral for conservative management. A physician knowledgeable about MSD/CTD and familiar with risks within the workplace is able to treat and rehabilitate injuries optimally for both the worker and the employer (11,12).

Evaluation of a Clinical Case or the Individual Patient

For the sake of argument, suppose that the difficulties inherent in epidemiologic studies could be overcome and that a definitive analysis of a particular job is carried out so that the proportion of cases of carpal tunnel syndrome (CTS) that are attributable to the exposure at work could be precisely determined. Whereas this type of information may be useful to an occupational safety officer, it would be of little value to the clinician treating an affected worker. Because epidemiologic data are statistical in nature, how these data might apply to a particular case cannot be determined. Even if a patient experiences symptoms only at work, the clinician is still unable to determine the extent to which the patient's CTS is related to the job. Quantitative understanding of intrinsic risk factors and their relationship to exposure to extrinsic factors at work is imperfect. The epidemiologic data are of only limited use to the clinician; at best, epidemiologic data might define the odds ratios for CTS between two jobs and the odds ratios between these and a matched sample of nonworking persons but can contribute little to analyzing the etiology of a specific case.

It is unfortunate that workers' compensation determinations must be made in individual clinical cases, because it is currently impossible to quantify the contribution of the job to the clinical problem. The proper arena for workers' compensation issues with regard to the etiology or causation of CTS and similar MSD conditions is at the statistical level, where surveillance, intervention, and regulation can be carried out in a meaningful way through prevention (13).

Six Tasks for the Occupational Health Care Provider

The administration of timely and effective treatment for CTD is important (13,14). Six critical tasks for the occupational health provider are outlined below.

1. Diagnosis: The occupational health care provider should try to identify the injured tissue and determine the nature and site-specific location of the injury. If the symptoms and signs do not allow for a specific anatomy-based diagnosis, the term *pain in limb* should be used for the diagnosis (11).

2. Contributing Factors: Once a diagnosis is made, the contributing factors must be evaluated, including intrinsic factors (anatomic abnormalities, metabolic disorders) as well as extrinsic factors (the nature of the patient's job, his or her avocations) (15).

3. Treatment: A treatment program must be selected that includes modified work during conservative treatment and continuation of return to work (16). If lack of improvement occurs from standard medical management, timely treatment may include surgery and early return to work. Early return to work with modified work can improve the individual's outcome from treatment and increase work survivability (17–21). Possible permanent job accommodation may be appropriate (21).

4. Legal: A reasonable determination should be made as to whether the condition is "caused" by the job; this requirement is not a medical mandate but rather a bureaucratic one. Such a determination is "medically" impossible. Nevertheless, physicians should be committed to improving the understanding of CTD to help patients cope with the medical and social issues that surround this condition, which has been called a "modern plague" (2).

5. Prevention: Prevention is the best treatment through early identification of persons at risk before they reach the need for medical care. The occupational physician and staff, using well-designed work evaluation protocols, must be willing to assist industry in the risk evaluation of new workers, the design and institution of programs to prevent worker injuries, and the rehabilitation of injured workers. Through programs focused on the workplace, physicians, supported by a staff of ergonomists, hand therapists, and occupational health care providers, can assist both the worker and employer by reducing the costs and numbers of injuries (22,23). If business perceives that medicine does not or will not have the answers for CTD, business will turn to the paramedical industry for help.

6. Education: The occupational physician will need to assume the role of a teacher to help the employer understand the multifactorial etiology of CTD. Education of the employer and employee is key to displacing the many myths about CTD that are currently recycled by the media. Sound education and valid information provide the best opportunity for the physician to reduce CTD risks in the workplace. Unfortunately, the response of many employers to an increase in CTD injuries has been denial (24). Predictably, many employers attempt to "cure" what they perceive as motivational inadequacies by providing incentive pay to their employees. The workers, even while experiencing the symptoms of CTD, often delay seeking appropriate medical treatment, thereby increasing their symptoms and further complicating their medical conditions. Ultimately, the employee may increase costs to their employers and, possibly, risk permanent disability.

CTD INTERVENTION PROGRAM

Injury-reduction programs in the workplace are not new. Traditional programs focused heavily on ergonomics and manipulation of the physical environment (8–10) and little on identifying the person at risk (25). Current outcome-based models, which may use prospective cohort (26), metanalysis (27), decision analysis (28), and cost-effectiveness analysis (29), suggest that the most effective injury reduction occurs with prevention programs that integrate the individual's risk level and appropriate application of ergonomics in the workplace (2,13,14,22,30,31).

Realizing the effectiveness of these outcome-based prevention programs and in an effort to help employers develop CTD intervention programs, NIOSH has provided an outline in the document *Elements of Ergonomics Programs* (32). These NIOSH "elements" include eight steps for the development and implementation of an intervention program:

Challenges of Intervention

First, the physician must be knowledgeable about CTD, familiar with risks within the workplace, and willing to take the challenge of an intervention program. He or she must be able to treat and rehabilitate injuries optimally for both the worker and the employer.

Multidisciplinary Approach

Second, ergonomics requires a multidisciplinary, task force approach (33). Communication breakdown among disciplines within the organization, self-interest, or noncommitment of a work group and a general lack of ergonomic and job knowledge within the segment of the organization making ergonomic decisions will interfere with workplace risk reduction (34). A common barrier is a management attitude favoring the "quick fix" or "band-aid approach" rather than investing time, manpower, and dollars necessary to implement a full-scale intervention (35–39).

Problem Identification

Third, problem identification is required. The existence of a problem and the need for intervention frequently are identified by the employer. Injury incidence is available for review using employee medical records. A medical health questionnaire provides the first phase of health screening. The questionnaire or risk identification instrument is used to enable identification of at-risk workers: those with existing symptoms and those who work in high-risk areas within the workplace. Many outcome-assessment instruments and risk-identification questionnaires are available (25,40–53). The employers' health services can add a clinical examination to supplement the questionnaire. Persons who are symptomatic and determined to be at increased risk can be referred to a health care provider for early conservative treatment and education. If improvement does not occur, standard medical management can be provided that may include surgery and early return to work. Possible permanent job accommodation may be required (21).

Establishment of Protocols

Fourth, preestablished protocols for prevention, job analysis, workstation-modifica-

tion methods, possible workplace physical design or redesign, ongoing evaluation by employer task group, core curriculum education for worker biomechanics, CTD etiology, and ergonomics should be developed in advance of the implementation.

Change Considerations

Fifth, recommendations for change must be made with careful consideration. Recommendations must be cost effective, feasible, and practical. In general, major risk reductions can be obtained through relatively simple, inexpensive adjustments. Many times, major stresses are eliminated completely as a result of minor changes (54). Changes that do not entail major financial implications in terms of time, equipment, and productivity costs are easily accepted and implemented. More costly equipment and redesign of tools and physical workstations, when cost effective, should not be overlooked. In instances where risk factors are evaluated against a history of CTD among workers, cost effectiveness is readily measured (33,55).

Education Programs

Sixth, the effectiveness of education programs in reducing musculoskeletal injuries has been proven (14). Training must be broadened beyond fundamental issues of safe work practices. Management and workers should be involved in training designed to identify job hazards and to develop problem-solving skills so they can participate in hazard-control activities (56).

Ergonomic Issues

Seventh, engineers and design staff are key players in ergonomic changes. Workplace design influences body postures during the job, force required for tool use, materials handling, rate, temperature, and vibration. Engineers must be included in ergonomics education to achieve the desired change in existing and new operations (57–66).

Total Quality Management (TQM) Principles

Finally, repeating the evaluation of the intervention program for CTD (outcome assessment, evaluation, implementation) creates a cycle consistent with total quality management principles. Several studies have described a benefit to cost saving of 3.4 to 9 dollars for every dollar spent on prevention (43,67–70).

Although the eight NIOSH elements are all inclusive, many employers have found them difficult to implement. The conversion of abstract risk concepts to daily application can be difficult. In an effort to improve implementation, the following five-step Intervention Program Model, part of the C+d MAP™ (Cumulative Trauma Disorders Monitorial Assessment Program) Risk Prevention Program©, was developed (13). Individual companies may use this intervention model or develop their own. This five-step program meets all the current suggestions provided by the NIOSH Elements of Ergonomics Programs (32).

Five-step C+d MAP™ Intervention Program Model

Below is a brief outline of the five-step C+d MAP™ program with details provided for each step.

1. Organization
   Employer commitment
   Intervention task force
   Medical consultants
2. Risk identification
   Select risk assessment instrument
   Establish individual risk factors
   Establish employer or workplace risk factors
3. Establish CTD risk reduction program protocols for
   Ergonomic
   Medical
   Education
   Use individual risk assessment
   Collect data
4. Risk analysis
   Review of risks
   Analysis of effects
   Problem identification
   Review of protocols
5. Risk resolution plan
   Recommendations
   Implementation of change
   Ergonomics
      Engineering modification
      Design changes
   Medical
   Educational
   Repeat steps 3, 4, and 5 for TQM.

Organization

- A commitment from the employer and an understanding from management that they truly do want to reduce work injuries is essential. It is helpful to have a 1- or 2-year commitment in writing in advance.
- The development of a task force using as many of the employer's staff as possible is critical. The employer's group may need to be supplemented with representatives from physical medicine and internal medicine; therapy for occupational, physical, and sports medicine; an ergonomist; a design engineer; nursing; insurance management; and hospital administration.
- Ergonomics requires a multidisciplinary approach (71). Staff with experience in ergonomics and workplace design are necessary. Ergonomics does not require a complete workplace make-over to reduce risk when the individual's risk levels can be used to modify traditional approaches for methods, materials, machines, and environment (35–39).

Selection of Risk-assessment Instrument

- A medical health questionnaire provides the first phase of health screening. The questionnaire or risk-identification instrument is used to enable identification of the at-risk worker. The at-risk worker may already have symptoms or may be the person who has increased individual risk factors based on age, gender, inherited characteristics, and psychosocial issues.

- Many outcome-assessment instruments and risk-identification questionnaires are available (25,40–53). The employer's health services can add a clinical examination to supplement the questionnaire. Additional information on outcome-assessment instruments follows this section.

Data Collection and Protocols

- The existence of a problem and the need for intervention are frequently identified by the company. Injury incidence is documented in company medical records, such as the Occupational Safety and Health Administration (OSHA) 200 log.
- Preestablished protocols for prevention, job analysis, work station modification methods, possible plant physical design or redesign, ongoing evaluation by in-plant task group, core curriculum education for worker biomechanics, CTD etiology, and ergonomics should be developed in advance of the implementation. These protocols will be modified as new data are collected using an "outcomes, effectiveness, and accountability" format.

Risk Analysis

- Individuals who are symptomatic or determined to be at increased risk can be referred to a health care provider for early conservative treatment and education. Should a lack of improvement occur, standard medical management can be provided that may include surgery and early return to work. Possible permanent job accommodation may be required (21).

Risk-resolution Plan

- Recommendations for change must be made with careful consideration. Recommendations must be cost effective, feasible, and practical. In general, major risk reductions can be obtained through relatively simple and inexpensive adjustments. Many times, major stresses are completely eliminated as a result of minor changes (54). Changes that do not entail significant financial implications in terms of time, equipment, and productivity costs are easily accepted and implemented. More costly equipment and redesign of tools and physical workstations when they are cost-effective should not be overlooked.

- The effectiveness of training programs in reducing musculoskeletal injuries has been proven (14). Key elements in the development of training include (a) involvement of both management and workers in identifying job hazards and (b) development of problem-solving skills to promote participation in hazard control activities (56).

- The role of engineers and design staff to achieve ergonomic change in existing and new operations is important because of the influence of workplace design related to issues such as body postures during the job, force required for tool use, materials handling, rate, temperature, and vibration (57–66).

- Repeating the CTD intervention program cycle at appropriate intervals allows for TQM. Several studies have demonstrated a benefit-to-cost saving of 3.4 to 9 dollars for every dollar spent on prevention (43, 67–70).

Requirements of Outcome-assessment Instruments

Outcome instruments must meet several requirements:

- *Sensibility*: Does the instrument make sense, and does it fit with common sense and a reasonable knowledge of pathophysiology and clinical condition?
- *Reliability*: Does the instrument provide the same answer or same results when the measure is repeated by the same or different clinicians on different occasions? Statistical methods to measure reliability include internal consistency using Cronbach's alpha $\geq$

0.8 or test–retest using Kappa's coefficient >0.75–0.80);

- *Validity*: Does the instrument provide the right answer and measure what is truly purports to measure? For most health measures, there is no "gold standard" or criterion. Therefore, construct validity is obtained by hypothesizing the relationship with other measures and testing them (construct validity correlations of 0.4 to 0.6 are appropriate).
- *Responsiveness*: Does the instrument measure change that is accurately reflected in true clinical change?

Examples of Outcome Assessment

Below are brief summaries of MSD-related outcomes studies that cover a broad range of predictive, clinical, and surveillance assessments.

Carpal Tunnel Syndrome Surgery Outcome

The outcomes after surgery were compared for wrist range of motion, power pinch, grip strength, pressure sensibility, and dexterity by several instruments (the Medical Outcomes Study 36-item short-form health survey (72), the Arthritis Impact Measurement Scale (73), and a self-administered questionnaire for the assessment of severity of symptoms and functional status in CTS (74)). In general, the standardized questionnaires were more sensitive to the clinical change produced by carpal tunnel surgery than many commonly performed physical measures of outcome. The condition-specific questionnaire was more sensitive to change than were more generic questionnaires (75).

Predictors of Work Disability

Several instruments, such as the Fibromyalgia Impact Questionnaire (FIQ) (76) and the Modified Stanford Health Assessment Questionnaire (SHAQ) (77), have been used to compare symptoms, signs, grip strength, and passive wrist flexion angle with predictors of work disability. The FIQ and SHAQ scores were significantly correlated with objective measures of upper-extremity function and were more valid measures of work disability than were symptoms or physical signs (78).

Workplace Surveillance for Carpal Tunnel Syndrome

Several screening procedures for CTS were evaluated in workers in a manufacturing plant. Nerve-conduction testing, considered the "gold standard," was used to compare the sensitivity and positive predictive value of a symptom survey, physical examination, limited electrodiagnostic testing at the wrists, quantitative vibratory threshold testing, two-point discrimination, palmar pinch, grip, and hand-grip strength testing. The positive predictive value of physical examination findings and quantitative test procedures were no better than, and usually worse than, the results on the symptom survey alone. Therefore, in the absence of electrodiagnostic testing, the simplest test and the procedure with the highest sensitivity and positive predictive values for CTS is a symptom survey alone. Quantitative test procedures (vibrometry, pinch-grip strength, hand-grip strength) and physical examination for findings consistent with CTS (e.g., Phalen's test, Tinel's test, thenar muscle wasting, two-point discrimination) appear to contribute little, if any, additional information when screening subjects in the work setting (79).

Self-reported Carpal Tunnel Syndrome

A self-administered symptom severity and functional status questionnaire was compared with measurements of grip, pinch, abductor pollicis brevis strength, two-point discrimination, and monofilament testing. Responsiveness was calculated with the standardized response mean and the effect size. The symptom severity scale was four times as responsive, and the functional status and activities of daily living scales were twice as responsive as the measures of strength and sensibility. Self-administered symptom severity and functional status scales are much more responsive to clinical improvement than measures of neuromuscular impairment and should serve as primary outcomes in clinical studies of therapy for CTS (80).

Shoulder Surgery Outcomes

The shoulder questionnaire provides a measure of outcomes for shoulder operations. It is short, practical, reliable, valid, and sensitive to clinically important changes (81).

Carpal Tunnel Syndrome Outcomes

A questionnaire was compared with a hand-symptoms diagram and physical measurements. The mean scores of items regarding sensory symptoms were significantly higher in patients with classic or probable CTS compared with patients with possible or unlikely CTS (p <.0001). The scores were similar for patients with CTS and for patients without CTS on the functional status subscale. The diagnosis of CTS could be made by questionnaire and hand-symptoms diagram alone (82).

Review of Applicable or Existing Functional Status Measures to the Study of Workers with MSD of the Neck and Upper Limbs

Twelve domains were identified as the major areas of life affected by workers' neck and upper-extremity disorders: work, household and family responsibilities, self-care, transportation/driving, sexual activity, sleep, social activities, recreational activities, mood, self-esteem, financial impact, and iatrogenic effects of assessments and treatment. Fifty-two functional status instruments were identified. Of these, 21 met the specified criteria as potentially relevant and were rated on the three-point scale for relevance and comprehensiveness for each domain. None of the instruments covered all 12 domains adequately (83).

Perceived Exertion as a Function of Physical Effort

To what extent can a worker's perception of exertion be used to establish what is an acceptable level of work? The increasing body of knowledge suggests that safe levels of work can be established using psychophysical and psychoscaling tools to assess the worker's perception of exertion (84). Recently, the variables of exertion, discomfort, and effort involved in work performances have been investigated (85). Studies indicate that individuals are capable of reliably estimating their endurance in a physical task and that there is a strong positive correlation between the objective and subjective aspects of a fatigue state (86,87). Interest in psychophysical assessment emanates from industry demands for guidelines or limits designed to prevent CTD; because of the difficulties inherent in assessing upper-extremity work, the use of more objective approaches is important (88).

Modems DASH

The American Academy of Orthopaedics Surgeons, in support of the Council of Musculoskeletal Specialty Societies and the Institute for Work and Health, developed the Disability of the Arm, Shoulder, and Hand (DASH) outcome instrument. The DASH is designed to evaluate upper-extremity functional loss. It is currently being used as a research instrument to evaluate medical treatment and to develop a data-driven medical practice (89).

Reliability and Validity Testing of the Michigan Hand Outcomes Questionnaire:

Psychometric principles were used to develop an outcomes questionnaire capable of measuring health state domains important to patients with hand disorders. These domains were hypothesized to include (a) overall hand function, (b) activities of daily living, (c) pain, (d) work performance, (e) aesthetics, and (f) patient satisfaction with hand function (90).

Other outcome studies continue to provide data on musculoskeletal pain in the workplace (21,23,27,41,46,60,79,91–104). In general, disease-specific outcome instruments are more sensitive to change and therefore are better for evaluating and measuring the changes in response intervention (105). Comparisons of outcome instruments have shown that certain diagnoses are better assessed by using different combinations of data (106, 107). For example, the questionnaire alone is the more sensitive outcome measure for change in persons who have been diagnosed as having CTS and tendinitis, whereas the combination of questionnaire and physical measures is a more sensitive outcome measure for change in persons diagnosed with shoulder injuries or fractures.

Because most outcome instruments were developed for use in the clinical setting and usually to evaluate a specific body area, an MSD/CTD outcome instrument was developed for use in the workplace. This instrument was designed to be disease specific for MSD/CTD and to examine the multifactorial etiology of MSD/CTD, which includes age, gender, inherited characteristics, workplace, nonwork environment, and psychosocial elements. To allow for decision analysis, a global scaling was selected instead of multiple scaling. Decision analysis is used in science to allow for a systematic approach to decision making under conditions of uncertainty. Decision analysis has three key features: (a) *explicit*: the problem must be explicitly defined and disaggregated into data, timing, and values of outcomes; (b) *quantitative*: everything must be expressed numerically, including subjective, but important, issues like anxiety, risk attitude, and quality of life; and (c) *prescriptive*: gives the solution preferred by a "rational" decision maker and does not replicate the processes of an unaided decision maker (108–110). After completion of several research studies with this MSD/CTD instrument, the research study group determined that the CTD MAP could serve a broad population and address the specific concerns of business, industry, and government (14,22,25).

HOW TO SELECT AN OUTCOME INSTRUMENT

The CTD Intervention Task Force will need to select the appropriate risk assessment or outcome instrument as the key driver for each of the health screening models. The best outcome instrument may not be the same for every company. The task force should review the assessment or outcome instrument for (a) *sensibility*: face and content validity compared with intended purpose (includes relevant items and excludes irrelevant items) is suited to the company's invention program (such as individual vs. group data or individual and group data) and appropriate for employee population; (b) *setting*: on site for employer, offsite, other, phone versus written versus computer; (c) *feasibility*: ease of use, ease of understanding, appropriate length, self-administered versus interviewer, no special equipment versus requiring special equipment, no training of staff versus training of staff, cost to administer, scoring, results easy to use and easy to interpret, easy to develop protocols or repeat evaluation; (d) *reliability*: internal consistency, interrater reliability, intrarater reliability; (e) *validity*: correlation with other outcome measures and ability to predict future events; and (f) *responsiveness*: able to detect subtle but relevant change.

Five-step CTD Intervention Program Model

Using the models of the five-step CTD Intervention program as outlines, employers can develop their own CTD intervention program. These models summarize the information provided above in a useful diagram format for a better understanding and easier "how to" integration of the health screening and the development of ergonomic, medical and educational protocols.

APPLICATIONS OF CTD INTERVENTION PROGRAMS

Several examples will be used to illustrate how a risk reduction program using an

MSD/CTD specific outcome assessment instrument can be effective in risk reduction for the individual employee and cost savings for the employer. The first step in development and application of a CTD Intervention Program is to assemble an intervention task force. In the second step, the intervention task force must select a risk assessment or outcome instrument using the criteria above. The third step is to develop data collection needs and protocols that are company specific. In the following examples, the MSD/CTD assessment instrument used was the Ctd MAP developed by Map Managers, Inc., of Wichita, Kansas (13). The fourth step is to analyze the data and review protocols. The final step is to recommend and implement changes. Examples of risk reduction programs are briefly outlined below.

Tools and Ergonomic Program Design

A prospective study with random sampling of 212 workers of an 8,000-member workforce were assigned randomly to the one of four primary factor groups: vibration-damped rivet guns, standard rivet guns (control group), ergonomic training, and exercise training. Risk assessment was performed at the start of the study and at 7 and 15 months. Ergonomics training included an awareness of early warning signs of CTD, methods for controlling risk factors, techniques to apply forces with less stress or strain, and correct posture and stance to improve balance and absorb forces. Exercise training included muscle relaxation and gentle stretching of muscles and tendons. Tools included vibration-dampening rivet (recoilless) gun or standard rivet gun, training and practice using those tools, and conventional bucking bars. A study model was developed, and the program was implemented. Risk assessment was repeated and additional data reviewed. At 15 months, the results showed ergonomic training to be the only main factor that was statistically significant. Additional reduction of risk occurs with ergonomic training for the covariates of dominant hand, time spent in an awkward po-

sition, and number of standard rivets bucked. Exercise training demonstrated a risk-reduction benefit for the covariates of dominant hand, number of parts routed, and number of parts ground. Vibration dampening riveting provided risk reduction for new employees but increased risk for current employees. Vibration dampening riveting increased the risk for the covariates of number of rivets bucked. The employees benefited from ergonomic training and exercise training with decreased complaints of work-related musculoskeletal pain; the employer's estimated savings was $4 million for the first 15 months (14).

General Safety Improvement Program Using Ergonomic Protocols

A prospective study of a plastic products manufacturer was developed to establish a continuous safety program, identify areas and individuals at risk, develop a prevention plan for each area and individual, and review the effectiveness of the program on a quarterly basis. Using the Health Screen Ergonomic Protocols Model, each job was reviewed for work requirements by methods, materials, machines, environment, and people and by workplace "stressors" of repetition, force, posture, work duration, contract stress, vibration, and low temperatures. Individual risk assessment was completed for each employee and linked to his or her job, department, group, and plant. Using the individual risk range of 1 (low) to 7 (high), the risk for each extremity was used to establish each individual's exercises and ergonomic training based on the established protocols. Population information (the average risk for job, department, and group) was used to develop decision trees for ergonomic modification of the production processes, including methods, materials, machines, and workplace environment. Ergonomic review of jobs, departments, and groups with relative higher risk for the employer were reviewed for workplace stressors. Risk-resolution planning was completed and recommendations implemented. At the end of the first 2 years, the company's risk level was reduced from 4.79 to 3.95. The modifications to the production process resulted in increased production of 8.5%, a decrease in rework of 4.7%, and an increase in profits of 15%. The company estimated savings of $234,000 the first year and $953,000 the second year in their Workers' Compensation expenses and a benefit-to-cost of 215% (2,13,30).

General Safety Improvement Program Using Education Protocols

A prospective study of a metal products manufacturer was developed to establish a continuous safety program, identify individuals at risk, and develop a prevention plan for the company based on education protocols. Using the Health Screen Education Protocols Model, all 96 employees were risk-assessed. Risk-level–specific educational protocols had been developed in advance. The intervention task force met individually with each employee who was considered to be at increased risk (level 5–7). During the meeting, education regarding the facts and myths of CTD (15), appropriate warmup exercises (111), and general education for possible workplace stressors of repetition, force, posture, work duration, contact stress, vibration, and low temperature were reviewed (14). Employees were encouraged to share concerns about musculoskeletal pain. Because the product manufactured did not change, no changes were made in the methods, materials, machines, or workplace environment during the 1-year study. The effectiveness of the Education Protocols Model was measured by a 12.3% increase in production, a 4.1% decrease in rework, and a 11% increase in profits with a company estimated cost-to-benefit of 294% (16).

Risk Prevention in New Hires

A prospective study for risk prevention in new hires was developed for an aircraft manufacturer with a employee population of 5,600. Using OSHA 200 logs for recordable CTD cases, the employer identified jobs that were at relatively higher risk for the occurrence of CTD. The employer elected to implement a prevention program based on the Health Screen Medical Protocols Model. All post-hire preplacement employees for the relatively higher risk jobs were evaluated by the risk assessment program and by a physician. The occupational physician reviewed the individuals' risk levels and, using establish protocols, provided work guides for the specific job. For individuals with level 7 risk, an ergonomic education program was also provided. After several weeks of accommodated work for the high-risk employee group, most employees were advanced to regular work without restrictions. During the first 2 years, 1,010 new employees were hired. Using the selection criteria of relatively high-risk jobs, 754 were individually risk assessed, and 256 with relatively lower risk jobs became the control study group. Retrospective data were collected for the previous 1,010 "new" employees before the start date of the CTD intervention program into a matching groups of 754 and 256 for age, gender, and job. The preprevention and postprevention groups of 1,010 were compared for the number of surgeries performed under the workers' compensation system and number of lost work hours. In the preprevention group, 14 of 754 new employees in relatively higher-risk jobs had surgery (rate of 20.4 per 1,000 employees), and three of 256 in the control group (relatively lower-risk jobs) had surgery (rate of 11.7 per 1,000 employees). In the postprevention group, one of 754 had surgery (a rate of 1.3 per 1,000 employees) and two of 256 in the control group (rate of 7.8 per 1,000 employees) had surgery. The total lost work hours for the year before the study was 3,009 compared with the first year of the study at 1,011 and the second year of the study 975. This decrease occurred despite an increase in the workforce of 1,010 employees and an increase in total man-hours of 14.3% in the first year and 17.1% in the second year. The company estimated their savings at $1.3 million for the first year and $1.8 for the second year and a benefit-to-cost of 300% (2,13,22,112).

Effects of Risk Intervention Programs on the Reporting of CTD in the Workplace a Preliminary Report

A prospective study (currently under review for publication) designed to review the effects and possible impact of workplace screening for MSD and CTD on the number of OSHA 200 injuries was started in 1997 in response to many employers who have expressed concern regarding workplace screening or risk assessment, despite being encouraged to do workplace screening by NIOSH and OSHA. The employer implemented an individual risk-screening program, education, and employee awareness for randomly assigned groups of employees in an effort to stimulate their awareness and possible reporting of musculoskeletal pain associated with the workplace. Currently, no increase has been seen in the incidence of work-related musculoskeletal pain or OSHA 200 reportable cases. This study would suggest that employers should be encouraged to develop, implement, and use screening programs because they provide the best opportunity for prevention of CTD and do not appear to increase the risk for reporting of CTD in the workplace.

screens, clinical examinations, and, when indicated, early referral for conservative management. Because NIOSH (7) has concluded that MSD/CTD are inherently preventable disorders that can be identified and controlled by health screening and intervention programs, physician involvement in risk reduction intervention programs should increase. With more information about risk prevention and with a better understanding of how the workplace interacts with the individual's unique risk factors, the occupational physician can work with business and industry to implement intervention programs. Task forces using intervention protocol models with specific risk assessment instruments that consider the total individual for anatomic, physiologic, functional, social, emotional, and satisfaction factors as they relate to the workplace can make appropriate ergonomic recommendations and see a direct decrease in the number and severity of MSD/CTD cases. At the same time, these intervention programs will benefit the employer by increasing production, decreasing costs, and improving profits. Ultimately, these prevention programs can reduce the national costs of MSD/CTD and reduce the impact of this "modern plague."

SUMMARY

If the prediction that 50% of the American workforce will have occupational injuries by the year 2000, physicians and their health care colleagues need to be involved in the decision-making process, the analysis, and the implementation of risk prevention in the workplace. Although traditional approaches to risk and injury reduction in the workplace have focused heavily on ergonomics and methods of effecting change through manipulation of the physical environment have resulted in some improvement, the number of cases and costs have continued to increase (3,8–10). Beyond ergonomics and education, medical consultation broadens the scope of intervention to include active surveillance of the worker population by means of health

ACKNOWLEDGMENTS

This manuscript was reviewed by Peggy Gardner, Ph.D., Executive Director, Research Via Christi Health System. Reference support was from the Via Christi Medical Libraries, and funding was from The Hand Center, Kansas.

REFERENCES

1. Kelsey JL, Pastides H, Kreiger N. *Upper extremity disorders: a survey of their frequency and cost in the United States*. St. Louis: Mosby, 1980, pp. 1–355.
2. Melhom JM. Identification of individuals at risk for developing CTD, In: Spengler DM, Zippieri JP, eds. *Workers' compensation case management: a multidisciplinary perspective*. Rosemont, IL: American Academy of Orthopaedic Surgeons, 1997:41–51.
3. Brady W, Bass J, Royce M, Anstadt G, Loeppke R, Leopold R. Defining total corporate health and safety

costs—significance and impact. *J Occup Med* 1997; 39:224–231.

4. Melhorn JM. Prevention of CTD in the workplace. In: *Workers' comp update 1998*. Walnut Creek, CA: Council on Education in Management, 1998, pp. 101–124.

5. U.S. Bureau of Labor Statistics. *Survey of occupational injuries and illnesses in 1994*. Washington, DC: U.S. Department of Labor, U.S. Government Printing Office, 1996 pp. 1–379.

6. American Academy of Orthopaedic Surgeons. *Repetitive motion disorders of the upper extremity*. Rosemont, IL: American Academy of Orthopaedic Surgeons, 1995.

7. U.S.Department of Health and Human Services. *Musculoskeletal disorders and workplace factors: a critical review of epidemiologic evidence for work-related musculoskeletal disorders of the neck, upper extremity, and low back*. Cincinnati, OH: NIOSH, 1997.

8. Hackman JR, Oldham GA. *Work redesign*. Reading, MA: Addison Wesley, 1980, pp. 1–80.

9. Nordin M, Franklin VH. Evaluation of the work place an introduction. *Clin Orthop* 1989;221;85–88.

10. Grandjean E. *Fitting the task to the man: an ergonomic approach*. London: Taylor and Francis, 1980.

11. Melhorn JM. Three types of carpal tunnel syndrome: the need for prevention. *ARMS News* 1996;5:18–24.

12. Melhorn JM. Understanding the types of carpal tunnel syndrome. *Journal of Workers' Compensation* 1998;7: 52–73.

13. Melhorn JM. Cumulative trauma disorders and repetitive strain injuries: the future. *Clin Orthop* 1998;351: 107–126.

14. Melhorn JM. A prospective study for upper-extremity cumulative trauma disorders of workers in aircraft manufacturing. *J Occup Environ Med* 1996;38:1264–1271.

15. Melhorn JM. CTD: Carpal tunnel syndrome, the facts and myths. *Kans Med* 1994;95:189–192.

16. Melhorn JM. Management of work related upper extremity musculoskeletal disorders. In: *Kansas Case Managers Annual Meeting*. Wichita: Wesley Rehabilitation Hospital, 1998:16–25.

17. Devlin M, O'Neill P, MacBride R. Position paper in support of timely return to work programs and the role of the primary care physician. *Ontario Medical Association* 1994;61:1–45.

18. Melhorn JM. CTD injuries: an outcome study for work survivability. *Journal of Workers' Compensation* 1996; 5:18–30.

19. Goodman RC. An aggressive return-to-work program in surgical treatment of carpal tunnel syndrome: a comparison of costs. *Plast Reconstr Surg* 1989;89:715–717.

20. Kasdan ML, Vender MI, Lewis K, Stallings SP, Melhorn JM. Carpal tunnel syndrome: effects of litigation on utilization of health care and physician workload. *J Ky Med Assoc* 1996;94:287–290.

21. Melhorn JM. CTD injuries: an outcome study for work survivability, In: Amadio PC, Hentz VR, eds. *Yearbook of hand surgery 1997*. St. Louis: Mosby, 1997: 261–262.

22. Melhorn JM, Wilkinson LK. *CTD solutions for the 90's: A comprehensive guide to managing CTD in the workplace*. Wichita, KS: Via Christi, 1996, pp. 1–45.

23. Melhorn JM. Cumulative trauma disorders: how to assess the risks. In: Amadio PC, Hentz VR, eds. *Yearbook of hand surgery 1997*. St. Louis: Mosby, 1997:258–259.

24. Gelberman RH. *The wrist*. New York: Raven Press,

25. Melhorn JM. Cumulative trauma disorders: how to assess the risks. *Journal of Workers' Compensation* 1996; 5:19–33.

26. Laupacis A, Rorabeck CH, Bourne RB, et al. Randomized trials in orthopaedics: why, how, and when? *J Bone Joint Surg Am* 1989;71A:535–543.

27. Melhorn JM. CTD solutions for the 90's: prevention. *Seventeenth Annual Workers' Compensation and Occupational Medicine Seminar*. Boston: Speak, 1997: 234–245.

28. Kassirer JP, Moskowitz AJ, Lau J, Pauker SG. Decision analysis: a progress report. *Ann Intern Med* 1987;106: 275–291.

29. Detsky AS, Naglie IG, Aagaard H. A clinician's guide to cost-effectiveness analysis. *Ann Intern Med* 1990;113: 147–154.

30. Melhorn JM. CTD's: risk assessment applications in the workplace, In: *Science symposium*. McPherson: McPherson College, Kansas, 1985:1–12.

31. Brown RE, Zook EG, Russell RC, Smoot EC, Kucan JO. Fingernail deformities secondary to ganglions of the distal interphalangeal joint (mucous cysts). *Plast Reconstr Surg* 1991;87:718–725.

32. Rosenstock L. *Elements of ergonomics programs: a primer based on workplace evaluations of musculoskeletal disorders*. Washington, D.C: U.S. Government Printing Office, 1997.

33. Liker JK, Joseph BS, Armstrong TJ. From ergonomic theory to practice: Organizational factors affecting the utilization of ergonomic knowledge, In: Henrick J, Brown JA, eds. *Human factors in organizational design and management*. New York: Wiley, 1984:1–256.

34. Hendrick HW, Brown O Jr. Human factors in organization designs and management. In: *Human factors*. Amsterdam: New Holland, 1984:99–155.

35. Chatterjee DS. Workplace upper limb disorders: A prospective study with intervention. *J Occup Med* 1992; 42:129–136.

36. Pravikoff DS, Simonowitz JA. Cumulative trauma disorders: developing a framework for prevention. *AAOHN J* 1994;42:164–170.

37. Orlandi MA. Health promotion technology transfer: organizational perspectives. *Can J Public Health* 1996;87: S28–33.

38. Stock SR, Cole DC, Tugwell P, Streiner D. Review of applicable or existing functional status measures to the study of workers with musculoskeletal disorders of the neck and upper limb. *Am J Ind Med* 1996;29:679–688.

39. Herbert R, Plattus B, Kellogg L, et al. The union health center: a working model of clinical care linked to preventive occupational health services. *Am J Ind Med* 1997;31:263–273.

40. Silverstein BA, Fine LJ, Armstrong TJ. Occupational factors in carpal tunnel syndrome. *Am J Ind Med* 1987; 11:343–358.

41. Nathan PA, Meadows KD, Doyle LS. Occupations as a risk factor for impaired sensory conductions of the median nerve at the carpal tunnel. *J Hand Surg* 1988;13B: 167–170.

42. National Safety Council. *Control of cumulative trauma disorders*. Washington, D.C.: U.S. Government Printing Office, 1994, pp. 1–457.

43. Melhorn JM. Occupational injuries: the need for preventive strategies. *Kans Med* 1994;95:248–251.

44. Cohen JE, Goel V, Frank JW, Gibson ES. Predicating risk of back injuries, work absenteeism, and chronic disability: the shortcomings of preplacement screening. *J Occup Med* 1994;36:1093–1099.

45. Bigos SJ, Battie MC, Spengler DM, Fisher LD. A prospective study of work perceptions and psychosocial factors affecting the report of back injury. *Spine* 1991;16:1–6.

46. Day DE. Preventive and return to work aspects of cumulative trauma disorders in the workplace. *Ergonomics Health* 1988;1:1–22.

47. Linton SJ, Kamwendo K. Risk factors in the psychosocial work environment for neck and shoulder pain in secretaries. *J Occup Med* 1989;31:609–613.

48. DeKrom M, Kester ADM, Knipschild PG, Spaans F. Risk factors for carpal tunnel syndrome. *Am J Epidemiol* 1990;132:1102–1110.

49. Rayan GM. *Compression neuropathies, including carpal tunnel syndrome.* Summit, NJ: Novartis, 1997, pp. 1–32.

50. Gerwatowski LJ, McFall DB, Stach DJ. Carpal tunnel syndrome: Risk factors and preventive strategies for the dental hygienist. *Dental Health* 1992;31:5–10.

51. Young VL, Seaton MK, Feely CA. Detecting cumulative trauma disorders in workers performing repetitive tasks. *Am J Ind Med* 1995;27:419–431.

52. Keyserling WM, Armstrong TJ, Punnett L. Ergonomic job analysis: a structured approach for identifying risk factors associated with over-exertion injuries and disorders. *Appl Occup Env Hyg* 1991;6:353–363.

53. Rystrom CM, Eversmann WW Jr. Cumulative trauma intervention in industry: a model program for the upper extremity, In: Kasdan ML, ed. *Occupational hand and upper extremity injuries & diseases.* Philadelphia: Hanely & Belfus, 1991:489–506.

54. Silverstein BA, Armstrong TJ, Buckle P, et al. Can some upper extremity disorders be defined as work-related? [Letter]. *J Hand Surg* 1932;21A:727–729.

55. Sell RG. Success and failure in implementing changes in job design. *Ergonomics* 1980;23:809–816.

56. Viegas SF. Extension block pinning for proximal interphalangeal joint fracture dislocations: preliminary report of a new technique. *J Hand Surg* 1992;17A: 896–901.

57. Nathan PA, Keniston RC. Carpal tunnel syndrome and its relation to general physical condition. *Hand Clinics* 1993;9:253–261.

58. Stevens JC, Sun S, Beard CM. Carpal tunnel syndrome in Rochester, Minnesota, 1961 to 1980. *Neurology* 1988;38:134–138.

59. Hadler NM. Arm pain in the workplace: a small area analysis. *J Occup Med* 1992;34:113–119.

60. Feuerstein M, Callan-Harris S, Hickey P, Dyer D, Armbruster W, Carosella AM. Multidisciplinary rehabilitation of chronic work-related upper extremity disorders: long-term effects. *J Occup Med* 1993;35:396–403.

61. Armstrong TJ, Buckle P, Fine LJ, et al. A conceptual model for work-related neck and upper-limb musculoskeletal disorders. *Scand J Work Environ Health* 1993;19:73–84.

62. Luopajarvi T, Juorinka I, Virolainen M, Holmberg M. Prevalence of tenosynovitis and other injuries of the upper extremities in repetitive work. *Scand J Work Environ Health* 1979;5:48–55.

63. Biering-Sorensen F. A prospective study of low back pain in a general population: I. Occurrence, recurrence and aetiology. *Scand J Rehabil Med* 1983;15:71–79.

64. Millar JD, Myers MD. Occupational safety and health. Progress toward the 1990 objective for the nation. *Public Health Rep* 1983;98:324–336.

65. Kelsey JL. *Epidemiology of musculoskeletal disorders.* New York: Oxford University Press, 1982, pp. 574–579.

66. Pransky GS, Snyder TB, Himmelstein JS. Organizational factors and cumulative trauma disorders. In: Sauter SI, Moon S., eds. *Psychosocial aspects of office-related cumulative trauma disoders.* Philadelphia: WB Saunders, 1997:1–89.

67. Golaszewski T, Snow D, Lynch W, Yen L, Solomita D. A benefit-to-cost analysis of a work-site health promotion program. *J Occup Med* 1992;34:1164–1172.

68. Hochanadel CD, Conrad DE. Evolution of an on-site industrial physical therapy program. *J Occup Med* 1993;35:1011–1016.

69. Cohen MS, Hastings H II. Acute elbow dislocation: evaluation and management. *J Am Acad Orthop Surg* 1998;6:15–23.

70. Warner KE, Smith RJ, Smith DG, Fries BE. Health and economic implication of a work-site smoking-cessation program: a simulation analysis. *J Occup Med* 1996;38: 981–992.

71. Gellman H, Nichols D. Reflex sympathetic dystrophy in the upper extremity. *J Am Acad Orthop Surg* 1997;5: 313–322.

72. Ware JE Jr. *SF-36 physical & mental health summary scales: a user's manual.* Boston: The Health Institute, 1994, pp. 121–130.

73. Meenan RF, Gertman PM, Mason JM. Measuring health status in arthritis: The arthritis impact measurement scales. *Arthritis Rheum* 1980;23:146–152.

74. Levine DW, Simmons BP, Koris MJ, et al. A self-administered questionnaire for the assessment of severity of symptoms and functional status in carpal tunnel syndrome. *J Bone Joint Surg Am* 1996;75A:1585–1592.

75. Amadio PC, Silverstein BA, Ilstrup DM, Schleck CD, Jensen LM. Outcome assessment for carpal tunnel surgery: the relative responsiveness of generic, arthritis-specific, disease-specific, and physical examination measures. *J Hand Surg* 1996;21A:338–346.

76. Burckhardt CS, Clark SR, Bennett RM. The fibromyalgia impact questionnaire: development and validation. *J Rheumatol* 1991;18:728–733.

77. Pincus T, Summery JA, Soraci SA, Wallston KA, Hummon NP. Assessment of patient satisfaction in activities of daily living using a modified Stanford Health Assessment Questionnaire. *Arthritis Rheum* 1983;26: 1346–1353.

78. Friedman PJ. Predictors of work disability in work-related upper-extremity disorders. *J Occup Med* 1997;39: 339–343.

79. Franzblau A, Werner RA, Valle J, Johnston EC. Workplace surveillance for carpal tunnel syndrome: a comparison of methods. *J Occup Med* 1993;3:1–14.

80. Katz JN, Gelberman RH, Wright EA, Lew RA, Liang MH. Responsiveness of self-reported and objective measures of disease severity in carpal tunnel syndrome. *Mass Med Care* 1994;32:1127–1133.

81. Dawson J, Fitzpatrick R, Carr AJ. Questionnaire on the perception of patients about shoulder surgery. *J Bone Joint Surg Br* 1996;78B:593–600.

82. Atroshi I, Breidenbach WC, McCabe SJ. Assessment of the carpal tunnel outcome instrument in patients with nerve-compression symptoms. *J Hand Surg* 1997;22A: 222–227.

83. Bell MJ, Bombardier C, Tugwell P. Measurement of functional status, quality of life, and utility in rheumatoid arthritis. *Arthritis Rheum* 1996:591–601.

84. Engin AE. On biomechanics of the shoulder complex. *J Biomechem* 1980;13:570–590.

85. Jones LA. Perception of force and weight: theory and research. *Psychol Bull* 1986;100:29–42.

86. Hosman J. *Adaptation to muscular effort*. Stockholm: University of Stockholm, 1967.

87. Eason RG. Electromyographic study of local and generalized muscular impairment. *J Appl Physiol* 1960;15: 479–482.

88. Lloyd AJ. Subjective and electromyographic assessment of isometric muscle contractions. *Ergonomics* 1970;13:685–691.

89. American Academy of Orthopaedic Surgeons. *Upper Limb—DASH outcomes data collection questionnaire*. Des Plaines, IL: Musculoskeletal outcomes data evaluation and management system, 1998, pp. 1–11.

90. Chung KC, Pillsbury MS, Walters MR, Hayward RA. Reliability and validity testing of the Michigan hand outcomes questionnaire. *J Hand Surg* 1998;23A: 575–587.

91. Ditmars DM Jr, Houin HP. Carpal tunnel syndrome. In: Kasdan ML, ed. *Hand clinics*. Philadelphia: WB Saunders, 1986:525–532.

92. Nathan PA, Meadows KD, Doyle LS. Relationship of age and sex to sensory conduction of the median nerve at the carpal tunnel and associations of slowed conduction with symptoms. *Muscle Nerve* 1988;11: 1149–1150.

93. Nathan PA, Keniston RC, Myers LD. Longitudinal study of median nerve sensory conduction in industry: relationship to age, gender, hand dominance, occupational hand use, and clinical diagnosis. *J Hand Surg* 1992;17A:850–851.

94. Lorig D, Draines RG, Byron MS. A workplace health education program that reduces outpatient visits. *Med Care* 1985;23:1044–1054.

95. Tanaka S, Seligman PJ, Halperin W. Use of worker's compensation claims data for surveillance of cumulative trauma disorders. *J Occup Med* 1988;30:488–492.

96. Muto T, Sakurai H. Relation between exercise and absenteeism due to illness and injury in manufacturing companies in Japan. *J Occup Med* 1994;35:995–999.

97. Farid I, Nathan PA. Carpal tunnel syndrome (CTS): its causes, treatment, and prevention, In: *American College of Occupational and Environmental Medicine Annual Meeting*. Arlington Heights, IL: American College of Occupational and Environmental Medicine, 1996: 75–76.

98. Armstrong TJ, Chaffin DB. Carpal tunnel syndrome and selected personal attributes. *J Occup Med* 1979;21: 481–486.

99. Louis DS. Evolving concerns relating to occupational disorders of the upper extremity. *Clin Orthop* 1990; 254:140–143.

100. Nathan PA, Keinston RC, Meadows KD. Keyboarding as a risk factor for carpal tunnel syndrome: comparing clerical workers to managers in eight industries. In: *American Society for Surgery of the Hand Annual Meeting*. Englewood, CO: American Society for Surgery of the Hand, 1993:78–79.

101. Lechner L, Vries HD. Participation in an employee fitness program: Determinants of high adherence, low adherence, and dropout. *J Occup Med* 1995;37:429–436.

102. Naso SJ, Watford P, Payseur G. Reduction of cumulative trauma disorders with a stretch fitness program. *J Occup Med* 1995;37:517–518

103. Lindstrom I, Ohlund C, Nachemson A. Validity of patient reporting a predictive value of industrial physical work demands. *Spine* 1994;19:888–893.

104. Melhorn JM. CTD in the workplace treatment outcomes, In: Speak, ed. *Seventeenth Annual Workers' Compensation and Occupational Medicine Seminar*. Boston: Speak, 1997:168–178.

105. Stewart AL, Hays RD, Ware JE Jr. The MOS Short-form general health survey. Reliability and validity in a patient population *Med Care* 1988;26:724–735.

106. Guyatt GH, Bombardier C, Tugwell PX. Measuring disease-specific quality of life in clinical trials. *Can Med Assoc J* 1986;134:889–895.

107. Feinstein AR, Josephy BR, Wells CK. Scientific and clinical problems in indexes of functional disability. *Ann Intern Med* 1986;105:413–420.

108. Sox H, Blatt M, Higgins M. *Medical decision making*. Massachusetts: Butterworths, Stoneham, 1988.

109. Weinstein M, Fineberg H. *Clinical decision analysis*. Philadelphia: WB Saunders, 1980.

110. Francis K. Decision analysis using a spreadsheet. *Phys Ther* 1988;68:1409–1410.

111. Melhorn, JM. Hand injuries diagnosis and treatment. Published via Christi Regional Medical Centers, Wichita, Kansas, 1997;1:1–11.

112. Melhorn JM. Physician support and employer options for reducing risk of CTD. In: Spengler DM, Zippieri JP, eds. *Workers' Compensation case management: a multidisciplinary perspective*. Rosemont, IL: American Academy of Orthopaedic Surgeons, 1997:21–34.

PART V

Postacute Occupational
Musculoskeletal Disorders

Occupational Musculoskeletal Disorders
edited by T. G. Mayer, R. J. Gatchel, and P. B. Polatin.
Lippincott Williams & Wilkins, Philadelphia © 2000.

22

Diagnostic Imaging

William Charles Watters III

Department of Orthopedic Surgery, Baylor College of Medicine, Houston, Texas 77030

The acute phase of a musculoskeletal injury normally lasts 4 to 8 weeks. Patients who remain symptomatic beyond this time can be considered to be in the postacute phase of injury. Most clinicians consider the postacute phase of injury to last up to 4 months, although for some injuries this might extend up to 6 months. During this postacute period, the majority of patients will come under the care of a musculoskeletal specialist and the potential exists for greatly increasing the cost of patient care. This potential results not only from the added financial burden of specialist care but also from the cost of additional diagnostic imaging and testing. In addition, costly care options, including surgery, often need to be applied to these more difficult treatment problems. This chapter is not intended for radiologists but rather for practicing clinicians. It is the clinicians' challenge to provide the best health care available to their patients within the varied contexts of the numerous occupational medicine systems in our country. In an era of cost consciousness, treating physicians are obliged to be prudent and thoughtful in their use and choice of diagnostic imaging in the postacute injury phase of injuries. To help fulfill this goal, three germane concepts will be discussed prior to consideration of the diagnostic options by skeletal region: the concept of validity in diagnostic testing, the value added by diagnostic imaging, and the role of treatment guidelines.

VALIDITY IN DIAGNOSTIC TESTING

Inherent in the process of diagnostic testing and imaging in human disease is the concept of validity (1–3). *Validity* is the ability of a diagnostic test to correctly identify those individuals who have a disease and those who do not. The more valid a test is, the better that test is at separating test-positive from test-negative individuals. Both the test's sensitivity and its specificity are used to assess its validity. Test *sensitivity* is defined as the probability of a test's being positive when a disease state is present. The closer that probability is to 1, the more sensitive the test is and the more likely that the disease, if present, will be identified. If a test fails to identify the disease when in fact it is present, the test result is referred to as false-negative. Test *specificity* is defined as the probability that individuals without a given disease will be identified as not having that disease. The closer to 1 that the specificity is, the less likely will an individual without the disease be misclassified as having the disease. When a test incorrectly identifies the disease as being present, the test result is referred to as false-positive. Because no test is perfect, that is, completely sensitive and completely specific, medical decisions are often made based on test results that may be false-negative and/or false-positive. When missing a diagnosis can have dire consequences for a patient, tests with high sensitivity are preferred. When the risks and costs of evaluating false-positive results are prohibitive, then tests with high specificity are preferred (1–3).

The need for diagnostic imaging beyond routine x-ray examination depends on both the amount of time that has passed since the injury and the severity of the patient's clinical condition. If the patient's clinical condition is severe, certain tests may be performed sooner than would normally be considered. While most advanced imaging techniques, beyond routine radiographs, would not be applied to an injury in the acute phase, there are instances when the use of these imaging modalities is dictated by the clinical situation. An example of this is the ordering of magnetic resonance (MR) imaging in a patient suspected of having a disc herniation with progressive neurologic change. This patient should have the MR scan done emergently as opposed to a patient suspected of having a herniated disc with simple radiculopathy. This latter patient has an 80% chance of resolution of symptoms in a relatively short time without surgical intervention, and obtaining a MR scan can be deferred or often eliminated.

Finally, it must be remembered that imaging studies do not test for pain. Rather, they identify structural abnormalities that may or may not correlate with the production of pain, such as a herniated disc irritating a nerve root. Thus, imaging studies have poor specificity for pain but are highly sensitive to structural abnormalities that can potentially cause pain (4). It is emphasized that the presence of a structural abnormality is only a potential cause of pain. Many research reports have demonstrated a relatively high incidence of structural abnormalities, such as a rotator cuff tear, disc herniation, or spondylolisthesis, seen on various imaging studies in asymptomatic individuals (4–12). Therefore, it is necessary for clinicians to take a careful history and perform a thorough physical examination to arrive at a differential diagnosis before ordering an imaging study to confirm or exclude a specific diagnosis (13). An imaging study ordered to confirm a specific diagnosis can provide considerable clinical

information, even when negative, and may be helpful in guiding the clinical investigator to the correct diagnostic conclusion. However, ordering an imaging study such as a MR or computed tomography (CT) scan to screen for pathology and using it alone to generate or exclude a diagnosis can only lead to many incorrect and costly conclusions. The misuse of diagnostic testing is more fully discussed in Chapter 15.

VALUE ADDED IN DIAGNOSTIC TESTING

The concept of validity is an important one for clinicians to keep in mind when deciding which is the appropriate diagnostic imaging study to evaluate a postacute musculoskeletal injury. Equally important to remember but more difficult to quantitate is the value that a particular diagnostic test adds to the clinical evaluation and treatment of patients (14). The newest imaging and testing techniques in modern medicine seem almost always to come at an increasingly higher cost. While many contemporary, sophisticated imaging technologies give astounding results in the appropriate clinical situation, it certainly is not a given that the more costly a diagnostic procedure is, the more useful it is in every clinical situation. In many situations, an appropriately chosen, though less expensive or less sophisticated, test will add as much or more value to the diagnostic process than a more sophisticated but inappropriate test. In addition, appropriate timing of a test can increase or decrease the value that it adds to a patient's diagnosis and treatment.

To illustrate this further, let us return to the example above of the patient with a suspected disc herniation in somewhat more detail. This patient is a 38-year-old employee who suffered the acute onset of lower back pain while lifting a heavy object at work. The worker was seen by a physician several days later, given light duty at work, and started on a nonsteroidal antiinflammatory drug and physical therapy. Over the next 3 weeks, the patient's lower back pain resolved partially, but increasingly severe right leg pain and numbness developed. This worker, now 4 weeks after her initial injury, was referred to a musculoskeletal specialist for further evaluation. A carefully taken history in the context of an occupational injury will usually reveal a short list of diagnostic possibilities. In this example, this might include a herniated disc, spondylolisthesis, or possibly a facet syndrome. The list can be further narrowed by a physical examination focused by the history on the diagnostic possibilities and, if indicated, routine radiographs. To extend this example further, let us assume that the injured worker has normal routine lumbar radiographs, a positive straight leg-raising test, and an absent ankle reflex, strongly suggesting the probability of a herniated disc. These physical findings add even more information for arriving at the diagnosis. In this and many similar examples of work-related injuries, for the cost of a specialist's office visit, most of the information needed to correctly and specifically diagnose and initially treat the patient was obtained. In fact, in this example, the treating physician can be more than 90% confident that the diagnosis of a disc herniation is correct (15). And because the conservative care of even a proven disc herniation has an 80% chance of being successful without surgery, obtaining an MR scan at this point would add little or no value to this patient's treatment. Only if a course of conservative care fails and surgery is being considered will MR imaging add value to the diagnosis and care of this patient by confirming the diagnosis and indicating the correct anatomic level for surgical intervention. MR imaging is highly sensitive and specific for detecting disc herniation (see "Imaging the Axial Skeleton in the Postacute Injury" below), and in this example it would have been ordered at the correct time, adding great value to the patient's treatment. A bone scan, on the other hand, has little sensitivity when applied to this patient's differential diagnostic list and would not have been useful in this clinical situation, adding no value to the diagnostic process. Testing beyond the positive MR scan with CT-myelography and/or CT-discography, both highly specific tests, just to confirm clear-cut MR findings not only would have been costly but also would have added no value to the diagnostic process. In the treatment of musculoskeletal injuries, it is important for treating physicians to limit diagnostic imaging to only those tests most sensitive and specific for the diagnoses being considered, and to time the ordering of those tests to maximize the value added to the diagnosis and care of the patient.

ROLE OF TREATMENT GUIDELINES

Practicing clinicians have the demanding task of keeping a multitude of historical facts and physical findings in mind while trying to select the most appropriate and cost-effective diagnostic and treatment options for patient care. Even if they have knowledge of the relative validity of the various testing modalities and the value that each brings to the treatment decision, this knowledge most likely assumes a secondary role in their goals for patient care. Treatment guidelines can aid physicians in decision making and increase the quality and cost effectiveness of care given to injured patients. A treatment guideline, whether in algorithmic form, an executive summary or a narrative text, is not meant to establish a "standard of care" or be a "cookbook" for the practice of medicine. Rather, the goal of a treatment guideline is to guide clinicians through the care of a musculoskeletal injury, indicating the appropriate timing and selection of diagnostic and treatment choices based on the best available knowledge while also allowing a choice in clinical decision making or treatment "style." In other words, a clinical guideline should reflect how a good physician would approach the diagnosis and treatment of an injury with the world's literature on that subject at his or her disposal. Use of evidence-based medicine in this manner allows the rich scientific background of clinical medicine to be applied directly to patient care. Chapter 39 deals with the subject of clinical guidelines in more detail.

IMAGING OF THE AXIAL SKELETON IN THE POSTACUTE INJURY

The diagnosis and treatment of postacute musculoskeletal injuries of the axial skeleton consume a disproportionately large amount of the occupational injury treatment dollar (16). This is partly a result of the incompleteness of knowledge about the etiology of many of the pain complaints associated with axial skeletal injuries. The source of these incapacitating complaints, which are often vague and inconsistent, is frequently sought with sophisticated and expensive diagnostic imaging. Frequently, the more ambiguous the complaint is, the more numerous and often overlapping the diagnostic imaging will be. Only by considering the validity of each test in its clinical context and its added value to the diagnostic process and by using a consistent diagnostic approach can treating physicians use these diagnostic modalities in a beneficial and cost-effective manner for patient care.

Magnetic Resonance Imaging

Currently, MR imaging is usually the first test utilized beyond routine radiographs of the spinal column (17–21). This is the result of MR imaging's ability to clearly image soft tissues, such as the intervertebral disc and neural structures, giving it the highest diagnostic sensitivity and specificity of spinal imaging modalities. MR imaging uses pulsed electromagnetic waves of a defined radiofrequency, which cause a portion of the protons in the body to jump to a higher energy state. When a proton goes to a higher energy state, it absorbs energy. As the electromagnetic field collapses with each pulse, protons return to a lower energy state and give off energy in a specific radiofrequency range. An antenna detects these radiofrequency signals, and a computer is used to process variations in these signals into an image. An added benefit of MR imaging is that its diagnostic abilities come without the need to expose patients to an invasive procedure or ionizing radiation. No harmful side ef-

fects of MR imaging have been demonstrated. There are, however, several absolute contraindications to MR imaging. These include the presence of ferromagnetic cerebral aneurysm clips or ferromagnetic cochlear implants, cardiac pacemakers, dorsal column stimulator leads, or metallic foreign bodies in the eye orbits. Relative contraindications include pregnancy, transcutaneous nerve stimulators, severe claustrophobia, or the presence of ferromagnetic spinal implants that can distort images.

Spinal Radicular Syndromes

MR imaging is the test of choice for evaluating radicular complaints in the postacute injury period that have failed to respond to conservative care (17–21). Its high sensitivity and specificity make it clearly superior to other modalities in evaluating the spinal column for the presence of disc herniation (Fig. 1). In ad-

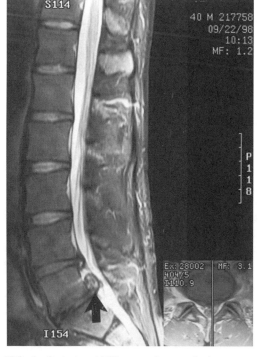

FIG. 1. A: Lateral MR scan demonstrates an extruded disc herniation at L5-S1.

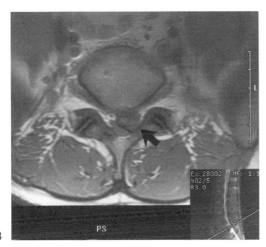

B

FIG. 1. *Continued.* **B:** Transaxial MR image at L5-S1 in the same patient shows a large extruded fragment.

dition, current levels of resolution allow excellent evaluation of central and lateral spinal stenosis as a potential source of neural compression. The facet joints can be well evaluated on cross-sectional views for the presence of hypertrophy and inflammatory changes, as can the sacroiliac joints. Finally, when enhanced with gadolinium contrast medium, MR imaging is unsurpassed in its ability to distinguish between a recurrent disc herniation and postoperative scarring in patients who have had previous spinal surgery.

Spinal Column Pain

MR imaging for back or neck pain without radicular complaints in the postacute injury phase must be approached not as a screen for spinal pathology but rather with a well defined differential diagnostic list in mind. This list of possible pathologic conditions should be based on the history, physical examination, findings on routine radiographs, and response to conservative care. The sensitivity of MR imaging for detecting anatomic changes, such as disc degeneration, combined with the lack of proven specificity of

many of these changes in the production of back or neck pain, can lead to many costly and ineffective treatment decisions. There is, however, a definite role for MR imaging in the evaluation of spinal column pain in the postacute injury phase (16,19,21). The presence of a symptomatic annular tear, as manifested by a high-intensity zone (HIZ) on a T2-weighted disc image, is felt by some authorities to represent a source of continuing back pain in the postacute phase (22,23). A HIZ on MR scan, though not common, may lend itself to conservative care and is important to identify (Fig. 2). Suspected spondylolysis as a source of continuing lower back pain not clearly imaged on radiographs can be identified by MR imaging. The ability of T1-weighted MR images to detect hypointense areas in the pars interarticularis has been reported in one series to allow earlier detection of a spondylolysis than with any other imaging modality (24,25). Finally, MR imaging has a role in the evaluation of chronic back and neck pain complaints of longer duration near the end or even beyond the end of the postacute phase of injury. MR imaging's ability to evaluate the internal structure of the intervertebral discs and the uncovertebral joints can be utilized to select appropriate pathologic and control sites for investigation by invasive, diagnostic injection techniques (see "Diagnostic Injections" below).

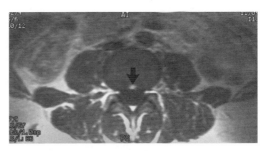

FIG. 2. Transaxial MR scan shows a high-intensity zone consistent with a potentially painful annular tear at L4-5.

Computed Tomography

High-resolution CT of the axial spine is a noninvasive test of high sensitivity but does not manifest the same high degree of specificity associated with MR imaging (13,17,18,21,26). In CT, a tightly collimated beam of radiation is passed through the body in multiple circumferential cuts. A computer then processes the resulting tomographic axial images into continuous coronal and sagittal images. Most contemporary machines can also format continuous images into any oblique tomographic projection or even into three-dimensional (3-D) images. High-resolution CT scans provide excellent spatial resolution and detail of calcified or osseous structures but are more limited than MR imaging in the ability to discriminate among soft tissue structures. In particular, intrathecal discrimination with CT is suboptimal in comparison to that with MR imaging and further exposes patients to ionizing radiation. For example, a typical radiation exposure from a CT scan of the lower three lumbar spine segments is a skin dose of 3 to 5 rad (0.03 to 0.05 Gy), which is equivalent to that of a routine lumbar spine series.

Spinal Radicular Syndromes

Unless MR imaging is not available, CT scan is not the test of choice for evaluating radiculopathy, for the reasons noted above.

Spinal Column Pain

In patients in the postacute injury phase with primarily back or neck pain, CT scan also plays a minor role, limited primarily to the more detailed evaluation of suspicious changes in the bony architecture of the spine or pelvis seen on routine radiography.

Myelography

Until relatively recently, myelography was considered the "gold standard" for the evaluation of the spinal column. MR imaging and high-resolution CT have now surpassed it in both sensitivity and specificity (17,19,26). Furthermore, myelography carries the added disadvantages of a higher ionizing-radiation dose than MR imaging or CT and the risks associated with an invasive procedure. These risks include headache, bleeding into the central nervous system (CNS), infection, seizure, and possible anaphylactic reaction to the myelographic dye.

Spinal Radicular Pain

In the evaluation of a radiculopathy, there is a limited role for myelography in selected patients, especially if combined with CT scan. In patients presenting with a valid clinical picture consistent with radiculopathy for whom MR imaging is not available, ambiguous, or contraindicated, a CT-myelogram can be useful. The combination of nerve root enhancement by the myelographic dye and the excellent resolution of bony structures by CT can provide useful information in these selected patients. However, myelography, even when combined with CT, cannot be considered a primary imaging study for investigating radiculopathy when MR imaging is available and not contraindicated.

Spinal Column Pain

Myelography does not play any clear role in the evaluation of postacute injury spinal column pain without radiculopathy (27).

Nuclear Scintigraphy

Bone scans of various types are notable for high sensitivity but poor specificity in skeletal imaging. In bone scintigraphy, a radioactive tracer is administered, usually intravenously, and taken up selectively by the target tissue (bone), which then emits concentrated levels of gamma radiation. The distribution of the radioactive tracer in the bone is detected by a gamma camera, and this distribution is felt to correlate with changes in physiologic activity in the bone. Technetium-99m pertechnetate is the most common tracer used to evaluate bone, but others are also available for specific imaging requirements. More recently, cross-sectional tomographic imaging has been applied to bone scans. Single-photon emission computed tomography provides improved spatial localization of abnormalities on bone scan.

Spinal Radicular Syndromes

There is no clear indication for the use of bone scintigraphy in the evaluation of radiculopathy.

Spinal Column Pain

Though much less expensive than MR imaging, bone scans suffer from the nonspecificity of their results. With the advent of generally available MR imaging, bone scans are used much less frequently than in the past in the evaluation of axial skeletal pain in the postacute injury phase of an occupational injury. One recent review questions the utility of bone scans in the evaluation of any spinal condition (28). Sacroiliac joint pain, a difficult diagnostic entity, has been evaluated by bone scan, but again the nonspecificity of bone scan findings in this clinical entity makes it usefulness limited (29).

Diagnostic Injections

As already noted, abnormalities on MR imaging, CT, and myelography associated with clinical symptoms have also frequently been reported in asymptomatic individuals (4–12). The incidence of these asymptomatic abnormalities, as well as degenerative findings, increases with the age of the population studied, thus making sound clinical judgments based on the imaging findings alone hazardous. In cases of prolonged axial skeletal pain, with or without a referred or radicular component, the history, physical findings, and imaging studies can often yield confusing and conflicting results. In such cases, selective injection techniques may be indicated.

Injection studies in the axial skeleton are bridging techniques that bring together both imaging and invasive, provocative diagnostic investigations. For an injection study to be considered a valid test of the pain-generating potential of a pathologic finding seen on imaging, several criteria must be met:

- The precise localization of the injection in close proximity to the pathologic lesion must be documented.
- Injection of the pathology must provoke a pain response and reproduce the patient's pain syndrome (concordant pain response).
- Injection of an anesthetic must provide relief of the pain response in a time of onset and for a duration consistent with the type of anesthetic used.
- Injection at a normal spinal segment should give a negative (nonconcordant) pain response.

Ideally, repetition of the test at another time or with an anesthetic of a different duration of onset and action (double-injection technique) should give consistent results. When these criteria are strictly adhered to, diagnostic injections can be an important adjunct to diagnostic imaging in axial skeletal pain (30).

Discography

When combined with CT scan, discography presents a clear picture of the integrity of an intervertebral disc. By application of the criteria for a valid injection technique, disc disruption or degeneration can be tested as a potential source of spinal pain (27, 30–36). While early reports raised concerns about the safety of the procedure, improvements in technique and contrast agents in the last two decades have greatly reduced these concerns (37). Using a double-needle technique and a lateral approach, contemporary discography is a safe technique that approaches 100% validity in its ability to image disc pathology (38). Starting with a study by Holt (39), however, the validity of the provocative aspect of this test has been questioned and has generated much heated debate. Published in 1968, Holt's study has frequently been referenced as evidence of the unreliability of discograms; however, more contemporary authors have voiced many criticisms of this study's design, methods, and conclusions. Simmons et al. (40) noted important methodologic errors in the study's design. They further pointed out that discograms are now obtained in a much more refined and reproducible manner than at the time of Holt's study. Several authors have shown that when the imaging and provocative pain-response data of discograms are combined, as is currently the norm, the test's reliability approaches 100% (27,32, 35,37,41). Furthermore, Walsh et al. (38) reproduced Holt's study with contemporary imaging and reporting techniques and found a false-positive rate of zero and a specificity of almost 100%. These contemporary reports suggest that a properly performed discogram, combining both the radiographic findings and the provocative pain-response data, can be a helpful procedure in the evaluation of axial skeletal pain (37).

Several investigators have shown that a positive discogram is highly correlated with the findings of disc degeneration on MR imaging (so-called "dark discs" on true T2-weighted images) and negatively correlated with normal-appearing discs on MR imaging (33,35,42,43). Thus, MR imaging is useful in deciding which discs are to be investigated by discography. According to one study, the discogram is likely to provide highly specific information on the presence of a painful lumbar disc when

• The patient has had unremitting lower back pain resistant to conservative care for more than 6 months;
• Issues of psychosocial dysfunction are not prominent;
• All degenerated discs and one normal disc by MR imaging are injected;
• The results of the appropriately and carefully performed provocative and imaging tests are combined (44).

While most contemporary research supports the specificity of a carefully done discogram in identifying a painful disc, this same literature is less clear that a positive discogram will predict a good outcome, even in a successfully fused motion segment (30,33,41,45,46). The reasons for persistence of spinal pain throughout the postacute phase can be multiple and complex. A decision to fuse a motion segment based only on a positive discogram alone is inappropriate. However, a positive discogram combined with information gained from the history, physical findings, response to conservative care, and other diagnostic results can aid the musculoskeletal specialist in arriving at an appropriate treatment decision. Colhoun et al. (41) showed that when the discogram is used in this manner, as an integral part of the treatment decision process, there is a marked improvement in the outcomes of surgical arthrodesis in discogram-positive patients compared to patients who had no provocative pain on discogram (Fig. 3).

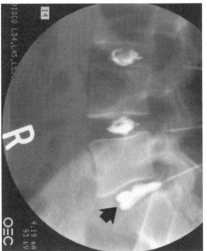

A

FIG. 3. A: Lateral discogram demonstrates disruption of the L5-S1 disc with a concordant pain response. L3-4 and L4-5 are normal.

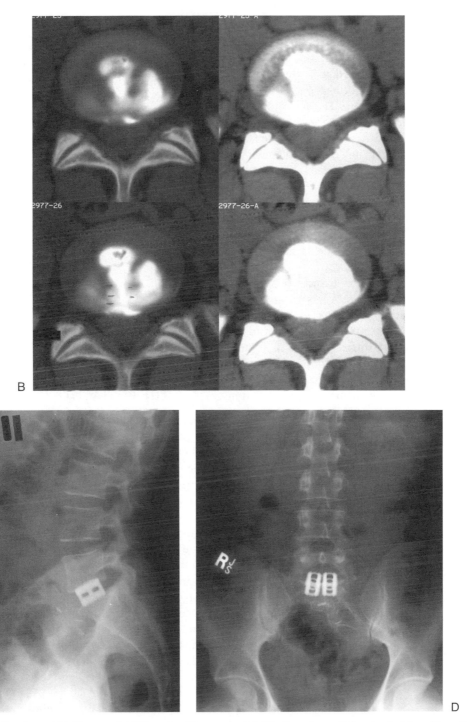

FIG. 3. *Continued.* **B:** Transaxial CT scan of the same L5-S1 disc shows the extent of the disruption. **C:** Postoperative lateral radiograph in the same patient treated with endoscopic interbody fusion by autologous bone graft and titanium cages. **D:** Postoperative anteroposterior radiograph in same patient shown in part **C**.

Facet Injections

Diagnostic injection and imaging of the uncovertebral, costovertebral, and zygapophyseal (collectively referred to as facet) joints allow evaluation of the posterior spinal column as a source of pain. The facet joint is a true synovial joint and has been postulated to become overloaded, degenerated, swollen, and thus painful in the unstable spine, in much the same way as does the cruciate-deficient and unstable knee. While this is an appealing analogy and a compelling argument for the pain-generating potential of the facet joints, testing of this postulate to date has been limited, and the predictive value of facet blocks in treatment decisions has not been completely determined. In a prospective study by Carette et al. (47), facet joints identified by injection as pain generators in the lumbar spine were no better treated with steroid injection than with a saline placebo. In a retrospective study, Esses and Moro (48) failed to show that facet injections were predictive of a good surgical result in lumbar spinal fusion for lower back pain. Nonetheless, many authors feel that the facet joints may be a source, though uncommon, of persistent axial skeletal pain (47–50). Recently, in a well controlled, prospective study using contemporary injection protocols, Lovely and Rastogi (50) showed a successful prediction of good surgical outcomes in lumbar spinal fusion. As the validity of this test has yet to be firmly established, some authors have argued that positive results should be retested at a separate time as a source of internal validation. While the results of facet joint injections must be interpreted with caution, they do appear to have a role in the evaluation of axial skeletal pain persisting through the postacute injury phase.

Sacroiliac Joint Injections

The sacroiliac (SI) joints have been noted to be a source of axial skeletal pain and can also be investigated by diagnostic injection. Schwarzer et al. (29) found that with the exception of groin pain, there was no consistent difference between pain patterns reported by patients with a spinal pain source compared to those with a SI pain source. Furthermore, they were able to demonstrate that within the limits of their study population, their patients' back pain symptoms actually appeared to arise from the SI joint with a prevalence between 13% and 30%. Thus, in patients with unremitting lower back pain extending through the postacute phase and remaining enigmatic after the usual diagnostic imaging, diagnostic SI joint injections may be indicated. While the sensitivity of SI joint injections appears to be high, no studies have definitively proven their reliability as a predictor of treatment outcomes. Therefore, as with discograms and facet joint injections, the results of SI joint injections must be interpreted in the context of all the information available about a patient.

IMAGING OF THE UPPER EXTREMITY IN THE POSTACUTE INJURY

Many occupational injuries of the upper extremity involve fractures of the arm, forearm, and hand, as well as dislocations of associated joints. Many specialized views and techniques have been developed to evaluate these injuries acutely by routine radiography. Most injuries are usually best followed by routine radiographs into rehabilitation in the postacute phase. Soft tissue injuries, however, that result from an acute insult or from repetitive motion and that remain symptomatic into the postacute phase often require advanced imaging techniques to better define and treat the source of persistent symptoms. Many of these persisting soft tissue complaints are confusing and difficult diagnostic problems that demand a thoughtful choice of diagnostic imaging on the part of treating physicians. As in the spine, investigations of imaging studies in the upper extremities, as well as some postmortem studies, have indicated a surprising number of pathologic findings in asymptomatic individuals (9–11,51). The musculoskeletal specialist must have a differential diagnostic list in mind that dictates the use of one or more of these advanced imaging studies prior to utilizing them. To order a sensitive study, such as an MR imaging, just as a screen for pathology can only lead to many costly and ineffective treatment choices.

Magnetic Resonance Imaging

MR imaging is notable for its high sensitivity and specificity in imaging soft tissue planes. It can also image in cross-section, with nonionizing radiation, to evaluate the upper extremity compartments and clearly visualize the inside of joints. These abilities have given MR imaging a dominant role in evaluating the upper extremities. In the evaluation of the joints in particular, MR imaging alone and combined with intraarticular injection of gadopentetic acid (Gd-DTPA) (MR arthrography) is more sensitive than even CT arthrography for evaluating inner joint structure (52).

Shoulder

Soft tissue injuries of the shoulder are common occurrences in the workplace. Because of its sensitivity, specificity, and ability to evaluate the entire shoulder, MR imaging is the best choice for evaluating a painful shoulder in the postacute injury. It is excellent for identifying labral and capsular lesions in the shoulder. These types of lesions occur in the context of falling onto the outstretched arm or with a severe traction injury that results in an often subtle tearing of the superior labrum from anterior to posterior (SLAP lesion). Tears of the superior labrum can also occur as a result of repetitive trauma secondary to throwing types of motion, while tear or fraying of the anterior labrum can result from an anterior instability pattern in repetitive-motion injuries (53) (Fig. 4). Anterior or posterior instability patterns can also produce subtle subscapularis tendon tears with resultant tendon retraction, which are well defined by MR imaging. MR imaging of these intraarticular injuries yields better findings than CT arthrography, with a sensitity and specificity of 88% and 93%, respectively (52,54).

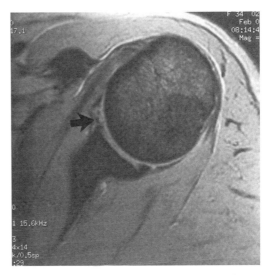

FIG. 4. MR image of the shoulder demonstrates a tear of the anterior labrum from anterior instability.

Acute trauma, as well as overuse, can lead to rotator cuff impingement and tendonitis, as well as varying degrees of frank rotator cuff tear. MR imaging evaluates the rotator cuff with a sensitivity ranging from 69% to 100% and a specificity ranging from 84% to 100%

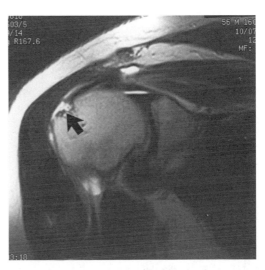

FIG. 5. MR scan of the shoulder in the anteroposterior plane demonstrates a complete rotator cuff tear. Note the subacromial signal consistent with fluid.

(54) (Fig. 5). It has been shown to be superior to arthrography and CT arthrography in demonstrating cuff tendinosis and partial cuff tears, as well as the size of a cuff tear (54–56).

MR arthrography using Gd-DTPA and fat-suppression T1-weighted imaging approaches 100% sensitivity and 100% specificity in the shoulder. While MR arthrography is not routinely required, it is specifically indicated if anterior instability is present and the history suggests an anterior labroligamentous periosteal sleeve avulsion (57). This lesion is difficult to detect in the chronic state by any other technique, including arthroscopy (58). In addition, MR arthrography is especially useful in the previously operated shoulder as long as no ferromagnetic implants or debris are present.

Elbow

While MR imaging is useful in detecting bone contusions and occult fractures about the elbow, as can occur at the radial head, these injuries rarely remain symptomatic into the postacute period of injury. MR imaging has become a major diagnostic tool, however, to investigate soft tissue injuries at the elbow (59). These ligamentous and capsular injuries can be overlooked or underdiagnosed in the acute stage and remain symptomatic for a long time. Ruptures, even incomplete, of the distal biceps tendon, partial triceps tendon ruptures, and tears of the medial or lateral collateral ligament complex are well imaged on MR scans (Fig. 6). Patients who experience repetitive valgus stress injuries of the medial elbow often present with persistent and vague work-related complaints at the medial elbow that can be confused with medial epicondylitis; however, these injuries do not respond to the usual treatment. These patients will often demonstrate capsular disruption and fluid within the medial collateral ligament on T2-weighted sagittal images (60). Both medial and lateral epicondylitis have characteristic low-intensity changes at the epicondyle on T2-weighted images, but usually MR imaging is not needed to makes these diagnoses (59) (Fig. 7). MR imaging of the medial elbow can

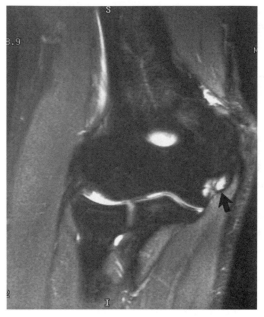

FIG. 6. MR image of the elbow in the anteroposterior plane demonstrates a midsubstance tear of the ulnar collateral ligament.

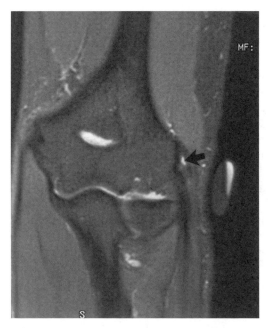

FIG. 7. MR scan shows lateral epicondylitis with signal changes at the origin of the lateral collateral ligament of the elbow.

also evaluate subluxation and entrapment and enlargement of the ulnar nerve, which is often traumatized in medial elbow injuries and presents with late symptoms. Finally, after the knee, the elbow is the second most common site for loose bodies. Unlike the knee, routine radiographs often do not image these bodies very well. Because of its multiplanar capability, MR imaging is an excellent modality for demonstrating loose bodies in the elbow (61). In difficult cases, MR arthrography may be required.

Wrist and Hand

MR imaging is used less extensively in the wrist and hand than in the shoulder or even the elbow. This is partly the result of the compact bony relationships seen in the wrist and hand that have given rise to numerous clever and useful radiographic views and techniques that take advantage of subtle changes occurring in these relationships with trauma and degeneration. In addition, MR imaging protocols for the hand and wrist are still evolving, along with improved technology such as smaller coils for this specialized type of imaging. Nonetheless, MR imaging has already proven useful in certain well defined clinical settings. One recent study using MR imaging to evaluate chronic dorsal wrist pain of unknown etiology found that 79% of the patients studied had occult dorsal wrist ganglions (62). MR scan had a positive predictive value of 100% in this study. The high sensitivity of MR imaging for marrow changes and edema allows the detection of the subtle marrow changes of ulnar impaction syndrome, as well as the early marrow changes of avascular necrosis of the scaphoid or other carpal bones as sequelae of trauma (Fig. 8). MR imaging is the best modality for evaluating the tendons and synovial sheaths of the wrist and hand, if clinically indicated. Finally, some centers have reported good imaging of the triangular fibrocartilage and intercarpal ligaments, but such high-resolution scanning is not yet generally available (63).

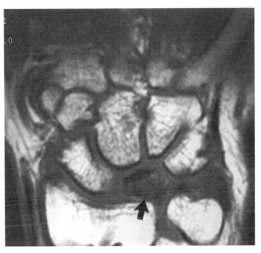

FIG. 8. MR image of an old lunate fracture demonstrates avascular necrosis of the proximal pole.

Arthrography

Until recent improvements in the resolution of MR imaging, the arthrogram was the "gold standard" in the evaluation of joint complaints in the upper extremities. In arthrography, the joint is injected with a contrast medium that is opaque to ionizing radiation, and multiple radiographs in various projections are obtained. The injected contrast material will leak out of an injured joint, as in a rotator cuff tear, and will be demonstrated on these routine radiographs in areas where it had not originally been injected. When combined with CT, arthrography can also give highly specific information about damage to the cartilage and ligaments inside a joint or about loose bodies in a joint.

Shoulder

Arthrography of the shoulder is a sensitive test for demonstrating rotator cuff tears. As noted above, MR imaging is a more sensitive test for detecting partial tears and estimating the size of a rotator cuff tear, but arthrography remains a valuable test when MR imaging is not available or is contraindicated or ambiguous. An arthrogram does not, however, give much useful information about tendinosis or impingement, unless combined with CT. In addition, when it is combined with CT, the internal structure of the glenohumeral joint can be imaged, and tears of the labrum can be identified. As noted above, however, MR imaging, if available, is a more sensitive test for these injuries.

Elbow

Arthrography is primarily useful for detecting capsular tears and loose bodies in the elbow. It is most effective when combined with CT (64). MR imaging, however, has become the diagnostic test of choice for most soft tissue injuries of the elbow.

Hand and Wrist

Arthrography remains the most reliable means of assessing the integrity of the intrinsic carpal ligaments, the triangular fibrocartilage, and the surrounding capsule (63,65). As in the shoulder, leakage of contrast medium from one compartment into another signifies a communicating defect consistent with a ligamentous injury. Multiple injections into all three compartments have been recommended as necessary for evaluating the wrist. Levinsohn et al. (66) demonstrated that up to one-third of communicating defects in the wrist are unidirectional secondary to a flap on the tear. Thus, they showed that a single injection (without injecting all three compartments) of the wrist will fail to demonstrate 24% of triangular fibrocartilage defects.

Computed Tomography

The excellent resolution of bony detail that CT affords makes it invaluable in assessing complex fractures and dislocations of the elbow and hand (especially with 3-D reconstruction), as well as in detecting occult fractures throughout the upper extremity. These needs occur most often in the acute phase of an injury, however. As well as its role as an adjunct to arthrography, CT in the postacute phase of an occupational injury is essentially limited to the evaluation of undetected and symptomatic hand fractures (e.g., hook of the hamate) and loose bodies in a joint and the late evaluation of complex fracture deformities.

Nuclear Scintigraphy

Bone scans are a sensitive but nonspecific means of evaluating bony lesions. The sensitivity of the bone scintigraphy made it valuable in the past for detecting suspected sequelae of traumatic bony lesions, such as avascular necrosis of the scaphoid. The availability, sensitivity, and specificity of MR imaging, however, diminished the role of bone scans in the evaluation of bony lesions of the upper extremity. Currently, bone scans are most useful when MR imaging is either not available or contraindicated.

Ultrasonography

The use of ultrasound in the evaluation of the upper extremity has its advocates, particularly in the shoulder. The advantage of ultrasonography is that it is associated with high sensitivity and specificity in certain areas while being noninvasive and much less expensive than MR imaging. The disadvantage of this technique is that it is very operator-dependent and good, reproducible results are usually only obtained by highly skilled operators with the latest equipment (58). Consequently, ultrasonography has not gained wide usage in the examination of the upper extremity.

Shoulder

Ultrasound examination of the shoulder is useful for identifying abnormalities of the rotator cuff, subacromial bursa, and long head of the biceps tendon. With real-time ultrasonography, a sensitivity and specificity of more than 90% have been reported from some centers in detecting partial and full-thickness tears of the rotator cuff (67–69). Unlike MR imaging, however, ultrasound cannot be used to evaluate other abnormalities of the shoulder that might have caused the cuff tear or might be contributing to the patient's complaints. In addition, a negative ultrasound in a patient with persistent symptoms of impingement requires MR imaging of the subacromial area for osseous changes and of joint structures for lesions associated with instability.

Wrist and Hand

The role of ultrasonography in the wrist and hand is limited, but one report advocated its usefulness in detecting nonradiopaque foreign bodies in the hand (70).

IMAGING OF THE LOWER EXTREMITY IN THE POSTACUTE INJURY

Routine radiographs remain the mainstay in the evaluation of acute injuries of the lower extremities. Complex or suspected occult fractures of the pelvis, hip, knee, and ankle require early evaluation by CT in most cases. In difficult diagnostic cases, early use of MR imaging has revealed contusions (microfractures) of the subchondral bone or even microfractures that have explained previously enigmatic joint pain after a traumatic event involving the joint. In most cases of lower extremity occupational injuries, however, advanced imaging is reserved for cases that remain symptomatic into the postacute period.

Magnetic Resonance Imaging

As in the rest of the musculoskeletal system, MR imaging has become the most important imaging modality in the postacute period of lower extremity injuries. Its high degree of sensitivity and specificity, as well as general availability, have allowed it to replace more traditional specialized imaging such as arthrography and bone scintigraphy in most clinical situations. In addition to its usefulness in the evaluation of joints, it is very helpful in the acute evaluation of musculotendinous ruptures hidden by swelling and pain, as well as muscular contusions that are slow to respond to treatment.

Hip

Hip pain without localized findings that persists beyond the acute injury period suggests a limited number of diagnoses: occult or stress fracture, early osteonecrosis of the femoral head, internal derangement of the hip, musculotendinous tears outside of the hip capsule, or exacerbation of an inflammatory arthritis of the joint. MR imaging best detects all of these conditions. Because of the associated marrow changes seen in an occult or stress fracture, MR imaging is highly sensitive and specific for making this diagnosis (71,72). In this clinical setting, MR imaging has also been shown to lead to the detection of undiagnosed, radiographically occult pelvic fractures, as well as associated soft tissue injuries (73). Significant hip trauma, as can occur in a work-related fall or vehicular accident, may result in osteonecrosis of the hip. In this condition, early diagnosis is critical for making a successful attempt to save the femoral head, and most authors agree that MR imaging is now the most sensitive and specific means of making this diagnosis (74). In patients in whom this diagnosis is suspected and radiographs are normal, MR imaging has the best probability of making an early diagnosis (Fig. 9). Within the hip joint, injuries of the acetabular labrum have been inconsistently identified by arthrography as a source of continued pain. MR imaging and MR arthrography with Gd-DTPA have proven more

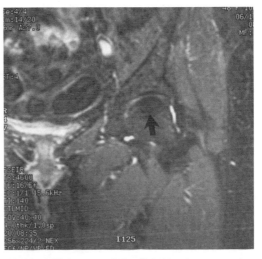

FIG. 9. MR image of the left hip demonstrates extensive avascular necrosis 3 months after a fall. Radiographs were normal.

useful in establishing this diagnosis (75). Outside the joint, musculotendinous injuries are clearly evaluated by abnormal signal intensity, discontinuities in anatomic structures in partial tears, and retraction of these structures in complete tears on T2-weighted images (74). Finally, plain radiographs best assess arthritis of the hip joint. However, exacerbation of a preexisting arthritic hip by an occupational injury can be well assessed by MR imaging findings of increased joint fluid, loose bodies, and tears of the labrum.

Knee

Perhaps more than in any other joint, MR imaging has proven of paramount importance in the diagnosis of injuries of the knee. Although plain radiographs remain the initial test of choice to evaluate a knee injury, MR imaging is often employed early in the acute phase to evaluate the knee for possible surgical intervention. Many less traumatic knee injuries, however, result in subtle internal derangements and ligamentous injuries that remain symptomatic into the postacute period of injury and require MR imaging. The timing of MR imaging of the knee depends on the clinical presentation of the

knee injury and the judgment of the treating physician. Damage to the menisci is common in work-related injuries of the lower extremities, and these meniscal injuries often occur in conjunction with other ligamentous and capsular knee injuries. MR imaging has replaced arthrography of the knee and is an excellent means of evaluation because virtually the entire anatomic structure of the knee can be evaluated in one study (Fig. 10). With respect to the meniscus, the accuracy of MR imaging approaches 100% (76). Currently, however, MR imaging remains more sensitive for tears in the medial meniscus but more specific for tears in the lateral meniscus (77). Partial or complete tears of the anterior and posterior cruciate ligaments or the medial and lateral collateral ligaments usually appear clearly on MR imaging and are to be sought, especially in a patient with a documented meniscal tear. Such ligamentous injuries are often associated with a meniscal injury. Also seen on MR imaging—and a common source of persistent knee pain—is the medial plica synovialis, which can mimic an internal derangement. On MR imaging, the plica appears as a thickened band of synovium, located anteromedially, and, if looked for, is readily seen (78). Another source of persistent

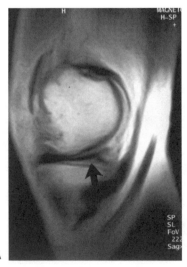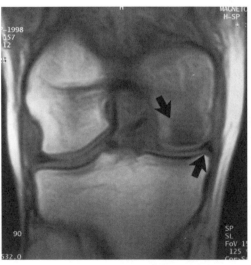

A

B

FIG. 10. A: Lateral MR scan of a painful knee 2 months after a slip and fall onto the knee demonstrates a torn posterior horn of the medial meniscus. **B:** Anteroposterior MR image of the posterior aspect of the same knee demonstrates the torn posterior horn of the medial meniscus. Note the associated osteochondral defect in the medial femoral condyle.

enigmatic knee pain readily seen on MR imaging is microfractures of the tibial plateau and femoral condyles. More severe knee trauma, as in the hip, can result in osteonecrosis, usually occurring in the medial femoral condyle and most accurately detected by MR imaging (79) (see Fig. 10). Outside the joint, partial quadriceps tendon ruptures and patellar tendinopathy (jumper's knee), which can go undetected as sources of anterior knee pain for a long time, are well demonstrated by MR imaging (Fig. 11). Although a chronic bursitis is usually obvious on clinical grounds, MR imaging can be valuable for differentiating a pes anserine bursitis or a tibial collateral ligament bursitis, whose treatment is usually nonsurgical, from a meniscal tear. Finally, popliteal cysts, which are the frequent sequelae of internal knee derangements and a source of posterior knee pain, are clearly delineated by MR imaging.

MR imaging in the previously operated knee is best done with intraarticular Gd-DTPA for enhanced contrast between scarring and new injuries. A contraindication to MR imaging in the previously operated knee is the presence of ferromagnetic implants or vascular clips.

Foot and Ankle

Persistent pain in work-related foot and ankle injuries is not uncommon and often difficult to diagnose. MR imaging has come to play an important role in the evaluation of these complaints. Acutely, 25% of Achilles tendon ruptures are inaccurately diagnosed on physical examination, and persistent tendon pain may result from this injury, as well as from tenosynovitis, tendinosis (degeneration), partial rupture, entrapment, and subluxation (80). These entities are distinguishable on MR imaging and are of course not limited to the Achilles tendon. Information on the condition of all the tendons of foot and ankle, as well as the plantar fascia, can be obtained with MR imaging (81). Imaging of the ankle ligaments is less precise but nonetheless has been shown to be useful in the assessment of chronic ankle pain (82,83). The sensitivity of MR imaging for the detection of subtle bone edema makes it the test of choice for evaluating occult bone contusions and fractures, as well as early osteonecrosis. The changes of a bone contusion, or microfracture, should be positive within minutes of a traumatic event and usually revert to normal in 12 weeks (81). The changes of osteonecrosis occur long after a traumatic injury, but MR imaging detects these changes earlier and with more specificity than any other imaging modality (74). MR imaging's ability to demonstrate hyaline cartilage combined with its sensitivity to bone marrow edema makes it superior to CT for the evaluation of osteochondral lesions, especially in the early stage (84) (Fig. 12). Finally,

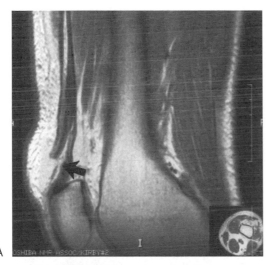

A

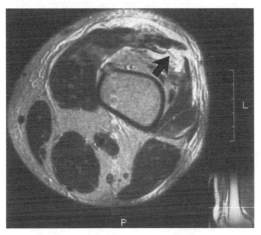

B

FIG. 11. A: Lateral MR scan demonstrates a chronic partial quadriceps tendon rupture still symptomatic 5 months after a fall on stairs while at work. **B:** Transaxial MR image of the same knee.

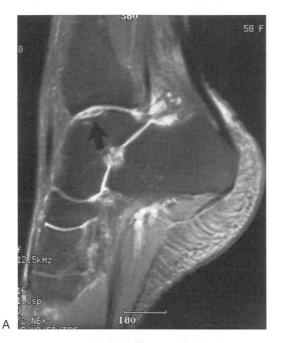

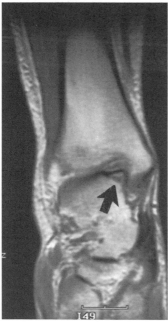

FIG. 12. A: Lateral MR scan of the foot and ankle still painful 2 months after a fall onto the foot 4 feet from a ladder. Note the osteochondral defect of the talar dome. **B:** Anteroposterior MR image of the same patient.

the exquisite sensitivity of MR imaging allows detection of subtle fluid collections in the foot and ankle secondary to traumatic and infectious synovitis and traumatic ganglia, which can be sources of persistent, enigmatic foot pain.

Computed Tomography

CT's excellent resolution of bony detail makes it a critical means of evaluating complex fractures of the hip and pelvis, tibial plateau fractures, and complex fractures of the foot and ankle, especially when augmented by 3-D reconstruction software. The advent of spiral scanning has made possible the rapid evaluation of difficult fractures and increased the speed with which these can be treated. In the postacute injury period, MR imaging has largely supplanted CT in diagnosis. The general availability of CT, however, makes it useful in evaluating questions of pseudarthrosis in complex fracture healing, occult or stress fractures, and loose bodies in the posttraumatic hip joint.

Arthrography

MR imaging has essentially eliminated the long tradition of arthrographic evaluation of lower extremity joint injuries. Knee arthrography still has a limited use, however, when MR imaging is either not available or contraindicated. When combined with CT, arthrography gains additional sensitivity in the evaluation of internal derangements, loose bodies, and lesions of the joint cartilage surface.

Nuclear Scintigraphy

Bone scan is very sensitive to occult or stress fractures and, though not as specific as MR imaging, remains an excellent and cost-effective choice when clinical suspicion is high in an area such as the tibia or the metatarsals of the foot. Beyond this limited indication, there is little use for bone scintigraphy in the evaluation of occupational injuries.

Ultrasonography

One limited use for ultrasonography in the lower extremities is the evaluation of a popliteal mass when MR imaging is not available or contraindicated.

REFERENCES

1. Eisenberg MJ. Accuracy and predictive values in clinical decision-making. *Cleve Clin J Med* 1995;62:311–316.
2. Obuchowski N. Decision model for choosing the best diagnostic test strategy with application to patients presenting with radiculopathy. *Semin Spine Surg* 1997;9: 9–17.
3. Sox H, Stern S, Owens D, et al. *Assessment of diagnostic technology in health care: rational, methods, problems and directions.* Washington, DC: National Academy Press, 1989.
4. Buirskie G, Silberstein M. The symptomatic lumbar disc in patients with low back pain: magnetic resonance imaging appearances in both symptomatic and control populations. *Spine* 1993;18:1808–1811.
5. Boden SD, Davis DO, Dina TS, Patronas NJ, Wiesel SW. Abnormal magnetic resonance scans of the lumbar spine in asymptomatic subjects. *J Bone Joint Surg Am* 1990;72:403–408.
6. Boos N, Rieder R, Schade V, Spratt KF, Semmer N, Aebi M. The diagnostic accuracy of magnetic resonance imaging, work perception, and psychosocial factors in identifying symptomatic disc herniations. *Spine* 1995; 20:2613–2625.
7. Hitzelberger WE, Witten RM. Abnormal myelograms in asymptomatic patients. *J Neurosurg* 1968;20:204–206.
8. Jenson M, Brant-Zawadski M, Obuchowski N, Modic MT, Malkasian D. MR of the lumbar spine in the asymptomatic patient. *N Engl J Med* 1994;331:69–73.
9. Erickson SJ, Cox HJ, Hyde JS, Carrera GF, Strandt JA. Effect of tendon orientation on MR imaging signal intensity: a manifestation of the "magic angle" phenomenon. *Radiology* 1991;181:389–392.
10. Davis SJ, Teresi LM, Bradley WG, Ressler JA. Effect of arm rotation on MR imaging of the rotator cuff. *Radiology* 1991;181:265–268.
11. Neumann CH, Holt RC, Steinbach LS, Jahnke AH, Peterson SA. MR imaging of the shoulder. *AJR* 1992;158: 1281–1287.
12. Wiesel SW, Tsourmas N, Feffer HL, Citron CM, Patronas N. A study of computer-assisted tomography. 1. The incidence of positive CAT scans in an asymptomatic group of patients. *Spine* 1984;9:549–551.
13. Herzog RJ. The radiological assessment for a lumbar disc herniation. *Spine* 1996;21(24 Suppl):S19–S38.
14. Boos N, Lander PH. Clinical efficiency of imaging modalities in the diagnosis of low back pain disorders. *Eur Spine J* 1996;5:2–22.
15. Spangfort E. Lumbar disc herniation: a computer-aided analysis of 2,504 disc operations. *Acta Orthop Scand Suppl* 1972;142:1–93.
16. Frymoyer JW, Durrett CL. The economics of spinal disorders. In: Frymoyer JW, ed. *The adult spine: principles and practice*, 2nd ed. Philadelphia: Lippincott–Raven, 1997, pp.143–150.
17. Albeck MJ, Hilden J, Holtas S, et al. A controlled comparison of myelography, computed tomography and magnetic resonance imaging in clinically suspected lumbar disc herniation. *Spine* 1995;20:443–448.
18. Forristall RM, Marsh HO, Pay NT. Magnetic resonance imaging and contrast CT of the lumbar spine: comparison of diagnostic methods and correlation with surgical findings. *Spine* 1988;13:1049–1054.
19. Hashimoto K, Akahori O, Kitano K, Nakajima K, Higashihara T, Kumasaka Y. Magnetic resonance imaging of lumbar disc herniation. *Spine* 1990;15:1166–1169.
20. Herzog RJ, Guyer RD, Graham-Smith A, Simmons E. Contemporary concepts in spine care: magnetic resonance imaging. Use in patients with low back pain or radicular pain. *Spine* 1995;20:1834–1838.
21. Modic MT, Masaryk TJ, Ross JS. *Magnetic resonance imaging.* Chicago: Year Book Medical Publishers, 1989.
22. Aprill C, Bogduk N. High-intensity zone: a diagnostic sign of painful lumbar disc on magnetic resonance imaging. *Br J Radiol* 1992;65:361–369.
23. Schellhas KP, Pollei SR, Gundry CR, Heithoff KB. Lumbar disc high intensity zone: correlation of magnetic resonance imaging and discography. *Spine* 1996; 21:79–86.
24. Ito M, Incorvaia KM, Yu SF, Fredrickson BE, Yuan HA, Rosenbaum AE. Predictive signs of discogenic lumbar pain on magnetic resonance imaging with discography correlation. *Spine* 1998;23:1252–1260.
25. Yamane T, Yoshida T, Mimatsu K. Early diagnosis of lumbar spondylolysis by MR. *J Bone Joint Surg Br* 1993;75:764–768.
26. Jackson RP, Cain JE, Jacob RR, Cooper BR, McManus GE. The neuroradiographic diagnosis of lumbar herniated nucleus pulposis. II. A comparison of computed tomography (CT), myelography, CT-myelography and magnetic resonance imaging. *Spine* 1989;14: 1362–1367.
27. Grubb SA, Lipscomb HJ, Guilford WB. The relative value of lumbar roentgenograms, metrizamide myelography and discography in the assessment of patients with chronic low back pain syndrome. *Spine* 1987;12: 282–286.
28. Esses S, Seymour M. The use of bone scanning in the diagnosis of spinal disorders. Presented at North American Spine Society annual meeting in Vancouver, British Columbia, Canada; October, 1966.
29. Schwarzer AC, Aprill CN, Bogduk N. The sacroiliac joint in chronic low back pain. *Spine* 1995;20:31–37.
30. Bogduk N, Modic MT. Lumbar discography. *Spine* 1996;21:402–404.
31. Antti-Poika I, Soini J, Tollroth K, Yrjonen T, Konttinen YT. Clinical relevance of discography combined with CT scanning: a study of 100 patients. *J Bone Joint Surg Br* 1990;72:480–485.
32. Bernard TN. Lumbar discography followed by computed tomography: refining the diagnosis of low back pain. *Spine* 1990;15:690–707.
33. Greenspan A, Amparo EG, Gorczyca DP, Montesano PX. Is there a role for diskography in the era of magnetic resonance imaging? Prospective correlation and quantitative analysis of computed tomography-diskography, magnetic imaging and surgical findings. *J Spinal Disord* 1992;5:26–31.
34. Sachs BL, Vanharanta H, Spivey MA, et al. Dallas discogram description: a new classification of CT/

discography in low back disorders. *Spine* 1987;12: 287–294.

35. Simmons JW, Emery SF, McMillin JN, Landa D, Kimmich SJ. Awake discography: a comparison study with magnetic resonance imaging. *Spine* 1991;16(6 Suppl): S216–S221.

36. Vanharanta H, Sachs BL, Spivey MA, et al. The relationship of pain provocation to lumbar disc deterioration as seen by CT/discography. *Spine* 1987;12: 295–298.

37. Guyer RD, Ohnmeiss DD. Lumbar discography: position statement from the North American Spine Society diagnostic and therapeutic committee. *Spine* 1995;20: 2048–2059.

38. Walsh TR, Weinstein JN, Spratt KF, Lehmann TR, Aprill C, Sayre H. Lumbar discography in normal subjects: a controlled, prospective study. *J Bone Joint Surg Am* 1990;72:1081–1088.

39. Holt JP. The question of lumbar discography. *J Bone Joint Surg Am* 1968;50:720–726.

40. Simmons JW, Aprill CN, Dwyer AP, Brodsky AE. A reassessment of Hlot's data on: "The question of lumbar discography." *Clin Orthop* 1988;237:120–124.

41. Colhoun E, McCall IW, Williams L, Pullicino C. Provocation discography as a guide to planning operations on the spine. *J Bone Joint Surg Br* 1988;70:267–271.

42. Schneiderman G, Flannigan B, Kingston S, Thomas J, Dillin WH, Watkins RG. Magnetic resonance imaging in the diagnosis of disc degeneration: correlation with discography. *Spine* 1987;12:276–281.

43. Zuckeran J, Derby R, Hsu K, et al. Normal magnetic resonance imaging with abnormal discography. *Spine* 1988; 13:1355–1359.

44. Schwarzer AC, Aprill CN, Derby R, Fortin J, Kine G, Bogduk N. The prevalence and clinical features of internal disc disruption in patients with chronic low back pain. *Spine* 1995;20:1878–1883.

45. Parker LM, Murrel SE, Boden SD, Horton WC. The outcome of posterolateral fusion in highly selected patients with discogenic low back pain. *Spine* 1996;21: 1909–1916.

46. Rhyne AL, Smith SE, Wood KE, Darden BV. Outcome of unoperated discogram-positive low back pain. *Spine* 1995;29:1997–2000.

47. Carette S, Marcoux S, Truchon R, et al. A controlled trial of corticosteroid injections into facet joints for chronic low back pain. *N Engl J Med* 1991;325:1002–1007.

48. Esses S, Moro JK. The value of facet joint blocks in patient selection for lumbar fusion. *Spine* 1993;18: 185–190.

49. Jackson RP. The facet syndrome: myth or reality? *Clin Orthop* 1992;279:110–121.

50. Lovely TJ, Rastogi P. The value of provocative facet blocking as a predictor of success in lumbar spine fusion. *J Spine Disord* 1997;10:512–517.

51. Neer CS. Impingement Lesions. *Clin Orthop* 1983;173: 70–77.

52. Chandnani VP, Yeager TD, Deberardiro T, et al. Glenoid labral tears: prospective evaluations with MR imaging, MR arthrography, plus CT arthrography. *AJR* 1993;161: 1229–1235.

53. Pagnani M, Galiant B, Warren R. Glenohumeral instability. In: DeLee J, Drez D, eds. *Orthopedic sports medicine: principles and practice*, vol 1. Philadelphia: WB Saunders, 1994:580–622.

54. Iannotti J, Zlatkin MB, Esterhai JL, Kressel HY, Dalinka MK, Spindler KP. Magnetic resonance imaging of the shoulder: sensitivity, specificity and predictive value. *J Bone Joint Surg Am* 1991;73:17–29.

55. Stiles R, Otte M. Imaging of the shoulder. *Radiology* 1993;188:603–613.

56. Zlatkin MB, Bjorkengren AG, Gylys-Morin V, Resnick D, Sartoris DJ. Cross-section imaging of the capsular mechanism of the glenohumeral joint. *AJR* 1988;150: 151–158.

57. Neviaser TJ. The anterior labroligamentous periosteal sleeve avulsion lesion: a cause of anterior instability of the shoulder. *Arthroscopy* 1993;9:17–21.

58. Tirman PFJ, Steinbach LS, Belzer JP, Bost FW. A practical approach to imaging of the shoulder with emphasis on MR imaging. *Orthop Clin North Am* 1997;28: 483–515.

59. Herzog RJ. Magnetic resonance imaging of the elbow. *Magn Reson Q* 1993;9:188–201.

60. Murphy BJ. MR imaging of the elbow. *Radiology* 1992; 184:525–529.

61. Quinn SF, Haberman JJ, Fitzgerald SE, Traughber PD, Belkin RI, Murray WT. Evaluation of loose bodies in the elbow with MR imaging. *J Magn Reson* 1994;4: 169–172.

62. Vo P, Wright T, Hayden F, Dell P, Chidgey L. Evaluating dorsal wrist pain: MR diagnosis of occult dorsal wrist ganglion. *J Hand Surg [Am]* 1995;20:667–670.

63. Schreibman KL, Freeland A, Gilula LA, Yuming Y. Imaging of the hand and wrist. *Orthop Clin North Am* 1997;28:537–582.

64. Mink JH, Eckhardt JJ, Grant TT. Arthrography in recurrent dislocation of the elbow. *AJR* 1981;136:1242–1244.

65. Yin Y, Evanoff BA, Gilula LA, Littenberg B, Dilgran TK, Kanterman RY. Surgeons' decision making in patients with chronic wrist pain: role of bilateral three-compartment arthrography: prospective study. *Radiology* 1996;200:829–832.

66. Levinsohn EM, Palmer AK, Coren AB, Zinberg E. Wrist arthrography: the value of the three-compartment injection technique. *Skeletal Radiol* 1987;16:539–544.

67. Bretzke CA, Crass JR, Craig EV. Ultrasonography of the rotator cuff: normal and pathological anatomy. *Invest Radiol* 1985;20:311–315.

68. Drakeford MK, Quinn MJ, Simpson SL, Pettine KA. A comparative study of ultrasonography and arthrography in evaluation of the rotator cuff. *Clin Orthop* 1990;253: 118–122.

69. Mack LA, Matson FA. US evaluation of the rotator cuff. *Radiology* 1985;157:205–209.

70. Bray PW, Mahony JL, Campbell JP. Sensitivity and specificity of ultrasound in the diagnosis of foreign bodies in the hand. *J Hand Surg [Am]* 1995;20:661–666.

71. Deutsch AL, Mink JH, Waxman AD. Occult fractures of the proximal femur: MR imaging. *Radiology* 1989;170: 113–116.

72. Quinn SF, McCarthy JL. Prospective evaluation of patients with suspected hip fracture and indeterminate radiographs: use of T-1 weighted MR images. *Radiology* 1993;187:469–471.

73. Bogost GA, Lizerbaum EK, Crues JV. MR imaging in evaluation of suspected hip fracture: frequency of unsuspected bone and soft-tissue injury. *Radiology* 1995;197: 263–267.

74. Hayes CW, Balkissoon ARA. Current concepts in imag-

ing of the pelvis and hip. *Orthop Clin North Am* 1997; 28:617–642.

75. Czerny C, Hofmann S, Neuhold A, et al. Lesions of the acetabular labrum: accuracy of MR imaging and MR arthrography in detection and staging. *Radiology* 1996; 200:225–230.

76. Gray SD, Kaplan PA, Dussault RG. Imaging of the knee: current status. *Orthop Clin North Am* 1997;28:643–658.

77. Justice WW, Quinn SF. Error patterns in the MR imaging evaluation of menisci of the knee. *Radiology* 1995; 196:612–615.

78. Nakanishi K, Inoue M, Ishida T, et al. MR evaluation of the mediopatellar plicae. *Acta Radiol* 1996;37:567–571.

79. Reicher MA, Bassett LW, Gold RH. High-resolution magnetic resonance imaging of the knee joint: pathologic correlations. *AJR* 1985;145:903–909.

80. Hochman MG, Min KK, Zilberfarb JL. MR imaging of the symptomatic ankle and foot. *Clin Orthop North Am* 1997;28:659–683.

81. Kier R. Magnetic resonance imaging of plantar fasciitis and other causes of heel pain. *Magn Reson Imaging Clin N Am* 1994;2:97–108.

82. Chandnani VP, Harper MT, Fickle JR, et al. Chronic ankle instability: evaluation with MR arthrography, MR imaging and stress radiography. *Radiology* 1994;192: 189–194.

83. Schneck FG, Mesgarzadeh M, Bonakdarpoor A. MR imaging of the most commonly injured ankle ligaments. II. Ligament injuries. *Radiology* 1992;184:507–512.

84. Anderson IF, Crichton KJ, Grattan-Smith T, Cooper RA, Brazier D. Osteochondral fractures of the dome of the talus. *J Bone Joint Surg Am* 1989;71:1143–1152.

Occupational Musculoskeletal Disorders
edited by T. G. Mayer, R. J. Gatchel, and P. B. Polatin.
Lippincott Williams & Wilkins, Philadelphia © 2000.

23

Electromyography in Occupational Medicine

Andrew J. Haig and *Alejandro Pérez

*The Interdepartmental Spine Program, University of Michigan Health Center,
Ann Harbor, Michigan 48108; *Department of Physical Medicine and Rehabilitation,
University of Michigan Hospitals, Ann Harbor, Michigan 48108*

Is electromyography (EMG) the appropriate test for carpal tunnel syndrome (CTS)? For back pain? Can it prove the cause of a nerve lesion? The answer is: wrong question. It is like asking, "Is occupational medicine a good treatment for repetitive trauma disorder?" EMG is not a test. It is a medical specialty called electrodiagnostic medicine (1). An understanding of this specialty—not a simple test—is necessary for appropriate use of this resource in the management of occupational musculoskeletal disorders. The best orientation to this chapter is a discussion about the first question—about CTS.

Of persons referred for electrodiagnostic evaluation for CTS, 10% to 20% actually have a cervical radiculopathy or an ulnar neuropathy instead of or in addition to CTS (2,3). A similar percentage have problems explained by a musculoligamentous disorder (4). Of persons with CTS, 50% have bilateral findings. However, in a prospective study, an extensive history and physical examination by an expert physician missed the appropriate diagnosis in 20% to 30% of persons referred for electrodiagnostic testing for an upper extremity nerve disorder (5).

Testing for CTS can be provided by an experienced board-certified subspecialist or a neophyte with 2 weeks exposure in a neurology residency. A "home-grown" technician can perform nerve conduction studies (NCS) before a physician even sees a patient. Yet the number of nerves tested by an expert has been shown to correlate with the number of past hospitalizations, the length of the medical problem list, and the ambiguity of the patient's complaint information, which the technician may not appreciate or interpret appropriately (5).

More than 30 different NCS can evaluate CTS. Current knowledge of the sensitivity and specificity of these different tests is quite different from the information available a decade ago, but the surgical literature often relies on the earlier, more insensitive tests. With the addition of more tests to a simple protocol, sensitivity is increased, but the false-positive rate is also increased unless the tests are carefully chosen and the combination of tests is studied (6).

This does not even begin to discuss the use of electrodiagnostic testing in screening for CTS, comparison with other modes of testing, or determining the severity, age, or prognosis of a lesion. Nor does it begin to discuss cost effectiveness, risk–benefit ratio, or the legal stature of electrodiagnostic testing in disability determination. And this is just for CTS. In a single chapter intended for nonelectromyographers, there must be limits.

This chapter introduces the basic science behind the clinical field. It explores the utilization of various specific tests for specific disorders. However, it also provides an understanding of the specialty itself and the way in which the practitioners of electrodiagnostic medicine provide answers to the questions of their colleagues who deal with occupational neuromuscular disorders.

QUESTIONS TO ASK

An electrodiagnostic medicine consultation can provide a diagnosis, but, if needed, it can often provide a wealth of other information. Lesion severity, its prognosis, and even its relative age can often be ascertained. Such information relates directly to occupational medicine questions about objectifying the illness or injury and determining the extent of impairment, its permanency, and causation.

Electrodiagnostic testing detects lesions of the anterior horn cell, nerve root, plexus, nerve, neuromuscular junction, or muscle. It can assess the presence of sensory nerve deficits and several autonomic nerve lesions. Testing can detect spasticity, tremors, and other movement disorders. While techniques such as somatosensory evoked potentials or electroencephalography can evaluate central nervous system (CNS) disorders, these are beyond the scope of this chapter, and electrical assessment of the CNS is not generally considered part of an electrodiagnostic medicine consultation.

Most clinicians dealing with occupational disorders have some knowledge of electrodiagnostic testing. Some preconceived notions about electrodiagnostic testing need to be identified:

- Does a patient have to wait for 1 month after an injury to get an electrodiagnostic consultation?
- Does EMG really have no false-positives?
- What about false-negatives?
- Can EMG detect effort? Fatigue? Force? Pain?
- What about the severity of a lesion? its age? its prognosis?
- If there are so many variables to consider, how can one tell whether an EMG was done well?

The rest of the chapter addresses the science behind these questions and then provides some specific answers.

ELECTRODIAGNOSTIC TESTING

Electrodiagnostic testing is commonly performed to evaluate the physiologic integrity of the peripheral nervous system. The typical electrodiagnostic evaluation consists of NCS of motor and sensory axons and needle EMG of selected muscles.

Nerve Conduction Studies

The basic concept of NCS is that electrical stimulation of nerves initiates an action potential that travels in both directions from the point of stimulation. Sensory, motor, and mixed (sensorimotor) axons are evaluated by these techniques.

Sensory Nerve Conduction

When sensory nerves or sensory axons of a mixed nerve are examined the sensory nerve action potential (SNAP) is recorded. Stimulating and recording electrodes are placed along the distribution of the selected nerve, and an impulse is generated and recorded. Figure 1 illustrates a number of measurements taken from the SNAP. The length of time between stimulation at a standardized site and the beginning or onset of the SNAP is termed *onset latency* and is determined by the speed of conduction of the fastest conducting nerve fibers (7). The peak latency of the SNAP is often measured. Prior to modern electronic advances, this was the most reliable measure from this small wave (8). When the latency has been recorded, the conduction velocity (CV) in meters per second can be calculated using the formula:

$$CV = D/T$$

D is the distance between stimulation and recording electrodes in millimeters and *T* is the time in milliseconds. The amplitude of the SNAP is measured from peak to peak in microvolts. The amplitude is an estimation of the number of nerve fibers activated during the stimulation.

Normal values for latency, amplitude, and CV are given elsewhere (9).

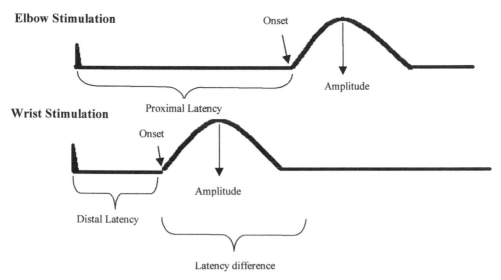

FIG. 1. A model motor nerve action potential. Conduction velocity equals the measured distance between the wrist and the elbow stimulation points divided by the latency difference.

Motor Nerve Conduction

The basic principles of stimulating and recording motor nerve conduction are similar to those for sensory nerves. One major difference from sensory NCS is that the recording electrode in motor NCS is placed over a muscle supplied by the nerve being studied (10). The evoked response generated by the impulse is called the compound muscle action potential (CMAP) (Fig. 2). It is typically in the 5000-μV range, in contrast to sensory responses, which are in the 10- to 20-mV range. Table 1 shows typical values for the various parameters of motor and sensory NCS along with other parameters discussed in this chapter.

The latency and amplitude in motor NCS are affected not only by the nerve being studied but also by the neuromuscular junction between the nerve and the muscle. The distal motor latency is measured at the onset of the evoked response, and depending on the lab, the amplitude is measured from peak to peak or baseline to peak. To calculate the CV, the nerve has to be stimulated at two different sites, proximal and distal, and the CV is calculated indirectly (9):

CV (meters per second) = distance between proximal and distal stimulating sites (millimeters) divided by (the proximal latency minus) the distal latency (milliseconds).

Other NCS techniques are frequently used by electromyographers. Long-latency NCS include the H-reflex, which is the physiologic equivalent of the Achilles tendon reflex; from the stimulation site in the popliteal space, it travels up sensory fibers, across a synapse, and

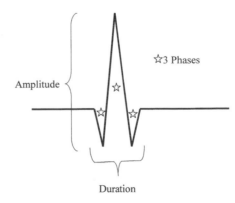

FIG. 2. A normal motor unit action potential.

TABLE 1. *Information recorded on a typical electrodiagnostic medicine consultation*

Parameter	Units	Normal findings
Needle examination		
Insertional activity	Normal, increased, or decreased	Normal
Spontaneous activity	0–4+ positive waves, fibrillations, complex repetitive discharges, or other rare findings	0
Paraspinal spontaneous activity	Mini-PM (paraspinal mapping) score	0–2
Motor-unit amplitude	Microvolts	800–4000 µV, depending on the muscle
Motor-unit duration	Milliseconds	Between 5 and 10 ms.
Motor-unit configuration	Phases, turns, baseline crossings	80% of motor units sampled have <4 phases
Motor-unit recruitment (decreased)	Firing rate of the first motor unit when a second unit begins to fire	0–20 Hz
Motor unit recruitment (increased)	Subjective sense that too many motor units are firing for the force generated	Not increased
Nerve conduction studies (NCS)		
Amplitude	Microvolts or millivolts	Highly dependent on the specific nerve and technique used: typically: motor NCS 2–10 mV, sensory NCS 5–50 µV
Latency	Milliseconds; sensory measured to onset or peak of response; motor measured to onset	Dependent on the nerve and technique used
Conduction velocity	Meters per second	Lower extremity, <40 m/s; upper extremity, 50 m/s
Temperature	Degrees centigrade	Skin temperature <32°C requires warming or correction
Repetitive stimulation	Percentage decrease in motor amplitude between the first and fourth stimulation when stimulated at 2 Hz	<5%

down motor fibers. It has some use in evaluating S-1 radiculopathies and polyneuropathies. The F-wave involves stimulation of motor fibers, resulting in retrograde transmission to the anterior horn cell, where the stimulation bounces around and returns down the same axon. Compared to the H-reflex, the F-wave's advantage is that it can be obtained in any nerve; however, it seldom detects a lesion not found on standard NCS or needle examination. The F-wave is useful in evaluating polyneuropathy but is typically confirmatory in the case of a focal nerve lesion or radiculopathy.

Repetitive stimulation of a motor nerve results in fatigue of the neuromuscular junction. Diseases affecting the synapse, such as myasthenia gravis, the paraneoplastic Eaton-Lambert myasthenic syndrome, or botulism, can be detected with this technique.

Needle Electromyography

Needle EMG helps differentiate between neurogenic and myogenic pathology. EMG examination consists of four basic steps. Inserting a needle (recording electrode) into healthy muscle tissue and advancing it in quick and short intervals create brief bursts of electrical potentials referred to as *insertional activity* (11). The electrode detects changes in the electrical stability of the muscle membrane when the muscle is at rest, termed *spontaneous activity*. When a patient contracts the muscle gently, the electrical activity generated by the discharges of the multiple muscle fibers driven by a single anterior horn neuron creates a motor unit action potential (MUAP). Finally, by gradually increasing the force, the patient allows the electromyographer to determine whether some motor units are not responding by measuring the recruitment rate.

Insertional activity can be normal, decreased, or increased. Decreased insertional activity is consistent with substitution of normal muscle by fibrotic tissue. Increased insertional activity occurs when there is active nerve damage or the muscle membrane is unstable, as in inflammatory muscle disease.

After inserting the needle, the electromyographer listens and watches the oscilloscope to evaluate the electrical activity when the needle and the muscle are at rest. The presence of any electrical activity when the muscle is at rest (*spontaneous activity*) is usually abnormal. Many types of abnormal spontaneous activity have been described. The most common are fibrillation potentials, positive sharp waves, and fasciculations. Fibrillation potentials and positive sharp waves arise from a single muscle fiber that is disconnected from its axon (9,11–13).

A fasciculation potential is the result of an involuntary spontaneous discharge of a single motor unit (consisting of perhaps hundreds of muscle fibers related to a single nerve cell) (8,13). Complex repetitive discharges and myokymic discharges are among the many other types of uncommon abnormal spontaneous activity, some of which are characteristic of certain diseases.

To obtain a true representation of the actual state of a given muscle, insertional activity and spontaneous activity are elicited from needle insertions in a number of different directions and depths. The electromyographer may test insertional activity in only a token way, thus missing pathology. In the paraspinal muscles and foot, a small amount of insertional activity and spontaneous activity occur in asymptomatic persons (14,15). Thus, the extent of exploration of insertional activity found in these muscles should be carefully recorded.

The third step of the EMG examination evaluates the MUAP during muscle contraction. The electromyographer looks for abnormalities in the amplitude, duration, and number of phases in the MUAP (Fig. 3). *Polyphasic* motor units imply pathology. Large-amplitude and long-duration polyphasic motor units imply that some axons have sprouted to incorporate the muscle cells of neighboring denervated muscle cells—a healing nerve injury. Small polyphasic motor units imply that there are absences in the hundreds of muscle cells that should be a part of the motor unit—a muscle disease.

The last step of the EMG examination analyzes the *recruitment pattern* of additional motor units. Abnormal recruitment is characterized as increased or decreased, terms that do *not* denote opposites. Nerve problems can cause decreased recruitment. This recruitment parameter can be quantified as the firing rate of the first motor unit seen (in hertz) when another motor unit jumps in to help out. If the second nerve cell is not firing, then the first motor unit fires abnormally fast before help (actually the third motor unit in the normal firing sequence) arrives. Decreased recruitment is detected the second a nerve injury occurs. Thus, if clinically relevant, EMG can objectify a moderately severe partial nerve

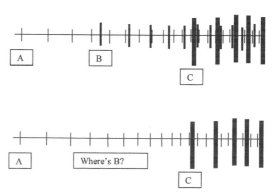

FIG. 3. Normal and decreased recruitment. **Top:** Small motor unit *A* begins firing, followed by *B*, then *C*. **Bottom:** Motor unit *B*'s neuron is damaged so *A*'s firing rate is very fast before another motor unit begins to fire.

injury immediately after it occurs. This is contrary to the truism that one should wait weeks or a month for electrical testing after an injury.

Increased recruitment occurs with muscle disease. If one expects three biceps motor units to be firing when the arm is bent 45 degrees to gravity but instead eight motor units appear on the screen, obviously the muscle cells themselves are not doing their work. This parameter is seldom objectified on clinical EMG, but it is meant to indicate that the amount of electrical activity on the oscilloscope screen is out of proportion to the force generated by the muscle. Thus, a person with a muscle and a nerve disease may demonstrate both increased and decreased recruitment in the same area.

PATHOPHYSIOLOGY

The physiologic factors of sex, age, digit circumference, height, and temperature can affect the interpretation of NCS (16,17). The electromyographer should be aware of the effects of these factors when performing and interpreting an electrodiagnostic examination.

Electrophysiologic abnormalities of the nerve fibers are usually divided into *axonal degeneration* and *segmental demyelination* (18). Most often, these two abnormalities coexist. In axonal degeneration, there is a decrease in impulse conduction in the axons distal to the site of injury. The SNAP or CMAP will be absent or abnormally decreased. Needle EMG will show abnormal spontaneous activity if there is active denervation, as in an acute injury. Changes in MUAP amplitude and duration will be observed, depending on the age of the lesion or illness. Recruitment abnormalities may also be observed. In demyelinating disorders, the main abnormalities in NCS are prolonged latencies and decreased CV. If the demyelinating process is severe enough, it will cause axonal damage, and similar EMG findings of axonal involvement will be observed during the needle examination.

Compression Neuropathies

In an industrial setting, nerve injuries are very common (19). They are secondary to acute trauma or a result of chronic repetitive microtrauma (19,20). Three basic categories describe nerve injuries: neurapraxia, axonotmesis, and neurotmesis (21).

Neurapraxia is a mild degree of neuronal insult resulting in blockage of impulse conduction across the affected segment (conduction block). It is marked by a focal demyelination at the site of injury and no axonal loss. Conduction slowing in unblocked fibers across the segment is observed. Weakness and paresthesias are common in this type of injury, but prognosis for recovery is excellent because there is axonal continuity.

In *axonotmesis*, the axon is injured, but the supporting neural structures are intact. Wallerian degeneration (death of the axon down to the muscle) occurs distal to the site of the injury. Active denervation (fibrillation potentials and positive sharp waves) is observed in the muscles innervated by the injured nerve distal to the lesion. NCS show decreased or absent SNAP or CMAP amplitude distal to the injury site. Fair to good recovery is expected because the nerve is grossly in continuity. Among the denervated muscles, function returns in a proximal to distal fashion, based on axon growth of about 1 mm per day.

Neurotmesis is the greatest degree of nerve injury. It results in complete disruption of the axon and its supporting connective tissue structures. Denervation potentials and absent CMAP and SNAP are observed. Symptoms are similar to axonotmesis, but prognosis is poor, even when surgical intervention is undertaken.

SPECIFIC NERVE SYNDROMES

Median Nerve

Median mononeuropathy at the wrist, or CTS, is the most recognized peripheral nerve injury (19,20). CTS involves entrapment of the median nerve as it passes through the carpal tunnel canal. Compression is mainly caused by the transverse carpal ligament.

Nerve conduction of sensory and motor axons is routinely evaluated. CVs are calculated for sensory and motor NCS. Even though sensory NCS are more sensitive than motor NCS, motor studies are performed to document lesion severity (22). CTS is a bilateral entity in close to 50% of individuals, even when no symptoms are present in the contralateral hand; therefore, some authorities recommend bilateral studies (23). An additional or alternative condition such as ulnar mononeuropathy, C8-T1 radiculopathy, lower trunk plexopathy, or an underlying polyneuropathy may occur in at least 10% to 20% of patients (3,5,24). Thus, ulnar nerve NCS are commonly performed to evaluate these possibilities (25).

Needle EMG examination is not absolutely necessary, but it is very useful for prognosis and determination of a lesion's age. Muscles distal to the lesion, such as the abductor pollicis brevis, should be evaluated to document the presence or absence of active denervation. Median-innervated muscles proximal to the lesion, cervical paraspinal muscles, and distal nonmedian-innervated muscles are routinely examined to rule out alternative diagnoses (22,26).

Anterior interosseous syndrome is another median nerve lesion. The median nerve divides into two branches after it passes under the pronator teres muscle: the main branch and the purely motor anterior interosseous branch. This latter branch can be entrapped at the tendinous origin of the deep head of the pronator teres, at the flexor digitorum superficialis, or by trauma to the forearm (27,28). Typical complaints are pain in the forearm, hand weakness, and clumsiness. NCS are typically normal, but EMG shows denervation of the three muscles supplied by the nerve: pronator quadratus, flexor pollicis longus, and flexor digitorum profundus.

Other possible entrapment syndromes of the median nerve are the pronator teres syndrome and the supracondylar syndrome with median nerve entrapment at the ligament of Struthers, which is found in 0.7% to 2.7% of individuals.

Ulnar Nerve

Entrapment of the ulnar nerve at the cubital tunnel in the medial epicondyle is a common neuropathy. Activities requiring heavy lifting, repetitive lifting, and prolonged upper extremity flexion may predispose to cubital tunnel syndrome (20). Symptoms range from neuropathic sensations in the forearm and hand to clawing of the hand secondary to flexor digitorum profundus and lumbrical muscle weakness. The main electrodiagnostic finding will be a conduction block at the medial epicondyle area. Needle EMG will show denervation potentials in the ulnar-innervated forearm and hand muscles.

The ulnar nerve might be entrapped or traumatized at the wrist as it passes through Guyon's canal. Repetitive trauma from holding or operating power tools at the workplace is a common cause of this neuropathy (29). Entrapment of the nerve causes numbness of the ulnar-supplied digits, hypothenar eminence weakness, and, if severe enough, intrinsic muscle atrophy and weakness. Electrodiagnostic examination is very helpful in the diagnosis of this neuropathy. Prolonged distal latencies and decreased or absent SNAP or CMAP are frequently observed. Needle EMG will show denervation of the ulnar-innervated muscles distal to Guyon's canal.

Radial Nerve

The posterior interosseous branch of the radial nerve is a purely motor branch that might be entrapped or truncated at the level of the elbow (30). This syndrome is commonly confused with lateral epicondylitis of the elbow (31). NCS may show slowing of CV across the injured segment, but typically the studies are normal (32). EMG is the most helpful technique and will show denervation potentials in the radial-innervated muscles distal to site of entrapment.

Other radial nerve lesions occur with direct trauma behind the humerus ("Saturday night palsy") or with compression of the superficial radial sensory nerve in the forearm ("handcuff palsy"). Because of its nerve distribution to the thumb and index finger, handcuff palsy can mimic CTS.

Lower Extremity Entrapment Syndromes

The femoral, obturator, peroneal, and tibial nerves can all be cause of entrapment or traumatic neuropathies in the lower extremity. The most common of these is a peroneal neuropathy at the fibular head. Sciatic neuropathies can mimic radiculopathy. Tibial nerve lesions in the foot (tarsal tunnel syndrome, or Morton's neuroma) may be detected by electrodiagnostic consultants who have a special interest in these areas.

Miscellaneous

Electrodiagnostic studies, especially needle EMG, are helpful in the diagnosis of peripheral nerve injuries in the proximal upper extremity. Musculocutaneous, suprascapular, and axillary neuropathy uncommonly occur as a result of heavy lifting or other trauma. Brachial plexus injuries are amenable to electrodiagnostic evaluation.

Radiculopathies

Electrodiagnostic testing is useful in diagnosing radiculopathies. Typically, testing involves needle EMG of at least five lower extremity muscles or seven upper extremity muscles spanning the roots in question and the paraspinal muscles. A NCS is typically done to rule out a polyneuropathy. This protocol is quite adequate in diagnosing radiculopathies, but an H-reflex can also detect rare S-1 lesions that appear normal on needle EMG. The F-wave does not appear to add sensitivity to the workup for a radiculopathy. Somatosensory evoked potentials are not typically useful, although they may have a place in the diagnosis of spinal stenosis.

Classic proof of a radiculopathy is demonstrated if there are abnormalities in two muscles sharing the same root but different nerves and in the paraspinal muscles, assuming that other testing does not detect a more diffuse process. Adjacent muscles supplied by different nerve roots should be spared unless the pathology is a polyradiculopathy (33). Importantly, the cervical paraspinal muscles appear to have a lower sensitivity for radiculopathies, and some data suggest that pure S-1 lesions may not involve the paraspinal muscles (34).

In the evaluation of radiculopathies, sensory NCS are usually normal because the lesion is typically proximal to the dorsal root ganglion, sparing the peripheral sensory cell. Motor NCS may show decreased CMAP. Needle EMG is the single most useful procedure for evaluating radiculopathies and has a higher diagnostic yield than other techniques (35).

After plain x-ray examination, electrodiagnostic testing was the first objective diagnostic test used in the diagnosis of spinal disorders. The early literature established the test as useful, since it correlated with surgical findings as well as or better than myelography or physical examination (36). With the advent of computed tomography (CT) and magnetic resonance (MR) imaging, as well as increased sophistication in research methodology, this early literature became less relevant, and EMG's role in spinal disorders was questioned. But evidence that imaging studies demonstrate a high rate of disk pathology in asymptomatic persons (37–40) led to a more critical look at the use of these anatomic tests without some physiologic correlates.

Attempts to modernize EMG techniques for radiculopathy have been highly successful. The lumbar paraspinal multifidus muscles have recently been shown to be innervated by single nerve roots (41). A needle placement technique in these muscles has been anatomically validated, and a codified technique resulting in nonsubjective scores has been developed (42,43). The technique was tested in a blinded protocol to demonstrate that asymptomatic persons indeed have normal or nearly normal scores (14). The technique, called MiniPM for Mini Paraspinal Mapping, has been further refined and simplified in a large diverse population of patients (34,44). Data show a high sensitivity and specificity. The scores correlate with the severity of the lesion on imaging tests. Recently, evidence was provided that the S-1 nerve root may not be innervated by the paraspinal muscles (34) and that the paraspinal muscles can indeed detect the anatomic level of a lesion (45). Similar research in the cervical region is not available, but it appears that the cervical paraspinal muscles are more complex.

Evidence suggests that EMG could be used as a first-line test in diagnosing radiating back pain. It is less expensive than MR imaging or CT and, despite concerns about pain, is tolerated as well as MR imaging (14). However, given the relatively easy access to imaging studies, the additional information that they provide on soft tissues, and the current variability in the quality of electrodiagnostic testing, it is likely that EMG will remain a second-line test. More reasonably, electrodiagnostic consultation should be considered when imaging studies do not make sense, for example, when MR imaging is positive in a person with nonradiating pain or negative in a person with radiating pain, or when MR imaging shows ambiguous multilevel findings.

Polyneuropathies

Electrodiagnostic studies are useful in the diagnosis of polyneuropathies. Occupational exposure to several agents can cause polyneuropathies. Mercury, lead, arsenic, and gold are few of these agents (46). Even though electrodiagnostic studies will not give a specific diagnosis, they will delineate whether the neuropathy is axonal or demyelinating, or has characteristics of both types. They will also reveal whether the neuropathy is predominantly sensory or motor. With this information, clinicians can narrow the differential diagnosis and, in combination with the patient's history, make the correct diagnosis.

Complete electrodiagnostic examination of a polyneuropathy requires both motor and sensory NCS. Multiple nerves in the upper and lower extremities should be evaluated. Bilateral studies are recommended to demonstrate the characteristic symmetry of the abnormality. Electrodiagnostic studies help differentiate a peripheral neuropathy from radiculopathies, myopathies, or a compressive neuropathy.

Neuromuscular Junction Disorders

Electrodiagnostic studies are helpful in the diagnosis of other neuromuscular disorders. Neuromuscular junction disorders such as myasthenia gravis, myasthenic syndrome (Eaton-Lambert syndrome), and botulism, as well as primary muscular disorders such as myotonic dystrophy, may be diagnosed with electrodiagnostic studies (47).

Screening for Nerve Injuries

CTS is the most prominent of the neuromuscular disorders that may be amenable to screening in the work environment. Several studies with long-term follow-up looked at whether abnormal slowing of the median nerve in active workers could predict whether CTS is more likely to develop (32). These studies showed that symptoms of CTS did not necessarily develop in patients with slowing of median nerve conduction. Furthermore, even when the prevalence of nerve conduction slowing increases with long-term follow-up, the prevalence of symptoms remains the same or decreases. Even when CTS has been diagnosed, there is a tendency for the prevalence of symptoms to decrease. In one study, CTS was no more likely to develop in workers with slowed median nerve conduction but no symptoms than workers with normal nerve conduction (32).

Slowing of median nerve conduction has to do in part with the aging process (18,48). Based on published data and the natural progression of median nerve CVs, NCS should be used with caution, if at all, to screen workers for CTS. Electrodiagnostic testing may be better used as a diagnostic tool for workers with symptoms of CTS.

Sensory NCS of the median nerve are typically more sensitive for diagnosing CTS.

When specialized techniques are used, such as the maximum latency differences as described by Ross and Kimura (26), the sensitivity of the test may be close to 87% and the specificity close to 83%, with a positive predictive value of nearly 70% and negative predictive value of 90%.

The more commonly used techniques have sensitivity and specificity close to 75%. In general, the sensitivity and the specificity of any electrodiagnostic test used to diagnose of any neuromuscular disorder depend on the technique used and the skill of the electrodiagnostician.

PRACTICAL ANSWERS

This discussion of the techniques of electrodiagnostic specialists and of the conditions commonly investigated has provided the background for further understanding of some of the clinical decisions made by these specialists. Based on this information, this section builds on the questions posed at the beginning of the chapter. The goal of this discussion is a more appropriate referral of patients and more sophisticated referral questions.

In earlier days, it was suggested that electrodiagnostic testing could not detect lesions in the first days after an injury. Indeed, the discussion of spontaneous activity shows that it will not appear for days to weeks after an injury, depending on the distance from the nerve injury to the muscle that the nerve innervates. However, NCS and motor unit recruitment rates are abnormal the instant that an injury occurs. Because spontaneous activity abnormalities are better for evaluating subtle lesions and the need to prove the existence of most lesions immediately after they occur is not common, waiting 3 to 4 weeks after onset to test is still recommended in most cases.

It has been said that a properly performed electrodiagnostic test has few or no false-positives (33). This statement is more true than not true, but it obviously bears some clarification related to specific disorders. Clearly,

the statistical cutoff for normal in a protocol such "as median and ulnar nerve sensory latency comparison" is based on a distribution of findings in an asymptomatic population, and that distribution can intersect with the population of persons who have symptoms. The normal values for NCS are not bell-shaped curves, despite the reporting of normal values in most EMG texts as ± 2 standard deviations.

False-positives occur in needle EMG of foot muscles (15) and the paraspinal muscles (14) of persons with no complaint or other pathology. However, most diagnostic questions can be answered without needling of the foot muscles, and the extent of abnormalities in the paraspinal muscles of asymptomatic persons is very low, compared with that in persons with known pathology (34,44).

False-negatives also occur. It is clear that a finite number of persons with clinically defined ulnar neuropathy at the elbow or lumbar radiculopathy have normal EMG studies (25,48,49). Testing of certain nerves (e.g., lateral femoral cutaneous nerve in meralgia paresthetica) is not reliable enough to make or reject the diagnosis. Fortunately, these cases are less common when the consultant is careful. Steroid myopathies and a few other peripheral disorders do not show up on EMG.

Occasionally, it is thought that electrodiagnostic testing can detect several lesions that are not directly related to the nervous system. Trauma or illness involving bone, ligament, tendon, or joint is not detected by such testing. As alluded to above, musculoskeletal problems are very commonly the cause of complaints that result in a electrodiagnostic medicine consultation. A thorough consultant will detect such problems in the history and physical examination and, while reporting electrodiagnostic findings, will weigh the nerve pathology in light of the musculoskeletal pathology.

Pain is another entity not proven by electrodiagnostic testing alone. EMG cannot directly assess pain, and it is an incorrect assumption to believe that evidence for nerve damage on electrodiagnostic testing means pain. For example, many diabetics and some persons with disc problems have painless radiculopathies. Experiments with needle EMG in fibromyalgia and with surface EMG in low back pain suggest some relation (50), but neither test is sensitive or specific enough for practical use (51,52).

Actually, EMG can detect force, fatigue, and effort in certain circumstances. Multichannel kinesiologic protocols, special signal processing to find the integrated amplitude of the EMG signal, and other signal manipulations to find the mean frequency of the EMG signal can determine some of these parameters. Although many modern clinical electromyographs can perform these calculations, the biomechanical and physiologic uses of EMG are actually beyond the experience of most clinical electrodiagnostic specialists, who focus on detection of nerve pathology.

The severity of a lesion can be documented. The amplitude of the nerve conduction response in comparison to the normal range relates to the loss of nerve cells. More gross severity information can be obtained from quantifying the recruitment rate of motor units on needle EMG. The presence of spontaneous activity almost always implies a lesion of some kind, but spontaneous activity alone is not a good measure of severity.

Prognosis can be determined to some extent from the course of recovery during serial EMG studies. The presence of any motor units in a given distribution suggests that the nerve is grossly in continuity across the lesion and that recovery is possible in the months and years to follow. A finding of no ability to recruit motor units suggests a severe lesion, but unless the lesion is more than 1 or 2 years old, there is still hope for recovery.

Sensory NCS can be extremely helpful in establishing the prognosis for a plexus injury. If a patient cannot feel in one area but weeks after the injury the sensory nerve amplitude is still intact, then the lesion occurred between the dorsal root ganglion and the spinal cord, and recovery is exceedingly rare. If the sensory amplitude declines after the injury, then the prognosis is indeterminate, but the presence of any motor units on needle EMG suggests that recovery is possible. For this reason, sensory NCS is advocated in the first days in

TABLE 2. *Typical sequence of findings in an incomplete but significant nerve lesion that does not completely recover*

Time	Nerve studies	Needle examination
Onset	Conduction block No amplitude drop if stimulated distal to the lesion F wave and H reflex abnormal	Normal spontaneous activity Decreased recruitment Normal motor-unit morphology
2–4 weeks	Amplitude drop Apparent mild conduction slowing, due to loss of some of the fastest fibers	Large positive waves and fibrillation potentials (100–500, μV) Decreased recruitment Few normal amplitude, very polyphasic motor units
1–12 months	Motor amplitude may increase due to collateral sprouting of axons to denervated muscle cells Sensory amplitude: no change	Positive waves and fibrillations shrink Decreased recruitment Fewer phases; large-duration, taller polyphasic motor units
1–10 years	Stable amplitude and velocity	Small (<50 μV) positive waves and fibrillations Decreased recruitment Some normal-duration, large-amplitude polyphasics
>10 years	Stable	Very small or absent positive, waves and fibrillations Decreased recruitment Large, slightly long motor units, but no longer polyphasic

the intensive care unit for any patient with a suspected severe brachial plexus injury.

The age of a lesion can be determined grossly from EMG testing. Immediately after an injury, there are no fibrillation potentials at all. Within weeks, an acute injury has large (100 to 500 μV) fibrillation potentials and positive waves, but a lesion older than 1 year typically has small (less than 50 μV) fibrillation potentials. Motor unit morphology changes over time. Immediately after an injury, the surviving motor units appear normal. Within days, a few small, polyphasic, inascentî potentials will appear. No recovery may be assumed, but within weeks, as a result of collateral sprouting of nerves to denervated muscle cells, there are large, polyphasic motor units. Over months to years, the collateral sprouts develop myelin and mature, resulting in very large motor units that are not polyphasic.

Thus, in the uncommon case of a person with a premorbid nerve problem more than 1 year old (e.g., an old unrelated radiculopathy in a person with a new back problem), electrodiagnostic consultation within days followed by repeat testing 2 to 3 months later can demonstrate whether any new nerve damage has resulted. Subjectively, talented consultants can find mixed old and new findings, suggesting superimposed lesions.

Table 2 illustrates the time sequence of electrodiagnostic findings in an incomplete lesion.

JUDGING THE QUALITY OF AN ELECTROMYOGRAPHIC REPORT

Room for variability in electrodiagnostic consultation is substantial. A consultant may be well trained and up-to-date or may be practicing based on a minimum of 3 months in a physiatry residency or 2 weeks or less in a neurology residency. Consultants' history and physical examination can vary in completeness, and the differential diagnosis generated may vary. For any given diagnosis, there is variation regarding which tests to use, the actual performance of the testing procedure, the interpretation of individual results, and the integration of the findings from multiple tests into a unified diagnostic impression (44,53). In short, electrodiagnostic medicine consultations can vary in quality.

How does a referring physician judge whether or not a consultation was acceptable? Frankly, it is sometimes hard to tell. The greater the knowledge of the anatomy, of the sensitivity and specificity of different tests, and of the procedures themselves that the referring physician has, the more sophisticated his or her judgment can be. However, some guidelines can be of assistance, regardless of the specific diagnosis involved. Table 3 outlines questions one might ask to ascertain the quality of an electrodiagnostic consultation, regardless of the diagnosis.

An electrodiagnostic medicine consultation may be excellent or poor, regardless of the questions in Table 3, but a tendency or trend can give hints to occupational physicians regarding the adequacy of a consultation. Certain items require some comment. Physicians without certification from the American Association of Electrodiagnostic Medicine may become quite proficient at electrodiagnostic testing. Although some of the best laboratories avoid the use of technicians altogether, others do use good-quality technicians. While substantial information may be lost if a technician begins testing with a set protocol prior to the physician's evaluation, the information provided will often enough be sufficient to answer the clinical question subsequently posed by the electrodiagnostic medicine specialist. The patient's recall of what happened during the test may not be fully accurate, and there are valid reasons why a physician may not have fully studied both spontaneous activity and motor unit changes in each muscle.

Report formats for electrodiagnostic medicine consultations vary widely. Some clinicians do not go through the exercise of documenting their history and physical examination or the differential diagnosis, but would rather just report the test conclusion. Still, a record of the electrodiagnostician's strategy in preparing the examination strategy adds greatly to the referring physician's confi-

TABLE 3. *Assessing the quality of the electrodiagnostic consultation*

From the electrodiagnostic medicine consultant
  ABEM board-certified?
  Technicians (if used) ABET-certified?
  What is the physician's testing schedule? (a typical consultation requires 1 hour or more per patient)
  Does the laboratory have a quality-assurance program (physician peer review or outcome-based quality
    check?)
From the patient
  Were nerve conduction studies performed by the physician or by an ABET-certified technician *after* the
    physician's history and physical examination?
  Did the physician's needle examination include exploration of each muscle in different directions?
    (adequate inspection for spontaneous activity)
  Did the physician have the patient gradually tense each muscle with the needle still in it?
    (adequate inspection for motor unit configuration and recruitment)
From the report
  Was an appropriate history and physical examination performed?
  Was an appropriate differential diagnosis listed?
  Was the skin temperature recorded or the extremity warmed prior to nerve conduction studies?
  Did the report format allow the physician flexibility to test patients differently, depending on their clinical
    situation? (e.g., a pretyped form with a few muscles or nerves already listed and little room for additional
    muscles or nerves to be added is suspect)
  Did the report record specific quantified data for each parameter for each muscle tested as listed in Table 2?
    (in contrast a report that lists muscles and simply indicates "Nl" or "0" after the first muscle with a line
    through the column to indicate that other muscles were also normal)
  Did the report discuss which test results were judged abnormal and how those results led to the final
    conclusion in exclusion of the other differential possibilities?

ABEM, American Board of Electrodiagnostic Medicine; ABET, American Board of Electrodiagnostic Technologists.
Nl, normal.

dence that his or her referral questions were addressed thoughtfully. While it is technically possible to take images of the actual EMG and NCS waveforms from the computer screen, it can be appreciated that such images are of limited value. In NCS, these images do not reflect the location of nerve stimulation or electrode placement or the sufficiency of the stimulation. In needle EMG, volumes of pictures would be needed to portray a single muscle, even if the needle was in the right muscle in the first place.

Clinicians may not record all the information listed in Table 1 with a numeric score, or even certain types of data listed there. However, computerized report generators are now common. They allow shorthand recording of detailed technical information, making it less common that an excellent electromyographer will simply scribble "wnl" in a column.

While the questions posed in Table 3 can help the uninitiated guess about the quality of a consultation, regardless of the specific question, electrodiagnostic medicine specialists look at other matters that occupational physicians may struggle to evaluate, depending on their knowledge. One aspect in which occupational physicians may become quite expert is anatomy. This comes into play when the electrodiagnostician evaluates whether isolated abnormalities could actually be due to a more broad diagnosis. For example, fibrillation potentials in the abductor pollicis brevis that the tester attributed to CTS might also be due to a proximal median lesion, a lower trunk brachial plexus lesion, a C-8 or T-1 radiculopathy, or a polyneuropathy. However, if the flexor digitorum superficialis (also median-innervated but proximal to the carpal canal), the first dorsal interosseous (also lower trunk–innervated but via the ulnar nerve), the cervical paraspinal muscles (with C-8 and T-1 innervation but proximal to the brachial plexus), and the sural nerve (the most sensitive nerve for a polyneuropathy and unaffected by upper body lesions) are all normal, the reviewer is more confident that the lesion is indeed at the wrist.

Finally, it seems that some aspects of the quality of testing will always be beyond the expertise of physicians who are not specialists in the field. It is difficult even for specialists within the field to keep up with the growing body of information in this area. A complete review of new findings in electrodiagnosis is immediately dated but can illustrate the point. Dillingham et al. (4) showed that a cervical radiculopathy workup should test at least seven muscles, covering C-5 to T-1 and a variety of nerves. A lumbar radiculopathy workup needs to test at least five muscles, spanning L-3 to S-1. Our group demonstrated that the 0-to-4+ scoring system commonly used in the extremities is not adequate for assessment of the lumbar paraspinal muscles (54). The MiniPM protocol described above is more appropriate. Robinson et al. (6) recently showed that the best sensitivity and specificity values come from adding the results of three of the most sensitive test results.

CONCLUSION

Occupational physicians frequently hears nerve and muscle complaints. Often, electrodiagnostic testing is seen as a method of arriving at a specific diagnosis. The technology and science involved in electrodiagnostic testing are substantial, but occupational physicians should understand that "ordering an EMG" is a consultation with a specialist, not just a technical evaluation.

REFERENCES

1. American Association of Electrodiagnostic Medicine. *Who is qualified to practice electrodiagnostic medicine? Position statement.* Rochester, MN: American Association of Electrodiagnostic Medicine, 1998.
2. Roija LN, Schneider LB, Ahmad BK. EMG referral patterns for cervical radiculopathy: the role of the primary care physician in a large multispecialty healthcare system. Presented at the American Association of Electrodiagnostic Medicine annual meeting in Minneapolis, MN; October, 1996.
3. Danner R. Referral diagnosis versus electroneurophysiological findings. Two years electroneuromyographic consultation in a rehabilitation clinic. *Clin Neurophysiol* 1990;30:153–157.
4. Dillingham TR, Lauder TD, Kumar S, Andary MT, Shannon SR. Musculoskeletal disorders in referrals

for suspected cervical radiculopathy. Presented at the American Association of Electrodiagnostic Medicine annual meeting, San Diego, CA; September 1997.
5. Haig AJ, Tzeng H-M, LeBreck DB. The value of electrodiagnostic consultation for patients with upper extremity nerve complaints: a prospective comparison with the history and physical examination. *Arch Phys Med Rehabil* 1998.
6. Robinson LR, Micklesen PJ, Wang L. Strategies for analyzing nerve conduction data: superiority of a summary index over single tests. *Muscle Nerve* 1998;21: 1166–1171.
7. Buchtal F, Rosenthal CAA. Evoked action potentials and conduction velocity in human sensory nerves. *Brain Res* 1966;3:1–122.
8. Robinson LR. In: Braddom RL, ed. *Physical medicine and rehabilitation.* Philadelphia: WB Saunders, 1996: 132–152.
9. DeLisa JA, Lee HJ, Baran EM, Ka-Siu L, Spielholz N. *Manual of nerve conduction velocity and clinical electrophysiology*, 3rd ed. New York: Raven Press, 1994.
10. Hodes R, Larabee MG, German W. The human electromyogram in response to nerve stimulation and the conduction velocity of motor axons. *Arch Neurol Psychiatry* 1948;61:340–365.
11. Dumitru D. *Electrodiagnostic medicine.* Philadelphia: Hanley and Belfus, 1995.
12. Dumitru D, DeLisa JA. Volume conduction. *Muscle Nerve* 1991;14:605–624.
13. Denny-Brown D, Penybacker JB. Fibrillation and fasciculation in voluntary muscle. *Brain* 1938;61: 311–332.
14. Haig AJ, LeBreck DB, Powley SG. Paraspinal mapping: quantified needle electromyography of the paraspinal muscles in persons without low back pain. *Spine* 1995;20:715–721.
15. Gatens PF, Saeed MA. Electromyographic findings in the intrinsic muscles of normal feet. *Arch Phys Med Rehabil* 1982;63:317–318.
16. Dumitru D. In Braddom RL, ed. *Physical medicine and rehabilitation.* Philadelphia: WB Saunders, 1996: 104–130.
17. Denys EH. *AAEM minimongraph #14: the influence of temperature in clinical neurophysiology.* Rochester, MN: American Association of Electrodiagnostic Medicine, 1991.
18. Kimura J. *Electrodiagnosis in diseases of nerve and muscle: principles and practice*, 2nd ed. Philadelphia: FA Davis Co, 1989.
19. Bernard BP, ed. *Musculoskeletal disorders and workplace factors.* Washington, DC: U.S. Department of Health and Human Services. NIOSH publication 97-141.
20. Levy BS, Wegonan DH, eds. *Occupational health: recognizing and preventing work related disease*, 3rd ed. Boston: Little, Brown & Company, 1995.
21. Seddon H. Three types of nerve injury. *Brain* 1943;66: 237–288.
22. Clarke SJ. *AAEM minimongraph #26: the electrodiagnosis of carpal tunnel syndrome.* Rochester, MN: American Association of Electrodiagnostic Medicine, 1987.
23. Bendler EM, Grenspun B, Yu J, et al. The bilaterality of carpal tunnel syndrome. *Arch Phys Med Rehabil* 1977; 58:362–364.
24. Blakeslee MA, Simmons Z, Logigian EL, Koghari MJ.

Does an electrodiagnostic study change clinical management? *Muscle Nerve* 1996;19:1225.

25. Jablecki CK. Andary MT, So YT, Wilkins DE, Williams FH. Literature review of the usefulness of nerve conduction studies and electromyography for the evaluation of patients with carpal tunnel syndrome. American Association of Electrodiagnostic Medicine Quality Assurance Committee. *Muscle Nerve* 1993;16:1392–414.

26. Ross MA, Kimura J. *AAEM case report #2:* the carpal tunnel syndrome. Rochester, MN: American Association of Electrodiagnostic Medicine, 1995.

27. Wertsch JJ. *AAEM case report #25:* anterior interosseous nerve syndrome. Rochester, MN: American Association of Electrodiagnostic Medicine, 1992.

28. Stern MB. The anterior interosseous nerve syndrome. *Clin Orthop* 1984;187:223–227.

29. Campbell WW. *AAEM case report #18: ulnar neuropathy in the distal forearm.* Rochester, MN: American Association of Electrodiagnostic Medicine, 1989.

30. Moss SH, Switzer HE. Radial tunnel syndrome: a spectrum of clinical presentations. *J Hand Surg* [Am]1983;8:411–420.

31. Roles NC, Maudsley RH. Radial tunnel syndrome: resistant tennis elbow as a nerve entrapment. *J Bone Joint Surg Br* 1972;54:449–508.

32. Rosen J, Werner CO. Neurophysiological investigation of posterior interosseous nerve entrapment causing lateral elbow pain. *Electroencephalogr Clin Neurophysiol* 1980;50:125–133.

33. Wilbourn AJ, Aminoff MJ. *AAEM minimonograph #32: the electrophysiologic examination in patients with radiculopathies.* Rochester, MN: American Association of Electrodiagnostic Medicine, 1988.

34. Haig AJ. Clinical experience with paraspinal mapping. I. Neurophysiology of the paraspinal muscles in various spinal disorders. *Arch Phys Med Rehabil* 1997;78:1177–1184.

35. Aminoff MJ. Clinical electromyography. In: Aminoff MJ, ed. *Electrodiagnosis in clinical neurology*, 2nd ed. New York: Churchill Livingstone, 1986:231–263.

36. Knuttson B. Comparative value of electromyographic, myelography, and clinical neurological examination in the diagnosis of lumbar root compression syndrome. *Acta Orthop Scand Suppl* 1961;49:1–35.

37. Wiesel SW, Tsourmas N, Feffer HL, Citrin CM, Patronas N. 1984 Volvo award in clinical sciences: a study of computer-assisted tomography. I. The incidence of positive CAT scans in an asymptomatic group of patients. *Spine* 1984;9:549–551.

38. Jensen MC, Brant-Zawadzki MN, Obuchowski N, et al. Magnetic resonance imaging of the lumbar spine in people without back pain. *N Engl J Med* 1994;331:69–73.

39. Boden SD, Davis DO, Dina TS, et al. Abnormal magnetic resonance scans of lumbosacral spine in asympto-

matic subjects: a prospective investigation. *J Bone Joint Surg Am* 1990;72:403–408.

40. Hitselberger WE, Witten RM. Abnormal myelograms in asymptomatic patients. *J Neurosurg* 1968;331:69–73.

41. MacIntosh JE, Valencia F, Bogduk N, Munro RR. The morphology of the human lumbar multifidus. *Clin Biomech* 1986;1:196–204.

42. Haig AJ, Moffroid M, Henry S, Pope MH. AAEM young investigator award: a technique for needle localization in the paraspinal muscle with cadaveric confirmation. *Muscle Nerve* 1991;14:521–526.

43. Haig AJ, Talley C, Grobler LJ, LeBreck DB. Paraspinal mapping: quantified needle electromyography in lumbar radiculopathy. *Muscle Nerve* 1993;16:477–484.

44. Haig AJ. Clinical experience with paraspinal mapping. II. A simplified technique that eliminates three-fourths of needle insertions. *Arch Phys Med Rehabil* 1997;78:1185–1190.

45. Haig AJ, Yamakawa K. Can paraspinal muscles determine nerve root level on EMG? Evidence from MiniPM in high lumbar disk lesions. *Muscle Nerve* 1998.

46. Donofrio PD, Albers JW. *AAEM minimonograph #34: polyneuropathy: classification by nerve conduction studies and electromyography.* Rochester, MN: American Association of Electrodiagnostic Medicine, 1990.

47. Keesey JC. *AAEM minimonograph #33: electrodiagnostic approach to defects of neuromuscular transmission.* Rochester, MN: American Association of Electrodiagnostic Medicine, 1989.

48. Dorfman LJ, Robinson LR. AAEM minimonograph #47: normative data in electrodiagnostic medicine. *Muscle Nerve* 1997;20:4–14.

49. Kothari MJ, Heistand M, Rutkove SB. Three ulnar nerve conduction studies in patients with ulnar neuropathy at the elbow. *Arch Phys Med Rehabil* 1998;79:87–89.

50. Triano JJ, Schultz AB. Correlation of objective measures of trunk motion and muscle function with low back disability ratings. *Spine* 1987;12:561–565.

51. Haig AJ, Gelblum JB, Rechtien JJ, Gitter A. Technology assessment: the use of surface EMG in the diagnosis and treatment of nerve and muscle disorders. *Muscle Nerve* 1996;19:392–395.

52. Hubbard DR, Berkoff GM. Myofascial trigger points show spontaneous needle EMG activity. *Spine* 1993;18:1803–1807.

53. Fuglsang-Frederiksen A, Johnsen B, Vingtoft S, et al. Variation in performance of the EMG examination at six European laboratories. *Electroencephalogr Clin Neurophysiol* 1995;97:444–450.

54. Haig AJ, Levine JW, Ruan CM, Yamakawa K. An evaluation of spontaneous activity reporting in the paraspinal muscles: is the Mayo 0–4+ grading system adequate? *Am J Phys Med Rehabil* 1998.

Occupational Musculoskeletal Disorders
edited by T. G. Mayer, R. J. Gatchel, and P. B. Polatin.
Lippincott Williams & Wilkins, Philadelphia © 2000.

24

Nonoperative Treatment for Postacute Spinal and Extremity Disorders

Vert Mooney

Department of Orthopaedics, University of California, San Diego, San Diego, California 92103

A postacute disorder can be defined as a soft tissue injury that has failed to heal spontaneously within 3 to 4 weeks and has escaped verifiable anatomic definition. Thus, it encompasses sprains, strains, and overuse complaints that constitute the largest proportion of musculoskeletal workers' compensation claims. In addition, in the context of industrial injuries, these are problems that have not been persistent for 6 months and have apparently not developed the habituation to disability that routinely occurs when poorly defined problems of the spine and extremities linger in the limbo of unresolved claims and continued disability. It is assumed therefore that these are injuries that do not require surgery. Imaging studies do not offer a clearcut objective definition of the mechanical incompetence. Nonetheless, diminished function created by pain prevents workers from returning to normal activity.

What unifying therapeutic theme could be applied to this type of ailment that would be appropriate for the extremities as well as the spine? The answer is easy: Look to the athletic model. What happens when a professional athlete has a function-limiting soft tissue injury? He or she receives some modalities to fool the nervous system. Perhaps, some massage is used to enhance fluid exchange. Most important, the athlete is placed on a therapeutic exercise program.

Every professional team has a training room that has specific exercise equipment. This equipment is generally focused at strength training at various joints and is generally under the supervision of a trainer. Thus, the theme of the following discussion is: If it's good enough for expensive professional athletes, why not the industrial athlete—the injured worker?

The themes to be discussed for individual anatomic sites concern the value of movement therapies. Again, obviously this type of treatment is to be applied to injuries that have not resulted in ligament and capsular tears that can be identified by physical examination or imaging studies. In the more common grade II injuries (in the context of ankle sprain), gradual progressive activity makes intuitive, as well as, scientific sense. A good example of this is the recent 1995 Quebec Task Force report on whiplash injuries (1). This report documented that activation either by manipulation or exercise was the most rational treatment program. The theme of this discussion is self-generated activity therapy as a reasonable and appropriate approach. An associated theme is that this exercise can and should be measured. It can be progressed rationally, based on previous performance and expected goals. That of course is the training event for injured athletes alluded to above.

SHORT HISTORY OF MEASURED THERAPEUTIC EXERCISE

The most reasonable evaluation method for the musculoskeletal system would be the measurement of strength and range. This could best be done in a comparative manner if some tool were available that could measure this more precisely than a clinician's estimate. In fact, the need for comparative measurement was probably even greater even before the objective definition available from x-ray examinations became common practice after the turn of the twentieth century. Indeed, there was such a system known as Zander equipment, called "medical mechanical therapy" (2). Zander developed a series of large pieces of equipment that isolated various joint systems. This equipment measured range and documented strength, based on resistance moved. Thus, the exercise was measured (Fig. 1). In fact, med-

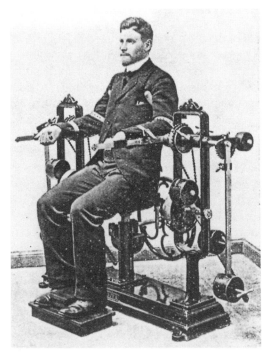

FIG. 1. One of the 40 pieces of Zander equipment that allowed resistance exercises in a measured manner during the latter nineteenth century.

ical mechanical institutes with associated gymnastic hall and circuit machines were developed and actually were similar to today's health clubs (Fig. 2). By the turn of the twentieth century, there were more than 200 facilities around the world with these training circuits (3). They fell out of favor for many reasons, but one reason was the emergence of the concept of prolonged rest as a therapeutic tool for musculoskeletal diseases. In addition, at that time, hospitals became workshops for serious medical care, and proper hygiene and supportive nursing were the theme. Assisted rest treatment for all disabilities was the norm. This was carried to what now seems an illogical extreme when by the 1930s the usual postpartum care for a young mother was rest in the hospital for 1 week to 10 days.

The same concepts of rest therapy were applied to cardiac care as well. Not until the 1950s did the idea emerge that exercises was helpful for the cardiac system (4). And not until improved technology, such as the Holter monitor, became available could documentation of the benefits of exercise, as well as its progress, be determined (5). The same rationale generates the need for having some method to monitor progress in training of the extremities, as well as the spine.

One of the first studies bringing back the concepts of progressive exercise into the medical model documented the benefit of treating joint injuries with progressive resistance exercise (PRE) (6). Dr. Tom Delorme transferred the concepts utilized by competitive weightlifters to injured joints. It was the start of modern-day rehabilitation. The value of exercise equipment itself was rediscovered by Arthur Jones (7) with the invention of Nautilus equipment. The publication of his work in *Iron Man Magazine* underlined the fact that there was—and is—much more enthusiasm for PREs in the health club culture than in the medical model.

With the arrival of commercially manufactured equipment and the lack of medical support for therapeutic exercise, the concept of training at health clubs emerged. The exercise circuit on specific equipment similar to that

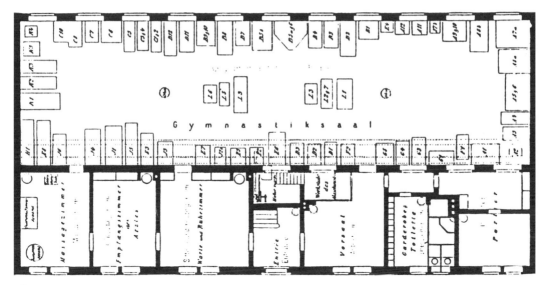

FIG. 2. Proposed layout for a Zander medical mechanical therapy center in the 1890s. The training circuit is reminiscent of modern health clubs.

first proposed by Zander was rediscovered. Thus, attractive centers for exercise with mirrors and chrome replaced the dingy workout gymnasiums of old YMCAs and basements of high schools. Those facilities had the barbells, hand weights, and medicine balls that had entertained enthusiasts of strength training in the past. Nonetheless, the new health club facilities were still distant from medical supervision. However, modern health clubs are now more attractive to men and women focused on health maintenance and not necessarily bodybuilding. And, thus, the most important question relative to exercise therapy is: When do efforts to improve health by exercise become medical care?

A new type of equipment that did attract the interest of the medical community was an innovation of isokinetic exercise. This type of equipment controlled the speed of joint function but did not limit resistance. It was felt to provide a more specific approach to exercise training [8]. This indeed was first felt to be a more precise system of exercise, and at first it was not conceived to be a test tool. Later, use of this equipment as a test tool began to overshadow its function as an exercise tool. Thanks to computers and VCRs, a graphic

display of specific patterns of joint function emerged. Numeric representation of functional measurement of peak torque and average torque could be computed. Although it is expensive, it could be tolerated in the medical model when abundant insurance coverage was available.

Later, specific equipment was designed for spine testing [9], and other technologies emerged for spine testing that became progressively more complex [10,11]. Although initially there was considerable enthusiasm for equipment that could do spinal testing, it was not especially useful for physical training and gradually fell out of favor, probably because there was an insufficient cost–benefit ratio [12].

These computerized systems for functional testing failed to gain support from the medical and scientific communities because of a lack of credibility [13,14]. Newton and Waddel [13] pointed out that the failure of computerized systems was due to the absence of standardized test protocols and the use of derived variables such as power, work, and agonist–antagonist ratios, which were not sufficiently defined to be accepted as scientific and reliable. In other words, if measurement becomes too sophisticated and does not offer sufficient insight into enhanced therapy, it may not be worth the effort.

In summary then, it is clear that measured progressive exercise is a reasonable therapeutic tool, certainly well established in rehabilitation as evidenced by the training rooms of all sports teams. The benefit of measurement, as evident in cardiac rehabilitation, is that it can guide a physical training program that is both safe and effective. The development of exercise as a therapeutic tool in the medical model is relatively recent and currently presents a somewhat blurred boundary between medical care and health maintenance.

With this background, discussion now turns to the use of exercise therapy for soft tissue injuries of the extremities and cervical and lumbar spine. In all settings, modalities are useful to distract the nervous system. Heat and massage are common, but active exercise programs are now also becoming accepted as the standard of care. A recent statement from the Zenith Insurance Company to workers' compensation providers sets the stage: "A maximum of 12 PT [physical training] visits for active exercise in the first month will be reimbursed only if appropriate. Passive treatment (no active patient participation) alone will not be compensated" (15).

GENERAL PRINCIPLES OF THERAPEUTIC EXERCISE

The consistent theme for nonoperative care of industrial soft tissue injuries of the extremities and the spine is active care. As noted above, passive care alone has become insufficient to be acceptable for physical treatment. And, of course, this is consistent with the analogy of the training room of any athletic team. Along with this analogy, other passive approaches are used.

Certainly, soft tissue injuries are painful and medication is appropriate. There is, however, little scientific support for any specific type of analgesic or antiinflammatory drugs. In the last 20 years, the family of antiinflammatory drugs has been growing due to an ap-

parent, more specific effect on inflammation than just pain reduction.

When an injury occurs, circulating monocytes infiltrate injured tissue and differentiate into macrophages. Cellular infiltrates release lysosomes to break down the damaged tissue. There are subsequent increases in circulating interleukin-1 and prostaglandin (PG) E_2 (16). PGE_2 has multiple effects on inflammation. It increases lysosome activity and is probably responsible for sensitizing afferent nerves (17). Inhibition of the PGE_2 is the main role of antiinflammatory drugs and is thought to be beneficial (18).

Of course, these drugs have many other effects. In a recent review of their effect on muscle function, it was found that antiinflammatory drugs acting on injured muscles initially protect the contractual proteins but later are associated with a functional loss (19). Therefore, diminished function may be expected in association with antiinflammatory agents. Certainly, the full effects of this broad array of medications are unknown. It would seem that retarding the inflammatory process may be counterproductive in that this process is needed for soft tissue healing. As a demonstration of this process, it has been shown that new bone formation in fracture healing or around implants is retarded by antiinflammatory drugs (20).

Another typical modality used in association with active exercise programs is manual massage. This is usually comforting and may even break up palpable muscle spasms. Certainly, the beneficial effects of massage have an ancient history, but very little evidence is available when what is actually done is examined. When objective measurement is available, it is clear that in spite of expectation massage does not affect muscle blood flow, irrespective of the massage method (21).

Although modalities are commonly applied in acute injuries, there is very little scientific evidence of their therapeutic role. In the most recent studies reviewing the literature relative to various physical treatments for soft tissue injuries, no credible evidence could be identified. This is true both in the most recent

Agency for Health Care Policy and Research literature review for low back pain (22), as well as for its predecessor, the Quebec Task Force report (23). Thus, the guidelines outlined by the insurance company notification quoted above seems justified.

What is appropriate active treatment? Certainly, a soft tissue injury hinders joint movement, and efforts to return the joint to normal range of motion are the appropriate first steps. Often, this is accomplished manually in a passive manner or in an active, assisted manner. Manipulative care in the form of high-velocity adjustments provided by chiropractors or osteopaths has been utilized for decades. The efficacy of manipulative care is discussed elsewhere in this volume by those who are expert in it.

One problem with manual therapy in the form of manipulation is that it tends to be a craft. The feel for tissues and for the amount of force to use that is effective but not destructive has to be learned and cannot be quantified. It is apparently justifiable that chiropractic training takes 4 years. This unmeasurable characteristic makes it difficult to determine what is accomplished in an episode of manipulation that is structural rather than charismatic or placebo.

Once mechanisms to improve range of motion have been appropriately applied, it is reasonable to turn next to resolution of the weak link that has been created by an industrial soft tissue injury. Usually, it is unknowable whether this is a deficiency of the muscle itself, the attachment within the capsule or ligaments of the joint, or the annulus of an intervertebral disc. Of course, it must be assumed that physical examination and appropriate studies have confirmed that the joints involved are stable and do not require surgical repair. However, in industrial soft tissue injuries as in sports injuries, the great majority of injuries fall into the nonsurgical treatment area.

It is certainly clear that, with rest, connective tissue becomes stiffer, weaker, and noncompliant, compared to the same joint when moved (24). With immobilization or rest, additional cross-linking develops between collagenous fibers, and slowly contractures develop. Early motion must be achieved both actively and passively. For therapeutic exercise, the active program should be a progressive strengthening exercise plan.

Again, in sports injuries, there are principles that are typically carried out in the training room when a competitive athlete sustains a workplace injury. The effectiveness of strength training programs depends on several factors, including frequency and amount (sets × repetitions × resistance). The mode is by free weights or variable-resistance machines, by dynamic or isometric exercises, and by concentric or eccentric contractions. A certain amount of clinical judgment is necessary in defining the optimal balance of these factors.

Obviously, strength training for an injured segment should not be of the same intensity as for bodybuilding. Strength training is often defined as range of motions, which means "repetition maximum." A one range of motion would be the maximum weight (resistance) that could be used for one repetition but could not be repeated due to fatigue. This is obviously far too severe a test for an injured segment.

Generally, 15 to 20 repetitions before fatigue occurs are appropriate for an injured segment. It must be remembered that strength training is different from endurance training and the exercise needs to be carried out in a slow, purposeful manner to enhance strength performance. Injury is less likely to occur if an exercised joint is stabilized in some manner. Sudden, rapid repetition that brings into play uncontrollable forces of inertia, as in the use of free weights, is to be avoided in the early stages of therapeutic exercise.

Compliance with an active exercise program is also an important aspect of therapeutic exercise. Motivation for a progressively strenuous program may be limited if there is too great discomfort or intrusion on time. In the past, when bodybuilding strengthening was the object, it was felt that multiple sets of exercise to the same joint system were appropriate. However, recent information indicates that a single set is just as reliable and less intrusive on time (25). This is currently the guideline for the American College of Sports Medicine (26). Ideally, single-set exercises should be applied to various joints related to the injured joint. Warming up and ranging the injured joint with associated aerobic efforts are also appropriate before progressive exercises.

Another aspect of strength training concerns frequency. There must be a rest period to allow for muscle recuperation after much training or injury to the muscle–tendon combination. On the other hand, too much rest between training sessions will result in detraining. Generally it is accepted that a 48-hour rest period between training sessions is appropriate (27). This usually translates into 3 days a week of exercises. Even that much time may not be necessary for some muscle groups. It has been determined that for the cervical and lumbar spine twice a week is as good as three or four times a week (28,29). These guidelines are all consistent with the most recent consensus in the sports medicine community (30).

Discussion now turns to the application of the principles of therapeutic exercise, both manual and active, to the various joint systems that are frequently injured in industrial accidents.

THERAPEUTIC EXERCISE: SHOULDER

A frequent workplace injury is marked by the sudden onset of pain in the shoulder secondary to a sudden overload or infrequent strenuous physical activity. Such injuries most commonly involve middle-aged workers because of degenerative changes about the rotator cuff. The term *impingement syndrome* was popularized by Neer (31) in the 1970s. It covers a wide array of abnormalities within the shoulder, often defined as stage I, II, or III (32).

Stage I is characterized by acute bursitis with subacromial edema and hemorrhage. This stage is usually observed in patients who are 30 to 40 years old who have continued irritation of the subacromial structures as the result of abnormal contact with the underlying soft tissues and loss of the ability to lubricate and protect the underlying rotator cuff. On this basis, a stage II abnormality develops, marked by reactive inflammation in the cuff known as tendinitis. This stage is characterized by edema and is often seen on magnetic resonance (MR) imaging studies. As the process continues, the anterior aspect of the acromion begins to impinge on the greater tuberosity of the humerus. If sufficient irritation occurs, eventually the supraspinous tendon will develop a full-thickness rotator cuff tear—stage III. Bigliani et al. (33) described the morphology of the acromion and its relationship to rotator cuff tear. A type I acromion is flat, a type II curved, and a type III hooked. It is felt that the more severely hooked or bent the acromion is, the greater a predisposition to impingement syndrome might be.

With the ability of today's diagnostic procedures, including arthroscopy and MR imaging, a specific anatomic diagnosis can frequently be made. In the workers' compensation setting, with its excellent funding for surgical repair, early surgery is often advocated. Will therapeutic exercise be a benefit?

Actually, even though the shoulder is one of the most complex anatomic structures, there is an excellent rationale for therapeutic exercise that is more self-evident than for most joints. Perry (34) described the depressor effect and downward-shear component of the subscapularis, infraspinatous, and teres minor muscles during active contraction. Thus, this gives justification for a reasonable exercise program. Strengthening these opposing muscle components to bring balance to the glenohumeral joint during subluxation by the overpowering deltoid seems a very reasonable approach. Can it be successful?

Hawkins and Dunlop (35) followed 33 patients who had proven full-thickness rotator cuff tears, providing them with a specific home exercise program to increase the strength of the external and internal rotators. Only 12 patients opted to have surgery after being followed for nearly 4 years. The program involved resistance exercise using rubber tubing.

In the more common simple impingement syndrome, the diagnosis is made by a positive impingement sign. This sign is characterized by the production of pain in the lateral region of the deltoid when the affected extremity is forcibly elevated with the scapula stabilized and the humerus is internally rotated. This causes impingement of the supraspinous tendon beneath the humeral head and the anterior aspect of the acromion. The pain can be obliterated by injection local anesthetic into this space.

A recent study documented the efficacy of an exercise program for impingement syndrome (36). In this series, a group of 616 patients with all the characteristics of an impingement syndrome but no evidence of arthritis were placed into a specific exercise program. Sixty-seven percent of the patients had satisfactory results, and only 20% felt that they had to go on to have surgery. The exercise program used elastic cuffs, specifically focused at strengthening the rotator cuffs (Fig. 3).

In this study, the classic routine for therapeutic exercise for an injured joint was initiated. Initially, to reduce the pain, inflammation was brought under control with antiinflammatory drugs, local anesthetic injections, and modalities (ultrasound, hot packs, etc.) Under therapist supervision, patients performed stretching exercises at home. These exercises were not initiated till full range of motion was possible. The strengthening program consisted of initial isometric external rotation performed against the resistance of an opposite hand, and then isometric internal rotation. Force was exerted for 10 seconds, followed by 2 seconds of rest. This was repeated for 10 repetitions. Internal- and external-rotation exercises were alternated until three sets of 10 repetitions could be performed. Once forceful, isometric exercises were tolerated with minimal pain, light isotonic exercises were introduced using Theraband or surgical tubing. In this situation, the arm was started in an externally or internally rotated position, brought to the neutral position for 10 seconds, and then rested for 2 to 3 seconds for 10 repetitions. Resistance was such that when the patient reached the tenth repetition on the third set, he or she was unable to hold the position for a full 10 seconds; resistance was adjusted to allow for that. The exercise program took 10 to 15 minutes per day. Once this was possible, the same exercise was performed through an arc of −30- to +30-degrees rotation, with emphasis on the eccentric phase of contraction (3 seconds concentric, 7 seconds eccentric). The deltoid was relaxed during this period, because the object was to avoid its being lifted upward. To assist in eliminating reduced effort, patients were made to hold a magazine between the lateral

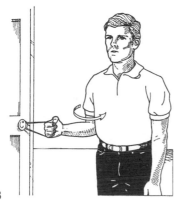
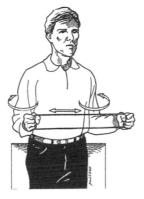

A,B

FIG. 3. One proposed method for strengthening the internal **(A)** and external **(B)** rotator as treatment for impingement syndrome. Gradually increasing resistance is needed.

chest wall and the inner surface of the upper arm.

These exercise programs lasted 6 weeks. It generally took 4 to 6 weeks for patients to achieve pain relief with these exercises. If they had not responded by that time, the exercise protocol was judged as probably not beneficial, and surgical care was considered. Compliance was enhanced by frequent reevaluation by the therapist either at home or in the office.

Of patients who had successful results from the exercise therapy, 18% had a recurrence, but the symptoms resolved with rest and repetition of the exercise program. Although most patients had a type III acromion, the success rate was about the same for all types. These studies have been repeated by other authors (37).

It is of interest that most of the patients in the study by Morrison et al. (36) had previous physical therapy with the usual hot packs, massage, and ultrasound. For most, a functional, specific exercise program was not prescribed. On the other hand, a patient's failure with physical therapy elsewhere had no bearing on the response to the specific exercise protocol. Overall, 70% of those whose previous treatment had apparently failed had a successful outcome rate with conservative management. In addition, a patient's failure to comply with this specific program could easily mark them as poor candidates for surgical care.

Few pieces of equipment are specifically designed for external–internal rotation strengthening of the shoulder. Better results may require a health club setting in which it can be done. It may be more reasonable to do it this way, although more costly. Certainly, the simple, conservative exercise program described above is reasonable. It does indicate the need for compliance and enthusiasm on the part of both supervising physicians and patients.

THERAPEUTIC EXERCISE: ELBOW

Epicondylitis is a common diagnosis made relative to workplace overuse syndromes. Pain and tenderness at many anatomic sites in both the upper and the lower extremities are classed as "tendinitis" because they appear to be related to tendons. This discussion of epicondylitis should serve as an example of the principles of care for upper and lower extremity overuse syndromes.

The true pathology in epicondylitis is poorly understood. In a recent symposium on repetitive motion disorders of the upper extremity, conducted by the American Academy of Orthopaedic Surgeons, only one histologic study was reported (38). In that study, Nirschl (39) made the specific point that epicondylitis is not an inflammatory process as has been assumed. Essentially, the histology represents a failure of repair of disrupted connective tissue. Disorganized collagen without appropriate orientation was interspersed with haphazardly oriented undifferentiated mesenchymal cells. Vascular buds without appropriate organization were present with incomplete lumina and insufficient elastin, representing the angiogenetic process. The picture was one of a mesenchymal process with a poor potential for healing. Apparently, insufficient material was available in these studies to carry out a biochemical analysis. Excessive matrix tissue, however, was a consistent finding.

Generally, it is difficult to obtain biopsies of tendons unless surgery is performed. However, one type of tendinitis can be biopsied without a true surgical procedure or significant tissue disruption. The relatively large size of the Achilles tendon makes it possible to carry out punch biopsies in the areas of tendinitis. In a study by Rolf et al. (40) using ultrasound to identify involved areas, punch biopsies were performed, obtaining sufficient material to do not only histologic but also biochemical analyses. The histology was quite similar to that described by Nirschl (39) for epicondylitis biopsies; however, a consistent increase in proteoglycans was also demonstrated—as much as 40 times more per unit area than in normal tendons. Proteoglycan molecules "soak up" water, creating swelling; and it is this swelling with associated distention that, when squeezed, creates pain and tenderness. As in Nirschl, there was a distinct absence of inflammatory cells and of an organized fibroblast response with associated angiogenesis. Excessive proteoglycan apparently hinders normal collagen formation. It is yet unknown which is cart and which is horse in this disorganized tissue. There is evidence, however, that it is not an inflammation related to the normal repair process. All these syndromes are more appropriately called tendinoses.

In light of this, what is an appropriate treatment program for epicondylosis? Certainly, there is no consensus. There are very few truly comparative studies. The literature really does not support any specific treatment program (41). An example of this confusion is seen in a randomized, prospective study by Verhar et al. (42) comparing steroid injection to deep massage. Initially, injection had a higher success rate, but by 1 year the success rate was only 50% and 30% of both groups required surgery. In a similar study by Solveborn et al. (43) involving steroid injection, the success rate at 6 months was only 50%, with 30% complaining of significant pain. An alternative method of achieving pain relief using extracorporeal shock waves yielded a favorable outcome in 48% at 24 weeks compared to 6% for the placebo group (44).

My colleagues and I have tried an alternative approach to therapy for the typical overuse syndrome using a specific manual massage method known as Active Release Therapy (45). It is based on the assumption that the source of pain is relative anoxia and secondary adhesions. Thus, tension is applied to the painful tissues, with passive and active stretching against the tension causing breakup of the adhesions. At 3 months, this procedure had an excellent success rate of 75%, but a recurrence rate began to be noted. Most patients who previously had received the usual forms of medical treatment felt that this technique was better. The study was carried out by an athletic trainer using techniques taught him by a chiropractor, Michael Leahy, the innovator of this technique. The problem of recurrence diminishes the early success of many treatment programs. Because of the high incidence of recurrence and variable results, Pransky and Himmelstein (46) in the most recent survey of this field acknowledged that "the long-term advantages of physical treatment are still unknown."

The only comparative long-term follow-up study of any mode of treatment for lateral epicondylitis was conducted by Pienimäki et al. (47). This is actually the only controlled study in the literature of the effects of exercise on the treatment of chronic epicondylitis. In the past, various authors have recommended exercise—but without any specific scientific justification; this of course has led to the current state of variable and inconsistent treatments (48). Pienimäki et al.'s (47) study involved 39 patients randomized into two groups: one undertaking therapeutic exercise and the other receiving pulsed ultrasound. This second group was meant to serve as placebo, because pulsed ultrasound has been demonstrated to have a success rate no better than placebo ultrasound (49).

The exercise program was a four-step training program done at home. Patients were instructed in the program and followed up weekly at home by a physical therapist. The program started with flexion and extension stretching exercises with resistance using an elastic band, then came resistance using more complex exercises, and finally repeated functional activity such as transferring buttons from one cup to another. It was a graduated program in which patients performed the exercise four to six times daily with 10 repetitions done in two to three sets. The treatment program lasted 6 to 8 weeks; follow-up continued for 3 years. Strength increased 45% in the exercise group but decreased 4% in the ultrasound group; grip strength increased 12% in the exercise group, and remained unchanged in the ultrasound group. At 3-year follow-up, five patients in the ultrasound group were operated on because of persistence of symptoms, whereas one patient in the exercise group required surgery. At follow-up, the visual analog pain score was 1.5 for the exercise group and 2.7 for the ultrasound group. No data emerged from this study regarding compliance with the exercise program, however. Results might have been better with better exercise compliance. In our study of Active Release Therapy, only 50% the patients performed the active stretching program that they were taught (45).

This discussion serves to emphasize several points about current evidence-based knowledge about the nonoperative care of soft tissue injuries. There are very few reliable comparative studies, and understanding of the pathophysiology involved is very poor. The only reliable concept, which indeed now has some scientific support, is that active exercises are the most positive influence on the disease process.

THERAPEUTIC EXERCISE: KNEE

Work-related soft tissue injuries involving the knee are strains insufficient to create instability. Therefore, postoperative therapy for meniscal tears and anterior cruciate ligament tears will not be discussed here. Instead, the focus is on the appropriate therapeutic exercise program for the injured knee.

Delorme's (6) reintroduction of exercise therapy into the medical context emerged from his experience as a doctor in the military caring for U.S. Navy trainees at Gardiner General Hospital in Chicago. At that time, personnel with knee injuries that now would be considered totally resolvable were being released from the service because of inability to participate. The reason for this was the prevailing medical custom of treatment of these knee injuries that required many weeks of rest and a long leg cast. Delorme, an Olympic-level weightlifter, transferred the competitive-weightlifting training principle of progressive increases in loads to the now well known PREs. These PREs utilized weights attached to the shoes. What his concept contributed was the value to muscle strengthening of significant resistance and a standardized protocol that minimized the number of repetitions while emphasizing the amount of resistance relative to an individual's maximum functional capacity for a particular joint—one repetition maximum. He advocated these exercises specifically in contradiction to the usual

program at the time (and at present) of bicycling and stair climbing, which he observed frequently caused swelling. He also emphasized the safety of this concept, based on experience with 300 patients: "We have never produced chronic muscle sprains or failed to achieve return of muscle power."

Controversy continues as to the appropriate exercise routine. This argument is crystallized by the question of open-chain versus closed-chain exercise. The concept of a biomechanical chain was introduced by Steindler (50). He defined a kinetic chain as a combination of successfully arranged joints constituting a complex motor unit. He observed that when the foot or hand meets considerable resistance, muscular recruitment and joint motion occurs differently from what is seen when the foot or hand is free to move without restriction. Thus, a closed-chain exercise is performed with the terminal segment of a limb fixed, such as doing a squat or a leg press. Conversely, an open-chain exercise is done with the terminal segment free to move, such as a knee extension with a weight on the foot, as originally proposed by Delorme.

Many studies have tried to analyze the relative benefits and disadvantages of each exercise mode. It must be recognized that normal knee function has variable amounts of open-chain versus closed-chain activity (e.g., swing versus stance phase of gait), and with increasing speed of function, such as running, the amount of stance phase gradually diminishes. Wilk et al. (51) did extensive analysis of myoelectric activity versus joint forces in the knee during various exercises with supernormal subjects (weightlifters). Their study showed that closed-chain exercises, as might be expected, put more compressive loads on the joint, while open-chain exercises put more shear forces in the joint that could be transferred to the cruciate ligaments—more to the posterior cruciate ligament with 10- to 40-degree knee flexion, and more to the anterior cruciate with 40- to 0-degree flexion and extension. With 0- to 30-degree knee flexion, myoelectric activity was somewhat reciprocal for both closed- and open-chain exercises.

Open-chain exercises allowed the most quadriceps function, whereas closed-chain had the least quadriceps function, and the reverse was true with 60- to 90-degree flexion. Our studies have indicated a significant increase in fatigue resistance by myoelectric analysis in open-chain exercises compared to closed-chain in normal subjects (52). Moreover, it has been demonstrated that the more specific the muscle stimulation either consciously or with electrical stimulation, the greater the percentage of strengthening will be (53). This particular study indicated that closed-chain kinetic exercises alone did not provide adequate stimulation to quadriceps function to achieve normal function in the knee.

On the other hand, there are practical measures. Closed-chain training can be accomplished with minimal equipment. Open-chain training usually requires some sort of instrument that can isolate knee function. This of course was the initial device that introduced isokinetic exercises in the form of the Cybex machine. New equipment has become progressively more sophisticated, but no studies have specifically documented the benefit of computerization other than improved feedback to clients, therapists, and supervising entities such as insurance companies and physicians.

In view of this, what is a rational approach to therapeutic exercise of the knee? Once again, methods to achieve pain control and improve range of motion are necessary. Resistance exercises are inappropriate while there is still effusion and tenderness. Some preliminary rest is appropriate. Perhaps, steroid injection to control the inflammation of the synovitis may be appropriate. Passive and active range of motion should be initiated. Once this is achieved, then PREs are applied to the injured knee joint.

In our view, neuromotor inhibition occurs as a result of noxious stimuli in the injured joint. Therefore, initial closed-chain exercises and other muscles will substitute around the injured quadricep–hamstring relationship and excessively facilitate the hip and lower leg

musculature (e.g., leg press). Therefore, early training should be an isolated PRE program. At our center, we use equipment that incorporates expected norms for knee function in a computer readout (Fig. 4). The muscle strength of the injured knee can be measured as isometric strength at various points in the range, and thus a pattern of performance can be defined as well. The computer readout provides excellent feedback to patients as to their early level of performance, as well as the goal of training.

It is unknown how much sophistication is necessary in exercise training. It is clear, however, that unless some feedback of performance is available, the efficacy of training is unknown. Clinically, one frequently sees patients for whom conservative care has failed, but there is no definition of what that care might have been. The modalities for controlling pain, such as massage and ultrasound, are usually not measurable and, as suggested above, of unknown benefit. Seldom do reviewing physicians have the benefit of any statement of baseline performance or changes that have occurred on repeated exercise attempts. This is basically why reliable data are lacking as to most appropriate therapeutic approach for soft tissue injuries not only in the

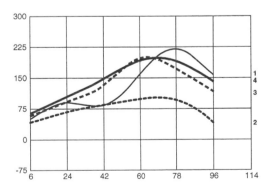

FIG. 4. Isometric strength testing of the quadriceps on a MedX machine. Pattern *1* is strength at the conclusion of training; pattern *2* is test strength at the onset of training; pattern *3* is tested strength on the uninvolved side; and pattern *4* is average quadriceps strength for an individual of this sex and age group.

knee but also in the extremities and spine. Function is not measured. Pain is the only criterion for treatment, and therapeutic protocols are not standardized to allow comparison or measurement of progress.

THERAPEUTIC EXERCISE: CERVICAL SPINE

Workplace cervical spine problems fall into two categories: They are secondary to either chronic postural problems, as can occur from prolonged work in front of video display terminals, or sudden overload that occurs during a fall in an unguarded moment. Some of the most complex neck problems are related to hyperextension–flexion (whiplash) injuries sustained in vehicular accidents.

The interrelationship between neck problems and the chronic postural problems of the upper extremity that are so typical of our current sedentary workplace has not been thoroughly investigated. Fatigue of the cervical spine musculature is clearly related to arm and shoulder problems. One-half of individuals presenting for medical care of overuse syndromes of the upper extremity in one study also complained of neck pain (43). When the myoelectric activity of the neck versus the shoulders was examined, a distinct relationship emerged. Using the power spectrum analysis technique, persons with painful shoulders were shown to experience muscle fatigue more quickly than those with nonpainful shoulders (54). This study showed that positioning of the arm in various constant-posture positions rapidly fatigues the neck. On the other hand, persons with neck complaints in the workplace showed an even more rapid fatiguing of the injured spot, but on the musculature of the shoulder (55). The obvious treatment for this is a strengthening program, which will be discussed later.

A more definable workplace injury is the sudden overload often described as a whiplash injury. In the context of workers' compensation claims, such an injury is certainly more readily definable because a specific date of injury can be documented.

Whiplash injuries are extremely common soft tissue injuries in both the workers' compensation and the personal-injury medicolegal contexts.

In the long term, whiplash injuries progress to degenerative change, and some studies have reported significant postinjury absence of lordosis (56,57), although other studies have shown no relationship of degenerative changes to an earlier injury in follow-up (58,59). Of course, this lack of consensus is the lifeblood of continuing litigation.

The varied pain patterns after cervical soft tissue injuries probably have some relationship to the site of injury. It is clear from pathologic studies of severe auto accidents in which extensive trauma resulted in death that in most cases tears occur at the junction of the annulus with the vertebral body (rim lesions). These pathologic studies also show tears of the facet capsule and occasionally disc herniation (60). Whether the pain in a postacute neck injury originates from a disc or a facet really cannot be defined by clinical examination.

In the first study of referred pain syndromes in cervical discs by Cloward (61), the distribution of pain from the discs was defined. The pain patterns lateralized to the site of injection but were significantly distal to the level of injection. The same pain patterns were more precisely defined by injection into the facet joints (62). The distribution of pain patterns was varied and overlapping, and thus diagnosis of a specific injured site was often difficult. Headache and radiation of pain into the shoulders occurred, probably on a referred basis as well (Fig. 5). Without any evidence of progressing neuropathic problems, however, there is no reason to suggest that surgery is necessary, and a program of therapeutic exercise can be initiated.

At least some evidence exists for the rational treatment of acute hyperextension–flexion injuries, in addition to analgesics, rest, and collars. In a study by McKinney (63), patients were advised to rest and keep the neck immobilized with a brace or instructed in a McKenzie-like activity program of mobilization.

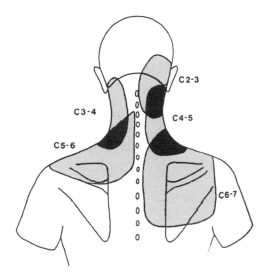

FIG. 5. Referral patterns from specific facet joint irritation. (From ref. 62, with permission.)

Short-term results and those at 2-year follow-up showed that earlier mobilization was superior to rest and collar immobilization in resolution or return of symptoms. A similar study corroborated these results (64). Early in the postacute phase, traction was frequently prescribed, but comparative studies have shown that it is less successful than mobilization (65). Although helpful for pain control, various other passive treatments, such as transcutaneous nerve stimulation, ultrasonography, diathermy, ice, and massage, have frequently been prescribed, but comparative studies have not shown them to be effective. In fact, there is no evidence to support the benefit of passive therapy alone in alleviating the symptoms of whiplash. A comprehensive literature review known as the Quebec Task Force report on whiplash-associated injuries failed to find any significant benefit of passive care (1).

Chiropractic manipulation is often applied in these types of injuries. No specific comparative studies appear to be available. On the other hand, clinical practice indicates that patients frequently go early to a chiropractor and find some benefit. (More specific details about chiropractic and manipulation are described in other chapters in this volume.) Certainly, chiropractic care is an important component of postacute cervical and lumbar injuries. Recently, Jacob (66) paraphrased guidelines for chiropractic quality assurance and practice parameters; these guidelines are quite consistent with reliable principles for postacute nonsurgical care of soft tissue injuries:

- The rehabilitation phase should be reached as rapidly as possible, and dependence on passive forms of therapy to obtain the optimal result should be minimized.
- Complete resolution of pain is often not possible until patients begin to focus on increasing the number and kinds of activities in which they participate.
- Elements that should be addressed include persuasion from pain behavior, body mechanics education, and supervised training for flexibility, stability, strength, coordination, and endurance.
- When signs of deconditioning or chronicity are present, simply handing out a list of exercises will not do.
- Early return to activity is associated with reduced disability and symptoms.
- Chronicity should be prevented whenever possible.
- Repeated use of acute care measures alone generally fosters chronicity, physician dependence, and overutilization.
- Pain behavior and illness conviction are best managed with focus on what patients are able to do. Understanding that movement is safe and healthful, even if not comfortable, needs to be emphasized.
- Rehabilitation should be emphasized as a means of improving quality of life, and reducing suffering can result in a significant reduction of secondary somatization.

The McKenzie mechanical treatment of cervical soft tissue injuries represents a contrasting approach to that of chiropractic. It expects that a specific method of evaluation will identify pain patterns related to specific exercise performance. On the basis of these pain patterns and changes in them, the goals of centralizing pain and improving cervical range, especially in extension, are advocated. It likewise is quite reliable and consistent and has the advantages of creating most of the treatment as self-directed on the part of patients and requiring no treating individual to achieve mobilization maneuvers. Retractions are a hallmark of this type of treatment (Fig. 6).

For more prolonged pain, especially that associated with fatigue, or for chronic recurrent pain indicating the obvious persistence of a weak link, a specific strengthening program appears to be a rational approach. Recent work in our center has demonstrated that with chronic neck pain, as in postwhiplash phenomenon, the lumbar muscles attempt to take over and substitute to stabilize the cervical spine (67) (Fig. 7). With appropriate physical training, the strength of the cervical spine increases, and the participation of the lumbar spine decreases. This study also emphasizes a reliable principle of neurophysical function: strong muscles will also try to substitute for weak muscles. Perhaps, this also explains why it is so common for back pain to develop after a whiplash type of injury.

Once improved range of motion is available and acute pain is reduced, it is appropriate to progress to a therapeutic exercise program that includes strengthening. As in any strengthening program, baseline strength and performance are valuables piece of information. The standard is fairly easily achieved in the extremities, especially if only one side is

injured, because comparison with the other, normal side offers a significant amount of information. Clearly, such comparison is not obtainable for the cervical spine. Isolated testing should be an ideal way to achieve documentation of deficit, as well as a mechanism to monitor progress. In a recent survey of measurement devices for the lumbar spine, only one type of commercially available isolated measurement equipment appeared to be viable (12). One reason for this may be the complexity of measuring dynamic motion in the cervical spine. There is a reasonable fear of injury when rapid flexion–extension maneuvers are undertaken against resistance, as would be the case in isokinetic testing in a patient with cervical injury and possible instability. Use of equipment that can measure isometric strength at various points in the full available range is a more reasonable measurement system (MedX, Inc., Ocala, Florida). Norms have been identified for isometric cervical extension strength (68). In addition, the ideal amount of exercise to obtain the most sufficient strength training has likewise been established at twice per week rather than one or three times per week (28).

A clinical study using this formatted treatment also demonstrated the efficacy of twice-a-week strength training using isolated resistance training of the cervical extensor musculature (69). In this study, 70 patients with cervical strain were evaluated and treated; all had diminished cervical extensor strength and associated pain, and most also had diminished range of motion. The average improvement was from 25 nm to 32 nm in a 16-session exercise program over 8 weeks. All had reduced pain, patient satisfaction was high, and there were no injuries. The exercise program for the lumbar extensors used a variable-resistance mechanism and a standardized protocol of progressive resistance once 20 repetitions of slow, variable-resistance, eccentric/concentric exercises had been performed. The weight was generally increased by 5%.

Documenting that such results are not specifically equipment-related, a similar study was conducted using a custom-made

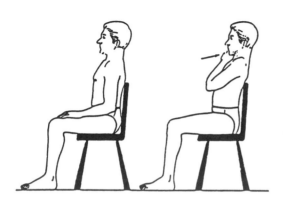

FIG. 6. Traction maneuvers typical of one phase of McKenzie cervical treatment.

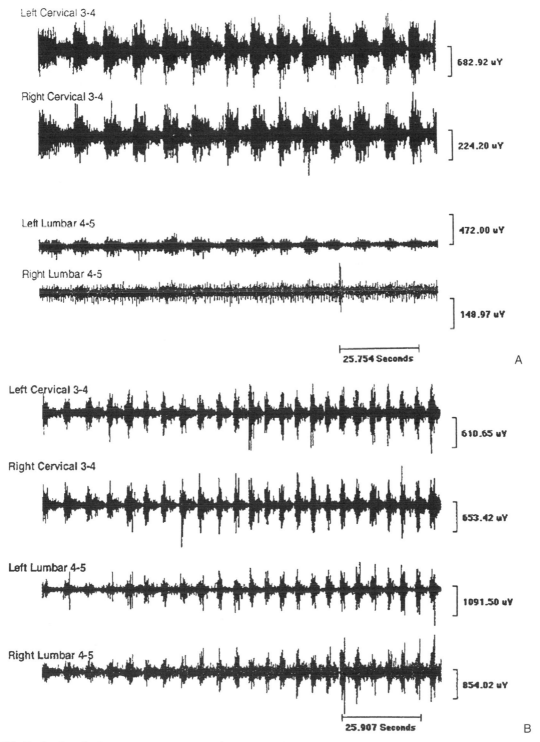

FIG. 7. A: Cervical and lumbar myoelectric activity in a postwhiplash patient at the beginning of strengthening exercises on the MedX cervical equipment. Although the back is not moving in these exercises, the lumbar muscles are active. **B:** Cervical and lumbar myoelectric activity at the conclusion of the strengthening program. Lumbar activity increases with increasing amplitude toward the end of exercise as the cervical musculature begins to fatigue. Again, the back is not moving. Cervical amplitude actually has decreased, although resistance has increased, associated with the physical training program on equipment that isolates musculature.

cervical extensor strengthening device in 17 female workers with chronic neck pain (70). They exercised twice a week for 8 weeks using three sets of 12 repetitions. Again, resistance was progressed as they met performance levels each week. Strength increased about 10% to 15%, and all patients reported significant reduction in pain. There were no injuries.

It appears then that an exercise program can very reasonably be applied in cervical strains. If it is measurable on specialized equipment, the results become more comfortable. Any setting that allows gradual PREs, especially involving the cervical extensors, should be reliable. Certainly, early motion has been demonstrated to be more effective than rest. The most important theme in the treatment of workplace cervical soft tissue injuries is that once it is clear that there is no significant instability, a progressive therapeutic exercise program similar to those for athletes should be initiated.

THERAPEUTIC EXERCISE: LUMBAR SPINE

Statistically, the lumbar spine is the most common area of work-related pain complaints and injuries, and thus ultimately the most expensive workers' compensation ailment. Many attempts have been made to try to reduce the incidence of lumbar spine injuries. It was once felt that preemployment testing would be able to predict them. However, in one study involving classification of job demand by the PDC (Physical Demand Capacity) levels among shipyard workers in physically demanding jobs, we found no relationship between back strength and the severity of job physical demands (71). Baseline testing was performed on all subjects, all of whom were at least 3-year veterans at their various jobs and had no back pain claims. At follow-up 2 years later to see whether any back pain claims had been filed, review of the 12 claims made revealed that 10 of these workers had originally tested as average or slightly above average on isometric testing over the full range of motion;

only two of the 12 workers had slightly below-average strength testing initially.

On the other hand, there is a difference between workplace back claims and the incidence of back pain. In another study that we conducted in a strip mine, about one-third of the workers had back pain complaints, although currently not making claims (72). In an effort to reduce a significant rate of back injury claims, a specific once-a-week training program for lumbar extensor strengthening was instituted. Only one-half of the workers volunteered for this program, but most (80%) had some back pain that nearly completely resolved after 20 weeks. Compliance with the exercise program was 95%, which is somewhat unique in workplace exercise programs. Most important, over the following year, the injury rate fell from 1.5 per month to one incident, a total of 1 day off work in the whole year. This demonstrates that a workplace exercise program can be beneficial in preventing workplace injuries.

One might challenge these studies because neither had an anatomic definition of the cause of back pain. However, in two extensive surveys—one in 1985 (73) and the other in 1992 (74)—undertaken to ascertain the current scientific state of knowledge regarding low back pain, the review committees could not identify any method that could consistently diagnose a structural/anatomic abnormality. Of course, radiculopathy can be confirmed by imaging studies as originating from a definable anatomic source, but this occurs only in 1% or 2% of cases. Certain factors of the dynamic anatomy of the lumbar spine may be important in causing persistent back pain. For years, it was felt that the abdominal muscles were important. This had emerged from Williams' (75) concept that reversal of lumbar lordosis would give more room in the neuroforamen and thus be a positive event. Now that it is possible to specifically measure the strength of the extensors versus the flexors of the spine, some correction in this unproved theory is possible. In one study, persons with chronic back pain showed less extensor strength and less density of extensor muscles than pain-free subjects (76). These findings are confirmed in other studies using electromyography and MR imaging (77). It also has been demonstrated by signal changes in MR imaging that the most vigorously used muscles in active lifting are the multifidus muscles of the lumbar extensors (78). In a clinical study using isokinetic equipment, it has been shown that the lumbar extensors in patients with back pain were weaker than the abdominals (79).

The low back appears to have a unique neuroanatomic characteristic. Selective atrophy in the lumbar extensors develops in patients with persistent back pain. This has been demonstrated by MR imaging as increased fatty infiltration in these muscles compared to all other muscles visualized (80,81). Our study also used myoelectric analysis to evaluate the lumbar extensors (81). It demonstrated that for people with persistent back pain, a twice-a-week physical training program for 8 weeks emphasizing lumbar extensor strengthening could improve strength 40% on average but could significantly reduce the myoelectric amplitude for the same resistance from the beginning to the conclusion of the training program. In addition, resistance to fatigue improved significantly (Fig. 8). More information related to the lumbar extensors has been demonstrated by a comparison of myoelectric activity in the lumbar extensors to that in the abdominal muscles during lifting activities. Only the lumbar extensors correlated with resistance (82).

The focus on lumbar extension relates not only to strength training but also to range of motion. The value of improving extensor range in individuals with back problems has been demonstrated by the McKenzie (83) method. It is a very specific training program with specific goals of enhanced range, especially in extension, and elimination of pain from the extremities. It can clearly identify responders from nonresponders in a short time (84). In an extensive study of 319 consecutive patients, Rath and Rath (85) demonstrated a greater than 80% success rate in individuals with no pain below the knee. Even about 47%

of patients with neurologic signs demonstrated good or excellent results. When patients were seen acutely before 7 days, the results for 83% were successful; only 6.7% had poor results. On the other hand, when they were seen after 7 weeks, the success rate diminished slightly, with about 46% having excellent and 34% good results. The average duration of treatment was six visits, but those with poor results had on average only 2.3 visits, documenting the efficacy of the evaluation system in predicting success and failure. This system is sufficiently standardized so that research studies can be carried out. It is used in a standardized manner around the world. For instance, a recent study from Sweden documented that continued self-care reduced the incidence of recurrent pain after 5 years compared to that in the nontreatment group (86).

For postacute lumbar pain, chiropractic care is the most commonly used alternative method. Although a prospective study carried out at a health maintenance organization in Seattle and supervised by Cherkin has not been published as of this date, a 2-year follow-up report was presented as an abstract at the September 1997 McKenzie Institute International Conference (87). This prospective, randomized study comparing chiropractic to the McKenzie method involved more than 300 patients with postacute back pain at least 2 weeks postonset or with no previous history of back pain. The study showed that both groups were more effectively treated than the placebo group at 6 weeks. The cost was similar for both treatment methods. However, at 3 months and in continuing follow-up for 2 years, the efficacy of treatment was about the same in all three groups. It is of interest that at the end of 2 years, 50% of the patients in this particular population sought medical attention once more for their back pain regardless of what treatment mode had been used. This study therefore demonstrates that recurrences cannot be prevented with a subacute treatment program focused at mobilization alone. However, compliance with a home stretching program typical of McKenzie treat-

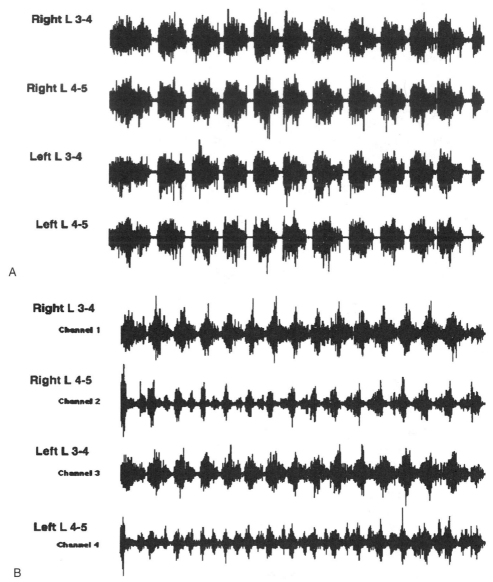

FIG. 8. A: Pretraining lumbar exercise dynamic electromyogram (EMG). Myoelectric signals are recorded by surface electrodes at the L3-4 and L4-5 levels on both the right and left. The peak of each burst of electrical activity represents the effort at full extension range. (This is the position of least mechanical efficiency for paraspinal lumbar extensors.) The absence of electrical activity represents initiation of the next extension–flexion cycles. These patterns point out that eccentric motor activity (the later phase of each bursts) requires less electrical activity for the same resistance than concentric function. **B:** Posttraining lumbar exercise dynamic EMG. Myoelectric activity is recorded for the same resistance as was used at the initiation of the training program. Thus, 8 weeks later, the training program has created a reorganization of effort so that the L3-4 level is working harder than the L4-5. The total amount of electrical activity seems to be less, compared with pretraining.

ment concepts was not identified in this study.

There is no question that the fitness of both connective tissue and muscle tone is an important factor in back pain prevention. The classic Cady et al. (88) study demonstrated that persons in poor physical condition but still working had a greater incidence of back pain.

An alternative exercise program to McKenzie stretching is known as a stabilization program, in which patients are taught strengthening exercises to obtain dynamic "corset" muscle control to maintain a neutral position (89). There are no comparative studies to demonstrate its efficacy. The exercises are progressively more demanding, and patient compliance may be a factor in the continued use of this type of treatment.

As noted earlier, lumbar extensors are the most demonstrable weak link in persistent back pain. It must be recognized that range of motion exercises have the advantage of improving fluid exchange in connective tissue, especially the disc, but may not have an affect on muscle strength. A generic type of device used to enhance lumbar extensor strengthening is known as the Roman chair. It has been demonstrated that deficit in maintaining an unsupported torso in the prone position (Sorenson test) is a predictor of low back pain (90). These devices can also be used for exercise, for which there are various models (Fig. 9).

The greatest specificity in lumbar extensor strengthening can only be achieved by a system that truly isolates the lumbar spine from the pelvis and legs. This is not possible with simple equipment, and a more complex device, such as that developed by MedX, is required to do this. Such a device was demonstrated to be cost-effective compared to no treatment (91). This study showed that people deteriorated both physically and psychologically when persistent chronic back pain went untreated by an active exercise program. However, motivation to be involved in this particular strengthening exercise program is not universal. In an extensive study of 895

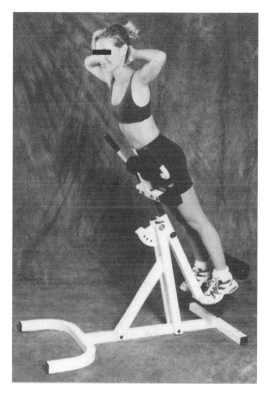

FIG. 9. A type of Roman chair that has the advantage of variable angles to start exercising to allow increasing demand as the patient becomes stronger.

consecutive chronic low back pain patients, only 627 (70.1%) completed the appropriate program (92). On the other hand, all of these patients had failed previous physical therapy programs, and among them 76% reported good or excellent results, with only 8% registering a poor result.

The bottom line for any treatment program related to workplace injuries is measurement of the need to reutilize the health care system. In a study of 412 persistent back pain patients, we compared treatment at two centers using the same equipment and protocol (93). We also evaluated the patients at 1 year for maintenance of improvement and reutilization of the system. Maintenance of the strength achieved at discharge from the program was consistent when testing was performed at 1-year follow-up, and the reutilization rate was

11%. Clearly, recurrences can be avoided by compliance with a strength training program.

CONCLUSION

The purpose of this chapter was to draw a parallel between the concepts of soft tissue rehabilitation currently advocated for professional athletes and available concepts for industrial athletes— injured workers. The only physical treatment that can be measured, however, is activity in various range-of-motion and strengthening exercises. Barriers to the efficacy of this type of treatment, however, relate to a human attitude problem: whether injury patients wish to merely feel better or to get better. If structural incompetence has been created by a soft tissue injury and spontaneous healing has not occurred within several weeks, the only known physiologic maneuver by which improvement may result is a strengthening–ranging program. However, according to the evidence-based system of care known as the medical model, very little true scientific evidence favors this approach. Some of that information has been presented. Nonetheless, far less support is available for the alternative systems of physical treatment. Only by measurement can systems be compared. Until they can be compared, systems will probably continue to be built on consensus rather than evidence.

REFERENCES

1. Spitzer WO, Skovro N, Salmir L, et al. Scientific monograph on the Quebec task force on whiplash-associated injuries. *Spine* 1995;20(suppl):1S–58S.
2. Zander G. OM Medico-Mekaniska Instituteti Stockholm. *J Nord Med Arch* 1872;4:42–52.
3. Levertin A, Heligenthal F, Schutz G, Zander G, eds. *The leading features of Dr. G. Zander's medico-mechanical gymnastic method and its use.* Wiesbaden, Germany: Rossel, Schwarz & Co, 1906.
4. Brummer P, Linko K, Kasanen A. Myocardial infarction treated by early ambulation. *Am Heart J* 1956;52:269–272.
5. Bruce RA. Principles of exercise testing. In: Naughton JP, Hellerstein HK, eds. *Exercise testing and exercise training in coronary heart disease.* New York: Academic Press, 1973:45–62.
6. Delorme TL. Restoration of muscle power by heavy resistance exercises. *Am J Bone Joint Surg* 1945;27:645–667.
7. Jones A. A totally new concept in exercise and equipment. *Iron Man Magazine* 1970;Nov:32–34.
8. Thistle H, Hislop, H, Moffroed M, Perrine JJ. Isokinetic contraction: a new concept of resistive exercise. *Arch Phys Med Rehabil* 1967;48:279–282.
9. Mayer T, Smith S, Keely J, Mooney V. Quantification of lumbar function. Part 2: sagittal plane trunk strength in chronic low back pain patients. *Spine* 1985;10:765–772.
10. Seeds R, Leven J, Goldberg H. Normative data for isostation B-100. *J Orthop Sports Phys Ther* 1987;9:141–155.
11. Seeds R, Levene J, Goldberg H. Abnormal patient data for the isostation B-100. *J Orthop Sports Phys Ther* 1988;10:121–133.
12. Mooney V. Physical measurements of the lumbar spine. *Phys Med Rehabil Clin N Am* May 1998;9(2):391–410.
13. Newton M, Waddell G. Trunk strength testing with iso-machines. Part 1: review of a decade of scientific evidence. *Spine* 1993;18:801–811.
14. Newton M, Thow M, Somerville D, Henderson I, Waddell G. Trunk strength testing with iso-machines. Part 2: experimental evaluation of the Cybex II back testing system in normal subjects and patients with chronic low back pain. *Spine* 1993;18:812–824.
15. *Calif Orthop Assoc Rep* 1998;11(June):10.
16. Smith LL. Acute inflammation: the underlying mechanism in delayed onset muscle soreness. *Med Sci Sports Exerc* 1991;23:542–551.
17. Brooks PM, Day RO. Nonsteroidal antiinflammatory drugs: differences and similarities. *N Engl J Med* 1991;324:1716–1725.
18. Vane JR. Inhibition of prostaglandin synthesis as a mechanism of action for aspirin-like drugs. *Nature N Biol* 1971;231:232–235.
19. Mishra DK, Fréden J, Schmitz MC, Lieber RL. Anti-inflammatory medication after muscle injury. *J Bone Joint Surg Am* 1995;77:1510–1519.
20. Friedman RJ, Acurio MT, Davis R, et al. Effects of growth factors and indomethacin on fracture healing. *Trans Orthop Res Soc* 1992;17:421.
21. Shoemaker JK, Tiidus PM, Mader R. Failure of manual massage to alter limb blood flow: measures by Doppler ultrasound. *Med Sci Sports Exerc* 1997;29:610–614.
22. Agency for Health Care Policy and Research. *Acute low back problems in adult treatment.* Agency for Health Care Policy and Research, Washington, D.C., 1994. AHCPR publication 95-0643.
23. Spitzer WO. Scientific approach to the assessment and management of activity-related spinal disorders: a monograph for clinicians. Report of the Quebec task force. *Spine* 1987;12(suppl):1–59.
24. Akeson WH, Amiel D, Abel MF. Effects of mobilization of joints. *Clin Orthop* 1987;219:28–37.
25. Stowers T, McMillan J, Scala D, et al. The short-term effects of three different strength-power training methods. *Natl Strength Conditioning Assoc J* 1983;5(3):24–27.
26. American College of Sports Medicine. *Guidelines for exercise testing and prescription,* 5th ed. Baltimore: Williams & Wilkins, 1995.
27. Fleck SJ, Kraemer WJ. *Designing resistance training programs.* Champaign, IL: Human Kinetics, 1987.
28. Pollock ML, Graves JE, Bamman MM, et al. Frequency and volume of resistance training: effect of cervical extension strength. *Arch Phys Med Rehabil* 1993;74:1080–1086.

29. Graves JE, Pollock ML, Foster D, et al. Effect of training frequency and specificity on isometric lumbar extension strength. *Spine* 1990;15:504–509.
30. American College of Sports Medicine. The recommended quantity and quality of exercise for developing and maintaining cardiorespiratory and muscular fitness in healthy adults. *Med Sci Sports Exerc* 1990;22:265–274.
31. Neer CS II. Anterior acromioplasty for the chronic impingement syndrome in the shoulder: a preliminary report. *J Bone Joint Surg Am* 1972;54:41–50.
32. Neer CS II. Impingement lesions. *Clin Orthop* 1983; 173:70–77.
33. Bigliani LJ, Morrison DS, April EW. The morphology of the acromion and its relationship to rotator cuff tears. *Orthop Trans* 1986;10:228.
34. Perry J. Biomechanics of the shoulder. In: CR Rowe, ed. *The Shoulder* New York: Churchill Livingstone, 1988: 1–15.
35. Hawkins R, Dunlop R. Nonoperative treatment of rotator cuff tears. *Clin Orthop* 1995;321:178–188.
36. Morrison DS, Frogameni AD, Woodworth P. Non-operative treatment of subacromial impingement syndrome. *J Bone Joint Surg Am* 1997;79:732–737.
37. Ellman H. Diagnosis and treatment of incomplete rotator cuff tears. *Clin Orthop* 1990;254:64–74.
38. Gordon S, Blair S, Fine L, eds. *Repetitive motion disorders of the upper extremity.* American Academy of Orthopaedic Surgeons, Chicago, IL, 1994.
39. Nirschl PR. Elbow tendinosis/tennis elbow. *Clin Sports Med* 1992;11:851–870.
40. Rolf C, Movin T. Etiology, histopathology, and outcome of surgery in achillodynia. *Foot Ankle Int* 1997;18: 565–569.
41. Labelle H, Guibert R, Joncas J, Newman N, Fallaha M, Rivard CH. Lack of scientific evidence for the treatment of lateral epicondylitis of the elbow. J Bone Joint Surg Br 1992;74:646–561.
42. Verhar JAN, Waldenkamp GHIM, Van Mameren H, Kester ADM, Van Der Linden AJ. Local corticosteroid injection versus Cyriax-typ physiotherapy for tennis elbow. *J Bone Joint Surg Br* 1996;78:128–132.
43. Solveborn SA, Buch F, Mallmin H, Adalberth G. Cortisone injection with anesthetic additives for radial epicondylalgia (tennis elbow). Clin Orthop 1995;316: 99–105.
44. Rompe JD, Hopf C, Küllmer K, Heine J, Bürger R. Analgesic effect of extracorporeal shock-wave therapy on chronic tennis elbow. *J Bone Joint Surg Br* 1996;78: 233–237.
45. Schiottz-Christensen B, Mooney V, Azad S, Selstad D, Gulick J, Bracker M. Protocol-driven treatment for overuse syndromes of the upper extremity. *J Occup Rehab* 1999.
46. Pransky G, Himmelstein J. Overview of complete patient management in upper extremity repetitive motion disorders of the upper extremity. In: Gordon S, Blair S, Fine L, eds. *Repetitive motion disorders of the upper extremity.* Chicago, IL American Academy of Orthopaedic Surgeons, 1994:539–549.
47. Pienimäki TT, Tarvainen TK, Siira PT, Vanharanta H. Progressive strengthening and stretching exercises and ultrasound for chronic lateral epicondylitis. *Physiotherapy* 1996;82:522–530.
48. Leach RE, Miller JK. Lateral and medial epicondylitis of the elbow. *Clin Sports Med* 1987;6:259–272.
49. Haker E, Lundeberg T. Pulsed ultrasound treatment in lateral epicondylitis. *Scand J Rehabil Med* 1991;3: 115–118.
50. Steindler A. *Kinesiology of the human body under normal and pathological conditions.* Springfield, IL: Charles C Thomas, 1955.
51. Wilk KE, Excamilla RF, Fleisig GS, et al. The comparison of tibiofemoral joint forces and electromyography during open and closed kinetic chain exercises. *Am J Sports Med* 1994;22:44–56.
52. Wallace J, Gulick J, Mooney V. Isolated versus integrated strengthening of vastus medialis. (*Submitted for pub.*)
53. Snyder-Mackler L, Delitto A, Bailey S, Stralka S. Strength of the quadriceps femoris muscle and functional recovery after reconstruction of the anterior cruciate ligament. *J Bone Joint Surg Am* 1995;77: 1166–1173.
54. Herberts P, Kadefors R, Broman. Arm positioning in manual tasks: an electromyographic study of localized fatigue. *Ergonomics* 1980;23:655–665.
55. Suurküla J, Hägg GM. Relations between shoulder/neck disorders and EMG zero crossing shifts in female assembly workers using the test contraction method. *Ergonomics* 1987;30:1553–1562.
56. Norris SH, Watt I. The prognosis of neck injuries resulting from rear-end collisions. *J Bone Joint Surg Br* 1983;65:608–611.
57. Watkinson A, Gargan MF, Bannister GC. Prognostic factors in soft tissue injuries of the cervical spine. *Injury* 1991;22:307–309.
58. Hildingson C, Toolanen G. Outcome after soft-tissue injury of the cervical spine: a prospective study of 93 car accidents. *Acta Orthop Scand* 1990;61:357–359.
59. Pennie B, Agambar L. Patterns of injury and recovery in whiplash. *Injury* 1991;22:57–59.
60. Twomey LT, Taylor JR. The whiplash syndrome: pathology and physical treatment. *J Manual Manipulative Ther* 1993;1:26–29.
61. Cloward R. Cervical discograms. *Ann Surg* 1959;150: 34–42.
62. Aprill C, Dwyer A, Bogduk N. Cervical zygapophyseal joint pain patterns. II. A clinical evaluation. *Spine* 1990; 15:458–446.
63. McKinney LA. Early mobilization and outcome in acute sprains of the neck. *BMJ* 1989;299:1006–1008.
64. Mealy A, Brennan H, Feneing C. Early mobilization of acute whiplash injuries. *BMJ* 1986;292:956–957.
65. Zylebergold RS, Piper MC. Cervical spine disorders: a comparison of three types of traction. *Spine* 1985;10: 867–871.
66. Jacob G. Rehabilitating chiropractic. *J of McKenzie Institute* 1998;6:24–26.
67. Herstoff R, Gulick J, Mooney V, et al. Electrical activity of the cervical and lumbar muscles during isotonic cervical extension exercise. American Orthopaedic Association Annual Meeting abstract. Sun Valley, ID, 1999, p. 70.
68. Leggett SH, Graves JE, Pollock ML, et al. Quantitative assessment and training of isometric cervical extension strength. *Am J Sports Med* 1991;19:653–659.
69. Highland TR, Dreisinger TE, Vie LL, et al. Changes in isometric strength and range of motion of the isolated cervical spine after eight weeks of clinical rehabilitation. *Spine* 1992;17:577–582.

70. Berg HE, Berggren G, Tesch PA. Dynamic neck strength training effect on pain and function. *Arch Phys Med Rehabil* 1994;75:661–655.

71. Mooney V, Kenney D, Leggett S, Holmes B. Relationship of lumbar strength in shipyard workers to workplace injury claims. *Spine* 1996;21:2001–2005.

72. Mooney V, Kron M, Rummerfield P, Holmes B. The effect of workplace-based strengthening on low back injury rates: a case study in the strip mining industry. *J Occup Rehabil* 1995;5:157–167.

73. LeBlanc FE, Spitzer WO, Dupuis M. Report of the Quebec task force on spinal disorders. *Spine* 1987;12 (suppl):S1–S8.

74. *Acute low back problems in adults: assessment and treatment.* U.S. Department of Health and Human Services, Agency for Health Care Policy and Research, Washington D.C., 1994. AHCPR publication 95–0643.

75. Williams PC. *The lumbar sacral spine emphasizing conservative management.* New York: McGraw-Hill, 1965.

76. Hultman G, Nordin M, Saraste H, Ohlsen H. Body composition, endurance, strength, cross-sectional area, and density of MM erector spinae in men with and without low back pain. *J Spinal Disord* 1993;6:114–123.

77. Parkkola R, Rytokoski R, Kormano M. Magnetic resonance imaging of the discs and trunk muscles in patients with chronic low back pain and healthy control subjects. *Spine* 1993;18:830–836.

78. Flicker PL, Fleckenstein JL, Ferry K, et al. Lumbar muscle usage in chronic low back pain. *Spine* 1993;18:582–586.

79. Shiado O, Kaneda K, Ito T. Trunk-muscle strength during concentric and eccentric contraction: a comparison between healthy subjects and patients with chronic low back pain. *J Spinal Disord* 1992;5:175–182.

80. Alaranta H, Tallroth K, Soukka A, Heliovaara M. Fat content of lumbar extensor muscles and low back disability: a radiographic and clinical comparison. *J Spinal Disord* 1993;6:137–140.

81. Mooney V, Gulick J, Perlman M, et al. Relationships between myoelectric activity, strength, and MRI of lumbar extensor muscles in back pain patients and normal subjects. *J Spinal Disord* 1997;10:348–356.

82. Ross EC, Parnianpour M, Martin D. The effects of resistance level on muscle coordination patterns and movement profile during trunk extension. *Spine* 1993;18:1829–1838.

83. McKenzie RA. *Treat your own back.* Waikaniae, New Zealand: Spinal Publications, 1980.

84. Donelson R, Silva G, Murphy K. The centralization phenomenon: its usefulness in evaluating testing referred pain. *Spine* 1990;15:211–213.

85. Rath W, Rath JD. Outcome assessment in clinical practice. *McKenzie Inst J* 1996;4:9–16.

86. Stankovic R, Jonell O. Conservative treatment of low back pain: a prospective randomized trial: McKenzie method of treatment versus patient education in "mini back school." *Spine* 1990;15:120–123.

87. Battie G, Cherkin D, et al. McKenzie therapy chiropractic manipulation or an education booklet: which is most cost-effective treatment for low back pain. Proceedings of the fifth McKenzie Institute international conference, September, 1997:12–14(abst); pp. 969–974.

88. Cady LD, Bischoff DP, O'Connel ER, et al. Strength and fitness in subsequent back injuries in fire fighters. *J Occup Med* 1979;21:269–272.

89. Saul JA, Saul JS. Nonoperative treatment of herniated lumbar intervertebral disc with radiculopathy and outcomes study. *Spine* 1989;14:431–439.

90. Biering-Sorenson F. Physical measurements as risk predictors for low back trouble over a one period. *Spine* 1984;9:106.

91. Risch SV, Norvell NK, Pollock ML, et al. Lumbar strengthening in chronic low back pain patients: physiologic and psychologic benefits. *Spine* 1993;18:232–238.

92. Nelson B, O'Reilly E, Miller M, Hogan M, Wegner J, Kelly C. Focus on the spine: the clinical effects of intensive, specific exercise on chronic low back pain: a controlled study of 895 consecutive patients with 1-year follow-up. *Orthopaedics* 1995;18:971–981.

93. Leggett S, Mooney V, Matheson LN, et al. Restorative exercise for clinical low back pain: a prospective two-center study with one-year follow-up. *Spine* 1999;24:889–898.

Occupational Musculoskeletal Disorders
edited by T. G. Mayer, R. J. Gatchel, and P. B. Polatin.
Lippincott Williams & Wilkins, Philadelphia © 2000.

25

Manipulative Therapy for Postacute Occupational Musculoskeletal Disorders

Scott Haldeman and *Paul D. Hooper

Department of Neurology, University of California, Irvine, Santa Ana, California, 92701;
*Department of Principles and Practice, Los Angeles College of Chiropractic, Whittier, California 90609

Over the past 30 years, spinal manipulative or manual therapy in its various forms has become one of the most widely utilized approaches to the treatment of occupational musculoskeletal injuries. The growth in interest in these treatment methods has been driven by several factors:

- High patient demand for and satisfaction with manipulative therapy;
- Need for a "low-tech," low-cost, readily available method of treating common musculoskeletal pain;
- Increasing amount of research demonstrating a positive effect of manipulation on musculoskeletal pain and disability;
- Failure of any other treatment method to provide a low-cost, effective means of resolving these problems.

ROLE OF MANIPULATION

Manipulative therapy represents the best example of the legitimization of a controversial modality for the treatment of spinal disorders (1). The past several decades have seen attitudes toward the use of manipulative therapy change from one of suspicion and disdain to one of cautious endorsement. Reimbursement for spinal manipulation is now almost universal in the workers' compensation insurance programs of Western industrialized nations. Recent government treatment guidelines in the United States (2), Canada (3), and

Great Britain (4) include manipulation as a reasonable method of treating patients with low back and/or neck pain.

With the changing face of today's health care system, there is an increasing demand for evidence-based, cost-effective treatment methods with a high level of patient satisfaction. The new managed care system of health care is increasingly directing patients to the least expensive professional who can get the job done most efficiently (5). It is therefore necessary to review current evidence supporting the use of each of the treatment approaches to occupational musculoskeletal disorders to place them in perspective. This chapter attempts to achieve this goal for the manipulative therapies.

Definition of Manipulation

Considerable confusion exists in the literature about what constitutes or should be included under the terms *manipulation* and *spinal manipulative therapy* (SMT). This is primarily because several different health professionals use manipulative procedures. Chiropractors, osteopathic physicians, physical therapists, medical doctors, and others who fall into the category of licensed or unlicensed massage therapists and lay manual therapists offer various forms of manipulative or manual treatments.

No universal agreement exists among these various groups regarding what manipulation actually accomplishes and which procedures are best. Even within a particular profession, there may not be agreement regarding the mechanisms or the techniques that should be used or the clinical indications for treatment. Theories regarding the effect of manipulation range from repositioning of misaligned vertebrae to removing spinal fixations (i.e., joint restrictions), reducing intervertebral disc herniations, relaxing muscles, and removing pressure from spinal nerves. For example, chiropractic manipulative procedures include the use the classic high-velocity, low-amplitude thrust techniques to increase spinal motion, mechanically assisted, handheld adjusting devices (e.g., activator adjusting instrument), traction–distraction methods to reduce disc herniation, and triggerpoint therapies to relax muscles. On the other hand, physical therapists often rely more on nonthrust techniques that may be referred to as mobilization, whereas osteopathic physicians utilize muscle energy or sacrooccipital techniques and incorporate these procedures into a rehabilitative program, often with prescription medication. It is therefore very difficult to compare the results of clinical trials of different methods that are described as manipulation or manual therapy.

Several authors have attempted to define and classify the various types of manipulation. Anderson et al. (6) described manipulation "as a procedure of manual therapy in which the operator applies a sudden thrust into a joint in order to cause it to move through a restrictive barrier into the para-physiological space." Shekelle (7) used a similar approach when he defined SMT as "the high-velocity, low amplitude movement of a joint past its usual end range of motion but not its anatomical range." The recently published Agency for Health Care Policy and Research guidelines for the management of acute low back pain (LBP) adopted a more general definition of manipulation as "manual loading of the spine using short or long leverage methods" (2). It is, however, more common to consider manipulative therapy as one form of manual therapy. Other forms of manual therapy include mobilization, manual traction, and massage. A useful classification of the different manual therapies is outlined in Table 1.

Manipulable Lesions

Confusion also exists among professional groups regarding the nature of the lesion that is the target of SMT. It has been variously referred to as a vertebral fixation, vertebral blockage, spinal dysfunction, vertebral subluxation, or osteopathic lesion (8) (Table 2). Most practitioners identify the lesion primarily through manual palpation or some form of biomechanical analysis. While this is a somewhat subjective procedure, several studies have shown reasonable agreement regarding the location of the lesion (9–11). Others have shown that some aspects of these palpation procedures are reliable while others are not (12), with perhaps the most reliable palpation finding being tenderness (13).

TABLE 1. *Types of manual therapies*

Joint manipulation procedures
    Mobilization (articulation/oscillation procedures): not associated with audible release
    High-velocity, low-amplitude adjustments/manipulation: usually associated with audible release
    Manual traction
    Flexion/distraction procedures
    Instrument-aided manipulation (e.g., activator adjusting instrument)
Soft tissue mobilization and manipulation procedures
    Pressure-point techniques (e.g., trigger-point therapy)
    Therapeutic massage
    Therapeutic muscle stretching
    Myofascial release techniques
    Strain/counterstrain techniques

From ref. 8, with permission.

TABLE 2. *Functional and/or structural disorders of synovial joints*

Subluxation (orthopedic definition)
  Partial or incomplete dislocation
Subluxation (chiropractic definition)
  Spinal misalignment (historical definition)
  Aberrant relationship between two adjacent
    structures
  May have functional or pathologic sequelae
Joint dysfunction
  Altered joint mechanics
  Functional disturbances without structural
    or pathologic changes
Somatic dysfunction (osteopathic definition)
  Impaired or altered function of related components
    of the somatic system
Osteopathic lesion (also referred to as a facilitated
    segment)
  Disturbance of musculoskeletal structure and/or
    function
  May include accompanying disturbances of other
    biologic mechanisms
Joint fixation
  Partial immobilization of a joint in a position that it
    may normally occupy during any phase of normal
    movement
  Partial limitation or restriction of joint movement

From ref. 8, with permission.

CLINICAL EFFICACY

Low Back Pain

Acute and Subacute Low Back Pain

By far the most common reason for SMT is pain in the lower back. It has been estimated that somewhere between 30% and 50% of all spinal manipulations delivered each year are for LBP (14,15). As a result, most research efforts have been directed at the effectiveness of SMT in patients with LBP.

Several metaanalyses of this research have now been published. Kocs et al. (16) identified 36 randomized, controlled trials comparing SMT with a number of other treatments. Of these, 12 trials included patients with acute LBP only. Five reported positive results, four reported negative results, and three reported positive results in a subgroup of the study population. The authors concluded that there are indications that manipulation is effective for certain subgroups of patients with LBP, but they cautioned that the final conclusion regarding the efficacy of SMT for pa-

tients with acute or chronic LBP requires a greater number of studies with better design. In another metaanalysis, Shekelle et al. (17) analyzed all the controlled trials on manipulation published prior to 1992. They assigned quality scores on the published research designs and selected seven papers that had either used single outcome measures or assessed outcome measures independently. They then developed differences in probability of recovery from LBP for each of the studies (Fig. 1). In this study, SMT increased the probability of recovery at 2 or 3 weeks after the start of treatment, indicating that manipulation hastens recovery from acute uncomplicated LBP.

In a prospective, randomized trial published after Shekelle et al.'s (17) metaanalysis, Hsieh et al. (18) compared the effect of SMT, transcutaneous muscle stimulation, massage, and corset use in patients with subacute LBP. The manipulation group showed the greatest improvement in flexion and pain after 3 weeks. Patient confidence was also greatest in the manipulation group. In another study, patients with acute and subacute LBP were randomized to two treatment groups: manual therapy (i.e., manipulation, specific mobilization, and muscle stretching) and steroid injections (19). Patients receiving manual therapy had significantly less pain and disability in both the early phase and at 90 days' followup. The manual therapy group also had a faster rate of recovery and lower drug consumption.

In a recent study involving patients with LBP without sciatica, Cherkin et al. (20) compared the use of physical therapy (i.e., McKenzie method), chiropractic manipulation without other standard chiropractic treatment methods, and a minimal intervention consisting of the provision of an educational booklet. Both the McKenzie method and chiropractic treatment were provided for 1 month, and patients were followed for 2 years. At 4 weeks, the chiropractic group had less severe symptoms than the booklet group, and the authors reported a trend toward less severe symptoms in the McKenzie treatment group. At 1 year, differences in dysfunction ap-

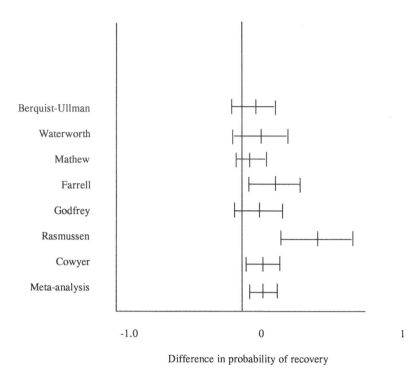

FIG. 1. Difference in probability of recovery in seven trials of manipulation. (From ref. 17, with permission.)

proached significance, with greatest dysfunction in the booklet group. Patient satisfaction, however, was much greater in the manipulation and McKenzie method groups. The tight restrictions of this study, however, make it difficult to extrapolate to common practice. These studies raise the question as to the importance of patient satisfaction in the selection of a treatment protocol and the reasonableness of the costs involved in manual treatment methods.

This study is in conflict with one by Meade et al. (21), who compared the effects of treatment provided in a hospital-based, outpatient physical therapy department to chiropractic care delivered in a typical private practice setting. Patients were followed up for 2 years. Unlike the study by Cherkin et al. (20), this study placed minimal limits on the type of treatment given to the two groups of patients. It demonstrated that chiropractic treatment is more effective than hospital-based physical therapy, particularly for patients with chronic or severe LBP. According to the authors, the

benefit of chiropractic treatment became more evident throughout the follow-up period. In a second follow-up study, Meade et al. (22) compared the effectiveness of chiropractic treatment with hospital outpatient management at 3 years. According to Oswestry scores, improvement was 29% greater in chiropractic than in hospital-treated patients. Similarly, Koes et al. (23) conducted a randomized, controlled trial of 256 patients with nonspecific back and neck complaints of at least 6 weeks' duration. They concluded that manipulative therapy and physiotherapy are both more effective than either general practitioner care or placebo treatment and that manipulative therapy is slightly better than physiotherapy after 12 months.

Belief is widespread that LBP is a self-limiting disorder, and most patients will eventually recover without any treatment. A recent 1-year follow-up study on the course of LBP in general practice suggests, however, that the clinical course for most patients is not as favorable as expected (24). This study monitored patients from 15 general practitioners over a 2-year period. Of 443 patients included in the study, 269 completed the follow-up. In general, patients who did not complete the study were identified as having less serious LBP. Thirty-five percent of the patients still had LBP at 12 weeks. In addition, a significant number suffered one or more relapses within 1 year.

Chronic Low Back Pain

While many of the early studies of SMT focused on patients with acute LBP, there is a growing interest in SMT's effect on patients with chronic problems. In one of the first studies of SMT for patients with recurrent or chronic LBP, Waagen et al. (25) showed a statistical benefit from chiropractic manipulation at 2 weeks compared to a sham adjustment group. Using patients as their own controls in a crossover-design clinical trial, Evans (26) showed diminished codeine use in patients undergoing manipulation. A trial by Ongley et al. (27) demonstrated that a group that received both rotational manipulation and proliferant injections showed significant improvement.

In a blinded, randomized trial of patients with chronic back and neck complaints, Koes et al. (23) found that manual therapy compared favorably to physiotherapy, treatment by a general practitioner, and a placebo therapy. The patients in the manipulation group showed a faster and greater improvement in physical functioning, and manipulative therapy was slightly better than physiotherapy after 12 months. In a second comparison of manipulation and mobilization of the spine with physiotherapy (i.e., exercises, massage, heat, electrotherapy, ultrasound, and short-wave diathermy) for patients with chronic conditions (i.e., duration of 1 year or longer), Koes et al. (28) again demonstrated that improvement was greater in those treated with manual therapy. In a comparison of SMT with back education programs for patients with chronic LBP, Triano et al. (29) noted greater improvement in pain and activity tolerance in the ma-

nipulation group. Bronfort (30) compared 5 weeks of SMT to nonsteroidal antiinflammatory drug therapy followed by an additional 6 weeks of supervised exercise alone for chronic LBP in a randomized, observer-blinded clinical trial. Each therapeutic regimen was associated with similar and clinically important improvement over time that was considered superior to the expected natural history of long-standing chronic LBP. In addition, there appeared to be a sustained reduction in medication use at the 1-year follow-up in the SMT and trunk-strengthening exercise group.

Not all studies have demonstrated a superior effect following manipulation. Timm (31) compared the effects of different approaches to the management of patients with chronic LBP. The purposes of the study were (a) to investigate the effects of the treatments, (b) to track the length of relief obtained, and (c) to determine the cost-effectiveness of the treatments. A total of 250 patients with chronic LBP following an L-5 laminectomy were randomly assigned to manipulation, low-tech exercise, and high-tech exercise. The author concluded that low-tech and high-tech exercises were the only effective treatments and that low-tech exercise produced the longest period of relief. Gibson (32) similarly failed to show a positive effect following osteopathic manipulation.

In separate reviews of the literature, Koes et al. (16) and van Tulder et al. (33) identified several randomized, controlled trials on chronic LBP of sufficiently high quality that demonstrate a positive effect of SMT. These studies suggest that SMT can now be considered a reasonable approach for patients with chronic LBP and that the effect might be greater if combined with exercise. This appears to be the growing consensus among both researchers and clinicians.

Sciatica

Although the number of significant randomized clinical trials on the use of SMT for patients with sciatica and radiculopathy remains small, several reports and case studies suggest that SMT may be useful for patients with these symptoms.

Several authors have reported improvement in certain outcome measures following manipulation in patients with sciatica (34–36). The significance of these studies is not clear, as they did not have very strict controls. Uncontrolled studies by Chrisman et al. (37) and Cassidy et al. (38) suggest that patients with demonstrated disc herniation and sciatica do less well following manipulation than patients with back pain alone, although a number of these patients report pain relief.

Many clinicians who recommend manipulation to patients with disc herniation and sciatica or radiculopathy prefer a modified manipulation technique. The most popular of these is a combination of flexion–distraction methods and side posture manipulation (39–42). In contrast, Polkinghorn and Colloca (40) used a mechanical device (i.e., activator adjusting instrument) to provide a manipulative force. However, in a review of data from a back pain clinic at the Royal University Hospital in Saskatoon, Saskatchewan, Cassidy et al. (43) concluded that side posture manipulation (i.e., high-velocity, low-amplitude thrust) is both safe and effective for lumbar disc herniations.

There are two published case series on manipulation of patients with sciatica. Stern et al. (44) studied 71 patients who presented in a postgraduate teaching chiropractic clinic with LBP and radiating leg pain, clinically diagnosed with lumbar disc herniations. Outcomes that were assessed included subjective improvement reported by the patient, range of motion, and nerve root tension signs. Ninety percent of the patients who received a course of treatment reported improvement. The authors concluded that manipulation may be a safe, effective nonoperative treatment of back and radiating leg pain. Ben-Eliyahu (45) reported on a prospective study of 27 patients with magnetic resonance imaging–documented, symptomatic disc herniations of either the cervical or lumbar spine. Twenty-two (81%) of the patients reported a good clinical outcome, and either a reduction or complete resorption of the disc was seen in 17 (63%). Unfortunately, there was no control group, and it is impossible to state whether the resorption was the direct result of the manipulation.

In the absence of controlled trials, it is not possible to state unequivocally that SMT is an effective treatment for disc herniation and sciatica. On the other hand, no studies have suggest that disc herniation or sciatica are contraindications to manipulation.

Neck Pain

Patients with neck pain represent the second largest population seeking manipulation or manual therapy. The number of controlled clinical trials on neck pain, however, is not as large as for LBP, making conclusions more difficult.

Several studies have reported decreased neck pain following SMT compared with analgesics or no treatment (46,47). Howe et al. (47) also described improvement in cervical rotation following manipulation. In contrast, Sloop et al. (48) failed to show improvement in neck pain following a single manipulation. There are also a few case reports of patients with confirmed cervical disc herniation that responded to cervical manipulation (49,50).

Several authors have attempted to analyze the literature on the conservative management of neck pain with SMT. Hurwitz et al. (51) identified articles on the efficacy and complications of SMT in the cervical spine using a structured search of four computerized bibliographic databases. Of the three randomized, controlled trials identified, two showed a short-term benefit for cervical mobilization in patients with acute neck pain. In patients with subacute or chronic neck pain, an improvement of pain at 3 weeks was shown for manipulation compared with muscle relaxants or other nonmanipulation forms of care. The authors suggested that SMT and mobilization of the cervical spine provide at least short-term benefits for some patients with neck pain and headaches.

A more extensive analysis of all forms of treatment for neck pain was carried out by Aker et al. (52). They concluded that there had not been sufficient studies to adequately prove the effectiveness of any treatment approach. However, they noted a positive effect following manipulation at 1 to 4 weeks, when they combined the results of five trials on manual methods (Fig. 2). Similar conclusions were reached by Gross et al. (53) following an overview of conservative treatments (i.e., drug therapy, manual therapy, patient education, and physical modalities) in reducing mechanical neck pain. They identified 24 randomized, controlled trials and eight before–after studies that met their selection criteria. Twenty of the randomized, controlled trials were rated moderately strong or better. The authors concluded that, within the limits of methodologic quality, the best available evidence supports the use of manual therapies in combination with other treatments for short-term relief of neck pain.

Attempts to isolate the most effective combination of manipulative treatment have yielded conflicting results. Cassidy et al. (54) compared the immediate results of SMT to mobilization in patients suffering from unilateral neck pain with referral to the trapezius muscles. One hundred consecutive patients received either a single high-velocity, low-amplitude, rotational manipulation (n=52) or mobilization in the form of muscle energy technique (n=48). Manipulation was shown to have a significantly greater effect on pain intensity, with 85% of SMT patients and 69% of mobilization patients reporting pain immediately after treatment. The decrease in pain intensity was greater (1.5 times) in the manipulated group. Both treatments increased cervical range of motion. On the other hand, Jordan et al. (55) conducted a randomized, prospective clinical trial to compare the relative effectiveness of intensive training of the cervical musculature, a physiotherapy regimen, and chiropractic treatment. This study included 119 patients with neck pain of greater than 3 months' duration. Although these three treatment interventions demonstrated meaningful improvement in all primary effect parameters, there was no single treatment approach that stood out as superior.

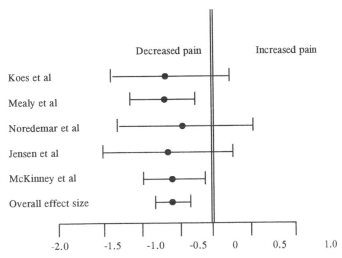

FIG. 2. Pooled effect size of pain reduction for five similar trials that used manual treatment in combination with either drug treatment, education, or physical medicine methods at 1 to 4 weeks of treatment. (From ref. 52, with permission.)

Headache

In addition to disorders of the back and neck, head pain is a significant problem for many workers, accounting for an estimated 150 million lost workdays and $57 billion in lost productivity and medical expenses annually (56). While many individuals are content to treat their conditions with a variety of medications, both prescribed and over-the-counter (OTC), some patients opt for alternative approaches such as manual therapy or SMT. It has been reported that head pain is a primary symptom in up to 35% of all patients presenting to a chiropractor (14). While caution must be taken with head pain patients to rule out metabolic or intracranial pathologies, some headaches appear to have a cervicogenic component (57). Several recent controlled, clinical trials have looked at the effect of SMT in common headache syndromes.

In a systematic review of the literature, Hurwitz et al. (51) assessed the evidence for both the efficacy and complications of manipulation and mobilization of the cervical spine for the treatment of headache. A total of five randomized, controlled trials, 10 case series, and 19 case reports specifically addressed the use of SMT for headache. Of these, one randomized, controlled trial and two case reports addressed migraine sufferers. The randomized, controlled trials ranged in quality from 36 to 77 out of a possible 100 points, making them similar in quality to the studies of SMT for LBP. The authors concluded that manipulation and mobilization may be beneficial for muscle tension headaches.

In one randomized, controlled trial reviewed by Hurwitz et al. (51), patients with chronic migraine were randomized into three treatment groups: general mobilization of the cervical spine, SMT performed by physiotherapists or physicians, or high-velocity, low-amplitude thrust performed by chiropractors. Patients treated with high-velocity, low-amplitude manipulation techniques had the greatest reduction in symptoms and pain relief at the end of the treatment period, but all three groups reported further improvement at follow-up 20 months later (58).

Several authors have reported significant improvement compared to controls in some parameters such as headache severity and frequency (58–60), but not all (61). In a recently published study, Boline et al. (62) randomized patients with tension-type headaches to SMT plus moist heat (two times weekly for 6 weeks) and amitriptyline taken daily for 6 weeks. No statistical differences were reported at 6 weeks. At 10 weeks, however, the manipulation group had improvements in headache intensity (32%), frequency (37%), use of OTC medications (37%), and functional status (16%). The amitriptyline group reported improvements of less than 6% in all categories.

In addition to a small number of controlled trials, there are several case studies suggesting a positive response to manipulation in patients with headaches following manipulation (63–70).

Carpal Tunnel Syndrome

Recently, claims have been made that manual therapies may play a role in the treatment of carpal tunnel syndrome (CTS). Several case series have suggested that a conservative approach, including manipulation, may be beneficial for certain patients with CTS (71–74). While these were not controlled studies, improvements were described for range of motion, strength, pain, and distress levels, as well as electromyographic findings.

A single randomized, controlled trial has been published, comparing the use of manipulative therapy with ibuprofen for CTS (75). Patients were randomized into two groups consisting of ibuprofen or chiropractic treatment. The ibuprofen group received 800 mg three times a day for 1 week, 800 mg twice a day for 1 week, and 800 mg as needed to a maximum daily dose of 2,400 mg for 7 weeks. Chiropractic treatment included manipulation of the soft tissues and bony joints of the upper extremities and spine (three treatments per week for 2 weeks, two treatments per week for 3 weeks and one treatment per week for 4 weeks) and ultrasound over the carpal tunnel. Both groups were provided with nocturnal wrist supports. Outcome measures were pre- and postassessments of self-reported physical and mental distress, nerve conduction studies, and vibrometry. Significant improvement in perceived comfort and function, nerve conduction, and finger sensation was seen overall. However, no significant differences between the groups were seen. The complication rate with ibuprofen, however, was greater than in the manipulation group. Ten patients (22%) receiving ibuprofen reported some intolerance within the first 2 weeks, and five of these experienced marked intolerance (i.e., acute gastrointestinal intolerance, headache, and/or nausea) and were unable to continue taking the medication. One chiropractic subject complained of a temporary sore neck linked to manipulation.

PHYSICAL AND SOCIAL OUTCOME MEASURES

Most randomized, controlled trials on the effectiveness of SMT have relied on outcomes in the form of pain or disability scores with relatively little emphasis on more objective outcome measures. The growing acceptance of manipulative therapy, however, requires that other physical and social outcomes be investigated. Several studies have attempted to look at these issues.

Physical Measurements

Several authors have described an increase in range of motion following manipulation. Rasmussen (76) found an improvement in spinal range of motion (i.e., C-7 to S-1 difference on standing and forward flexion) following SMT. Hviid (77) and Jirout (78) both reported an increased cervical range of motion following manipulation; however, significant change in range of motion was not seen by Nilsson et al. (79).

At the same time, several authors have demonstrated an increase in straight leg raising in patients with LBP following manipulation (80–83). Grice (84) and Diebert and Eng-

land (85) both reported changes in surface electromyographic activity in spinal muscles, while Zhu et al. (86) noted that cerebral evoked potentials on magnetic stimulation of paraspinal muscles returned to normal amplitude following a period of time after the application of SMT. In view of the small number of patients studied and the methods used to record change, further trials will be necessary to determine what effect, if any, manipulation has on muscle activity.

Cyriax (87) suggested that SMT was effective because of its ability to reduce intervertebral disc herniations. This theory was based partially on the observations of Matthews and Yates (88), who utilized epidural venography before and after manipulation. Others have also proposed that manipulation has a positive effect on the intervertebral disc (41,42,45,89), but evidence is not yet available that changes in the size of a disc herniation represent more than normal resorption with time.

Patient Satisfaction

In addition to providing clinically meaningful care, managed care organizations are interested in providing care that is acceptable to their enrollees. This has greatly increased the importance of patient satisfaction as an outcome measure.

Several studies have looked at patient satisfaction, and all showed a high level of satisfaction following manipulation (20,90–96). Furthermore, when seeking chiropractic care, patients appear to be largely more satisfied with their care, with the ability of the doctor to treat their conditions, and with the explanations provided.

Some authors have tried to isolate the patient who is most likely to show high satisfaction with SMT. In an attempt to examine changes in pain, functional activity, and patient satisfaction, Verhoef et al. (97) demonstrated that pain relief and functional changes were greatest among patients whose initial level of pain or disability was moderate or severe, whose condition was acute, and who was only seen by a chiropractor. In addition, pain relief was highest among men, those who perceived themselves to be in good or excellent health, and those who had completed treatment in 6 weeks. In a study to identify patient characteristics that might predict satisfaction, Sawyer and Kassak (95) stated that women were slightly more satisfied than men with care received and a patient's perception of treatment outcome was the most important predictive variable.

Cost

With skyrocketing health care costs, greater attention is being devoted to cost effectiveness. While no studies have looked at the cost of SMT in and of itself, several studies have looked at the cost of chiropractic care.

In a review of the literature, Johnson et al. (98) identified 17 studies comparing the cost effectiveness of chiropractic treatment for patients receiving workers' compensation. Chiropractic care was lower in cost in 14 of the studies reviewed. In a follow-up study of workers with back and neck injuries, Johnson et al. (99) showed lower disability costs, provider costs, and compensation payments for chiropractic patients. Mean disability compensation paid was $264 for those treated by chiropractors, $618 for those treated by physicians, and $1,565 for osteopathic patients. Average provider costs for chiropractors and physicians were $223 and $352, respectively. In addition, compensated days lost from work were less for patients treated by chiropractors. According to the authors, in general, fewer workdays were lost and lower amounts of disability compensation and provider costs were paid when chiropractic was included in the care pattern. However, in many of these studies, it is difficult to tell whether patients seeking chiropractic and medical care were identical.

Jarvis (100) and Jarvis et al. (101) looked at total costs for a group of patients with similar reported diagnoses. Costs for compensation of chiropractic patients were $68.38 and $668.39 for patients treated by medical doctors. Treatment costs were more similar between providers, with $527 for chiropractors and $684 for physicians. Stano (102) reported that the average insurance payment to chiropractors was $573, compared to $1,112 for medical doctors. For episodes lasting more than 1 day, the payments to chiropractors were $870 and those to physicians were $2,141. A recent study by Smith and Stano (103) compared health insurance payments and patient outcomes for recurrent episodes of care for low back conditions initiated with chiropractic treatment versus episodes initiated with medical treatment. A total of 7,077 patients were involved in 9,314 episodes of care. Outcome measures included total insurance payments, total outpatient payments, length of episodes (both initial and recurrent), consistent use of initiating providers for recurrent episodes, and time lapsed between episodes. Total insurance payments were substantially greater for medically initiated episodes; however, there was no significant difference of time lapse between episodes. The authors stated that using analysis of recurrent episodes as measures of patient satisfaction, chiropractors retain more patients for subsequent episodes. Both chiropractic and medical patients were comparable on measures of severity; however, the chiropractic group included a greater proportion of chronic cases. Patients who changed providers for multiple episodes were more likely to return to chiropractic providers, suggesting that chronic, recurrent cases may gravitate to chiropractic over time.

This may explain the results of a study of workers' compensation claimants in Oregon by Nyiendo (104), who noted that those attending chiropractors were found to have more treatments over a longer duration and at greater cost than claimants seeking care from medical physicians. The findings were attributed to (a) a higher proportion of chiropractic claimants with low-back risk factors influencing recovery, (b) differences in age and sex, (c) the different nature of physician–patient contact, (d) differences in the therapeutic modalities employed, and (e) allowance of physician reimbursement under Oregon workers' compensation law.

A review of the workers' compensation system of New South Wales, Australia, looked at average chiropractic and medical treatment per case, total compensation payments, and assessments of related indirect costs (105). Approximately 30% of the total reported injuries were back problems. Chiropractic services represented 12% of the total utilization rate for these injuries, with payments of more than $25.2 million (2.4%) for chiropractic and physiotherapy treatments. Analysis of 20 randomly selected cases revealed an average chiropractic treatment cost of $299.65 compared to $647.20 for average medical costs. Shekelle et al. (17) attributed some of these differences to the high cost of diagnostic procedures, hospitalizations, and surgery in the medical group.

The lower cost of chiropractic care in studies, however, may be due to a preapproval program required of chiropractic physicians to control costs in an environment where medical costs escalated in the absence of price controls. A recently published study investigated the effect of managed care preapproval on the cost of workers' compensation claims in Utah (106). Treatment costs between 1986 and 1989 increased 12% for cases managed by chiropractors and 71% for cases managed by physicians, while compensation costs (i.e., wage replacement) increased 21% and 114%, respectively.

If one leaves the workers' compensation field, the results are much less dramatic. Carey et al. (107) noted that the costs for chiropractic care for patients with LBP in general practice were greater than those for care by a primary care practitioner or health maintenance organization physician, and approximated those of an orthopedic surgeon. Similarly, Cherkin et al. (20) demonstrated a higher cost for McKenzie-type physical therapy and chiropractic care compared with the handing out of an informational booklet for only modest long-term effects. Both these studies again showed a high patient satisfaction rate for chiropractic care, which may have driven up the costs by encouraging higher utilization rates.

Return to Work

Several studies have shown that patients receiving chiropractic care recover more quickly and have an overall reduction in time lost from work. In 16 of the 17 studies reviewed by Johnson et al. (98), patients treated by chiropractors had lower time loss from work, compared to those treated by conventional methods. In a comparison of medical and chiropractic management in the Australian workers' compensation system, Ebrall (108) showed that patients receiving chiropractic care had 25% fewer lost workdays, compared to those receiving medical treatment. In the studies by Jarvis (100) and Jarvis et al. (101), the average number of compensation days was 2.7 for patients treated by chiropractors and 20.7 for those seen by medical doctors. Similarly, Nyiendo and Lamm (109) reported that lost work time was less for chiropractic patients compared to patients of medical doctors (9 days versus 34.5 days). Only one study has shown that disability days and costs were greater for patients seen by chiropractors than for those seen by medical doctors or osteopaths (110). The recent study by Cherkin et al. (20) showed no significant difference between the number of days lost from work and reduced activity in the chiropractic group compared with the handing out of a pamphlet, which raises the possibility that medical care in the prior studies actually prolonged disability in the workers' compensation system.

CONCLUSION

Manipulative therapy is a widely utilized approach to patients with occupational musculoskeletal disorders, with the majority of this care offered by chiropractors. Based on controlled clinical trials on the effectiveness of manipulation, it appears to be of benefit in patients with acute LBP and subacute or chronic neck pain. There is a growing body of evidence that manipulation may be effective in treating chronic LBP and headaches, whereas the effectiveness in patients with intervertebral disc herniation with sciatica and radiculopathy is based primarily on noncontrolled case series. One controlled trial showed that manipulation was no more effective than ibuprofen in the treatment of CTS, although there were fewer side effects with manipulation.

An analysis of objective and social outcome measures following SMT are more difficult to analyze. The claims that SMT can increase spinal range of motion, increase straight leg raising, reduce muscle spasm, and cause resorption of herniated intervertebral discs are based primarily on small, noncontrolled case series or reports and have yet to be proven. On the other hand, there is no controversy that patients express a high level of satisfaction with manipulative or chiropractic care that exceeds most other treatment methods. The relative cost of manipulation or chiropractic care appears to depend on the frequency and number of treatments given to patients, whether care is given within the workers' compensations system, and the alternative care to which it is being compared.

REFERENCES

1. Haldeman S, Hooper PD, Phillips RB, Scaringe JG, Traina AD. Spinal manipulative therapy. In: Frymoyer JW, ed. *The adult spine: principles and practice*, 2nd ed. Philadelphia: Lippincott–Raven, 1997, pp. 1837–1861.
2. Bigos SJ. *Acute low back problems in adults.* Rockville, MD: U.S. Department of Health and Human Services, Agency for Health Care Policy and Research, 1994.
3. Scientific approach to the assessment and management of activity-related spinal disorders: a monograph for clinicians. Report of the Quebec task force on spinal disorders. *Spine* 1987;12(7 suppl):S1–S59.
4. Waddell G. *Clinical guidelines for the management of acute low back pain:* clinical guidelines and evidence review. London: Royal College of General Practitioners, 1996.
5. White AH. Integration of chiropractic into managed care in a multidisciplinary setting. *J Manipulative Physiol Ther* 1995;18:626–627.
6. Anderson R, Meeker WC, Wirick BE, Mootz RD, Kirk DH, Adams A. A meta-analysis of clinical trials of spinal manipulation. *J Manipulative Physiol Ther* 1992;15:181–194.
7. Shekelle PG. Spine update: spinal manipulation. *Spine* 1994;19:858–861.
8. Bergmann TF, Peterson DH, Lawrence DJ. *Chiropractic technique*. New York: Churchill-Livingstone, 1993.
9. Dvorak J, Dvorak V, Schneider W. *Manual medicine*. Berlin: Springer-Verlag, 1985.
10. Johnson WL, Allan BR, Hendra JL, et al. Interexaminer study of palpation in detecting location of spinal segmental dysfunction. *J Am Osteopath Assoc* 1983; 82:839–845.
11. Maltezopoulos V, Armitage N. A comparison of four chiropractic systems in the diagnosis of sacroiliac malfunction. *Eur J Chiropr* 1984;32:4–42.
12. Wiles MR. Reproducibility and interexaminer correlation of motion palpation findings of the sacroiliac joints. *J Can Chiropr Assoc* 1980;24:59–69.
13. Hubka MJ. Palpation for tenderness: a reliable and accurate method for identifying the target of spinal manipulation. *Chiropr Tech* 1994;6:5–8.
14. Breen AC. Chiropractors and the treatment of back pain. *Rheumatol Rehabil* 1977;16:46–53.
15. Nyiendo J, Phillips RB, Meeker W, Kunsler G, Jansen R, Menon M. A comparison of patients and patient complaints at six chiropractic college teaching clinics. *J Manipulative Physiol Ther* 1989;12:79–85.
16. Koes BW, Assendelft WJ, van der Heijden GJ, Bouter LM. Spinal manipulation for low back pain: an updated systematic review of randomized clinical trials. *Spine* 1996;21:2860–2871.
17. Shekelle PG, Adams AH, Chassin MR, Hurwitz EL, Brook RB. Spinal manipulation for back pain. *Ann Intern Med* 1992;117:590–598.
18. Hsieh CY, Phillips RB, Adams AH, Pope MH. Functional outcomes of low back pain: comparison of four treatment groups in a randomized controlled trial. *J Manipulative Physiol Ther* 1992;15:4–9 .
19. Blomberg S, Svardsudd K, Tibblin G. A randomized study of manual therapy with steroid injections in low-back pain: telephone interview follow-up of pain, disability, recovery and drug consumption. *Eur Spine J* 1994;3:246–254.
20. Cherkin DC, Deyo RA, Battie M, Street J, Barlow W. A comparison of physical therapy, chiropractic manipulation, and provision of an educational booklet for the treatment of patients with low back pain. *N Engl J Med* 1998;339:1021–1029.
21. Meade TW, Dyer S, Browne W, Townsend J, Frank AO. Low back pain of mechanical origin: randomised comparison of chiropractic and hospital outpatient treatment. *BMJ* 1990;300:1431–1437.
22. Meade TW, Dyer S, Browne W, Frank AO. Randomised comparison of chiropractic and hospital outpatient management for low back pain: results from extended follow-up. *BMJ* 1995;311:349–351.
23. Koes BW, Bouter LM, van Mameren H, et al. Randomized clinical trial of manipulative therapy and physiotherapy for persistent back and neck complaints: results of one-year follow-up. *BMJ* 1992;304: 601–605.
24. van den Hoogen HJ, Koes BW, van Eijk JT, Bouter LM, Deville W. On the course of low back pain in general practice: a one-year follow-up study. *Ann Rheum Dis* 1998;57:13–19.
25. Waagen GN, DeBoer K, Hansen J, McGhee D, Haldeman S. A prospective comparative trial of general practice medical care, chiropractic manipulative therapy and sham manipulation in the management of patients with chronic or repetitive low back pain. Presented at the meeting of the International Society for the Study of the Lumbar Spine, Boston, 1990.
26. Evans DP, Burke MS, Lloyd KN, Roberts EE,

Roberts GM. Lumbar spinal manipulation on trial. Part 1: clinical assessment. *Rheumatol Rehabil* 1978; 17:46–53.

27. Ongley MJ, Klein RG, Droman TA, Eck BC, Hubert LJ. A new approach to the treatment of low back pain. *Lancet* 1987;2:143–146.

28. Koes BW, Bouter LM, van Mameren H, et al. A randomized clinical trial of manual therapy and physiotherapy for persistent back and neck complaints: subgroup analysis and relationship between outcome measures. *J Manipulative Physiol Ther* 1993;16: 211–219.

29. Triano JJ, McGregor M, Hondras MA, Brennan PC. Manipulative therapy versus education programs in chronic low back pain. *Spine* 1995;20:948–955.

30. Bronfort G. Effectiveness of spinal manipulation and adjustment. In: Haldeman S, ed. *Principles and practice of chiropractic*. Norwalk, CT: Appleton & Lange, 1992:415–441.

31. Timm KE. A randomized, controlled study of active and passive treatments for chronic low back pain following L5 laminectomy. *J Orthop Sports Phys Ther* 1994;20:276–286.

32. Gibson T, Grahame R, Harkness J, et al. Controlled comparison of short-wave diathermy treatment with osteopathic treatment in non-specific low back pain. *Lancet* 1985;1:1258–1260.

33. van Tulder MW, Koes BW, Bouter LM, Metsemakers JF. Management of chronic nonspecific low back pain in primary care: a descriptive study. *Spine* 1997;22: 76–82.

34. Nwuga VC. Relative therapeutic efficacy of vertebral manipulation and conventional treatment in back pain management. *Am J Phys Med* 1982;61:273–278.

35. Coxhead CE, Inskp H, Meade TW, North WR, Troup JD. Multicentre trial of physiotherapy in the management of sciatic symptoms. *Lancet* 1981;1:1065–1068.

36. Edwards BC. Low back pain and pain resulting from lumbar spine conditions: a comparison of treatment results. *Aust J Physiother* 1969;15:104–110.

37. Chrisman OD, Mittnacht A, Snook GA. A study of the results following rotatory manipulation in the lumbar intervertebral-disc syndrome. *J Bone Joint Surg Am* 1964;46:517–524.

38. Cassidy JD, Kirkaldy-Willis WH, McGregor M. Spinal manipulation for the treatment of chronic lowback and leg pain: an observational study. In: Buerger AA, Greenman PE, eds. *Empirical approaches to the validation of spinal manipulation*. Springfield, IL: Charles C Thomas, 1985:119–148.

39. Bergmann TF, Jongeward BV. Manipulative therapy in lower back pain with leg pain and neurological deficit. *J Manipulative Physiol Ther* 1998;21:288–294.

40. Polkinghorn BS, Colloca CJ. Treatment of symptomatic lumbar disc herniation using activator methods of chiropractic technique. *J Manipulative Physiol Ther* 1998;21:187–196.

41. Cox JM, Hazen LJ, Mungovan M. Distraction manipulation reduction of an L5-S1 disk herniation. *J Manipulative Physiol Ther* 1993;16:342–346.

42. Hession EF, Donald GD. Treatment of multiple lumbar disk herniations in an adolescent athlete utilizing flexion-distraction and rotational manipulation. *J Manipulative Physiol Ther* 1993;16:185–192.

43. Cassidy JD, Thiel HW, Kirkaldy-Willis WH. Side posture manipulation for lumbar intervertebral disk herniation. *J Manipulative Physiol Ther* 1993;16:96–103.

44. Stern PJ, Cote P, Cassidy JD. A series of consecutive cases of low back pain with radiating leg pain treated by chiropractors. *J Manipulative Physiol Ther* 1995; 18:335–342.

45. Ben-Eliyahu DJ. Magnetic resonance imaging and clinical follow-up: study of 27 patients receiving chiropractic care for cervical and lumbar disc herniations. *J Manipulative Physiol Ther* 1996;19:597–606.

46. Brodin H. Cervical pain and mobilization. *Manual Med* 1982;20:90–94.

47. Howe DH, Newcombe RG, Wade MT. Manipulation of the cervical spine: a pilot study. *J R Coll Gen Pract* 1983;33:574–579.

48. Sloop PR, Smith DS, Boldenberg SRN, Dore C. Manipulation for chronic neck pain: a double-blind controlled study. *Spine* 1982;7:532–535.

49. Ben-Eliyahu DJ. Chiropractic management and manipulative therapy for MRI-documented cervical disk herniation. *J Manipulative Physiol Ther* 1994;17: 177–185.

50. Polkinghorn BS. Treatment of cervical disc protrusions via instrumental chiropractic adjustment. *J Manipulative Physiol Ther* 1998;21:114–121.

51. Hurwitz EL, Aker PD, Adams AH, Meeker WC, Shekelle PG. Manipulation and mobilization of the cervical spine: a systematic review of the literature. *Spine* 1996;21:1746–1760.

52. Aker PD, Gross AR, Goldsmith CH, Peloso P. Conservative management of mechanical neck pain: systemic overview and meta-analysis. *BMJ* 1996;313:1291–1296.

53. Gross AR, Aker PD, Quartly C. Manual therapy in the treatment of neck pain. *Rheum Dis Clin North Am* 1996;22:579–598.

54. Cassidy JD, Lopes AA, Yong-Hing K. The immediate effect of manipulation versus mobilization on pain and range of motion in the cervical spine: a randomized controlled trial. *J Manipulative Physiol Ther* 1992;15: 570–575.

55. Jordan A, Bendix T, Nielsen H, Hansen FR, Host D, Winkel A. Intensive training, physiotherapy, or manipulation for patients with chronic neck pain: a prospective, single-blinded, randomized clinical trial. *Spine* 1998;23:311–318.

56. *Business and health special report:* controlling headache costs. Montvale, NJ: Medical Economics Publishing, 1992.

57. Hubka MJ, Hall TA, Taylor JAM, Hubka MA, Brantingham JW. A new look at the classification of headaches. *Chiropr Tech* 1994;6:49–56.

58. Parker GB, Tupling H, Pryor DS. A controlled trial of cervical manipulation of migraine. *Aust N Z J Med* 1978;8:589–593.

59. Hoyt WH, Schafter F, Bard DA, et al. Osteopathic manipulation in the treatment of muscle contraction headache. *J Am Osteopath Assoc* 1979;78:325–332.

60. Jensen OK, Nielsen FF, Vosmar L. An open study comparing manual therapy with the use of cold packs in the treatment of post-traumatic headache. *Cephalgia* 1990;10:241–250.

61. Bitterli J. Zur Objektivierung der manuellen therapeutischen Beeinflussbarkeit des spondylogenen Kopfschmerzes. *Nervenarzt* 1977;48:259–262.

62. Boline PD, Kassak K, Bronfort G, Nelson C, Anderson

AV. Spinal manipulation vs. amitriptyline for the treatment of chronic, tension-type headaches: a randomized clinical trial. *J Manipulative Physiol Ther* 1995; 18:148–154.

63. Droz J, Crot F. Occipital headaches. *Ann Swiss Chiropr Assoc* 1985;8:127–133.

64. Jirout J. Comments regarding the diagnosis and treatment of dysfunctions in the C2-C3 segment. *Manual Med* 1985;2:16–17.

65. Lewit K. Pain arising in the posterior arch of the atlas. *Eur Neurol* 1977;16:263–269.

66. Livingstone M. Spinal manipulation: a one-year follow-up study. *Can Fam Phys* 1969;15:35–39.

67. Mennell JM. The validation of the diagnosis of joint dysfunction in the synovial joints of the cervical spine. *J Manipulative Physiol Ther* 1990;13:7–12.

68. Schultz D. Occipital neuralgia. *J Am Osteopath Assoc* 1977;76:335–343.

69. Turk Z, Ratkolb O. Mobilization of the cervical spine in chronic headaches. *Manual Med* 1987;3:15–17.

70. Vernon H. Chiropractic manipulative therapy in the treatment of headaches: a retrospective and prospective study. *J Manipulative Physiol Ther* 1982;5: 109–112.

71. Bonebrake AR, Fernandez JE, Marley RJ, Dahalan JB, Kilmer KJ. A treatment for carpal tunnel syndrome: evaluation of objective and subjective measures. *J Manipulative Physiol Ther* 1990;1:507–520.

72. Brzovic Z. Nerve compression syndromes of the arm. *Acta Med Iugosl* 1989;43:373–395.

73. Sucher BM. Myofascial release of carpal tunnel syndrome. *J Am Osteopath Assoc* 1993;93:92–94.

74. Mariano KA, McDougle MA, Tanksley GW. Double-crush syndrome: chiropractic care of an entrapment neuropathy. *J Manipulative Physiol Ther* 1991;14: 262–265.

75. Davis PT, Hulbert JR, Kassak KM, Meyer JJ. Comparative efficacy of conservative medical and chiropractic treatments for carpal tunnel syndrome: a randomized clinical trail. *J Manipulative Physiol Ther* 1998;21: 317–326.

76. Rasmussen GG. Manipulation in low back pain: a randomized clinical trial. *Manuelle Med* 1977;1:8–10.

77. Hviid H. The influence of chiropractic treatment on the rotary mobility of the cervical spine: a kinesiometric and statistical study. *Ann Swiss Chiropr Assoc* 1971;5:31–34.

78. Jirout J. The effect of mobilization of the segmental blockade on the sagittal component of the reaction on lateroflexion of the cervical spine. *Neuroradiology* 1972;3:210–215.

79. Nilsson N, Christensen HW, Hartvigsen J. Lasting changes in passive range of motion after spinal manipulation: a randomized, blind, controlled trial. *J Manipulative Physiol Ther* 1996;19:165–168.

80. Fisk JW. A controlled trial of manipulation in a selected group of patients with low back pain favoring one side. *N Z Med J* 1979;90:288–291.

81. Bergquist-Ulman M, Larsson U. Acute low back pain in industry. *Acta Orthop Scand Suppl* 1977;170: 1–117.

82. Hoehler FK, Tobis JS, Buerger AA. Spinal manipulation for low back pain. *JAMA* 1981;245:1835–1838.

83. Mathews JA, Mills SB, Jenkins VM, et al. Back pain and sciatica: controlled trials of manipulation, traction, sclerosant and epidural injections. *Br J Rheumatol* 1987;26:416–423.

84. Grice AA. Muscle toning changes following manipulation. *J Can Chiropr Assoc* 1974;19(4):29–31.

85. Diebert PW, England RW. Electromyographic studies. I. Consideration in the evaluation of osteopathic therapy. *J Am Osteopath Assoc* 1982;72:221–223.

86. Zhu Y, Haldeman S, Starr A, Seffinger MA, Su SH. Paraspinal evoked cerebral potentials in patients with unilateral low back pain. *Spine* 1993;18:1096–1102.

87. Cyriax J. *Textbook of orthopaedic medicine:* diagnosis of soft tissue lesions, vol 1, 6th ed. London: Bailliere Tindall, 1971.

88. Matthews JA, Yates DAH. Reduction of lumbar disc prolapse by manipulation. *BMJ* 1969;3:696–697.

89. Cox JM. *Low back pain*, 3rd ed. Fort Wayne, IN: 1980. (Self-published.)

90. Cherkin DC and MacCormack FA. Patient evaluation of low back pain care from family physicians and chiropractors. *West J Med* 1989;150:351–355.

91. Manga P, Angus DE, Papadopoulos C, Swan WR. A study to examine the effectiveness and cost-effectiveness of chiropractic management of low back pain. Ontario Ministry of Health, Ottawa, 1993.

92. Pope MH, Phillips RB, Haugh LD, Hsieh CY, MacDonald L, Halderman S. A prospective randomized three-week trial of spinal manipulation, transcutaneious muscle stimulation, massage and corset in the treatment of subacute low back pain. *Spine* 1994;19: 2571–2577.

93. Sanchez JE. A look in the mirror: a critical and exploratory study of public perceptions of the chiropractic profession in New Jersey. *J Manipulative Physiol Ther* 1991;14:165–176.

94. Sandhu DJ, Schoner B. *Images of and attitudes toward B.C. health professionals:* a study prepared for the B.C. *Chiropractic Association.* Vancouver, BC, 1992. (Unpublished.)

95. Sawyer CE, Kassak K. Patient satisfaction with chiropractic care. *J Manipulative Physiol Ther* 1993;16: 25–32.

96. Wardwell WI. The Connecticut survey of public attitudes toward chiropractic. *J Manipulative Physiol Ther* 1989;12:167–173.

97. Verhoef MJ, Page SA, Waddell SC. The chiropractic outcome study: pain, functional ability, and satisfaction with care. *J Manipulative Physiol Ther* 1997;20: 76–82.

98. Johnson MR, Ferguson AC, Swank LL. Treatment and cost of back or neck injury: a literature review. *Res Forum* 1985(spring):68–78.

99. Johnson MR, Schultz MK, Ferguson AC. A comparison of chiropractic, medical and osteopathic care for work-related sprains and strains. *J Manipulative Physiol Ther* 1989;12:335–344.

100. Jarvis KB. Cost per case analysis of Utah industrial back injury claims: chiropractic management versus medical management for diagnostically equivalent conditions. Datatrace Publications. *DC Tracts* 1989;1: 67–79.

101. Jarvis KB, Phillips RB, Morris EK. Cost per case comparison of back injury claims of chiropractic versus medical management for conditions with identical diagnostic codes. *J Occup Med* 1991;33:847–852.

102. Stano M. A comparison of health care costs for chiro-

practic and medical patients. *J Manipulative Physiol Ther* 1993;16:291–299.

103. Smith M, Stano M. Costs and recurrences of chiropractic and medical episodes of low-back care. *J Manipulative Physiol Ther* 1997;20:5–12.

104. Nyiendo J. Disabling low back Oregon workers' compensation claims. Part III: diagnostic and treatment procedures and associated costs. *J Manipulative Physiol Ther* 1991;14:287–297.

105. Tuchin PJ, Bonello R. Preliminary findings of analysis of chiropractic utilization and cost in the workers' compensation system of New South Wales, Australia. *J Manipulative Physiol Ther* 1995;18:503–511.

106. Jarvis KB, Phillips RB, Danielson C. Managed care preapproval and its effect on the cost of Utah worker compensation claims. *J Manipulative Physiol Ther* 1997;20.372–376.

107. Carey TS, Garrett J, Jackman A, McLaughlin C, Fryer J, Smucker DR. The outcomes and costs of care for acute low back pain among patients seen by primary care practitioners, chiropractors, and orthopedic surgeons. The North Carolina Back Pain Project. *N Eng J Med* 1995;333:913–917.

108. Ebrall PS. Mechanical low-back pain: a comparison of medical and chiropractic management within the Victorian workcare system. *Chiropr J Aust* 1992;22:47–53.

109. Nyiendo J, Lamm L. Disabling low back Oregon workers' compensation claims. Part I: methodology and clinical categorization of chiropractic and medical cases. *J Manipulative Physiol Ther* 1991;3:177–184.

110. Greenwood JG. *Report on work-related back and neck injury cases in West Virginia:* issues related to chiropractic and medical costs. West Virginia Workers' Compensation Fund, Charleston, WV, 1983.

Occupational Musculoskeletal Disorders
edited by T. G. Mayer, R. J. Gatchel, and P. B. Polatin.
Lippincott Williams & Wilkins, Philadelphia © 2000.

26

Injection Procedures

*Carl Edward Noe, †Noor M. Gajraj, and †Akshay S. Vakharia

*Eugene McDermott Center for Pain Management; †Department of Anesthesiology and
Pain Management, University of Texas Southwestern Medical Center, Dallas, Texas 75235*

Injections are common procedures in the occupational medicine setting (1) and may be performed at a number of anatomic sites (Table 1). They may be used not only therapeutically but also diagnostically to identify pain generators and prognostically to predict the outcome of more invasive procedures. This chapter discusses common injections (Table 2) with reference to relevant studies that have changed clinical opinion or practice significantly.

Various needles and medications are used, but as optimal techniques have not been established by well designed clinical studies, choices are largely determined by physician preference. The use of insulated needles during selective nerve blocks and subsequent stimulation may facilitate accuracy. Neurologic examination before and after blocks is sometimes helpful; pain relief without motor or sensory changes indicates that the sympathetic pathway may be responsible for pain transmission. Performing the blocks on separate occasions using local anesthetics (LAs) with different durations of action is also

TABLE 2. *Injection procedures*

Peripheral nerve blocks
Selective nerve root block
Medial branch blocks
Continuous brachial plexus block
Neurolysis of the dorsal root ganglion
Sympathetic nerve blocks
Cervical sympathetic nerve blocks
Thoracic sympathetic nerve blocks
Lumbar sympathetic nerve blocks
Percutaneous neurolytic lumbar sympathetic
  procedure
Percutaneous neurolytic thoracic sympathetic
  procedure
Piriformis injection
Joint injections
Sacroiliac joint injections
Facet joint blocks
Lumbar facet injections
Cervical facet injections
Cervical facet denervation
Lumbar facet denervation
Bursae injections
Tendon injections
Trigger-point and tender-point injections
Epidural steroid injections
Intrathecal baclofen (Lioresal) injections

sometimes helpful. Common problems with injection procedures include low efficacy in the presence of high patient expectations and lack of an interdisciplinary approach.

Neurolytic blockade has recently received increased critical interest. Analgesia following prognostic nerve blocks with LA has been shown to correlate poorly with relief of chronic pain following nerve resection (2). Numerous mechanisms exist to account for the discrepancy (3). Interpretation of diagnos-

TABLE 1. *Anatomical sites for injection*

Peripheral nerve
Nerve plexus
Dorsal root ganglion
Sympathetic nerve
Muscle, joint, tendon, and bursae
Epidural space
Subarachnoid space

tic blocks is frequently confounded by placebo responses, responses to sedation, systemic analgesia from LAs, and other, less defined neurologic phenomena.

AGENTS AND TECHNIQUES

Saline, LAs, opioids, and corticosteroids have been used for a variety of injections into and around muscles, tendons, joints, bursae, neuromas, peripheral nerves, and the epidural and subarachnoid spaces. More recently, sodium hyaluronate, ketorolac tromethamine (Toradol), clonidine hydrochloride (Catapres), botulinum toxin, and a variety of other agents have also been injected for pain relief.

LAs block sodium channels in nerves, preventing depolarization and conduction of nociceptive impulses. The longest-acting LAs only last for hours, and high concentrations of LA may be neurotoxic. However, the duration of analgesia often far exceeds the LA's duration of action.

Corticosteroids have an antiinflammatory effect by inhibiting phospholipase A_2, and they may inhibit neuronal excitation directly (4). There has been some evidence that prostaglandins enhance neurotransmitter release from primary afferent neurons and play a role in spinal sensitization for pain. These and related actions may occur both peripherally and centrally.

Alcohol and phenol have been used for a variety of neurolytic procedures. Alcohol dehydrates nerves and extracts cholesterol and phospholipids, while phenol coagulates proteins. Both alcohol and phenol produce nonselective nerve damage and wallerian degeneration. Alcohol neuritis is a potential complication. The block produced by phenol tends to be less profound and of shorter duration than that produced by alcohol.

Cryoneurolysis involves freezing a peripheral nerve, leaving the perineurium intact so that regeneration can occur. Gas is expanded through an orifice producing a temperature drop by the Joule-Thompson effect. Gas-expansion cryoprobes usually produce temperatures of $-70°C$ to $-80°C$, and nitrous oxide is most commonly used. Cryoprobe lesions are not nearly as well controlled as radiofrequency (RF) lesions.

RF thermocoagulation utilizes alternating electrical current in the 1-MHz range. Current movement generates heat as it passes through tissues. A large surface electrode is placed on the skin, and care is taken to avoid passage of current across electrically sensitive structures such as the heart. High (sensory) and low (motor) frequency stimulation can be performed prior to thermocoagulation to ensure accurate placement of a lesion. The active tip of the RF probe is placed along the axis of a nerve to be lysed. The tissue temperature can be monitored during lesion formation. In addition to the length and diameter of the active probe tip, temperature is among primary determinants of lesion size. At a given temperature, the size of the lesion plateaus after about 60 seconds. The lesion is relatively well circumscribed compared to that made with older, direct-current or other neurolytic techniques. Temperatures greater than 90°C should be avoided to prevent tissue boiling and adherence to the probe tip.

COMPLICATIONS

Several principles are important to minimize the risk of complications and other adverse outcomes. A needle should be placed directly onto the target with the minimum of failed attempts. When injections are performed around the neural axis, fluoroscopy may be used to minimize complications, especially when LAs or neurolytic agents are used. Intravenous access and monitoring of vital signs and oxygen saturation are necessary when LA is injected around the neural axis, when large doses of LA are injected, or when intravenous sedation is administered. Aspiration is performed prior to any injection to avoid intravascular or subarachnoid placement. Correct needle placement is also facilitated by the use of radiopaque nonionized dye. To avoid major complications during blind injections (without radiographic guidance) at the level of the pleura, foramen magnum, or cranial nerve foramen, relatively short needles are recommended.

Neurologic complications following injection of neurolytic solutions include neurologic deficits due to intravascular and intrathecal spread. Epidural abscess, hematoma, arachnoiditis, and total spinal blocks are uncommon but very real risks with spinal procedures. Overdose of LA, steroid, or sedative is another serious concern. Adequate monitoring and resuscitation equipment are essential. The incidence of neuritis and catastrophic complications due to spread of neurolytic solutions is probably reduced by the use of RF thermocoagulation and cryoneurolysis.

PERIPHERAL NERVE BLOCKS

Peripheral nerve blocks are frequently used as diagnostic maneuvers with peripheral nerve entrapments, particularly in the upper extremity (Fig 1). Common peripheral nerve entrapment syndromes include carpal tunnel syndrome, median nerve entrapment, ulnar nerve entrapment at the elbow, ulnar nerve entrapment at the wrist, radial nerve entrapment, thoracic outlet syndromes, digital nerve entrapments in the hand, sciatic nerve entrapment, peroneal nerve entrapment, tarsal tunnel syndrome, and lateral femoral cutaneous nerve entrapment. Injection responses correlate poorly with outcomes following ablative procedures (2). Neuroma injections are commonly per-

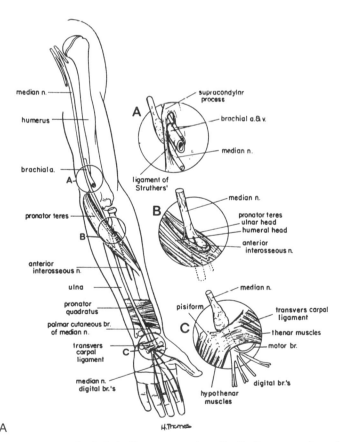

FIG. 1. Nerve entrapments particularly in the upper extremity. **A:** Common sites of median nerve entrapment: A, supracondylar; B, pronator teres; C, carpal tunnel. *(Continued on next page)*

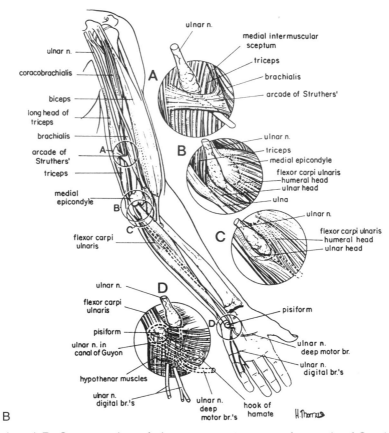

FIG. 1. *Continued.* **B:** Common sites of ulnar nerve entrapment: A, arcade of Struthers; B, cubital tunnel; C, flexor carpi ulnaris; D, Guyon's tunnel. *Continued.*

formed on both a diagnostic and a therapeutic basis with variable results. Peripheral nerve blocks are best performed with small-gauge needles after skin wheal placement with LA. Paresthesias should be avoided, and neuromuscular stimulation is sometimes helpful.

Carpal tunnel syndrome is a diagnosis being made with increasing frequency. Injections have been shown to be helpful for predicting outcomes following decompression (5). The ulnar bursa may be injected with LA and corticosteroid rather than injecting the carpal tunnel and risking injection or trauma to the median nerve.

Cryoneurolysis of the ilioinguinal nerve has been shown to reduce pain and opioid consumption, as well as improving mobility and return-to-work status following herniorrhaphy (6). Cryoneurolysis has been used for ilioinguinal neuralgia following inguinal herniorrhaphy and for a variety of peripheral neuralgias affecting predominately sensory nerves, including neuromas of the occipital and lateral femoral cutaneous nerves. Although intercostal cryoneurolysis has been shown to be inferior to thoracic epidural fentanyl following thoracotomy (7), the postthoracotomy syndrome will sometimes respond well to intercostal nerve blocks with LA and corticosteroid.

SELECTIVE NERVE ROOT BLOCKS

Selective nerve root blocks have been shown to correlate with surgical findings better than myelography in patients treated previously with surgery (8). Selective nerve root blocks should be performed under fluoro-

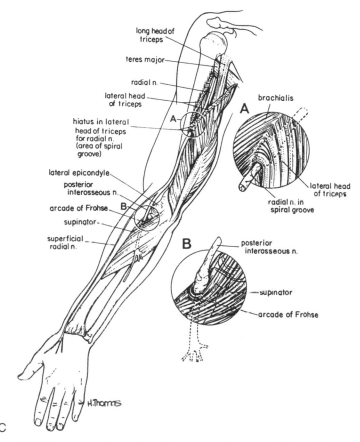

FIG. 1. *Continued.* **C:** Common sites of radial nerve entrapment: A, spiral groove; B, arcade of Frohse. (From Ruskin A. *Current therapy and physiatry*. Philadelphia: WB Saunders Co, 1984:309, 312, 314; with permission.).

scopic visualization, with care being taken to avoid nerve trauma with the needle or volume of injectate. After confirmation of needle placement with fluoroscopy and radiographic contrast injection, a small volume and dose of short-acting LA can be injected together with a small dose of aqueous corticosteroid. Aspiration and contrast injection are particularly important, as the subdural space may follow the nerve root laterally to the foramen. Selective nerves may be blocked with the patient in the prone position for thoracic and lumbar levels, and with the patient supine for cervical levels. The approach is similar for facet injections, the needle being directed more anteriorly toward the posterosuperior aspect of the neural foramen. Paresthesias should be avoided, and aspiration test and contrast injection are important. The S-1 nerve root can be blocked via the posterior S-1 foramen.

Medial Branch Blocks

The medial branch of the dorsal primary ramus of the spinal nerves supplies the facet joint and the supraspinous and interspinous ligaments. Medial branch blocks can be performed at the mediosuperior aspect of the transverse process at the thoracic and lumbar levels, at the sacral ala and superior aspect of the S-1 foramen at the lumbosacral junction, and at the midbody of a cervical vertebral body posterior to the neural foramen at the cervical levels. Patient positioning and the use of fluoroscopy are similar for facet joint injections at the respective level. Neuromuscular stimulation is useful to confirm accurate needle placement and minimize the volume of LA required for a diagnostic medial branch block.

Continuous Brachial Plexus Block

Placement of a catheter in the axillary sheath allows continuous analgesia for upper extremity pain. This technique is a good alterative to epidural analgesia and is associated with fewer complications. Catheter dislodgement can occur, as with interscalene catheters and other percutaneous infusion techniques. A Crawford epidural needle can be advanced toward the palpated axillary artery in the axillary sheath, with the bevel of the needle inverted to prevent traumatic damage. An initial skin and superficial subcutaneous puncture with a sharp needle of the same size is necessary to allow easy passage of the Crawford needle into the axillary sheath, where resistance will be experienced. The inverted Crawford needle can be bluntly advanced into the sheath without trauma to the contents of the sheath. After a negative aspiration test, a catheter can be advanced into the axillary sheath and secured with suture laced along the catheter. Continuous infusion with bupivacaine 0.125%, 5 to 10 mL per hour, will provide sympathetic blockade and significant analgesia for the distal upper extremity with minimal risk from LA toxicity.

Neurolysis of Dorsal Root Ganglion

Dorsal root ganlgionotomies are performed only after more conservative interventional therapies have failed. They are usually reserved for either radiculopathy or pain related to a specific and well defined dermatome and should be preceded by diagnostic selective nerve root blocks.

Ganglionotomies may be performed at the cervical, thoracic, lumbar, and sacral levels. In a study of patients with cervicobrachialgia, RF thermocoagulation of the cervical spinal dorsal ganglia produced significant reduction of pain scores. However, no difference was shown between a lesion produced at 40°C versus 67°C (9). An important potential advantage of the 40°C lesions is that nerve damage related side effects may be reduced, although the study did not demonstrate this. Contralateral hemiparesis has been reported with this technique and was thought to be caused by a steal syndrome (10).

Sympathetic Nerve Blocks

Reflex sympathetic dystrophy or complex regional pain syndrome is frequently treated with sympathetic blockade. While many would advocate the early use of sympathetic blockade for this disorder, strong data supporting this practice are lacking. Nevertheless, cervical sympathetic blocks are frequently associated with pain relief from sympathetically maintained pain involving the head and upper extremity. Upper thoracic sympathetic blocks are also useful in some patients with upper extremity sympathetically maintained pain. For sympathetically maintained pain involving the knee, lumbar sympathetic blocks at the L-2 level may be helpful. It is frequently necessary to perform a block at the L-4 and L-5 levels for sympathetically maintained pain involving the foot.

Cervical Sympathetic Block

The paratracheal approach for cervical sympathetic block is recommended. Intravenous access is necessary for both the treatment of complications and the provision of sedation. Appropriate monitoring includes pulse oximetry, continuous electrocardiography, and blood pressure monitoring. The patient is positioned in the supine position with the cervical spine extended.

A skin wheal of LA can be placed one fingerbreadth inferior to the cricoid cartilage, lateral to the trachea. Fluoroscopic guidance may be reserved for patients with morbid obesity or other anatomic abnormalities. A 1.5-inch, 25-gauge needle is advanced toward the C-7 vertebral body at a slightly medial direction. Bony contact should be made at a depth of 2.5 to 3.2 cm. If bony contact is not made, then the needle should be withdrawn, as it may be too lateral and therefore too close to the nerve roots and vertebral artery. The angle of insertion should be approximately 15 degrees medial. Once bony contact is made, the needle should be withdrawn approximately 2 mm to place the needle tip anterior to the longus coli muscle. If blood or clear fluid is aspirated prior to injection, then the procedure should be repeated using a fresh needle or postponed until another day; 5 mL of ropivacaine 0.2% (Naropin) or 1% lidocaine (Xylocaine) may be injected for the block.

Thoracic Sympathetic Block

Thoracic sympathetic blocks should be performed using fluoroscopy with the patient in the prone position. Following the injection of LA and intravenous sedation, an intravenous cannula is directed toward the space between the lateral aspect of the spine and the pleura. A blunt-tipped needle can then be advanced through the cannula to the lateral aspect of the vertebral body. This procedure must be performed using fluoroscopy, and the risk of pneumothorax is relatively high on the right side. Injection of radiographic contrast following aspiration is important prior to the placement of approximately 3 mL of LA for a diagnostic block.

Lumbar Sympathetic Block

Lumbar sympathetic block is also performed using fluoroscopy with the patient in the prone position. A 7-inch, 22-gauge needle can be advanced from a skin entry point 6 to 8 cm lateral to the midline. The needle can be advanced just inferior to the transverse process at the respective level to pass superior to the nerve root at that level. Oblique fluoroscopic visualization allows placement to the anterolateral aspect of the vertebral body with a minimal amount of redirection attempts. Radiographic contrast injections should be performed with fluoroscopic visualization in

the anteroposterior and lateral projections to ensure placement along the lumbar sympathetic chain distribution. For the block, 3 to 10 mL of 0.2% ropivacaine or 0.25% bupivacaine can be injected in 3-mL increments. If multiple levels require blockade, the volume of LA should be reduced at each level to avoid LA toxicity.

Percutaneous Neurolytic Lumbar Sympathetic Procedure

In a comparison of phenol neurolysis to RF thermocoagulation for percutaneous lumbar sympatholysis, phenol was associated with more effective sympatholysis but was also associated with a higher incidence of postsympathectomy neuralgia (11). However, a modified technique with a more extensive pattern of lesions produced results comparable to phenol neurolysis (12).

Lumbar sympathetic RF thermocoagulation is performed with the patient in the prone position. Under local anesthesia a 15-cm RF probe with a 10-mm exposed active electrode is inserted. The skin entry point should be made 7 to 8 cm lateral to the midline just inferior to the transverse process at the lumbar levels. Lesions are most commonly placed at the L-2, L-3, and L-4 levels. The L-2 level is particularly important if knee pain is present. In patients with distal leg pain, a lesion may be required at the L-5 level. Oblique fluoroscopic visualization is helpful to minimize the number of passes and avoid medial placement within the spine or lateral placement into the kidney. Lateral fluoroscopic viewing facilitates placement of the probe inferior to the transverse process and superior to the neural foramen. This is thought to significantly reduce the incidence of lumbar nerve root paresthesia. The probe is advanced, but the tip should not pass anterior to the vertebral body. Low-frequency stimulation at 2 Hz is important to rule out neuromuscular activity in the lower extremities resulting from any cracks in insulation that could cause a nerve root lesion. Aspiration and contrast injection should be performed routinely, and 1 mL of LA should be injected for anesthesia prior to lesion formation. A single lesion at 80°C for 1 minute is adequate for each lumbar level. Corticosteroid and LA may be injected following lesion placement and may reduce the incidence of postsympatholysis neuralgia.

Percutaneous Neurolytic Thoracic Sympathetic Blockade

RF lesioning of the sympathetic chain was pioneered by Wilkinson (13), who reported on his extensive experience with the thoracic chain in patients with palmar hyperhidrosis and sympathetically maintained pain. His original technique has been modified to place a series of two to three lesions along the axis of the thoracic sympathetic chain at the T-2 and T-3 levels. The procedure is performed with the patient in the prone position. The skin entry point is made just lateral to the vertebral body between the ribs. Care is needed to avoid pleural puncture, especially on the right side where the pleura is more medial. A cannula is used to guide an electrode with a 10-mm active, blunt tip to the lateral aspect of the vertebral body. The thoracic sympathetic chain sits in a posterior position at a point near the junction of the anterior two-thirds of the body with the posterior one-third. Aspiration, contrast injection, and low-frequency (2 Hz), high-voltage (4 V) stimulation should be performed prior to lesion formation.

Piriformis Injection

Piriformis syndrome is a benign myofascial pain disorder that may mimic other causes of low back pain (14,15). The piriformis muscle arises from the inner aspect of the sacrum, stretches over the sciatic notch, and crosses the sciatic nerve to insert into the greater trochanter. The sciatic nerve may be compressed within the buttock by the muscle, resulting in pain that is increased by muscular contraction, palpation, or prolonged sitting. The muscle may be injected with the patient in the lateral position with the affected side up. The tender area may be identified by

transrectal palpation. A spinal needle is placed into the buttock toward the identified area, which may be injected using 5 mL of 0.25% bupivacaine.

JOINT INJECTIONS

Intrarticular injections with LAs and corticosteroid are performed on most joints. Hyaluronate is approved for injection for osteoarthritis of the knee. In many cases, fluoroscopy and arthrography are necessary for accurate needle placement. A systematic review on steroid injections for shoulder disorders indicates that the evidence for their efficacy is scarce and what there is shows poor effect (16).

Sacroiliac Joint Injections

Sacroiliac joint injections may be increasing, as there has been increased interest in this joint as a source of pain. However, Dreyfus et al. (17) found a poor correlation between history and physical examination findings and analgesia with LA injected into the sacroiliac joint. The "gold standard" for diagnosing sacroiliac joint pain remains elusive.

With the patient in the prone position, fluoroscopy is used to confirm accurate delivery of LA and steroid; 10 to 20 degrees of contralateral rotation may facilitate visualization of the joint space. A 3.5-inch, 22-gauge spinal needle is advanced into the lower one-third of the joint. For each joint, 3 mL of 0.25% bupivacaine and 40 mg of methylprednisolone are adequate. It is not clear whether intraarticular spread is necessary to achieve efficacy. Pain relief after injection may actually be related to infiltration of the sacroiliac ligament or sacrospinalis muscle.

Facet Blocks

Facet or zygapophyseal joint injections remain controversial (18,19). Patterns of pain from spinal joints have been described for atlantooccipital, lateral atlantoaxial, cervical, thoracic, and lumbar facet joints (20–23) (Fig 2.)

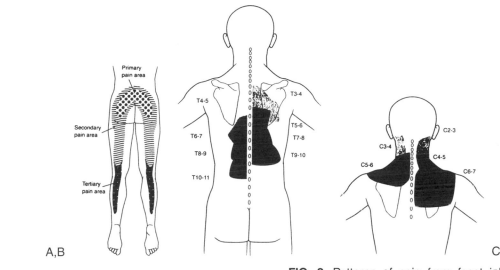

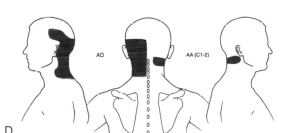

A,B

C

D

FIG. 2. Patterns of pain from facet joints. **A:** Lumbar zygapophyseal. **B:** Thoracic zygapophyseal. **C:** Cervical zygapophyseal. **D:** Atlantoaxial joint pain distribution. **B–D:** Sketches of the average pain referral patterns reported by volunteers subjected to provocative injections. (From Cousins MJ, Bridenbaugh PO, eds.: *Neural blockade in clinical anesthesia and management of pain.* Philadelphia: Lippincott–Raven Publishers, 1998; with permission.)

Lumbar Facet Injections

Injections have been shown to be ineffective in most patients with chronic low back pain (24). However, in patients who experienced relief of low back pain with LA medial branch blocks, subsequent steroid injection produced significant analgesia at 6-month follow-up as compared with saline controls. Responses to facet injection have been shown to correlate poorly with both operative arthrodesis and nonsurgical management (25).

Cervical Facet Injections

Cervical facet injections can be performed with the patient in the supine or prone position. Some physicians prefer the supine position whenever possible because of easier airway access when sedation is required. In the supine position, oblique fluoroscopic images allow visualization of the facet joint, as well as the neural foramen. Skin entry points are made directly lateral to the axis of the joints. A 1.5-inch, 25-gauge needle is suitable for most patients, and it can be directed medially using intermittent fluoroscopy in the oblique view. It is suggested that the image intensifier be oriented so that the radiation source is anterior to the patient and the beam passes from a point anterolateral to the cervical spine on the ipsilateral side, along an axis directed posteromedially away from the operator. Bony contact with the joints is usually made at a depth of 2.5 to 3.2 cm. Anteroposterior fluoroscopic viewing should be performed to ensure that the needle has not passed medially into the vertebral artery or subarachnoid space. Care should be taken while the needle is advanced using the oblique view to ensure the needle does not pass into the neural foramen. Following a negative aspiration test, 1 mL of 0.25% bupivacaine with 10 mg of methylprednisolone may be injected into each joint.

Cervical Facet Denervation

In a study of patients who were followed-up for 8 months or more, RF facet denervation was shown to produce superior analgesia, compared with a sham procedure (26). This study reported a refined technique requiring parasagittal and oblique lesions. However, 5 (42%) of 12 patients had sensory deficits following the procedure.

Lumbar Facet Denervation

Lumbar facet denervation seems to be relatively safe, and cryoneurolysis is probably a safe alternative to RF denervation at the lumbar level. Lumbar facet denervations should not be performed based on responses to facet joint injections, but rather only after interpretation of selective medial branch blocks. It is easier to place an effective lesion at the medial aspect of the transverse process using cryoneurolysis. However, effective results can be obtained using RF thermocoagulation, and the smaller-sized RF probe has advantages. The procedure is performed with the patient in the prone position. Noninvasive monitoring should be applied including pulse oximetry before intravenous sedation is administered.

With cryoneurolysis, the exact angle of approach to the medial branch is less important because the cryoprobe lesion is larger than a RF thermocoagulation lesion. However, with the RF technique, the needle should enter the skin inferomedial to the medial branch on a particular transverse process. This approach will align the axis of the nerve with the RF probe, resulting in a longer lesion. High-frequency (50 Hz), low-voltage (1 V) stimulation may be performed to reproduce the patient's chronic pain. More important, low-frequency (2 Hz) stimulation at up to 4 V is used to rule out neuromuscular activity in the lower extremity. This will minimize the risk of a nerve root lesion. In contrast to the undesirability of neuromuscular activity in the lower extremities, neuromuscular activity in the paraspinous muscles is desired prior to

lesion formation because the medial branch innervates them. Following an injection of 0.5 mL of 1% lidocaine, a lesion at 80°C for 1 minute is recommended. Corticosteroid and LA may be injected following lesion placement, which may reduce the incidence and severity of neuritis.

At the lumbosacral junction, lesions should be placed at the sacral ala and at points between the L5-S1 facet joints and the posterior S-1 foramen. RF probes with curved tips may improve results at these sites because the segmental lesion is relatively short when the active tip is placed perpendicular to the nerve.

BURSA INJECTIONS

Common bursae that may be injected include the subacromial, trochanteric, ischial, prepatellar, infrapatellar, olecranon, calcaneal, and retrocalcaneal bursa (Fig. 3).

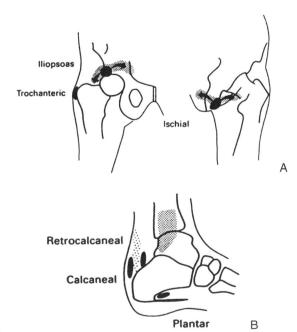

FIG. 3. Common bursa injections. **A:** Hip. **B:** Hindfoot. *Continued.*

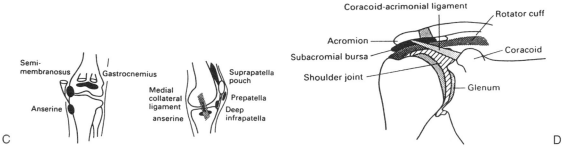

FIG. 3. *Continued.* **C:** Knee. **D:** Coronal section of the shoulder. (From Hutton C. Regional problems of the arm and leg in adults. Maddison PJ, Isenberg PW, Glass DN, eds. *Oxford textbook of rheumatology.* Oxford: Oxford University Press, 1993; pp. 70–77, with permission.)

TENDON INJECTIONS

Tendinitis commonly involves the rotator cuff, biceps, Achilles, or de Quervain's tendons. Medial and lateral epicondylitis, stenosing tenosynovitis, iliotibial band syndrome, and plantar fasciitis are other common syndromes sometimes treated with injections.

TRIGGERPOINT AND TENDER-POINT INJECTIONS

Myofascial triggerpoints and fibromyalgia tender points have been injected with a variety of substances but most commonly with LAs (27). Triggerpoint injections should be performed after sterile preparation of the skin. The triggerpoint should be palpated with one fingertip. The triggerpoint is the most tender point in a muscle, not a point of muscle contraction that may also be tender. A 30-gauge needle can be introduced next to the operator's finger at an angle to produce placement immediately under the fingertip to the triggerpoint. A twitch response immediately adjacent to the muscle is thought to be a good sign. Although all LAs have a similar therapeutic effect, 1 mL of 0.25% bupivacaine is commonly injected as a bolus, or 1 to 2 mL can be infiltrated to ensure analgesia of the triggerpoint. Care should be taken when triggerpoint injections involve the thoracic body wall. Pneumothorax can be produced, especially in patients who are thin. Using a 1.5-inch, 30-gauge needle, directing the needle at an oblique angle, and using superficial injections can minimize the risk of pneumothorax.

EPIDURAL STEROID INJECTIONS

A large percentage of injection procedures are related to spinal pain. Epidural steroids have been used in a number of conditions producing radicular pain, including lumbar disc disease, spinal stenosis, and the postlaminectomy syndrome. Pain relief is achieved by a reduction of nerve root inflammation. Although studies support the beneficial effect of this procedure (28–30), it still remains controversial (31). Bush and Hillier (32) demonstrated clinical improvement of sciatica at 1 month and 12 months following caudal epidurals. Epidural steroids have been shown to be moderately effective in relieving radicular pain in acute lumbar disc herniation (33). In this study, epidural steroid injections were associated with an improvement in sensory function and reduced medication use. However, the study did not show a reduction in the percentage of cases proceeding to surgical therapy. The use of depot preparations for epidural steroid injections has been controversial. However, there is thought to be a sufficient amount of clinical experience with methylprednisolone acetate (Depo-Medrol) to justify its continued use. As with most treatments for midline spinal pain with a radicular component, epidural steroids seem to be most effective for the radicular component. Factors associated with failure of lumbar epidural steroid injections include prolonged duration of symptoms, nonradicular diagnosis, lack of employment, and smoking (34).

This procedure may be performed via the sacral hiatus (caudal approach) or at the lumbar, thoracic, or cervical levels. In a study of patients with neck pain, epidural steroid injections produced good or very good pain relief in 76% (35). Epidural steroid injections may be performed with the patient in the sitting, lateral, or prone position. The prone position is preferable if fluoroscopic guidance is necessary. Fluoroscopic guidance is particularly useful in obese patients and those who have had previous back surgery. The lateral view, as well as the use of contrast injection, may be helpful. A loss-of-resistance technique is preferred. This technique requires advancement of the epidural needle with one hand while the other hand is firmly compressed against the patient's back. This technique avoids movement of the back and stabilizes the operator's hand and needle. The risk of sudden increases in needle depth is therefore minimized. The operator intermittently and gently attempts to inject fluid through the needle. While the needle tip is placed in ligament, advancement of the plunger will be countered by a consistent resistance. Once the needle tip is advanced into the epidural space, this consistent resistance is lost, hence the name of the technique. Fluid in the syringe can be either saline or air. The principal advantage of using air is that flow of cerebrospinal fluid is not misidentified as saline. The disadvantage of using air is that air injected in the subdural space may produce headache in some patients. Injection of air could theoretically introduce infection and may also cause venous air embolism. Methylprednisolone acetate at a dose of approximately 1 mg/kg is commonly injected.

INTRATHECAL BACLOFEN INJECTION

Intrathecal baclofen (Lioresal) may be used for spasticity associated with spinal cord in-

jury, cerebral palsy, or head injury when oral therapy has been unsuccessful in terms of efficacy or side effects. A trial is performed by injecting a test dose of 50 to 75 µg. The decrease in spasticity is assessed using the Ashworth scale, and the degree of motor weakness is also assessed (36). Continuous intrathecal baclofen via an implanted catheter and pump may then be considered.

FUTURE DIRECTIONS

Injection procedures are well incorporated into the practice of occupational medicine. However, with a growing trend toward evidence-based medicine, clinical practice will reflect the results of well designed clinical trials. The effect of procedures on long-term patient outcome is likely to receive particular attention.

Neurolytic blockade should continue to be reserved for patients who not only respond profoundly to prognostic blockade but also have also been thoroughly evaluated; they should have complied with and failed more conservative treatment. Comprehensive evaluation should include a medical assessment of both the sensory and emotional component of pain. More conservative treatment includes pharmacotherapy and neuroaugmentation. An interdisciplinary pain management evaluation is likely to identify significant opportunities to improve quality of life and functional status.

Prolonged neural blockade with LA can be performed with infusion techniques, and in the future there may be injectable, biodegradable drug delivery systems such as microspheres (37).

Several other percutaneous procedures are quite popular but are both controversial and costly. Discography is problematic, as it is difficult to interpret this provocative test. Trials of spinal opioid injections need to be performed meticulously. There are no conclusive studies demonstrating superior efficacy over other treatments. Percutaneous trials of dorsal column stimulation have been shown to reduce failure rates from implanted dorsal column stimulators. However, without a specific lesion, implanted dorsal column stimulators have been shown to be superior only to rhizotomy and surgical reexploration.

Interdisciplinary pain evaluations should be performed on a more frequent basis than is currently the practice for patients who are being evaluated for implantable devices or major procedures. Additionally, until better data are available, caution should be employed in the interpretation of responses to percutaneous procedures as dictating the need for more expensive and invasive procedures.

REFERENCES

1. Falco FJ. Lumbar spine injection procedures in the management of low back pain. *Occup Med* 1998;13: 121–149.
2. Noordenbos W, Wall PD. Implications of the failure of nerve resections and graft to cure chronic pain produced by nerve lesions. *J Neurol Neurosurg Psychiatry* 1981;44:1068–1073.
3. Hogan QH, Abram SE. Neural blockade for diagnosis and prognosis: a review. *Anesthesiology* 1997;86: 216–241.
4. Johansson A, Hao J, Sjolund B. Local corticosteroid application blocks transmission in normal nociceptive C-fibers. *Acta Anaesthesiol Scand* 1990;34:335–338.
5. Green DP. Diagnostic and therapeutic value of carpal tunnel injection. *J Hand Surg [Am]* 1984;9:850–854.
6. Wood GJ, Lloyd JW, Bullingham RES, Britton BJ, Finch DRA. Postoperative analgesia for day-case herniorrhaphy patients: a comparison of cryoanalgesic, paravertebral block and oral analgesia. *Anaesthesia* 1981;36:603–610.
7. Gough JD, Willliams AB, Vaughan RS. The control of post-thoracotomy pain: a comparative evaluation of thoracic epidural fentanyl infusions and cryoanalgesia. *Anaesthesia* 1998;43:780–783.
8. Haueisen DC, Smith BS, Myers SR, Pryce ML. The diagnostic accuracy of spinal nerve injection studies: their role in the evaluation of recurrent sciatica. *Clin Orthop* 1985;198:179–183.
9. Slappendel R, Crul B, Braak G, et al. The efficacy of radiofrequency lesioning of the cervical spinal dorsal root ganglion in a double-blinded randomized study: no difference between 40% centigrade and 67% centigrade treatments. *Pain* 1997;73:159–163.
10. Konig HM, Koster HG, Niemijer RPE. Ischemia spinal cord lesion following percutaneous radiofrequency spinal rhizotomy. *Pain* 1991;45:161–166.
11. Haynsworth RF, Noe CE. Percutaneous lumbar sympathectomy: a comparison of radiofrequency denervation versus phenol neurolysis. *Anesthesiology* 1991;74: 459–463.
12. Noe CE, Haynsworth RF. Lumbar radiofrequency sympatholysis. *J Vasc Surg* 1993;17:801–806.
13. Wilkinson HA. Percutaneous radiofrequency upper thoracic sympathectomy. *Neurosurgery* 1996;38:715–725.
14. Steiner C, Staubs C, Ganon M, Buhlinger C. Piriformis syndrome: pathogenesis, diagnosis, and treatment. *J Am Osteopath Assoc* 1987;87:318–323.
15. Parziale JR, Hudgins TH, Fishman LM. The piriformis syndrome. *Am J Orthop* 1996;25:819–823.
16. Van der Heijden GJ, van der Windt DA, Kleijnen J, Koes BW, Bouter LM. Steroid injections for shoulder disorders: a systematic review of randomized clinical trials. *Br J Gen Pract* 1996;46:309–316.
17. Dreyfuss P, Michaelsen M, Pauza, K, et al. The value of medical history and physical examination in diagnosing sacroiliac joint pain. *Spine* 1996;21:2594–2602.
18. Dreyfuss PH, Dreyer SJ, Herring SA. Lumbar zygapophysial (facet) joint injections. *Spine* 1995;20: 2040–2047.
19. Maldjian C, Mesgarzadeh M, Tehranzadeh J. Diagnostic and therapeutic features of facet and sacroiliac joint injection: anatomy, pathophysiology, and technique. *Radiol Clin North Am* 1998;36:497–508.
20. Dreyfuss P, Michaelsen M, Fletcher D. Atlanto-occipital and lateral atlanto-axial joint pain patterns. *Spine* 1990;19:1125–1131.
21. April C, Dwyer A, Bogduk N. Cervical zygapophysial joint pain patterns. II. A clinical evaluation. *Spine* 1990;15:453–461.
22. Dreyfuss, P, Tibiletle C, Dreyer S. Thoracic zygapophysial joint pain patterns: a study in normal volunteers. *Spine* 1994;19:807–811.
23. Boas R. Facet joint injections. In: Stanton-Hicks M, Boas R, eds. *Chronic low back pain*. New York: Raven Press, 1982:199–211.
24. Carette S, Marcoux S, Truchon R, et al. A controlled trial of corticosteroid injections into facet joints for chronic low back pain. *N Engl J Med* 1991;325: 1002–1007.
25. Esses SI, Moro JK. The value of facet joint blocks in patient selection for lumbar fusion. *Spine* 1993;18: 185–190.
26. Lord SM, Barnsley L, Wallis BJ, et al. Percutaneous radiofrequency neurotomy for chronic cervical zygapophyseal joint pain. *N Engl J Med* 1996;335: 1721–1726.
27. Han SC, Harrison P. Myofascial pain syndrome and trigger-point management. *Reg Anesth* 1997;22:89–101.
28. Benzon HT. Epidural steroid injections for low back pain and lumbosacral radiculopathy. *Pain* 1986;24: 277–295.
29. Watts RW, Silagy CA. A meta-analysis on the efficacy of epidural coticosteroids in the treatment of sciatica. *Anaesth Intensive Care* 1995;23:564–569.
30. Weinstein SM, Herring SA, Derby R. Epidural steroid injections. *Spine* 1995;20:1842–1846.
31. Koes BW, Scholten RJ, Mens JM, Bouter LM. Efficacy of epidural steroid injections for low-back pain and sciatica: a systematic review of the literature. *Pain* 1995;63:279–288.
32. Bush K, Hillier S. A controlled study of caudal epidural injections of triamcinolone plus procaine for the management of intractable sciatica. *Spine* 1991;16: 572–575.
33. Carette S, LeClaire R, Marcoux S, et al. Epidural corticosteroid injections for sciatica due to herniated nucleus pulposus. *N Engl J Med* 1997;336:1634–1640.

34. Hopwood MB, Abram SE. Factors associated with failure of lumbar epidural steroids. *Reg Anesth* 1993:18:238–243.

35. Stav A, Ovadia L, Sternberg A, Kaadan M, Weksler N. Cervical epidural steroid injection for cervicobrachialgia. *Acta Anaesthesiol Scand* 1993;37:562–566.

36. Coffey JR, Cahill D, Steers W, et al. Intrathecal baclofen for intractable spasticity of spinal origin: results of a long-term multicenter study. *J Neurosurg* 1993;78:226–232.

37. Curley J, Costillo J, Hotz J, et al. Prolonged regional blockade: injectable biodegradable bupivacaine/polyester microspheres. *Anesthesiology* 1996;84:1401–1410.

Occupational Musculoskeletal Disorders
edited by T. G. Mayer, R. J. Gatchel, and P. B. Polatin.
Lippincott Williams & Wilkins, Philadelphia © 2000.

27

Surgical Treatment of Spinal Disorders

Robert J. Benz and Steven R. Garfin

Department of Orthopaedics, University of California, San Diego, San Diego, California 92103

This chapter provides an overview of the surgical treatment of common degenerative spinal disorders. This is a broad topic. The pathoanatomy, diagnosis, surgical indications, surgical techniques, and expected results of the more common procedures are reviewed. Brief descriptions of the common surgical procedures and some of the more controversial issues in spinal surgery are outlined.

CERVICAL SPINE

Pathoanatomy of Cervical Degenerative Disorders

With aging of the cervical spine the intervertebral disc undergoes biochemical and structural changes that affect its mechanical characteristics. Proteoglycan content alters and a gradual desiccation of the disc occurs. These changes occur in both the nucleus pulposus and in the annulus. The normal circumferential orientation, as well as the structure, of the annular fibers become disrupted, allowing the nucleus and portions of the degraded annular fibers to herniate as a soft disc herniation. The degradation of the normal disc structure also results in decreased disc height and alters the forces experienced by the vertebral endplates and facet joints. Over time, chondroosseous spurs develop in response to these new forces, leading to impingement on the vertebral canal as well as to narrowing of the vertebral foramina. Spurring occurs mostly at the uncovertebral joints but also occurs at insertion of the annular fibers. Ossification and thickening of the

posterior longitudinal ligament also result in narrowing of the vertebral canal, culminating in stenosis (Fig. 1).

Indications for Surgical Intervention

The decision to proceed with surgery should be based on a quality-of-life decision by the patient. The type of surgery and prognosis relate to an accurate diagnosis as determined by the patient's history and physical examination, which are confirmed by imaging studies and possibly by electrodiagnostic studies. Patients presenting with radiculopathy should undergo a course of nonoperative therapy, including antiinflammatory medications, activity modification, or physical therapy as indicated. Most patients improve without surgical intervention. Some, however, do not and have sufficient pain, weakness, or numbness to consider surgical intervention. The length of time nonoperative care should be pursued in terms of possibly jeopardizing surgical success has not been evaluated well in the cervical spine. Progressive neurologic deficits and loss of bowel or bladder function are relative emergent indications for surgical decompression once confirmatory imaging studies have been obtained (1). Patients presenting with myelopathy tend to have a gradual progression, and decompression of the spinal cord is often recommended to limit permanent neurologic damage (2). The role of surgical intervention in patients presenting with neck pain only is much more limited.

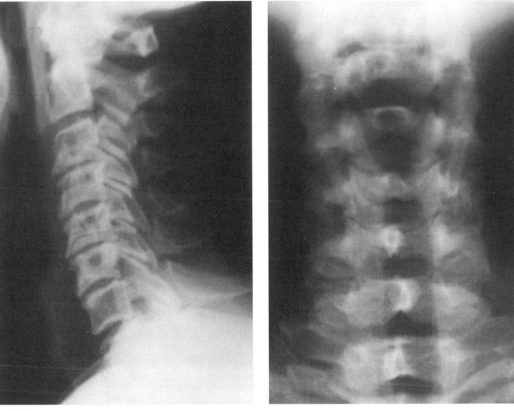

A B

FIG. 1. A: Lateral radiograph of 65-year-old man with degenerative changes of the cervical spine including osteophytes and cystic changes. **B:** Anteroposterior radiograph of a degenerative cervical spine demonstrating osteophytic changes in the uncovertebral joints. (From Gore RG. Radiological evaluation of the degenerative cervical spine. In: *The cervical spine*, 3rd ed. Philadelphia: Lippincott-Raven Publishers, 1998:766–767.)

Once the decision to proceed with surgical intervention has been made, the operative plan must be addressed. The need to approach the spine anteriorly or posteriorly, the need for arthrodesis, and the need for instrumentation all must be assessed. We generally prefer to approach cervical disc herniations anteriorly. Lateral herniations, however, may be approached posteriorly with laminotomy, foraminotomy, and discectomy. Patients with spondylosis and radiculopathy, central discs (hard or soft), or myelopathy are best and more reliably approached anteriorly, which allows for direct removal of offending disc and osteophytic material along with arthrodesis of the motion segment to prevent recurrence

(3–6). If large osteophytes extending along the posterior aspect of the vertebral body are present, or if the posterior longitudinal ligament is ossified and causing neural compression, a partial or complete corpectomy with strut grafting is indicated (7–11). Posterior decompression through laminectomy must be used with caution in these situations because of possible postlaminectomy instability with resultant kyphosis (12). Posterior arthrodesis should be considered to supplement laminectomy if preoperative kyphosis is present. An alternative to full laminectomy is laminoplasty, which also should not be routinely performed in a kyphotic cervical spine. Laminoplasty leads to increased canal area and acceptable improvement in neurologic function in patients who do not have significant anterior disease. This procedure involves opening the lamina while maintaining the ligamentous and paraspinal musculature attachments (13–20).

ANTERIOR CERVICAL SURGICAL PROCEDURES

Surgical Approach to the Anterior Cervical Spine

The anterolateral approach as described by Robinson and Smith (21) is typically used. Superficial landmarks serve as a guide to the appropriate level of the skin incision (Fig. 2) The patient's neck should be extended and the head rotated away from the surgical side. Head halter traction or Gardner-Wells tongs may be used to apply traction. A transverse skin incision in Langer's lines is made from near the midline to lateral to the anterior border of the sternocleidomastoid muscle. The platysma muscle and superficial fascia are identified and split longitudinally or transversely. The deep fascia has three sublayers: a superficial layer surrounding the sternocleidomastoid, a middle layer surrounding the carotid sheath and pretracheal structures, and a deep vertebral layer. The superficial portion of the deep fascia then is incised along the anterior border of the sternocleidomastoid. The dissection is developed in the interval be-

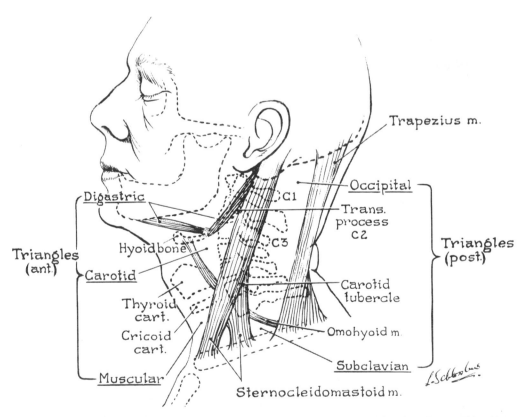

FIG. 2. Landmarks for planning surgical incisions. C2–3 found at lower border of mandible. C-3 at the level of the hyoid. C4 at the level of the thyroid cartilage. C5 at the level of the cricoid cartilage. C6 at the level of the carotid (Chassaignac's) tubercle. (From Whitecloud TS, Kelley LA. Anterior and posterior surgical approaches to the cervical spine. In: Frymoyer JW, ed. *The adult spine*, 2nd ed. Philadelphia: Lippincott–Raven Publishers, 1997:1181.)

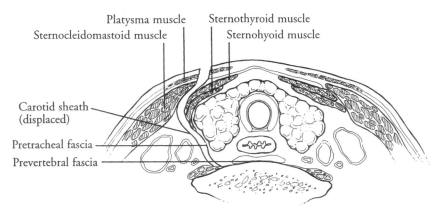

FIG. 3. Coronal view of the anterior approach to the cervical spine. (From Fellrath RF, Hanley EN. Anterior cervical discectomy and arthrodesis for radiculopathy. In: *The cervical spine*, 3rd ed. Philadelphia: Lippincott-Raven Publishers, 1998:789.)

tween the carotid sheath laterally and the trachea and esophagus medially to the spinal column. The prevertebral fascia should be divided in the midline to allow a spinal needle to be placed in a disc space for a confirmatory lateral radiograph. The longus coli muscle on each side of the spine is elevated a few millimeters laterlly with electrocautery (Fig. 3).

Anterior Cervical Discectomy and Arthrodesis: Surgical Technique

Once the desired level of the anterior cervical spine is exposed, discectomy is performed. A retractor with a smooth blade placed medially and a serrated blade laterally can be used. Some surgeons strongly recommend only handheld retractors to avoid excessive pressure on surrounding structures. Disc excision is performed by cutting the edges of the annulus with a scalpel. Dissection past the uncinate processes should be avoided, as injury to the vertebral arteries is possible. The bulk of the disc can be removed with curettes and pituitary rongeurs. Lamina spreaders or screwpost distraction may be used to open the disc space and to allow visualization of the posterior longitudinal ligament (PPL). If osteophytic compression of the vertebral canal or foramen is present, burrs, curettes, and small Kerrison punches can be used to aid in the de-

compression. Some surgeons feel decompression of bone spurs is not critical as these will resorb after fusion is obtained. The author, however, prefers to take down these osteophytes. The endplates then are abraded down to bleeding subchondral bone. The resultant height and depth of the space are measured. The tricortical anterior iliac crest graft is harvested using an oscillating saw (22). The graft is gently tapped into place and should be slightly countersunk to prevent dislodgment. We generally do not recommend anterior instrumentation for single-level anterior discectomy. For multilevel discectomies, however, we recommend anterior plating to prevent graft dislodgment and presumably lower the pseudarthrosis rate. Postoperative immobilization consists of a hard collar for 6 to 12 weeks, followed by a soft collar for an additional period, depending on radiographic evidence of graft consolidation.

In addition to the Smith-Robinson technique described above, several other graft configurations have been advocated (Fig. 4), one of which is the Keystone technique. With this technique, an upward bevel is created with osteotomes at the superior aspect of the graft and a downward bevel created inferiorly. This construct results in improved interlocking and prevents graft migration. Another technique is the Cloward Dowel technique,

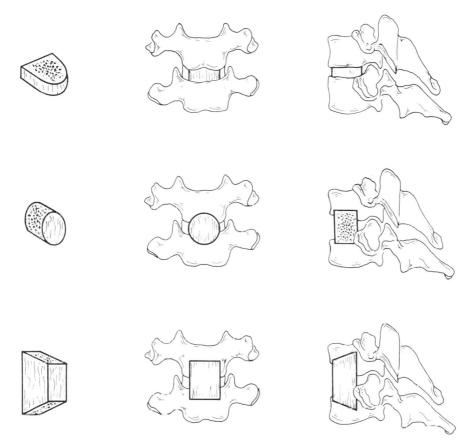

FIG. 4. Arthrodesis techniques for the cervical spine. **Top:** Smith-Robinson iliac crest technique. **Middle:** Cloward dowel technique. **Bottom:** Bhalla Keystone technique. (From Rappoport LH, O'Leary PF. Cervical disc disease. In: Bridwell KH, DeWald RL, eds. *The textbook of spinal surgery*, 2nd ed. Philadelphia: Lippincott-Raven Publishers, 1997:1,386.)

which uses special guarded drills to drill the disc space within 1 mm of the posterior cortex. The posterior cortex is removed while leaving the PLL intact. A bicortical dowel graft is harvested from the anterior superior iliac crest using a dowel cutter, which is tamped in place (23). The latter technique does not have the mechanical strength, or distracting ability, of the former two.

Arthrodesis Versus Nonarthrodesis and Graft Choice

The available literature does not clearly answer the question of whether to perform arthrodesis along with anterior cervical discectomy. Insertion of structural bone graft prevents further development of osseous spurs, leads to the regression of existing spurs, relieves radicular symptoms through distraction, and prevents advancement of painful spondylosis. Arthrodesis, however, tends to accelerate degenerative changes at adjacent disc spaces, although these are not necessarily clinically significant. To avoid these changes, as well as pain at the donor site and complications related to the graft (dislodgment, fractures, pseudarthrosis), some physicians prefer discectomy without arthrodesis. Osseous union occurs in 50% to 70% of patients undergoing anterior cervical discectomy without arthrodesis, whereas the nonunion rate of single-level anterior discectomy with arthrodesis is about 5% to 10%. This difference in arthrodesis rate may have an effect on the clinical outcome. Pseudarthrosis may contribute to treatment failure if instability becomes a problem and may contribute to neck pain (24–26). We routinely perform an arthrodesis using bone graft in association with anterior cervical discectomy (27). Graft-site morbidity usually does not constitute a long-term problem, but it does add to hospital costs and early morbidity. An ideal solution would be arthrodesis with an inexpensive material that consistently resulted in successful arthrodesis without added morbidity (28).

Multilevel Cervical Disc Disease

If multiple intervertebral levels are causing significant canal compromise, surgical options include multilevel discectomy and arthrodesis, vertebrectomy and strut grafting, or a posterior procedure. The pseudarthrosis rate of anterior discectomy and interbody arthrodesis increases with the number of levels performed. Successful arthrodesis rates are greater than 90% for one level, 80% for two levels, and 70% for three levels (3,27,29–31). With multilevel disease, corpectomy and strut grafting is a viable option because there are fewer healing "points" and the fusion rate for strut grafting is in the range of 80% to 90%. Other indications for corpectomy and strut grafting include spinal stenosis that occurs behind the vertebral body, large bony spurs on the endplates, especially if there is an associated free disc fragment located behind the vertebral body, and spondylolisthesis or severe kyphosis with cord compression (32).

Cervical Corpectomy: Surgical Technique

The standard anterior approach of Southwick and Robinson (33) as already described is used to expose the cervical spine. When two or more vertebral bodies are to be removed, it is recommended that a longitudinal incision paralleling the anterior medial border of the sternocleidomastoid muscle belly be used. Once the prevertebral fascia is incised and the surgical level confirmed radiographically, the longus colli musculature is elevated bilaterally to expose the central vertebral bodies. A scalpel is used to enter the disc spaces, and a combination of pituitary rongeurs and curettes are used to excavate the disc material. The uncinate processes serve as a landmark to limit lateral resection. Lateral resection usually should not exceed a total width of 15 mm at C-3 to 19 mm at C-6 to allow a safety margin of not entering the foramen transversarium (34) (Fig. 5)

After disc excision is initiated to identify levels, rongeurs and burrs are used to create a longitudinal trough in the vertebral bodies to the posterior cortex. Bone wax should be used to control bony bleeding. Small curettes and Kerrison rongeurs can be used to remove the thinned posterior cortex, disc material, and posterior longitudinal ligament to complete the decompression. The superior and inferior endplates to be fused then are decorticated. If plating is to be performed, the graft may be placed flush with the endplates. If no plating is used, the graft and endplates may be fashioned into locking troughs to help secure the graft.

Cervical Corpectomy: Graft Selection and Instrumentation

The choices for anterior strut grafting are typically autograft or allograft. The reported rate of successful arthrodesis varies greatly in the literature from 60% to 100% (27,35–37). Therefore, it is difficult to recommend one graft source over another. It appears, however, that appropriately processed allograft has an arthrodesis rate similar to autograft but perhaps a slightly slower rate of consolidation.

Anterior cervical plating has been investigated with the hope that it would increase the successful arthrodesis rate of strut grafting and minimize deformity and settling. Proponents of anterior internal fixation cite several

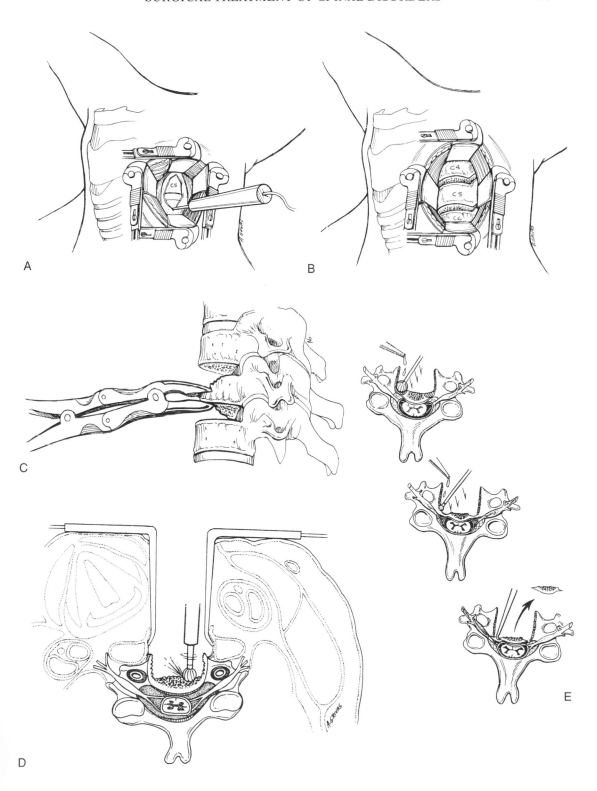

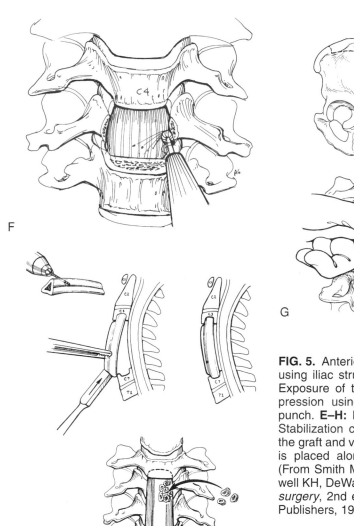

F

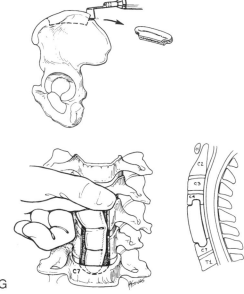

G

H

FIG. 5. Anterior cervical corpectomy and fusion using iliac strut graft or fibular strut graft. **A,B:** Exposure of the involved levels. **C–F:** Decompression using rongeurs, burrs, and Kerrison punch. **E–H:** Iliac crest graft or fibula is used. Stabilization can be improved with notching of the graft and vertebral bodies. Excess bone graft is placed along the edges of the strut graft. (From Smith MD. Cervical spondylosis. In: Bridwell KH, DeWald RL, eds. *The textbook of spinal surgery*, 2nd ed. Philadelphia: Lippincott-Raven Publishers, 1997:1410–1411.)

theoretic advantages of plating, including adding immediate stability of the reconstructed segment, improving the rate of arthrodesis, preventing graft dislodgment, and obviating the need for halo-vest immobilization postoperatively (38). Animal studies have shown decreased vascularity beneath anterior cervical plates and have not shown an increased rate of arthrodesis with plating after a three-level interbody arthrodesis (39).

Graft dislodgment occurs in 1% to 2% of interbody arthrodeses and in 6% to 30% of strut grafts (40–42). The use of a buttress plate may prevent graft dislodgment but does introduce the added risks of anterior hardware and increased operative time and expense. Anterior cervical plating has been used successfully with a low rate of complications and is preferred by many surgeons because of immediate stability and a decreased need for external immobilization, resulting in earlier return to work (30,43–48).

Anterior Cervical Plating Techniques

A wide assortment of anterior cervical plates are now available. Plating systems are designed for both bicortical and unicortical screw fixation. Most unicortical plating systems use a locking screw to prevent screw backout (Fig. 6). Biomechanical testing of constructs using bicortical and unicortical locking fixation systems found no significant difference between the two techniques (49,50).

Once the cortical bone graft, after either discectomy or corpectomy, has been placed, the appropriate-length plate is selected. The plate is contoured to fit on the anterior vertebral column, centered in the mediolateral plane. Preset depth drill bits are available to control the depth of drilling. Screws are inserted in either a unicortical or bicortical fashion as dictated by the system. Image intensification may be helpful, especially for bicortical screw placement. Screws should not violate the endplates. Screws may be placed in the strut grafts to help lock the graft in position.

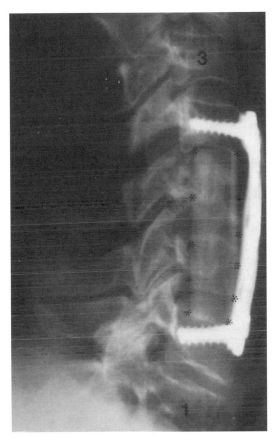

FIG. 6. Lateral radiograph of C-5 and C-6 corpectomies, strut graft, and anterior plating. (From ref. 32, with permission.)

Posterior Cervical Surgical Procedures

Degenerative conditions of the cervical spine may be addressed surgically by one of many posterior cervical procedures. Posterior procedures on the upper cervical spine include occipitocervical arthrodesis and atlantoaxial arthrodesis. Posterior procedures on the subaxial cervical spine range from laminotomies and discectomies, to laminoplasty, to full laminectomies and arthrodesis. The decision to go posteriorly should be based on the pathology. In general, anterior pathology should be approached anteriorly.

Posterior Cervical Decompression

For a lateral disc herniation, a keyhole laminotomy is performed by burring the adjacent borders of the superior and inferior laminae at the correct interspace. The ligamentum flavum is removed by using Kerrison rongeurs. If the offending pathology is a soft disc herniation, the affected nerve root can be gently elevated and the disc fragment removed. Kerrison rongeurs also can be used to perform foraminotomies at this level if indicated. Visualization is best achieved through a microscope.

Full laminectomies also can be performed if indicated. The decompression should span the width of the spinal canal while minimizing injury to the facets. Foraminotomies can be performed with Kerrison rongeurs; however, as little of the facet joint as possible should be removed to decrease the risk of late postoperative instability (41). Often at least 25% to 50% of the facet must be removed to achieve adequate decompression; however, resection of greater than 50% of the facet compromises shear strength of the motion segment and increases the risk for development of postoperative instability (51).

Laminoplasty

An alternative to laminectomy is laminoplasty. This technique was developed to increase the anteroposterior (AP) dimensions of the cervical spinal canal while leaving the posterior elements partially intact to prevent postoperative instability (52). Indications for laminoplasty include multilevel spondylotic myelopathy with a relatively narrow canal of less than 13 to 14 mm of AP diameter (11,53). Myelopathy resulting from single- or two-level disease without significant congenital stenosis is best treated from an anterior approach. One relative contraindication for laminonplasty is cervical kyphosis (54).

Many techniques have been described, but the basic premise is to create a full-thickness defect at the junction of the lamina and facet joints on one side and then create a partial-thickness defect on the opposite side at the lamina–facet junction. The laminae are opened by creating a greenstick fracture through the partial-thickness defect. Then the laminae are held open by suture, bone graft, or metal plates (19) (Fig. 7). An alternative is to split the lamina open through the spinous process and lamina–facet junction hinges.

Postoperative imaging studies have shown an increase in the canal area of up to 48%. This increase in canal area appears to be maintained in long-term follow-up (20). In addition, there has been documented posterior

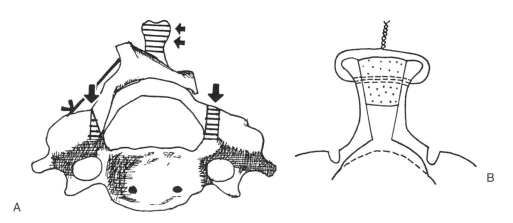

FIG. 7. Laminoplasty techniques. **A:** The lamina may be open on one side and held open with bone graft, plates, or sutures. **B:** Alternatively, the spinous process may be split and bone graft used to keep the lamina open. (From Kawai S. Indications and techniques for cervical laminoplasty. In: Bridwell KH, DeWald KH, eds. *The textbook of spinal surgery*, 2nd ed. Philadelphia: Lippincott-Raven Publishers, 1997:1422,1424.)

migration of the spinal cord, allowing for relative anterior decompression. Neurologic improvement has occurred in 50% to 84% of patients (13,15,19,53). Although not as severe as with laminectomy, laminoplasty has been associated with loss of cervical lordosis (15). Other complications include loss of neck motion, especially extension, and neck pain (14,55). A comparison study between laminoplasty and anterior discectomy and arthrodesis for soft disc herniation showed no significant difference in outcome between the two groups, although follow-up was 5 years longer in the anterior discectomy group. The complication rate was significantly higher in the anterior discectomy group (56).

Posterior Cervical Arthrodesis Techniques

Anatomically, arthrodesis can be divided into occipitocervical, atlantoaxial, and subaxial. Hardware types can be divided into wiring techniques, plate and screw techniques, and transarticular techniques. The choice of which method to use is based on the bony anatomy, the patient's pathology, and surgeon experience and preference.

Occipitocervical Arthrodesis

Indications for occipitocervical arthrodesis include occipitocervical instability due to trauma, congenital disorders, inflammatory

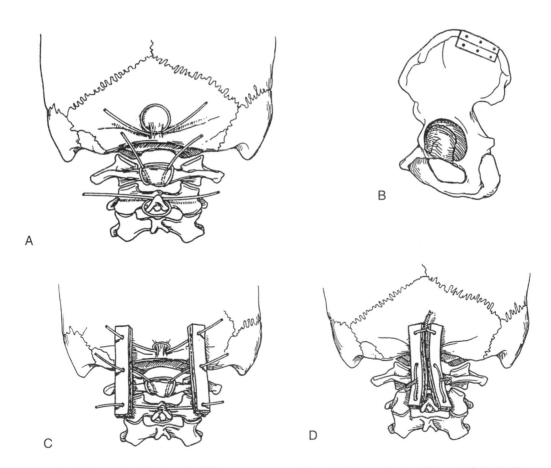

FIG. 8. Occipitocervical fusion. **A:** Wires are passed through the occiputs, C-1 and C-2. **B:** Bone grafts are harvested from the iliac crest. **C:** Wires are passed through holes drilled in the grafts. **D:** The grafts are secured in place. (From An HS, Coppes M. Cervical spine instrumentation. In: An HS, ed. *Principles and techniques of spine surgery.* Baltimore: Williams & Wilkins, 1998:659.)

arthropathies, infection, and tumor. The goal of this surgery is to decompress the neural elements, if necessary, and to achieve a solid bony union to prevent further neurologic injury, reestablish stability, and relieve pain.

Occipitocervical arthrodesis is performed through a posterior, midline incision from the occipital protuberance to the fourth cervical spinous process. The dissection is carried down onto the occiput and lamina in a subperiosteal fashion. A 20-gauge wire can be passed through the external occipital protuberance without violating the inner table of bone. A trough then is burred along each side of the protuberance to lessen the mass effect of the wires. The wire is looped over the protuberance and taken back through the protuberance. Separate wires are passed under the lamina of C-1 and through the spinous process of C-2. Corticocancellous bone grafts then are harvested from the iliac crest and holes are drilled in the grafts corresponding to the level of the wires. The occipital cortex and the laminae of C-1 and C-2 are decorticated. The bone graft is laid down and the wires tightened sequentially. The patient then is immobilized with a halo vest for 10 to 12 weeks (Fig. 8). Other wiring techniques exist, as do fixation techniques using cables (57–59).

Plate and screw fixation devices have been advocated by numerous researchers (60). A computed tomography (CT) scan is strongly recommended to confirm the local anatomy when planning these procedures. The exposure for plating is the same as for wiring techniques, although the dissection must be carried out further laterally to expose the lateral masses of C-2 and possibly C-3. Reconstruction plates or specially designed plates can be used for the arthrodesis. The plates are fashioned to match the contour of the occipitocervical junction. The plates then are secured to C-2 with pedicle screws and to C-3 if needed by using lateral mass screws. Alternatively, the C-2 screw can be a transarticular C1–2 screw (61). Bicortical screws are placed in the occiput below the nuchal line on each side of the midline. Corticocancellous

bone graft is placed across the arthrodesis levels on each side of the midline (Fig. 9).These procedures produce solid constructs but are technically demanding and have obvious associated risks related to screw placement and failure. In rheumatoid patients, plate fixation has had superior rates of arthrodesis and improved rates of neurologic recovery compared with wiring techniques (62–65), and plating techniques frequently obviate the need for halo immobilization, an important result.

Atlantoaxial Arthrodesis

Although the main indication for atlantoaxial arthrodesis is trauma, other indications for arthrodesis of C1–2 include inflammatory arthropathies, congenital anomalies, tumors, and infections. In the trauma situation, an atlantodens interval of 3 to 5 mm indicates incompetence of the transverse ligament, and an atlantodens interval greater than 5 mm indicates rupture of the transverse and accessory ligaments (66). In the rheumatoid patient, the space available for the cord on flexion and extension films should be used to assess the need for arthrodesis. A space smaller than 14 mm available for the cord should be considered for decompression and arthrodesis (67); this tends to correlate with an atlantodens interval (ADI) of greater than 10 mm and a posterior ADI of less than 10 to 13 mm.

Surgical technique depends on the patient's pathology, local anatomy, and surgeon preference. If halo-vest immobilization is planned postoperatively, the halo can be placed preoperatively and used for distraction/positioning intraoperatively. If a reduction is needed, it should be done with the patient awake. A posterior midline longitudinal incision is used to expose from the occiput to C-3. Several wiring techniques have been described that involve sublaminar wires at C-1 and sublaminar or spinous process wires at C-2 (68–71). Corticocancellous bone grafts are incorporated into the construct to promote arthrodesis. These constructs generally require supplemental halo-vest immobilization.

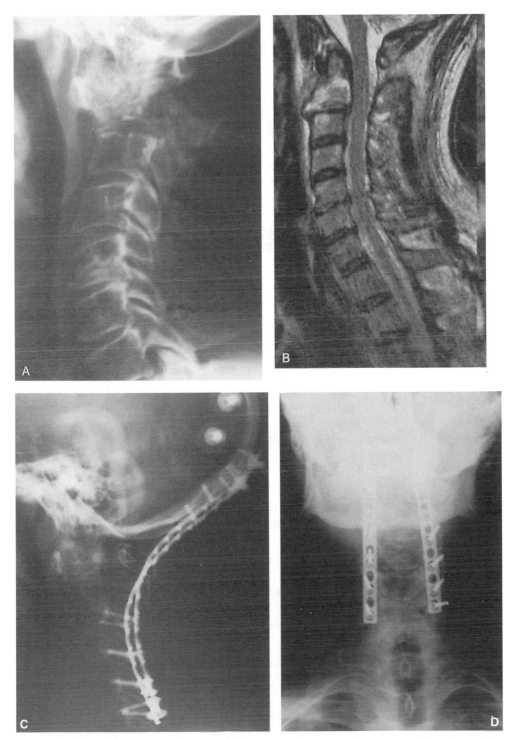

FIG. 9. A 60-year-old man with increasing neck and low back pain of 6 months' duration. **A,B:** Radiographs and magnetic resonance imaging show destruction at C-2. **C,D:** The patient underwent occipital cervical fusion using the Synthes Anderson plate. (From Montesano PX. Anterior and posterior screw and plate techniques used in the cervical spine. In: Bridwell KH, DeWald RL, eds. *The textbook of spinal surgery*, 2nd ed. Philadelphia: Lippincott-Raven Publishers, 1997:1757.)

In addition to wiring techniques, other techniques have been developed for C1–2 arthrodesis, including the Halifax interlaminar clamps and transarticular C1–2 screws (72,73). Transarticular screws do not rely on the integrity of the posterior elements and do not require postoperative halo-vest immobilization; however, transarticular screws do depend on the competency of the C-2 lateral masses (74). C1–2 transarticular arthrodesis is performed through a posterior midline incision from the occiput to C-5. The lateral masses of C-2 and C-3 are exposed, taking care not to injure the vertebral artery or strip the C2–3 facet capsule. The starting point of the screw is 3 mm cephalad and 2 mm lateral to the lower medial edge of the caudad articular process. Image intensification in two planes is used to guide the drill into the lateral mass of C-1 exiting anteriorly. The first drill bit is left in place to stabilize the joint while the second hole is drilled. Screws then are placed through the facet joints into the lateral masses of C-1 (Fig. 10).

Long-term results using mostly wiring techniques have been good. Ghanayem et al. reported on 13 of 14 patients with long-term follow-up who achieved a solid arthrodesis; the remaining patient had an asymptomatic fibrous union (75). The Magerl transarticular technique has produced the greatest rotational stability of the C1–2 fixation techniques (74). The incidence of malpositioning of the screws has been about 15%, with screw complications in 6% of patients. The pseudarthrosis rate of C1–2 transarticular screws is reported to be 0.6% (74).

Subaxial Cervical Arthrodesis Technique

In instances where the posterior decompression results in potential instability, a lateral mass arthrodesis may be added to prevent late kyphosis. In failed anterior cervical arthrodesis, posterior spinal arthrodesis has shown higher arthrodesis rates than repeat anterior arthrodesis with anterior plating (76).

Posterior fixation of the lower cervical spine uses wiring techniques or lateral mass plating. Determination of technique depends on the integrity of the posterior elements, patient anatomy and needs, and surgeon experience.

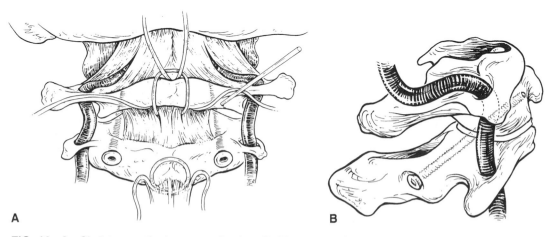

A   **B**

FIG. 10. A: Cl–2 transarticular screw fixation. **B:** The screw should be started caudally enough to transfix the facet joint. Posterior fixation and fusion may be added. (From Moskovich R. Cervical Instability. In: Bridwell KH, DeWald, eds. *The textbook of spinal surgery,* 2nd ed. Philadelphia: Lippincott-Raven Publishers, 1997:996.)

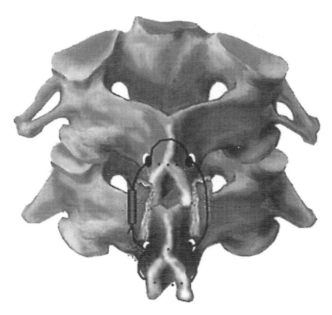

FIG. 11. Rogers' wiring technique. Corticocancellous grafts are secured underneath the intervertebral sections of the wires. (From Weis JC, McAfee PC. Lower cervical spine arthrodesis wiring techniques. In: *The cervical spine*, 3rd ed. Philadelphia: Lippincott-Raven Publishers, 1998:493.)

Rogers' Wiring Technique

The involved levels are exposed through a posterior midline approach. Levels are confirmed by lateral radiograph. Using a burr, holes are made through the cortex at the junction of the spinous process and lamina at each level on both sides. The holes at each level are connected with a towel clip. Using an 18-gauge wire or flexible cable, one end of the fixation device is passed through the uppermost hole, looped over the cephalad border of the spinous process, and then passed back through the hole again. In cases of multilevel fusion, both ends of the wire or cable are passed through the middle level spinous process holes in opposite directions. At the most caudal level, one end of the cable or wire is looped around the caudal side of the spinous process, which results in both ends of the fixation device ending up on the same side of the spine, ready for tightening and fixation. Decortication of the laminae, spinous processes, and facet joints is followed by placing corticocancellous bone grafts on each side of the spine beneath the longitudinal portion of the cable or wire (Fig. 11).

Triple Wiring Technique

A standard posterior midline approach is used to expose the intended levels. A lateral radiograph is obtained to confirm the vertebral levels. The dissection is carried laterally to expose the facet capsules and lateral masses. A hole is created at the base of the spinous processes of the superior and inferior levels using a burr. A 20-gauge wire then is passed through both holes and tightened. An additional wire is placed through each of the holes. Decortication of the laminae, facets, and lateral masses is performed. Two corticocancellous grafts from the iliac crests are harvested and fashioned with drill holes to match the spinous process wires. The bone grafts then are tightened in place with the wires. Care must be taken to avoid injuring adjacent facet capsules or placing bone graft in adja-

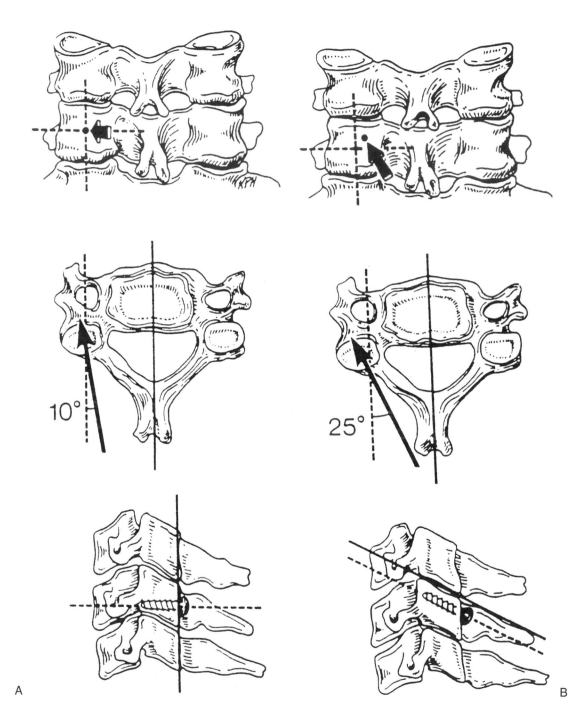

FIG. 12. A: The Roy-Camille technique can potentially injure the neurovascular structures and un-affected facet joints. **B:** The Magerl technique can potentially injure the superior nerve root. (From McGuire RA. Cervical spine arthrodesis. In: *The cervical spine*. 3rd ed. Philadelphia: Lippincott-Raven Publishers, 1998:506.)

cent interspaces to prevent unwanted adjacent level arthrodesis.

Robinson-Southwick Technique

In the postlaminectomy patient with deficient posterior elements, this technique allows stable fixation to the facets. Twenty-gauge wires are passed through drill holes in the facets. The wires then are looped through corticocancellous grafts and tightened.

Lateral Mass Plating

Lateral mass plating may be substituted for wiring techniques and is especially useful if the posterior elements are deficient. Multiple plating systems are available, and different techniques have been described for screw orientation. The approach is through a standard posterior midline approach. Once the lateral masses are exposed, a burr is used to penetrate the lateral mass cortex. The starting point ranges from the center point of the lateral mass to medial and cephalad. Recommendations for drill orientation range from straight ahead (*tout-droit*), to 10 to 30 degrees laterally and 0 to 15 degrees cranially (Fig. 12). Palpation of the facets with an elevator can guide insertion further. The drill is advanced carefully until the far cortex is reached or penetrated. Most surgeons prefer unicortical fixation, but bicortical fixation can be used. Bicortical screws can be placed through the plate into the lateral masses. Lateral mass plates may be extended up to C-2 using pedicle screws and down into the thoracic spine using pedicle screws. The Magerl hook plate also may be used for stabilization to C-7 using lateral mass screws at C-6 and above and C-7 laminar hooks. Once the hardware is in place, decortication is performed and bone graft is placed. Once again, care must be taken not to injure adjacent facet capsules and not to place bone graft at nonfused levels.

Postoperative immobilization for wiring techniques may require halo-vest immobilization. Lateral mass plating usually can produce enough stability that a rigid collar suffices. Complications with wiring techniques usually are related to failure of the construct. Hardware complications associated with lateral mass plating include nerve-root impingement, vertebral-artery injury, and hardware failure. Both techniques produce excellent rates of arthrodesis (77,78).

THORACIC SPINE

As with the cervical spine, this section focuses on degenerative disorders of the thoracic spine. Thoracic disc herniations represent fewer than 1% of all disc herniations and fewer than 2% of all disc operations (79–81). Thoracic disc herniations are most common in the lower levels of the thoracic spine, with 75% occurring below T-8 (79). The pathophysiology of thoracic disc disease is not unlike that in other regions of the spine; however, the rib cage appears to provide a stabilizing mechanism that helps protect the thoracic discs from forces that may cause herniation (82). Pain patterns with thoracic herniations tend to be less specific than in the cervical or lumbar spine and may cause local pain; cause radiating pain around the trunk, legs, or groin; or mimic visceral pain, such as cardiac disease (83). Pain tends to be exacerbated by overhead activities and twisting motions. Neurologic deficits include lower-extremity numbness or weakness, spasticity, ataxia, or bowel and bladder disturbances. Because of these nonspecific findings, the diagnosis of thoracic disc herniation often is delayed.

Physical examination should include the Adam's test (forward bending with the arms extended) for spinal asymmetry suggesting scoliosis along with checking for focal kyphosis suggestive of Scheuermann's kyphosis. Geographic tenderness, including muscle spasms and triggerpoints, should be assessed. A thorough neurologic examination that includes sensory examination of the thorax and abdomen along with neurologic examination of the lower extremities is indicated. Assessment for the presence of any pathologic long-tract reflexes, such as the Babinski or clonus, should be performed. Evidence of upper motor-neuron abnormalities in the lower extremities with a normal upper-extremity examination is suggestive of thoracic pathology.

Clinical suspicion of a herniated thoracic disc should be confirmed by an imaging study. Plain radiographs may show signs of degenerated discs with collapse and endplate spurring. Of the advanced imaging studies, including CT myelography and magnetic resonance (MR) imaging, the preferred method is MR imaging, because it gives more information about the surrounding soft tissue and neural elements and because it is noninvasive. As with other regions of the spine, imaging studies must correlate with clinical findings, because there is a high incidence of abnormal findings on MR imaging in asymptomatic persons. One MR imaging study that evaluated the thoracic spines of 90 asymptomatic persons found some abnormality in 73% of patients, disc herniation in 37%, and spinal cord deformation in 29% (84). In rare instances, patients who have persistent thoracic pain will have negative imaging studies and may be considered for discography (85). If a single painful disc can be localized, an arthrodesis may be considered (85).

Thoracic spinal stenosis is much less common than stenosis in the cervical or lumbar spine. Causes of canal stenosis include degenerative changes of the disc, facets, or congenital narrowing of the canal. Although the thoracic motion segments are relatively protected by the rib cage, degenerative changes do occur, resulting in osteophyte formation with resultant neural impingement. Workup of stenosis includes the usual imaging modalities of radiographs and MR imaging or CT myelography.

Surgical Indications

Failure of nonoperative modalities to achieve adequate relief of patient symptoms is the indication for decompressive surgery. Initial treatment for thoracic pain symptoms include nonsteroidal antiinflammatory medications and activity modification. A trial of steroids also may be useful for radicular symptoms. As discussed in previous chapters, treatment should progress to aerobic conditioning and strengthening of the paraspinal musculature. If no progress is made and the level of discomfort is unacceptable to the patient, surgical intervention may be considered. In patients with myelopathy and documented neurologic compression, decompressive surgery is indicated sooner rather than later.

Surgical Approaches to the Thoracic Spine

The numerous approaches to the thoracic spine include conventional open techniques as well as minimally invasive techniques. The common open approaches to the thoracic spine include transthoracic–transpleural, laminectomy, transpedicular–transfacetal, and posterolateral–extrapleural approaches. With the development of improved instrumentation, video-assisted thoracoscopic surgery (VATS) is gaining popularity. As with the cervical and lumbar spine, the indicated approach is dependent on the site of the pathology, patient anatomy, and surgeon experience. If the compression is purely posterior, laminectomy and partial facetectomy are indicated. If disc pathology is the main culprit, a posterolateral or anterior approach is indicated. Compression from vertebral endplate osteophytes is best addressed from an anterior approach.

Posterior Thoracic Surgical Approaches

Posterior Laminectomy

This technique is similar to laminectomies in the cervical spine. A dorsal midline incision is used. The dissection is carried down to the tips of the spinous processes. The paraspinal musculature is stripped in a subperiosteal fashion to the lamina. After obtaining a confirmatory radiograph, the involved levels are decompressed. Care is taken to avoid removing more than 50% of the facet joint on each side to avoid iatrogenic instability. Care also must be used to avoid injury to adjacent

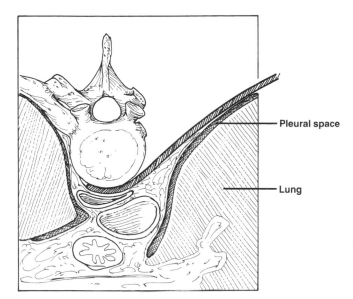

FIG. 13. Costotransversectomy approach to the posterolateral thoracic spine. (From ref. 88, with permission.)

facet joint capsules to avoid iatrogenic spondylosis.

Posterior laminectomy and discectomy in the thoracic spine has largely been abandoned because of the high incidence of neurologic injury. Paraplegia rates of up to 40% have been reported in relatively large series of patients (83,86,87).

Transpedicular–Transfacetal Approach

This approach involves removing the facet joint posterior to the involved disc herniation and the superior half of pedicle inferior to the disc space. The disc space is entered lateral to the spinal cord. Alternatively, a true transpedicular approach may be used. In this approach, the medial wall and possibly the lateral wall of the pedicle should be left intact, and curettes are used to enter the vertebral body. This technique is useful for biopsy of vertebral body tumors (88).

Costotransversectomy

This approach is useful for centrolateral herniations, especially in patients who cannot tolerate a thoracotomy. The patient is placed

in a slight lateral position, and an outward convex paramedian incision is used; 8 to 15 cm of the rib leading to the affected disc space are removed. The pleura and lung are retracted anteriorly. The transverse process and pedicle are visualized by removing the head of the rib, thereby exposing the disc space and anterolateral aspect of the cord tracing through the neuroforamen (Fig. 13). The posterior aspect of the disc can be removed.

Anterior Thoracic Approaches

Debate exists as to whether a transthoracic–transpleural approach or a costotransversectomy is better for performing thoracic discectomies. The thoracotomy approach allows access to the entire disc. Pulmonary function compromise is the greatest disadvantage of thoracotomy. Deciding whether to use a left-sided or right-sided approach depends on the level of the spine involved and the position of the herniation. A right-sided approach is suggested for the upper thoracic spine to avoid the heart and great vessels. In the middle and lower thoracic spine, a left-sided approach is suggested because the aorta is more resistant to injury than the vena cava.

Anterior Thoracotomy

The anterior thoracic approach is performed with the patient in the lateral decubitus position. A double-lumen endotracheal tube is used to allow for selective deflation of one lung. The rib intersecting the involved disc space is dissected subperiosteally and removed. The pleura then is opened and the lung deflated. A segment of the proximal rib and rib head is removed to allow visualization of the lateral pedicle and the costovertebral joints. Depending on the pathology, the whole pedicle of the inferior vertebral body or a portion of it is taken down using a burr or Kerrison. The dissection is then carried into the posterior portion of the vertebral body with burrs. The dissection in the vertebral body is carried up through disc space into the superior vertebral body. Once the posterior cortex of both vertebral bodies are identified, they are carefully perforated and removed with curettes. This technique creates an island of bone and disc material that can be safely removed from the spinal canal and off the dura (89) (Fig. 14). Arthrodesis can be performed if necessary. If only the posterior portion the disc and a small amount of posterior end plate is removed, fusion may not be necessary.

Arthrodesis following thoracic discectomy is also debated; however, indications for arthrodesis are not well defined. It is argued that arthrodesis will prevent kyphotic deformity (83). Others argue that routine arthrodesis is not indicated unless excessive bone resection is performed (90). It would seem logical to elect for arthrodesis when there is a large component of back pain and when an abundant disc resection has been performed.

Thoracic Decompression Surgical Results

The results of surgical decompression depend largely on patient selection. As with other regions of the spine, neurologic compressive symptoms have better outcomes than local pain. Less precise diagnoses tend to result in less predictable outcomes (90–96). Complications with thoracic decompression are those related to the thoracotomy, residual neural compression, and iatrogenic neural injury. Spinal cord injury is the most feared complication; however, this occurrence can be minimized with careful meticulous technique.

Thoracoscopic Techniques

A great deal of enthusiasm has been generated about minimally invasive techniques as a result of the recent advances in videoscopic equipment and spinal instrumentation. These techniques offer many advantages over open techniques, including minimizing incisional trauma to the patient, providing visualization to the entire operative team, and potentially decreasing rehabilitation and hospitalization time. These techniques are demanding, and the importance of practicing in a cadaver or animal laboratory cannot be overemphasized. It is also advisable to have an experienced endoscopic thoracic surgeon or laparoscopic surgeon present until the surgeon gains considerable experience in the technique.

The indications for thoracoscopic techniques are expanding rapidly. As more experience is gained, larger procedures are being attempted and performed successfully. Thoracoscopic techniques are well suited to biopsy of vertebral body lesions from T2–12, excision and arthrodesis of degenerative discs, and thoracic vertebrectomy with strut graft arthrodesis (93,97–111). In addition, instrumentation systems are becoming available that will allow anterior instrumentation using minimally invasive techniques. Contraindications to its use include patients who are unable to tolerate single-lung ventilation, severe or acute respiratory insufficiency, and pleural symphysis. Previous chest-tube placement and previous thoracotomy are relative contraindications.

A right- or left-sided approach may be used, depending on the site of the pathology. The ipsilateral lung is deflated by using a dual-

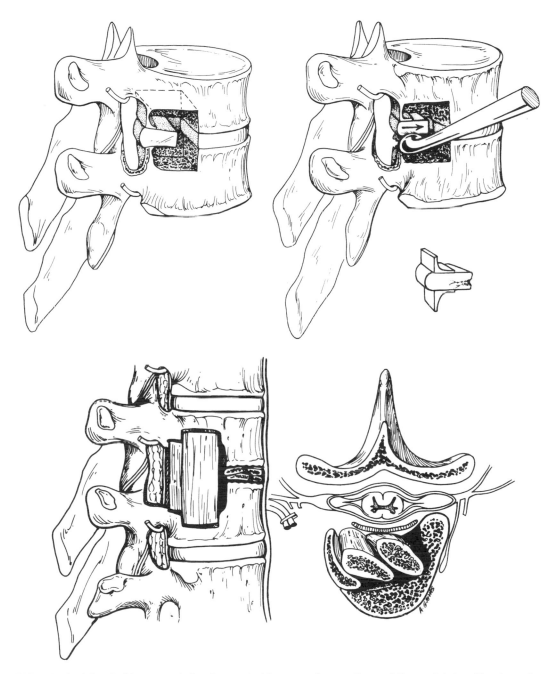

FIG. 14. An island of bone and disc is created by removing portions of the endplates. The bone island is safely removed by curretting away from the spinal cord. Corticocancellous bone graft can then be placed. (From ref. 89, with permission.)

lumen endotracheal tube. Anteroposterior fluoroscopic views are useful for determining the correct level. The specific instrumentation needed is beyond the scope of this text (99,110). Typically, three portals, each 15 to 20 mm long, are made in the intercostal spaces. The first portal is placed in the sixth or seventh intercostal space to avoid injury to the diaphragm. The portals are spaced to allow triangulation of the surgical instruments. Tilting the patient forward can help deflate the ipsilateral lung; however, fan retractors are usually needed to keep the lung retracted. The parietal pleura is taken down either sharply or with electrocautery, and then segmental vessels are controlled using vascular clips. A wide variety of spinal instruments are available for performing the bony work, including decompressions and biopsies (Fig. 15).

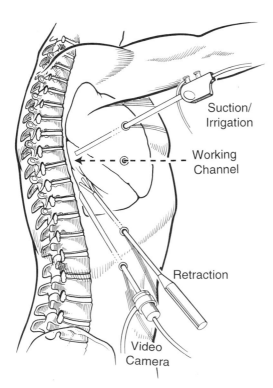

FIG. 15. Routine thoracoscopic portals. Patient is in lateral decubitus position with single lung ventilation. (From Regan JJ. Endoscopic spinal surgery anterior approaches. In: Frymoyer JW, ed. *The adult spine*, 2nd ed. Philadelphia: Lippincott-Raven Publishers, 1997:1673.)

Thoracoscopic techniques have proved safe and effective. A multicenter study of the first 100 patients undergoing thoracolumbar endoscopic procedures resulted in a low incidence of complications, with only two patients requiring conversion to an open procedure (106). Animal models have demonstrated the equivalency of anterior releases performed thoracoscopically versus through traditional open techniques (107). The results of decompressive anterior thoracic procedures performed thoracoscopically are comparable to open procedures and have lower morbidity rates (104). As experience is gained in these techniques, operating time, blood loss, complications, and hospitalization time continue to decrease.

LUMBAR SPINE DISEASE

Lumbar Disc Diseases

Low back pain has an enormous socioeconomic cost to the Western world. Low back pain is second only to respiratory illness in reason for visits to primary care physicians. At some point during their lifetimes, 60% to 80% of all people will be afflicted with low back pain (112–115). Ninety-five percent of the people who experience low back pain will return to work; however, 85% of medical costs are spent on the remaining 5% of patients who are unable to return to work (116). Most of these patients are able to return to gainful employment, but if disability persists for longer than 1 year, the likelihood of returning to work is less than 20% and approaches zero if disability is extended for 2 years (117).

Because of this socioeconomic impact, a great deal of effort has been devoted to understanding the pathoanatomy of the lumbar disc. The intervertebral disc is composed of the nucleus pulposus surrounded by the annulus fibrosis. The young, healthy nucleus is composed of proteoglycan units and type II collagen that is well hydrated, having a water content of 85%. This allows the disc to act as a viscoelastic material that is superb for shock absorption. As the disc ages and degenerates, the proteoglycan content decreases, and consequently hydrostatic forces are decreased. The disc loses its viscoelastic properties as well as its function of force distribution. With further degeneration, the nuclear material is replaced with fibrocartilage and the distinction between the nucleus and annulus decreases (118). The annulus fibrosis consists of collagen lamellae arranged at 30-degree angles to the vertebral endplates. This orientation improves the functional ability of the annulus to withstand torsional and axial loads (119). With disc desiccation, the disc collapses and this architecture is lost, resulting in weakening of the annulus. The combination of these changes produces defects and degeneration of the annulus and the nucleus, which can result in disc herniation with associated neural compression.

Clinical Presentation and Evaluation

About 5% of all persons will experience sciatica sometime after the age of 35 years (120). Patients with lumbar disc disease often present with low back pain and may or may not have classic radicular symptoms. The pain is usually intermittent and brought on by strenuous physical activity. The pain often is exacerbated by prolonged sitting, bending, or twisting. Radicular symptoms usually are increased by valsalva maneuvers such as coughing, sneezing, or straining. Often the symptoms can be relieved with recumbency or rest. The history obtained from the patient should include the relative proportion of leg versus back pain, because patients with mostly back symptoms are less likely to have neural compression and are less likely to benefit from surgical intervention.

True radicular pain is classically described as sharp, lancinating pain that is in a specific pattern. The location of radicular symptoms is well documented (121). Muscle weakness should be evaluated to help in confirming the diagnosis. Inquiries also should be made as to any bowel or bladder symptoms. Cauda equina syndrome is one of the few surgical emergencies in degenerative spinal surgery

with a high rate of residual dysfunction, even if addressed emergently.

It is important to determine whether an injury initiated the patient's symptoms and where the injury occurred. Determining whether there are litigation issues or workers' compensation claims is extremely important in assessing the patient's motivation for getting better. It is wise to proceed cautiously in these patients, because the results of all treatments are diminished by up to one third in this group (122–125). Waddel noted several signs that strongly indicate the involvement of psychosocial factors, including nonanatomic superficial tenderness, axial loading and rotation simulation tests, distraction tests such as seated straight leg raising, nonanatomic weakness or sensory loss, overreaction, verbalization, or muscle tremor (125). If three or more of these signs are present, the patient's suitability for surgery must be questioned.

The differential diagnosis of low back pain is broad but can be narrowed by sorting back pain into age groups. In children, back pain is unusual and seldom is discogenic in origin. Back pain in this age group is more likely to be caused by discitis, spondylolysis, or various neoplastic disorders, such as osteoid osteoma, osteoblastoma, or eosinophilic granuloma. In the age group over 50 years, malignant processes and infection should be considered.

Much information can be obtained by observing the patient walking into the examination room. The patient's posture can hint at the underlying diagnosis. Patients who walk with a flexed posture may have spinal stenosis, whereas listing to one side can indicate a contralateral disc herniation (126). In addition, the patient's overall mannerisms can help to elucidate underlying motivations. Physical examination should include looking for any unusual skin markings or hair patches that would indicate diagnoses such as neurofibromatosis or spinal dysraphism. The midline spinal structures should be carefully palpated, as should the paraspinal musculature. Range of motion of the spine and hips should be checked. A root-specific neurologic examination of the upper and lower extremities, including graded motor examination, sensory examination, deep tendon reflexes, and pathologic reflexes, should be performed. Tension signs such as the straight leg raise test, contralateral straight leg raise test, and femoral nerve traction tests should be evaluated. A vascular examination also should be performed to rule out vascular claudication.

Once a thorough history and physical examination are completed and the diagnosis of herniated disc suspected, plain radiographs can be obtained. Plain films, however, are most useful to rule out neoplastic conditions and infection and to assess the general condition and alignment of the spine. If the patient's symptoms are of recent onset, it is reasonable to delay obtaining films until after an initial nonoperative treatment regimen has been unsuccessful for 4 to 6 weeks (127). If the patient's symptoms warrant surgical intervention, an axial imaging study should be obtained. MR imaging scanning is preferred; however, CT myelography can provide adequate information if a MR imaging is unobtainable or equivocal (128–130).

Operative Indications

Patient selection is crucial to contributing to a successful outcome. The axiom that "we operate on patients, not diagnostic studies" certainly holds true for patients with low back disorders. Rates of disc abnormalities on MR imaging in asymptomatic patients are extremely high, up to 63% in some series (131,132). If nonoperative therapies have failed to control symptoms for longer than 6 weeks, a patient may become a surgical candidate. Patients with sciatica predominating over back pain, with a positive straight leg raise or contralateral straight leg raise, neurologic deficit, and an imaging study consistent with the clinical findings are ideal candidates for surgery. Leg pain, however, is the primary indication for disc surgery independent of neurologic findings if the symptoms are consistent, persistent, and correlate with the imaging studies.

In two situations, however, surgery should not be considered elective. The first is progressive neurologic deficit, and the second cauda equina syndrome, fortunately a rare occurrence. Spangfort reported a 1.2% incidence of cauda equina syndrome in his series of 2,500 operative cases and an overall incidence of this syndrome in 2.5% of patients with disc herniation. The L4–5 level is usually involved in most series (133). Kostuik et al. reported on 31 patients with cauda equina syndrome caused by central disc herniation (134). The classic presentation of bilateral sciatica, saddle dysesthesia, motor weakness in the lower extremities, and bladder or bowel dysfunction did not occur in most of their patients. Seventeen of the 31 patients had unilateral sciatica. Patients with bilateral sciatica and saddle dysesthesia also had decreased anal sphincter tone and perianal sensory loss. All patients developed urinary retention before surgery. Eight had sexual dysfunction. The onset of symptoms and signs was rapid in 10 patients and gradual in 17 patients. The L5–S1 level was most frequently involved followed by the L4–5 level. Motor recovery occurred fully in most cases; however, bladder function fared poorer in those with an acute onset. The authors recommended that surgery be performed as soon as possible, although not necessarily considered an absolute emergency, to maximize recovery (134). Other reports also suggested that decompression within 48 hours of presentation improves the chance of bladder function recovery (135).

Assuming that the patient does not have a cauda equina syndrome or progressive weakness, the question of when surgery should be performed must be addressed. Weber prospectively studied surgically and nonoperatively treated patients with lumbar disc herniations. At 1 year, 92% of the surgical patients improved, whereas only 60% of the nonoperatively treated patients demonstrated improvement. At the end of 4 years, however, the surgery group remained at 90% and the nonoperatively treated group improved to 85% satisfactory results (136). These results indicate the early advantage of surgery and that a gradual improvement will occur in the nonsurgically treated group over time. Hakelius reported similar findings in his retrospective review of more than 500 patients with lumbar disc herniation. In this study, the nonoperatively treated group reported, after 7 years, more low back pain, more restricted sport activity, and more time off work than the surgical group (120). In reviewing these studies, it does not appear that delaying surgery for 3 to 6 months negatively influences the final outcome. It should be emphasized that in Weber's 10-year follow-up, the improvement in muscle weakness, sensory dysfunction, and reflex loss was not statistically improved in the surgery group compared with the nonoperative group.

In general, decompressive surgery for leg pain is highly successful if the patient is selected properly. Multiple series have demonstrated success rates of greater than 90% for relieving leg pain with lumbar discectomies (137). These studies also have shown a suprisingly high rate of improvement in back pain symptoms in the same population (138).

Recurrent Disc Herniation

The reported incidence of recurrent disc herniation ranges from 3% to 6%, and in 45% to 69% of cases, the herniation is at the same level (138–140). Enhanced MR imaging is the most useful study for differentiating scar from recurrent herniated disc (141–143). It is important to differentiate recurrent disc herniation from epidural scar formation, because surgery for scar excision has a low success rate (141,144,145). Haglund et al. reported on a series of 55 carefully selected patients who underwent repeat microdiscectomy at the same level as the first surgery and reported a success rate of 86% (146). Other studies found lower success rates for reoperation (60% to 70% successful), especially in multiply reoperated patients for recurrent herniated discs (147,148). Silvers et al. found that recurrent disc herniations at the same level and same side have a worse prognosis than recurrent disc herniations at other levels (124). It appears, as with primary hernia-

tions, that patient selection is the key to successful outcomes.

Role of Arthrodesis in Discectomy

Another controversy in lumbar spinal surgery is the role of arthrodesis following lumbar discectomy, especially after recurrent disc herniation. The rate of successful outcome in multiple large studies comparing primary discectomy with and without arthrodesis showed no significant benefit of arthrodesis (149,150). Generally, arthrodesis for the first recurrent disc herniation is also not recommended (148). Situations do exist where concomitant arthrodesis appears beneficial. Recurrent disc herniations at the L4–5 level are exposed to greater biomechanical stresses and may benefit from arthrodesis (151). Patients with gross instability as diagnosed by flexion and extension films showing greater than 4 mm of translation or more than 10 degrees of angular change are also candidates for arthrodesis (152). If back pain is a significant component of the patient's symptoms and concordant pain is produced with discography, arthrodesis may be indicated. Finally, removal of a significant portion of the facet joints during surgery is an indication for arthrodesis.

Degenerative Spinal Stenosis

The three-joint complex of the spine plays a role in the development of spinal stenosis. As the intervertebral disc degenerates, increased forces are placed on the facet joints (153). These degenerative changes manifest as disc bulges and herniations, bony osteophyte formation, facet enlargement, and ligament thickening and buckling. These changes result in narrowing of the spinal canal and neural foramina (154). The normal lumbar canal has an anteroposterior diameter of at least 12 mm and a cross-sectional area of 77 +/– 13 mm^2 (155,156). The critical area of the lumbar spine is not well established, but cadaveric studies show that a 50% compromise of the canal area results in significant increase in pressure experienced by the cauda equina (157–159). In addition to the cross-sectional area of the canal, the canal shape also appears to play a role in the etiology of stenosis. Spinal canals are classified as round, oval, or trefoil in shape, with the trefoil shape tending to produce more nerve-root compression in the lateral recesses (160–165).

Clinical Presentation and Examination

Degenerative spinal stenosis usually presents in the sixth or seventh decade of life and is more common in women than in men (166). Patients typically present with leg pain either in a radicular pattern or with neurogenic claudication. Neurogenic claudication is indicative of central canal stenosis, whereas lateral recess stenosis more commonly produces radicular symptoms. Neurogenic claudication typically radiates to the buttocks and progressively radiates down the legs to the feet. Patients may have pain, numbness, cramping, weakness, or tingling. Symptoms are exacerbated with spine extension, such as during walking or standing, whereas flexion of the spine tends to relieve symptoms (167). Bladder dysfunction is present in only 3% to 4% of cases. The differential diagnosis of neurogenic claudication includes vascular claudication and peripheral neuropathy such as that caused by diabetes.

Physical examination should include examination of gait, posture, palpation of the spine and pelvis, and a thorough neurologic examination of the lower extremities. Patients may have a flexed posture with mild tenderness over the sacroiliac joints and sciatic notch. The neurologic examination may be normal. Deficits in the L4–5 levels are most common. With long-standing disease, especially if significant lateral recess stenosis is present, muscle weakness and atrophy may develop. Straight leg raising is often unremarkable, as is the reflex examination.

If patient symptoms are significantly impairing function, radiologic examination is indicated. Plain radiographic findings include disc-space narrowing, facet arthrosis, degener-

ative spondylolisthesis or scoliosis, and spinous-process settling (168–170). Flexion and extension films are useful in assessing spinal stability. Axial images with either MR imaging or CT myelography should be obtained to confirm the diagnosis and plan surgical decompression if indicated. Little difference in sensitivity or specificity is noted between CT myelography and MR imaging for diagnosing spinal stenosis. Because of the noninvasive nature of MR imaging, most authors recommend it over CT myelography (129). Care must be taken to correlate imaging studies to clinical findings, because there is a high rate of abnormal imaging findings in asymptomatic patients who undergo MR imaging (131).

Spinal Stenosis Treatment

Nonoperative treatment for spinal stenosis includes general aerobic conditioning, avoidance of symptom-inciting activities, physical therapy, and careful medication use. Strengthening the paraspinal musculature along with physical therapy-type modalities may relieve symptoms. Aerobic conditioning, including stationary biking or swimming, may increase endorphin production and decrease symptoms. Narcotic pain medications should be used sparingly in this population. An alternative to narcotics may be antidepressants, which may help to restore a more normal sleep cycle and reduce symptoms of depression. Additionally, antidepressants alter nerve-membrane conductors and may help decrease radicular pain. A more thorough discussion of this topic was presented in previous chapters (19,20,23).

The decision of when to proceed with operative intervention generally depends on how severely the symptoms are affecting the patient's lifestyle. If a patient has not shown improvement after 3 to 6 months of nonoperative therapy, surgery should be considered.

Surgical Indications

The following are indications for surgery in the patient with documented spinal stenosis:

1. Significant limitation of walking ability because of neurogenic claudication or leg pain
2. Progressive neurologic dysfunction
3. Restriction of lifestyle that is unacceptable to the patient
4. Medical condition allowing surgery

Surgical Outcomes

Operative treatment for spinal stenosis is successful in 60% to 90% of cases (138,171–176). As in surgical decompression for a herniated disc, the primary goal for surgical decompression for spinal stenosis is relief of leg pain. A metanalysis by Turner et al. showed a success rate of 64% for surgical intervention for lumbar stenosis (177). Early success rates with lumbar decompression for spinal stenosis tend to deteriorate over time. An initial success rate of 88% at 6 weeks postoperatively was reported for 86 patients with spinal stenosis who underwent decompression. This rate dropped to 71% at an average follow-up of 5 years (178).

Complications occurring with decompression for spinal stenosis include dural tear, pulmonary emboli, hematoma causing cauda equina compression, and postoperative slipping (iatrogenic spondylolisthesis). Postoperative slipping appears to be the most common problem occurring with decompressive laminectomy, followed by dural tears. Some consideration for arthrodesis in appropriate patients should be made to avoid the former problem.

Indications for Arthrodesis

The criteria for spinal arthrodesis in conjunction with decompression were previously outlined by Wiltse et al. (179):

1. Patient 60 years of age or younger, with degenerative spondylolisthesis when total facetectomy has been performed
2. Patient 55 years of age or younger with degenerative spondylolisthesis
3. Patient younger than 50 years of age with isthmic spondylolisthesis

It is difficult to base a decision purely on age because so many other factors must be considered. The incidence of postoperative slip after decompression for degenerative spinal stenosis ranges from 2% to 30% in published series (171,180–184). Patients with degenerative spondylolisthesis preoperatively have a higher incidence of postoperative slippage, up to 73% in one series (171). Patients who develop postoperative spondylolisthesis have an increased rate of poor clinical outcome (171,180,181). Patients with preexisting spondylolisthesis who have increased slip postoperatively tend to have a better clinical outcome than patients who develop new spondylolisthesis postoperatively, however, possibly because of the better adaptability of the nerve roots in patients with preexisting slips (181). Factors that may influence postoperative slippage in degenerative spinal stenosis and spondylolisthesis include the extent of the decompression, the amount of slip present preoperatively, the gender of the individual, the severity of spondylosis of the anterior column, the number of levels decompressed, abnormal frontal or lateral plane alignment, abnormal motion on preoperative flexion/extension radiographs, and, finally, penetration of a disc space at the time of decompression.

Clinical outcome from lumbar arthrodesis following decompression for degenerative spinal stenosis has been mixed. Zdeblick's review of the literature on spinal stenosis revealed multiple studies that showed significantly better outcomes in patients undergoing spinal arthrodesis along with decompression than patients who did not undergo fusion (181,185–187). This view is not universal, however. The literature review by Turner et al. identified four studies that compared arthrodesis to nonarthrodesis. Three of the four studies showed no advantage of arthrodesis (177). Lee et al. reported that arthrodesis following decompression for spinal stenosis should be the exception rather than the rule (182).

Review of the available literature showed that the following trends appear to help predict postoperative instability:

1. A person with a preoperative slip has a greater risk of developing increased postoperative slippage.
2. Postoperative slip does not necessarily correlate with development of symptoms.
3. Decompression across disc space of normal height may lead to postoperative slip.
4. Excision of more than 50% of both facets at the same level increases the risk of slip.
5. Increasing the levels of decompression increases the risk of slip.
6. Penetration of the disc space at a decompressed level increases the risk of slip.
7. Women are at a higher risk than men for development of postoperative slip.

In general, arthrodesis should be considered with decompressive lumbar surgery if the following conditions are present:

1. *Spinal stenosis*
   a. Multiple-level decompression (three or more) with minimal anterior column degeneration
   b. Surgical disruption of more than 50% of each facet joint at the same level
   c. Prior decompression at the same level
2. *Degenerative spondylolisthesis*
   a. Documented preoperative progressive slip
   b. Minimal anterior column degeneration at the level of decompression
   c. High lumbosacral angle
   d. Sacralization of L5 (L4–5 spondylolisthesis)
   e. Surgical disruption greater than 50% of each facet joint at the same level
   f. Prior decompression at the same level
   g. Penetration of the disc space at the time of decompression
3. *Degenerative scoliosis with spinal stenosis*
   a. Larger curve (mean of 36 degrees)
   b. Decompression within the apex of the curve
   c. Lateral spondylolisthesis
   d. Decompression along the length of the curve with minimal anterior column degeneration
   e. Curve progression prior to surgery

Instrumentation for Lumbar Arthrodesis

Instrumentation of the lumbar spine has evolved greatly over the past 80 years. The Harrington rod revolutionized instrumentation of the thoracolumbar spine. Modifications and refinements of these early devices led to multiple fixation systems for the lumbar spine. Today both anterior and posterior fixation systems exist. Posterior systems consist of rod or plate systems using pedicle screws or laminar hooks for attachment to the spine. Anterior systems include rod or plate designs with screw fixation to the vertebral bodies and, more recently, arthrodesis cages.

The results of noninstrumented spinal arthrodesis have reported arthrodesis rates of 46% to almost 100% (188–192). Because of this high failure rate, instrumentation systems have been used to improve arthrodesis rates. Zdeblick performed a prospective randomized study that compared posterolateral lumbar arthrodesis rates using autologous bone graft only, autologous bone graft with a semirigid pedicle screw/plate system, or autologous bone graft with a rigid pedicle screw/rod system. Arthrodesis rates were significantly higher in the rigidly instrumented group (95% for rigid pedicle screw/rod system, 77% for the semirigid system, and 65% for the noninstrumented group) (192). Although other studies have supported higher arthrodesis rates in the lumbar spine when instrumentation is used (193,194), this finding is not universal. Thomsen et al., in a randomized prospective study of 130 patients receiving posterolateral lumbar arthrodesis either with or without instrumentation, found no significant difference in arthrodesis rates (195). In addition, concerns about instrumentation-related stress shielding osteopenia and an accelerated rate of adjacent level disc degeneration have been raised.

Arthrodesis for Low Back Pain

A new interest in arthrodesis for low back pain has developed, possibly as a result of the evolution of minimally invasive arthrodesis techniques. Classic teaching, based on multiple studies, advocated a high rate of clinically unsatisfactory results. Success rates of only 50% to 60% have been reported for lumbar arthrodesis for back pain, and successful results have not always correlated with radiographic arthrodesis (172,196,197). More recent studies reported higher success rates when arthrodesis levels were based on concordant pain with discography (198–200). Discography in the lumbar spine has been a reliable test for discogenic pain, with false-positive rates of 5% or less (201,202). MR imaging, unfortunately, has not been specific enough to determine clinically important disc disruption leading to back pain (203–206). Arthrodesis may be considered in a young patient (under age 45) who has an abnormal MR imaging examination and concordant pain production on discography at one or, at most, two levels. Successful results with lumbar arthrodesis have been reported in up to 89% of such patients (198,199).

Debate also exists about which arthrodesis procedure is best for discogenic pain. Anterior disc excision and interbody arthrodesis, posterior lumbar interbody arthrodesis, circumferential arthrodesis, and posterolateral arthrodesis all have been advocated (133,192,199, 207–213). Most studies have a wide variety of patients with varying pathology. Thus, outcome comparison of these techniques is nearly impossible. We advise that arthrodesis for discogenic back pain be approached with caution. Candidates for this procedure must have failed extensive nonoperative therapy, must have concordant pain on discography, and possibly most importantly, must have stable psychosocial situations. Currently, anterior fusion with titanium mesh or threaded cages (bone dowels, titanium) or bone wedges appears useful.

Lumbar Surgical Techniques

Lumbar Decompression

Multiple techniques are available for lumbar decompression, ranging from standard laminectomy and decompression to minimally invasive techniques using arthroscopic technology. Decompression can be performed ante-

riorly or posteriorly, depending on the pathology present. A thorough discussion of these techniques is obviously beyond the scope of this chapter; however, an attempt is made to cover the basic principles as well as the advantages and disadvantages of each technique.

Lumbar Laminectomy/Laminotomy

Positioning for posterior lumbar surgery is important to help decrease bleeding and thereby aid in visualization at surgery. In general, we use a kneeling position with the abdomen free and noncompressed, which helps to decrease intraabdominal and inferior vena cava pressure and also to decrease the amount of blood in the epidural vascular system. The kneeling position places the spine in some degree of extension; however, with the decompression performed in this position, the result is more likely to be adequate when the patient is in a flexed or neutral position.

A standard laminectomy is performed through a midline posterior incision down to the fascia. The fascia then can be stripped subperiosteally to the facet joints. For a single-level disc herniation, the approach need only be performed on the affected side. For spinal stenosis or a large central disc, the dissection should be performed bilaterally. Hemostasis, using electrocoagulation, should be performed at each tissue level, beginning at the subcutaneous tissues down to the interlaminar spaces. The surgical levels are confirmed with a lateral radiograph. The appropriate interlaminar spaces should be debrided of soft tissue using curettes and rongeurs. Again, hemostasis is essential. The ligamentum flavum, spanning the interlaminar space, can be separated from the inferior aspect of the cephalic lamina with a small curette. The ligamentum flavum can be teased off distally and sharply excised while protecting the dura with a small elevator. For a single-level discectomy, the laminotomy should be widened if necessary to visualize the lateral aspect of the involved nerve root using rongeurs and Kerrison punches. At this point, the proximal and distal aspects of the root can be packed off with a small cottonoid and the nerve root retracted medially, which provides good exposure to the disc space and the protruded and free disc fragments. It is important to emphasize that the laminotomy should extend lateral to the nerve root to avoid inadvertent injury to the nerve root while trying to limit the bony resection.

For decompression for spinal stenosis, bilateral laminectomies are required (Fig. 16). The laminectomies should extend across all levels of compromise observed on the preoperative imaging studies. The laminectomies should be performed using rongeurs and Kerrison punches, completing the midline canal decompression from distal to proximal and then working laterally. Finally, each nerve root should be explored to ensure that it is free in tension and compression. A dural elevator should pass easily anterior and posterior to the nerve root, out the foramen. If evidence of residual compression exists, more bone or disc should be removed and the foraminotomy extended until the root is free. Throughout the procedure, 3.5 loupe magnification and headlights should be worn to improve visualization and to help identify the nerve root, the disc margins, and the epidural vessels. Alternatively, an operating microscope may be used. In the epidural space, hemostasis should be obtained using bipolar electrocautery. If necessary, Gelfoam, Surgicel, and Avitene can be used to help control bleeding. Drains are used to minimize the risk of a postoperative cauda equina syndrome developing from a hematoma.

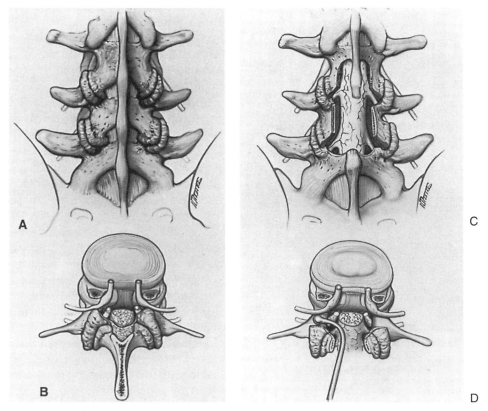

FIG. 16. A,B: Degenerative spinal stenosis with facet hypertrophy and thickened ligamentum. **C:** Typical decompression for spinal stenosis with medial facetectomy and foraminotomy. **D:** Probe is placed in the foramen to document adequate decompression. (From Whiffen JR, Neuwirth MG. Spinal stenosis. In: Bridwell KH, DeWald RL, eds. *The textbook of spinal surgery,* 2nd ed. Philadelphia: Lippincott-Raven Publishers, 1997:1562,1567.)

Postoperative Management

In general, patients can be mobilized early. Assuming no complications or dural tears occur, the patient can be allowed out of bed on the day of surgery or the next day, depending on the magnitude of surgery. We ask patients to minimize sitting for a week, other than bathroom privileges, and avoid driving a car for 2 to 3 weeks. Aerobic exercise is encouraged at 2 to 3 weeks, but twisting activities, such as golf or tennis, are best avoided for 3 months. These general guidelines are empirically derived. By following these broad recommendations, we have noted a less than average incidence of failed back syndrome and recurrent leg and back pain.

Posterior Lumbar Spinal Arthrodesis

Numerous techniques exist for lumbar arthrodesis, including anterior arthrodesis, posterior arthrodesis, posterolateral arthrodesis, posterior lumbar interbody arthrodesis, and instrumented arthrodesis, including anterior arthrodesis cages.

Posterolateral Lumbar Arthrodesis

A posterolateral arthrodesis can be added to the decompression if indicated. The transverse processes, pars interarticularis, and facet joints are included in the arthrodesis bed by clearing soft tissues and decorticating the osseous surfaces. Corticocancellous bone graft, obtained from the posterior iliac crest through the same incision or a separate incision, then is placed. Some advocate excising the facet joints at the arthrodesis levels and placing corticocancellous grafts in them. The paraspinal musculature falls in over the arthrodesis site, providing a rich blood supply to the graft.

Posterior Lumbar Interbody Fusion

Posterior lumbar interbody fusion (PLIF) was described by Jaslow in 1946 (214). The technique offers the advantages of total disc excision, restoration of disc-space height, en-

hanced foraminal decompression, and a high rate of arthrodesis. Unfortunately, disadvantages have included graft migration and neurologic injury (215–218). The procedure is performed following a complete laminectomy (Fig. 17). The nerve roots and cauda equina are retracted medially and the disc is completely excised using osteotomes, curettes, and burrs. Rectangles of corticocancellous bone are placed from posterior to anterior into the disc space. Some researchers advocate undercutting anterior to the posterior vertebral body cortex to help prevent graft retropulsion.

Posterior Lumbar Spinal Instrumentation

From the first report of spinal instrumentation by Hadra in 1889, great advances have been made in instrumentation systems for the lumbar spine. Laminar hooks were first used in 1964, and Harrington's rod system became popular in the late 1960s (219,220). Segmental fixation techniques using sublaminar wires were described by Resina and Alves in 1977 and by Luque in 1982 (221,222). Sublaminar wires allow good control of rotational forces and are used mainly in the neuromuscular scoliosis population. In 1984 the Cotrel-Dubousset instrumentation system was introduced. This system uses multiple laminar, pedicle, and transverse process hooks in the thoracolumbar spine to achieve control of the spine without the dangers of passing sublaminar wires. In addition, this system allows for control of compression and distraction along the length of the rod (223–226). The next advancement in posterior spinal fixation was the pedicle screw. The pedicle screw is placed from posterior to anterior into the vertebral body and thus allows three-dimensional control of the vertebrae (227,228). A multitude of instrumentation systems are now available that use pedicle screws or hooks to anchor the spine to rods or plates. Many systems have only small variations between them. It is more important to understand the principles of stabilization rather than the nuances of each system.

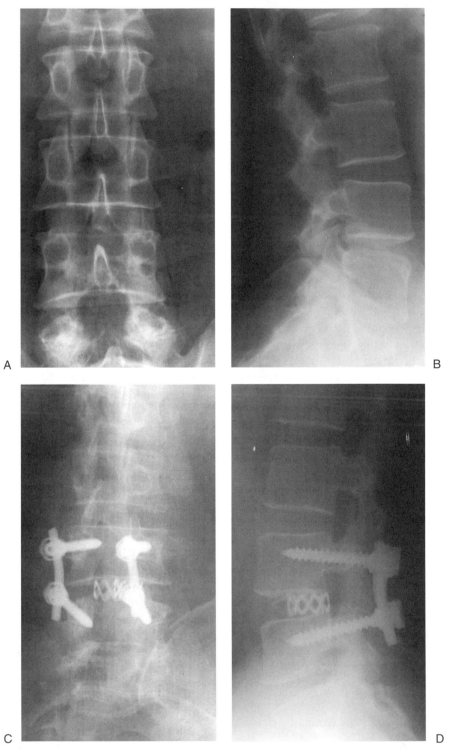

A   B   C   D

FIG. 17. A,B: A 50-year-old man who failed a previous laminectomy. The patient had significant back pain, instability, and recurrent stenosis. **C,D:** The patient underwent repeat decompression and posterior lumbar interbody fusion (*PLIF*) using a titanium mesh cage with iliac crest bone graft supplemented by instrumented posterolateral fusion.

The starting points for pedicle screws are made with a burr at the intersection of a transverse line that runs through the middle of the transverse process and a vertical line along the center of the facet (Fig. 18). Angulation of the screw depends on the region of the spine. In the thoracic spine, the screw should be angled from posterolateral to anteromedial. This angulation varies from 14 degrees at T-4 to 0 degrees at T-12 (229). The lumbar pedicle screw should be angled in the same direction, varying from 5 degrees at L-1 to 25 degrees at L-5 (230). Of course, these are guidelines. Screw placement should be based on preoperative planning using MR imaging or CT scans as well as blunt-tipped probes or curettes intraoperatively to determine the course of the pedicle. Markers should be placed and lateral radiographs obtained before placing the screws. Even using all these techniques, however, screw malposition may occur. Studies using CT to evaluate pedicle screw placement postoperatively found pedicle cortex disruption in up to 40% of the screws, with up to 29% penetrating the medial pedicle cortex. The incidence of clinically significant screw malposition was less than 1% (231,232). Other reports found rates of clinically significant pedicle screw malposition to be as high as 5% (233). Plain radiographs have been shown to underestimate significantly the rate of malpositioned screws; therefore, CT with thin cuts should be used to evaluate patients with postoperative nerve-root dysfunction (232,234).

Percutaneous Lumbar Discectomy

In 1975 Hijikata et al. reported the use of a percutaneous technique using a 5-mm cannula from a posterolateral approach to enter the disc space and remove nuclear material. The success rate was approximately 80% (235). Kambin advocates using a bilateral posterolateral percutaneous technique to allow visualization of the disc space and direct observation of nuclear material. Success rates of up to 87% were reported using these techniques (236–238). As technology advanced, smaller instruments that allow visualization and disc ablation through a single instrument have been developed. Laser disc ablation also has been advocated. Success rates using laser disc decompression range from 50% to 84% (239,240). Success of these techniques is highly dependent on patient selection. Patients with extruded or sequestered disc fragments are not candidates for these techniques. In addition, if lateral recess stenosis resulting from bony osteophytes is present, these techniques will be of limited use. Because of the minimally invasive nature of these procedures, it is tempting to stretch the indications; however, strict selection criteria must be followed.

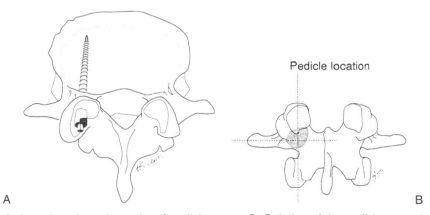

FIG. 18. A: Location of starting point of pedicle screw. **B:** Relation of the pedicle screw to surrounding structures. (From Haher TR, Felmly WT, O'Brien M. Thoracic and lumbar fractures: diagnosis and management. In: Bridwell KH, DeWald RL, eds. *The textbook of spinal surgery*, 2nd ed. Philadelphia: Lippincott-Raven Publishers, 1997:1786,1787.)

Anterior Lumbar Procedures

Anterior Lumbar Interbody Fusion

Anterior lumbar interbody fusion (ALIF) can be used to provide anterior column stability without the technical problems of inserting an interbody graft through a posterior laminectomy. Relative indications for ALIF include the following (241):

1. Revision of pseudarthrosis of previously failed posterolateral lumbar arthrodesis, or PLIF
2. Extension of arthrodesis to degenerative levels adjacent to previous arthrodesis
3. Severely osteoporotic bone in which adequate pedicle screw purchase cannot be obtained
4. Correction of deformity requiring anterior release, osteotomy, discectomy, or corpectomy

5. Low back pain that correlates with a degenerative disc on MR imaging and discography

The T-12 through the L-5 region can be accessed through an anterolateral retroperitoneal approach, exploiting the interval between the visceral peritoneum and the posterior muscular wall. This procedure usually is performed from the left side to limit the risk of injuring the vena cava and avoid retracting the liver (Fig. 19). Access to the L5–S1 interspace is more challenging but can be reached from an anterior transperitoneal or anterior retroperitoneal approach (242). Complications of the anterior approach include great vessel injury, visceral injury, sympathetic plexus injury, and possible cord ischemia.

The indications for anterior instrumentation are developing. Schlegel et al. list the fol-

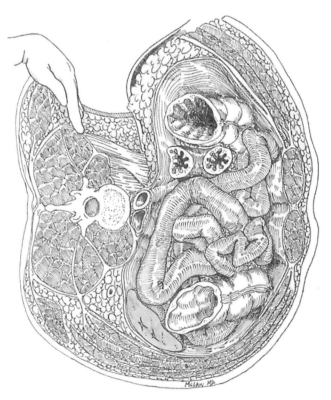

FIG. 19. Planes of dissection for the retroperitoneal approach. The kidney, ureter, and retroperitoneal fat are retracted anteriorly. (From ref. 242, with permission.)

lowing indications for anterior lumbar instrumentation:

1. Symptomatic posttraumatic kyphosis
2. Iatrogenic lumbar kyphosis (flat back syndrome)
3. Painful lumbar degenerative scoliosis

These authors list their relative indications for anterior instrumented arthrodesis as (a) revision of posterior pseudarthrosis, (b) instability secondary to wide laminectomy, (c) spondylolisthesis, and (d) spinal osteotomy (243).

A wide variety of plate/screw and rod/screw instrumentation systems are available for anterior instrumentation. Some of these devices are relatively high profile and should be placed on the right side of the thoracic spine to avoid contact with the pulsatile vessels. Interbody devices also are becoming much more popular. Titanium mesh cages can be filled with autologous bone graft and serve as a strut to provide anterior column stability. More recently, threaded interbody arthrodesis cages and titanium and allograft and allograft wedges/cylinders have become popular. These are filled with autograft. A great deal of recent attention has been given to placing intervertebral threaded cages through laparoscopic techniques.

Anterior Minimally Invasive Fusion Techniques

The Bagby and Kuslich (BAK) cage originated from the equestrian world, where it was used for cervical arthrodesis in the early 1980s (244–246). The original device was modified, and several versions of threaded interbody cages are now available. The indications for use include degenerative disc disease at one or two levels that causes chronic disabling low back pain unresponsive to nonoperative therapy. The cages can be inserted anteriorly using either open or laparoscopic techniques or from a posterior approach (PLIF or transforaminal). A skilled laparoscopic surgeon uses the anterior laparoscopic approach. The laparoscopic technique involves either a transperitoneal or retroperitoneal approach. The anterior approach involves marking the midline of the disc space and confirming it with fluoroscopy. Entrance holes are drilled on the left and right sides of midline. Properly sized plugs then are inserted in the holes. The hole is tapped and the cage filled with cancellous bone graft. The cage is then screwed into place. The spacer plug is removed from the contralateral side, and the cage is placed in the same manner (Fig. 20). The posterior approach involves a standard midline approach. The dura over the disc space is exposed by removing as much of the posterior elements as necessary to place drill guides and dural retractors. Special instrumentation is used to retract the neural structures. The threaded cages are placed in the same manner as outlined for the anterior approach (247).

An arthrodesis rate of 87% in 58 patients who underwent anterior arthrodesis with threaded cage implants with 2-year follow-up was reported (247). In addition, pain relief has been significant with continued improvement throughout the course of the follow-up (247). The possibility of multiple complications exist with this procedure. Fortunately, the rate of complications has been low and has been associated with the usual learning curve. In a multicenter study involving 22 laparoscopic BAK lumbar arthrodesis procedures, only one patient required conversion to an open procedure as a result of an iliac vein injury (106). Implant migration has occurred in 1.25% of implants, all within the first 3 postoperative months (247).

Role of Bone Morphogenetic Protein in Spinal Arthrodesis

Urist et al. first isolated osteoinductive proteins in 1973 (248). Individual BMPs have since been isolated, sequenced, and cloned, making possible recombinant production. The most promising of these proteins appears to be (rh) BMP-2 and BMP-7. These proteins

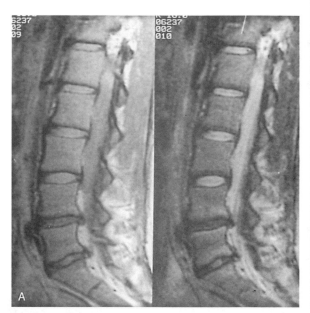

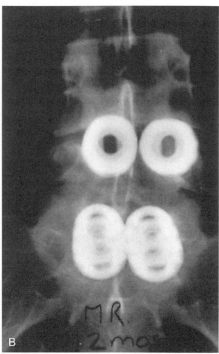

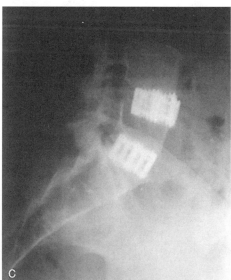

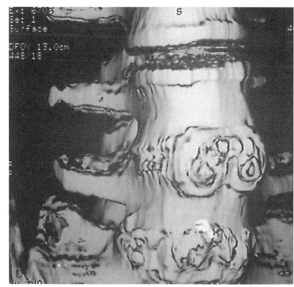

FIG. 20. A: Preoperative magnetic resonance (MR) imaging scan of a 34-year-old woman with chronic low back pain. MR imaging shows degenerative discs at L4–5 and L5–S1. Discography produced concordant pain. **B:** One year after anterior implantation of the Bagby and Kuslich (*BAK*) fusion cages. **C:** Lateral view 1 year after arthrodesis shows evidence of fusion. **D:** Three-dimensional computed tomography (*CT*) scan shows fusion at both levels. (From Kuslich SD. Anterior interbody fusion of the lumbar spine using a bone graft containing hollow, rigid, interbody device: the Bagby and Kuslich method of spinal fusion. In: Bridwell KH, DeWald RL, eds. *The textbook of spinal surgery*, 2nd ed. Philadelphia: Lippincott-Raven Publishers, 1997:2253.)

are currently undergoing investigational studies and are pending approval of the U.S. Food and Drug Administration. Animal studies have been promising, with extremely high rates of arthrodesis (249–251). Concerns of arthrodesis of adjacent levels and ossification of soft tissues will need to be investigated more fully.

REFERENCES

1. Whitecloud T. Complications of anterior cervical fusion. *Instr Course Lect* 1978;27:223–227.
2. Clarke E, Robinson P. Cervical myelopathy: a complication of cervical spondylosis. *Brain* 1956;79:483.
3. Bohlman HH, Emery SE, Goodfellow DB, Jones PK. Robinson anterior cervical discectomy and arthrodesis for cervical radiculopathy: long-term follow-up of one hundred and twenty-two patients. *J Bone Joint Surg Am* 1993;75:1298–1307.
4. Gore DR, Sepic SB. Anterior cervical fusion for degenerated or protruded discs: a review of one hundred forty-six patients. *Spine* 1984;9:667–671.
5. Simmons EH, Bhalla SK. Anterior cervical discectomy and fusion. A clinical and biomechanical study with eight-year follow-up. *J Bone Joint Surg Br* 1969;51:225–237.
6. White AA, Southwick WO, Deponte RJ, Gainor JW, Hardy R. Relief of pain by anterior cervical-spine fusion for spondylosis: a report of sixty-five patients. *J Bone Joint Surg Am* 1973;55:525–534.
7. Emery S, Bolesta M, Bohlman H. Anterior decompression and fusion for cervical spondlotic myelopathy: two to seventeen year follow-up. *Othop Trans* 1994–1995;18:1135.
8. Hanai K, Fujiyoshi F, Kamei K. Subtotal vertebrectomy and spinal fusion for cervical spondylotic myelopathy. *Spine* 1986;11:310–315.
9. Okada K, Shirasaki N, Hayashi K, Oka S, Hosoya T. Treatment of cervical spondylotic myelopathy by enlargement of the spinal canal anteriorly, followed by arthrodesis. *J Bone Joint Surg Am* 1991;73:352–364.
10. Saunders RL, Bernini PM, Shirreffs TG Jr, Reeves AG. Central corpectomy for cervical spondylotic myelopathy: a consecutive series with long-term follow-up evaluation. *J Neurosurg* 1991;74:163–170.
11. Yonenobu Y, Fuji T, Ono K, Okada Y, Yamamoto T, Harada N. Choice of surgical treatment for multisegmental cervical spondylotic myelopathy. *Spine* 1985;10:710–716.
12. Mikawa Y, Shikata J, Yamamuro T. Spinal deformity and instability after multilevel cervical laminectomy. *Spine* 1987;12:6–11.
13. Baba H, Chen Q, Uchida K, Imura S, Morikawa S, Tomita K. Laminoplasty with foraminotomy for coexisting cervical myelopathy and unilateral radiculopathy: a preliminary report. *Spine* 1996;21:196–202.
14. Baba H, Maezawa Y, Furusawa N, Imura S, Tomita K. Flexibility and alignment of the cervical spine after laminoplasty for spondylotic myelopathy. A radiographic study. *Int Orthop* 1995;19:116–121.
15. Baba H, Uchida K, Maezawa Y, Furusawa N, Azuchi M, Imura S. Lordotic alignment and posterior migration of the spinal cord following en bloc open-door laminoplasty for cervical myelopathy: a magnetic resonance imaging study. *J Neurol* 1996;243:626–632.
16. Hirabayashi K, Bohlman HH. Multilevel cervical spondylosis. Laminoplasty versus anterior decompression. *Spine* 1995;20:1732–1734.
17. Kawano H, Handa Y, Ishii H, Sato K, Oku T, Kubota T. Surgical treatment for ossification of the posterior longitudinal ligament of the cervical spine. *J Spinal Disord* 1995;8:145–150.
18. Kimura S, Homma T, Uchiyama S, Yamazaki A, Imura K. Posterior migration of cervical spinal cord between split laminae as a complication of laminoplasty. *Spine* 1995;20:1284–1288.
19. Lee TT, Manzano GR, Green BA. Modified open-door cervical expansive laminoplasty for spondylotic myelopathy: operative technique, outcome, and predictors for gait improvement. *J Neurosurg* 1997;86:64–68.
20. Satomi K, Nishu Y, Kohno T, Hirabayashi K. Long-term follow-up studies of open-door expansive laminoplasty for cervical stenotic myelopathy. *Spine* 1994;19:507–510.
21. Robinson RA, Smith GW. Anterolateral cervical disc removal and interbody fusion for cervical disc syndrome. *Bull Johns Hopkins Hospital* 1955;96:223–224.
22. Jones AA, Dougherty PJ, Sharkey NA, Benson DR. Iliac crest bone graft. Osteotome versus saw. *Spine* 1993;18:2048–2052.
23. Wood EGd, Hanley EN Jr. Types of anterior cervical grafts. *Orthop Clin North Am* 1992;23:475–486.
24. Riley LH Jr, Robinson RA, Johnson KA, Walker AE. The results of anterior interbody fusion of the cervical spine: review of ninety-three consecutive cases. *J Neurosurg* 1969;30:127–133.
25. Gaetani P, Tancioni F, Spanu G, Rodriguez Y, Baena R. Anterior cervical discectomy: an analysis on clinical long-term results in 153 cases. *J Neurosurg Sci* 1995;39:211–218.
26. Pointillart V, Cernier A, Vital JM, Senegas J. Anterior discectomy without interbody fusion for cervical disc herniation. *Eur Spine J* 1995;4:45–51.
27. Zdeblick TA, Ducker TB. The use of freeze-dried allograft bone for anterior cervical fusions. *Spine* 1991;16:726–729.
28. Murphy MG, Gado M. Anterior cervical discectomy without interbody bone graft. *J Neurosurg* 1972;37:71–74.
29. Robinson R, Walker A, Ferlic D, Wieking D. The results of anterior interbody fusion of the cervical spine. *J Bone Joint Surg Am* 1962;44:1569–1587.
30. Swank ML, Lowery GL, Bhat AL, McDonough RF. Anterior cervical allograft arthrodesis and instrumentation: multilevel interbody grafting or strut graft reconstruction. *Eur Spine J* 1997;6:138–143.
31. Zdeblick TA, Cooke ME, Wilson D, Kunz DN, McCabe R. Anterior cervical discectomy, fusion, and plating. A comparative animal study. *Spine* 1993;18:1974–1983.
32. Cheney RA, Herkowitz HJ. Anterior cervical corpectomy and fusion for radiculopathy. In: Clark CR, ed. *The cervical spine*. Philadelphia: Lippincott-Raven, 1998:805–816.

33. Southwick W, Robinson R. Surgical approaches to the vertebral bodies in the cervical and lumbar regions. *J Bone Joint Surg Am* 1957;39:631–644.

34. Vaccaro AR, Ring D, Scuderi G, Garfin SR. Vertebral artery location in relation to the vertebral body as determined by two-dimensional computed tomography evaluation. *Spine* 1994;19:2637–2641.

35. Bernard TN Jr, Whitecloud TSd. Cervical spondylotic myelopathy and myeloradiculopathy. Anterior decompression and stabilization with autogenous fibula strut graft. *Clin Orthop* 1987:149–160.

36. Boni M, Cherubino P, Denaro V, Benazzo F. Multiple subtotal somatectomy. Technique and evaluation of a series of 39 cases. *Spine* 1984;9:358–362.

37. Fernyhough JC, White JI, LaRocca H. Fusion rates in multilevel cervical spondylosis comparing allograft fibula with autograft fibula in 126 patients. *Spine* 1991;16:S561–S564.

38. Herkowitz H. Internal fixation for degenerative cervical spine disorders. *Semin Spine Surg* 1995;7:57.

39. Zdeblick T. Biomechanical evaluation of cervical spine fixation. *Semin Spine Surg* 1995:7:20.

40. Villas C, Martinez-Peric P, Preite R, Barrios RH. Union after multiple anterior cervical fusion: 21 cases followed for 1–6 years. *Acta Orthop Scand* 1994;65:620–622.

41. Wetzel FT, Hoffman MA, Arcieri RR. Freeze-dried fibular allograft in anterior spinal surgery: cervical and lumbar applications. *Yale J Biol Med* 1993;66:263–275.

42. Zdeblick TA, Bohlman HH. Cervical kyphosis and myelopathy. Treatment by anterior corpectomy and strut-grafting. *J Bone Joint Surg Am* 1989;71:170–182.

43. Bose B. Anterior cervical fusion using Caspar plating: analysis of results and review of the literature. *Surg Neurol* 1998;49:25–31.

44. Herman JM, Sonntag VK. Cervical corpectomy and plate fixation for postlaminectomy kyphosis. *J Neurosurg* 1994;80:963–970.

45. Katsuura A, Hukuda S, Imanaka T, Miyamoto K, Kanemoto M. Anterior cervical plate used in degenerative disease can maintain cervical lordosis. *J Spinal Disord* 1996;9:470–476.

46. McLaughlin MR, Purighalla V, Pizzi FJ. Cost advantages of two-level anterior cervical fusion with rigid internal fixation for radiculopathy and degenerative disease. *Surg Neurol* 1997;48:560–565.

47. Paramore CG, Dickman CA, Sonntag VK. Radiographic and clinical follow-up review of Caspar plates in 49 patients. *J Neurosurg* 1996;84:957–961.

48. Shapiro S. Cauda equina syndrome secondary to lumbar disc herniation. *Neurosurgery* 1993;32:743–747.

49. Abitbol J, Zdeblick TA, Kunz DN, McCabe RP, Cooke ME. A biomechanical analuysis of modern anterior and posterior cervical stabilization techniques. In: *Cervical Spine Research Society Meeting.* Palm Desert, CA: 1992.

50. Grubb MR, Currier BL, Bonin V, Grabowski JJ, Chao EYS. Biomechanical evaluation of anterior cervical spine stabilization in a porcine model. In: *Cervical Spine Research Society Meeting.* Palm Desert, CA: 1992.

51. Herkowitz HN. A comparison of anterior cervical fusion, cervical laminectomy, and cervical laminoplasty for the surgical management of multiple level spondylotic radiculopathy. *Spine* 1988;13:774–780.

52. Hirabayashi K, Satomi K. Operative procedure and results of expansive open-door laminoplasty. *Spine* 1988;13:870–876.

53. Yonenobu K, Hosono N, Iwasaki M, Asano M, Ono K. Laminoplasty versus subtotal corpectomy: a comparative study of results in multisegmental cervical spondylotic myelopathy. *Spine* 1992;17:1281–1284.

54. Yonenobu K, Yamamoto T, Ono K, Laminoplasty for myelopathy. In: Clark CR, ed. *The cervical spine.* Philadelphia: Lippincott-Raven, 1998:849–864.

55. Hosono N, Yonenobu K, Koizumi M, Ono K. Axial symptoms in cervical spondylotic myelopathy. *Rinsho Shinkeigaku* 1993;28:405.

56. Iwasaki K, Ebara S, Miyamoto S, Wada E, Yonenobu K. Expansive laminoplasty for cervical radiculomyelopathy due to soft disc herniation. *Spine* 1996;21:32–38.

57. Crockard A. Evaluation of spinal laminar fixation by a new, flexible stainless steel cable (Sof'wire): early results. *Neurosurgery* 1994;35:892–898.

58. Robinson RA, Southwick WO. Surgical approaches to the cervical spine. *Instr Course Lect* 1960;17:299–330.

59. Starr J, Eismont F, Scuderi G. Posterior occipitocervical fusion for non-rheumatoid instability. In: *Annual meeting of the Cervical Spine Research Society.* Desert Springs, CA: 1992.

60. Abumi K, Kaneda K. Pedicle screw fixation for non-traumatic lesions of the cervical spine. *Spine* 1997;22:1853–1863.

61. Grob D. Unisegmental three dimensional stabilization of C1–C2: report on a new surgical technique. In: *Annual Meeting of the Cervical Spine Research Society.* Washington, DC: 1987.

62. Grob D, Dvorak J, Panjabi M, Froehlich M, Hayek J. Posterior occipitocervical fusion: a preliminary report of a new technique. *Spine* 1991;16:S17–S24.

63. Grob D, Dvorak J, Panjabi MM, Antinnes JA. The role of plate and screw fixation in occipitocervical fusion in rheumatoid arthritis. *Spine* 1994;19:2545–2551.

64. Sasso RC, Jeanneret B, Fischer K, Magerl F. Occipitocervical fusion with posterior plate and screw instrumentation: a long-term follow-up study. *Spine* 1994;19:2364–2368.

65. Smith MD, Anderson P, Grady MS. Occipitocervical arthrodesis using contoured plate fixation: an early report on a versatile fixation technique. *Spine* 1993;18:1984–1990.

66. Fielding JW, Hawkins RJ, Ratzan SA. Spine fusion for atlanto-axial instability. *J Bone Joint Surg Am* 1976;58:400–407.

67. Boden SD, Dodge LD, Bohlman HH, Rechtine GR. Rheumatoid arthritis of the cervical spine: a long-term analysis with predictors of paralysis and recovery. *J Bone Joint Surg Am* 1993;75:1282–1297.

68. Brooks AL, Jenkins EB. Atlanto-axial arthrodesis by the wedge compression method. *J Bone Joint Surg Am* 1978;60:279–284.

69. Gallie WE. Fractures and dislocations of the cervical spine. *Am J Surg* 1939;46:495–499.

70. Grob D, Crisco JJD, Panjabi MM, Wang P, Dvorak J. Biomechanical evaluation of four different posterior atlantoaxial fixation techniques. *Spine* 1992;17:480–490.

71. Savini R, Parisini P, Cervellati S. The surgical treatment of late instability of flexion-rotation injuries in the lower cervical spine. *Spine* 1987;12:178–82.

72. Magerl F. Spondylodesen an der oberen halwirbelsaule. *Acta Chir Aust* 1982;(Suppl):43–69.

73. Moskovich R, Crockard HA. Atlantoaxial arthrodesis using interlaminar clamps: an improved technique. *Spine* 1992;17:261–267.

74. Grob D, Jeanneret B, Aebi M, Markwalder TM. Atlanto-axial fusion with transarticular screw fixation. *J Bone Joint Surg Br* 1991;73:972–976.

75. Ghanayem AJ, Leventhal M, Bohlman HH. Osteoarthrosis of the atlanto-axial joints: long-term follow-up after treatment with arthrodesis. *J Bone Joint Surg Am* 1996;78:1300–1307.

76. Lowery GL, Swank ML, McDonough RF. Surgical revision for failed anterior cervical fusions: articular pillar plating or anterior revision? *Spine* 1995;20:2436–2441.

77. Anderson PA, Henley MB, Grady MS, Montesano PX, Winn HR. Posterior cervical arthrodesis with AO reconstruction plates and bone graft. *Spine* 1991;16:S72–S79.

78. Weiland DJ, McAfee PC. Posterior cervical fusion with triple-wire strut graft technique: one hundred consecutive patients. *J Spinal Disord* 1991;4:15–21.

79. Arce CA, Dohrmann GJ. Herniated thoracic disks. *Neurol Clin* 1985;3:383–392.

80. Love JG, Schorn VG. Thoracic disk protrusions. *Rheumatism* 1967;23:2–10.

81. McBeath AA, Keene JS. The rib-tip syndrome. *J Bone Joint Surg Am* 1975;57:795–797.

82. Agostini E, Mognoni G, Tori G, Miserocki G. Forces deforming rib cage. *Respir Physiol* 1956;2:105.

83. Errico TJ, Stecker S, Kostuik JP. Thoracic pain syndromes. In: Frymoyer JW, ed. *The adult spine: principles and practice.* Philadelphia: Lippincott-Raven, 1997:1623–1637.

84. Wood KB, Garvey TA, Gundry C, Heithoff KB. Magnetic resonance imaging of the thoracic spine: evaluation of asymptomatic individuals. *J Bone Joint Surg Am* 1995;77:1631–1638.

85. Mixter WJ, Barr JS. Rupture of the intervertebral disc with involvement of the spinal cord. *N Engl J Med* 1934;211:210–215.

86. Schellhas KP, Pollei SR, Dorwart RH. Thoracic discography: a safe and reliable technique [see comments]. *Spine* 1994;19:2103–2109.

87. Perot PL Jr, Munro DD. Transthoracic removal of midline thoracic disc protrusions causing spinal cord compression. *J Neurosurg* 1969;31:452–458.

88. Kostuik JP. Surgical approaches to the thoracic and thoracolumbar spine. In: Frymoyer JW, ed. *The adult spine: principles and pratice.* Philadelphia: Lippincott-Raven, 1997:1437–1470.

89. Smith MD. Thoracic disc disease. In: An HS, ed. *Principles and techniques of spine surgery.* Baltimore: Williams & Wilkins, 1998:413–423.

90. Bohlman HH, Zdeblick TA. Anterior excision of herniated thoracic discs. *J Bone Joint Surg Am* 1988;70:1038–1047.

91. Albrand OW, Corkill G. Thoracic disc herniation: treatment and prognosis. *Spine* 1979;4:41–46.

92. Currier BL, Eismont FJ, Green BA. Transthoracic disc excision and fusion for herniated thoracic discs. *Spine* 1994;19:323–328.

93. Horowitz MB, Moossy JJ, Julian T, Ferson PF, Huneke K. Thoracic discectomy using video assisted thoracoscopy. *Spine* 1994;19:1082–1086.

94. Maiman DJ, Larson SJ, Luck E, El-Ghatit A. Lateral extracavitary approach to the spine for thoracic disc herniation: report of 23 cases. *Neurosurgery* 1984;14:178–182.

95. Otani K, Yoshida M, Fujii E, Nakai S, Shibasaki K. Thoracic disc herniation: surgical treatment in 23 patients. *Spine* 1988;13:1262–1267.

96. Rogers MA, Crockard HA. Surgical treatment of the symptomatic herniated thoracic disk. *Clin Orthop* 1994:300;70–78.

97. Buff HU. Thoracoscopic operations of the spine. *Ther Umsch* 1997;54:529–532.

98. Caputy A, Starr J, Riedel C. Video-assisted endoscopic spinal surgery: thoracoscopic discectomy. *Acta Neurochir (Wien)* 1995;134:196–199.

99. Dickman CA, Apfelbaum RI. Thoracoscopic microsurgical excision of a thoracic schwannoma: case report. *J Neurosurg* 1998;88:898–902.

100. Dickman CA, Rosenthal D, Karahalios DG, et al. Thoracic vertebrectomy and reconstruction using a microsurgical thoracoscopic approach. *Neurosurgery* 1996;38:279–293.

101. Holcomb GW III, Mencio GA, Green NE. Video-assisted thoracoscopic diskectomy and fusion. *J Pediatr Surg* 1997;32:1120–1122.

102. Huang TJ, Hsu RW, Liu HP, Liao YS, Hsu KY, Shih HN. Analysis of techniques for video-assisted thoracoscopic internal fixation of the spine. *Arch Orthop Trauma Surg* 1998;117:92–95.

103. Ikard RW, McCord DH. Thoracoscopic exposure of intervertebral discs. *Ann Thorac Surg* 1996;61:1267–1268.

104. Mack MJ, Regan JJ, McAfee PC, Picetti G, Ben-Yishay A, Acuff TE. Video-assisted thoracic surgery for the anterior approach to the thoracic spine. *Ann Thorac Surg* 1995;59:1100–1106.

105. McAfee PC, Regan JR, Fedder IL, Mack MJ, Geis WP. Anterior thoracic corpectomy for spinal cord decompression performed endoscopically. *Surg Laparosc Endosc* 1995;5:339–348.

106. McAfee PC, Regan JR, Zdeblick T, et al. The incidence of complications in endoscopic anterior thoracolumbar spinal reconstructive surgery: a prospective multicenter study comprising the first 100 consecutive cases. *Spine* 1995;20:1624–1632.

107. Newton PO, Cardelia JM, Farnsworth CL, Baker KJ, Bronson DG. A biomechanical comparison of open and thoracoscopic anterior spinal release in a goat model. *Spine* 1998;23:530–535.

108. Newton PO, Wenger DR, Mubarak SJ, Meyer RS. Anterior release and fusion in pediatric spinal deformity: a comparison of early outcome and cost of thoracoscopic and open thoracotomy approaches. *Spine* 1997;22:1398–406.

109. Regan JJ, Guyer RD. Endoscopic techniques in spinal surgery. *Clin Orthop* 1997:122–139.

110. Regan JJ, Yuan H, McCullen G. Minimally invasive approaches to the spine. *Instr Course Lect* 1997;46:127–141.

111. Wall EJ, Bylski-Austrow DI, Shelton FS, Crawford AH, Kolata RJ, Baum DS. Endoscopic discectomy increases thoracic spine flexibility as effectively as open

discectomy: a mechanical study in a porcine model. *Spine* 1998;23:9–16.

112. Frymoyer JW, Cats-Baril WL. An overview of the incidences and costs of low back pain. *Orthop Clin North Am* 1991;22:263–271.

113. Frymoyer JW, Pope MH, Clements JH, Wilder DG, MacPherson B, Ashikaga T. Risk factors in low-back pain: an epidemiological survey. *J Bone Joint Surg Am* 1983;65:213–218.

114. Horal J. The clinical appearance of low back disorders in the city of Gothenburg, Sweden: comparisons of incapacitated probands with matched controls. *Acta Orthop Scand Suppl* 1969;118:1–109.

115. Lawrence JS. Disc degeneration. Its frequency and relationship to symptoms. *Ann Rheum Dis* 1969;28:121–138.

116. Fischgrund JS, Montgomery DM. Diagnosis and treatment of discogenic low back pain. *Orthop Rev* 1993;22:311–318.

117. Andersson GB, Svensson HO, Oden A. The intensity of work recovery in low back pain. *Spine* 1983;8:880–884.

118. Eckert C, Decker A. Pathologic studies of the intervertebral discs. *J Bone Joint Surg* 1947;29A:447–454.

119. Silveri CP, Simeone FA. Lumbar disc disease. In: An HS, ed. *Principles and techniques of spine surgery*. Baltimore: Williams & Wilkins, 1998:425–441.

120. Hakelius A. Prognosis in sciatica: a clinical follow-up of surgical and non-surgical treatment. *Acta Orthop Scand Suppl* 1970;129:1–76.

121. Hoppenfeld S. *Orthopedic neurology*. Philadelphia: JB Lippincott, 1977.

122. Herron LD, Turner JA, Novell LA, Kreif SL. Patient selection for lumbar discectomy with a revised objective rating system. *Clin Orthop* 1996;325;48–55.

123. Milette PC, Fontaine S, Lepanto L, Dery R, Breton G. Clinical impact of contrast-enhanced MR imaging reports in patients with previous lumbar disk surgery. *AJR Am J Roentgenol* 1996;167:217–223.

124. Silvers HR, Lewis PJ, Asch HL, Clabeaux DE. Lumbar diskectomy for recurrent disk herniation. *J Spinal Disord* 1994;7:408–419.

125. Waddell G, Kummel EG, Lotto WN, Graham JD, Hall H, McCulloch JA. Failed lumbar disc surgery and repeat surgery following industrial injuries. *J Bone Joint Surg Am* 1979;61:201–207.

126. Bell G. Diagnosis of lumbar disc disease. *Semin Spine Surg* 1994;6:186–195.

127. Liang M, Komaroff AL. Roentgenograms in primary care patients with acute low back pain: a cost-effectiveness analysis. *Arch Intern Med* 1982;142:1108–1112.

128. Albeck MJ, Hilden J, Kjaer L, Holtas S, Praestholm J, Henriksen Ogjerris F. A controlled comparison of myelography, computed tomography, and magnetic resonance imaging in clinically suspected lumbar disc herniation. *Spine* 1995;20:443–448.

129. Bischoff RJ, Rodriguez RP, Gupta K, Righi A, Dalton JE, Whitecloud TS. A comparison of computed tomography-myelography, magnetic resonance imaging, and myelography in the diagnosis of herniated nucleus pulposus and spinal stenosis. *J Spinal Disord* 1993;6:289–295.

130. Janssen ME, Bertrand SL, Joe C, Levine MI. Lumbar herniated disk disease: comparison of MRI, myelography, and post-myelographic CT scan with surgical findings. *Orthopedics* 1994;17:121–127.

131. Boden SD, Davis DO, Dina TS, Patronas NJ, Wiesel SW. Abnormal magnetic-resonance scans of the lumbar spine in asymptomatic subjects: a prospective investigation. *J Bone Joint Surg Am* 1990;72:403–408.

132. Boos N, Rieder R, Schade V, Spratt KF, Semmer N, Aebi M. 1995 Volvo Award in clinical sciences: the diagnostic accuracy of magnetic resonance imaging, work perception, and psychosocial factors in identifying symptomatic disc herniations. *Spine* 1995;20:2613–2625.

133. Spangfort EV. The lumbar disc herniation. A computer-aided analysis of 2,504 operations. *Acta Orthop Scand Suppl* 1972;142:1–95.

134. Kostuik JP, Harrington I, Alexander D, Rand W, Evans D. Cauda equina syndrome and lumbar disc herniation. *J Bone Joint Surg Am* 1986;68:386–391.

135. Shapiro S. Banked fibula and the locking anterior cervical plate in anterior cervical fusions following cervical discectomy. *J Neurosurg* 1996;84:161–165.

136. Weber H. Lumbar disc herniation: a controlled, prospective study with ten years of observation. *Spine* 1983;8:131–140.

137. Hirsch C, Nachemson A. The reliability of lumbar disc surgery. *Clin Orthop* 1963;29:189–195.

138. Garfin SR, Glover M, Booth RE, Simeone FA, Rothman RH. Laminectomy: a review of the Pennsylvania hospital experience. *J Spinal Disord* 1988;1:116–133.

139. Cauchoix J, Ficat C, Girard B. Repeat surgery after disc excision. *Spine* 1978;3:256–259.

140. Frymoyer JW, Matteri RE, Hanley EN, Kuhlmann D, Howe J. Failed lumbar disc surgery requiring second operation: a long-term follow-up study. *Spine* 1978;3:7–11.

141. Fandino J, Botana C, Viladrich A, Gomez-Bueno J. Reoperation after lumbar disc surgery: results in 130 cases. *Acta Neurochir (Wien)* 1993;122:102–104.

142. Georgy BA, Hesselink JR, Middleton MS. Fat-suppression contrast-enhanced MRI in the failed back surgery syndrome: a prospective study. *Neuroradiology* 1995;37:51–57.

143. Tullberg T, Grane P, Rydberg J, Isacson J. Comparison of contrast-enhanced computed tomography and gadolinium-enhanced magnetic resonance imaging one year after lumbar discectomy. *Spine* 1994;19:183–188.

144. Fiume D, Sherkat S, Callovini GM, Parziale G, Gazzeri G. Treatment of the failed back surgery syndrome due to lumbo-sacral epidural fibrosis. *Acta Neurochir Suppl (Wien)* 1995;64:116–118.

145. Jonsson B, Stromqvist B. Repeat decompression of lumbar nerve roots. A prospective two-year evaluation. *J Bone Joint Surg Br* 1993;75:894–897.

146. Haglund MM, Moore AJ, Marsh H, Uttley D. Outcome after repeat lumbar microdiscectomy. *Br J Neurosurg* 1995;9:487–495.

147. Baba H, Chen Q, Kamitani K, Imura S, Tomita K. Revision surgery for lumbar disc herniation. An analysis of 45 patients. *Int Orthop* 1995;19:98–102.

148. Herron L. Recurrent lumbar disc herniation: results of repeat laminectomy and discectomy. *J Spinal Disord* 1994;7:161–166.

149. Gurdjian E. Herniated lumbar intervertebral discs—an analysis of 1176 operated cases. *J Trauma* 1961;1:158.

150. LaMont RL, Morawa LG, Pederson HE. Comparison of disk excision and combined disk excision and spinal fusion for lumbar disk ruptures. *Clin Orthop* 1976:212–216.

151. Tollison CD, Satterthwaite JR. Multiple spine surgical failures: the value of adjunctive psychological assessment. *Orthop Rev* 1990;19:1073–1077.

152. Hanley EN, David SM. Who should be fused? In: Frymoyer JW, ed. *The adult spine: principles and practice.* Philadelphia: Lippincott-Raven Publishers, 1997: 2157–2174.

153. Lorenz M, Patwardhan A, Vanderby R Jr. Load-bearing characteristics of lumbar facets in normal and surgically altered spinal segments. *Spine* 1983;8:122–130.

154. Lancourt JE, Glenn WV Jr, Wiltse LL. Multiplanar computerized tomography in the normal spine and in the diagnosis of spinal stenosis: a gross anatomic-computerized tomographic correlation. *Spine* 1979;4: 379–390.

155. Schonstrom N, Hansson T. Pressure changes following constriction of the cauda equina: an experimental study *in situ. Spine* 1988;13:385–388.

156. Schonstrom N, Lindahl S, Willen J, Hansson T. Dynamic changes in the dimensions of the lumbar spinal canal: an experimental study in vitro. *J Orthop Res* 1989;7:115–121.

157. Olmarker K, Holm S, Rosenqvist AL, Rydevik B. Experimental nerve root compression: a model of acute, graded compression of the porcine cauda equina and an analysis of neural and vascular anatomy. *Spine* 1991;16:61–69.

158. Olmarker Y, Rydevik B, Holm S, Bagge U. Effects of experimental graded compression on blood flow in spinal nerve roots: a vital microscopic study on the porcine cauda equina. *J Orthop Res* 1989;7:817–823.

159. Rydevik BL, Pedowitz RA, Hargens AR, Swenson MR, Myers RR, Garfin SR. Effects of acute, graded compression on spinal nerve root function and structure: an experimental study of the pig cauda equina. *Spine* 1991;16:487–493.

160. Eisenstein S. The trefoil configuration of the lumbar vertebral canal. A study of South African skeletal material. *J Bone Joint Surg Br* 1980;62:73–77.

161. Eisenstein S. Lumbar vertebral canal morphometry for computerised tomography in spinal stenosis. *Spine* 1983;8:187–191.

162. Lee CK, Rauschning W, Glenn W. Lateral lumbar spinal canal stenosis: classification, pathologic anatomy and surgical decompression. *Spine* 1988;13: 313–320.

163. Postacchini F, Ripani M, Carpano S. Morphometry of the lumbar vertebrae: an anatomic study in two caucasoid ethnic groups. *Clin Orthop* 1983;172:296–303.

164. Rauschning W. Normal and pathologic anatomy of the lumbar root canals. *Spine* 1987;12:1008–1019.

165. Winston K, Rumbaugh C, Colucci V. The vertebral canals in lumbar disc disease. *Spine* 1984;9:414–417.

166. Rosenberg NJ. Degenerative spondylolisthesis: predisposing factors. *J Bone Joint Surg Am* 1975;57: 467–474.

167. Lipson SJ. Spinal stenosis. *Rheum Dis Clin North Am* 1988;14:613–618.

168. Jones RA, Thomson JL. The narrow lumbar canal. A clinical and radiological review. *J Bone Joint Surg Br* 1968;50:595–605.

169. Kirkaldy-Willis WH, Paine KW, Cauchoix J, McIvor G. Lumbar spinal stenosis. *Clin Orthop* 1974;99: 30–50.

170. Tsukamoto Y, Onitsuka H, Lee K. Radiologic aspects of diffuse idiopathic skeletal hyperostosis in the spine. *AJR Am J Roentgenol* 1977;129:913–918.

171. Fox MW, Onofrio BM, Onofrio BK, Hanssen AD. Clinical outcomes and radiological instability following decompressive lumbar laminectomy for degenerative spinal stenosis: a comparison of patients undergoing concomitant arthrodesis versus decompression alone. *J Neurosurg* 1996;85:793–802.

172. Johnsson KE, Willner S, Pettersson H. Analysis of operated cases with lumbar renal stenosis. *Acta Orthop Scand* 1981;52:427–433.

173. Nasca RJ. Surgical management of lumbar spinal stenosis. *Spine* 1987;12:809–816.

174. Paine KW. Results of decompression for lumbar spinal stenosis. *Clin Orthop* 1976;115;96–100.

175. Spengler DM. Lumbar discectomy: results with limited disc excision and selective foraminotomy. *Spine* 1982;7:604–607.

176. Tile M, McNeil SR, Zarins RK, Pennal GF, Garside SH. Spinal stenosis: results of treatment. *Clin Orthop* 1976:115;104–108.

177. Turner JA, Ersek M, Herron L, et al. Patient outcomes after lumbar spinal fusions. *JAMA* 1992;268:907–911.

178. Javid MJ, Hadar EJ. Long-term follow-up review of patients who underwent laminectomy for lumbar stenosis: a prospective study. *J Neurosurg* 1998;89: 1–7.

179. Wiltse LL, Kirkaldy-Willis WH, McIvor GW. The treatment of spinal stenosis. *Clin Orthop* 1976:115; 83–91.

180. Johnsson KE, Redlund-Johnell I, Uden A, Willner S. Preoperative and postoperative instability in lumbar spinal stenosis. *Spine* 1989;14:591–593.

181. Johnsson KE, Willner S, Johnsson K. Postoperative instability after decompression for lumbar spinal stenosis. *Spine* 1986;11:107–110.

182. Lee CK. Lumbar spinal instability (olisthesis) after extensive posterior spinal decompression. *Spine* 1983;8: 429–433.

183. Nachemson A. Lumbar spine instability: a critical update and symposium summary. *Spine* 1985;10:290–291.

184. Spengler DM. Degenerative stenosis of the lumbar spine. *J Bone Joint Surg Am* 1987;69:305–308.

185. Bolesta MJ, Bohlman HH. Degenerative spondylolisthesis. *Instr Course Lect* 1989;38:157–165.

186. Herkowitz HN, Kurz LT. Degenerative lumbar spondylolisthesis with spinal stenosis: a prospective study comparing decompression with decompression and intertransverse process arthrodesis. *J Bone Joint Surg Am* 1991;73:802–808.

187. Zdeblick TA. The treatment of degenerative lumbar disorders. A critical review of the literature. *Spine* 1995;20:126S–137S.

188. Boucher H. A method of spinal fusion. *J Bone Joint Surg Br* 1959;41B:248–259.

189. Lenke LG, Bridwell KH, Bullis D, Betz RR, Baldus C, Schoenecker PL. Results of *in situ* fusion for isthmic spondylolisthesis. *J Spinal Disord* 1992;5:433–442.

190. Stauffer RN, Coventry MB. Posterolateral lumbar-spine fusion. Analysis of Mayo Clinic series. *J Bone Joint Surg Am* 1972;54:1195–1204.

191. Watkins M. Posterior lateral fusion in pseudarthrosis and posterior element defects of the lumbosacral spine. *Clin Orthop* 1964;35:80–85.

192. Zdeblick TA. A prospective, randomized study of lumbar fusion. Preliminary results. *Spine* 1993;18:983–991.

193. Jacobs RR, Montesano PX, Jackson RP. Enhancement of lumbar spine fusion by use of translaminar facet joint screws. *Spine* 1989;14:12–15.

194. Schwab FJ, Nazarian DG, Mahmud F, Michelsen CB. Effects of spinal instrumentation on fusion of the lumbosacral spine. *Spine* 1995;20:2023–2028.

195. Thomsen K, Christensen FB, Eiskjaer SP, Hansen ES, Fruensgaard S, Bunger CE. 1997 Volvo Award winner in clinical studies: the effect of pedicle screw instrumentation on functional outcome and fusion rates in posterolateral lumbar spinal fusion: a prospective, randomized clinical study. *Spine* 1997;22:2813–2822.

196. Flynn JC, Hoque MA. Anterior fusion of the lumbar spine. End-result study with long-term follow-up. *J Bone Joint Surg Am* 1979;61:1143–1150.

197. Sorensen KH. Anterior interbody lumbar spine fusion for incapacitating disc degeneration and spondylolisthesis. *Acta Orthop Scand* 1978;49:269–277.

198. Colhoun E, McCall IW, Williams L, Cassar Pullicino VN. Provocation discography as a guide to planning operations on the spine. *J Bone Joint Surg Br* 1988;70:267–271.

199. Newman MH, Grinstead GL. Anterior lumbar interbody fusion for internal disc disruption. *Spine* 1992;17:831–833.

200. Simmons EH, Segil CM. An evaluation of discography in the localization of symptomatic levels in discogenic disease of the spine. *Clin Orthop* 1975:57–69.

201. Milette PC, Melanson D. A reappraisal of lumbar discography. *J Can Assoc Radiol* 1982;33:176–182.

202. Walsh TR, Weinstein JN, Spratt KF, Lehmann TR, Aprill C, Sayre H. Lumbar discography in normal subjects: a controlled, prospective study. *J Bone Joint Surg Am* 1990;72:1081–1088.

203. Horton WC, Daftari TK. Which disc as visualized by magnetic resonance imaging is actually a source of pain? A correlation between magnetic resonance imaging and discography. *Spine* 1992;17:S164–S171.

204. Ito K, Incorvaia K, Yu S, Fredrickson B, Yuan H, Rosenbaum A. Predictive signs of discogenic lumbar pain on magnetic resonance imaging with discography correlation. *Spine* 1998;23:1252–1260.

205. Schneiderman G, Flannigan B, Kingston S, Thomas J, Dillin WH, Watkins RG. Magnetic resonance imaging in the diagnosis of disc degeneration:correlation with discography. *Spine* 1987;12:276–281.

206. Simmons JW, Emery SF, McMillin JN, Landa D, Kimmich SJ. Awake discography: a comparison study with magnetic resonance imaging. *Spine* 1991;16:S216–S221.

207. Blumenthal SL, Baker J, Dossett A, Selby DK. The role of anterior lumbar fusion for internal disc disruption. *Spine* 1988;13:566–569.

208. Chow SP, Leong JC, Ma A, Yau AC. Anterior spinal fusion or deranged lumbar intervertebral disc. *Spine* 1980;5:452–458.

209. Fredrickson BE, Baker D, McHolick WJ, Yuan HA, Lubicky JP. The natural history of spondylolysis and spondylolisthesis. *J Bone Joint Surg Am* 1984;66:699–707.

210. Fujimaki A, Crock HV, Bedbrook GM. The results of 150 anterior lumbar interbody fusion operations performed by two surgeons in Australia. *Clin Orthop* 1982:164–167.

211. Grubb SA, Lipscomb HJ. Results of lumbosacral fusion for degenerative disc disease with and without instrumentation: two- to five-year follow-up. *Spine* 1992;17:349–355.

212. Knox BD, Chapman TM. Anterior lumbar interbody fusion for discogram concordant pain. *J Spinal Disord* 1993;6:242–244.

213. Linson MA, Williams H. Anterior and combined anteroposterior fusion for lumbar disc pain: a preliminary study. *Spine* 1991;16:143–5.

214. Jaslow IA. Intercorporal bone graft in spinal fusion after disc removal. *Surg Gynecol Obstet* 1946;82:215–218.

215. Cloward RB. Spondylolisthesis: treatment by laminectomy and posterior interbody fusion. *Clin Orthop* 1981:74–82.

216. Hutter CG. Spinal stenosis and posterior lumbar interbody fusion. *Clin Orthop* 1985:103–114.

217. Lin PM, Cautilli RA, Joyce MF. Posterior lumbar interbody fusion. *Clin Orthop* 1983:180;154–168.

218. Simmons JW. Posterior lumbar interbody fusion with posterior elements as chip grafts. *Clin Orthop* 1985;193:85–89.

219. Harrington PR. The history and development of Harrington instrumentation. *Clin Orthop* 1973;93:110–112.

220. Knodt H, Larrick R. Distraction fusion of the spine. *Ohio State Med J* 1964;60:1140–1142.

221. Luque ER. The anatomic basis and development of segmental spinal instrumentation. *Spine* 1982;7:256–259.

222. Resina J, Alves AF. A technique of correction and internal fixation for scoliosis. *J Bone Joint Surg Br* 1977;59:159–165.

223. Cotrel Y, Dubousset J, Guillaumat M. New universal instrumentation in spinal surgery. *Clin Orthop* 1988;227:10–23.

224. Denis F. Cotrel-Dubousset instrumentation in the treatment of idiopathic scoliosis. *Orthop Clin North Am* 1988;19:291–311.

225. Ecker ML, Betz RR, Trent PS, et al. Computer tomography evaluation of Cotrel-Dubousset instrumentation in idiopathic scoliosis. *Spine* 1988;13:1141–1144.

226. Gurr KR, McAfee PC. Cotrel-Dubousset instrumentation in adults. A preliminary report. *Spine* 1988;13:510–520.

227. Richards BS, Birch JG, Herring JA, Johnston CE, Roach JW. Frontal plane and sagittal plane balance following Cotrel-Dubousset instrumentation for idiopathic scoliosis. *Spine* 1989;14:733–737.

228. Harrington PR, Tullos HS. Reduction of severe spondylolisthesis in children. *South Med J* 1969;62:1–7.

229. Roy-Camille R, Saillant G, Berteaux D, Salgado V. Osteosynthesis of thoracolumbar spine fractures with metal plates screwed through the vertebral pedicles. *Reconstr Surg Traumatol* 1976;15:2–16.

230. Vaccaro AR, Rizzolo SJ, Allardyce TJ, et al. Placement of pedicle screws in the thoracic spine. Part I: morphometric analysis of the thoracic vertebrae. *J Bone Joint Surg Am* 1995;77:1193–1199.

231. Humphreys SC, An HS. Posterior Instrumentation of the thoracolumbar spine. In: An HS, ed. *Principles and techniques of spine surgery*. Baltimore: Williams & Wilkins, 1998:675–691.

232. Castro WH, Halm H, Jerosch J, Malms J, Steinbeck J, Blasius S. Accuracy of pedicle screw placement in lumbar vertebrae. *Spine* 1996;21:1320–1324.

233. Laine T, Makitalo K, Schlenzka D, Tallroth K, Poussa M, Alho A. Accuracy of pedicle screw insertion: a prospective CT study in 30 low back patients. *Eur Spine J* 1997;6:402–405.

234. Farber GL, Place HM, Mazur RA, Jones DE, Damiano TR. Accuracy of pedicle screw placement in lumbar fusions by plain radiographs and computed tomography. *Spine* 1995;20:1494–1499.

235. Hijikata S. Percutaneous nucleotomy: a new concept technique and 12 years' experience. *Clin Orthop* 1989;238:9–23.

236. Kambin P. Diagnostic and therapeutic spinal arthroscopy. *Neurosurg Clin North Am* 1996;7:65–76.

237. Kambin P, McCullen G, Parke W, Regan JJ, Schaffer JL, Yuan H. Minimally invasive arthroscopic spinal surgery. *Instr Course Lect* 1997;46:143–161.

238. Kambin P, Zhou L. Arthroscopic discectomy of the lumbar spine. *Clin Orthop* 1997;337:49–57.

239. Casper GD, Mullins LL, Hartman VL. Laser-assisted disc decompression: a clinical trial of the holmium:YAG laser with side-firing fiber. *J Clin Laser Med Surg* 1995;13:27–32.

240. Liebler WA. Percutaneous laser disc nucleotomy. *Clin Orthop* 1995;30:58–66.

241. Whitecloud TS, Wolfe MW, Indications for internal fixation and fusion in the degenerative lumbar spine. In: Bridwell KH, DeWald RL, eds. *The textbook of spinal surgery*. Philadelphia: Lippincott-Raven, 1997:1581–1600.

242. McLain RF. Surgical approaches to the lumbar spine. In: Frymoyer JW, ed. *The adult spine: principles and practice*. 1997, Philadelphia: Lippincott-Raven, 1997:1723–1742.

243. Schlegel JD, Yuan HA, Fredricksen BE. Anterior interbody fixation devices. In: Frymoyer JW, ed. *The adult spine: principles and practice*. Philadelphia: Lippincott-Raven: 1997:2205–2223.

244. Bagby GW. Compression bone-plating: historical considerations. *J Bone Joint Surg Am* 1977;59:625–631.

245. Bagby GW. Arthrodesis by the distraction-compression method using a stainless steel implant. *Orthopedics* 1988;11:931–934.

246. DeBowes RM, Grant BD, Bagby GW, Gallina AM, Sande RD, Ratzlaff MH. Cervical vertebral interbody fusion in the horse: a comparative study of bovine xenografts and autografts supported by stainless steel baskets. *Am J Vet Res* 1984;45:191–199.

247. Kuslich SD, McAfee PC, Regan JF. Spinal instrumentation. In: Regan JF, McAfee MF, eds. *Atlas of endoscopic spinal surgery*. St. Louis: Quality Medical Publishing, 1995, pp. 293–332.

248. Urist MR, Iwata H, Ceccotti PL, et al. Bone morphogenesis in implants of insoluble bone gelatin *Proc Natl Acad Sci U S A* 1973;70:3511–3515.

249. Boden SD, Martin GJ Jr, Horton WC, Truss TL, Sandhu HS. Laparoscopic anterior spinal arthrodesis with rhBMP-2 in a titanium interbody threaded cage. *J Spinal Disord* 1998;11:95–101.

250. Fischgrund JS, James SB, Chabot MC, et al. Augmentation of autograft using rhBMP-2 and different carrier media in the canine spinal fusion model. *J Spinal Disord* 1997;10:467–472.

251. Helm GA, Sheehan JM, Sheehan JP, et al. Utilization of type I collagen gel, demineralized bone matrix, and bone morphogenetic protein-2 to enhance autologous bone lumbar spinal fusion. *J Neurosurg* 1997;86:93–100.

Occupational Musculoskeletal Disorders
edited by T. G. Mayer, R. J. Gatchel, and P. B. Polatin.
Lippincott Williams & Wilkins, Philadelphia © 2000.

28

Surgical Treatment for Upper Extremity Disorders

J. Mark Melhorn and *Joseph P. Zeppieri

*Section of Orthopaedics, Department of Surgery, University of Kansas School of Medicine, Wichita, Wichita, Kansas, 67208; *Orthopaedic Surgery/Plastic Hand Department, Lawrence and Memorial Hospital, New London, Connecticut 06320*

This chapter is written as a practical guide for upper-extremity disorders that cause workers to seek medical attention and is designed as a reference for nonmedical readers and as a review for medical readers. Musculoskeletal disorders can be thought of as occurring in specific body locations or by the type of organ system involved. This chapter takes the latter approach to provide a unique approach for general understanding and then a more detailed look at specific diagnoses.

Musculoskeletal disorders have a multifactorial etiology, as discussed in other chapters. Musculoskeletal pain can occur in response to a change in the neurologic system, soft-tissue system (e.g., muscle, tendon, skin), vascular system, and skeletal system (bone, joint, ligament). For a musculoskeletal disorder to be considered work related, the injury must meet specific requirements as outlined by the workers' compensation system of the state where the worker resides. These requirements are legal rather than medical (1).

This chapter deals with the musculoskeletal disorders of the International Classification of Diseases (ICD)-9. For each organ system, a general discussion of the system is followed by specific diagnoses for injuries that occur to that organ system. The specific diagnoses are reviewed, beginning with the most common and including a review of the history of onset (symptoms), physical findings (clinical examination), treatment options (nonsurgical intervention, surgery, after surgery), return to work, and expected outcome from treatment.

Occupational health care requires complex decision making. Confronted with a musculoskeletal problem, physicians draw on their understanding of basic medical and surgical principles, their experiences, and their familiarity with the literature to formulate a reasonable plan for diagnosis and treatment. All decisions are necessarily influenced by nonscientific considerations, such as limited facilities, patient noncompliance, financial constraints, psychosocial issues, economic issues, and the current limitations of the workers' compensation system (employer, insurer, legal, legislative, and medical). The clinical approach to diagnosis is described, with strong emphasis on outcome and return to work. Obviously, this chapter cannot and should not be a comprehensive text for the surgical treatment of all disorders of the upper extremities that might be work related.

CLINICAL EVALUATION OF THE INJURED WORKER

Physicians are asked to evaluate patients with occupational disorders for different reasons. They may be the treating physician, or they may be asked to carry out an independent medical evaluation for the employer, insurance company, or attorney, and each role is different. As the treating physician, the doctor's role is to treat the patient's medical problem, to work closely with allied health professionals, and to return the patient to the workplace. The role of an independent medical examiner is to examine the patient and to make determinations regarding return to work, treatment options, causal relationship to the job, and a permanent impairment if the patient's recovery has reached maximum medical improvement. The distinction between physical *impairment* and *disability* must be clearly understood. *Impairment* measures functional loss based on deformity, loss of motion, weakness, and other physical determinations. The percent of impairment is based on the American Medical Association (AMA) *Guidelines to the Evaluation of Permanent Impairment* (2). Physical impairment is determined by physicians. In contrast, *disability* is a legal determination and is based on factors such as education, job skills, and other socioeconomic considerations. Disability is awarded by judges or other legal authorities (3).

Patient Categories

Upper-extremity work-related injuries result in four types of work-related impairment: (a) acute traumatic injuries, (b) acute-onset nontraumatic, (c) chronic with return to work likely, and (d) chronic with return to work unlikely.

Acute Traumatic

Acute traumatic injuries would include sprains, strains, contusions, lacerations, fractures, and amputations. The symptoms and the injuries have a direct relationship and occur at the same time. The etiology and relationship to the job are easily determined. Treatment involves standard care or repair of the injured structures. Return to work usually depends on the severity of the injury. Treatment outcomes are usually good.

Acute-onset Nontraumatic

Musculoskeletal pain with acute onset can occur without a history of a traumatic event. The symptoms and the injury may have a direct relationship, but the date of specific onset may be difficult to determine. Examples would include tendinitis, synovitis, bursitis, joint inflammation, and nerve entrapment. The symptoms and the injury may be straightforward, but on occasion their relationship may be difficult to establish. The etiology and relationship to the job may be difficult to determine. Conventional treatment can include standard nonsurgical and surgical treatment. Continuing work or early return to work is usually possible. When these conditions become chronic or recurrent, the physician should evaluate job and psychosocial issues to determine possible influences before repeating surgical treatment.

Chronic Onset with Return to Work Likely

Musculoskeletal pain that has a history of multiple acute nontraumatic onsets or no history of acute onset is more likely to become chronic musculoskeletal pain. If this group of patients also has few secondary-gain issues, the motivation to return to work is high, and if employment issues are favorable, patients are more likely to be able to return to work. The physician must evaluate the disorder and the job to determine whether surgical intervention is reasonable or job modification or rehabilitation would be preferable. The surgical judgment in these cases is critical and often difficult. The physician traditionally has been called on to make a decision regarding surgery to alleviate pain or improve function. When treating the worker, the physician must consider not only whether the surgery will relieve pain and improve function but also whether it will allow the patient (employee) to return to work. Patients should be informed of the anticipated outcome of surgery and the likelihood of being able to return to previous work activities. Reasonable expectations on the part of the patient will improve the outcome from treatment.

Chronic Onset with Return to Work Unlikely

This group has a similar onset of chronic pain, but unlike the previous group, these patients have many secondary-gain issues, a low motivation to return to work, and unfavorable employment issues. As the result of these additional factors, this group is less likely to be able to return to work. This group often is described as having *chronic dysfunction pain*, because symptoms are disproportionate to the findings on physical examination (4). The treating physician in these cases becomes more of a medical manager and patient care facilitator than a traditional health care provider. Although opinions vary regarding physician involvement in legal issues, such as vocational rehabilitation or complicated return-to-work issues, physician involvement is both appropriate and helpful. In cases in which conflict exists between the insurer, employer, or attorney, the physician often is the best qualified to advise the patient (i.e., the worker). When there is mutual trust between the physician and worker, the patient can voice fears, frustrations, and anger. Whereas the employer, insurer, and attorney often have specific agendas, the physician's one concern is the total well-being of the patient (5,6).

Occupational Evaluation of the Injured Worker

The complexity or thoroughness of the occupational history will vary with the specific case and its requirements. When occupational issues are few and impairment is minor, the evaluation is straightforward. When issues such as causality, return to work, and the degree of impairment arise, the history becomes extremely important. The occupational history has several components.

The initial history should be accurate and detailed because of the many issues (medical and legal) that will need to be considered. Obviously, if an acute injury has occurred, the history should focus on the events that caused the injury. If the worker developed an acute

tendinitis or sustained a laceration or crush injury to the hand, the details of the event should be recorded and a copy of the emergency room record obtained, if possible. In addition to the obvious questions regarding the mechanism of the injury and the type of instrument that caused the injury, inquiry should be made about the machine or the work factors being used at the time of the injury. This information might be important later from a legal standpoint, and it is wise to have an initial detailed record. Such a record may be necessary when determining return-to-work issues and when causal relation issues are raised later.

In chronic work-related disorders or long-standing cases, a plethora of reports come from other treating physicians, therapists, evaluating physicians, and lawyers. The patient may have had physical-capacity evaluations, psychological evaluations, and multiple consultations. The physician must allow adequate time to study these reports. A frequent problem occurs when a worker who comes in for a physician visit has a large folder of medical reports that must be evaluated and inadequate time has been scheduled. The physician's office staff should determine the complexity of the case before the patient is seen so that adequate time can be allowed for consultation.

It is important to allow the patient time to describe the injury and the job in detail, which can be time consuming and seemingly nonproductive, depending on how articulate the patient is. When the job is technical or the worker uses unfamiliar terms, it may be difficult for the physician to comprehend clearly the demands of the job. If the physician takes the time to listen, however, insight often will be gained about the daily tasks the patient is required to perform. Some specific facts need to be ascertained during the history, including repetition (job cycle), force (grip, lift, carry), posture (standing, sitting, awkward position, twisting, wrist flexion–extension, elbow flexion, overhead work), vibration (from tool or to body), temperature (how long, to what level), contact stress (how objects or materials are held), and unaccustomed activities (new job, new product, new employee). In addition to understanding the specific job, it must be determined whether there will be opportunities to adjust the job. Is job rotation, job enlargement, or light-duty work available to the worker? If the job is incentive pay or machine paced, can these factors be adjusted? What is the company's policy regarding injured workers, and what other job opportunities exist for alternate work in the company? How long has the worker been employed there, and does he or she like the job and wish to return to the same company? When complicated return-to-work situations occur or job descriptions are limited, the therapist or vocational rehabilitation counselor can help the physician determine appropriate job recommendations. It is essential to emphasize that the treating or evaluating physician directs the multiple parties to help the patient.

Patients also should have the opportunity to describe in detail what they believe caused their current disability. When the physician takes the time to listen, a positive relationship is established and the patient feels the physician cares. It is important that the physician realize that the patient often embellishes the history because of his or her need to emphasize or prove a point, but this situation may give the physician an opportunity to understand some of the emotions surrounding the injury. It is wise for the physician to inquire about the patient's personal life as well. A simple question such as "How are things at home?" may release a flood of emotion and sometimes tears resulting from frustration and depression associated with the injury as well as confusion and anger with the workers' compensation system.

In these complicated situations, the rehabilitation specialist can be valuable in providing additional information. In addition to assisting the physician in understanding the complicated physical, social, and employment issues, the rehabilitation specialist facilitates the development of a strong and positive doctor–patient relationship, which is so important in these complicated cases. Although some physicians and patients are resistant to working with rehabilitation specialists, thinking that they represent the employer or insurer, these specialists can be used to communicate, coordinate the myriad bureaucratic issues, aid the physician by explaining and reinforcing recommendations, assist in obtaining and scheduling treatment, and help the employee return to work.

Return-to-Work Issues

Return-to-work guides or work restrictions are probably the most frustrating requirements for the occupational physician who is seeing the patient with a work-related musculoskeletal disorder. Little or no formal training occurs during residency training regarding work guides or work restrictions. Often the patient wants to negotiate the work guidelines or simply refuses to return to work, which often results in a "no-win" situation. It is important for the occupational physician to regain or remain in control. Work guides are simply *guides*, however and are not "written in stone" but rather should be flexible and adjusted as the individual patient's symptoms respond to treatment. An understanding of the symptoms, signs, job description, essential functions of the job, accommodation options, employer willingness, employee willingness, previous work guides (family physician, company physician, or other), response to previous modified work activities, and current work status are required to provide reasonable work guides.

Temporary or permanent work guides (not postsurgical) should include the level of work (sedentary work = maximum lift/carry of 10 lbs and occasional lift/carry combined for right and left upper extremity; light work = maximum 20 lbs or less, frequent 10 lbs; light medium work = maximum 35 lbs or less, frequent 20 lbs; medium work = maximum 50 lbs or less, frequent 25 lbs; medium heavy work = maximum 75 lbs or less; frequent 35 lbs; and heavy work = 100 lbs or less, frequent 50 lbs), work frequency (limited = 0% to 12% of time, occasional = 0% to 33%, frequent = 34% to 66%, constant = 67% to 100%), work characteristics (total hours per day of repetitive grasping, pushing/pulling, fine manipulation, vibratory tools, power tools, hand over shoulders, task rotation, or job rotation), length of workday in hours, and use of aids (splint, casts, wraps, bands, or protective aids).

Expectations for return to work after surgery should be discussed before surgery. When a patient elects to consider surgery, the physician should discuss the expectations from surgery, traditional informed-consent issues, postoperative care, and the plan for returning the patient to work. This plan should include specific guides and a specific date for return to work. An example summary of post-surgical work guides follows: before surgery, the same work pattern; after surgery, return to modified light work the day after surgery (maximum of 20 lbs or less lift/carry: frequently at 10 lbs), possibly with a cast or dressing on, using no large power or vibratory tools and limiting the use of the extremity on the operated side. The workday should be 8 hours or less for 5 days per 7-day week. Work production initially may be decreased during the postoperative period. In general, activities both at home and at work should be decreased. These guides should be given to the employer before the surgery is done. The patient signs the agreement after reviewing the guides with the physician (7).

Outcome studies show that early return to modified or regular activities improves the outcome from treatment and increases the likelihood of being employed for 2 years without any increased risk of recurrence (8–25). Returning the employee back to the employer as a productive employee is the primary objective of treating work-related musculoskeletal disorders. Early return to work is a "win–win" situation for both employee and employer.

NEUROLOGIC SYSTEM

The neurologic system consists of all peripheral and central nerve tissue. The upper-extremity peripheral nerve system originates from the cervical and thoracic nerve roots (C-5, C-6, C-7, T-1) and is called the *brachial plexus*. Three major peripheral nerves develop from the brachial plexus: the median, ulnar, and radial nerves. Peripheral nerve compression or entrapment is the most common form of nerve injury in the upper extremity. Each of the peripheral nerves of the upper extremities has several locations at which the compression can occur. Starting at the proximal end (the upper part of the arm), for the median nerve the locations are at the ligament of Struthers, anterior interosseous of forearm, lacertus, pronator teres, superficialis arch, and carpal tunnel wrist. For the ulnar nerve, the locations are at the thoracic outlet (thoracic outlet syndrome, or TOS), arcade of Struthers, cubital tunnel at elbow, and Guyon's canal at the wrist. For the radial nerve, the locations are above the elbow, the posterior interosseous syndrome at forearm, and the distal forearm (Wartenberg syndrome) (26–28).

Peripheral nerve compression lesions in the upper extremity can be difficult to localize. Many lesions are *idiopathic* (of unknown cause), but other types of pathology must be excluded in each lesion. The patient's general medical condition, the possibility of trauma, the existence of any inflammatory condition, symptoms of generalized neuropathy, or the possibility of tumor should be assessed. Symptoms may be nonspecific. Heaviness, weakness, aching, and pain, particularly after exertion of the extremity, are common complaints. Night pain and specific areas of sensory loss or specific motor weakness are more discrete signs that may help to localize the level of compression. General physical examination as well as careful examination of the limb in question should be made. A compressed nerve is irritable, and palpation or percussion in the injured area will elicit tenderness or paresthesias. The course of the nerve should be palpated for tenderness, masses, and provocation of symptoms. Maneuvers to increase pressure on the nerve, such as Phalen's test, may help to localize the level. Pulses also should be checked for concomitant vascular compression. Radiographs may reveal certain bony and soft-tissue abnormalities. Posttraumatic changes in the elbow or at the wrist may be the cause of nerve compression. A cervical rib may be associated with lower plexus lesions. Electrodiagnostic studies may help to confirm and localize a peripheral nerve compression, because compression may occur at more than one level in the same nerve. Prolonged latency in conduction velocity suggests that damage to the myelin sheaths of the nerve fibers is sufficient to interfere with conduction. Electromyography (EMG) may be useful primarily in motor nerves to document either denervation or recovery. Abnormal nerve conduction velocity or EMG is corroborative evidence of pathology; a normal study does not exclude a compression lesion. Localization of the level of compression requires an understanding of the anatomy of the upper extremity and the sites of potential compression neuropathy. Careful, repeated examinations using provocative maneuvers are the key to a correct diagnosis. Anatomic variations, such as Martin-Gruber connections, should be kept in mind. Once the probable location of compression is identified, other causes of nerve injury must be excluded (e.g., tumor, infection, inflammation, vascular malformation, congenital anomalies, trauma, degenerative changes). Correctable problems should be addressed (27). Symptoms of nerve compression represent a continuum of injury. By the time sensory loss and motor weakness are present, significant damage has occurred. Paralysis of muscles supplied by a pure motor nerve (i.e., anterior or posterior interosseous nerve) indicates long-standing pathology and a relatively poorer prognosis. The risk of not treating a compression neuropathy is that ultimately the compression may result in a neuroma with no chance of spontaneous recovery (29–32).

Carpal Tunnel Syndrome

History

The patient complains of pain, burning, paresthesias, or numbness involving the thumb or the index or middle finger. The symptoms usually are worse at night, while driving, holding a telephone, or fixing the hair. As symptoms progress, the patient may complain of clumsiness, loss of dexterity, and dropping things. As a work-related condition, the patient frequently complains of pain with any work activity. Often the patient will shake his or her fingers or rub the hands because to do so makes feeling return for a short period (33,34).

Examination

Signs on the physical examination include paresthesias or numbness in the median nerve distribution (thumb, index, middle finger) accentuated by provocative tests (Phalen's, reverse Phalen's, percussion, direct pressure, and pronator test), altered two-point or monofilament testing, and possible thenar muscle atrophy. The diagnosis can be supported by appropriate radiographs, nerve-conduction tests, and the patient's response to conservative treatment (35–38).

Nonsurgical Intervention

Nonsurgical treatment is appropriate when symptoms are mild, of recent onset, or aggravated by pregnancy. This treatment includes education about nerve entrapment and expectation from treatment, nonsteroidal anti-inflammatory drugs (NSAIDs), splinting, steroid injection, and modification of activities (both in the workplace and at home). Estimated duration of treatment is up to 3 months (39).

Surgery

Failure of nonsurgical treatment, progression of symptoms, objective loss of sensibility, intolerable numbness or pain, or thenar atrophy are indications for surgery. Surgical options include release of the transverse carpal ligament by open (mini versus standard) or endoscopic surgery, usually on an outpatient basis, using a regional block. The benefits of each technique have been debated, but several studies show outcomes to be similar at 6 months for the mini-open and endoscopic procedures. There does appear to be a slightly greater initial risk from the endoscopic method as a result of the learning curve that is required (40–44). Estimated duration of treatment is up to 12 months (45,46).

After Surgery

The method and time of immobilization vary with the physician. In addition to return to work, scar management and therapy start around 2 to 14 days postoperatively (47).

Return to Work

Modified light work with Band-Aid or cast on, depending on the job, may be the day after surgery. As pain decreases, activities may be gradually increased (8,9).

Outcome

Decrease or elimination of paresthesias, decreased pain, improved sensation, improved thenar motor function, pillar pain decreases over 6 months. Symptoms recur in about 5% of patients (48–51), and most patients can return to regular work activities with some modifications (9,21,25,52–54).

Cubital Tunnel Syndrome

History

The patient complains of numbness or tingling in the ring and little finger. Pain may radiate down the forearm from the elbow to the hand. The patient complains of decreased grip

and pinch strength. The onset of symptoms may be slower and less noticeable to the patient (55,56).

Examination

Signs on the physical examination include increased pain or numbness with the flexion test of the elbow or percussion of the ulnar nerve elbow. Sensory testing shows decreased light touch and two-point sensation and possible clawing of fingers with loss of intrinsic muscle mass. The diagnosis can be supported by radiographs and nerve-conduction studies (26).

Nonsurgical Intervention

Nonsurgical treatment is appropriate when symptoms are mild or of recent onset. This treatment includes education, NSAIDs, splinting, steroid injection, and modification of activities. Estimated duration of treatment is up to 6 months (32).

Surgery

Failure of nonsurgical treatment, progression of symptoms, objective sensibility loss, intolerable numbness or pain, or intrinsic atrophy are indications for surgery. Options include decompression of the cubital tunnel, subcutaneous transposition of the ulnar nerve, submuscular transposition of the ulnar nerve with or without medical epicondectomy, usually done as outpatient surgery using a regional block. Estimated duration of treatment is up to 12 months (57).

After Surgery

A Band-Aid, a soft dressing, a splint, or a soft cast may be used. Scar management and therapy start around 2 to 14 days postoperatively. The time of immobilization varies with the physician.

Return to Work

Modified light work wearing a Band-Aid or cast, depending on the job, may be done on the day after surgery. As pain decreases, activities may be increased gradually.

Outcome

Decrease or elimination of paresthesias, pain improvement, improved sensation, and improved motor function may be achieved. Patients sometimes experience a numb area at the medial epicondyle below the level of the incision (55).

Thoracic Outlet Syndrome

History

The patient complains of pain in the neck, shoulder, and upper limb, often accompanied by paresthesias and numbness that may have a predilection for the medial aspect of the arm, forearm, and hand; alternatively, the entire limb may be affected. Often the patient complains of nocturnal paraesthesias, and activities that involve lifting or the use of the limb at shoulder level or above may produce symptoms. Sometimes holding the arms out in front of the body as might be done while steering an automobile also may cause pain. Patients may complain of weakness in the hand. All these symptoms are manifestations of compression of the lower trunk of the brachial plexus at the level of the first rib. Intermittent swelling of the arm may result in front compression of the subclavian vein or artery. Rarely, symptoms stemming from thrombosis may occur, resulting from compression of the nerves and vessels that supply the upper limb within the area of the thoracic outlet. This space extends from the axilla to the neck and encompasses the area between the clavicle and the first rib. Because it is adjacent to and intimately associated with the shoulder complex, it is not unexpected that the two areas are mutually influential. Unfortunately, TOS is the subject of great controversy regarding pathogenesis and treatment, and it tends to be included in the general topic of cervicobrachial syndromes (58,59).

Examination

The diagnosis is made by history and physical examination. The position of the scapula is an important part of the pathology. Despite the fact that early interest focused on the scalene muscles, anatomic variations within the thoracic outlet continue to be important. Many patients have postural abnormalities as the major cause rather than definable cervical ribs or bands. This postural abnormality serves as both the common denominator and the explanation for the occurrence of TOS in the industrial population. It may result from a wrenching injury that alters the supporting structures of the shoulder girdle, or it may be caused by repetitive weight-bearing motions or by long periods of static shoulder loading. The actual incidence of TOS in the industrial population is difficult to establish but has been suggested as high as 18% (32,58).

The ability to reproduce the symptoms by positioning the arm in abduction and external rotation with the shoulder braced has been the most consistently useful test. The pulse is usually occluded at the wrist with this maneuver, but pulse obliteration by itself should not be taken as a positive test. Often subtle findings of neurologic loss in the hand, usually limited to the muscles supplied by T-1 and C-8, as well as the sensory territory of the ulnar aspect of the forearm and hand, are present. In long-standing compression, particularly when there is a congenital band compressing the nerves, atrophy of the hand muscles may be severe.

In all cases of suspected TOS, the patient should have a radiograph of the cervical spine and chest to look for long transverse processes at C-7 or the cervical ribs. The chest film is important in ruling out the possibility of a Pancoast tumor of the lung. Magnetic resonance (MR) imaging and computed tomography (CT) scanning have not contributed materially to the diagnosis of TOS. Electrodiagnostic studies are usually unreliable in confirming the diagnosis of TOS. These studies are most applicable in cases where a double-crush syndrome is suspected or in the differential diagnosis with a more peripheral lesion of the median or ulnar nerves. The use of both noninvasive and invasive studies of the vascular system to establish the diagnosis of TOS have limited benefit, because the symptoms of TOS are usually the result of neural compression, not vascular compression. Furthermore, because it is possible to occlude the pulse in many totally asymptotic and normal young women, it seems inadvisable to perform invasive vascular testing on those suspected of having TOS unless there is evidence of an aneurysm of the subclavian artery (60).

Nonsurgical Intervention

In most cases of TOS, the initial treatment is nonoperative unless significant and objective neural loss, impending vascular catastrophe, or documented failure of a carefully supervised program of exercise therapy is present. All other patients are treated by using an exercise routine to strengthen the shoulder girdle suspensory muscles and to correct any postural malalignments. If patients are overweight, losing weight is advised. Wherever possible, some adjustment in the working conditions is attempted as an alternative to surgery, particularly with overhead work or heavy lifting. Fewer cases of TOS have occurred in heavy laborers, and it is considerably more common in women than men. As the composition of the workforce continues to change, this group of manual laborers with TOS will be interesting to follow. Modification of activities can be helpful, along with exercises that strengthen the trapezius. Estimated duration of treatment is up to 12 months (61).

Surgery

If conservative treatment has failed after 4 to 6 months, and significant motor loss with atrophy or persistent and annoying vascular problems occur, surgery in the form of exploration of the thoracic outlet with resection of the first thoracic rib and any adventitious bony or soft tissues that can be seen to be causing compression is indicated. Surgery is done on an inpatient basis, often with the patient under general anesthesia. Estimated duration of treatment is up to 12 months (62).

After Surgery

Therapy is started a few days after surgery and is increased to tolerance (62).

Return to Work

The patient is often able to return to regular activities by 1 month (58).

Outcome

If the diagnosis is correct and a specific etiology is found at the time of surgery, the outcome is good to fair in well-motivated workers. The possibility of secondary gain in continued postoperative complaints of pain is difficult to interpret. Assuming all goes well, however, most clerical workers should be able to resume full duties within 2 to 3 months. The return to work of heavy manual laborers is somewhat problematic. If no cause is found at the time of surgery, the outcome is often fair to poor (62).

SOFT-TISSUE SYSTEM (MUSCLE, TENDON, SKIN, AND OTHERS)

The soft-tissue system consists of the muscles, tendons, fatty tissue, connective tissue, and skin (63). Injury to these structures can occur as tendinitis, inflammation, synovitis, masses, and ganglions. *Tendinitis* is defined as inflammation in the tendon or tendon cover (the *tendon sheath*). Any tendinitis disorder can cause pain and disability. Tendinitis can be caused by performing a new activity or by performing an activity that is more physically demanding than usual. Onset can be acute or gradual. The pain is localized and generally improves with modification of activities. The most common types are listed by their location. For the hand and wrist, trigger finger, or thumb, there may be tendinitis of the thumb (de Quervain's), flexor carpi ulnaris tendinitis, extensor carpi ulnaris tendinitis; for the elbow, lateral epicondylitis, medial epicondylitis, triceps tendinitis, biceps tendinitis; for the shoulder, rotator cuff tendinitis, shoulder impingement, and biceps tendinitis. Subluxation of a tendon or tendon rupture also can cause pain. An example of the more common disorders are listed in the order of frequency.

Trigger Finger or Thumb

History

The patient complains of a painful, limited range of motion of the digit, with possible popping or snapping with movement. The patient may feel a mass on the flexor surface of the digit that is painful to direct pressure. Triggering is more common in persons aged over 40 years. Heat sometimes allows the digit to move without catching (64).

Examination

The examination demonstrates tenderness in the palm over the tendon pulley of the involved digit. The classic picture is of "locking" at the level of the first annular pulley with the digit in flexion and difficulty extending the proximal interphalangeal joint. If triggering does not occur spontaneously, it may be elicited by putting pressure on the pulley with the examiner's own finger. The examiner should check the range of motion carefully; fixed flexion deformities or diffuse flexor tenosynovitis can be a common complication of prolonged triggering and may be an indication for earlier surgical intervention. A limited range of motion in flexion and or extension also implies osteoarthritis, which should be considered in the differential diagnosis in this age group. Radiographs should be obtained for patients who have a limited range of motion.

Nonsurgical Intervention

For mild or early onset, nonsurgical treatment would include NSAIDs (which rarely yield significant results), splints, steroid injection, and modification of activities. Estimated duration of treatment is about 6 months (65).

Surgery

With failure of nonsurgical treatment, pain interfering with activities, an inability to use the hands, or digits locked that will not open, surgery should be considered. The results of surgical release of the pulley are so good that the patient may opt for that treatment rather than prolonging the course with several injections and a period of impairment. The two types of surgery, open and percutaneous, usually are done as outpatient surgery using a regional or local block (66,67). The estimated duration of treatment is up to 4 months.

After Surgery

A Band-Aid or a soft dressing may be worn. Modified light work may be done the next day after surgery, depending on the job. As pain decreases, activities should be increased. Scar management and therapy are started around 2 to 4 days postoperatively (68,69).

Outcome

Outcome would be expected to be good to excellent for a complete recovery barring the occurrence of multiple trigger fingers or significant osteoarthritis. Pain reduction or relief is quite common. Restoration of motion without triggering is common. Most workers are able to return to heavy work, although to do so may take somewhat longer after surgery because of a tender palmar (64).

De Quervain's

History

The patient complains of local tenderness and swelling over the extensor retinaculum of the wrist at the level of the first dorsal compartment. De Quervain's is more common in women over the age of 40 (70).

Examination

The Finkelstein's test is used to confirm the diagnosis of de Quervain's. On examination, crepitus or squeaking with movement of the thumb is often found. Radiographs are helpful to exclude scaphoid fractures and arthrosis of the radiocarpal or intercarpal joints (71).

Nonsurgical Intervention

With mild symptoms, the use of NSAIDs, local steroid injection, or thumb and wrist splinting may provide temporary relief, but symptoms often return with activities (70). The estimated duration of treatment is up to 3 months.

Surgery

Surgery is indicated if nonsurgical treatment or limitation of activities fails. Release of the first dorsal compartment of the wrist (which includes the abductor pollicis longus and the extensor pollicis brevis) as an outpatient surgery using regional or local block allows return to near regular activities the next day, limited only by pain (70). The estimated duration of treatment is up to 3 months.

After Surgery

A Band-Aid, a soft dressing, a splint, or a soft cast may be worn. Scar management and therapy may be started around 2 to 14 days postoperatively. The duration of immobilization varies with the physician.

Return to Work

Modified light work while wearing a Band-Aid or a cast, depending on the job, may be done the next day. As pain decreases, activities may be increased gradually. Outcome studies show that early return to modified work and early return to regular activities improve outcome and increase the likelihood of being employed at 2 years without any increased risk of recurrence (8).

Outcome

Recurrence with nonsurgical treatment is high. With surgery, expectations for a complete recovery are good to excellent, barring other musculoskeletal disorders requiring surgery at the same time. Pain reduction or relief is common with restoration of motion. Most workers will be able to return to heavy work (64).

Intersection Syndrome

History

History may include symptoms of pain and swelling at 4 cm proximal to the wrist crease at the level of the muscle bellies of the abductor pollicis longus and the extensor pollicis brevis. This condition is probably more common than generally recognized (70).

Examination

Signs on examination include pain, swelling, redness, or crepitus at the muscle bellies on the forearm. Pain increases with direct pressure or movement of the thumb and direct pressure on muscles.

Nonsurgical Intervention

For mild symptoms, treatment includes NSAIDs, steroid injection at the level of the muscle bellies, heat or cold, exercise, and modification of activities. Unfortunately, these treatments often provide only temporary relief of pain (70). Estimated duration of treatment is up to 3 months.

Surgery

If nonsurgical treatment fails, release of the deep fascia and the second dorsal compartment extensor carpi radialus longus and brevis can be done on an outpatient basis using regional or local block. This surgery often allows the patient to return to near-normal activities the next day, limited only by pain (70). The estimated duration of treatment is up to 3 months.

After Surgery

A Band-Aid, a soft dressing, a splint, or a soft cast may be worn. Scar management and therapy is started around 2 to 14 days postoperatively. The duration of immobilization varies with each physician.

Return to Work

Modified light work while wearing a Band-Aid or cast, depending on the job, may begin the next day. As pain decreases, gradually increasing activities should be encouraged. Outcome studies show that early return to modified work and early return to regular activities improve the outcome and increase the likelihood that the patient will be employed 2 years postoperatively without any increased risk of recurrence (8).

Outcome

The recurrence rate with nonsurgical treatment is high but good to excellent for a complete recovery barring other musculoskeletal disorders requiring surgery at the same time. Pain reduction or relief is common with restoration of motion. Most workers should be able to return to heavy work.

Lateral Epicondylitis

History

Lateral epicondylitis (tennis elbow) is the most common musculoskeletal disorder of the elbow and pain the most common symptom. The pain may be associated with gripping activities, particularly if the elbow is extended and the wrist flexed. Repeated forced supina-

tion and the presence of vibration also seem to be aggravating workplace stressors. Pathology is suggested to be secondary to tearing of the common extensor tendon, inflammation at the point of attachment of the common extensor tendon to bone (periosteum), or synovitis over the radial head (72). Regardless of the cause, the symptoms involve pain over the lateral aspect of the elbow that is sharply localized to the area of the lateral epicondyle and joint line in the area of the radial head. Occasionally, pain radiates into the lateral forearm, which can cause confusion with the radial tunnel syndrome. Grip strength is often weakened because of pain. True radicular pain that radiates into the forearm should not occur (58,70).

Examination

The physical examination should elicit tenderness directly over the lateral epicondyle, common extensor tendon, or radial head. Discomfort increases with elbow extension and wrist flexion, by stretching the extensor musculature, and by resisted extension of the wrist and finger extensors. There is commonly a permanent flexion contracture if symptoms last for some time. The diagnosis is made by physical examination. Routine radiographs are indicated, and the presence of calcific deposits in the area of the common extensor tendon confirms the diagnosis. EMG and nerve-conduction studies may be carried out to rule out the radial entrapment syndromes (70).

Nonsurgical Intervention

If onset of symptoms is mild or early, nonsurgical treatment includes modification of activities or rest by means of a sling or splint, hot or cold applications, NSAIDs, and physical therapy modalities, such as ultrasound, are commonly used in the conservative treatment of the acute phase of this condition. Stretching exercises to eliminate permanent flexion contracture of the elbow as well as muscle-strengthening exercises for the wrist and finger extensors are important later. Steroid injections in the painful areas are commonly used. It is important not to inject a steroid into the elbow joint itself but rather into the tendon and periosteal area of the epicondyle. Injections of this type can be used several times over a few months, but they should not be used longer (70). Although workplace ergonomic changes are most important in the prevention of this condition, medical preventive techniques include work-hardening activities to prevent permanent flexion contractures and to increase finger and wrist extensor muscle strength. Occasionally, it is helpful to use a pressure splint that places pressure over the lateral extensor muscle mass just distal to the common extensor tendon and radial head during work activities. Resistant tennis elbow may be due to posterior interosseous nerve or radial tunnel syndrome. The estimated duration of treatment is up to 6 months.

Surgery

Surgery is reserved for the most resistant cases and involves releasing the common extensor tendon at the lateral epicondyle with or without exploration of the lateral compartment of the elbow joint. Usually, this surgery is done on an outpatient basis using a regional block. The major benefit of these procedures is elimination of scarring caused by the inflammatory reaction. The estimated duration of treatment is up to 9 months.

After Surgery

A Band-Aid, soft dressing, splint, or a soft cast may be worn. Scar management and therapy should be started around 2 to 14 days postoperatively. The duration of immobilization varies with each physician.

Return to Work

The time until return to work will vary with the individual physician and patient. Return to activities is gradual, pain being the limiting factor. Job modification or education regard-

ing modified work techniques is key, which may include changing tools, work environment, work methods, and machines.

Outcome

If the condition is chronic, a large element of operant conditioning may be involved in the patient's total symptoms. This effect can be elicited by inconsistent physical findings, which may help the treating physician in both the diagnosis and treatment, in particular the avoidance of surgery. Such inconsistent physical findings are patterned along the lines of those outlined by Waddell for evaluation of industrial chronic low back pain and include tenderness above rather than at the lateral epicondyle, increased pain with resisted finger and wrist flexion, pain being the same with the elbow flexed or extended when the wrist is held in flexion, and tenderness over the olecranon (73).

Shoulder Impingement (Rotator Cuff Tendinitis)

History

The clinical presentation of the patient with a rotator cuff problem depends on the stage of the pathology, although in all cases there is pain as the arm is elevated or abducted. Pain may be in the subacromial area or often is felt as a vague ache in the upper lateral arm at the level of the deltoid tuberosity. The discomfort on examination is usually present in only part of the arc of range of motion. With the arm at the side, there is little pain, but as the arm is brought into a horizontal position and then rotated medially rotated, pain occurs (74).

Examination

On physical examination, abduction, and external rotation, the humeral head impinges into the acromion and the rotator cuff is compressed. There is a variable amount of crepitus and possible weakness of the shoulder muscles. The diagnosis can be confirmed by injection of local anesthetic beneath the acromion, which abolishes the pain if it is due to impingement. Radiographs can be supportive if acromial humeral height is less than 7 mm, a type II or III acromion is present, or the acromial clavicluar joint demonstrates osteoarthritic spurs. Although it is an invasive and occasionally painful procedure, the most reliable means of demonstrating a complete tear of the rotator cuff is contrast arthrography. MR imaging, CT, and ultrasonographic studies are gradually replacing arthrography (74).

Nonsurgical Intervention

The nonsurgical treatment is based on the level or stage of rotator cuff involvement. Treatment for stage I impingement is conservative, and modification to activities is key. Attempts to limit shoulder motions that might be contributing to the impingement irritation of the rotator cuff are reasonable. The use of NSAIDs can be of benefit, but to prescribe them on a long-term basis is unjustified, as is the use of multiple intrabursal injections of cortisone and local anesthetic. The differentiation of stage II impingement from a tear of the cuff is clarified by diagnostic maneuvers, but some patients do not appear to have complete tears and yet continue to be disabled by their symptoms of pain whenever they do anything but light activities or use their arms overhead. The modalities of therapy for delivering heat to the shoulder are useful for symptomatic relief, but in established lesions, they do not promote healing. They can be useful as an adjunct to active range-of-motion and strengthening exercises, but even these exercises are not to be continued if they cause persistent pain or do not effect significant improvement within a month or so. Maintenance of gentle range of motion is done until surgery can be scheduled. These patients sometimes have partial tears with notable symptoms, and ultimately they are unable to function. To continue physical therapy indefinitely in patients who do not demonstrate im-

provement is often demoralizing to all concerned. The estimated duration of treatment is up to 6 months (75,76).

Surgery

If nonsurgical treatment and limiting activity fail, or the patient cannot elevate the arm posttraumatically, surgery is indicated. Surgery of the rotator cuff is tailored to the pathology found at the time of surgery. For the patient with an intact cuff, a significant bursitis, and evidence of impingement, treatment should be an anterior acromioplasty with or without resection of the coracoacromial ligament. It is important to avoid detaching deltoid muscle during surgery, because to do so will result in considerable impairment and weakness of the deltoid. The estimated duration of treatment is up to 12 months (77,78).

After Surgery

Recovery is slower than other after upper-extremity surgery. A formal physical therapy program starting with Codeman exercises and progressing to active range of motion with strengthening exercises is required.

Return to Work

The patient may return to light work while wearing a sling (no overhead activities allowed) 4 to 7 days after surgery. As strength returns and pain decreases, it is appropriate to increase activities. Permanent work guides for limiting hand-over-shoulder activities are required.

Outcome

The prognosis for recovery of the patient with rotator cuff derangement depends on the degree and duration of the pathology and the future occupational demands that will be placed on the shoulder (77,79).

Dorsal Wrist Ganglions

History

Dorsal wrist ganglions are common problems that may be either work related or not. They present as prominent cystic masses of varying sizes located over the dorsum of the wrist and often are painful. This problem occurs more often in women than in men and often is associated with ligamentous wrist laxity. The cystic mass invariably arises from the dorsal scapholunate interosseous ligament. The ganglion may be asymptomatic or associated with dorsal wrist pain that is usually activity related. As the ganglion enlarges, it becomes more painful and interferes with joint motion

Examination

The patient complains of an enlarging mass that is often painful and interferes with joint motion. The mass can be tender on direct pressure and is usually soft and freely movable; it transilluminates and varies in size with activities. Routine radiographs are usually normal, as are stress radiographs done to look for scapholunate instability. Bone scans are sometimes hot (i.e., they show increased activity), and a wrist arthrogram may show dye entering the ganglion. In general, the diagnosis is made by the clinical examination and is confirmed by aspiration or ultrasound studies (80).

Nonsurgical Intervention

If the mass is small, slow growing, or asymptomatic and the patient has no history of trauma, the mass can be treated by observation, NSAIDs, aspiration with or without steroid injection, splints, and modification of activities. The estimated duration of treatment is up to 6 months.

Surgery

If nonsurgical treatment is not effective, the mass continues to enlarge, or the patient experiences unusual pain or limitation of function, surgery is indicated. Surgery is designed to remove the mass and to close the origin of the mass from the joint; the mass then is reviewed by pathology. The estimated duration of treatment is up to 3 months.

After Surgery

May include on a Band-Aid up to a soft cast. Scar management and therapy started around 7 to 14 days postoperative.

Return to Work

Modified light work with Band-Aid or cast on and depending on job may be the day after surgery. As pain decreases encourage gradual increasing activities.

Outcome

Pain reduction or relief are achievable. The postsurgical recurrence rate is about 10% and after aspiration 25% to 90% (70).

Volar Wrist Ganglions

The second most frequent ganglion is located over the volar (flexor) radial side of the wrist. It protrudes from the radiocarpal joint, the trapeziometacarpal joint, or the scaphotrapezial–trapezoid joints. In the last two cases, it dissects along the flexor carpi radialis tendon sheath and presents adjacent to this tendon. The signs and symptoms are similar to those of dorsal ganglion, with onset after a wrist injury or after a change in activity. These ganglions also may be asymptomatic and may change in size, depending on the patient's activity. The differential diagnosis is similar to that of dorsal wrist ganglion and radial artery problems. Routine radiographs are usually normal; however, ganglions may be associated with arthritic conditions, which can be confirmed by radiograph. A wrist arthrogram may communicate with the volar wrist ganglion. Treatment is similar to that for dorsal wrist ganglions and includes NSAIDs, splinting, job modification, and injection. Surgical excision is reserved for persistent symptomatic ganglions. Surgery is not without complications. The radial sensory nerve, palmar cutaneous nerve, terminal portions of the lateral antebrachial cutaneous nerves, and the radial artery must be avoided. When the ganglion arises from the scaphotrapezial–trapezoid joint or the carpometacarpal joint, the flexor carpi radialis tendon sheath must be opened and the ganglion dissected to its base. If the ganglion does not represent a significant arthritic process in the carpometacarpal joint, the scaphotrapezial–trapezoid joint, or wrist joint, the prognosis for full recovery should be good. If other conditions are present, however, they can influence the final outcome (70).

Flexor Carpi Ulnaris (FCU) Tendinitis

Patients present with acute-onset or chronic pain over the volar ulnar side of the wrist. This condition sometimes is seen when the patient begins a new job that requires increased wrist flexion or after a brief episode of heavy lifting. It also can occur spontaneously. Examination shows tenderness over the FCU tendon, especially at the insertion. Pain is associated with resisted wrist flexion and passive wrist extension. In acute situations, mild swelling or erythema may be present. A radiograph may show calcification within the FCU tendon. In most cases, conservative treatment using a wrist splint in slight ulnar deviation and neutral wrist flexion is helpful. NSAIDs alleviate the acute inflammation. Sometimes a steroid injection is indicated. Some patients develop a chronic FCU tendinitis, however, and have recurrent bouts of pain. Most patients have one bout of FCU tendonitis, which never recurs. If the condition becomes chronic or the patient has repeated bouts of acute FCU tendonitis associated with the job, modification to a less repetitive job might be curative. Occasionally, surgical excision of calcific deposits is necessary. The prognosis for complete recovery is good (70).

Extensor Carpi Ulnaris (ECU) Tendinitis

Patients present with acute or chronic pain over the extensor surface at the ulnar side of the wrist. Pain is exacerbated by active extension and ulnar deviation. Diagnosis, treatment, and outcome are similar to those of FCU (70).

Extensor Carpi Ulnaris Tendon Subluxation

Patients present with a painful snapping of the ECU that is noted with ulnar deviation and rotation. Onset can be from a traumatic event in which the wrist was in supination and extension and was forced into flexion and ulnar deviation, which causes an acute rupture of the ECU retinactilum. In these cases, the history suggests the diagnosis. Patients also may present with a chronic subluxation that becomes symptomatic. Some patients have a congenital subluxation of the ECU that becomes inflamed, especially when increased wrist motions are carried out. On physical examination, it should be possible to see the ECU tendon sublux out of the ulnar grove as the patient rotates the wrist. In acute or inflamed cases, pain may be associated with motion. No tests are available to confirm the diagnosis; rather, the diagnosis is a clinical one. For acute ruptures of the ECU sheath, casting in a pronated, dorsiflexed, and radial deviated position may be attempted to determine whether the sheath will heal. If subluxation persists despite the casting, reconstruction of the ruptured tendon sheath is advised, although it may require the use of a strip of either the palmaris longus tendon, ECU tendon, or extensor retinaculum. A similar type of reconstruction is required for patients who have a chronic ECU tendon subluxation and have repeated episodes of inflammation. Reconstruction of the ECU tendon sheath is usually quite successful, and in most cases patients are able to return to repetitive wrist activities. Obviously, not all patients have this outcome, and job modification may be necessary for some patients (70).

Distal Biceps Tendon Ruptures

Ruptures of the distal end of the biceps occur as a sudden injury with maximum contraction of the biceps. Discomfort is felt in the anterior elbow, physical findings are nonspecific, and radiographs are negative; so the acute diagnosis is often missed. Elbow flexion strength remains intact because of brachialis function, but supination is significantly weaker. There is loss of prominence of the biceps tendon and tenderness over the anterior elbow to deep pressure. Because of the unusual anatomic prominence of the bicipital tuberosity, fraying of the biceps tendon may occur on pronation and supination, with rupture occurring with less than a maximal flexion/supination effort. This condition may be confused with median nerve entrapment syndromes, but there should be no positive Tinel's sign or any sensory or motor changes. No good confirmatory tests exist, although MR imaging is occasionally helpful in localizing the pathology to the area of the biceps tendon and bicipital tuberosity. Rarely, there may be an avulsion fracture of the bicipital tuberosity with this injury that is visible on plain radiographs. Conservative treatment consisting of immobilization of the elbow in flexion for a period of 4 to 6 weeks allows healing, although flexion and supination strength is permanently weakened and the muscle will have an abnormal shape. In the younger worker, operative repair also may yield good results. Late repairs requiring a tendon graft may be worthwhile. Surgery is extensive and rehabilitation lengthy, up to 6 to 12 months, but the worker can expect to return to the original employment, including heavy work (70).

Medial Epicondylitis

Less common than lateral epicondylitis, medial epicondylitis has many of the same features as lateral epicondylitis but is less common. Anatomically, the joint–ligament–tendon relationship is less complicated than on the lateral side because of the absence of the radial head. Physical examination reveals tenderness directly over the medial epicondyle or medial collateral ligament. Pain may be accentuated by resisted flexion of the fingers and wrist, although this physical sign is not as predictable as on the lateral side. Because the ulnar nerve lies immediately posterior as it courses the cubital canal, some confusion between medial epicondylitis and the cubital canal syndrome may occur. Medial epicondylitis can be confirmed by the presence of point tenderness over the medial epicondyle or ulnar collateral ligament of the joint line (but not distally), a lack of tenderness over the ulnar nerve or soft tissues distal to the medial epicondyle, and an absence of any subluxation of the ulnar nerve on flexion. Surgical treatment is less common, and the outcome is better than for lateral epicondylitis.

Triceps Tendinitis

Pain over the posterior aspect of the elbow is the hallmark of this diagnosis, which is associated with activities involving frequent pushing with the arms or lifting over the head. Occasionally, it is a secondary condition superimposed over other elbow joint pathology. Physical findings include point tenderness over part of the attachment of the triceps tendon into the olecranon. Localized swelling may occur in this area. Pathology usually includes either minor tearing of the triceps tendon or a traumatic inflammatory reaction secondary to irritation at the point of maximal tenderness. Permanent flexion contracture may occur when symptoms have been present for some time, either by an impinging spur formation at the tip of the olecranon or from protective muscular spasm. Routine radiographs, particularly the lateral view, often confirm the diagnosis by showing the presence of calcium at the area of maximal tenderness. Without such evidence, however, only the physical findings noted above are available to make the diagnosis. Symptoms abate, and motion and muscle-strengthening exercises are gradually instituted but must progress slowly so as not to cause symptoms to recur. Steroid injections have been used but may cause further degeneration in the tendon if injected directly. Repeat injections are not indicated. In general, the diagnosis is readily apparent, treatment is often successful, and return to work is common. Occasionally, activities may need to be modified. Surgery sometimes is performed to remove calcium deposits or to debride part of the olecranon if it is blocking full extension (70).

Proximal Biceps Tendinitis

Pain over the anterior aspect of the shoulder at the location of the long head of the biceps is uncommon (81). The pain of bicipital tendinitis usually is associated with anterior glenohumeral instability, lesions of the glenoid labrum in the absence of instability, and impingement or tear of the rotator cuff. Even when the presenting complaint is an acute rupture of the long head of the biceps, acute onset of pain in the shoulder and sudden retraction of the muscle, which gives a "Popeye" appearance to the arm usually are caused by an associated rotator cuff tear that has resulted from attrition. If instability, other labral lesions, and rotator cuff derangements have been ruled out, a biceps rupture in most cases can be treated conservatively, without operative tenodesis in the bicipital groove. Usually, the pain subsides spontaneously, and the patient may resume the use of the shoulder as comfort determines, depending on occupational demands.

Frozen Shoulder and Adhesive Capsulitis

The patient with a stiff, painful shoulder should not be immediately labeled as having a frozen shoulder or adhesive capsulitis, because several different entities may present similarly; in addition, the term also may convey an inappropriate sense of negativism to the treatment, which can prove costly. Adhesive capsulitis is a distinct entity that occurs uncommonly in manual workers and far more commonly in persons who have a sedentary lifestyle. The etiology is unknown. The typical patient's age is 40 to 60 years, and the condition occurs most commonly in the dominant arm. Although presentation is variable, there is usually no history of trauma. Pain is the presenting complaint, and the pain is often severe. Usually, the pain diminishes over a few weeks and is gradually replaced by increasing stiffness. The diagnosis is confirmed by arthrogram, which shows decreased capsule space. Treatment includes NSAIDs, range-of-motion exercises, and modalities. Seldom is manipulation under general anesthesia indicated, and surgery is performed only in patients who do not regain a useful range of motion. The prognosis is fair, and range of motion is often limited, but recurrence is rare (81).

Occupational Cervicobrachial Disorder

The term *occupational cervicobrachial disorder* (OCD) is used to describe pain in the neck, paracervical musculature, and shoulders of workers who are doing either repetitive motions of the shoulders and arms or who must maintain a constant position of the neck and shoulders while performing stereotyped tasks with the wrists and hands. It is a most unfortunate and imprecise term that will survive on the basis of the large amount of literature that has come mostly from Japan, where the term originated, and Australia, where it is known as *repetitive strain injury* (RSI). No specific anatomic or pathologic criteria for the diagnosis of OCD exists, other than symptoms of discomfort in the general location of the neck with radiation down the arms. The lack of a specific anatomic cause makes comparison and study almost impossible. A better approach is to shift from the term OCD to the ICD-9 pain in limb (other code 729.58). Education, treatment (exercise and physical conditioning), efforts at prevention in the workplace, and reduction in the incidence of pain in limb therefore can take place without the emotional term OCD (82,83). The prognosis for recovery from pain in a limb is extremely difficult to predict, although, as might be expected, the more severe the degree of impairment, the longer it is likely to persist.

Hypothenar Muscle Contusion

Patients have acute or chronic pain over the hypothenar region. The patient usually has a history of direct injury or chronic overuse. Tenderness over the muscles is demonstrated, and pain with resisted abduction of the fifth digit is noted. Other causes of pain are excluded. Discoloration or swelling may be noted when an acute injury has occurred. The diagnosis is a clinical one, and no tests to diagnose it exist. Conservative treatment includes rest, splinting, NSAIDs, and alteration of the activity. The prognosis is good, especially when the condition is associated with an acute injury or with chronic overuse and the activity can be adjusted.

VASCULAR SYSTEM

The vascular tissue system consists of the veins, arteries, and lymphatic system. Work-related vascular injuries are usually acute. Several examples of nonacute arterial injuries are reviewed.

Hypothenar Hammer Syndrome

The condition of impact or vibratory ulnar artery thrombosis is commonly called *hypothenar hammer syndrome*. The initial traumatic event may not have been noted. Gradual increasing coolness of the ring and little fingers is associated with possible blue discoloration or numbness. On occasion, swelling in the hypothenar palm area may occur. The physical examination can confirm the diagnosis by using Allen's test for arterial patency. MR imaging or ultrasound also can confirm the diagnosis. Treatment is surgical removal of the thrombosis, which occasionally requires arterial repair or grafting. The prognosis is usually good. Return to regular activities with modification of impact on the hand is recommended (84).

False (Pseudo) Aneurysms

False aneurysms may follow any type of penetrating trauma, but perhaps the most typical situation is one in which a narrow, long, sharp object, such as a piece of glass or a knife, perforates the skin over an artery to an unknown depth. The profuse bleeding that follows the injury is controlled by pressure, the skin wound is closed, and the patient is sent on his or her way. Within the next few weeks or months, a pulsatile mass appears beneath the skin wound. The best treatment is surgical removal of the false aneurysm and repair or replacement of the artery. The prognosis is good, and recurrence is unusual (84).

Vibration White Finger

Vibration white finger is defined as both a vascular and a neurologic injury. It comprises digital blanching and loss of sensation that occurs with exposure to cold. *Vibration* is the motion that starts at a reference point and then moves in a horizontal, vertical, or lateral direction (*linear motion*), or in pitch, yaw, or roll (*rotational motion*). The actual pathophysiology of nerve damage is not clear but is likely to be multifactorial. Histologic changes in the peripheral nerves may result from vibration, including demyelination, axonal degeneration, and perineural and endoneural fibrosis. Reduction of grip strength probably results from a combination of factors that include nerve involvement, vessel involvement, and a direct effect of vibration on the muscles. Diagnosis rests on history, chronic exposure to vibration, and the presence of secondary Raynaud's phenomenon in the absence of any other cause (85–88).

Raynaud's Phenomenon and Related Occlusive and Vasospastic Problems

This group of diagnoses is difficult to relate directly to work activities, although some states have legislated their inclusion for coverage under the workers' compensation system. Raynaud's phenomenon is a pallor of the digits with or without cyanosis on exposure to cold. The thumbs are usually spared. Paresthesias or hyperesthesias are common in the involved digits. After an attack and during rewarming, an intense hyperemia is followed by a gradual return to normal. Characteristically, the hands are normal between attacks. The phenomenon may occur because of one of three situations: (a) blood pressure decreases and blood flow ceases when a critical closing pressure of the vessel is reached; (b) vessel constriction reaches a point where blood flow ceases; or (c) an increase in blood viscosity causes sluggish flow. Raynaud's disease is seen mainly in young women, who have attacks precipitated by cold exposure and, often, by emotional upset. Treatment includes education, limiting cold exposure, oral steroids, steroid injections, calcium channel blockers, biofeedback, and muscle relaxation. On occasions, the digits may become ischemic, with or without trophic changes, suggesting consideration of a partial palmar sympthectomy. The outcome is fair to poor. Permanent work guides are required (58,84).

SKELETAL SYSTEM (BONES, JOINTS, AND LIGAMENTS)

The bone and joint system consists of the bones, joints, ligaments, and the attachment of muscles and tendons (63). Activities can cause stress and strain to this system. An injury to this system can be acute, such as a fall, a sudden twist, or a blow to the body, or chronic, such as activities that accumulate over time. The result of the injury is usually the onset of pain. Specific terms used to describe these injuries are defined in the following sections.

Sprains

The joints of the body are supported by *ligaments*, which are strong bands of connective tissue that connect one bone to another. When a ligament stretches or tears, the result can be a sprain (partial or complete). A sprained wrist can occur when the hand is bend backwards, as in a fall. The recommended treatment for a sprain is usually "RICE" (i.e., rest, ice, compression, and elevation). If the ligament is torn, surgery may be required to repair the injury.

Strains

The bones are supported by a combination of muscles and tendons. Tendons connect muscles to bones. A strain is the result of an injury to either a muscle or a tendon. The strain may be a simple stretch in the muscle or tendon, or it may be a partial or complete tear in the muscle and tendon combination. The recommended treatment for a strain is the same as for a sprain: RICE, followed by simple exercises to relieve pain and restore mobility. For a serious tear, surgical repair may be required.

Contusions

A contusion is a bruise caused by a blow to the muscle, tendon, or ligament. The bruise is caused when blood pools around the injury and discolors the skin. Most contusions are mild and respond well to rest, ice, compression, and elevation of the injured area.

Bursitis

A *bursa* is a sac filled with fluid and is located between a bone and a tendon or muscle. The bursa allows the tendon to slide smoothly over the bone. Repeated small stresses and overuse can cause the bursa in the shoulder or elbow to swell. The swelling and irritation are called bursitis, and many people experience it in association with tendinitis. Bursitis usually is relieved by rest and possibly by NSAIDs. Persistent bursitis may require an injection of steroid and occasionally removal of the bursa.

Fracture

Fractures, defined as breaks in the normal structure of the bone (89), can occur as acute or chronic (*stress*) injuries. Acute fractures are caused directly from physical overload of the bone resulting in mechanical failure. Chronic or stress fractures are caused by an accumulative load applied to the bone over time that results in fatigue and eventual mechanical failure of the bone. Fractures are classified as *open* (bone exposed through skin) and *closed* (skin intact). Fracture treatment varies from splint immobilization to open reduction and internal fixation.

Arthritis of the Basilar Joint of the Thumb

History

Most patients are women over age 40 who complain of pain in the thumb with use. Swelling at the base of the thumb with activities and possible history of fracture are common. Over time, the swelling is constant. Function is decreased for pinching and grip using the thumb (90).

Examination

Common clinical signs are tenderness and subluxation of the carpometacarpal joint of the thumb, an axial grind test that reproduces the pain, a decrease in the span of the thumb–index finger web space, and reduced pinch and grip strength. Radiographs are appropriate to support diagnosis and provide insight into the amount of degenerative changes.

Nonsurgical Intervention

If involvement is mild or no previous treatment has been provided, NSAIDs, thumb spica splint, steroid injections, heat or cool modalities, and activity modification may be considered. The estimated duration of treatment is up to 3 months.

Surgery

Failure to respond to nonoperative treatment, progressive symptoms, disabling pain, limitation of motion, adduction contracture of the basilar joint, or unstable carpometacarpal joint are indications for surgery. Several options are available: total or partial trapezium excision with soft-tissue interposition arthroplasty with or without capsular or ligamentous reconstruction, silicone implant, or arthrodesis surgery, usually performed on an outpatient basis using regional anesthetic block.

After Surgery

Cast immobilization for 6 to 8 weeks is usual with soft-tissue surgery. If arthrodesis if performed, splinting may take up to 6 months. The estimated duration of treatment is up to 6 months.

Return to Work

Depending on the job, the patient may return to modified light work within in a few days after surgery but will wear a cast. As pain decreases, activities may be increased gradually.

Outcome

Usually pain reduction, possible improved range of motion, increased strength, and some improvement in appearance are achievable (90).

Rotator Cuff Derangement or Tear

History

In 1934 E.A. Codman (91) wrote, "Complete rupture of the supraspinatus is the most common cause of prolonged disability from industrial accidents to the shoulder.... The incomplete form accounts for the majority of shoulder disabilities." Codman first brought the pathology of the rotator cuff of the worker to the attention of both the medical profession and the workers' compensation authorities. Despite considerable attention to this condition, controversy about its etiology continues.

Two explanations are mutually complementary. First, the vascular anatomy of the rotator cuff has been proposed as a reason for the pathology of cuff tear and the poor healing once rupture has occurred. The second is based on biomechanical studies confirmed by the fact that the shoulder muscles, particularly the supraspinatus and infraspinatus, are heavily loaded when the arm is elevated; this tonic contraction would result in high intramuscular pressures that, in turn, accentuate the hypovascularity of the supraspinatus tendon and contribute to its fibrosis and ultimate cuff tear. Three stages of derangement are described. *Stage I* consists of edema and hemorrhage in the cuff. In *stage II*, the subacromial bursa becomes thickened and scarred. In *stage III*, the cuff tears.

Examination

The clinical presentation of the patient with a rotator cuff problem depends on the stage of the pathology, although in all cases pain is felt as the arm is elevated or abducted. Pain may be in the subacromial area or felt as a vague ache in the upper lateral arm at the level of the deltoid tuberosity. On examination, the discomfort is usually present in only part of the arc of range of motion. With the arm at the side, little pain is felt, but as the arm is brought to the horizontal plane and then medially rotated, pain occurs. As the horizontal plane is passed, pain is caused by forced upward elevation of the humerus against the acromion and is confirmed by injection of local anesthetic beneath the acromion, which abolishes the pain if it is due to impingement. The amount of crepitus is variable. With a complete tear, the lift of sign (i.e., the patient cannot lift the hand away from the low back) is positive. A late sign is the inability to hold the arm out to the side. Most patients with rotator cuff tears do not have significant stiffness, although some do; particularly in longstanding large tears, atrophy of the muscles develops in the supraspinous and infraspinous fossae. The arthrogram is the gold standard for confirming the diagnosis, but the test is invasive and painful. This test is being replaced by MR imaging and sonography.

Nonsurgical Intervention

If symptoms are mild or do not interfere with activities, the rotator cuff tear can be treated with modification of activities, NSAIDs as needed, steroid injections, heat, cold, and physical therapy. As symptoms progress or interfere with activities and the examination and supporting tests are diagnostic, surgery is a reasonable option.

Surgery

Surgical repair is appropriate if nonsurgical treatment is ineffective, if the pain interferes with activities, or if the tear is acute. Surgical options include the open technique (traditional deltoid pectoral or minideltoid splitting) or the arthroscopic technique (closed or combined with minideltoid splitting). Each technique has specific advantages and disadvantages, depending on the size and location of the tear and the associated soft-tissue or bone derangement (77,78).

After Surgery

Recovery is slower than with other upper-extremity surgery. A formal physical therapy program is important and should start with Codeman exercises. The general therapy program should be written out for the patient and provided to the patient before surgery. The patient must understand the commitment of time and effort on his or her part necessary to improve the postsurgical outcome. Modifications to the therapy program are appropriate based on the operative findings.

Return to Work

Return to light work with the patient wearing a sling (with no overhead activities) 4 to 7 days after surgery is reasonable. Activities may be increased gradually as strength returns and pain decreases. Permanent work guides for limiting hand-over-shoulder activity is required.

Outcome

The prognosis for recovery of the patient with rotator cuff derangement depends on the degree and duration of the pathology. Future occupational demands may require permanent modification (77,79).

Osteoarthritis of the Distal Interphalangeal Joint

The most common osteoarthritic joints (Heberden's nodes) of the hand are at the distal interphalangeal (DIP) joint and the thumb interphalangeal joint. The clinical picture is the same as that seen at the proximal interphalangeal (PIP) joint level. Mucous cysts are common. Radiographs and an arthritis screen are sufficient to confirm the diagnosis. Conservative treatment is the same as for the PIP joint. When conservative treatment fails, arthrodesis should be considered. It is excellent for relieving pain and correcting deformity, obviously at the cost of motion. Patients rarely complain of stiffness, however. Small mucous cysts require no treatment. If they are large and the skin over them is thin, the potential for rupture is high. With rupture, infection can occur and may involve the DIP joint. It is best to treat these cysts surgically to avoid more significant problems. The prognosis is guarded, although many variables must be considered. Modification of the job may be required.

Osteoarthritis of the Proximal Interphalangeal Joint

After the distal interphalangeal and thumb carpometacarpal joint, the PIP joint (osteoarthritic changes called Bouchard's nodes) is most commonly affected by osteoarthritis, usually in patients over 45 years of age. It is considerably more common in women than men over 50 years of age, but it is slightly more common in men than in women in persons younger than 50. There is a real question of causality, especially in patients who do not perform heavy manual labor, because it occurs fairly commonly in the population at large. Patients present with complaints of pain, deformity, or stiffness. Examination may reveal synovitis with swelling, limitation of motion, and deformity, frequently in the ulnar direction. Radiographs usually confirm the diagnosis, especially in the younger age group. An arthritis screen (laboratory testing) to rule out rheumatoid arthritis and other systemic disorders is appropriate. Treatment includes education, NSAIDs, modification of activities, heat or cool as needed, splinting, and possibly steroid injections. None of these modalities will correct the deformity. If the patient is sufficiently symptomatic or the rehabilitation consultant, patient, and physician believe that surgery may enable a return to the job, it should be undertaken. The surgical alternatives include arthrodesis or arthroplasty. In general, arthrodesis is suggested for border fingers and arthroplasty for middle and ring fingers. This general guide must be modified based on age, activities, quality of other fingers, and deformity. Although arthroplasty is effective in relieving pain, deformity may persist or recur, and the range of motion will remain limited. Whereas arthrodesis will reduce the pain, loss of motion occurs.

Radiocapitellar Arthritis

Posttraumatic arthritis of the radiocapitellar joint may occur after a fracture or simply may be part of a generalized degenerative arthritis of the elbow that becomes symptomatic in the radiocapitellar area because of repeated pronation and supination work activities. Usually, a permanent flexion contracture is present, and pronation and supination are limited. Crepitation may be present, and the patient may have a history of locking if loose bodies are present secondary to the arthritis. Mild arthritic changes consisting of early cartilaginous fraying, roughening, and splitting also may occur. These changes may be caused by heavy work activities, such as handling heavy vibrating tools like jackhammers. Discomfort is noted over the lateral aspect of the elbow, which is differentiated from lateral epicondylitis and the radial tunnel syndrome by its accentuation of symptoms with pronation and supination. Crepitation on range of motion may be present. All but the earliest stages (early chondral changes) of radiocapitellar arthritis are seen on plain radiographs, which also may show loose bodies. Standard conservative treatment for arthritis is appropriate and includes modification of activities, heat or ice, NSAIDs, steroid injections, and possible splinting. Arthroscopy may help with the diagnosis and with the treatment by means of a minimally invasive debridement. Prognosis is guarded. Return to work usually requires job modification.

Kienbock's Disease

Kienbock's disease, or avascular necrosis of the lunate, generally is thought to be caused by microfractures of the lunate associated with an abnormal blood supply. Usually, this condition is associated with a negative ulnar variance, which results in the concentration of abnormal forces across the lunate. The clinical findings vary and are related to the stage of the process and the severity of the disease. Initially, patients complain of aching and mild pain that is usually activity related. As the process worsens, the pain intensifies and eventually becomes constant. On examination, varying degrees of wrist stiffness, swelling, dorsal tenderness, crepitation, and weakness of grip strength are found. When dorsal tenderness is localized directly over the lunate, this diagnosis should be considered. The condition is not uncommon and is frequently seen in young men who do manual work. Depending on the stage of the disease, routine radiographs may confirm the condition. In early stages, increased density, sclerosis, and often a fracture line on the lateral radiograph may be seen. In more advanced stages, collapse and fragmentation and eventually arthritis are present. A negative ulnar variance is

commonly seen. It is now known that in the earliest cases routine radiographs may be completely normal. Bone scans sometimes show a "hot spot" localized to the lunate, and MR imaging is sometimes helpful in suggesting the diagnosis. Treatment is controversial but is somewhat related to the stages of the disease. Because of the incidence of silicone synovitis, the previously recommended lunate prosthesis is no longer used. Current suggestions include radial shortening, ulnar lengthening, or vascularized bone graft for cases in early stages that have no collapses (92). For advanced stages or in patients who have normal ulnar variance, intercarpal fusions are recommended to unload the lunate. For advanced stages with osteoarthritis, a limited wrist fusion can be considered. The prognosis is fair and depends on the stage of the disease. Most patients are able to return to a modified work routine with limitations on vibration, repetition, and impact.

Ligamentous or Capsular Injuries of the Digits

Soft-tissue injuries of the digital joints are sufficiently common at the metacarpalphalangeal (MCP), PIP, and DIP joints and can be discussed together. Acute injuries occur considerably more commonly at the PIP joint level than at the MCP or DIP joints. They are produced by a hyperextension mechanism that results from "jamming" the tip of the finger. Patients present with pain, swelling, or stiffness. The joint is usually stable on lateral stress. At the MCP level, the disorder is generally chronic. It occurs from repeated stress in a lateral, usually ulnar direction. Tenderness can be located over the base of the proximal phalanx or the metacarpal head. Pain can be elicited by stressing the radial collateral ligament, which is most efficiently done with the MCP joint in full flexion. In the thumb, especially if there is a history of an old injury, instability is more common. The hallmark for all these injuries is the slow rate of resolution. It is not uncommon for the pain to take 3 to 6 months to abate, and the patient still may be left with some swelling and stiffness, especially at the PIP levels. Radiographs are helpful in confirming the diagnosis. Treatment for these disorders is usually mechanical (edema control, intermittent splinting, buddy taping to the adjacent finger, joint protection, and range-of-motion exercises). NSAIDs occasionally help with the pain. If chronic instability is present, ligamentous reconstruction or arthrodesis may be indicated. The prognosis is good as long as the patient and employer realize that resolution may take several months. The time lost from work may be minimized if the worker can tolerate mild discomfort or the job can be modified to eliminate significant complaints.

Pisiform Fracture

A history of a direct blow to the palm of the hand usually is involved in this type of fracture. The patient demonstrates direct tenderness over the pisiform, and ulnar nerve function may be altered. Routine radiographs may not demonstrate the fracture; an oblique lateral is helpful. Treatment may include casting or splinting for 3 to 4 weeks. The prognosis is good for full recovery following casting. Sometimes excision is necessary. Most patients can return to their normal jobs as pain resolves.

Fracture of the Hook of Hamate

Most cases are associated with a fall on the outstretched hand or a direct blow; however, the hook of the hamate also can be fractured by indirect injury, for example, by holding on to a tool that is suddenly moved. The patient develops pain and tenderness over the hypothenar area of the palm, although dorsal pain also has been reported. Routine radiographs are always negative, and usually the diagnosis is missed initially. When a patient complains of pain over the hypothenar aspect of the palm and there is tenderness over the hook of the hamate, fracture should be suspected. Sometimes direct pressure over the

volar portion of the palm is not painful, but pressure over the ulnar side of the hook reproduces the symptoms. Again, the pain and tenderness are not always severe, and diagnosis may be delayed for months because it is missed by numerous physicians. Ulnar nerve symptoms or injury to the flexor tendons, especially to the small finger, may be seen. Carpal tunnel views or oblique views of the hand with the forearm supinated 45 degrees and the wrist dorsiflexed sometimes demonstrate the fracture. A CT scan best delineates the fracture. A bone scan is obviously positive over the hook of the hamate. If the diagnosis is made acutely, casting is often effective. The cast must include not only the fourth and fifth MCP joint but also the thumb to alleviate forces through the transverse carpal ligament. In cases of delayed diagnosis, most physicians recommend excision of the hook. In most cases, fracture healing or excision of the hook will restore the hand to essentially normal function and allow the worker to return to most jobs.

Distal Radioulnar Joint Instability

Acute and chronic tears of the triangular fibrocartilage complex can result in wrist pain. The diagnosis of this condition is often difficult. When the patient presents with an acute injury and there is in obvious fracture or dislocation of the distal radioulnar (DRU) joint, the diagnosis is obvious and treatment more straightforward. In most cases, however, the patient is seen several weeks or months after a twisting injury to the wrist or a combination hyperextension and hyperpronation injury and has persistent pain. When the patient is seen in an emergency room initially, the condition is diagnosed as a sprain after negative radiographs are obtained. The wrist is splinted, and the patient may be treated with an NSAID. When the problem continues, the worker presents with a persistently painful wrist and increasing pain associated with ulnar deviation and grip. The clinical findings are increased with supination and pronation of the wrist and concurrent ulnar deviation.

Sometimes a wiper sign or a click at the distal ulna is seen with stress testing. Radiographs may confirm the tear by position of the ulna. CT scans, MR imaging, and arthrography can all be helpful in making this difficult diagnosis. Treatment includes immobilization, NSAIDs, steroid injections, and therapy. If improvement does not occur, surgical repair by open or arthroscopic technique is possible. The prognosis is fair to good, with some residual pain likely. Work modification for supination, pronation, power tools, and vibratory tools is often required.

Olecranon Bursitis

The olecranon bursa is the most commonly inflamed bursa. The bursa lies between the subcutaneous tissue and the olecranon. Although inflammation can occur spontaneously, it usually is associated with single or multiple direct trauma and related to a job injury rather than to an activity, unless the job requires constant leaning on the elbows against a hard surface. The diagnosis is simple, because the condition creates a large swelling over the surface of the olecranon; the swelling usually causes only mild discomfort. If the injury involves a break in the skin, the bursitis may become septic, in which case there is considerably more pain and inflammatory reaction. Olecranon bursitis does not affect the triceps mechanisms or the elbow joint itself; so examination of these structures is negative. No confirmatory tests are necessary to make the diagnosis, which is obvious on physical examination, and the history will inform the examiner as to whether the changes are acute or chronic. The only diagnostic question is whether sepsis is present. Aspiration of bursal fluid for culture establishes the presence of sepsis. Aspiration as a treatment maneuver has limited success, and the incidence of recurrence is considerable. Often, aspiration is carried out once, with application of a pressure dressing and immobilization of the elbow in acute flexion to decrease the dead space. The major indication for this procedure is discomfort. If the condi-

tion persists or recurs frequently, surgical excision may be performed and is usually successful, although discomfort is felt over the area for many months when the patient leans that elbow on a hard surface. Prognosis for return to work is good; the only modification to the work environment that is necessary is to prevent chronic trauma to this area caused by leaning on hard surfaces. Padded surfaces or wearing pads over the elbows at work can prevent chronic trauma to the area by minimizing pressure on the area of the bursa even when leaning on hard surfaces.

Calcific Tendonitis and Bursitis of the Shoulder

The presence of a calcific deposit in a radiograph of the shoulder, usually in the supraspinatus tendon adjacent to the greater tuberosity of the humerus, may give rise to spurious conclusions about the relationship of that finding to the patient's symptoms or their etiology. Although it would be tempting to ascribe the lesion to a worker's job, it is generally agreed that such is not the case. Uhtthoff (93) reported that shoulder calfications are found in 20% of asymptomatic persons. Symptoms associated with the presence of a calcium deposit will depend on the location of that deposit. In most cases, it is located within the substance of the supraspinatus tendon, and because it constitutes a space-occupying lesion under the subacromial arch, it can produce symptoms of impingement. It is conceivable that, in this situation, if the employee was engaged in an activity involving continued overhead work that would ordinarily predispose to the development of the symptoms of impingement, then the presence of the calcification could enhance the effect of the overhead work on the rotator cuff; however, the work *per se* does not cause the deposit to form. The second expression of the calcific deposit is a reflection of the natural history of the lesion, which is that the deposit may work its way out of the tendon and ultimately rupture into the subacromial bursa, where it is irritating and produces severe but time-limited pain in the shoulder. It is important to obtain radiographs of the shoulder both in the anteroposterior plane with the arm medially and laterally rotated and in an axillary view to enable the calcific deposit to be located accurately. As previously stated, the supraspinatus tendon is suspected, but deposits can occur in other tendons. One must differentiate the scattered, small radiopacities adjacent to the greater tuberosity that are associated with chronic rotator cuff tear from calcific deposits, because they are different entities that require different treatment (94).

Treatment of the calcific deposit depends on the stage in its natural history. Because many calcific deposits about the shoulder are totally asymptomatic, they do not require treatment. If they are seen because of impingement on the subacromial arch, the pain occurs only during a specific arc in the range of motion, which is usually when the arm is forward flexed and then medially rotated. In these situations, treatment is the same as that of impingement, which includes rest and avoidance of the position that provokes pain. This treatment may require that the worker's job be changed temporarily, or, if that is not possible, the employee may need simply to stop working for a week or two. One or two subacromial injections of steroids and local anesthetic may be beneficial at this stage, as is the use of oral NSAIDs. Repeated injections into the shoulder are to be avoided, however. The worker who presents with an acute calcific bursitis has severe pain. The use of a sling and local applications of ice rather than heat are indicated. The pain is often severe enough to warrant oral narcotic analgesics. Occasionally, it is possible to aspirate a fluid deposit from the subacromial bursa, but in most cases, the severe pain disappears spontaneously over a few days as the deposit is absorbed. The prognosis for most patients with symptoms of either impingement or acute calcific bursitis is good. The symptoms subside within a few weeks with adequate rest and supportive treatment. For those who have either multiple recurrences or in whom the impingement continues to be a problem, surgery is indicated to remove the deposit and decompress the subacromial arch.

SUMMARY

Occupational health care requires complex decision making. Confronted with a musculoskeletal injury to neurologic system, soft-tissue system (muscle, tendon, skin, and others), vascular system, and skeletal system (bone, joint, and ligament), the physician draws from an understanding of basic medical and surgical principles, experience, and familiarity with the literature to formulate a reasonable plan for diagnosis and treatment. Included in the decision-making process is consideration for patient noncompliance, financial constraints, psychosocial issues, economic issues, and the current limitations of the workers' compensation system (employer, insurer, legal, legislative, and medical). Early return to work, without placing the patient at increased risk for recurrence, is in the patient's (the employee's) best interests. Successful outcomes for upper extremity disorders will require the employee, employer, and physician to work together.

REFERENCES

1. Melhorn JM. CTD, RSI and their relationship to work injury, In: Spengler DM, Zeppieri JP, eds. *Workers' compensation case management: a multidisciplinary perspective.* Rosemont, Il: American Academy of Orthopaedic Surgeons, 1997;1–25.
2. American Medical Association. *Guides to the evaluation of permanent impairment.* Chicago: American Medical Association, 1993.
3. Zeppieri JP. The physician's role in workers' compensation: changing the paradigm. In: Spengler DM, Zeppieri JP, eds. *Workers' compensation case management: a multidisciplinary perspective.* Rosemont, IL: American Academy of Orthopaedic Surgeons, 1998;3–8.
4. Amadio PC. Current concepts review pain dysfunction syndromes. *J Bone Joint Surg Am* 1988;70A:944–948.
5. Melhorn JM. Occupational injuries: the need for preventive strategies. *Kans Med* 1994;95:248–251.
6. Melhorn JM. Three types of carpal tunnel syndrome: the need for prevention. *ARMS* (Association for Repetive Motion Syndromes) *News* 1996;5:18–24.
7. Melhorn JM. Work restrictions for return to work, In: Zeppieri JP, Spengler DM, eds. *Workers' compensation case management: a multidisciplinary perspective.* Rosemont, IL: American Academy of Orthopaedic Surgeons, 1997;249–266.
8. Melhorn JM. CTD injuries: an outcome study for work

survivability. *Journal of Workers' Compensation* 1996;
5:18–30.

9. Cook AC, Birkholz S, King EF, Szabo RM. Early mobilization following carpal tunnel release: a prospective randomized study. *J Hand Surg Br* 1995;20B:228–230.

10. Melhorn JM, Wilkinson LK. *CTD solutions for the 90's: a comprehensive guide to managing CTD in the workplace.* Wichita, KS: Via Christi, 1996, pp.1–45.

11. Melhorn JM. CTD solutions for the 90's: prevention. In: *Seventeenth Annual Workers' Compensation and Occupational Medicine Seminar.* Boston: Speak, 1997; 234–245.

12. Melhorn JM. Identification of individuals at risk for developing CTD, In: Spengler DM, Zippieri JP, eds. *Workers' compensation case management: a multidisciplinary perspective.* Rosemont, IL: American Academy of Orthopaedic Surgeons, 1997;41–51.

13. Melhorn JM. Physician support and employer options for reducing risk of CTD. In: Spengler DM, Zippieri JP, eds. *Workers' compensation case management: a multidisciplinary perspective.* Rosemont, IL: American Academy of Orthopaedic Surgeons, 1997;21–34.

14. Ballard M, Baxter P, Bruening L, Fried S. Work therapy and return to work. *Hand Clin* 1986;2:247–258.

15. Bruce WC, Bruce RS. Return-to-work programs in the unionized company. *Journal of Workers' Compensation* 1996;Spring:9–17.

16. Burke SA, Harms-Constas CK, Aden PS. Return to work/work retention outcomes of a functional restoration program: a multi-center, prospective study with a comparison group. *Spine* 1994;19:1880–1885.

17. Centineo J. Return-to-work programs: cut costs and employee turnover. *Risk Management* 1986;33:44–48.

18. Day CS, McCabe SJ, Alexander G. Return to work as an outcome measure in hand surgery. *Annual meeting of the ASSH* (Baltimore American Society for Surgery of the Hand), 1993.

19. Devlin M, O'Neill P, MacBride R. Position paper in support of timely return to work programs and the role of the primary care physician. *Ontario Medical Association* 1994;61:1–45.

20. Gice JH, Tompkins K. Cutting costs with return-to-work programs. *Risk Management* 1988;35:62–65.

21. Goodman RC. An aggressive return-to-work program in surgical treatment of carpal tunnel syndrome: a comparison of costs. *Plast Reconstr Surg* 1989;89:715–717.

22. Groves FB, Gallagher LA. What the hand surgeon should know about workers' compensation. *Hand Clin* 1993;9:369–372.

23. Grunet BK, Devine CA, Smith CJ, Matloub HS, Sanger JR, Yousif NJ. Graded work exposure to promote work return after severe hand trauma: a replicated study. *Ann Plast Surg* 1992;29:532–536.

24. Kasdan ML, June LA. Returning to work after a unilateral hand fracture. *J Occup Med* 1993;35:132–135.

25. Nathan PA, Meadows KD, Keniston RC. Rehabilitation of carpal tunnel surgery patients using a short surgical incision and an early program of physical therapy. *J Hand Surg* 1993;18A:1044–1050.

26. Eversmann WW Jr. Entrapment and compression neuropathies. In: Green DP, Hotchkiss RN, eds. *Operative hand surgery.* New York: Churchill Livingstone, 1993; 1341–1385.

27. Mackinnon SE, Dellon AL. *Surgery of the peripheral nerve.* New York: Thieme Medical Publishers, 1988.

28. Mackinnon SE, Dellon AL. Carpal tunnel syndrome, In: *Surgery of the peripheral nerve.* New York: Thieme Medical, 1988;149–169.

29. Bucholz RW, Lippert III FG, Wenger DR, Ezaki M. *Orthopaedic decision making.* Saint Louis: CV Mobsy, 1984.

30. Feldman RG, Goldman R, Keyserling WM. Classical syndromes in occupational medicine: peripheral nerve entrapment syndromes and ergonomic factors. *Am J Ind Med* 1983;4:661–681.

31. Dawson DM, Hallett M, Millender LH. *Entrapment neuropathies.* Boston: Little, Brown and Company, 1990.

32. Gelberman RH, Eaton RG, Urbaniak JR. Peripheral nerve compression. *J Bone Joint Surg Am* 1993;75A: 1854–1878.

33. American Society for Surgery of the Hand. Carpal tunnel syndrome. *Clinic Guidelines* 1996;1:1–2.

34. Melhorn JM. Carpal tunnel syndrome. *Protector of Halstead Hospital* 1988;6:4–7.

35. Melhorn JM. Understanding the types of carpal tunnel syndrome. *Journal of Workers' Compensation* 1998;7: 52–73.

36. American Academy of Neurology. Practice parameter for electrodiagnostic studies in carpal tunnel syndrome [summary statement]. *Neurology* 1993;43:2404–2405.

37. American Academy of Neurology. Practice parameter for carpal tunnel syndrome [summary statement]. *Neurology* 1993;43:2406–2407.

38. Braun RM, Davidson K. Provocative testing in the diagnosis of dynamic carpal tunnel syndrome. *J Hand Surg* 1989;14A:195–197.

39. Duncan KH, Lewis RC, Foreman KA, Nordyke MD. Treatment of carpal tunnel syndrome by members of the American Society for Surgery of the Hand: results of a questionnaire. *J Hand Surg* 1987;12A:384–391.

40. Melhorn JM. Carpal tunnel release. A prospective, randomized assessment of open and endoscopic methods [letter; comment]. *J Bone Joint Surg Am* 1994;76A: 1273–1275.

41. Nathan PA, Keniston RC, Meadows KD. Carpal tunnel release a prospective, randomised assessment of open and endoscopic methods. *J Bone Joint Surg Am* 1994; 76:1272–1275.

42. Rowland EB, Kleinert JM. Endoscopic carpal-tunnel release in cadavera. *J Bone Joint Surg Am* 1994;76A: 266–268.

43. Szabo RM. Carpal tunnel syndrome—general, In: Gelberman RH, ed. *Operative nerve repair and reconstruction.* Philadelphia: JB Lippincott, 1991;869–888.

44. American Society for Surgery of the Hand. *Position statement on endoscopic carpal tunnel release.* Englwood: American Society for Surgery of the Hand, 1994, pp.28–29.

45. Adams ML, Franklin GM, Barnhart S. Outcome of carpal tunnel surgery in Washington State workers' compensation. *Am J Ind Med* 1994;25:527–536.

46. Atroshi I, Johnsson R, Ornstein E. Patient satisfaction and return to work after endoscopic carpal tunnel surgery. *J Hand Surg* 1998;23A:58–65.

47. Katz JN, Keller RB, Simmons BP, et al. Maine carpal tunnel study: outcomes of operative and nonoperative therapy for carpal tunnel syndrome in a community-based cohort. *J Hand Surg* 1998;23A:697–710.

48. Al-Qattan MM, Bowen V, Manktelow RT. Factors asso-

ciated with poor outcome following primary carpal tunnel release in non-diabetic patients. *J Hand Surg* 1994; 19B:622–625.

49. American Academy of Orthopaedic Surgeons. Carpal tunnel syndrome. *AAOS Clinical Policies* 1991;7: 11–13.

50. Bessette L, Keller RB, Liang MH, Simmons BP, Fossel AH, Katz JN. Patients' preferences and their relationship with satisfaction following carpal tunnel release. *J Hand Surg* 1997;22A:613–620.

51. Higgs PE, Edwards D, Martin DS, Weeks PM. Carpal tunnel surgery outcomes in workers: effect of workers' compensation status. *J Hand Surg* 1995;20A:354–359.

52. Katz JN, Keller RB, Fossel AH, et al. Predictors of return to work following carpal tunnel release. *Am J Ind Med* 1997;31:85–91.

53. Parenmark G, Alffram PA, Malmkvist AK. The signficance of work tasks for rehabilitation outcome after carpal tunnel surgery. *J Occup Rehabil* 1992;2:89–94.

54. Szabo RM, Madison M. Management of carpal tunnel syndome, In: Kasdan ML, ed. *Occupational hand and upper extremity injuries and diseases*. Philadelphia: Hanley & Belfus, 1991,341–351.

55. American Society for Surgery of the Hand. Cubital tunnel syndrome. *Clinic Guidelines* 1996;1:1–2.

56. Bernhardt M, Kuhn MP, Melhorn JM, Yang JH. Surgery for ulnar nerve entrapment at the elbow. *Kans Med* 1988;89:233–238.

57. Mackinnon SE, Dellon AL. Diagnosis of nerve injury. In: Mackinnon SE, ed. *Surgery of the peripheral nerve*. New York: Thieme Medical, 1988.65–88.

58. Millender LH, Louis DS, Simmons BP. *Occupational disorders of the upper extremity*. New York: Churchill Livingstone, 1992.

59. Fechter JD, Kuschner SH. The thoracic outlet syndrome. *Orthopaedics* 1993;16:1243–1251.

60. Leffert RD. Thoracic outlet syndromes. In: Rayan GM, ed. *Nerve compression syndromes*. Philadelphia: WB Saunders, 1992:285–298.

61. Totten PA, Hunter JM. Therapeutic techniques to enhance nerve gliding in thoracic outlet syndrome and carpal tunnel syndrome. In: Mackin EJ, Callahan AD, eds. *Frontiers in hand rehabilitation*. Phiadelphia: WB Saunders, 1991:505–520.

62. Leffert RD. Thoracic outlet syndrome. *J Am Acad Orthop Surg* 1994;2:317–325.

63. Warwick R, Williams PL. *Gray's anatomy*. Philadelphia: WB Saunders, 1973.

64. American Society for Surgery of the Hand. Trigger finger. *Clinic Guidelines* 1996;1:1–2.

65. Benson LS, Ptaszek AJ. Injection versus surgery in the treatment of trigger finger. *J Hand Surg* 1997;22A: 138–144.

66. Bain GI, Turnbull J, Roth JH, Richards RS. Percutaneous a1 pulley release: a cadaveric study. *J Hand Surg* 1995;20A:781–784.

67. Patel MR, Moradia V. Percutaneous release of trigger digit with and without cortisone injection. *J Hand Surg* 1997;22a:150–155.

68. Eastwood DM, Gupta KJ, Johnson DP. Percutaneous Release of the trigger finger: an office Procedure. *J Hand Surg* 1992;17:114–117.

69. Topper SM, Jones C, Klajnbart JO, Friedel SP. Trigger finger: the effect of partial release of the first annular pulley on triggering. *Am J Orthop* 1997;675–677.

70. Froimson AI. Tenosynovitis and tennis elbow. In: Green DP, Hotchkiss RN, eds. *Operative hand surgery*. New York: Churchill Livingstone, 1993;1989–2006.

71. Terrono AL, Millender LH. Evaluation and management of occupational wrist disoders. In: Millender LH, Louis DS, Simmons BP, eds. *Occupational disorders of the upper extremity*. New York: Churchill Livingstone, 1992:117–143.

72. Viikari-Juntura E, Kurppa K. Prevalence of epicondylitis and elbow pain in the meat processing factory. *Scand J Work Environ Health* 1991;17:38–45.

73. Simmons BP, Wyman ET. Occupational injuries of the elbow. In: Millender LH, Louis DS, Simmons BP, eds. *Occupational disorders of the upper extremity*. New York: Churchill Livengston, 1998;155–176.

74. Iannotti JP. *Rotator cuff disorders evaluation and treatment*. Park Ridge: IL, American Academy of Orthopaedic Surgeons, 1991, pp.17–29.

75. Burk JrDL, Karasick D, Kurtz AB, et al. Rotator cuff tears: prospective comparison of mr imaging with arthrography, sonography, and surgery. *AJR Am J Roentgenol* 1989;153:87–92.

76. Calvert PT, Packer NP, Stoker DJ, Bayley JIL, Kessel L. Arthrography of the shoulder after operative repair of the torn rotator cuff. *J Bone Joint Surg Br* 1986;68B: 147–150.

77. Bigliani L, Levine WN. Current concepts review: subacromial impingement syndrome. *J Bone Joint Surg Am* 1997;79A:1854–1868.

78. Budoff JE, Nirschl RP, Guidi EJ. Debridement of partial-thickness tears of the rotator cuff without acromioplasty: long-term follow-up and review of the literature. *J Bone Joint Surg Am* 1998;80A:733–748.

79. Grana WA, Teague B, King M, Reeves RB. An analysis of rotator cuff repair. *Am J Sports Med* 1994;22: 585–588.

80. American Society for Surgery of the Hand. Ganglions. *Clinic Guidelines* 1996;1:1–2.

81. Leffert RD. Disorders of the neck and shoulder in workers, In: Millender LH, Louis DS, Simmons BP, eds. *Occupational disorders of the upper extremity*. New York: Churchill Livingstone, 1993:177–202.

82. Melhorn JM. The history of cumulative trauma/repetitive strain injury. In: Zippieri JP, Spengler DM, eds. *Workers' compensation case management: a multidisciplinary perspective*. Rosemont, IL.: American Academy of Orthopaedic Surgeons, 1998:79–98.

83. Melhorn JM. Musculoskeletal disorders (CTD/RSI) and their relationship to work injury. In: Zeppieri JP, Spengler DM, eds. *Workers' compensation case management: a multidisciplinary perspective*. Rosemont, IL.: American Academy of Orthopaedic Surgeons, 1998:115–134.

84. Newmeyer WL. Vascular disorders. In: Green DP, Hotchkiss RN, eds. *Operative hand surgery*. New York: Churchill Livingstone, 1993:2251–2308.

85. Boyle JC, Smith NJ, Burke FD. Vibration white finger. *J Hand Surg* 1988;13B:171–176.

86. Halder NM. Vibration white finger revisited. *J Occup Environ Med* 1998;40:772–779.

87. International Organization for Standardization. *Mechanical vibration—guidelines for the measurement and the assessment of human exposure to hand transmitted vibration. [International Standard ISO 5349]*. Geneva: International Organization for Standardization, 1986.

88. Bernard BP, Nelson NA, Estill CF, Fine LJ. The NIOSH

review of hand-arm vibration syndrome: vigilance is crucial. *J Occup Environ Med* 1998;40:780–784.

89. Mish FC, Gilman EW. *Webster's ninth new collegiate dictionary.* Springfield, MA: Merriam-Webster, 1991, p.1510.

90. American Society for Surgery of the Hand. Care of human bites of the hand. *Clinic Guidelines* 1996;1:1–2.

91. Codman EA. *The shoulder.* Boston: Thomas Todd Company, 1934.

92. Shin AY, Bishop AT, Berger RA. Vascularized pedicled bone grafts for disorders of the carpus. *Techniques Hand and Upper Extremity Surgery* 1998;2:94–109.

93. Uhthoff HK. Calcifying tendinitis. In: Rockwood CA Jr, Matsen FA III, eds. *The shoulder.* Philadelphia: WB Saunders, 1998;774–775.

94. Winn RS, Melhorn JM, DeSmet AA. Layering of calcifications in synovial effusions. *J Can Assoc Radiol* 1981;32:66–68.

Occupational Musculoskeletal Disorders
edited by T. G. Mayer, R. J. Gatchel, and P. B. Polatin.
Lippincott Williams & Wilkins, Philadelphia © 2000.

29

Postoperative Treatment: Outpatient Medical Rehabilitation

Peter Barth Polatin, *James Rainville, †Thomas T. Haider, and ‡Nancy D. Kishino

*Department of Anesthesiology and Pain Management, University of Texas Southwestern Medical School, Dallas, Texas 75235; *Department of Spine Physiatry, The Spine Center, New England Baptiste Hospital, Boston, Massachusetts 02120; †Department of Orthopaedics, University of California, Riverside, California 92501; and ‡West Coast Spine Restoration Center, Riverside, California 92507*

In the past decade, there has been an increasing emphasis on the documentation of therapeutic outcomes after defined medical and surgical interventions. This emphasis has been fueled by the focus on cost efficiency by governmental and managed-care organizations in the United States and other countries where the health care dollar has been stretched by burgeoning indemnity expenditure. Low back pain, the most expensive benign condition in clinical practice, has been particularly targeted for scrutiny. Concerns about complications and limited effectiveness of surgery for lumbar spine dysfunction have generated a great deal of controversy. Which surgical procedure is most effective for a particular problem? What patient factors may be associated with good or bad outcomes after surgery? How, in fact, do we measure these outcomes? Should we rely primarily on self-reporting by the patient through instruments such as the "pain drawing," the Oswestry low back pain questionnaire, and the SF-36, or by more objective socioeconomic measures, such as return to work, subsequent health care utilization, and recurrent injury? Do functional and physical capacity measures have any relevance in determining outcomes? These questions are dealt with more comprehensively in Chapters 26, 29, and 35 of this

volume. Several recent studies suggest, however, that medically supervised rehabilitation following spine surgery greatly improves outcome measures (1–3). Taking a cue from the experience of knee surgeons, who, for several decades, have used postoperative rehabilitation techniques to restore function (4–7), Mayer et al. suggest that "poor surgical outcomes...may result from outmoded postoperative methods, rather than failures of patient selection or surgical technique" (1). Surgery may correct the anatomic dysfunction, but subsequent recovery and return to productivity will be governed by nonsurgical factors that are best addressed in a goal-oriented rehabilitation environment (8).

PARASPINAL MUSCLE ATROPHY IN THE POSTOPERATIVE PATIENT

Ischemia of paralumbar musculature has been shown during posterior lumbar surgery, related to retraction pressure, time, and extent of exposure (9). Kawaguchi et al. demonstrated abnormalities of multifidus muscle histology and elevations in serum creatinine phosphokinase MM isoenzyme activity immediately after surgery (10). See and Kraft found electromyographic (EMG) changes in the paraspinal muscles of postlaminectomy patients for up to 41 months after decompression for nerve root symptoms, even in the absence of recurrent radiculopathy (11). Rantanen et al. described residual atrophy in the lumbar multifidus muscle groups of individual patients even 5 years after surgery, the extent of which correlated with occupational activity. Because these changes were significantly less in subjects who had made a more adaptive work return, they were considered potentially reversible with adequate therapy (12). Scapinelli and Candiotto evaluated the paraspinal muscle area and density by computed tomography (CT) and magnetic resonance (MR) imaging in patients 7 months to 42 years after surgery for disc herniation; they found variable but significant atrophy and degeneration of muscle fibers with fibrofatty substitution, the severity of which correlated with the extent of the surgery (13). Mayer et al. correlated mechanical trunk strength performance with muscle density on CT scan in the postoperative period and found it to be invariably below normal (14). Kahanovitz et al. also demonstrated that patients who do not undergo aggressive rehabilitation after lumbar surgery are likely to have significant strength deficits thereafter (15).

HEALING AND RECOVERY TIME AFTER SPINE SURGERY

Recovery time is a relative term that refers to the expected duration of healing and convalescence after a surgical procedure, after which the patient can be expected to resume normal life activities. Recovery may be prolonged by medical factors such as age, concurrent medical disease, and postoperative complications as well as by psychosocial factors such as emotional distress, fear of reinjury, and secondary gain. Uncomplicated postsurgical recovery time varies from 6 weeks to 6 months, depending on the extent of the operative procedure. A simple removal of instrumentation may have little "down time," whereas a two-level lumbar laminectomy with posterior or posterior-lateral fusion may re-

quire 24 weeks or longer for recovery (16) (Table 1).

Recovery from surgery, however, does not occur in a vacuum. Prolonged postoperative bed rest increases the risk of such complications as thrombophlebitis, urinary tract infections, and muscle atrophy (8). Progression to early ambulation and independence in self-care activities is generally well tolerated. In

TABLE 1. *Recovery time for various spinal surgeries*

Surgery	Recovery time (wk)
Lumbar laminotomy/discectomy, one level	11
Lumbar laminotomy/disectomy, more than one level	12
Lumbar laminectomy/discectomy with posterior or posterior lateral fusion, one level	20
Lumbar laminectomy/discectomy with posterior or posterior lateral fusion, more than one level	24
Lumbar laminectomy/discectomy with posterior or posterior lateral fusion with instrumentation	23
Lumbar laminectomy/discectomy and interbody fusion, one level	20
Lumbar laminectomy/discectomy and interbody fusion, more than one level	22
Lumbar laminectomy/discectomy and interbody fusion with instrumentation	22
Lumbar laminectomy/discectomy/ interbody with cages	18
Anterior lumbar discectomy/fusion, one level	15
Anterior lumbar discectomy/fusion, more than one level	16
Anterior lumbar discectomy/fusion with instrumentation	17
Lumbar fusion, anterior/posterior, one level	19
Lumbar fusion, anterior/posterior, more than one level	21
Exploration of fusion	13
Removal of instrumentation, anterior	6
Removal of instrumentation, posterior	7
Reinsertion of instrumentation, anterior	12
Reinsertion of instrumentation, posterior	19

From the Texas Workers' Compensation Commission.

all but arthrodesis patients, mobilization may be initiated in the immediate postoperative period. A progressive algorithm of activation ensures the most optimal recovery for a patient after spine surgery.

EARLY IDENTIFICATION OF PROBLEM PATIENTS

The postoperative patient with extremely elevated pain complaints and reluctance to initiate physical activities may be difficult to assess during the first few months after surgery. Imaging may be misleading, because normal postoperative healing may confuse the differentiation of scar, deformity, or mass effect indicative of complicating or recurrent disease (17). Distortion of imaging from surgical hardware adds to this assessment problem. After efforts to eliminate anatomic reasons for pain complaints are completed, the focus should shift toward correcting these pain behaviors. Step one should be reassurance and the clearly stated expectation for function despite pain. Step two is the enforcement of progressive activation, even in the face of the patient's reluctance, under the direction of therapists who are comfortable with this treatment philosophy. "Backing down" from rehabilitation because of subjective pain or distress complaints, without a strong clinical suspicion of additional underlying structural pathology, will reinforce the patient's pain behaviors and jeopardize successful recovery.

Patients who have a potentially poor prognosis after surgery almost invariably have psychological or socioeconomic barriers to recovery that are influencing their behavior (18–22). Chapter 31 of this volume is devoted to an extensive discussion of these socioeconomic, psychosocial, and psychiatric factors. Behavioral "red flags" that may help to identify such patients include elevated pain complaints that defy clinical explanation, symptom magnification with nonorganic signs, oversolicitation of narcotics, extreme passivity without motivation for recovery, family discord centering on the patient's sick status,

noncompliance with treatment recommendations, overt emotional distress (particularly depression or anxiety), ambivalence about return to work or anger at the workplace, and a focus on disability. These signs are *not* synonymous with treatment failure, but they do indicate a need for a more extensive multidisciplinary evaluation (described in Chap. 32).

The proper use of mental health and social service resources in combination with physical therapy is essential and may follow one or more of the formats outlined here: (a) a mental health evaluation by a clinical psychologist, which involves an interview and psychological testing to render clinical hypotheses and treatment recommendations; (b) a psychiatric evaluation to determine the need for psychotropic medication management; (c) short-duration psychotherapy that uses primarily cognitive behavioral techniques (education, task assignments, relaxation training, biofeedback, coping strategies); (d) physical rehabilitation, with the overall purpose of implementing maximal physical recovery; (e) disability case management to address secondary gain issues through education and negotiation; and (f) vocational rehabilitation. Junge et al. (23) suggest that patients whose prognosis for recovery after surgery is particularly poor, as defined by sociodemographic and psychodiagnostic findings, should be considered for a tertiary-level pain management program instead of postsurgical rehabilitation, which is considered a less intensive, secondary level of health care utilization as defined by guidelines set forth by the North American Spine Society (24).

POSTOPERATIVE REHABILITATION: PRESURGICAL CONSIDERATIONS

The more information a patient has before surgery about what to expect in the postoperative period, the less likely it will be that he or she will experience unpleasant surprises that increase anxiety and precipitate mistrust of the treatment team. Carragee et al. suggest that a good preoperative orientation emphasizing the resumption of normal physical activities as soon as tolerated may preclude the need for postoperative rehabilitation after a discectomy (25). Even unusual complications, if they are addressed beforehand, do not undermine the patient's sense of well-being. The burden may be on the surgeon to provide this education and orientation, which also can be delegated to a spine rehabilitation team. Such an orientation should include the exact surgical procedure, its purpose, expected outcome, possible adverse effects and how they will be handled, postoperative pain and how it will be controlled, the projected schedule of postsurgical physical activation, and physical activities that may be constrained during the healing phase (particularly after fusions). A simple stretching and walking program might be prescribed before surgery to facilitate earlier initiation of postsurgical activation (26).

THE SURGICAL PROCEDURE DRIVES THE REHABILITATION SCHEDULE

A discectomy creates minimal disruption to the stability of the spine. Ambulation and remobilization therefore are inititiated almost immediately after surgery, and patients are discharged from the hospital on the day of surgery or on the first postoperative day. Patients may be able to progress back to normal activities without any postoperative intervention (25). Fusions are associated with increased blood loss, greater soft-tissue and bone trauma, and greater postoperative pain. The hospital stay after a fusion is therefore longer, and mobilization and activation are delayed because of prolonged healing time and protection required for the arthrodesis site even after normal soft tissue recovery. Decompressive procedures, sometimes with massive excision of vertebral posterior elements, still have far less blood loss than an arthrodesis, with more dramatic relief of pain once neural compression has been relieved. These patients, despite usually being older, typically begin ambulation and leave the hospital earlier than fusion patients (8). The

timetable for postsurgical rehabilitation will be different, depending on the surgery and the age of the patient, but will include the same general elements in the same sequence.

FUNCTIONAL GOAL SETTING IN POSTOPERATIVE REHABILITATION

There is fairly general agreement that early activation is desirable after a surgical procedure to the spine, but how much rehabilitation is necessary and what constitutes a therapeutic end-point are controversial. Do some patients fare better after posterior discectomies with open-ended instructions and benign neglect, so as not to encourage fear of reinjury (25)? Is it enough to focus on improving mobility and endurance, or should the residual weak link be corrected? How much trunk extensor strength and lifting capacity can be attained after a spinal arthrodesis? And what constitutes a safe endpoint for functional activities after such an operation? Is quantification of functional capacity useful in the rehabilitation of patients after spinal surgery, and if so what should be measured, and when can these tests be safely performed? Significant differences of opinion exist about the answers to these questions. To provide some perspective about varying postoperative rehabilitation philosophies, the protocols of several treatment centers are reviewed in this chapter.

DEFINING THE POSTOPERATIVE DECONDITIONING SYNDROME

All patients who have undergone lumbar surgery will have some degree of deconditioning, as defined by deficits of lumbar mobility, trunk strength, cardiovascular endurance, lifting capacity, and functional task tolerance (see Chap. 29). In subjects who have had a prolonged period of immobilization, these deficits may be extensive and fairly obvious. Even in relatively unimpaired patients who have regained a great deal of mobility and endurance, residual strength deficits may be demonstrated by the use of objective physical and functional quantification techniques (26,27).

Mobility

The measurement of true lumbar mobility by the dual inclinometer technique has been well described; however, the single inclinometer method to derive total lumbosacral motion may be more easily applied to clinical practice, because it is simpler to perform and requires no calculations (28). Lumbar flexion and extension are measured by placing the inclinometer on the T12–L1 interspace. Straight leg raising is recorded with the inclinometer below the tibial tuberosity and is a good clinical indicator of hamstring tightness. Initial measurement of mobility should begin when the patient is first referred to physical therapy for initial stretching and then is monitored on a weekly basis to document progress (Table 2).

Trunk Strength

Chapter 29 discusses the various options available to measure strength in the lumbar spine. Trunk extensor strength is the most relevant measurement from the point of view of clinical rehabilitation, as it has been clearly demonstrated that this is the most consistent and dramatic deficit in the postoperative patient (13–15). Trunk extensor strength testing will load the spine and should not be performed until adequate postoperative healing and consolidation of a fusion have occurred. Some clinicians do not perform trunk extensor testing on their postoperative patients, particularly after an arthrodesis. Trunk extensor testing would not be performed earlier

TABLE 2. *Normal values for lumbar sagittal motion/straight leg raise*

Total flexion	100–120 degrees
Total extension	25–40 degrees
SLR	75–85 degrees

SLR, straight leg raise, which is equivalent to hamstring mobility.

than 2 months after any spinal procedure or 4 months after a fusion. Its therapeutic application is as a beginning point to vigorous spinal rehabilitation aimed at maximizing residual functional capacity. Isokinetic testing is state of the art and also causes the least loading on the spine because the velocity can vary as dictated by clinical considerations; therefore, a less stressful test can be conducted at a higher speed. Such a unit is the Cybex Trunk Extensor-Flexor (TEF) device. Less expensive equipment also may be used to give a relative value for trunk extensor strength, which then can be monitored throughout rehabilitation. Timing a subject's sustained prone lumbar extension on a table with appropriate restraining straps for the lower extremities or on a Roman Chair has been described (29). Timing prone static positioning while holding the sternum off the floor and with a pillow under the abdomen to decrease lumbar lordosis also has been suggested for measuring extensor endurance (30). Another testing procedure uses the Cybex Eagle back-extension machine (Lumex Corporation; Ronkonkoma, NY) and is based on the maximum amount of weight a patient can lift in four repetitions. Testing begins with one plate (9.1 kg) and is progressed by protocol. If the initial weight is easy, two plates (18.2 kg) are added for the next four repetitions. If moderate difficulty is noted by the therapist, only one plate is added. If the subject appears to be significantly challenged, only half a plate (4.5 kg) is added. The testing continues until one of three endpoints is reached: (a) the patient declines further testing because of perceived inability, pain, or fear of injury (psychophysical endpoint); (b) the patient cannot maintain correct form in the test and uses compensatory movements (form endpoint); (c) the patient reaches a safe upper limit (100% of ideal body weight for women, 120% of ideal body weight for men), the safety endpoint (26). For trunk extensor strength, the goal would be 100% of ideal body weight for the postfusion patient but up to 120% of body weight for postdiscectomy men, using either the Cybex back-extension protocol or the isokinetic Cybex TEF device.

Cardiovascular Endurance

Standardized submaximal protocols using a stationary bicycle or treadmill and an upper-body ergometer (UBE) have been described extensively in the literature and are discussed in Chapter 29. Such a test is initiated at the beginning of rehabilitation.

Lifting Capacity

Isometric, isokinetic, and isoinertial lifting protocols also are discussed extensively in Chapter 29. The low-technology test most adaptable to a rehabilitatIon environment without expensive equipment is the Progressive Isoinertial Lifting Evaluation (PILE), which requires only a plastic crate, a shelf at 30 inches and another at 54 inches, and a quantity of 5-pound weights (31). Adequate postsurgical recovery and arthrodesis consolidation should take place before patients undergo lift testing, at 2 to 4 months after discectomy/laminectomy and 4 to 6 months after fusion surgery.

IMMEDIATE POSTSURGICAL CARE, INLAND EMPIRE SPINE CENTER, RIVERSIDE, CALIFORNIA

Simple Laminectomy and Discectomy

Normally, the patient is kept in the hospital for 1 or 2 days after surgery. The patient is encouraged to get out of bed on the first postoperative day and to walk in the hallway. On discharge, a daily walking program is implemented, with distance progressed as tolerated. For the first 6 weeks, no bending is permitted, and lifting is restricted to 10 lbs or less. It is recommended that a recliner be used when sitting, and an upright sitting posture should be avoided to prevent increased loading at the initially weakened surgical site. The patient has a postoperative appointment with the surgeon at 2 weeks, at which time the wound is examined and the sutures removed, and again at 6 weeks, when he or she is referred for rehabilitation.

Anterior Cervical Fusion

Patients who undergo anterior cervical discectomy and fusion normally stay in the hospital for 2 days after surgery. If the fusion is multilevel, hospitalization may be extended to 3 days. The patient is allowed to get out of bed and walk 1 day after surgery. After being discharged home, the patient is restricted to lifting less than 10 lbs and is placed in a cervical collar, which will be worn for 2 months. The patient may walk as much as can be tolerated and can perform routine light activities around the house. Because the neck is immobilized in a cervical collar, the patient is restricted from driving for 2 months.

At two weeks postoperatively, the patient is seen for suture removal and wound check, at 8 weeks for radiographs of the fusion mass, and then at about 14 weeks, after which the patient is referred for rehabilitation.

Lumbar Fusions

The patient remains in the hospital for 5 to 7 days after surgery. Typically, more aggressive pain management is required postoperatively: Intrathecal Duramorph may be used for the first night, and a PCA (patient controlled anesthesia) pump for 2 or 3 days thereafter, with oral analgesics started after the PCA pump is discontinued. A cooling blanket, which is a brace with cooling coils in it, may be used during the immediate postsurgical period while the patient is still in the hospital, for pain control and for mitigation of edema and bleeding. Ambulation still may begin on the first day after surgery and progresses as in other postsurgical protocols. A progressive walking program is continued once the patient is discharged home. The patient is expected to be walking a mile a day by 6 weeks after surgery and 2 miles a day at 3 months postoperatively. Bracing may be used for about 14 weeks after surgery to enforce the avoidance of active twisting movements that could disrupt the arthrodesis. In one- or two-level instrumented fusions, it may not be required. Lifting is limited to 10 lbs, and no bending or stooping is allowed. Once at home, the patient is instructed to sit in an upright position every day for an extended period of time. That patient is asked to time how long he or she is in that position and then to attempt to increase sitting tolerance by about 5 minutes every other day until he or she can sit upright for 2 hours straight. The purpose of this regimen is to stretch the trunk extensors while they are healing. Normally, these muscles shrink as they heal, and if they are not gently stretched during this process, their contracture may impair sitting tolerance later.

POSTOPERATIVE REHABILITATION, THE WEST COAST SPINE RESTORATION CENTER (WCSRC), RIVERSIDE, CALIFORNIA

The WCSRC is a therapist-directed rehabilitation facility that treats a large volume of postsurgical spine patients. Each referring physician may dictate his or her own preferences for rehabilitation progression for his particular patients and receives direct feedback from the treatment team. The postsurgical program is divided into preprogram and program phases and has separate tracks for younger and older patients, who differ in the intensity of the reconditioning offered (Table 3).

The postoperative preprogram is initiated at between 8 and 16 weeks after surgery, depending on the procedure (see Table 3), and continues for 2 to 6 weeks, as dictated by patient response. Supervised mobilization starts as a 1-hour session twice weekly and progresses to three times a week. The patient undergoes dual-inclinometer sagittal range of motion measurements before starting and then at regular intervals thereafter, but no other quantification testing is performed at the preprogram phase. Swiss ball stretches are used to begin the mobilization process, with progression to light dynamic stabilization exercises. Typically, manual stretches are not initiated until the next phase, but cardiovascular training on a treadmill or stationary bike is a standard part of this phase. Mobilization and walking in a therapy pool may also be offered.

Progression to the postoperative program is dictated by patient response in the preprogram but certainly will occur within 6 weeks. This phase lasts from 6 to 8 weeks, typically a longer program in fusion patients. At entry, additional quantification testing is performed, including a submaximal treadmill and UBE protocol, PILE, and material-handling tests, as described elsewhere. Trunk extensor testing is not performed. The patient then attends the program 5 days a week for 2 hours per day, during which period he or she performs regular restorative exercises. The patient also participates in physical therapy three times per week, consisting of treadmill, stationary bike, and UBE training to tolerance, aerobic and manual stretching sessions, and strength training on weight machines. The strengthening program is closely monitored: Patients begin at low weights and progress slowly (Table 4). Multilevel or multiple-procedure fusion patients are not given trunk extensor training, however; rather, they are treated with lumbar stabilization exercises (see Tables 5 and 6). Occupa-

TABLE 3. *Timetable for progression of postsurgical care (West Coast Spine Restoration Center)*

	Lumbar lami/dissect.	ACF	Lumbar fusion
Postop hospitalization	1–2 days	2–3 days	4–5 days
Walking program/ADLs	Day 1	Day 1	Day 1
Stretching preprogram	@6–8 wk	@14 wk	@12 wk
Rehabilitation	@8–10 wk	@16 wk	@14 wk
Therapy discharge	@5 mo	@6 mo	@6 mo

ACF, anterior cervical fusion.
ADL, activities of daily living.

TABLE 4. *Postoperative strengthening program (West Coast Spine Restoration Center)*

To begin: Leg press up to 30 lbs; all other weight
stations up to 20 lbs
Start with 2 sets of 10 repetitions for first week
2nd week, same weights
Increase to 3 sets of 10 repetitions
3rd week-increase weights at each station by
maximum of 10 lbs.
Drop to 2 sets of 10 repetitions
Progress weekly thereafter

TABLE 5. *Back extension guidelines (West Coast Spine Restoration Center)*

Back extension training	No back extension training
One-level fusion	Multiple levels
First surgery	Multiple surgeries

TABLE 6. *Substitution of back stabilization for back extension exercises*

Sets of 10:	Prone position, alternate arm/leg
	Quadriped, alternate arm/leg
	Bridging

tional therapy is provided twice a week and consists of functional activities training, particularly lifting drills, material handling, and positional activities related to work requirements. Lifting on the PILE has an upper limit that is determined by the time since surgery (Table 7). Additionally, educational back school is provided once a week on various relevant topics, including anatomy, body mechanics, nutrition, communication skills, lumbar stabilization exercises, stress management, benefits of exercise, and job readiness.

TABLE 7. *Postoperative lifting limitations on the PILE (West Coast Spine Restoration Center)*

Time after surgery (mos)	Males (lbs)	Females (lbs)
4–6	30[a]	15[a]
6–9	40[a]	20[a]
9–12	50[a]	25[a]
>12	Safety endpoint	

PILE, Progressive Isoinertial Lifting Evaluation.
[a]Plus an additional 3 lbs. for the basket.

Once a patient has completed a postoperative program, he or she is typically given work restrictions, initially with limited lifting and no repetitive bending or stooping. At that point, the patient may return to the job or go through vocational rehabilitation, which is offered to every injured worker in the state of California. The patient continues with regular follow-up with the surgeon for up to 2 years postoperatively and is encouraged to maintain a home-fitness program based on the exercise routines that were initiated during formal rehabilitation.

Simple Laminectomy/Discectomy

The preprogram is initiated between 6 and 8 weeks after surgery, and rehabilitation continues for about 2 months. Typically, the patient has completed the full program at 4 months after surgery.

Anterior Cervical Fusion

Initiation of the preprogram is delayed 10 to 14 weeks to allow some fusion to take place, so that no collapse of the bone graft or displacement of the bone plug, with resultant kyphotic deformity, will occur. Impact exercises are avoided during the rehabilitation of these patients. Therapy is completed in approximately 2 months, or 6 months after surgery.

Lumbar Fusion

These patients usually are referred to the preprogram 3 months postoperatively. Trunk rotation and side bending are restricted to limit shearing forces on the arthrodesis during initial mobilization. Activation begins at about 14 weeks postoperatively. Trunk extensor strength testing is not performed, and trunk extensor training is restricted as outlined above. Lifting is monitored closely and restricted.

Postsurgical Care in Patients Not Considered Appropriate for Vigorous Rehabilitation

Patients who are over age 55, have had multiple surgeries, or do not plan to return to work are progressed much less rigorously in rehabilitation, although the duration of their hospitalization and the initiation of walking and home activities proceed on the same timetable as in other postoperative patients. The same preprogram mobilization and cardiovascular phase is offered, followed by a 10-week program of primarily physical therapy for 1 hour a day consisting of pool exercises, Swiss ball stretches, and cardiovascular training on the treadmill, stationary bike, and UBE. Vigorous impact aerobics are avoided, and strength training with weights and iso-machines is not performed

NEW ENGLAND BAPTIST HOSPITAL POSTOPERATIVE SPINE REHABILITATION PROGRAM, BOSTON, MASSACHUSETTS

The New England Baptist Hospital has a rehabilitation facility that provides postoperative care for the patients of a number of spine surgeons. Spine physicians at the facility supervise therapists and provide medical management as well as feedback to the referring surgeons.

Lumbar Discectomy

As a general rule, lumbar discectomies are performed as day surgeries. Because most patients do extremely well postoperatively, rapid return to normal activities is the rule (25). Initially, patients are told to ambulate as tolerated and to keep lifting activities light. After several days, some patients return to their business or sedentary work activities for several hours per day and are allowed to increase these as tolerated. After 2 weeks, patients are allowed to increase activities further, including carrying daily household objects, such as laundry or a bag of groceries. By 2 or 3 weeks after surgery, most office and sedentary workers return to their regular work schedules. At 6 weeks, patients are encouraged to progress to normal recreational and social activities and to resume exercise. Patients with employment requiring manual labor are usually re-leased to full time, light to moderate duty work by 4 to 6 weeks. All work restrictions usually can be lifted over the next 1 to 2 months.

The use of rehabilitation services for post-discectomy patients varies according to the surgeon but usually is reserved for patients with special needs. At the 2-week postoperative visit, patients with significant residual pain, poor mobility, or extreme fearfulness about their backs may be referred to physical therapy. The purpose of therapy is to instruct the patient in appropriate exercises that will help to normalize back flexibility. After single inclinometer quantification of trunk range of motion and straight leg raising, stretches are initiated for the back, hip, and lower extremities. Only several therapy sessions are needed for most patients to complete this education, to ensure compliance, and to document progress. Therapists understand that their ultimate goals are (a) to improve the patient's confidence to return to normal activities and (b) to teach the patient that residual symptoms do not necessitate limited function.

Patients whose occupations require moderate to heavy lifting or who participate in aggressive sports activities may require more extensive rehabilitation to help reestablish high-level physical capacities and back strength. These patients usually begin an aggressive rehabilitation program 4 to 6 weeks after surgery and exercise three times per week for 2 to 3 hours per session under the guidance of a physical therapist. Exercises include aggressive stretching of the back and lower extremities, back strengthening on isoinertial exercise equipment, lifting training using a free lift style, and endurance training, including step aerobics. The goals of rehabilitation are documented normal lumbar flexibility, strength, and endurance and usually can be accomplished in 4 to 6 weeks. When the patient documents normal strength, full activities are encouraged. All patients are instructed to maintain their back strength and flexibility at ideal levels through continued exercise at home or in a fitness facility.

Anterior Cervical Fusion

When patients are discharged from the hospital, they wear a hard cervical collar, which they are instructed to use for 2 months. They are encouraged to resume activities as tolerated and to walk daily; they may do modest lifting. After the 2-month postoperative visit, patients are weaned from wearing the collars over a 2-week period, at which point most patients are told to return to all normal activities as tolerated. Some patients report residual symptoms of stiffness, pain, or fear of physical activities. This group, like the previously described problematic postlumbar discectomy patients, may be referred for a brief course of therapy using a similar approach to reaching the same goals. Following rehabilitation, participation in high-speed contact sports is discouraged, but no other limitations for activities are suggested.

Lumbar Fusion

All postfusion patients are ambulated on the day after surgery and are independent in self-care activities by day 6, when they are discharged from the hospital. They may be provided with narcotic medication initially after discharge and will be expected to follow a walking program with the goal of at least 2 miles per day by 2 months after surgery. A light, flexible brace may be prescribed postoperatively, but if the fusion is greater than three segments or considered at particular risk because of other patient factors such as osteoporosis, a molded polypropylene brace will be used. In patients with noninstrumented fusions, a thoracolumbar sacral orthosis with leg extension may be used (25). At 2 months, patients begin structured rehabilitation. Sessions occur once or twice a month and are instructional in nature. At the first visit, single inclinometer measurement of sagittal lumbar motion and straight leg raise is performed, and a home stretching program focusing on increasing lower extremity and hip flexibility is recommended. Patients are encouraged to perform these stretches at least twice a day. At follow-up visits, they are monitored by a therapist, with mobility measures taken at each visit to document progress. At 3 months, additional trunk extensor stretches are added as the patient is weaned from bracing. Walking is continued and light functional activities are resumed, but suggested lifting may be restricted to 10 lbs and 20 lbs during this period, and frequent bending or twisting is discouraged. At 4 months, instruction is given in floor exercises for initial abdominal and trunk exten-

TABLE 8. *New England Baptist Hospital postfusion protocol*

Time after surgery (mo)	Quantification	Activity initiated
0–2		Walking, up to 3 miles/day
2 (1–2 sessions)	ROM[a]	Hip and LE stretches
3 (1 session)	ROM	Trunk extensor stretches
4 (1–2 sessions)	ROM	Floor exercises for trunk strengthening
5 (1–2 sessions)	ROM	UE and LE strengthening
	Aerobic capacity[b]	CV fitness training
6 (solid fusion) (physical inhibition)	ROM	Intensive rehabilitation
	Aerobic capacity	
	Trunk extensor strength[c]	
	Lifting capacity[d]	
8	ROM	Discharge
	Aerobic capacity	
	Trunk extensor strength	
	Lifting capacity	

CV, cardiovascular; LE, leg extensor; ROM, UE, UBE, upper body ergometer
[a]Single inclinometer lumbar flexion/extension/SLR.
[b]Submax. treadmill or bike + UBE protocols.
[c]Cybex trunk extensor protocol to normal.
[d]Progressive Isoinertial Lifting Evaluation (PILE) protocol to maximum.

sor strengthening. At 5 months general upper- and lower-extremity strengthening exercises are initiated using resistive elastic bands for the arms and isometric floor exercises for the legs or isoinertial weight training equipment. Cardiovascular fitness training also is started at 5 months; aerobic capacity is quantified and then measured along with range of motion at each subsequent visit. At 6 months, if there is adequate fusion and the patient demonstrates sufficient need, an intensive rehabilitation program is initiated. Trunk extensor strength and lifting capacity are measured, along with follow-up measures of mobility and aerobic capacity. Patients then begin a 4- to 6-week protocol of vigorous and specific exercise at a frequency of three times per week, including advanced stretching, aerobic conditioning, general strengthening, and lifting drills. The goals are normalized functional capacities, regardless of residual symptoms, and the confidence to resume normal life activities. Release to full-time work, within established capacities, is the expectation of all patients at this point (Table 8).

SUMMARY

Patients who have undergone spinal surgery generally have better functional outcomes if they participate in a postoperative rehabilitation program that uses a sports medicine model of progressive activation. This is particularly true for patients who demonstrate overreactive pain behaviors in the early postoperative period. Such rehabilitation corrects the deconditioning that invariably results from the surgical damage to paraspinal muscles and the early postoperative physical restrictions, which are imposed to promote protected healing of spinal elements. Quantification of selected functional capacities can be helpful in guiding the rehabilitation process. Typically, range of motion will be measured earliest, followed by cardiovascular endurance, and then trunk extensor strength and lifting capacity, as the patient progresses from initial mobilization and endurance train-

ing to strengthening and functional activities training. There are differences of opinion about whether to quantify, particularly whether trunk extensor strength should be measured. Treatment programs vary in the intensity of their reconditioning protocols and the timing of the various phases of rehabilitation. With such latitude in the process, the spine clinician is best served by developing a progressive program with which he or she feels comfortable and that assists patients in their postsurgical recovery. As long as there is a process of functional recovery, good therapeutic outcomes will result. Patients who fail to progress as expected should be reassessed in a timely fashion, not only for unexpected recurrent disease, but also for psychosocial barriers that are delaying the recovery process. Such patients should be referred for a mental health assessment and considered for tertiary care.

REFERENCES

1. Mayer T, McMahon M, Gatchel R, Sparks B, et al. Socioeconomic outcomes of combined spine surgery and functional restoration in workers compensation spinal disorders with matched controls. *Spine* 1998;23: 598–606
2. Rainville J, Sobel J, Hartigan C. Does prior spine surgery affect outcomes of spine rehabilitation for chronic low back pain? Presentation. Annual meeting of the International Society for the Study of the Lumbar Spine, Helsinki, Finland, June 1995
3. Haider T, Kishino N, Gray T, Tomlin M, Daubert H. The effectiveness of functional restoration for post lumbar spine surgery patients: a comparison study [Poster presentation]. Annual meeting of the International Society for the Study of the Lumbar Spine, Brussels, Belgium, June 1998.
4. Shelbourne K, Nitz P. Accelerated rehabilitation after anterior cruciate ligament reconstruction. *Am J Sports Med* 1990;18:292–299.
5. Noyes F, Mangine R, Barber S. Early knee motion after open arthroscopic anterior cruciate ligament reconstruction. *Am J Sports Med* 1987;15:149–160.
6. Moffet J, Richard C, Malouin F, Bravo G, et al. Early and intensive physiotherapy accelerates recovery post-arthroscopic meniscectomy: results of a randomized controlled study. *Arch Phys Med Rehabil* 1994;75: 415–426.
7. Frndak P, Berasi C. Rehabilitation concerns following anterior cruciate ligament reconstruction. *Sports Med* 1991;12:338–346.
8. Mooney V. Surgery and postsurgical management of the patient with low back pain. *Phys Ther* 1979;59: 1000–1006.

9. Styf J, Willen J. The effects of external compression by three different retractors on pressure in the erector spine muscles during and after posterior lumbar spine surgery in humans. *Spine* 1998;23:354–358.

10. Kawaguchi Y, Matsui H, Tsuji H. Pack muscle injury after posterior lumbar spine surgery: a histologic and enzymatic analysis. *Spine* 1996;21:941–944.

11. See D, Kraft G. Electromyography in paraspinal muscles following surgery for root compression. *Arch Phys Med Rehabil* 1975;56:80–83.

12. Rantanen J, Hurme M, Falck B, Alaranta H, et al. The lumbar multifidus muscle five years after surgery for a lumbar intervertebral disc herniation. *Spine* 1993;18:568–574.

13. Scapinelli R, Candiotto S. Changes in the paravertebral musculature following a traditional herniated lumbar discectomy: a computed tomographic and magnetic resonance study. *Radiol Med (Torino)* 1994,88:209–215.

14. Mayer T, Vanharanta H, Gatchel R, Mooney V, et al. Comparison of CT scan muscle measurements and isokinetic trunk strength in postoperative patients. *Spine* 1989;14:33–36.

15. Kahanovitz N, Viola K, Gallagher M. Long-term strength assessment of postoperative discectomy patients. *Spine* 1989;14:402–403.

16. Texas Workers' Compensation Commission. *Spinal surgery questionnaire:* recovery times for various spinal *surgeries*, administered to Texas Spine Surgeons, 1997.

17. Dina T, Boden S, Davis D. Lumbar spine after surgery for herniated disk: imaging findings in the early postoperative period. *AJR Am J Roentgenol* 1995;164:665–671.

18. Dzioba R, Doxey N. A prospective investigation into the orthopedic and psychological predictors of outcome of first lumbar surgery following industrial injury. *Spine* 1984;9:614–623.

19. Penta M, Fraser R. Anterior lumbar interbody fusion: a minimum 10 year follow-up. *Spine* 1997;22:2429–2434.

20. Vaccaro A, Ring D, Scuderi G, Cohen D, et al. Predictors of outcome in patients with chronic back pain and low-grade spondylolisthesis. *Spine* 1997;22:2030–2035.

21. Greenough C, Taylor L, Fraser R. Anterior lumbar fusion: a comparison of noncompensation patients with compensation patients. *Clin Orthop* 1994;300:30–37.

22. Greenough C, Peterson M, Hadlow S, Fraser R. Instrumented posterolateral lumbar fusion: results and comparison with anterior interbody fusion. *Spine* 1998;23:479–486.

23. Junge A, Frohlich M, Ahrens S, Hasenbring M, et al. Predictors of bad and good outcome of lumbar spine surgery: a prospective clinical study with two years follow-up. *Spine* 1996;21:1056–1064.

24. Mayer T, Polatin P, Smith B, Smith C, et al. Contemporary concepts in spine care: spine rehabilitation-secondary and tertiary nonoperative care. *Spine* 1995;20:2060–2066.

25. Carragee E, Helms E, O Sullivan G. Are postoperative activity restrictions necessary after posterior lumbar discectomy? *Spine* 1996;21:1893–1897.

26. Sobel J, Hartigan C, Rainville J. Rehabilitation of the post-fusion patient. In: Margulies J, et al., eds. *Lumbosacral and spinopelvic fixation.* Philadelphia: Lippincott-Raven, 1996, pp. 837–849.

27. Mayer T. Physical assessment of the postoperative patient. *Spine:* State of the Art Reviews 1986;1:93–101.

28. Rainville J, Sobel J, Hartigan C. Comparison of total lumbosacral flexion and true lumbar flexion measured by a dual inclinometer technique. *Spine* 1994;19:2698–2701.

29. Biering-Sorenson F. Physical measures as risk indicators for low back trouble over a one year period. *Spine* 1984;9:106–119.

30. Ito T, Osamu S, Suzuki H, Takahashi M, et al. Lumbar trunk muscle endurance testing: an inexpensive alternative to a machine for evaluation. *Arch Phys Med Rehabil* 1996;77:75–79

31. Mayer T, Gatchel R. *Functional restoration for spinal disorders: the sports medicine approach.* Philadelphia: Lea & Febiger, 1988:166–167.

Occupational Musculoskeletal Disorders
edited by T. G. Mayer, R. J. Gatchel, and P. B. Polatin.
Lippincott Williams & Wilkins, Philadelphia © 2000.

30

Quantitative Physical and Functional Capacity Assessment

Tom G. Mayer

Department of Orthopedics, University of Texas Southwestern Medical School, Dallas, Texas 75235

While pain is the symptom that produces the majority of all initial medical contacts, increasing chronicity may cause pain report to reflect multiple obscure physiologic, psychomedical, and socioeconomic factors only marginally related to the inciting injury. As the definition of *injury* has broadened from one involving only obvious trauma, such as fractures, to arcane overuse and repetitive motion disorders, the importance of structural determinants has diminished. Most health providers continue to focus attention on pain and its alleviation, even in the face of compensation factors that promote increasing chronicity and illness behaviors (1,2). However, other stakeholders, including insurers, employers, and legislators, have determined on a course to provide an increasingly cost-conscious reimbursement system. At a time of treatment guidelines, standardized impairment methodology, and fee guidelines, symptomatic treatment alone is no longer sufficient medicine.

Pain control techniques, including manipulation, thermal modalities, narcotics, and immobilization, remain the basis of most acute care (3,4). There can be little dispute that postulated injury results in healing within a relatively short time. Many examples of imperfect healing abound (e.g., bone angulation, scar tissue, arthritic joints, etc.) that may lead to persistent symptoms through established biomechanical malalignments. However, modern imaging generally permits rapid identification of those correctable biomechanical defects, leading to surgical procedures that realign bone, remove impediments to joint mobility, decompress nerves/tendons, or correct musculoligamentous instabilities. In most cases, combinations of patience in awaiting musculoskeletal healing, and providing invasive, corrective procedures, can result in healing within a 4- to 6-month time frame. Thereafter, in an efficient medical system, attention must be centered elsewhere. After occupational injuries, disability helps narrow the focus because it is the central problem from which all others arise. Fortunately, in the workers' compensation system, medical treatment is linked to indemnity payments (as opposed to personal injury and long-term disability insurance programs), so that the medical system can be held accountable for persistence of disability. Lower productivity of individual injured workers certainly foreshadows major losses to society. Disability itself may lead to mental and physical dysfunction, which perpetuates itself and produces a general decline in human performance. As health providers dealing with occupational injuries as only a small proportion of our practices, we may sometimes become personally frustrated, ending up blaming patients for therapeutic failures caused by the lack of recognition of the secondary concomitants of their failure to respond to treatment.

Debilitation and/or *deconditioning* may be a response mediated physically by the injury, as well as psychosocially by a variety of secondary factors. Some of these may include injury-imposed inactivity, neurologically mediated spinal reflexes, iatrogenic medication dependence, nutritional disturbance, and psychologically mediated responses to prior psychiatric distress, vocational adjustment problems, and/or limited social coping resources (1,5–7). Over time, such factors may potentiate each other, particularly in view of a compensation system that encourages dependence while symptom complaints persist (2). These secondary factors may lead to the creation of the "disease" of work disability or incapacity by reinforcing a variety of factors within affected individuals. Additional factors at play in a compensation system may include the adversary employee–employer relationship, limited occupational alternatives, compensation factors (1,8), and family stressors. Thus, potentiation of debilitation may have both an endogenous and exogenous initiation.

Injury generally results in an inflammatory response that produces inhibition of function to the surrounding tissues. The longer healing is delayed because of injury severity, repetitive overuse/reinjury, poor local/systemic nutrition, or other factors, the more profound the inhibition will be. Inhibition of normal motion will impair both the normal healing process and the removal of substances associated with noxious stimuli, leading to an extremely prolonged period of regional symptoms. During this period of splinting, secondary contracture of apophyseal joint structures and muscle–tendon units can be expected to occur, gradually worsening with the passage of time. Sudden resumption of strenuous activities can be expected to increase symptoms by sudden overuse of these disused musculoskeletal structures.

Following soft tissue healing (which will routinely occur within a maximum of a few months if no systemic disease is present), scar tissue in any of the involved mesenchymal structures may continue to wreak mechanical havoc. Partial intrinsic contractures of annulus, joint capsule, or musculotendinous units may lead to retearing of these structures when uncontrolled motions and loads are applied without sufficient preparation of the tissues. In the spine, disc narrowing in the axial plane produces malalignment of apophyseal joints that contributes to facet joint degeneration and greater symptom report. Disc narrowing, particularly combined with postsurgical epidural scar, leads to *dynamic* foraminal narrowing, in that the stenosis may only be symptomatic when local tissue swelling, muscular tightness, or spasm produces sufficient foraminal narrowing to temporarily compress neural structures. In contrast to true stenosis, dynamic foraminal narrowing may be only intermittently symptomatic and thus much more difficult to diagnose and treat.

Nonspinal postinjury biomechanical defects occur with less frequency in occupational injury. Posttraumatic arthritis is common in lower extremity weightbearing joints, with secondary musculoligamentous problems (e.g., patellofemoral dysfunction) found as common sequelae. Upper extremity overuse commonly leads to tendinitis (medial/lateral epicondylitis) or tendinitis in which pulleys or other potential stenosis occur (e.g., shoulder tendinitis, de Quervain's tendinitis, trigger finger, etc.). Nerve compression in potentially stenotic or high-motion areas may result from direct injury or be insidiously related to a tourniquet effect promoting swelling in an extremity, as may occur with thoracic outlet syndrome. Stress and tension may create or interact with vascular factors to promote additional biomechanical disturbance (e.g., cervical tension headaches, reflex sympathetic dystrophy, etc.).

DECONDITIONING CASCADE

Loss of the capacity to perform physical tasks may be associated with both structural lesions and decrements in physical capacity. An example of the first factor is a tibial fracture, while an example of the second is the joint stiffness and muscle atrophy attendant on prolonged immobilization and pain-induced neural-inhibiting influences that in some cases may go on to chronic pain and dysfunction. This example delineates general principles of behavior of the human organism following musculoskeletal injury. Soon after injury, effects of the trauma on structural factors predominate. Inflammation leads to repair of the tissue with the original mesothelial elements or (in large defects) replacement with collagenous scar equivalents. In more significant trauma, the period of immobilization/inactivity may be prolonged and lead to dysfunctional behaviors, abetted by a variety of psychosocial and cultural factors. These dysfunctional behaviors may be succeeded by loss of physical capacity measured by deterioration of a variety of basic elements of performance (BEPs) such as motion, strength, endurance, and agility (9–11). The longer the period of inactivity, the greater will the opportunity be for disuse to create physical capacity deficits leading to decreased human performance. Ultimately, these changes lead to a variety of psychosocial and affective concomitants such as depression, medication abuse, and disability habituation. Pain may be a parallel factor, but its direct relationship to changes in muscles or other mesothelial structures remains a conundrum. While pain may be a potent distractor of attention and inhibitor of function through a variety of fear-mediated mechanisms, its very subjectivity may create a simultaneous excuse for patients to avoid recovery.

The passage of time is the critical factor. Physical capacity deficits are rarely a factor in human performance in the acute posttraumatic stages, but become a gradually increasing factor accompanying inactivity and disuse. As time progresses, functional deficits become the dominant physical impairment disabling the more chronic patient. Strength testing during the early posttraumatic period will be hampered by invalid measurements due to pain-induced neuromuscular inhibition. There is also some limited concern that overaggressive attempts at achieving performance might actually exacerbate the injury during acute phases of occupational injury.

Given usual soft tissue healing periods, such concerns should no longer be necessary 1 to 2 months posttrauma. While testing may be feasible from that point forward, deconditioning produced by inactivity is likely to make its appearance only after that acute time period. Epidemiologically, it could be anticipated that the majority of occupational musculoskeletal cases will have resolved spontaneously by then. However, even as the healing process approaches a plateau, the cascade of progressive joint immobility, muscle inhibition/atrophy, decreased cardiovascular conditioning, and musculotendinous contracture will routinely follow disuse associated with occupational musculoskeletal injury, if not actively dealt with. Many patients will recognize the problem and respond to gentle encouragement. Others will require consistent supervision and coaching on a group or individualized basis.

Does atrophy or contracture represent the whole problem? The term *deconditioning syndrome* has been applied to the cumulative disuse changes produced in chronically disabled patients suffering from spinal and other musculoskeletal chronic dysfunction. It is initially produced by the immobilization and inactivity attendant on injury and supplemented by disruption of spinal soft tissues and scarring resulting from degenerative change, surgical approaches, or repetitive microtrauma. As pain perception is enhanced, learned protective mechanisms lead to a dynamic vicious cycle of inactivity and disuse. As physical capacity decreases, the likelihood of fresh sprains/strains to unprotected joints, muscles, ligaments, and discs increases. The disruption of soft tissue homeostasis accelerates pain, and dysfunction is typically perceived by the patient as a "recurrence" or "reinjury," but it is really secondary to a cycle of healing contracture and deconditioning. The concept of joint and muscle *inhibition* must be introduced to account for much of the measured loss of human performance. In normal subjects, there is generally a level of activity specific to each individual that is tolerated without overuse symptoms. The point at which overuse pain is produced is related to age, sex, body size, and current status of physical capacity. The degree to which the *overuse threshold* is exceeded determines the degree of injury. In deconditioning, there is a progressive shift of the activity–symptom curve to the left, so that less and less activity is tolerated before overuse pain appears. This pain is perceived as "reinjury" by an already inhibited patient. Activity is further suppressed, and the level of physical capacity declines concomitantly. The relationship of activity and symptoms continues to shift until a steady state of relative inactivity and functional decline comes into balance. In certain individuals, such disability may involve simply eliminating a few home or recreational activities. In others, particularly those with heavier job demands and fewer transferable skills, the deconditioning may have devastating consequences, including total disability from work.

Moreover, as early chronicity of impairment and disability lead to greater stress, fear of injury, and disuse of the injured body part, there is a tendency to develop a "weak link" in the injured musculoskeletal functional unit. The low back that used to serve the patient so well now breaks down after 1 hour of weeding in the garden. The knee that confidently supported the college athlete now buckles frequently. For individuals in whom such problems develop, simple whole-person reconditioning is insufficient. Only by identifying the more specific BEPs primarily responsible for the weak link—whether tightness of musculoligamentous structures in the shoulder, rigidity of facet joints in the low back, or decreased muscular control of the patella—can an effective therapeutic plan be developed.

The recognition of deconditioning associated with knee meniscal injuries and surgery in World War II (and popularized by highly visible football players two decades later) led to a therapeutic revolution in combined surgical and rehabilitation treatment of the knee that goes on today. Though facilitated by easy visual access, the concepts translate nicely to spinal and upper extremity disorders. Inactiv-

ity leads to loss of general body functional performance ability, well recognized by any athlete, with uniform loss of *functional capacity*. On the other hand, the injured area sustains more profound loss of paraarticular soft tissue function, becoming progressively greater as the period of disuse and immobilization increases. These changes create a weak link in the localized extremity joint or spinal region whose *physical capacity* must be measured separately. What are the BEPs that are of value in characterizing extremity physiologic "functional units"? Range of motion (ROM), strength, neurologic status, and endurance, combined with whole-body aerobic capacity and activities of daily living measurements, are some of the major factors traditionally assessed.

Evaluation of extremity neurologic function (straight leg raising, lower extremity strength, and sensation and reflexes in dermatomal/myotomal patterns) is still viewed by the majority of clinicians as the ideal objective spine functional evaluation, but these neurologic characteristics may be irrelevant for several reasons. First, they are a measure of acute change when noted in relation to surgical pathology. In the chronic situation, persistence of neurologic changes generally reflects epidural fibrosis or other permanent, noncorrectable anatomic abnormalities. In addition, the neurologic deficits, though emanating from spinal structures, are perceived by the patient as *extremity abnormalities* producing pain, sensory changes, and weakness of arms or legs. In sum, what the clinician currently views as standard "objective" functional tests may provide no useful information to overcome spinal deconditioning.

In matters of musculoskeletal disability, the various psychosocial and socioeconomic components associated with the physical symptoms are likely to make self-report of pain symptoms an unreliable gauge of treatment progression. For this reason, indirect, objective assessment of function is necessary. In fact, such quantitative measures are a necessity for deriving any objective information in the spine, as compared to extremity rehabilitation, where functional tests may be an adjunct luxury only. Objective, quantitative measurements of function provide clinicians with a definition of patient physical capacity, while succeeding tests document changes in performance with treatment. Suboptimal effort demonstrates the degree to which barriers to recovery impede physical performance and lead to changes in psychosocial treatment interventions. Finally, at *maximum medical recovery,* the quantitative tests outline the patient's work capacity and the functional elements often required as part of impairment/disability evaluation.

PRINCIPLES OF HUMAN PERFORMANCE MEASUREMENT

Human performance measurement is the cornerstone for organizing *secondary-* and *tertiary-level rehabilitation programs* for disabled patients with occupational musculoskeletal disorders (5,6,12–15). Outcomes of such rehabilitation programs are critically dependent on quantitative assessment methods (12,16). Certain principles are critical to understanding some or all of these methods, and they are described in the sections that follow.

Accuracy, Reliability, and Validity

The term *accuracy* refers to how close a measured value approaches the "real" or "actual" value (9). It is limited by the precision of the measurement, which is determined by the smallest increment of measurement indicated by the scale on the device. *Reliability* or *reproducibility* refers to the ability of a clinical measurement to equal a previous or prior series of measurements. Reliability is a complex concept that depends on a multitude of factors. Reliability testing is the most common method for assessing the utility of a measurement system because it is easy to evaluate statistically. However, its disadvantage is that it originates from a somewhat imprecise social sciences conceptual framework rather than from physics-based measurement principles commonly used in engineering science. *Valid-*

ity is another social sciences concept that refers to the usefulness of a measurement system (as opposed to a device) in evaluating a clinical paradigm. It may consist of many types of validity (e.g., face validity, content validity, construct validity, consensual validity, etc.).

ROM is the oldest and most commonly measured musculoskeletal physical capacity variable, used both in extremity measures using two-armed goniometers and in spine measurements using inclinometers. Discussion of measurement concepts in conjunction with ROM measurement is illustrative. Considering all of the potential *sources of error,* ± 5 degrees is the commonly acknowledged variability that may be encountered before any real change in motion can be accepted as valid (17–19). Additionally, it is axiomatic that inclinometers or goniometers should be checked periodically against a *reference standard* such as a wall or floor. While device accuracy of a simple two-armed goniometer is usually limited only by its precision, its reliability in a measurement system is generally conceded to be good, although intertester reliability is usually less than intratester reliability. This appears to be more a function of test administrator training than an issue related to the device itself (19–23). Reliability testing for inclinometers provides a confusing mixture of impressions for the reader, since most investigators have failed to recognize that assessment of inclinometric measurements in a measurement system like the spine raises all the possible *sources of error* noted in Table 1.

The *device error* for inclinometers is usually found to be very low, with the device accuracy generally determined by its precision. This is usually about ± 5 degrees for inexpensive fluid-filled inclinometers, decreasing to 0.5 degrees for electronic inclinometers with optical-electronic scanners. Limitations in reliability testing noted in many clinical studies are usually on the basis of sources of error other than the device. Common pitfalls are improper identification of bony landmarks, inadequate warm-up of subjects, improper contact with the subject, and lack of recogni-

TABLE 1. *Factors important in testing reliability and clinical utility involving devices for human performance measurement*

Device accuracy/precision	The ability of the device to repeatably produce the same reading from measurement of the same angle, usually evaluated by a bench test
Human/device interface	The realibility component based on applying the device appropriately to the individual measured, depending commonly on factors such as bony landmarks, overlying soft tissues, parallax, skin adhesion, relationship between skin movement and underlying bony movement, etc
Test administrator training	The skill and training of the test administrator recognizing the multiple potential sources of error, usually evaluated by comparing intratester and intertester reliabilities
Normal human variability	Variability associated with factors such as age, sex, weight, occupation, training, and culture that can be anticipated even with perfect device and measurement validity
Errors unique to subjects undergoing impairment evaluation	Limited effort and cooperation; secondary gain for poor performance; effect of pain; threat of litigation and adversary environment

tion of the motion endpoint (24–38). In general, examiners interested in maximizing the reproducibility of their spinal measurement skills should concentrate on expertise with the device chosen, ability to find bony landmarks, and firm contact in the human–device interface.

In the measurement of isolated strength, the usual concern is the paraarticular musculature supporting a specific joint in a long bone, or a spinal region (cervical, thoracolumbar, etc.). In strength measurements, concepts of *accuracy, precision,* and *relevance* are similar to the principles involved in mobility measurement. However, such measurements are far more dependent on patient effort/compliance, with the examiner having less ability to detect effort levels. Moreover, functional inhibition leads to the additional problem of *recruitment deficits*, so that muscle deficits seem even more profound than mobility loss. Muscle performance is also affected by joint ROM and may be difficult to measure if the range permitted is too limited. Except perhaps for circumferential extremity measurements or magnetic resonance imaging estimates of muscle volume, there are no passive measurements of muscular performance. The measurement of whole-person task performance introduces even more variability, since higher level tasks involve many BEPs, including motion, strength, agility, and coordination. As such, these *functional ca-*

pacity measurements tend to have less ability to discriminate between normal and deconditioned subjects, with less pre- and posttreatment change (39,40). Because functional tests have high face validity in comparison to actual tasks of daily living, they are extremely relevant and there is a high demand for such services. However, most *functional capacity evaluations* are in reality *qualitative* observational responses to consumer demand, rather than scientifically based quantitative measurements.

Normal Human Variability and Databases

Age is definitely a factor in ROM. Due to intrauterine compression, significant alterations in ROM can be demonstrated in neonates, particularly in the shoulders, elbows, ankles, knees, and hips (41,42). Generally, mobility is higher in children than in adults, and progressively declines with age, depending on a number of factors including genetics, sex, training, trauma, and occupation (43–47). Age-related changes tend to occur symmetrically in the extremities if they are not accompanied by unilateral factors such as injury or arthritis. As such, the importance of age-related change is greater in the spine, where lack of contralaterality implies that quantitative impairment evaluation using ROM must rely on a normative database. Normal values depend on a multitude of factors, many of which have been assessed and demonstrated (30,31,48,49). Other studies have tested chronically disabled patients before and after rehabilitation to document the physical progress in overcoming *temporary impairment* to reach their final status of *residual permanent impairment* (39,50,51). Changes related to age have been well documented in the literature (27,52–55). Sex plays a surprisingly small role in mobility, except in cases of ligamentous laxity and normal human variability seen with training effect in women engaged in activities involving stretching. Cultural differences related to childhood positioning or customary postures (i.e., hunkering in many Asian cultures) are also related to significant variability of motion in certain lower extremity joints such as the hip and ankle (30,52,54).

Neutral Zero Method and Terminology

Two parallel goals in musculoskeletal quantitative evaluation are to achieve *objectivity* and *consistency.* One crucial factor in meeting these goals is standardized terminology and measurement protocols to enhance both intratester and intertester reliability. The *neutral zero* concept is the most generally accepted of these concepts (56,57). The principle begins with a *zero starting position,* equivalent to an individual standing erect with hands by the side in a *military attention* posture. All movement is then recorded from this starting position in the three planes intersecting at 90 degrees angles: *sagittal, coronal,* and *axial.*

The most common sagittal plane terms *flexion* and *extension* will be addressed first. This terminology may be confusing if one fails to recognize that there is a difference between the *neutral zero position* (from which the numeric starting point is derived) and the *supine anatomic position* (from which the named direction of motion is derived). The difference is only relevant in the upper extremity distal to the elbow. Beginning in the *supine anatomic position,* all sagittal motion is termed *flexion/extension.* One must view

the femur as the dividing line above which *flexion* increases as the volar angle decreases; distal to the femur, volar angle decrease is termed *extension.* All axial motion is termed *pronation/supination* or *rotation* (either left/right or internal/external). Coronal motion is described by a large number of terms, including *abduction/adduction, eversion/inversion, deviation* (e.g., ulnar/radial), or *lateral* bend (e.g., left/right spinal).

Regardless of direction of measurement, the neutral zero position *always* represents the 0-degree position, whether at end range or some intermediate point for the joint(s) or regions under consideration. Numeric values of ROM are generally expressed in the angle through which a joint passes from the neutral zero position to terminal movement. In some joints, such as the elbow, knee, and fingers, the neutral zero position is essentially in full extension, and all the recorded motion is in flexion. Loss of extension mobility is termed *flexion contracture.* In other joints, the neutral zero position is at some midpoint of the planar range. *Ankylosis* refers to complete joint immobility and is expressed as a specific angle in the terminology of the plane(s) involved (e.g., ankle ankylosed at 10 degrees plantar flexion). More commonly, some residual joint ROM persists but is limited in reaching the extreme of the range. Because it is generally acknowledged that impairment is greater when the neutral zero position can no longer be achieved, the presence of a flexion contracture in a joint such as the elbow, knee, or fingers is of greater significance than loss of terminal planar motion when the neutral zero position is preserved (e.g., retained cervical spine motion from 30-degree flexion to 30-degree extension). Contractures in joints with a midpoint neutral zero position may also be administratively termed *ankylosis* (18).

The term *hyperextension* connotes a potentially pathologic condition of *hypermobility* that may involve either a genetic predisposition to ligamentous laxity or a ligament and capsular injury creating residual posttraumatic joint instability (44,47). When an extremity is affected in terms of mobility, a contralateral normal side is often available for comparison. This is not true in the spine, so that a *normative database* must be developed if deviations from "normal" are to be identified. The need for quantitative rather than qualitative expressions of these deviations introduces the requirement of accounting for normal human variation in performance measurements, including such factors as age, sex, weight, and/or joint laxity. Even occupational variations can be identified in some joints; although it remains unclear whether the presumed occupational influence causes the mobility difference, there is an accompanying genetic predisposition selecting for the occupation or both (58).

ROM can be measured either actively (AROM) or passively (PROM). AROM, generally acknowledged as a *safer* method of measurement, requires the patient's voluntary cooperation using active muscle contraction. This method may have the unintended side effect of limiting terminal motion, as when a co-contraction is stimulated. PROM requires the intervention of the examiner moving a joint to a terminal position, which is generally considered more objective because the movement is free of control by the examinee. Distal extremity joints lend themselves more readily to this type of measurement. Even under conditions of maximum effort, AROM may be different from PROM as in the case of pain-inhibiting active (increased loading) motion or muscle weakness preventing full active motion against gravity. Whenever possible, both AROM and PROM should be described.

MEASUREMENT TECHNIQUES

Range of Motion

Quantitative measurement in most joints, particularly in the extremities, is facilitated by use of the simple, two-armed goniometer (59). As the goniometer is essentially a hinge, it is particularly useful whenever a typical hinge or ball-and-socket joint is being measured in a single plane. Measurement is also facilitated by the presence of a contralateral side, easy palpation of bony landmarks, and experience of the test administrators. In contrast, however, overlying soft tissue, obesity, lack of contralaterality, or regional movements (e.g., the spine) make use of the goniometer less preferable because of decreasing accuracy, relevance, and/or objectivity. For special situations, smaller, flat-surface goniometers have been developed (e.g., finger measurements). A large universal goniometer is available for measuring large extremity joints, although there is some question whether any significant difference between alternative devices can be demonstrated in reliability tests, since greater variability is produced by other factors (21).

Inclinometers are versatile tools that have evolved from the simple carpenter's level. Small, inexpensive versions of these devices with reasonable accuracy can be obtained at any hardware store. Convenience and expense are often comparable to two-armed goniometers. Since goniometry is ineffective in spine measurement, inclinometers are preferred for use in these regions (60–63). A dual-inclinometer technique has been developed for measuring each of the specific spinal regions. Subtraction of the motion of the lower inclinometer from the upper inclinometer leads to a *true* spinal motion measurement (30,31,62). It is customary to measure true cervical motion from the occiput to T-1, thoracic from T-1 to T-12, and lumbar from T-12 to the sacrum.

Beyond the simple tools, many other motion measurement devices have been devised. A magnetic compass may be utilized to measure inclination out of the gravitational plane (61,64,65). Flexicurves and kyphometers have been used for specialized spinal regional measurements, designed to overcome some of the limitations of other measurement tools in these areas (66,67). Various electrogoniometers or electronic inclinometers have been developed as tools for more accurately assessing spinal motion in a gravitational plane. Excellent device accuracy may be offset in routine spinal evaluation by human–device interface problems and training required to handle these instruments (31,68,69). Finally, various computerized goniometers have been utilized, primarily for research purposes, to obtain very precise motion measurements. These include devices such as three-dimensional digitizers, computerized inclinometers, optical scanners, video combined with light-emitting diodes, and various multiposition x-ray techniques. Expense precludes generalizability into the clinical environment (70–76).

Isolated Strength Measurements

Emerging technology has provided a number of accurate assessment devices for measuring strength of paraarticular muscles throughout the musculoskeletal system. Isometric protocols measure the maximal force that a muscle can generate in a contraction, felt by some investigators to be more accurate than other technologies. Isometric strength testing is generally used for assessing muscular function in which there is either minimal motion associated with joint excursion or for which dynamic technologies have not been developed. An example of the former is the variety of meters, using either spring-loaded or hydraulic devices, for measuring grip strength in the hand. The more comprehensive devices involve multiposition isometric grip measurement. An example of the latter device occurs in a number of handheld or stabilized devices for measuring cervical spine strength, in which the devices are held against a standard position on the head while forces are exerted in the sagittal and coronal planes. Isometric technology has also been used successfully in multiposition devices measuring sagittal strength in the lumbar spine.

Isokinetic measurement of both extremity joints and spinal regions is the dynamic standard for isolated physical capacity measurements of the paraarticular muscles. Over the past three decades, several manufacturers have developed devices for performing these measurements, characterized by dynamometers that can be set to a preselected speed (hence, *isokinetic*), measuring the torque around a defined fulcrum through simultaneous reciprocal (i.e., flexion/extension) movements. For the first 15 years of their existence, these devices measured only extremity joint strength, with right/left comparisons becoming the standard for measurement. However, with the advent of trunk strength measurements in the sagittal and axial planes, it was recognized that *normative databases* were necessary for comparison to patient performance. With greater experience, it has been recognized that chronic disability is frequently accompanied by bilateral extremity deconditioning, even when the injury only affects one side. Therefore, normative databases have become more widely used in dynamic measurements of extremity joint strength also. With more advanced computerization, the *work* and *power* measurements throughout a contraction sustained through a full ROM can be obtained from instantaneous torque measurements, providing a more comprehensive single measurement of muscle performance. Naturally, validity of these measures depends on *full effort,* which will usually be absent when chronic pain is a distraction or there is significant fear of injury. Muscle recruitment through overcoming inhibition can be demonstrated by improvements in serial testing, which often accompanies improvements in mental, as well as physical, health. An extensive literature on isokinetic testing with multiple devices is available in the literature (49,77–79). The validity of human performance strength measurements has been challenged in some reviews, but the purposes of such measurements may often be misunderstood (9,79–81).

Functional Capacity Tests

These tests have become very popular in recent years under the rubric *functional capacity evaluation* (FCE), originally described by Isernhagen (82). FCEs represent tests involving *motion time measurement* for simulating specific activities of daily living. In these whole-person tests, the evaluator attempts to assess the patient's ability to perform activities of daily living *relevant to the injured body part.* For example, if the injury involves the lumbar spine, relevant activities of daily living of greatest importance might include lifting from floor to waist, bending, or static sitting. If the injury involves the knee, FCE might include squatting, kneeling, running, or walking. In the shoulder girdle, reaching or lifting above shoulder height might be most relevant. In this way, a FCE must be individualized to the needs of the injured worker and can become quite cumbersome when there are multiple injury claims. Moreover, the state-of-the-art is still relatively qualitative, since few manufacturers have developed devices that can help identify activity of daily living human performance. Since such performance is dependent on the coordination of multiple body "functional units," there is considerably more normal human variability in functional task measurements than in physical capacity measurements. However, the demands of the occupational market for expert opinions regarding the evaluation of disability have led to an explosion of FCE performance requests and products.

The few standardized and quantitative FCEs available involve aerobic capacity (using bicycle or treadmill protocols), lifting capacity, or upper body endurance (using rotary ergometers). Each test serves a useful purpose, with quantification methodology and clinician experience continually increasing. Dynamic lift testing generally involves either *isokinetic* or *isoinertial* protocols. The isokinetic devices have the same advantages and limitations of the isolated joint/regional measurement devices. Isoinertial tests are inexpensive and relatively easy to perform, but are associated with significant human variability (40,83–88).

Effort Assessment

Effort may be assessed with variable success on each of the individual tests with a variety of techniques. On mobility measures, whether using goniometry or inclinometry,

consistency of the motion measurements is the single best method for determining effort. However, such reliance on a ±10% criterion is obviously not foolproof, particularly in the situation of a well prepared subject. Variability of 10% to 20% associated with good effort, with much higher variability in those showing poor effort, has been demonstrated for strength tests and lifting tests (79,89,90). In certain specific situations, comparison of one test to another may lead to effective effort validation, as in the case of comparing the supine straight leg raise to the standing hip flexion component in lumbar flexion (62,90). The isokinetic strength devices allow computerized comparison of curve replication throughout a dynamic range that is a more sophisticated version of the consistency test. All such consistency tests depend on the ability to recognize variations of 5% to 20%. In a disabled patient population, the tests may therefore be dependent on sufficient performance amplitude. Finally, use of normative databases comparing patients based on variables such as age, sex, weight, or height allow the identification of gross variation, which can often be assumed to represent limited effort. However, it must be recognized that the term *effort* must be used guardedly, since its use implies a voluntary aspect to low test performance. Unconscious barriers such as pain, stress, or joint/muscle inhibition may be the primary factors producing "low" effort. Consequently, the recognition of performance limitations in most patients is not well suited to single evaluations for determining faking or malingering. Rather, poor performance can be used to educate such patients and, through serial testing, motivate them to train and demonstrate higher levels of performance motivation. With maximum effort, such quantitative tests can be very useful in identifying patient return to a work capacity in which their physical performance is equivalent to that of other incumbent workers. Such databases are now being used to test large populations of workers involved in relatively heavy jobs, so that the preparedness for return to those jobs after treatment can be identified.

Implementation of Quantitatively Directed Therapeutic Exercise

Physical deconditioning and debilitation occur as a cascade that is both physically and psychologically mediated. Once they occur, therapeutic exercise requiring active participation on the part of the injured worker is the only rational treatment response. Education and limited pain control methods become adjuncts to stimulate adherence to an exercise program, which may involve some pain, as contracted joints are stretched and weak, irritable muscles tighten or spasm. Motivating patients to work through such pain is one of the important attributes of the measurement of function.

Few, if any, commercially available products standardize methodology and normalize multiple quantitative measurements into a single evaluation product. In certain clinical venues, such as at the Productive Rehabilitation Institute of Dallas for Ergonomics (PRIDE), each of the functional measurements alluded to above has been standardized according to protocol and is accompanied by normative data collected on large numbers of patients. These normative data are segregated based on age. For certain strength tests around weightbearing regions and joints, data are also normalized on the basis of a body weight variable (40,51,78,91–94). In some cases specific industrial databases have been developed (48,49,86). Computerized comparison of an individual patient's scores to the normalized values permits expression of each individual's performance on a given test as a *percent normal* of a performance level anticipated based on the normalizing variables. Knowledge of the additional factor of the patient's usual fitness based on job or recreational demands (i.e., heavy lifting work, high aerobic demand work, etc.) can aid in the interpretation of individual tests. For purposes of global comparison, a *cumulative score*, similar to the concept of a grade-point, average may assist the casual observer in comparing performance in a single individual from one measurement to the next or across patient populations without having to

take the normalizing variables into account. A medically interpreted summary, commenting on performance, areas of greatest deficit, and effort/validity, generally accompanies such a quantitative FCE report.

The next step is to utilize the functional measurement in guiding the therapeutic exercise approach. Without measurement of human performance, the clinician is essentially blind to the patient's real physical and psychologic status, having to rely entirely on verbal self-report. The level of exercise prescribed is subject to the concept of a *dose,* just as vital as in prescribing medication. These exercise concepts will be discussed further elsewhere, but it is important to note for the purposes of this chapter that the variability of the therapeutic exercise dose can be substantially narrowed by the results of the quantitative evaluation, particularly if performed serially. In the PRIDE facility, a computerized exercise progression program—broken into 75 step levels and normalized to various age, sex, and body weight variables—has evolved through use of a normative sample and been modified through experience. Each quantitative FCE sets a level of exercise that can generally be tolerated by most patients, after which the exercise level is progressed in steps according to the therapist's judgment of how successfully the patient accomplishes that day's task for each exercise machine or related group of machines. Localized *weak-link* injured areas are trained for strength and endurance by this method, as are the various activities of daily living tasks. Without the quantification of function, patients would tend to oscillate between doing far too little and performing excessively, triggering the fear/tension/pain cycle anew.

CONCLUSION

Injury to soft tissues in the musculoskeletal system leads to a dynamic, progressive debilitation and deconditioning cascade whose extent is determined by physically and psychosocially mediated mechanisms. Socioeconomic factors, including globalization of labor markets and politically inspired liberalization of injury definitions, contribute to the mix of body and mind factors recognized as the patient with a progressive deconditioning syndrome. As the injured area becomes a *weak link* in the more chronic, high-cost injured worker, decreases in efficiency of performing certain activities of daily living for which the injured area is critical may occur. This leads to a sequential loss of *functional capacity* and work performance. These losses are recognized as progressive *disability* by health providers observing the gradual deterioration of the worker. Recognition of debilitation alone, without recognition of severity of deficits or the role of psychologic inhibition, may act as an impediment to health providers in prescribing an appropriate dose of therapeutic exercise. Although the current state-of-the-art remains very much in flux, there has been a movement over the past several decades toward greater interest in functional measurement, and an accompanying but slower movement from qualitative to quantitative methods whenever possible. This process has been helped by the manufacturers of a variety of measurement devices but has been slowed by limited interest on the part of medical providers and researchers, many of whom have tended to view prescription of therapeutic exercise as an allied health responsibility, unworthy of their interest. Besides being used to direct therapeutic exercise levels and frequency, physical and functional capacity measurements have other uses. They may be employed to identify inhibition of function that leads to appropriate education and counseling on psychosocial issues. Persistent failure to progress or large discrepancies between exercise training levels and testing may provide evidence of motivational deficiencies, possibly related to financial *secondary gain*. On the other hand, achievement of normal physical and functional capacity after a period of disability, in which the treated patient performs at levels similar to those of successful incumbent workers, can provide *objective* evidence for the ability to perform the demands of the job to which the patient may wish to return. Finally, the measurement of *permanent impairment,* once temporary im-

pairment has been dealt with through surgical and rehabilitation treatment methods, may be individually determined in a fair fashion through use of selected, standardized physical capacity measures. The need for further research in this area cannot be overemphasized. Use of ROM for impairment measures has stimulated a great deal of research over the past decade. Similar interest in the development of normative databases, better effort assessment, and improved protocols for human performance should galvanize researchers over the next several years and improve the quality of nonoperative care, work capacity assessment, and impairment evaluation.

REFERENCES

1. Beals R. Compensation and recovery from injury. *West J Med* 1984;104:233–237.
2. Hadler N. *Occupational musculoskeletal disorders.* New York: Raven Press, 1993.
3. U.S. Department of Health and Human Services, Agency for Health Care Policy and Research. *Clinical practice guideline #14: acute low back problems in adults.* U.S. Department HHS, Washington, D.C. 1994.
4. North American Spine Society and American Academy of Orthopaedic Surgeons. *Clinical algorithm on low back pain, phase I.* Chicago: American Academy of Orthopaedic Surgeons, 1996.
5. Jordan K, Mayer T, Gatchel R. Should extended disability be an exclusion criterion for tertiary rehabilitation: socioeconomic outcomes of early vs. late functional restoration in compensation spinal disorders. *Spine* 1998;23:2110–2117.
6. Mayer T, McMahon M, Gatchel R, Sparks B, Wright A, Pegues P. Socioeconomic outcomes of combined spine surgery and functional restoration in workers' compensation spinal disorders with matched controls. *Spine* 1998;23:598–606.
7. Polatin P, Kinney R, Gatchel R, Lillo E, Mayer T. Psychiatric illness and chronic low back pain: the mind and the spine—which goes first? *Spine* 1993;18:66–71.
8. Polatin P. Affective disorders in back pain. In: Mayer T, Mooney V, Gatchel R, eds. *Contemporary conservative care for painful spinal disorders.* Philadelphia: Lea & Febiger, 1991:149–154.
9. Mayer T, Kondraske G, Beals S, Gatchel R. Spinal range of motion: accuracy and sources of error with inclinometric measurement. *Spine* 1997;22:1976–1984.
10. Kondraske G. Towards a standard clinical measure of postural stability. In: Kondraske G, Robinson C, eds. *Proceedings of the 8th annual conference of the IEEE Engineering in Medicine and Biology Society.* Fort Worth: TX, 1986;3:1579–1582.
11. Kondraske G. Human performance: measurement, science, concepts and computerized methodology. In: T. Munsat, ed. *Quantification of Neurologic Deficit.* Stoneham: MA, Butterworths 1989, pp.33–48.
12. Mayer T, Polatin P, Smith B, Smith C, Gatchel R, Herring S, et al. Contemporary concepts in spine care:

spine rehabilitation: secondary and tertiary nonoperative care. *Spine* 1995;20:2060–2066.

13. Mayer T, Gatchel R, Mayer H, Kishino N, Keeley J, Mooney V. A prospective two-year study of functional restoration in industrial low-back injury: an objective assessment procedure. *JAMA* 1987;258;1763–1767.

14. Hazard R, Fenwick J, Kalisch S, et al. Functional restoration with behavioral support: a one-year prospective study of patients with chronic low back pain. *Spine* 1989;14:157–161.

15. Garcy P, Mayer T, Gatchel R. Recurrent or new injury outcomes after return to work in chronic disabling disorders: tertiary prevention efficacy of functional restoration treatment. *Spine* 1996;21:952–956.

16. Hazard R. Spine update: functional restoration. *Spine* 1995;20:2345–2348.

17. American Medical Association. *Guides to the evaluation of permanent impairment*, 3rd ed. Chicago: American Medical Association, 1988.

18. American Medical Association. *Guides to the evaluation of permanent impairment*, 3rd ed rev. Chicago: American Medical Association, 1990.

19. Boone D, Azen S, Lin C-M, et al. Reliability of goniometric measurements. *Phys Ther* 1978;58:1355–1390.

20. Elveru R, Rothstein J, Lamb R. Goniometric reliability in a clinical setting: subtalar and ankle joint measurements. *Phys Ther* 1988;68:672–677.

21. Hamilton G, Lachenbruch P. Reliability of goniometers in assessing finger joint angle. *Phys Ther* 1969;49: 465–469.

22. Riddle D, Rothstein J, Lamb R. Goniometric reliability in a clinical setting: shoulder measurements. *Phys Ther* 1987;67:688–673.

23. Rothstein J, Miller P, Roettger R. Goniometric reliability in a clinical setting: elbow and knee measurements. *Phys Ther* 1983;63:1611–1615.

24. Boline P, Keating J, Haas M, Anderson A. Interexaminer reliability and discriminant validity of inclinometric measurement of lumbar rotation in chronic low-back pain patients and subjects without low-back pain. *Spine* 1992;17:335–338.

25. Capuano-Pucci D, Rheault W, Aukai J, Bracke M, Day R, Pastrick M. Intratester and intertester reliability of the cervical range of motion device. *Arch Phys Med Rehabil* 1991;72:338–340.

26. Clapper M, Wolf S. Comparison of the reliability of the orthoranger and the standard goniometer for assessing active lower extremity range of motion. *Phys Ther* 1988; 68:214–218.

27. Dvorak J, Panjabi M, Novotny J, Antinnes J. *In vivo* flexion/extension of normal cervical spine. *J Orthop Res* 1991;9:828–834.

28. Gajdosik R, Bohannon R. Clinical measurement of range of motion: review of goniometry emphasizing reliability and validity. *Phys Ther* 1987;67:1867–1872.

29. Gill K, Krag M, Johnson G, Haugh L, Pope M. Repeatability of four clinical methods for assessment of lumbar spinal motion. *Spine* 1988;13:50–53.

30. Keeley J, Mayer T, Cox R, Gatchel R, Smith J, Mooney V. Quantification of lumbar function, 5: reliability of range-of-motion measures in sagittal plane and *in vivo* torso rotation measurement techniques. *Spine* 1986;11:31–35.

31. Mayer T, Brady S, Bovasso E, Pope P, Gatchel R. Noninvasive measurement of cervical triplanar motion in normal subjects. *Spine* 1993;18:2191–2195.

32. Miller S, Mayer T, Cox R, Gatchel R. Reliability problems associated with the modified Schober technique for true lumbar flexion measurement. *Spine* 1992;17: 345–348.

33. Portek I, Pearcy M, Reader G, Mowat A. Correlation between radiologic and clinical measurement of lumbar spine movement. *Br J Rheumatol* 1983;22:197–205.

34. Reynolds P. A measurement of spinal mobility: a comparison of three methods. *Rheumatol Rehabil* 1975;14: 180–185.

35. Rheault W, Miller M, Nothnagel P, Straessle J, Urban D. Intertester reliability and concurrent validity of fluid-based and universal goniometers for active knee flexion. *Phys Ther* 1988;78:1676–1678.

36. Shirley F, O'Connor P, Robinson M, MacMillan M. Comparison of lumbar range of motion using three measurement devices in patients with chronic low back pain. *Spine* 1994;19:779–783.

37. Williams R, Binkley J, Bloch R, Goldsmith C, Minuk T. Reliability of the modified-modified Schober and double inclinometer methods for measuring lumbar flexion and extension. *Phys Ther* 1993;73:26–36.

38. Youdas J, Carey J, Garrett T. Reliability of measurements of cervical spine range of motion—comparison of three methods. *Phys Ther* 1991;71:98–106.

39. Kohles S, Barnes D, Gatchel R, Mayer T. Improved physical performance outcomes following functional restoration treatment in patients with chronic low back pain: early versus recent training results. *Spine* 1990;15: 1321–1324.

40. Curtis L, Mayer T, Gatchel R. Physical progress and residual impairment after functional restoration. III. Isokinetic and isoinertial lifting capacity. *Spine* 1994; 18:401–405.

41. Forero N, Okamura L, Larson M. Normal ranges of hip motion in neonates. *J Pediatr Orthop* 1989;9:391–395.

42. Hoffer M. Joint motion limitation in newborns. *Clin Orthop* 1980;148:94–96.

43. Baxter M. Assessment of normal pediatric knee ligament laxity using the Genucom. *J Pediatr Orthop* 1988; 9:546–550.

44. Cheng J, Chan P, Hui P. Joint laxity in children. *J Pediatr Orthop* 1991;11:752–756.

45. Roach K, Miles T. Normal hip and knee active range of motion: the relationship to age. *Phys Ther* 1991;71: 656–665.

46. Svenningsen S, Terjesen T, Auflem M, et al. Hip motion related to age and sex. *Acta Orthop Scand* 1980;60: 97–100.

47. Wynne-Davies R. Familial joint laxity. *Proc R Soc Med* 1971;64:689–690.

48. Mayer T, Gatchel R, Keeley J, Mayer H, Richling D. A male incumbent worker industrial database. I. Lumbar spinal physical capacity. *Spine* 1994;19:755–761.

49. Mayer T, Gatchel R, Keeley J, Mayer H, Richling D. A male incumbent worker industrial database. II. Cervical spinal physical capacity. *Spine* 1994;19:762–764.

50. Lowery W, Horn T, Boden S, Wiesel S. Impairment evaluation based on spinal range of motion in normal subjects. *J Spinal Disord* 1992;5:398–402.

51. Mayer T, Pope P, Tabor J, Bovasso E, Gatchel R. Physical progress and residual impairment quantification after functional restoration. I. Lumbar mobility. *Spine* 1994;19:389–394.

52. Dvorak J, Antinnes J, Panjabi M, Loustalot D, Bonomo M. Age and gender related normal motion of the cervical spine. *Spine* 1992;17(suppl):393–398.

53. Moll J, Wright V. Normal range of spinal mobility. *Ann Rheum Dis* 1971;30:381–386.

54. Sullivan M, Dickinson C, Troup J. The influence of age and gender on lumbar spine sagittal plane range of motion: a study of 1,126 healthy subjects. *Spine* 1994;19: 682–686.

55. Twomey L, Taylor J. Age changes in the lumbar articular triad. *Aust J Physiother* 1985;31:106–112.

56. Cave E, Robert S. A method for measuring and recording joint function. *J Bone Joint Surg* 1936;18:455–465.

57. Gerhardt J. *Documentation of joint motion*, 3rd ed rev. Portland, OR: Oregon Medical Association, 1992.

58. Reid D, Burnham R, Saboe L, et al. Lower extremity flexibility patterns in classical ballet dancers and their correlation to lateral hip and knee injuries. *Am J Sports Med* 1987;15:347–352.

59. Greene W, Heckman J. *The clinical measurement of joint motion*. Chicago: American Academy of Orthopaedic Surgeons, 1994.

60. Loebl W. Measurements of spinal posture and range in spinal movements. *AM J Phys Med* 1967;9:103–110.

61. MacRae I, Wright V. Measurement of back movement. *Ann Rheum Dis* 1969;28:584–589.

62. Mayer T, Tencer A, Kristoferson S, Mooney V. Use of noninvasive techniques for quantification of spinal range-of-motion in normal subjects and chronic low-back dysfunction patients. *Spine* 1984;9:588–595.

63. Troup J, Hood C, Chapman A. Measurements of sagittal mobility of the lumbar spine and hips. *Ann Phys Med* 1968;9:308–313.

64. Dillard J, Trafimow M, Andersson G, Cronin K. Motion of the lumbar spine: reliability of two measurement techniques. *Spine* 1991;16:321–324.

65. Mellin G. Method and instrument for noninvasive measurements of thoracolumbar rotation. *Spine* 1987;12: 28–31.

66. Burton A. Regional lumbar sagittal mobility: measurement by flexicurves. *Clin Biomech* 1986;1:20–26.

67. Hart D, Rose S. Reliability of a noninvasive method for measuring the lumbar curve. *J Orthop Sports Phys Ther* 1986;8:180–184.

68. Paquet N, Malouin F, Richards C, Dionne J, Comeau F. Validity and reliability of a new electrogoniometer for the measurement of sagittal dorsolumbar movements. *Spine* 1991;16:516–519.

69. Zaki A, Goldberg M, Khalil T, et al. Comparison between the one and two inclinometer techniques for measuring body ranges of motion using the Orthoranger II. In: Das B, ed. *Advances in industrial ergonomics and safety II*. Taylor and Francis, 1990:135–142.

70. Brown R, Burstein A, Nash C, Schock C. Spinal analysis using a three-dimensional radiographic technique. *J Biomech* 1976;9:355–365.

71. Dopf C, Mandel S, Geiger D, Mayer P. Analysis of spine motion variability using a computerized goniometer compared to physical examination: a prospective clinical study. *Spine* 1994;19:586–595.

72. Pearcy M. Measurement of back and spinal mobility. *Clin Biomech* 1986;1:44–51.

73. Pearcy M, Portek I, Sheperd J. The effect of low-back pain on lumbar spine movements measured by three-dimensional x-ray analysis. *Spine* 1985;10:150–153.

74. Salisbury P, Porter R. Measurement of lumbar sagittal mobility: a comparison of methods. *Spine* 1987;12: 190–193.

75. Stokes I, Wilder D, Frymoyer J, Pope M. Assessment of patients with low back pain by biplanar radiographic measurements of intervertebral motion. *Spine* 1980;6: 233–240.

76. Whittle M. Calibration and performance of a three-dimensional television system for kinematic analysis. *J Biomech* 1982;15:185–196.

77. Flores L, Gatchel R, Polatin P. Objectification of functional improvement after nonoperative care. *Spine* 1997; 22:1622–1633.

78. Brady S, Mayer T, Gatchel R. Physical progress and residual impairment quantification after functional restoration. II. Isokinetic trunk strength. *Spine* 1994;18:395–400.

79. Newton M, Waddell G. Trunk strength testing with iso-machines, 1. Review of a decade of scientific evidence. *Spine* 1993;7:801–811.

80. Newton M, Thow N, Somerville D, Henderson I, Waddell G. Trunk strength testing with iso-machines, 2. Experimental evaluation of the Cybex II back testing system in normal subjects and patients with chronic low back pain. *Spine* 1993;7:812–824.

81. Mayer T, Gatchel R, Keeley J, Mayer H. Optimal spinal strength normalization factors among male railroad workers. *Spine* 1993;18:239–244.

82. Isernhagen S. *The comprehensive guide to work injury management*. Gaithersburg, MD: Aspen Publishers, 1995.

83. Mayer T, Barnes D, Kishino N, et al. Progressive isoinertial lifting evaluation. I. A standardized protocol and normative database. *Spine* 1988;13:993–997.

84. Mayer T, Barnes D, Nichols G, et al. Progressive isoinertial lifting evaluation. II. A comparison with isokinetic lifting in a disabled chronic low-back pain industrial population. *Spine* 1988;13:998–1002.

85. Mayer T, Gatchel R, Barnes D, Mayer H, Mooney V. Progressive isoinertial lifting evaluation: an erratum notice. *Spine* 1990;15:5.

86. Mayer T, Gatchel R, Keeley J, Mayer H, Richling D. A male incumbent worker industrial database. III. Lumbar/cervical functional testing. *Spine* 1994;19:765–770.

87. Cady L, Bischoff D, O'Connel E, Thomas P, Allan J. Strength and fitness and subsequent back injuries in firefighters. *J Occup Med* 1979;21:269–272.

88. Schmidt A. Cognitive factors in the performance level of chronic low back pain patients. *J Psychosom Res* 1985;29:183–189.

89. Hazard R, Reid S, Fenwick J, Reeves J. Isokinetic trunk and lifting strength measurements: variability as an indicator of effort. *Spine* 1988;13:54–57.

90. American Medical Association. *Guides to the evaluation of permanent impairment*, 4th ed. Chicago: American Medical Association, 1993.

91. Smith S, Mayer T, Gatchel R, Becker T. Quantification of lumbar function, 1. Isometric and multispeed isokinetic trunk strength measures in sagittal and axial planes in normal subjects. *Spine* 1985;10:757–764.

92. Mayer T, Smith S, Keeley J, Mooney V. Quantification of lumbar function, 2. Sagittal plane trunk strength in chronic low back pain patients. *Spine* 1985;10:765–772.

93. Mayer T, Smith S, Kondraske G, Gatchel R, Carmichael T, Mooney V. Quantification of lumbar function, 3. Preliminary data on isokinetic torso rotation testing with myoelectric spectral analysis in normal and low back pain subjects. *Spine* 1985;10:912–920.

94. Kishino N, Mayer T, Gatchel R, et al. Quantification of lumbar function, 4: isometric and isokinetic lifting simulation in normal subjects and low back dysfunction patients. *Spine* 1985;10:921–927.

PART VI

Chronic Occupational Musculoskeletal Disorders

Occupational Musculoskeletal Disorders
edited by T. G. Mayer, R. J. Gatchel, and P. B. Polatin.
Lippincott Williams & Wilkins, Philadelphia © 2000.

31

Pain, Function, Impairment, and Disability: Implications for Workers' Compensation and Other Disability Insurance Systems

Allard E. Dembe

Center for Health Policy and Health Services Research, University of Massachusetts Medical School, Shrewsbury, Massachusetts 01545

Any modern society must confront the fundamental question of how to provide economic protection for people who are incapable of working because of some physical or mental problem and therefore unable to derive income through gainful employment. In the United States, several disability insurance systems have been developed for providing this kind of protection, the most prominent being workers' compensation insurance, Social Security disability insurance, and private short- and long-term disability insurance.

Each of these insurance arrangements has incorporated tests to determine whether or not a person is truly incapable of working and thus entitled to income protection benefits. In each system, medical judgments of a person's condition, as evaluated by physicians, therapists, and other health care professionals, play an important role in establishing both a person's eligibility for benefits and the amount of benefits to be provided.

While this arrangement sounds relatively simple, it is extremely complex in practice. There are at least four important complicating factors:

- Whether or not a person can potentially work is determined not only by his or her physical and mental health but also by a variety of nonmedical considerations, such as the availability of suitable work and the person's vocational skills;
- A person may have a substantial physical or mental problem that adversely affects his or her life but does not directly interfere with wage-earning capacity;
- A person suffering from a physical or mental problem might be able to engage in income-producing work, but at a diminished wage level or with fewer vocational opportunities;
- A person may suffer physical or mental harm that affects neither wage-earning capacity nor nonwork functioning but leaves the person with a permanent physical or mental abnormality that merits some form of compensation.

Resolving the above-mentioned complications involves economic and political decisions regarding the intended objectives and structure of the insurance plan. Even if such questions were able to be clarified sufficiently, the responsibilities of medical practitioners within these systems would be complex and difficult. One role for clinicians is the traditional one of establishing a diagnosis and prescribing appropriate treatment. But disability insurance systems typically also require a medical assessment to be made of claimants' physical and mental condition relative to some baseline criterion.

For example, a disability insurance system might require a doctor to determine whether a person's actual condition deviates from some ordinary functional state, physiologic norm, or usual anatomic status. To make those determinations, the doctor would need to measure the deviation between a customary expected state and the person's actual condition. Even under the best clinical circumstances, making such a determination is extremely complicated because it presupposes having a precise knowledge and description of the expected baseline state and sensitive, specific, and reliable clinical tests to measure the extent of deviation. There are few areas of medicine where sufficient evidence and techniques exist to make exacting assessments of this type.

Moreover, because disability insurance systems aim to compensate people for the adverse effect of medical problems on their income-producing capability, nonvocational functioning, and (sometimes) bodily or psychologic harm unrelated to function, medical practitioners could be asked to assess a person's condition relative to various nonmedical criteria. For example, a doctor may be required to assess the impact of a person's medical problem on his or her ability to perform a variety of everyday functions such as eating, dressing, walking, or driving a car. That requires a systematic evaluation of the deviation existing between a person's current condition and a baseline expectation of what is considered customary or normal. It is obvious that making such a determination is fraught with a host of methodologic complexities, such as whether the comparative baseline is established for a population as a whole or for a person of similar age, sex, medical and social history, and overall constitution.

In addition, owing to the vocational focus of disability insurance systems, doctors are frequently called on to evaluate the impact of a person's medical problem on his or her ability to engage in vocational activities, including the actual activities required by a particular job (e.g., the person's current job) and/or common vocational activities such as lifting, inspecting, carrying, climbing, and bending. Actually, measuring deviations between the person's existing condition and the baseline vocational criteria presupposes having a detailed evaluation of the person's present condition, a precise description of the expected job requirements or vocational functional norms, and valid measurement techniques for evaluating the type and magnitude of deviation. Here, too, such an undertaking would be fraught with numerous practical and theoretical perplexities, such as whether the comparative norms ought to be population-based or adjusted for a person of similar circumstances, whether the baseline norms adequately reflect all pertinent aspects of current and potential job function, and so forth.

From a practical standpoint, it is difficult to see how an individual medical doctor or health care practitioner would have the skills and tools necessary to make this complex assessment. At a minimum, it would require extensive knowledge and familiarity with the way that jobs are performed in various industries and occupations. Additionally, it requires an understanding of the precise relationship between particular physical and mental capabilities and job performance. Neither of these considerations is customarily covered in the training of medical practitioners. In fact, there is little credible scientific evidence describing and quantifying the relationship between physical capacities and actual labor market performance.

Despite these practical and theoretical difficulties, most disability insurance systems rely on medical evaluations to certify a claimant's request for income protection benefits, and use medical findings as a basis for determining the appropriate amount of benefits to award. Commentators have traced the medicalization of the current disability system to society's historical faith in doctors' ability to render objective, nonbiased decisions, the belief that the medical profession has reliable tests to screen out fraudulent claims, and politicians' conviction that it is administratively expedient to utilize medical judgments of disability as a qualifying procedure (1,2).

Despite the contemporary dependence on medical approaches to assessing disability, there is no theoretical reason why eligibility for disability insurance payments has to be medically based or determined by clinical evaluations. As pointed out in Deborah Stone's (1) *The Disabled State,* one could also conceive of disability as primarily a social, educational, or legal category to be ascertained, for instance, by judges or industrial labor experts. Alternatively, disability insurance payments could be granted according to preestablished criteria involving the type of medical problem (diagnosis) and occupation, presumptive standards (as in the federal black lung program), or an affected worker's own decision to utilize work-absence benefits available under a comprehensive employee benefits plan or collectively bargained benefits arrangement.

CONTROVERSIES REGARDING MEDICAL EVALUATION OF IMPAIRMENT AND DISABILITY

In practice, the need to develop a qualifying test for disability insurance benefits has spawned an elaborate system based on medical evaluations of impairment and/or disability. Doctors and other health care professionals in the United States spend considerable time conducting clinical evaluations of impairment and disability, often with little training in assessment methodologies or understanding of the underlying conceptual foundation of those concepts. Requests for performing such evaluations are frequently initiated by insurance claims adjusters, lawyers, or other administrative officials. This pulls doctors and other clinicians into a medical process with significant financial and legal ramifications that is unlike the customary caring relationship that characterizes the traditional doctor–patient encounter.

The present system is based on a supposed conceptual distinction between *impairment* and *disability,* predicated on the knowledge that disability assessment depends on social and economic as well as medical considerations. Impairment, according to this view, is a medical concept amenable to clinical evaluation, while disability is not. However, there is considerable evidence that doctors are not entirely clear about or consistent in their interpretation of this distinction and that in practice many clinicians evaluate disability instead of or in addition to impairment (3–5). Moreover, one could also question whether impairment is strictly a clinical issue, since it requires evaluation of an individual relative to baseline criteria of normal function or physiology that might not be completely appraisable through standard medical means.

According to the prevailing view, *impairment* is a loss or abnormality in functional capacity or bodily structure. A frequently cited definition of impairment is that adopted in the World Health Organization's (6) *International Classification of Impairments, Disabilities, and Handicaps*: "any loss or abnormality of psychological, physiological, or anatomical structure or function." *Disability* is usually conceived to be an inability to fully perform various common activities. Most definitions of disability generally follow the one used in the fourth edition of the American Medical Association's (7) *Guides to the Evaluation of Permanent Impairment* (AMA *Guides*): "a decrease in, or loss or absence of, the capacity of an individual to meet personal, social, or occupational demands, or to meet statutory or regulatory requirements."

Some of the practical difficulties inherent in clearly distinguishing the two concepts is evident from a close examination of these definitions. For example, many functional abnormalities may be detected and measured by observing a person's incapacity to meet activity demands. Do "personal and social demands" include breathing, eating, speaking, and other functions that are commonly part of an impairment assessment?

Many disability insurance systems have adopted different mechanisms for paying income protection benefits, depending on whether a claimant's disability is temporary or permanent. For example, in workers' compensation plans, income replacement benefits due to temporary work disability caused by a work injury are usually paid to beneficiaries as weekly indemnity payments based on a proportion of the wages lost during the period of incapacity. Other approaches, frequently involving lump sum payments, are used in various states to confer benefits to claimants for permanent disability related to a work injury (8,9). The Social Security disability insurance program only provides compensation for permanent disability or long-term disability that can be expected to persist for at least 12 months (10). Thus, another challenge for clinicians is to ascertain whether a person's medical problem creates a temporary, long-term, or a permanent physical or functional decrement. Many systems of medical impairment evaluation, including the AMA's, are directed only at identifying and assessing permanent, rather than temporary, incapacity.

The process of evaluating whether a condition creates a permanent rather than a temporary abnormality or functional incapacity is commonly referred to as determining whether *maximal medical improvement* (MMI) has occurred, where MMI is understood to be a static state in which no further recovery or restoration of function can be expected to take place with a reasonable degree of medical certainty (11). Even in serious cases involving gross structural loss or manifest physiologic change, it might be very difficult for a physician to predict accurately whether further functional improvement is possible, and this obviously introduces further uncertainty into the entire impairment evaluation process (12).

The current system of medical determination of impairment is predicated on the idea that clinicians can make assessments that are objective, reproducible, quantifiable, and supported by clinical measurements and tests. Impairment is presumed to be essentially a biologic phenomenon, manifested through observable physical signs and laboratory findings. Purely subjective complaints such as pain, fatigue, dizziness, and other symptoms unaccompanied by overt, observable evidence are generally considered to be unreliable indicators of impairment. According to the dominant paradigm, impairment is an objective, scientific phenomenon clearly distinguishable from disability that is determined not only by *tangible* impairment but also by a host of social, political, and contextual factors, as well as the individual's subjective responses.

The view described above, while widely adopted by practicing physicians and inculcated into the AMA *Guides* and medical texts, has provoked extensive controversy and criticism. Some of its internal inconsistencies and ambiguities are immediately evident. For example, the determination of impairment, as noted earlier, is a relative notion involving an abnormality that creates a deviation in function. Its evaluation, according to the AMA *Guides,* requires the physician to estimate the degree to which an individual's capacity to carry out daily activities has been diminished. On the surface, it is hard to see how evaluating a person's ability to "use a keyboard, travel by airplane, participate in 'desired' sexual activity, participate in group activities, participate in hobbies, drive a car, or have restful sleep," all of which are defined as "activities of daily living" in the AMA *Guides,* is any less subjective or more clinically precise than assessing a person's capacity to perform a particular job.

Apparently, practicing physicians also find this distinction confusing. Studies have revealed that physicians apply multiple factors when evaluating impairment related to low back pain, and the vast majority of them consider nonmedical factors such as the patient's education, motives, intelligence, personality, and social environment in determining the impairment rating (3,4). Moreover, many physicians report that they will base a finding of permanent impairment on a history of chronic low back pain in the absence of observable signs. These findings have compelled investigators to conclude that there are no purely "objective means" to rate low back impairment and that in practice most physicians actually rate disability rather than impairment as defined in the AMA *Guides* (3–5).

This confusion is perhaps inevitable, given the original intent behind creating the AMA impairment rating process, which was to provide a way for state workers' compensation agencies to make permanent partial disability (PPD) awards based on a systematic quantified assessment of the extent of harm resulting from a workplace injury (1,13). Currently, 42 states and jurisdictions in the United States use AMA-based impairment ratings in determining eligibility for PPD payments and/or calculating the amount of those awards (14). Five states, including Texas and Maine, base PPD benefits directly on the magnitude of the injured worker's AMA impairment rating. These practices obviously encourage both doctors and patients to think of impairment and disability as intimately connected.

Perhaps, the most serious continuing criticism of the present AMA impairment rating system is the absence of scientific and medical evidence on which to base the ratings. The development of the numeric schema in which percentages of permanent impairment are attributed to various observed clinical conditions is generally not founded on empiric data about the actual functional impact of those abnormalities but rather represents the combined subjective opinions of physicians selected to serve on the AMA *ad hoc* committees that authored the AMA *Guides.* The fourth edition of the AMA *Guides,* published in 1993, was drafted through the collective work of 71 persons (69 of whom were physicians) serving on 15 panels grouped according to organ system (7). The process by which these committees of "experts" reached "consensus" and derived the precise ratings has not been publicly documented by the AMA or subjected to external validation.

For some areas, such as pulmonary function evaluation, impairment ratings are based on available empiric data regarding population norms for spirometric testing of forced expiration, stratified by age, height, and sex. By contrast, there is virtually no empiric evidence available for deciding what an appro-

priate impairment rating might be for many musculoskeletal system complaints. No scientific justification, for example, is presented in the AMA *Guides* for its assertion that ankylosis of the ankle in the neutral position represents a 4% whole-body impairment. Even in the case of a measured deviation from population norms in forced expiration volume, the actual impact on an individual's functional capacity to perform daily activities might vary considerably, depending on the person's general health, conditioning, and other factors (12).

Moreover, the impairment rating process inevitably represents only a snapshot of a person's condition at a particular place and time, as assessed during a particular clinical encounter. In reality, the functional impact created by many chronic conditions fluctuates over time, thereby further clouding the validity of the calculated impairment ratings. Furthermore, a valid assessment of actual functional impairment of the musculoskeletal system requires a consideration of dynamic motions, as well as the static conditions constituting the focus of the impairment determination process outlined in the AMA *Guides* (13).

Further complicating the AMA *Guides'* process is its practice of translating an impairment of a system or body part into a so-called "whole-person" impairment. For example, the AMA *Guides* considers a 100% impairment of the great toe to represent a 5% impairment of the entire person. Here again, there is virtually no scientific basis or evidence for making this translation. The AMA's attempt to create such a category is not necessarily relevant from a diagnostic or therapeutic standpoint. It is only introduced into the impairment rating process because legal and insurance systems bestow compensation based on the person's capacity to function as a whole in performing work and other gainful activities. The introduction of a translation of segmental impairment into a "whole-person" rating, while posing as part of an objective clinical evaluation, really serves as a medicolegal expediency, further blurring the supposed distinction between the scientifi-cally pure impairment assessment process and the socially predicated determination of dis-ability.

Similarly, there is no empiric evidence un-derlying the AMA *Guides'* technique of com-bining various whole-person impairment val-ues for different body parts or systems into a single whole-person impairment rating. Un-der the system described in the AMA *Guides,* when two separate abnormalities are present, they are "combined" to provide a consoli-dated whole-person impairment rating ac-cording to a formula that always produces a "total" rating that is less than the sum of the individual ratings. For example, a 40% whole-person impairment related to a musculoskele-tal injury is combined with a 20% whole-per-son impairment due to a visual defect to yield a 52% total whole-person impairment. It is quite evident that the selection of 52% as the "correct" combined rating is a contrivance that is not supported by any clinical or epi-demiologic data. The goal of this technique is to account for multiple impairments in a way that will not result in a total impairment rating exceeding 100%, so as to have a workable quantified basis on which to award disability payments. Other than serving in that capacity, the concept of somehow "combining" differ-ent types of bodily impairments has no med-ical relevance, and it is not grounded on sci-entific fact.

In light of the foregoing considerations, it is perhaps not surprising that there is at pre-sent no convincing evidence demonstrating that physicians' impairment ratings have pre-dictive value with respect to actual functional capacity or work ability (15–17). Further-more, many physicians find it difficult to evaluate impairment accurately and reliably, and significant variations have been found with regard to both interrater and intrarater evaluation of impairment (15). Studies have shown that there is poor reproducibility of range of motion measurements, an important component of assessing musculoskeletal im-pairment (18,19). Physicians' use of incli-nometers to assess range of motion does not

significantly improve the reliability of mea-surement (20,21). Given the same informa-tion concerning a standardized clinical sce-nario, California physicians produced widely different disability ratings, ranging from 0% to 70% based on the California Disability Evaluation Schedule (22). Studies in Texas have found that about 50% of disabled work-ers receive multiple permanent impairment ratings from different doctors and that the av-erage deviation between their highest and lowest ratings is about 7% (23). Intracorp, a case management and utilization review com-pany, reviewed 615 cases in which impair-ment evaluations had been conducted and found 526 cases (86%) with errors in the way that permanent whole-person impairment was calculated, resulting in an average deviation of approximately 10.4 impairment rating per-centage points from what should have been determined (24).

Rather than being an objective and uniform process conforming to invariable standardized measures, impairment evaluation is actually highly variable and subjective, open to a con-siderable range of reasonable medical opin-ion. This allows room for the system to be manipulated by both physicians and patients, as well as for social biases about the disabil-ity insurance system to affect its outcome. Physicians are not immune from these influ-ences. A recent study in Texas found that im-pairment ratings determined by a patient's pri-mary treating physician varied significantly from those calculated by doctors representing workers' compensation insurance companies or appointed by the state workers' compensa-tion agency (25). Further variability is intro-duced by differences in perspective between general practitioners and subspecialists.

Not surprisingly, there is a high level of worker frustration and dissatisfaction with the present system. Disputes about impairment ratings and disability awards based on those ratings are responsible for an extensive amount of litigation. Many workers feel that the impairment evaluation process is unfair. Injured workers surveyed in Texas cited a va-riety of problems with the current system, including cursory examinations, biased doctors, inadequate information about how the ratings were determined, and improperly calculated ratings (14,26).

FUNCTIONAL CAPACITY EVALUATIONS

The present system for determining whether a person is incapable of working and thus entitled to income protection benefits rests on the edifice of doctors' putative ability to make an objective, clinical evaluation of impairment and functional limitations that can somehow be translated into an appropriate disability rating. As we have seen, there are many practical and theoretical difficulties in this arrangement, including physicians' inability to accurately assess various functional limitations in the clinical environment. Furthermore, there may be little scientific basis for thinking that the assessment of functional impairment performed in a doctor's office is directly relevant for evaluating the type of physical skills and capabilities that truly determine whether an individual has the capacity to do gainful work.

To address these deficiencies, instruments and procedures have been developed to evaluate more systematically a person's ability to perform the kind of functional tasks commonly found in an occupational context. So-called functional capacity evaluation (FCE) is designed to provide a standardized method to evaluate workers' capacity to perform vocational functions and activities. Functions typically assessed in a FCE include lifting, pulling, pushing, bending, sitting, climbing, reaching, and grasping. In a FCE, measurements may be taken of a person's strength, lifting capacity, endurance, aerobic uptake, standing range of motion, manual dexterity, and other selected indicators of work capacity. Special test instrumentation and mechanical devices for conducting FCEs have been developed by commercial vendors. These devices allow the measurement of isometric, isokinetic, isoinertial, and dynamic exertions to supplement the static assessments that are part of a more traditional clinical examination. It is common for FCEs to be conducted by physical or occupational therapists, rehabilitation specialists, exercise physiologists, ergonomists, or other allied health professionals who have been trained in the use of the relevant test procedures and instruments (27–30).

The fundamental idea behind FCEs is to bridge the gap between clinical assessment of impairment and a more meaningful and pertinent assessment of work capacity and disability. According to Leonard Matheson (27), a chief proponent of functional capacity testing, performing a FCE is critical because it provides a way "to translate the effect of impairment into disability." Backers of FCEs promote them as an objective, measurable, systematic, and direct means of estimating a person's functional capacity to perform occupational tasks.

FCEs are based on the concept of simulation: The tests and measurements composing a FCE permit the clinical assessment of key physical demands that are thought to simulate those that are essential for performing actual work. Just as physicians attempt to evaluate the ability to perform the activities of daily living through having patients simulate those activities during examination, FCEs permit an individual's work abilities to be simulated, and thus observed and measured, in a controlled clinical environment. FCEs are intended to provide a mechanism for incorporating knowledge of workplace conditions and job demands into the medical impairment evaluation process.

There are various types of FCE, depending on the intended specificity and scope of the evaluation. Some FCEs compare a person's functional capacities to a specific job (e.g., the patient's current job or anticipated job), while other FCEs measure the subject's capacity to perform general vocational activities (e.g., grasping, carrying, pulling, balancing) that might be applicable in a variety of different occupations. Although FCEs typically assess an individual's capacities at a particular point in time, the evaluation can also be conducted over an extended period of several days to gauge fluctuations in functional performance and the workers' ability to meet the demands of employment on a continuing basis. A FCE directed toward a general or specific job assessment typically lasts 2 to 6 hours and costs between $200 and $500 (28,30,31).

Although FCEs have been widely touted as a way of objectifying impairment assessment and linking functional incapacity with work disability, there are still significant practical and conceptual problems with this approach. As mentioned previously, to be of value in determining impairment or disability, a FCE must compare measured functional capacity either to the patient's preinjury baseline capacities or to population norms. From a practical standpoint, accurate measurements of a subject's preinjury capacities rarely exist, and clinician estimates of preinjury capabilities are notoriously inaccurate (31,32). Using population-derived norms as a baseline is also problematic because individuals can vary considerably from mean values, even after adjustment for age, height, weight, and sex. For example, an individual who originally had an especially large lifting capacity and lost a significant percentage of function due to injury may still have a "normal" lifting ability according to FCE (12). Moreover, many aspects of functional capacity decrease naturally with age, and appropriate evidence on which to base age adjustments is not always available or applied (31).

FCEs only provide a snapshot of a person's functional capacities as evaluated on a particular occasion. However, workers suffering or recovering from injuries or illnesses may have impairments that affect functionality in a variable fashion (33). Pain and a subject's health status have been shown to affect the variability of FCE results (34). Chronic pain presents a significant difficulty because of its potentially powerful impact on a person's functional capacity and tendency to fluctuate over time. For these reasons, some authorities recommend against administering FCEs when a person is in pain or impaired due to injury,

which obviously decreases the value of the procedure in the disability determination process (28).

The subject's motivation and reaction to the evaluation is also a major factor that can affect FCE test results (35). FCEs presuppose that the individual being tested will cooperate and will do the best he or she can when performing the various tasks involved. Baseline comparisons assume that the patient is exerting a "maximal effort"— FCEs cannot be used to study submaximal exertions (34,36). However, there are as yet no objective measures for determining a patient's true maximal performance, despite various attempts to concoct clinical tests for establishing the patient's "sincerity of effort" (34,36,37).

The aforementioned considerations have led authorities to question the reliability, accuracy, and validity of FCEs (32,33,37). Reliability is hampered by the absence of widely accepted standardized protocols for performing FCEs or agreement about the specific test equipment to use for various kinds of functional tests (31,36). Intratest and test–retest (interrater) reliability have been found to be dependent on various factors involving the evaluator's instructions and exhortations to the subject, as well as the evaluator's allowing patients to have an opportunity for practice sessions prior to performing the actual FCE (27,38). Moreover, there is considerable evidence showing that patients' performance on a FCE is reactive, meaning that measured performance changes because of the individual's experience of taking the test. Several studies have reported significant improvement in subjects' functional capacity subsequent to a FCE, suggesting that there is a "learning effect" involved in taking a FCE or that changes occur in patients' self-perception about their functional capabilities (27). The paucity of trained specialists having appropriate skills, experience, and knowledge in how to properly conduct a FCE further reduces the test's overall reliability (27).

Even if functional capacity measurements could be taken reliably, there would still be questions about the relevance of those results for accurately assessing a person's ability to perform real work. As observed by Matheson (27), "At the interface between the patient's physical abilities and the job's physical demands stand activities... that have a complex physiologic, psychologic, musculoskeletal, and environmental basis." At best, a FCE captures only some of those characteristics, and physical functional capacities, by themselves, will generally not provide a complete picture of a person's ability to perform a job. Empiric studies of FCEs' efficacy in predicting actual vocational outcomes are rare and provide little support for the tests' validity (27). Moreover, even if FCE results were found to be associated with patients' ability to undertake or resume work, additional questions and concerns could arise about the ability to pursue long-term safe employment without impact on wage-producing capacity, reinjury potential, or other social and economic outcomes (33).

Along with the aforementioned theoretical concerns about FCEs, various technical problems impede their widespread acceptance and use. For example, the tests themselves may cause injury and reinjury (34). FCEs are often requested by case managers, insurance representatives, and other nonclinicians who do not have the training and knowledge to interpret the results appropriately (28). Suitable test equipment may not be available or might be prohibitively expensive (27). The relatively lengthy time and expense involved in conducting FCEs might limit their application to only the more serious cases.

In theory, FCEs provide a way to more accurately and objectively assess the kinds of functional limitations that are most relevant for understanding the relationship between impairment and disability. They hold promise for expanding the arsenal of clinical approaches available for helping the medical profession contribute meaningfully to the process of determining eligibility for disability insurance benefits. However, they are clearly not the final answer, especially in the absence of compelling evidence for their validity in predicting successful work outcomes, and in the significant problems associated with their reliability and use.

ALTERNATIVE APPROACHES FOR AWARDING DISABILITY BENEFITS

The present system for conferring income protection insurance benefits is based on the medical determination of impairment and its translation into an assessment of disability status. Physicians and other medical professionals are being asked to function as system "gatekeepers," making clinical judgments that are ultimately used as the basis for legal, regulatory, and political decisions having substantial economic consequences. This system has been widely criticized by scholars, policymakers, lawyers, worker advocates, and the business community as unfair, potentially biased, and lacking scientific and medical justification. It is plagued by the illusion that doctors can consistently establish valid, objective, and meaningful assessments of impairment that are reliably associated with the inability to engage in gainful employment.

Although this system has been extensively criticized, there have been few attempts to propose a workable alternative. Even some of the most exhaustive scholarly analyses of the problems in the current scheme have failed to suggest viable solutions. Deborah Stone's (1) incisive examination in *The Disabled State* ends disappointingly with an admonition for government to "abandon the no-fault insurance model of compensation," implying unrealistically that a tort-based liability system would somehow solve these problems and be more manageable and fair than the current arrangement. Nortin Hadler (39), one of the foremost critics of the prevailing medically based disability paradigm, stridently beseeches policymakers to reform the system but offers only vague hints of how this might be accomplished through providing incentives for full employment and comprehensive health care (37), "reconstructing" the use of scheduled awards (40), and drawing on models used in other countries that he feels are "far less convoluted and expensive and far more compassionate than ours"(5).

While a complete abandonment of the current medically based model is unlikely and probably undesirable, there are specific steps that can be taken to make the system work better and more clearly define physicians' role. Potential reforms fall into two categories: those that maintain a system of basing disability awards on the medical determination of impairment and those that do not do so.

The most immediate way of improving the current system is to launch a concentrated national effort to conduct empiric research studying the relationship between injured workers' impairment evaluations, functional capabilities, and actual labor market experiences and outcomes. As noted earlier, there is at present little hard evidence underlying impairment assessments, their translation or combination into whole-person impairment ratings, or the value of those ratings for predicting whether a patient can perform various types of productive work. The present system will never be perceived as fair or entirely credible until such research is conducted. The AMA should take the lead to ensure that its impairment guides are clearly evidence-based (41,42).

The recent movement toward developing methods of more directly assessing vocational functionality through FCEs needs to be further refined and validated. Standardized protocols and test procedures should be adopted. A positive step in this direction was recently taken with the development and public dissemination of the California Functional Capacity Protocol, a standardized method to measure the work consequences of soft tissue musculoskeletal injury (31). However, until the reliability of FCEs is improved and their validity verified through empiric investigation, the value of FCEs in disability insurance systems will remain limited.

Various reforms are possible that would preserve the ability of injured workers to qualify for income protection benefits related to a medical problem while deemphasizing physicians' role in determining impairment and disability levels. This could potentially be accomplished in a variety of ways, described in the following sections.

Scheduled Awards

Several state workers' compensation systems use a predetermined schedule of allowable permanent partial disability payments for certain specific injuries. Typically, such schedules cover only the manifest physical loss of a part of the body, such as amputation of an arm or leg. But, conceivably, a system of predetermined PPD benefits could be established for any work-related injury or illness that creates a permanent impairment and can be objectively diagnosed. The advantage of such a system is that it circumvents the need for a (supposedly) precise medical assessment of the degree of impairment and functional incapacity. In a way, this would transfer part of the PPD benefit decision making from the clinical arena to the political process involved in establishing the scheduled benefits. An increased reliance on scheduled PPD awards was apparently one of the options Hadler (40) had in mind when he wrote:

> If we could improve the administrative algorithm, we could solve most of the shortcomings of disability determination as currently practiced. The [workers' compensation] listings and schedules could be reconstructed so they are comprehensive, multivariate instruments and their predictive value could be measured.

One of the principal problems with moving toward an increased reliance on scheduled PPD benefits is the difficulty in scheduling appropriate benefits for injuries and illnesses that are not plainly evident and precisely determinable, for example, soft tissue musculoskeletal conditions.

Presumptive Standards

A related approach is for the state to establish qualifying criteria for PPD benefits that can be applied even in the absence of a precise diagnosis or compelling medical evidence. So-called presumptive standards specify a set of conditions under which a claimant's burden of proof is considered to have been met (43). This approach is used by many states for compensating victims of occupational diseases for which it might otherwise be medically difficult or impossible to demonstrate a causal connection between the disease and workplace exposures. The federal Black Lung Act, for example, adopted a presumptive standard under which workers with specified clinical indicators of coal miner's pneumoconiosis and at least 10 years of work experience in a coal mine are presumed to be eligible for PPD benefits irrespective of whether or not a precise medical determination of causality or impairment has been made. In theory, similar presumptive criteria for disability benefits could be established for a host of other diseases and conditions based on the presence of certain preestablished clinical indicators of disease, work history, and exposure, without requiring a definitive medical assessment of impairment or disability status.

Wage Loss

One proposed system that has attracted considerable attention is predicated on the concept of awarding PPD benefits based on actual wage loss rather than on an estimation of potential impact of impairment on earning capacity. Under this approach, benefits could be paid either if a person's medical incapacity prevents him from working or if the individual returns to work at a diminished wage level. This system has the advantage of basing PPD benefits on demonstrable labor market experiences, thereby avoiding the pitfalls inherent in translating medical impairment ratings into a supposed disability effect. This kind of arrangement was used in Florida between 1979 and 1993. Despite some initial success in decreasing costs and streamlining the system, most commentators now believe that the Florida experiment was a failure because it created a strong disincentive for injured workers to return to productive employment and promoted increased litigation about patients' true work capabilities (44).

Hybrid System

Some authorities have advocated a hybrid approach that utilizes the traditional medical impairment model but provides injured workers additional options for obtaining PPD benefits if the impairment-based disability award is determined to be inappropriate or inadequate. The alternative award could be based on scheduled benefits or wage loss payments. This approach could potentially serve as a validation test for the clinically derived impairment rating. John F. Burton Jr (44), a leading workers' compensation theorist, recently advocated this kind of hybrid system:

> My view—which is also the position of others who have carefully studied this topic—is that a hybrid system is the best possible compromise for a PPD benefits system that will serve the multiple criteria of equity and efficiency. Such a system would begin with a period of PPD benefits based on the impairment approach, followed by a safety valve of wage-loss benefits for those workers whose actual labor market experience far exceeds the earnings losses predicted by an assessment of the extent of impairment.

Nonmedical Review Panels

It is conceivable that a disability insurance system could be established that determines benefits eligibility primarily through a legal or administrative process that supplements or replaces the need to rely on medical judgments. Hadler (45) described a system used in France, in which citizen panels with members representing government, labor, trade associations, employer representatives, and disability experts ultimately decide most cases. Panels of this sort could be charged with reviewing and establishing the initial PPD award or be utilized as part of an appeals process if the claimant or insurer feels that the determination is unfair. In this kind of system, medical evidence could be considered but would not necessarily be determinative. The advantage of this type of arrangement is that it places the decision-making process in the hands of a balanced group of informed individuals representing a variety of perspectives and it avoids relying solely on questionably "objective" medical determinations of impairment. However, unless it is designed and operated efficiently, such a scheme runs the risk of creating a relatively complex bureaucratic structure that could potentially slow the determination process, promote increased disputes and litigation, and increase system costs.

Comprehensive Benefit Plans

The aforementioned alternatives presuppose separate systems for compensating workers for different types of work disability. Workers' compensation insurance, for example, provides income protection benefits only for work absences that are the result of occupational injuries and illnesses. In reality, though, there are many reasons that individuals miss time away from work, including holidays, vacation time, sick leave for minor illnesses, family situations, and religious observances, as well as acute illness and injury, occupational disorders, and long-term and permanent impairment. Currently, most employers have benefit plans covering these work absences differently, with each having its own eligibility requirements. To some extent, employers need to do this because of prevailing laws, including the requirement that work injuries be handled according to state workers' compensation statutes. However, one could conceive of the possibility for employers to have flexibility in devising comprehensive plans covering a wide variety of work absences, especially in unionized situations where such arrangements could be developed and codified through a collective bargaining agreement. In a truly "comprehensive" benefits arrangement, a preestablished amount of compensation could be allocated for covering expected time away from

work, irrespective of its cause. For example, an employer that traditionally provided 3 weeks (15 days) vacation, 5 sick days, 3 "personal" days, and an average of 5 days annually for other reasons (including workers' compensation injuries) might create a plan whereby workers are entitled to payment for up to 28 days per year (15+5+3+5) of time away from work. If an individual uses less, the company could "buy back" those days, or the worker might be able to "bank" some of them for future use, thereby creating an incentive for minimizing work absences. Such a system would still need to have a "safety net" of long-term disability insurance for workers who truly need it. But a system of undifferentiated "flexible time off" would provide a number of advantages, insofar as it alleviates the need for making the often ambiguous determination of whether a person ought to count a particular day off as a sick day, a personal day, or a vacation day (e.g., when a child is sick) and it avoids the frequently contentious dilemma involved in deciding whether or not an injury (e.g., back pain) is truly work-related. Long-term disability and PPD benefits could also be built into such a plan, either through criteria embodied in the benefits plan or through eligibility provisions of the long-term disability insurance arrangement. In a collectively bargained environment, ultimate qualification for the long-term disability benefits could be invested in a labor–management panel or jointly designated review board.

Integrated System without Workers' Compensation Insurance

The considerations mentioned above raise questions about whether a separate workers' compensation system is really needed, and whether many of the problems involved in impairment and disability determinations might be minimized if there were a truly integrated health care system providing appropriate access to medical and rehabilitative services and income protection for all persons with injuries or illnesses, irrespective of whether or not their conditions are job-related. Much of the current controversy surrounding impairment and disability determination stems from the particular features of state workers' compensation systems, including the need to determine eligibility for available indemnity and PPD benefits, to assess readiness for return to work, and to verify patients' need for rehabilitative services, along with differentiating eligibility for workers' compensation benefits from similar benefits available through Social Security and private disability insurance. In a system that provides appropriate medical services and benefits to all workers and integrates health care with a plan for ensuring suitable income protection due to sickness and injury, many of these subtle nuances and the need for precise medical quantification of impairment could dissolve or at least become far less controversial. In envisioning a comprehensive system of this sort, it is important not to lose sight of the professed advantages of workers' compensation insurance, which include creating incentives for preventing workplace accidents and relieving both workers and employers from the need to establish negligence and fault for occupational mishaps.

Whether or not a new system evolves for impairment evaluation and the determination of disability insurance benefits, it is critical to remember that the best long-term approach for dealing with disability is for society to focus on better controlling its root causes. Improved housing, nutrition, economic conditions, education, medical care, and employment opportunities will help keep impairments from developing and reduce the likelihood that functional limitations will prohibit individuals from undertaking gainful employment. In the workplace, the optimal way to control disability is to create safer work environments, better labor–management relations, and expanded opportunities for using people's diverse skills in productive ways. These are the measures that may ultimately have the greatest impact on lightening the burden of physicians who must now serve as gatekeepers for disability benefits.

ACKNOWLEDGMENTS

I would like to thank Leslie Boden and Emily Spieler for their helpful comments during the preparation of this manuscript. This chapter has been written with the support of a grant from The Robert Wood Johnson Foundation.

REFERENCES

1. Stone D. *The disabled state.* Philadelphia: Temple University Press, 1984.
2. Greenwood JG. History of disability as a legal construct. In: Demeter SL, Andersson G, Smith G, eds. *Disability evaluation.* St. Louis, MO: Mosby, 1995:5–12.
3. Brand RA, Lehmann TR. Low-back impairment rating practices of orthopaedic surgeons. *Spine* 1983;8:75–78.
4. Greenwood JG. Low-back impairment-rating practices of orthopaedic surgeons and neurosurgeons in West Virginia. *Spine* 1985;10:773–776.
5. Hadler NM. *Occupational musculoskeletal disorders.* New York: Raven Press. 1993;249–262.
6. World Health Organization (WHO). *International classification of impairments, disabilities and handicaps.* Geneva: WHO, 1980.
7. American Medical Association. *Guides to the evaluation of permanent impairment,* 4th ed. Chicago: American Medical Association, 1993.
8. Burton JF Jr. Permanent partial disability benefits: a re-examination. *Workers Comp Monitor* 1996;9(4):1–15.
9. Durbin D, Kish J. Factors affecting permanent partial disability ratings in workers' compensation. *J Risk Insur* 1998;65:81–99.
10. Demeter SL. Disability evaluation. *Occup Med* 1998; 13:315–323.
11. Brigham CR, Babitsky S. Independent medical evaluations and impairment ratings. *Occup Med* 1998;13: 325–343.
12. Himmelstein JS, Pransky GS. Ability to work and disability evaluation. In: Levy BS, Wegman DH, eds. *Occupational health,* 3rd ed. Boston: Little, Brown and Company, 1995:221–239.
13. Mooney V. Impairment, disability and handicap. *Clin Orthop* 1987;221:14–25.
14. Ellenberger JN. Labor's perspective on health care cost reform. In: Greenwood J, Taricco A, eds. *Workers' compensation health care cost containment.* Horsham, PA: LRP Publications, 1992:245–259.
15. Rondinelli RD, Robinson JP, Scheer SJ, Weinstein SM. Industrial rehabilitation medicine: strategies for disability management. *Arch Phys Med Rehabil* 1997;78: S21–S27.
16. Rondinelli RD. Practical aspects of impairment rating and disability determination. In: Braddom R, ed. *Physical medicine and rehabilitation.* Philadelphia: WB Saunders, 1996:191–205.
17. Scheer SJ. The physician's responsibility in assessing vocational capacity. In: Scheer SJ, ed. *Medical perspectives in vocational assessment of impaired workers.* Gaithersburg, MD: Aspen Publishers, 1991:1–18.

18. Katz RT, Rondinelli RD. Impairment and disability rating in low back pain. *Occup Med* 1998;13:213–230.

19. Merritt JL, McLean TJ, Erickson RD, Offord KP. Measurement of trunk flexibility in normal subjects: reproducibility of three clinical methods. *Mayo Clin Proc* 1986;61:192–197.

20. Rondinelli RD, Murphy J, Esler A, Marciano T, Cholmakjian C. Estimation of normal lumbar flexion with surface inclinometry: a comparison of three methods. *Am J Phys Med Rehabil* 1992;71:219–224.

21. Bline PD, Keating JC, Haas M, Anderson AV. Interexaminer reliability and discriminant validity of inclinometric measurement of lumbar rotation in chronic low-back pain patients and subjects without low-back pain. *Spine* 1992;17:335–338.

22. Clark WL, Haldeman S, Johnson P, et al. Back impairment and disability determination: another attempt at objective, reliable rating. *Spine* 1988;13:332–341.

23. Texas Research and Oversight Council on Workers' Compensation. *An analysis of Texas workers with permanent impairments.* Austin: Texas Research and Oversight Council, 1996.

24. Intracorp. *Intracorp impairment rating review project.* Dallas, Texas: Intracorp, Inc., 1995.

25. Texas Research and Oversight Council on Workers' Compensation. Discrepancies in impairment ratings by types of doctors. *Texas Monitor* 1996;1(4):7–8.

26. Texas Research and Oversight Council on Workers' Compensation. Impairment ratings—the employee perspective. *Texas Monitor* 1996;1(4):5–6.

27. Matheson LN. Functional capacity evaluation. In: Demeter SL, Andersson G, Smith G, eds. *Disability evaluation.* St. Louis, MO: Mosby, 1995:168–188.

28. Kraus J. The independent medical examination and the functional capacity evaluation. *Occup Med* 1997;12:525–556.

29. Hart DL, Isernhagen SJ, Matheson LN. Guidelines for functional capacity evaluation of people with medical conditions. *J Sports Phys Therapy* 1993;18:682–686.

30. Little BE. Functional capacity evaluation. *On Workers Compensation* 1996;6:138–139.

31. Matheson LN, Mooney V, Grant JE, Leggett S, Kenny K. Standardized evaluation of work capacity. *J Back Musculoskel Rehabil* 1996;6:249–264.

32. Fishbain D, Khalil T, Abdel-Moty E, et al. Physician limitations when assessing work capacity: a review. *J Back Musculoskel Rehabil* 1995;5:107–113.

33. Vasudevan SV. Role of functional capacity assessment in disability evaluation. *J Back Musculoskel Rehabil* 1996;6:265–276.

34. Simonsen JC. Validation of sincerity of effort. *J Back Musculoskel Rehabil* 1996;6:289–295.

35. Jackson A, Ross RM. Methods and limitations of assessing functional work capacity objectively. *J Back Musculoskel Rehabil* 1996;6:265–276.

36. Harten JA. Functional capacity evaluation. *Occup Med* 1998;13:209–213.

37. Velozo CA. Work evaluations: critique of the state of the art of functional assessment of work. *Am J Occup Ther* 1993;47:203–209.

38. Newton M, Thow M, Somerville D, Henderson I, Waddell G. Trunk strength testing with iso-machines, 2. Experimental evaluation of the Cybex II back testing system in normal subjects and patients with chronic low back pain. *Spine* 1993;18:812–824.

39. Hadler NM. Work incapacity from low back pain. *Clin Orthop* 1997;336:79–93.

40. Hadler NM. *Medical management of the regional musculoskeletal diseases.* Orlando, FL: Grune & Stratton, 1984.

41. Spieler EA, Barth PS, Burton JF Jr, Himmelstein JS, Rudolph L. Statement of principles that should be used to prepare the fifth edition of the American Medical Association's *Guides to the evaluation of permanent impairment.* Morgantown: WV, *JAMA,* 1998 (*in press*).

42. Lipold AG. Use of AMA *Guides* as rating tool remains controversial as changes loom. *BNAs Workers Comp Rep* 1998;9:545–546.

43. Boden L. Presumptive standards: can they improve occupational disease compensation? In: Lee JS, Rom WN, eds. *Legal and ethical dilemmas in occupational health.* Ann Arbor, MI: Ann Arbor Science, 1982:317–330.

44. Burton JF Jr. Permanent partial disability benefits: the criteria for evaluation. *Workers Comp Monitor* 1997;10:10–31.

45. Hadler N. Disabling backache in France, Switzerland, and the Netherlands: contrasting sociopolitical constraints on clinical judgment. *J Occup Med* 1989;31:823–831.

Occupational Musculoskeletal Disorders
edited by T. G. Mayer, R. J. Gatchel, and P. B. Polatin.
Lippincott Williams & Wilkins, Philadelphia © 2000.

32

Psychosocial, Psychiatric, and Socioeconomic Factors in Chronic Occupational Musculoskeletal Disorders

*A. LaVonne Wesley, †Peter Barth Polatin, and *Robert J. Gatchel

*Department of Psychiatry and †Department of Anesthesiology and
Pain Management, University of Texas Southwestern Medical School, Dallas, Texas 75235

Occupational musculoskeletal disorders (MSDs) are the leading cause of work disability in the United States. In Chapter 15 by Melhorn of this text, the specific epidemiologic data of these costly disabilities have been presented. It is of no great surprise then that there is growing pressure on health care professionals to provide the most effective methods for determining the etiology and treatment of MSDs. In turn, this pressure has led to a great deal of research assessing the key factors involved in the initial development and/or exacerbation of MSDs. Initially, research focused primarily on possible ergonomic/biomechanical mechanisms as preeminent etiologic factors. However, recently, nonmechanical variables, such as psychosocial and socioeconomic factors, have been addressed as important in better understanding this complex biopsychosocial disability phenomenon. In fact, a workshop on work-related musculoskeletal injuries, hosted by the National Academy of Sciences in Washington, DC, in August 1998, concluded that there were psychologic, social, and organizational factors that could contribute to the development of MSDs. This chapter reviews these factors.

OVERVIEW

Traditional views of occupational MSDs and their treatment focused primarily on the mechanistic aspects of injury and tissue damage (1). However, purely mechanistic explanations failed to fully explain disparities discovered between physical pathology and self-report of pain and disability evident in chronic conditions (2,3). Further, treatments focusing only on the physiologic aspects of many chronically disabling conditions have had disappointing results (4). After the relatively limited treatment success of these conservative, physiologic approaches, investigators began to explore other possible mediating factors.

The role of psychosocial, psychiatric, and socioeconomic factors in the development and maintenance of chronic occupational MSDs has gained considerable attention in recent years. A good example of this broader perspective is the growing acceptance of the *biopsychosocial model* of chronic conditions (5). The biopsychosocial model integrates the physiologic, psychologic, and social elements of one's experience resulting in a multidimensional phenomenon. The pioneering work of Melzack and Wall (6) in the development of the *gate-control theory* of pain clearly demonstrates the utility of this model. Succinctly, the theory postulates that the experience of pain is more than the result of perception of sensory input resulting from tissue damage. The pain message, originating at the site of bodily damage or disease, passes through a mechanism in the central nervous system (CNS) that acts much like a gate. This mechanism can be partially or fully opened by psychologic factors such as motivational-affective and cognitive-evaluative variables, thus regulating the intensity of nerve signals to the CNS (7). Pain perception is modulated in part by one's thoughts (e.g., focusing on the pain, nonconstructive thinking) and emotional experience (e.g., depression, anger, anxiety, stress). Hence, from the biopsychosocial perspective, it is important to examine the interplay among biologic, psychologic, and social factors that may serve to initiate and maintain a chronic condition (5). Only from this multidimensional perspective can the interdependence of all the contributing variables be observed. This chapter reviews the psychosocial/psychiatric characteristics of the individual, as well as the socioeconomic aspects of the environment, found to be significantly involved in chronic occupational MSDs.

PSYCHOLOGIC/PSYCHIATRIC FACTORS

Many individual characteristics have been investigated to gain a better understanding of why patients vary in terms of the development of chronic occupational MSDs, as well as response to treatment. Personality, psychiatric syndromes, cognitive factors, and stress have all been implicated in these processes.

Personality

Personality comprises an integration of traits resulting in unique, characteristic response patterns. Included here are such variables as coping capacity, frustration tolerance, adaptability or flexibility, capacity for interpersonal relationships, ability to function autonomously, sense of mastery and competence, and so on. Each of these variables has a direct influence on every aspect of an individual's experience from the moment of sensory input to the final behavioral response. Therefore, personality factors are likely to have a

significant impact on a patient's experience of a chronic condition, beginning with the perception and interpretation of the condition and ending with the response to its treatment. Moreover, Millon (8) indicated that there are three major characteristics of individuals with personality disorders:

- Style of perceiving and relating to challenges tends to perpetuate and/or intensify preexisting difficulties;
- Coping styles leave them vulnerable under conditions of subjective stress;
- Actual coping strategies are few in number and appear to be protected rigidly.

Thus, a personality disorder may negatively affect an individual's coping ability and may be related to chronic pain problems. An evaluation of such disorders will therefore be important in successfully treating patients with chronic occupational pain disorders.

Recognizing the importance of exploring the role of personality in both the development and maintenance of chronic occupational MSDs, investigators have searched for personality types and traits that may help explain individual differences (9–11). While investigations have yielded inconsistent results with regard to one specific personality type or disorder, several consistencies have emerged. First, the presence of a personality disorder, regardless of type, has been found to be linked to chronic occupational MSDs, with prevalence rates ranging from 18% to 59% (12–14). Personality disorders are indicative of long-standing maladaptive and inflexible behavioral patterns that do not readily respond to attempts at intervention. Thus, the presence of a personality disorder is likely to negatively impact the course of treatment of chronic conditions due to interferences such as noncompliance with treatment recommendations, negative interactions with medical personnel, and behavioral inflexibility.

Second, specific personality traits have been investigated using a number of different psychologic measures in persons with chronic occupational MSDs. The Minnesota Multiphasic Personality Inventory (MMPI) is by far the most widely used measure and appears to have gleaned the most consistent results (11,15–21). Elevations on scales 1 (hypochondriasis), 2 (depression), and 3 (hysteria) are frequently found. This pattern of elevations is known as the "neurotic triad," indicative of persons who are somatically focused. These individuals typically display several physical complaints yet have little motivation for change, and are apt to be resistant to treatment. This is especially true in another common variation known as the "conversion V," in which scales 1 and 3 are elevated, while scale 2 is 10 or more T points below. The conversion-V configuration has been found to be associated with increased disability, as defined by physical measures such as range of motion and muscle strength in patients with chronic low back pain (16).

When traits are considered in conjunction with chronic conditions, it is important to remember that many studies have evaluated patients after chronicity has set in. The stress associated with a chronic condition has a negative impact on an individual's psychologic well-being. The MMPI has been found to be sensitive to pathologic states resulting from chronic conditions (22–24). For example, Barnes et al. (22) administered the MMPI to chronic pain patients before and 6 months after successful participation in an intensive rehabilitation program that resulted in return to work for the majority of the patients. Prior to treatment, elevations on the first three scales were revealed. However, scores on the same three scales were within the normal range at the 6-month follow-up. Hence, investigators suggested that the elevations found on the first three scales of the MMPI were indicative of a response to the stress associated with a chronic condition. In other words, perhaps a temporary *state* is being measured in these patients rather than a *trait*.

In summary, there is ample evidence to indicate that personality characteristics are potentially important risk factors for the development and maintenance of chronic pain disability. Indeed, Weisberg and Keefe (25) recently noted the need for more accurate diagnoses of personality disorders in chronic

pain patients. Moreover, Gatchel and Weisberg (26) carefully delineated the important personality factors associated with chronic pain conditions.

Psychiatric Disorders

Several studies have investigated the prevalence of psychiatric syndromes in chronic occupational MSDs (27–29). Psychiatric syndromes, other than personality disorders, found to have a significantly high incidence include depression (13,30,31), anxiety (13,32), somatization (30,33), and substance abuse (13,30,33,34). The method of determining psychiatric diagnosis in these studies varied considerably and did not always adhere to structured interviews designed to coincide with diagnostic criteria as delineated on axis I of the *Diagnostic and Statistical Manual of Mental Disorders* (DSM) (35,36). Further, it was not clear whether the psychiatric disturbance preceded or followed the onset of the chronic condition. This is an extremely important question in evaluating the role of psychiatric disturbance in chronic conditions.

Polatin et al. (14) attempted to address the aforementioned limitations in a study of 200 chronic back pain patients. Using the structured clinical interview for the DSM-III-R, patients were assessed for the presence of both current and lifetime psychiatric diagnoses. After excluding somatoform pain disorder, which is perceived as controversial, 77% of patients met lifetime diagnostic criteria, and 59% met current diagnostic criteria, for a psychiatric disorder. Major depression, substance abuse, and anxiety disorders were determined to be the most frequently occurring diagnoses, and all were determined to be significantly higher in prevalence than that found in the general population. Perhaps, the most significant finding of this study was that 94% of those with a preexisting history of substance abuse and 95% of those with a previous history of anxiety disorder experienced these syndromes *before* the onset of their back pain. These findings suggest that certain psychiatric syndromes (substance abuse and anxiety disorder) appear to precede chronic back pain. Indeed, work by Asmundson et al. (37) showed that anxiety sensitivity is a key factor in the maintenance of pain disability in patients with work-related MSDs.

The picture is more complicated for major depression. Polatin et al. (14) found that 54% of patients with a lifetime history of major depression experienced symptoms of depression *before* the onset of the back pain. Depression symptoms developed in the remaining patients subsequent to the pain. Thus, while depression may leave some more vulnerable to chronic pain, for others the experience of chronic pain itself is likely to deplete resources, resulting in the development of a reactive depression. Even though there is a relationship usually found between pain and depression (38), the nature of the relationship between the two variables remains inconclusive. Depression secondary to chronic pain develops in some, but not all, patients. Other individuals show depression as the primary syndrome, of which pain is a symptom. Moreover, factors that mediate the relationship between depression and pain remain largely unknown (39). Much more has been written on the relationship between chronic pain and depression, and a fuller discussion is beyond the scope of this chapter.

Cognitive Factors

People are not passive recipients of information. Sensory input is actively screened and interpreted by attempts to match new information with a preexisting schema to make sense of the input. Hence, when an individual is confronted with a chronic condition, the experience is modified by his or her appraisals, beliefs, and expectations regarding the condition, the situation, one's ability to cope, and treatment (40,41). Several studies have identified cognitive errors or negative distortions in persons with chronic occupational MSDs (42–45). Specific cognitive errors identified by Lefebvre (42) that appear frequently include selective abstraction (focusing on negative aspects of an experience),

overgeneralizing (overapplication of an idea from one experience to all experiences), personalization (misinterpretation resulting in the assumption of personal responsibility or meaning to negative events), and catastrophizing (misinterpreting an event as catastrophic or expectation of an extremely negative result in the future). Studies have suggested a significant role for cognitive errors in differences observed in patients with regard to disability (46), depression (47,48), and perceived pain intensity (47,49). For example, a patient who believes the pain experienced during physical therapy is associated with reinjury (catastrophizing) is less likely to cooperate with treatment regimens that include such exercises. An important issue for treatment then becomes addressing the fear and educating and reassuring the patient.

The aforementioned cognitive errors are likely to result in an exacerbation of stress level for the patient, accompanied by strong physiologic response as the sympathetic nervous system is activated. In fact, studies have demonstrated how just thinking about physical discomfort can result in significant physiologic arousal, including increases in muscle tension, heart rate, and skin conductance (50–52). Patients with a preponderance of cognitive errors are likely to be vulnerable to chronic muscle tension, which is likely to maintain or exacerbate the chronic condition.

Stress

The role of stress in the development and exacerbation of chronic conditions has been well documented. Stress associated with life changes (e.g., death of a loved one, relocation to a new area, job change) has been found to have particularly deleterious effects on health (32,53–56). For example, in one study, investigators found that future rates of injury and episodes of illness could be predicted in part by high self-report ratings of stress associated with life change, both on the job and outside of work, in a group of air traffic controllers (56).

In a more recent study, Lampe et al. (54) studied chronic back pain patients whose pain had a clear organic etiology and patients with pain of unknown origin (idiopathic group). Significantly more members of the idiopathic group had at least one highly stressful event preceding the most recent episode of elevated pain. Further, these patients reported more exhaustion and difficulties in active coping than the other group.

Patients suffering with a chronic occupational MSD endure many life changes, and adaptation may be hampered by any combination of the characteristics of the individual mentioned earlier. If other significant changes occur simultaneously, there is apt to be a cumulative effect that could impede treatment progress.

The type of stress associated with "overload," occurring when the level of demand exceeds one's coping capacity, can also negatively affect health (57–60). Within the context of the work environment, excessive responsibility, lack of support, time pressures, and unrealistic expectations from self or others are all factors that contribute to overwhelming stress levels. As mentioned previously, if stress becomes chronic, the result can be overactivation of the sympathetic nervous system, muscle hyperactivity, and eventual exacerbation of the symptoms associated with the chronic occupational MSD. It should also be noted that Melzack (61) recently proposed a *neuromatrix theory* of the interaction of pain and stress. Surprisingly, there had been no formal model proposed concerning the relationship between pain and stress. Melzack's theory has great potential for better understanding the underlying biopsychosocial mechanisms associated with stress that lead to chronic pain disability syndromes.

SOCIOECONOMIC FACTORS

As the focus broadens to include investigation of all types of mediating factors in chronic occupational MSDs, the role of social factors has come to the forefront. Patients with chronic conditions live within a social milieu. Different aspects of one's social system will either reinforce or discourage disability, and can be perceived as supportive or stressful by the patient. Thus, it is of considerable importance to increase understanding of the role of social factors. Studies designed specifically for identification of social variables that significantly contribute to rates of illness and injury are on the rise in an attempt to address issues related to prevention and treatment (5,56,62). Several social factors have emerged as playing a part in the development and maintenance of chronic occupational MSDs, including familial issues, occupational issues, and socioeconomic issues.

Family

Retrospective studies attempting to examine the role of family history in the development of chronic occupational MSDs have begun to emerge. These studies have uncovered higher incidences of chronic pain, depression, psychosomatic disorders, and alcoholism in the families of patients with chronic occupational MSDs (30,63). For example, Krishnan et al. (64) found that depression, alcoholism, and chronic back pain occurred with significantly high frequency in the first-degree relatives of chronic back pain patients. Further, patients with concurrent depression were more likely to have first-degree relatives with histories of depression. Thus, genetic and social learning factors are undoubtedly at work here.

Chronic occupational MSDs result in significant stress not only for the patient but also for the patient's family (32,65). Chronic disability is frequently accompanied with financial concerns, disruptions of family routine and familial roles, decreased intimate contact between partners due to pain and/or stress, and other negative changes within the context of the family. On the other hand, perceived positive change can also accompany chronic conditions (e.g., an increased sense of family cohesion as members respond to the crisis of disability, or an increased availability of the patient to family members). It is important under these circumstances to evaluate whether the family is serving to reinforce disability and dependent behaviors (66,67). The implications for treatment are clear. Families of patients with chronic occupational MSDs must be educated on how to meet their needs in positive, healthy ways and must learn to reinforce wellness behaviors in patients if there is to be long-term treatment success.

Occupational Issues

The work environment and work-related factors have been the focus of many investigations exploring the development and maintenance of chronic occupational MSDs. These studies have identified many variables that make intuitive sense in terms of at-risk job types, such as jobs involving heavy lifting, twisting, and bending (68,69), or repetitive movements (70,71). More covert work-related variables have also been identified. For example, stability of work history (72), previous low supervisory rating (68), perception of work as repetitive and boring, and an unpleasant, noisy work environment (72) have all been shown to be significant factors in chronic occupational MSDs.

The aforementioned studies suggest that job performance and satisfaction are very important. In fact, job dissatisfaction has repeatedly been found to be a significant factor in occupational MSDs (73–76). Linton and Warg (75) found that workers who reported dissatisfaction with their job were seven times more likely to be at risk for back pain. Yet while some studies espouse the predictive potential of job dissatisfaction, Skovron et al. (77) cautioned that job dissatisfaction is better thought of as an intervening variable, for example, by playing a role in determining the patient's response to perception of back pain (e.g., missing work). This is substantiated by a recent study that found that job satisfaction appears to serve a protective function, reducing the risk that an acute episode will evolve into a chronic one by providing an incentive to return to work (78).

Finally, the availability of work after chronic disability, and employers' attitudes regarding employees' attempting to return to work after long periods of disability leave, are important work-related variables to consider as well (79). In fact, Polatin et al. (80) found that the availability of a job after treatment contributed significantly to their model designed to predict success in response to participation in a functional restoration program for chronically disabled workers. Previously injured workers may be treated suspiciously by employers and coworkers. There may be an expectation of future injury or relapse. Such expectations could result in a self-fulfilling prophesy, sabotaging recovery. However, Garcy et al. (81) found no increased rates of recurrent or new injury after return to work among individuals with chronic low back pain disability who underwent a functional restoration treatment program.

The critical role that occupational factors play in the development and maintenance of chronic occupational MSDs is clear. In terms of prevention, neglecting evaluation of these factors is likely to result in missing at-risk patients and a chance at early intervention. After the onset of a condition, exacerbation of symptoms is likely if these occupational factors are not addressed.

Socioeconomic Issues

Compensation

The exponential growth of state workers' compensation programs in the United States has been identified by some as the most dramatic event of the twentieth century in U.S. civil justice (82). Since establishment of the compensation system, many studies have been conducted to examine the relationship between disability and compensation.

Concerns regarding financial disincentives that may serve as secondary gains have been described as barriers to treatment (79). Patients receiving financial assistance subsequent to injury on the job stand to lose that assistance once they are no longer medically restricted from work. Therefore, if the assistance is equivalent or nearly equivalent to their normal income, there is little incentive to cooperate with treatment and return to work. An early study substantiated this concern (83). In this study, two groups of patients with occupational MSDs, one receiving compensation and the other not receiving any compensation, were treated in the same facility using the same methods of treatment. Improvement was measured by patient's self-report and attained level of functioning. In the group receiving compensation, only 55.8% were considered improved, compared to 88.5% of patients not receiving compensation. Other studies have also demonstrated poorer treatment response in patients on compensation (84–86).

It has been suggested that the most dramatic change in disability occurs for some compensated patients after reaching a settlement in their case, because the result of this "greenback poultice" is frequently resolution of disability (87). Burry and Gilkison (88) suggested that some compensated patients would reap therapeutic benefits from a lump sum payment of compensation. Removing the reinforcing power of ongoing compensation could allow patients to move forward with their rehabilitation.

Compensation also appears to affect the frequency of reporting injuries. Beals (89) discovered broad discrepancies between reported rates of back injury as the cause for sciatica in three nations. Frequency rates were 22% in Sweden, 59% in Great Britain, and 92% in the United States. Beals attributed this discrepancy to the compensation laws in the United States that require an injury before compensation. It is suggested that if injury is not required for compensation, the incidence of injury is likely to be reduced.

The rate of compensation also appears to affect chronic occupational MSDs. For example, investigators have found that an increase in benefits results in an increase in disability claims, as well as duration of claims (90,91).

Regional Economic Factors

Finally, it is important to examine how socioeconomic factors in the broader context can affect disability claims. Examination of regional economic factors may reveal another important variable. One study investigated the impact of per capita income, unemployment rate, and percentage of population receiving food stamps on rate of back pain–related disability claims in the state of Washington for 3 years (92). These variables were found to account for approximately one-third of the variance in the rate of claims for 2 out of 3 years. The investigators suggested that job and economic insecurity in a region contributes to the likelihood that pain will become disabling. Disability was viewed by the authors as symptomatic of distress. Greenwood (93) suggested that in economically depressed regions with high unemployment, low per capita income, and frequent use of food stamps, compensation for disability may not be perceived as negatively as in other, more economically secure regions.

CONCLUSION

There now can be no doubt that psychosocioeconomic factors play important roles in the development of pain-related disability among injured workers. Indeed, Melamed (94) reviewed studies clearly demonstrating how psychosocial and physical disorders are "intertwined in a complex way." In a study of patients with low back pain by Gatchel et al. (95), the influence of psychosocioeconomic factors in the development of chronic disability was clearly highlighted. The study prospectively evaluated a large cohort of acute low back pain patients within 6 weeks of acute back pain onset. At 1-year follow-up evaluation, it was found that the following variables (assessed during the acute period) differentiated between those who had returned to work and those who had not done so because of the now chronic nature of their low back pain:

- High self-reported pain and disability,
- Elevated scores on scale 3 (hysteria) of the MMPI,

- Female sex
- Presence of a workers' compensation/personal injury insurance claim.

There were *no* significant differences between the two groups in terms of physician-rated severity of the initial back injury or the physical demands of the job that the patient had resumed.

What implications do such results have for the prevention of chronic occupational MSDs? Clinicians who treat such patients need to be aware of the potential role played by psychosocioeconomic disability factors in the development of chronic occupational MSDs, and make efforts to deal with such factors early in the treatment process.

REFERENCES

1. Turk DC. Biopsychosocial perspective on chronic pain. In: Gatchel RJ, Turk DC, eds. *Psychological approaches to pain management: a practitioner's guide.* New York: Guilford Publications, 1996:3–32.
2. Magora A, Schwartz A. Relation between the low back pain syndrome and x-ray findings. *Scand J Rehabil Med* 1980;12:9–15.
3. Waddell G, Main CJ. Assessment of severity in low back disorders. *Spine* 1984;9:204–208.
4. Turk DC, Flor H. Etiological theories and treatments for chronic back pain. II. Psychological models and interventions. *Pain* 1984;19:209–233.
5. Turk DC, Rudy TE. Towards a comprehensive assessment of chronic pain patients. *Behav Res Ther* 1987;25:237–249.
6. Melzack R, Wall P. Pain mechanisms: a new theory. *Science* 1965;150:971–979.
7. Melzack R, Casey KL. Sensory, motivational and central control determinants of pain: a new conceptual model. In: Kenshalo D, ed. *The skin senses.* Springfield, IL: Charles C Thomas, 1968:423–443.
8. Millon T. *Disorders of personality:* DSM-III, axis II. New York: John Wiley and Sons, 1981.
9. Blumer D, Heilbronn M. Chronic pain as a variant of depressive disease: the pain-prone disorder. *J Nerv Ment Dis* 1982;170:381–406.
10. Bradley LA, Haile JM, Jaworski TM. Assessment of psychological status using interviews and self-report instruments. In: Turk DC, Melzack R, eds. *Handbook of pain assessment.* New York: Guilford Publications, 1992:193–213.
11. Love AW, Peck CL. The MMPI and psychological factors in chronic low back pain: a review. *Pain* 1987;28:1–12.
12. Dworkin RH, Caligor E. Psychiatric diagnosis and chronic pain: DSM-III-R and beyond. *J Pain Symptom Manage* 1988;3:87–98.
13. Fishbain DA, Goldberg M, Meagher BR, Steele R, Rosomoff H. Male and female chronic pain patients categorized by DSM-III psychiatric diagnostic criteria. *Pain* 1986;26:181–197.
14. Polatin PB, Kinney RK, Gatchel RJ, Lillo E, Mayer TG. Psychiatric illness and chronic low back pain. *Spine* 1993;18:66–71.
15. Costello RM, Hulsey TL, Schoenfeld LS, Ramamurthy S. P-A-I-N: a four-cluster MMPI typology for chronic pain. *Pain* 1987;30:199–209.
16. Frymoyer JW, Rosen JC, Clements J, Pope MH. Psychologic factors in low back pain disability. *Clin Orthop* 1985;195:178–184.
17. Lawlis GF, McCoy CE. Psychological evaluation: patients with chronic pain. *Orthop Clin North Am* 1983;14:527–538.
18. Leavitt F, Garron DC. Validity of a back pain classification scale for detecting psychological disturbance as measured by the MMPI. *J Clin Psychol* 1980;36:186–189.
19. McCreary C. Empirically derived MMPI profile clusters and characteristics of low back pain patients. *J Consult Clin Psychol* 1985;53:558–560.
20. Schmidt JP, Wallace RW. Factorial analysis of the MMPI profiles of low back pain patients. *J Pers Assess* 1982;46:366–369.
21. Trief PM, Elliot DJ, Stein N, Fredrickson BE. Functional vs. organic pain: a meaningful distinction? *J Clin Psychol* 1987;43:219–226.
22. Barnes D, Gatchel RJ, Mayer TG, Barnett J. Changes in MMPI profile levels of chronic low back pain patients following successful rehabilitation. *J Spinal Disord* 1990;3:353–355.
23. Hendler N. Depression caused by chronic pain. *J Clin Psychiatry* 1984;45(3):30–36.
24. Sternbach RA, Wolf SR, Murphy RW, Akeson WH. Aspects of chronic low back pain. *Psychosomatics* 1973;14:520–526.
25. Weisberg JN, Keefe FJ. Personality disorders in the chronic pain population: basic concepts, empirical findings and clinical implications. *Pain Forum* 1997;6:1–9.
26. Gatchel RJ, Weisberg JN. *Personality characteristics and pain patients: recent advances and future directions.* Washington, DC: American Psychological Association Press (*in press*).
27. Flor H, Turk DC. Etiological theories and treatments for chronic back pain. I. Somatic models and interventions. *Pain* 1984;19:105–121.
28. Katon W, Sullivan MD. Depression and chronic mental illness. *J Clin Psychiatry* 1990;51:3–11.
29. Kinney RK, Gatchel, RJ, Polatin PB, Fogarty WT, Mayer TG. Prevalence of psychopathology in acute and chronic low back pain patients. *J Occup Rehabil* 1993;3:95–103.
30. Katon W, Eagan K, Miller D. Chronic pain: lifetime psychiatric diagnoses and family history. *Am J Psychiatry* 1985;142:1156–1160.
31. Magni G, Caldieron C, Rigatti-Luchini S, Mersky H. Chronic musculoskeletal pain and depressive symptoms in the general population: an analysis of the first national nutrition examination survey data. *Pain* 1990;43:299–307.
32. Feuerstein M, Sult S, Houle M. Environmental stressors and chronic low back pain: life events, family and work environment. *Pain* 1985;22:295–307.
33. Reich J, Tupin J, Abramowitz S. Psychiatric diagnosis of

chronic pain patients. *Am J Psychiatry* 1983;140: 1495–1498.

34. Sandstrom J, Anderson G, Wallerstedt S. The role of alcohol abuse in working disability in patients with low back pain. *Scand J Rehabil Med* 1984;16:147–149.

35. American Psychiatric Association. *Diagnostic and Statistical Manual of Mental Disorders* (DSM-III-R). American Psychiatric Association, Washington, D.C., 1987.

36. American Psychiatric Association. *Diagnostic and Statistical Manual of Mental Disorders* (DSM IV). American Psychiatric Association, Washington, D.C., 1994.

37. Asmundson GJG, Frombach IK, Hadjistavropoulos HD. Anxiety sensitivity: assessing factor structure and relationship to multidimensional aspects of pain in injured workers. *J Occup Rehabil* 1998;8:223–234.

38. Romano JM, Turner JA. Chronic pain and depression: does the evidence support a relationship? *Psychol Bull* 1985;97:18–34.

39. Turk DC, Rudy TE. Toward an empirically derived taxonomy of chronic pain patients: integration of psychological assessment data. *J Consult Clin Psychol* 1988; 56:233–238.

40. Jenson MP, Turner JA, Romano JM, Karoly P. Coping with chronic pain. a critical review of the literature. *Pain* 1991;47:249–283.

41. Turk DC, Rudy TE. Cognitive factors and persistent pain: a glimpse into Pandora's box. *Cogn Ther Res* 1992;16:99 112.

42. Lefebvre MF. Cognitive distortion and cognitive errors in depressed psychiatric low back pain patients. *J Consult Clin Psychol* 1981;49:517–525.

43. Smith T, Aberger FW, Follick MJ, Ahern DL. Cognitive distortion and psychological distress in chronic low back pain. *J Consult Clin Psychol* 1986;54:573–575.

44. Smith T, Follick MJ, Ahern DL, Adams A. Cognitive distortion and disability in chronic low back pain. *Cogn Ther Res* 1986;10:201–210.

45. Smith TW, Peck JR, Milano RA, Ward JR. Helplessness and depression in rheumatoid arthritis. *Health Psychol* 1990;9:377–389.

46. Flor H, Turk DC. Chronic back pain and rheumatoid arthritis: predicting pain and disability from cognitive variables. *J Behav Med* 1988;11:251–265.

47. Gil KM, Williams DA, Keefe FJ, Beckham JC. The relationship of negative thoughts to pain and psychological distress. *Behav Ther* 1990;21:349–352.

48. Slater MA, Hall HF, Atkinson JH, Garfin SR. Pain and impairment beliefs in chronic low back pain: validation of the Pain and Impairment Relationship Scale (PAIRS). *Pain* 1991;44:51–56.

49. Keefe FJ, Williams DA. New directions in pain assessment and treatment. *Clin Psychol Rev* 1989;9:549–568.

50. Barber T, Hahn KW. Physiological and subjective responses to pain-producing stimulation under hypnotically-suggested and waking-imagined analgesia. *J Abnorm Soc Psychol* 1962;65:411–418.

51. Jamner LD, Tursky B. Syndrome-specific descriptor profiling: a psychophysiological and psychophysical approach. *Health Psychol* 1987;6:417–430.

52. Rimm DC, Litvak SB. Self-verbalizations and emotional arousal. *J Abnorm Psychol* 1969;74:181–187.

53. Holmes TH, Rahe RH. The social readjustment rating scale. *J Psychosom Res* 1967;11:213–218.

54. Lampe A, Sollner W, Krismer M, et al. The impact of stressful life events on exacerbation of chronic low-back pain. *J Psychosom Res* 1998;44:555–563.

55. Murray JB. Psychological aspects of low back pain: summary. *Psychol Rep* 1982;50:343–351.

56. Niemcryk S, Jenkins CD, Rose RM, Hurst MW. The prospective impact of psychosocial variables on rates of illness and injury in professional employees. *J Occup Med* 1987;29:645–652.

57. Arena JG, Blanchard EB. Biofeedback and relaxation therapy for chronic pain disorders. In: Gatchel RJ, Turk DC, eds. *Psychological approaches to pain management: a practitioner's handbook.* New York: Guilford Publications, 1996:179–230.

58. Friedman M, Rosenman R, Carroll V. Changes in the serum cholesterol and blood clotting time in men subjected to cyclic variation of occupational stress. *Circulation* 1958;18:852–861.

59. Grayson R. Air controllers syndrome: peptic ulcer in the air traffic controller. *Ill Med J* 1972;142:111–115.

60. Magora A. Investigation of the relationship between low back pain and occupation. *Scand J Rehabil Med* 1973; 5:191–196.

61. Melzack R. Gate-control theory: on the evolution of pain concepts. *Pain Forum* 1996;5:128–138.

62. Mechanic D. Social psychological factors affecting the presentation of bodily complaints. *N Engl J Med* 1972; 286:1132–1139.

63. Chaturvedi SK. Family morbidity in chronic pain patients. *Pain* 1987;30:159–168.

64. Krishnan KRR, France RD, Houpt JL. Chronic low back pain and depression. *Psychosomatics* 1985;26:299–304.

65. Payne B, Norfleet MA. Chronic pain and the family: a review. *Pain* 1986;26:1–22.

66. Fordyce WE. *Behavioral methods for chronic pain and illness.* St. Louis, MO: Mosby, 1976.

67. Turk D, Flor H, Rudy, T. Pain and families. I. Etiology, maintenance and psychosocial impact. *Pain* 1987;30: 3–27.

68. Bigos SJ, Spengler DM, Martin NA, et al. Back injuries in industry: a retrospective study. II. Injury factors. *Spine* 1986;11:246–251.

69. Nachemson A. The lumbar spine: an orthopaedic challenge. *Spine* 1976;1:59–71.

70. Hybbinette CH, Mannerfelt L. The carpal tunnel syndrome: a retrospective study of 400 operated patients. *Acta Orthop Scand* 1975;46:610–620.

71. Szabol RM, Madison M. Carpal tunnel syndrome. *Orthop Clin North Am* 1992;23:103–109.

72. Frymoyer J, Cats-Baril, W. Predictors of low back pain disability. *Clin Orthop* 1987;221:89–98.

73. Bigos SJ, Battie MC, Spengler DM, et al. A prospective study of work perceptions and psychosocial factors affecting the report of back injury. *Spine* 1991;16:1–6.

74. Cats-Baril WL, Frymoyer JW. Identifying patients at risk of becoming disabled because of low-back pain: the Vermont Rehabilitation Engineering Center predictive model. *Spine* 1991;16:605–607.

75. Linton SJ, Warg L. Attributions (beliefs) and job satisfaction associated with back pain in an industrial setting. *Percept Mot Skills* 1993;76:51–62.

76. Papageorggiou AC, MacFarlane GJ, Thomas E, Croft PR, Jayson MIV, Silman AJ. Psychosocial factors in the workplace—do they predict new episodes of low back

pain? Evidence from the South Manchester Back Pain Study. *Spine* 1997;22:1137–1142.

77. Skovron ML, Szpalski M, Nordin M, Melot C, Cukier D. Sociocultural factors and back pain: a population-based study in Belgian adults. *Spine* 1994;19:129–137.

78. Williams RA, Pruitt SD, Doctor JN, et al. The contribution of job satisfaction to the transition from acute to chronic low back pain. *Arch Phys Med Rehabil* 1998; 79:366–374.

79. Mayer TG, Gatchel RJ. *Functional restoration for spinal disorders: the sports medicine approach.* Philadelphia: Lea & Febiger, 1988.

80. Polatin PB, Gatchel RJ, Barnes D, Mayer H, Arens C, Mayer TG. A psychosociomedical prediction model of response to treatment by chronically disabled workers with low back pain. *Spine* 1989;14:956–961.

81. Garcy P, Mayer TG, Gatchel RJ. Recurrent or new injury outcomes after return to work in chronic disabling spinal disorders: tertiary prevention efficacy of functional restoration treatment. *Spine* 1996;21:952–959.

82. Darling-Hammond L, Kniesner TJ. *The law and economics of workers' compensation.* Santa Monica, CA: The Institute for Civil Justice, 1980.

83. Krusen EM, Ford DE. Compensation factor in low-back injuries. *JAMA* 1958;166:1128–1133.

84. Hammonds W, Brena SF, Unikel IP. Compensation for work-related injuries and rehabilitation of patients with chronic pain. *South Med J* 1978;71:664–666.

85. Block AR, Kremer E, Gaylor M. Behavioral treatment of chronic pain variables affecting efficacy. *Pain* 1980; 8:367–375.

86. White AWM. Low back pain in men receiving workmen's compensation. *Can Med Assoc J* 1966;95:50–56.

87. Polatin PB. Predictors of low back pain. In: White AH, Anderson R, eds. *Conservative care of low back pain.* Baltimore: Williams & Wilkins, 1991:265–273.

88. Burry HC, Gilkison MS. The conceptualization of low back pain as compensable accident. In: Hadler NM, ed. *Clinical concepts in regional musculoskeletal illness.* New York: Grune & Stratton, 1987:317–332.

89. Beals R. Compensation and recovery from injury. *West J Med* 1984;104:233–237.

90. Butler RJ. Wage and industry rate responses to shifting levels of workers' compensation. In: Worrall JD, ed. *Safety and the workforce: incentives and disincentives in workers' compensation.* Ithaca, NY: ILR Press, 1983: 61–78.

91. Worrall JD, Appel D. The impact of workers' compensation benefits on low back claims. In: Hadler NM, ed. *Clinical concepts in regional musculoskeletal illness.* New York: Grune & Stratton, 1987:281–297.

92. Volinn E, Lai D, McKinney S, Loeser JD. When back pain becomes disabling: regional analysis. *Pain* 1988; 33:33–39.

93. Greenwood J. Socioeconomic factors in back pain and compensation systems. In: Mayer TG, Mooney V, Gatchel RJ, eds. *Contemporary conservative care for painful spinal disorders.* Philadelphia: Lea & Febiger, 1991:155–165.

94. Melamed BG. Introduction to the special section: the neglected psychological-physical interface. *Health Psychol* 1995;14:371–373.

95. Gatchel RJ, Polatin PB, Mayer TG. The dominant role of psychosocial risk factors in the development of chronic low back pain disability. *Spine* 1995;20: 2702–2709.

Occupational Musculoskeletal Disorders
edited by T. G. Mayer, R. J. Gatchel, and P. B. Polatin.
Lippincott Williams & Wilkins, Philadelphia © 2000.

33

Psychosocial Assessment of Chronic Occupational Musculoskeletal Disorders

Dennis C. Turk and *Robert J. Gatchel

*Department of Anesthesiology, University of Washington, Seattle, Washington 98195; *Department of Psychiatry and Rehabilitation, University of Texas Southwestern Medical School, Dallas, Texas 75235*

Despite major advances in the understanding of the nervous system, the development of potent analgesic preparations, and increasingly sophisticated surgical procedures, permanent amelioration of pain for patients with chronic pain has not been achieved. The inadequacy of surgical and pharmacologic treatment regimens has frustrated physicians, as many patients continue to report pain despite the disruption or blockage of putative pain pathways. For significant numbers of patients, no physical pathology can be identified using plain radiography, computed tomography, or electromyography to validate the report of pain severity (1). Moreover, advanced imaging procedures such as magnetic resonance imaging will reveal significant structural abnormalities in a substantial minority—up to 40%—of asymptomatic individuals (2,3).

Thus, we are confronted with a strange set of circumstances: pain reported in the absence of physical pathology, and no reports of pain in the presence of objective pathology. Further confusion is added when clinicians observe that patients respond quite differently to ostensibly the same syndrome and note widely varying benefits from identical treatment interventions. Finally, the extent of physical pathology is not predictive of return to work following an injury that occurred on the job (4,5).

Perplexed by these anomalies, physicians have turned to psychologists for assistance.

Referral questions from physicians to psychologists often include the following:

- Is the patient's reported pain real (organic) or psychogenic (functional)?
- Is the patient malingering (faking)?
- Is the patient at risk for the development of chronic disability?
- Does the patient have a psychiatric problem, a particular personality style, or characteristics that motivate or magnify the report of pain, if not initiating it in the first place?
- Did the psychologic problems identified predate the injury, or are they secondary (psychologic) factors affecting physical condition?
- Will the psychologic makeup of the patient influence his or her response to treatment?
- Are there any psychosocial factors that are contraindications to treatment?

Unfortunately, there is no evidence to support the predictive power of any psychologic test or procedure for determining the responses to any of these questions with complete certainty. Rather, psychosocial evaluation may be helpful in providing probabilistic statements regarding the relative likelihood of psychologic factors affecting symptom report or treatment response.

Psychosocial evaluation can be useful in all cases in which pain causes significant disability in normal functioning or has had a significant impact on interpersonal relationships, or in which a patient exhibits signs of significant psychologic distress such as depression or anxiety. A psychosocial evaluation is also indicated when disability greatly exceeds that expected on the basis of physical findings and when patients excessively use the health care system or persist in seeking diagnostic tests or treatments when not indicated. In addition, psychosocial assessment may provide some indication of whether a patient is at risk for the development of chronic disability following an injury.

The primary goals of this chapter are to provide an introduction to the concepts and process of the psychosocial evaluation of patients with persistent chronic pain. It also addresses the important issue of how to prepare patients for a psychologic evaluation. Finally, an illustrative strategy for comprehensive assessment, including psychologic and behavioral components, is described for use with all patients with chronic pain.

ASSUMPTIONS CONCERNING REFERRALS FOR PSYCHOSOCIAL ASSESSMENT

It is important to acknowledge that there are two fundamental and implicit assumptions on which classic referral questions for psychosocial evaluations are based:

- A common assumption is that pain can be readily dichotomized based on etiology into physical (somatic) or psychologic (psychogenic) pain.
- Referring physicians commonly assume that there can be a "psychologic overlay" to physically based pain (either preceding or succeeding an injury) that amplifies patient reports.

The acknowledgment of psychosocial mediators of the pain complaint raises assumptions about individual differences (traits), secondary gains (environmental reinforcers, attention, sympathy, avoidance of undesirable activities), and conscious motivation (malingering). These assumptions are derived from a sensoriphysiologic model of pain that has been dogma in medical training during the past two centuries.

The major premise of the sensoriphysiologic model of pain is that there is an isomorphic relationship between physical pathology and sensation of pain. It is assumed that the greater the tissue pathology, the greater the pain that *should* be experienced. Consequently, removal of the source of pain will eliminate the patient's report of pain. From this perspective, psychologic factors are treated as secondary and simply amplify the report of the objective sensory information. It is only when the physical cause of the pain cannot be identified, or is viewed as excessive, that the primary care physician typically considers a psychologic evaluation.

The failure to find a one-to-one relationship between the report of pain and tissue pathology has led some to believe that the report of pain is psychogenic ("is in the patient's head"). In this case, the emphasis is on the causal mechanisms underlying the report of pain. It is important to keep in mind that chronic pain extends over many months and years. Thus, regardless of the initial cause, as pain persists, it will affect all aspects of the individual's life—psychologic, familial, social, recreational, and occupational, as well as physical. We do not believe that psychologic factors are the cause of pain in the vast majority of patients. Moreover, we believe that it is important to evaluate the person and not just the pain (6).

Evaluation of an individual with an occupational musculoskeletal disorder (MSD) includes assessment of his or her current emotional status and appraisals, attributions, expectations, and fears regarding his or her plight, treatment, and future. All people experience pain, and it would be naive to assume that individual differences in personality, current mood states, attitudes, and beliefs are irrelevant when patients seek treatment for pain. Regardless of the initial cause of nociception, a range of personality, cognitive, and affective factors can modulate the experience and report of pain.

PRIMARY PURPOSES OF PSYCHOSOCIAL AND BEHAVIORAL EVALUATION

Most occupational MSDs represent a combination of contributing components in which both physical and psychologic influences are represented. That significant psychosocial factors contributing to pain problems can be identified does not preclude the existence of physical pathology, nor do positive physical findings necessarily imply the absence of significant psychologic or behavioral contributors to pain and subsequent disability. Although psychosocial evaluation can address the usual referral questions described earlier, it is more fruitful to think of a psychosocial evaluation as providing information critical to an understanding of the patient with an occupational MSD.

Psychologic evaluation can be crucial in identifying psychosocial and behavioral factors that influence reports of the nature, severity, and persistence of pain and disability. Regardless of whether an organic basis for pain can be documented or whether psychosocial problems preceded or resulted from pain, factors such as depression, anxiety, beliefs about the etiology of pain, and social reinforcement of pain behaviors can contribute to the maintenance of suffering and dysfunction. If ignored, these psychologic factors can impede a patient's recovery and interfere with his or her response to treatment and restoration of physical and psychologic functioning.

The primary purposes of a psychosocial evaluation are to:

- Determine specific psychologic and behavioral contributors to a patient's pain behaviors, disability, and suffering;
- Determine appropriate treatment targets and intervention strategies;
- Provide pertinent information on aspects of a patient's psychosocial history and current situation that may have a bearing on the pain problem (7).

In contrast, it is inappropriate to try to use psychologic evaluations to:

- Determine whether the pain is organic ("real") or functional (psychogenic),
- Identify malingers,
- Justify physician "dumping" of difficult patients,
- Predict an individual's response to a specific treatment.

This last point is especially worth emphasizing.

Prediction of Response to Treatment

One very prevalent type of chronic MSD involves the spine. For example, each year approximately 280,000 spinal surgeries are performed in the United States (8). Although many patients achieve significant improvements following such surgery, the results are not uniformly positive. Only about one-half to two-thirds of patients reported significant reductions in pain severity, and only about 20% of these patients return to work (9). Franklin et al. (10) examined the effects of lumbar surgery for injured workers receiving disability in the state of Washington. They found that 67.7% of patients operated on for back pain reported that the pain was worse following surgery, and 55.8% of the patients indicated that the quality of their lives was no better following surgery than it was prior to surgery. Reoperation is performed in 10% to 23% of these patients (10,11). Friedlieb (12) examined the outcomes for repeat lumbar surgery for injured workers in Ontario, Canada. For 20% of these workers, the pain was worse, for 60% the pain remained the same, and for only 20% was there any improvement in the pain; moreover, none of the injured workers was cured by the second lumbar surgery.

In recent years, there has been a growing interest in identifying patients who are at risk for having a poor response to surgery for the pain. If factors could be discovered, it might be possible to reduce the number of unsuccessful surgeries and thus the accompanying expenses associated with surgery and postsurgical complications. There is a growing body of literature demonstrating that among the strongest predictors of poor response to surgery are psychosocial factors, including a patient's personality, emotional state, and social and occupational environment. However, it should be pointed out that not all individuals being considered for surgery to alleviate pain should be referred for a complete psychosocial evaluation.

Turk and Marcus (13) reviewed the available literature and suggested that health care providers should focus on three general areas to determine whether a referral for comprehensive psychologic assessment was warranted—clinical, legal, occupational, and psychologic. They recommended a set of 20 screening questions that could be used as "red flags" (Table 1). Similar sets of predictors have been suggested by several clinicians (14,15). We have observed that if at least six or more of these are answered affirmatively, this is prognostically significant, and referral for a complete psychologic evaluation is recommended.

The most frequently used assessment measure to predict response to surgery is the Minnesota Multiphasic Personality Inventory (MMPI). Several studies have reported that the MMPI was a good predictor of surgical responses, although the results are not consistent (16). However, other instruments and procedures should be used as alternatives to or in conjunction with the MMPI.

A word of caution is needed here. A psychologic evaluation can identify risk factors for poor response to surgery, although it cannot lead to a precise prediction as to how well a particular patient will respond to surgery. For example, although several studies have demonstrated a moderate statistical association between various psychologic indices on the MMPI and surgical response (17), the strength of these associations is not sufficient to warrant reliance on such techniques for making surgical decisions in individual cases. The decision for or against surgery must be made on the basis of a patient's history, physical examination, and diagnostic test findings. A psychologic evaluation may be useful in identifying patients with psychologic charac-

TABLE 1. *Presurgical screening questions*

Clinical issues
  Has the pain persisted for 3 months or longer despite appropriate interventions and in the absence of a progressive disease?
  Does the patient report nonanatomic changes in sensations or symptoms that are inconsistent with objective signs of pathology?
  Does the patient seem to have unrealistic expectations of the surgeon or the treatment being considered?
  Does the patient complain vociferously about treatments received from previous health care providers?
  Does the patient have a history of previous painful or disabling medical problems?
  Does the patient have present or past history of substance abuse?
  Does the patient display many pain behaviors such as grimacing or moving in a rigid and guarded fashion?

Legal and occupational issues
  Is litigation pending?
  Is the patient receiving or seeking disability compensation?
  Was the patient injured on the job?
  Does the patient have a job to which he or she can return?
  Does the patient have a history of frequent changing of jobs?
  Does the patient have negative attitudes toward his or her employer, supervisor, or job?

Psychological issues
  Does the patient report any major stressful life experiences just prior to the onset or exacerbation of pain?
  Does the patient demonstrate inappropriate or excessive depressed or elevated mood?
  Is their a high level of marital conflict?
  Has the patient given up many activities (social, recreational, sexual, occupational, physical) because of the pain?
  Do the patient's significant others provide positive attention to pain behaviors such as taking over chores or rubbing the patient's back?
  Is there anyone else in the patient's family who has chronic pain?
  Does the patient have no plans for increased or renewed activities if the pain is reduced?

teristics that are associated with poor response to surgery. Such patients may benefit from psychologic treatment as an adjunct to medical and surgical management (15).

Prediction of Disability

Most would agree that interference with, and thereby prevention of, the transition from acute to chronic pain following an occupational MSD would be the most cost-effective way to proceed. Several studies have attempted to identify predictors of chronicity following acute pain onset (5,18). For example, Gatchel et al. (18) analyzed data from a large cohort of patients who were prospectively tracked. At 1 year after an initial evaluation (the structured clinical interview from the *Diagnostic and Statistical Manual of Mental Disorders* (DSM) III-R, the MMPI, and the Million Visual Pain and Disability Analogue Scale) administered within 6 weeks of acute back pain onset, 504 patients were available for a structured telephone interview to assess return-to-work status and any recurrence of back pain or a new back injury. In addition, complete information about workers' compensation or personal injury insurance status was also collected at this time. Logistic regression analyses applied to these data differentiated between patients who were back at work at 1 year afterward and those who were not back at work because of the original back injury. Results revealed the importance of four variables:

- Level of self-reported pain and disability,
- Score on scale 3 (hysteria) of the MMPI,
- Female sex,
- Workers' compensation or personal injury insurance status at 1 year.

Thus, the model isolated the characteristics of patients who were more likely not to be at work at 1 year: women who had workers' compensation/personal injury insurance–related injuries and scored high on self-reported pain and disability and on scale 3 of the MMPI during the initial evaluation. These results revealed the presence of a "psychosocial disability factor" associated with injured workers in whom chronic low back pain (LBP) disability problems were likely to develop at 1 year. It should also be noted that there were no significant differences between the return-to-work and no-return-to-work groups in terms of physician-rated severity of the initial back injury or in the physical demands of the jobs that the patients resumed. Such results again highlight not only that chronic pain disability reflects the presence of some physical symptomatology, but also that psychosocial characteristics make a significant contribution to characterizing which injured workers will progress to chronic LBP disability.

There needs to be a tradeoff here, because the vast majority of individuals who experience acute pain do not progress to a chronic pain condition. However, those who do progress can be recalcitrant to treatment, consume great amounts of health care resources, and account for a large percentage of indemnity costs. Providing comprehensive psychosocial assessment for all individuals with acute pain, however, would be prohibitively expensive and excessive. What is needed is the identification of a set of predictors that could identify those at risk for progression to chronic pain conditions, but the method of acquiring the information must be reasonably inexpensive.

Once valid predictors are identified, it would be possible to intervene appropriately. This of course assumes that the factors identified as predictors are modifiable. For example, age has repeatedly been shown to predict disability and failure to return to work (5), with older age associated with lower rates of return to gainful employment among those with work-related injuries. Unfortunately, there is little intervention that can be envisioned that will alter an injured worker's age. It might be useful, however, to acknowledge the role of age in making a decision for rehabilitation, retraining, or acceptance of early retirement. Conversely, identification of maladaptive coping, low job satisfaction, and poor marital relationships as predictors might suggest some intervention strategies.

Many studies have examined a variety of different predictors of disability, including demographic factors (e.g., age, sex, marital status, educational level, family income), physical pathology, pain severity, psychologic distress (e.g., history of anxiety, current depression, personality disorders, alcohol and substance abuse, maladaptive coping, stress, somatic preoccupation), and job factors (physical job demands, job dissatisfaction, wage replacement, compensation). These have been reviewed by Turk (5). Although there are methodologic limitations in most of these studies, all of these factors appear to have some predictive power, with the exception of physical pathology.

Based on their review of the available literature, Feuerstein and Turk (unpublished) developed a screening form designed to predict chronicity (Table 2). The predictive power of

---

TABLE 2. *Feuerstein and Turk predictors of disability*

I. **Demographics**
   A. **Age** [older]
   B. **Sex** [male]
   C. **Height** [>6 ft]
   D. **Weight** [20% over appropriate body weight]
   E. **Education** [less than high school]
   F. **Smoking history** [smokes/smoked more than 2 pack/day]
II. **Injury/symptoms**
   A. Current
      1. Severity of pain during the **past week**? [higher pain, poorer prognosis]
      2. Experience of pain, numbness, or tingling in legs during the **past week**? [yes, poorer prognosis]
      3. Did pain begin (1) suddenly or (2) slowly over days, weeks or months? [sudden onset, poorer prognosis]
   B. Prior:
      1. Before current injury, did the individual experience any of the following: back pain, previous workers' compensation injury, surgery; or was surgery recommended for pain, numbness, or tingling in legs? [yes, poorer prognosis]
      2. Before the current injury, how many times hospitalized for occupational musculoskeletal disorders? [once or greater poorer prognosis; worse as number increases]
      3. Before this recent injury, does the individual report feeling sick much of the time? [yes, poor prognosis]
III. **Family**
   A. Marital status [currently married, better prognosis]
   B. Current living situation: (1) alone, (2) with spouse, (3) with spouse and children, (4) with no spouse but children, (5) other? [living with spouse or spouse and children, better prognosis]
   C. Number of years living in the relationship you indicated above? [>5 years, better prognosis]
   D. Moved in the last 6 months? [yes, poorer prognosis]
   E. If yes to D, why? (1) to improve home or job position, (2) because of social or financial problems, (3) other. [if response is (2), poorer prognosis]
IV. **Work history**
   A. Current job title? [laborer, poorer prognosis]
   B. Length of time held current job? [>6 months, better prognosis]
   C. Hours of work at weekly job: (1) part time (<20 hr/week), (2) or full time (>20 hr/week)? [fulltime work, better prognosis]
   D. Current total monthly income (include both wages and other sources of income)? [higher income, better prognosis]
   E. Was the person employed immediately prior to the current job? [no, poorer prognosis]
   F. If not employed immediately prior to current job, length of time unemployed? [longer, poorer prognosis]
   G. Number of full-time jobs held since high school? [>5, poorer prognosis]
   H. If >5, were they different kinds of work? [if increased responsibility, better prognosis]
V. **Job characteristics**
   A. Member of a union? [yes, poorer prognosis]
   B. Employed in any of the following job types: construction, agriculture, or transportation? [yes, poorer prognosis]
   C. On-the-job use of equipment that vibrates, for example, power tools? [yes, poorer prognosis]

TABLE 2. Continued.

D. Does current job require sitting for extended periods without opportunities to get up? [yes, poorer prognosis]

E. Does current job involve any of the following materials handling tasks such as lifting, pushing/pulling, lifting objects overhead, twisting while lifting? [yes, poorer prognosis]

F. Frequency of lifting objects on job each hour? [higher number, poorer prognosis]

G. Number of people working for current employer? [>50, poorer prognosis]

VI. Perceptions of work environment

A. Does the individual enjoy the job tasks? [no, poorer prognosis]

B. Does the individual believe that an unsafe workplace contributed to or caused his or her pain? [yes, poorer prognosis]

C. Does the individual feel that he or she has little to say about job tasks or how fast they need to be done? [yes, poorer prognosis]

VII. Employer practices

A. Does the individual believe that his or her employer.

1. Provides and uses procedures to monitor and encourage supervisors to assist the return of injured workers to their jobs? [no, poorer prognosis]

2. Provide light-duty assignments, modified equipment, or reduced hours of work of help injured workers return to work? [no, poorer prognosis]

3. Encourage employees to participate in problem solving and decision making as a regular part of company operations? [no, poorer prognosis]

VIII. Psychologic factors—preinjury

A. Prior to the current musculoskeletal injury, did the individual feel that he or she had many life stresses? [yes, poorer prognosis]

B. Prior to the current injury, did the individual experience physical symptoms (problems) most of the time? [yes, poorer prognosis]

C. Prior to the current musculoskeletal injury, did the individual feel 'down' (blue, depressed) most of the time? [yes, poorer prognosis]

IX. Psychologic factors—postinjury

A. Does the individual feel stressed, anxious, or irritable since his or her current musculoskeletal problem? [yes, poorer prognosis]

B. Does the individual think that he or she will be back to his or her usual work within the next month? [no, poorer prognosis]

C. Does the individual believe that the work is too heavy for him or her? [yes, poorer prognosis]

D. Does the individual believe that the work makes or would make the pain worse? [yes, poorer prognosis]

E. Do any of the individual's relatives/friends think that the condition will get worse if he or she returns to work? [yes, poorer prognosis]

X. Coping

A. Since the current musculoskeletal injury how successful does the individual feel he or she has been in coping with stressful life situations (e.g., finances, spouse conflicts, children's behavior)? [if indicates not very successful, poorer prognosis]

XI. Miscellaneous

A. Has the individual consulted an attorney regarding a workers' compensation claim [yes, poorer prognosis]

B. How cooperative does the individual's supervisor feel the injured worker is? [if uncooperative, poor prognosis]

XII. Supervisor's ratings

A. Given past performance, how confident is the supervisor that this employee will return to his or her previous job in the next month? [low confidence, poor prognosis]

B. How soon: (1) 1 month or less, (2) 1–3 months, (3) 3–6 months, (4) >6 months? [3 months or longer, poor prognosis]

C. Does the supervisor believe that the employer: [no responses to these, poorer prognosis]

1. Provides an environment that encourages return to work?

2. Provides and uses procedures to monitor and encourage supervisors to assist the return of injured workers to their jobs?

3. Provides light-duty assignments, modified equipment, or reduced hours of work to help injured workers return to work?

4. Encourages employees to participate in problem solving and decision making as a regular part of company operations?

Each of the factors/questions given in this table has been shown to be related to return to work following a work-related injury this instrument is currently being evaluated. Recently, Linton and Hallden (19) developed a similar questionnaire. The Linton-Hallden instrument has been used to develop a set of "yellow flags" for use with LBP and is currently being evaluated in New Zealand within the workers' compensation system. At this point, it is too early to conclude that these screening instruments are adequate, but they appear promising. Results from large-scale, prospective studies are required before use of either the Feuerstein-Turk or Linton-Hallden instruments can be recommended.

Identification of Goals of Treatment

Psychologic evaluation can also aid in identifying specific goals of treatment. Often, patients, their families, and health care providers focus to such an extent on alleviation of pain that other related problems go unaddressed. Goals of treatment for occupational MSD patients depend on the needs of the individual patients and might include increasing activity levels, return to gainful employment, decreasing depression and family discord, and/or enhancing stress management and muscle relaxation skills, in addition to reduction of pain intensity. The evaluation can also provide information on the extent to which patients may be receptive to rehabilitation if total elimination of pain is not reasonable, allowing potential problems in compliance to be identified and, hopefully, prevented.

Fortunately, several standardized screening approaches specifically for back pain patients have appeared in the literature (20). It is important to acknowledge that these are only screening devices, and the response to any one question or examination procedure should only be used as a red flag. As the number of these red flags increases, the appropriateness of a comprehensive psychologic evaluation is justified. At this point, it is too early to conclude that any of the available screening instruments are adequate, but they appear promising.

PATIENT PREPARATION FOR PSYCHOLOGIC REFERRAL

Before the strategies used in psychosocial evaluations of patients with occupational MSDs are reviewed, it is important to consider preparation of the patient for referral to a psychologist. Patients with persistent pain are usually not very receptive of a referral to a psychologist. Such a referral may be seen as implying that they are psychologically disturbed or, worse, that they do not have a legitimate pain problem. Many patients fear that referral for a psychosocial evaluation implies that they can no longer be helped by the health care system and are therefore being abandoned. When compensation or litigation issues are present, patients may be concerned that they are being viewed as malingerers, and thus see the referral for psychologic evaluation as an attempt to "prove" that they do not have a legitimate pain problem. Patients usually believe that psychosocial assessment is not relevant to their pain problem, particularly if they have a significant degree of conviction that there is an undiagnosed medical disorder responsible for their pain.

Patients may be particularly defensive when referral to a psychologist is raised. Their defensiveness may be expressed in the form of reticence, hostility, or an overly positive presentation with the patient trying to project an image of psychologic health by denying even minimal psychologic distress or difficulties. Even if patients express no concern, the physician making the referral should assume that it is a problem and should inform the patient as to why a psychologic evaluation is being recommended, the specific nature of the referral question, how the results will be used, and who will have access to them (21).

It is also helpful for the physician to acknowledge the devastating effects that chronic pain can have on areas of patients' lives other than medical status, such as disruption of vocational, familial, and social functioning. This can provide an additional rationale for consultation. Patients are usually willing to acknowledge that pain has caused disruption across a number of areas of functioning. Such a discussion should alleviate some of the resistance, defensiveness, and hostility that patients feel and that may undermine the psychologic evaluation.

PSYCHIATRIC DIAGNOSES

Many physicians anticipate that a psychiatric diagnosis will be assigned to patients referred for psychologic evaluation. The most frequently used psychiatric diagnoses applied to occupational MSD patients are discussed below. Differential diagnoses among several psychiatric classifications are often particularly quite difficult to make. Preoccupation with pain, with or without a diagnosed medical condition, has been included in the DSM-IV (22). To be diagnosed as having a *pain disorder*, a patient's report of pain must be either inconsistent with the anatomic distribution of the nervous system, or if it mimics a known disease entity, it cannot be adequately accounted for by organic pathology after extensive diagnostic evaluation. Even in the presence of a medical condition that may cause pain, psychologic factors may be implicated, and thus the patient may receive a psychiatric diagnosis of "pain disorder associated with *both* psychologic factors and a general medical condition" (code 307.89). A cautionary note—the criteria for a diagnosis of pain disorder assumes that the true cause of all pain syndromes is known. However, this assumption seems unwarranted because the physical basis for many pain syndromes is unclear and recent advances in diagnostic radiology have pinpointed physical bases for syndromes that were thought to be of psychologic origin before the development of such sophisticated technology.

Factitious disorders, as presented in the DSM-IV, are characterized by physical or psychologic symptoms that are *intentionally produced* or feigned. The presentation of physical symptoms may be a total fabrication, self-inflicted, exaggeration, or exacerbation of a preexisting physical condition, or any combination of these. The presence of factitious physical or psychologic symptoms can coexist with true physical or psychologic symptoms. Unlike malingering (discussed below), there are no external incentives such as economic gain, better care, or physical well-being in factitious disorders. Only rarely is a diagnosis of factitious disorder identified in patients with persistent pain.

Malingering is of particular concern to physicians and insurance companies. It is not attributable to a mental disorder, although it may be a focus of psychiatric treatment. In considering malingering, clinicians must determine whether or not the symptoms are *intentionally* exaggerated and produced in pursuit of a goal that is obviously recognizable, given the person's environmental circumstances. Patients who are malingerers are characterized by the presence of external incentives that motivate symptom reporting, such as avoiding work, obtaining financial compensation, or obtaining drugs. Although patients produce symptoms intentionally in both factitious disorders and malingering, the two are distinguished by the goal of malingering being obviously recognizable when the environmental circumstances are known. By way of contrast, in factitious disorder, there is a psychologic need to assume the sick role, as evidenced by the absence of external incentives for the behavior. That is, assuming the sick role is rewarding to the patient.

Pain disorders, according to the DSM-IV, need to be distinguished from factitious disorders and malingering in that the symptom production is not intentional. Thus, although the symptoms of pain disorders are physical, the specific pathophysiologic processes involved are not demonstrable or understandable by existing laboratory procedures, and are conceptualized most clearly by means of psychologic constructs. The classification of pain disorders can be used to describe disorders that used to be referred to as psychosomatic or psychophysiologic.

According to the final report of the Social Security Administration (23) Commission on the Evaluation of Pain, outright malingering is rarely observed in chronic pain sufferers.

Symptom magnification (i.e., overreaction to symptoms), however, is frequently observed. Again, it is important to be cautious in labeling a patient's report as symptom magnification because this assumes that reasonable estimates of pain intensity related to specific pathology are known.

Conversion disorder (or hysterical neurosis, conversion type) is characterized by an alteration or loss of physical functioning that suggests a physical disorder but apparently is instead an expression of a psychologic conflict or need. The symptoms are not intentionally produced and, after appropriate investigation, cannot be explained by any physical disorder or known pathologic mechanism.

Hypochondriasis (or hypochondriacal neurosis) is characterized by a preoccupation with the fear or belief of having a serious disease, based on the person's interpretation of physical signs or sensations as evidence of physical illness. Physical examination, however, does not support the diagnosis of any physical disorder that can account for the physical signs or sensations or for the person's unwarranted interpretation of them. Although common among psychiatric patients, conversion disorders and hypochondriasis are rarely diagnosed in persistent pain patients.

These diagnoses, with the exception of malingering, focus on psychogenic factors; that is, psychologic factors play a causal role in the report of pain. A second set of psychiatric diagnoses focuses more on the role of psychologic disorders that are *secondary to physical diagnoses.* In persistent pain sufferers, a much more common diagnosis than those noted above is *psychologic factor affecting a physical condition.* To receive this diagnosis, (a) a physical condition should be identified, and (b) a temporal relationship should exist among the environmental stimuli, the meaning ascribed to them, and the initiation or exacerbation of the physical condition. This diagnosis is not used in cases of conversion disorder or other pain disorders, since they are regarded as disturbances whose specific pathophysiologic processes are not demonstrable by existing standard laboratory procedures, and that are conceptualized by psychologic constructs only. This category can apply to any physical condition to which psychologic factors are judged to be contributory.

Although vague and diffuse reports of pain are common among patients with diverse mood disorders without any physical illness, it is also quite common for patients with persistent pain to display *dysthymia* (or depressive neurosis) secondary to an illness or injury. Dysthymia is a chronic disturbance of mood present on the majority of days for at least 2 years. In contrast with major depression, chronic symptoms in dysthymia are relatively mild. The associated symptoms of dysthymia include poor appetite or overeating, insomnia or hypersomnia, low energy or fatigue, low self-esteem, poor concentration or difficulty making decisions, and feelings of helplessness. It is particularly difficult to diagnose dysthymia in patients with persistent pain because many of the associated features are readily attributable to medication use, physical deconditioning, and physical impairments that accompany persistent pain.

A common psychiatric diagnosis associated with persistent pain is *adjustment disorder.* Adjustment disorders are characterized by a patient's ongoing maladaptive reaction to an identifiable stressor. Typically, they are determined by the identification of an impairment in occupational functioning, social activities, and social relationships. This diagnosis is used when a patient's reactions are viewed as excessive. Several specific subtypes of adjustment disorders have been identified, based on specific features of the patient's response, such as anxiety and nervousness (adjustment disorder with anxious mood), depressed mood and feelings of hopelessness (adjustment disorder with depressed mood), or physical symptoms such as headache or backache that are not directly linked with a physical disorder or condition (adjustment disorder with physical complaints). It is important to acknowledge that the use of the diagnosis of adjustment disorder is predicated on identifying a significant source or sources of stress. Psychologists must make a subjective interpretation of the excessiveness of a patient's response(s) to the stressor.

ESTABLISHING A PSYCHIATRIC DIAGNOSIS

To determine whether or not a pain patient suffers from a psychiatric condition, and to arrive at a differential psychiatric diagnosis, a psychologist will make use of semistructured interviews and standardized assessment instruments. Among the most widely used assessment questionnaires is the MMPI, a true–false personality inventory containing 566 items. It has been argued that patients with persistent pain will show one of several profiles on the MMPI (24). Perhaps, the most prevalent profile reported for chronic pain patients is the so-called "conversion V." This profile is characterized by elevations on the hypochondriasis (scale 1) and hysteria (scale 3) scales, with a significantly lower score on the depression scale (scale 2)—hence, the *V*.

Several limitations exist to using standardized psychologic testing with chronically ill populations. For example, these instruments were never developed for or standardized on medical populations, and there is some suggestion that the MMPI items on the hypochondriasis and hysteria scales are associated with physical symptoms that may be characteristics of any individual with a physical condition (25). Naliboff et al. (26) used the MMPI with LBP, chronic illnesses, and migraine, concluding that in general the differences observed could be accounted for by the individual's self-rated functional limitations, emotional disturbance, and concomitant disruption of activities. Recently, a revised MMPI (the MMPI-2) has been designed to deal with some of the problems of the original version; however, this revision is too new to permit any definitive statements regarding its validity and utility.

Psychologists also rely on interviews to assess psychologic problems that may be causing, exacerbating, or maintaining reports of pain. Depression and anxiety are routinely assessed during interviews. Assessment of depression should cover the full spectrum of vegetative, affective, and cognitive symptoms because chronic pain patients often deny or minimize mood disturbance, while admitting to other symptoms of depression and anxiety such as persistent irritability, fatigue, muscle tension, and insomnia. However, these symptoms may be produced by pain, deactivation, excessive alcohol use, or opioid or sedative-hypnotic medication use, making diagnoses of depression and anxiety disorders difficult. Standardized psychiatrically focused questionnaires may bias in the direction of over-pathologizing and inflate estimates of psychologic distress (27). If pain onset was associated with a traumatic injury, ongoing fears and avoidance of situations in which trauma occurred may be of particular importance. During interviews, the psychologist will attempt to ascertain residual posttraumatic anxiety that may be present.

In some cases, alterations in psychologic functioning result from the impact of dealing with chronic pain, disability, and associated life changes; in others, psychologic dysfunction can predate pain onset and may be exacerbated by the pain problem or hamper efforts to cope with it. Current stressors in a patient's life may contribute to increased levels of muscle tension, illness behavior, and disability, as well as use of medications as coping strategies. Legal and financial problems secondary to pain can be a source of severe stress. During interviews, the psychologist should inquire about these areas.

Reliance on psychiatric diagnoses and psychologically based questionnaires (e.g., the MMPI) provides only a limited understanding of chronic pain patients. Conventional psychopathology measures may provide useful information in selected cases and should be used on a as-needed basis rather than as standard operating procedure. As will be discussed below, a comprehensive approach to pain assessment that examines the range of relevant factors should be undertaken if one wishes to prescribe treatments matched to patient needs.

Indeed, as Gatchel (28) emphasized, no one psychiatric device can reliably be used in the assessment process. A major misapplication of psychiatric measures in the field of medicine has been the assumption that one psychologic instrument can be used as a sole conclusive, predictive, or descriptive variable. Such data should be viewed as just one source of information to be used with other types of information in helping make a probability statement concerning the prediction of some behavior. It is extremely rare to be able to make a totally accurate prediction of some behavior based on a single psychologic instrument. Multiple sources of assessment data need to be used to appropriately interpret the "convergence" of signs or symptoms of a pain and disability problem.

It is also important to note that the perspective that one holds about pain will influence the referral questions raised and the nature of the assessment procedures performed. Up to this point, the emphasis has been on the dichotomous model of pain—pain is either physical or psychologic. From this perspective, the referral for psychologic evaluation is made to identify psychologic factors as causal in lieu of sufficient physical pathology. Alternative conceptualizations of pain have been posed that lead to rather different questions; for example:

- Do affective and cognitive factors magnify reports of pain?
- Are there environmental contingencies that reward the complaints of pain?
- Do patients avoid activity because they fear injury or exacerbation of pain and report high levels of pain because they have a limited coping repertoire and feel incapable of doing anything to control the pain?

The first question is linked to Melzack and colleagues' conceptualization of gate-control theory (29,30). The second question is likely raised by those who ascribe to the operant-conditioning formulation of pain (31). And the final set is related to the cognitive-behavioral perspective proposed by Turk and colleagues (21,32). Each of these conceptual models is briefly outlined below.

Gate-control Model

Melzack and colleagues' postulation of the gate-control model of pain emphasized the importance of both the central and peripheral nervous systems in reports of pain (29,30). According to this model, affective and cognitive factors, in addition to sensory phenomena, are important in reports of pain. The McGill Pain Questionnaire (MPQ) was designed to assess each of the three components of pain postulated by the gate-control model (33). The MPQ consists of 102 adjectives used by patients to describe their pain. The words are grouped into three subsets based on whether they describe sensory, affective, or evaluative aspects of pain. The words are further subdivided into 20 lists of adjective descriptors believed to describe pain. Ten sets of adjectives are designed to measure the sensory aspect of pain, five sets are affective descriptors, one set includes cognitive adjectives, and four set are composed of miscellaneous sets of descriptors. In this way, the distinct contribution of sensory, affective, and cognitive components to a report of pain can be determined.

Although the gate-control model has made a significant contribution by expanding the perspective of pain, it tends to focus only on psychologic contributors in the reporting of pain intensity. Chronic pain, however, is a longitudinal problem, and there are a number of psychologic as well as behavioral factors that contribute to reports of pain and need to be considered. The MPQ focuses largely on the intensity of pain rather than on the pain patient (33). A quite different perspective from the gate-control model is provided by the operant-conditioning model, which focuses exclusively on behavior of pain patients, completely ignoring pain intensity.

Operant-conditioning Model

Fordyce (31) noted that pain is a totally subjective state that cannot be objectively evaluated. He proposed that the only way anyone other than the patient knows about his or her pain is by means of overt communication of pain and suffering—so called "pain behaviors." According to Fordyce, pain behaviors include the following:

- Verbal complaints of pain and suffering;
- Nonlanguage, paraverbal sounds (e.g., moans, sighs);
- Body posturing and gesturing (e.g., limping, rubbing a painful body part or area, grimacing);
- Display of functional limitations or impairments (e.g., reclining for excessive periods of time—"downtime");
- Behaviors designed to reduce pain such as use of medication and the health care system.

Because pain behaviors are overt, they are particularly susceptible to conditioning and learning influences. Such behaviors are subject to influence by consequences that follow their occurrence. Patients experiencing persistent pain have many opportunities to learn that the display of pain behavior may lead to reinforcing consequences, such as attention from a solicitous spouse, delivery of pain medication, or the opportunity to avoid unwanted responsibilities in the home, work, or treatment settings. That is, a behavior becomes more likely to occur as a result of having been reinforced by positive consequences or the removal of aversive consequences. Thus, reinforcement contingencies, such as attention for the display of moaning, would lead to maintenance and potentially increased moaning, even when the original cause of nociceptive stimulation has resolved.

Pain behaviors in acute pain patients are likely to be directly related to actual tissue damage or nociception (activation of sensory transduction in nerves that convey information about tissue damage), where they may serve important adaptive functions. However, these same behaviors may lose their adaptive functions over time and may be maintained by the environment long after resolution of any pathologic process and the termination of nociceptive stimulation. In this manner, a vicious circle of pain behaviors (initiated during the acute phase) is created and perpetuated through contingent reinforcement during the chronic phase. From this perspective, pain behaviors, and not pain *per se*, become the target of assessment and subsequent intervention.

Assessment of Operant-learning Factors

The most systematic approach to the quantification of pain behaviors is reflected in the work of Keefe and colleagues. Keefe and Block (34) developed a coding system for the observation of five pain behaviors in back pain patients—grimacing, rubbing, bracing, guarded movement, and sighing—that occur under static and dynamic movement conditions. Patients are videotaped during the performance of each of a set of activities in both positions. The frequency of pain behaviors emitted during the specified activities is aggregated for each of the five categories under both conditions to create a total pain behavior score.

In a well designed series of studies, Keefe and colleagues showed that these behaviors can be reliably observed and correlated with patients' and observers' subjective pain ratings, that they change in the course of treatment, and that they are specific for chronic back pain, when compared to the behaviors of depressed and normal control groups. Keefe and Block's (34) original pain behavior observation system has been modified and extended to assess pain in patients suffering from rheumatoid arthritis (35) and osteoarthritis (36). Keefe et al. (37) reported that the original categorical system developed by Keefe and Block can be used with observation during physical examination without the cumbersome requirements of videotaping patients.

There is evidence that the frequency of pain behaviors during physical examination of patients presenting for neurosurgical evaluation is positively correlated with the presence of organic pathology. Thus, considerable caution needs to be exercised in interpreting pain behaviors solely as a response to reinforcement contingencies (38). Moreover, a patient may believe that he or she must convince the evaluator (psychologist) that the pain is real, and thus exaggerates symptoms in the evaluator's presence. Thus, the frequency of pain behaviors observed during an interview may not be related to the presence of these behaviors in a patient's usual environment.

In addition to quantifying pain behaviors, interviews with patients and their significant others can assist in identifying the controlling factors that reinforce and perpetuate pain behaviors. During an interview, psychologists observe patients' and significant others' interactions and nonverbal behaviors to identify antecedent stimuli that are consistently associated with emission of pain behaviors (e.g., certain topics of discussion). For example, the psychologist will attend to whether pain behaviors are displayed more frequently when the spouse is present. If the significant other is present when pain behaviors occur, how does he or she respond? How do others know when the patient has increased pain, and exactly how do others respond? How does the significant other infer the presence of pain, and what does he or she do? How do others respond to wellness behaviors. That is, are behaviors incompatible with disability? The psychologist will also be attentive to the presence of inconsistencies between patient or spouse report versus interviewer observation of pain behaviors and spouse response.

During the interview, the psychologist will ask questions related to the patient's prior learning history. Did the patient have a history of long illness or family role models who had chronic illnesses? Patients are asked to list specific activities that they less often or no longer do because of pain. Both patients and spouses are asked what activities they would engage in if the patient had no pain. Patients are asked specifically to describe the frequency of performance of each activity just prior to pain onset, as well as the extent to which they enjoyed the activity. Significant others should be asked the same questions to confirm and to identify disagreements. In most cases, a patient's degree of satisfaction with his or her current lifestyle will be con-

sistent with the extent of losses or gains in pleasurable activities.

Cognitive-behavioral Model

It is important to realize that cognitive processes reciprocally determine and redefine perception and patients' reports of unremitting pain. Moreover, it is important to consider the indirect as well as the direct effects of patients' thoughts on sensory processes. Because the experience of pain, and subsequently the fear of pain, are aversive, the expectancy of the occurrence of pain is a strong motivator for the avoidance of situations or behaviors expected to produce nociception. The belief that pain signals harm serves to further reinforce avoidance of activities believed to cause pain and increase physical damage. The persistence of such avoidance will reduce physical activity and consequently the opportunities for experiencing disconfirmations. In this way, cognitive processes contribute indirectly to reductions in muscle strength, endurance, and flexibility. More directly, perceptions of stress and maladaptive thoughts may induce muscular arousal that can initiate nociceptive stimulation (39).

According to the cognitive-behavioral model, it is a patient's perspective that interacts reciprocally with emotional factors, sensory phenomena, and behavioral responses. Moreover, the patient's behavior will elicit responses from significant others that can reinforce both adaptive and maladaptive modes of thinking, feeling, and behaving. Thus, a reciprocal model is proposed that does not include the linear causation postulated by unidimensional models such as the traditional sensoriphysiologic model and the operant model. Rather, it emphasizes the interaction between the patient and his or her environment.

The specific types of cognitive experiences relevant to pain perception are thought to include focus of attention, beliefs, attributions, expectations, coping self-statements, images, and problem-solving cognitions. The cognitive-behavioral perspective suggests that behavior and emotions are influenced by interpretations of events rather than solely by characteristics of the event itself. Thus, pain interpreted as signifying ongoing tissue damage or life-threatening illness is likely to produce considerably more suffering and behavioral dysfunction than if it is viewed as being the result of a minor injury, although the amount of nociceptive input in the two cases may be equivalent.

Although the gate-control and operant-conditioning models differ in their views of pain, they may be complementary. An important contribution of such a complementary, cognitive-behavioral model is the increased attention given to the attitudes and beliefs of patients regarding their understanding of their plight, the health care system, appropriate response to disease, their own capabilities, and their responses to stress.

The cognitive-behavioral model adopts a broad perspective on pain—one that focuses on the patient and not just the symptom. That is, persistent pain, like any chronic disease, extends over time and affects all domains of a patient's life: vocational, familial, marital, social, and psychologic, as well as physical. Rather than focusing on cognitive and affective contributions to the perception of pain in a static fashion, as in the gate-control view, or exclusively on behavioral responses and environmental reinforcement contingencies, a transactional view emphasizes the ongoing reciprocal relationships among physical, cognitive, affective, and behavioral factors. Recent studies have supported the cognitive-behavioral model and demonstrated the important role of cognitive distortions, coping strategies, and self-efficacy in the experience of pain (40,41).

From the cognitive-behavioral perspective, assessment of a patient with an occupational MSD resulting in persistent pain requires a more comprehensive strategy that examines a range of psychosocial and behavioral factors, in addition to the pathophysiology, subjective report of pain, and observable pain behaviors. The report of the Social Security Administration (23) Commission on the Evaluation of

Pain acknowledged that "pain is a complex experience, embracing physical, mental, social, and behavioral processes, which compromises the quality of life of many individuals."

Assessment of Cognitive-behavioral Factors

To understand and treat pain, consideration must be given to the role of cognitions (appraisals, attributions), emotions, and behavior, as well as sensory contributions, psychopathologic states, and conscious dissimulation, in the formation of perceptions of pain as they evolve over time. From this perspective, assessment needs to focus not only on psychologic contributors to pain intensity, as suggested by use of the MPQ (33), or solely on pain behaviors (31) but also on a range of cognitive and emotional factors that can mediate the experience and report of pain.

Several psychologic constructs have received attention in the assessment of patients with persistent pain (42,43). These are reviewed below. It is important to note that psychologic evaluation from the cognitive-behavioral perspective makes use of many of the strategies described above but attempts to integrate them with a wider set of relevant factors. When conducting an interview from this broad cognitive-behavioral perspective, the psychologist will focus on the patient's and significant other's thoughts and feelings and observe specific behaviors while attempting to obtain factual information (44). Table 3 summarizes some of the areas covered in this type of interview.

It is increasingly recognized that a patient's interpretation of the meaning of pain and the extent to which pain forms a focus of attention can have profound effects on the patient's response to pain. In light of this, it is important to gather information on patients' appraisals of their pain problems and their thoughts and images of what is happening in their bodies when they experience pain; it is similarly important to explore significant others' explanatory model for the cause and implications of pain. In many cases, patients have fears based on misinformation or faulty concepts of anatomy and medicine.

TABLE 3. *Targets covered in interview*

History of the problem from the point of view of the patient
Patient's concerns about problem (e.g., degeneration, reinjury, paralysis)
How the patient thinks about his or her problem and the health care system
Cognitive and behavioral antecedents that are consistently associated with fluctuations in pain (e.g., when certain topics are discussed)
Thoughts and feelings that precede, accompany, and follow exacerbation of pain
Problems that have arisen because of pain
How the patient expresses pain
How others react to the patient's pain and disability
What effect the patient believes the problem is having on others
Activity patterns
Learning history (prior history of pain or chronic illness)
Marital relationship, including sexual functioning
Current or recent life stresses
Vocational history and goals for return to work
Job satisfaction (employers, coworkers, job conditions)
Compensation-litigation status
Benefits from having pain and disability
Patterns of alcohol and medication use
Mental status examination, including anxiety and depression
What the patient has tried to do to alleviate the pain
Inconsistencies and incongruities between patient report and behavior or between patient and significant-other reports
Patient's and significant-other's goals for treatment

TABLE 4. *Entering the patient's perspective*

What do you think is wrong with you?
Why do you think your pain started when it did?
What do you think is happening to your body?
What do you think of the explanations given to you by others you have consulted?
Do you understand the explanation(s) and find it acceptable?
Do you have any fears about your pain?
What are the main problems that your pain has caused you?
What do your family, friends, and coworkers think about your pain?
Do you have any ideas or opinions on how this type of pain is treated?
What do you hope to gain from treatment?
If your pain is not entirely relieved by the treatment, what will you do?

Thus, patients told that they have degenerative disc disease may believe that their spine is fragile and unstable and that movement will hasten the process of degeneration and disability. Patients told that they have a pinched nerve or a "slipped disc" compressing a nerve may fear that they may damage their spinal cord and become paralyzed if they increase activity. If patients interpret persistent pain as a signal of ongoing and progressive tissue damage, it is understandable that they avoid any activities that increase pain. If a spouse has such fears, he or she is likely to reinforce pain behaviors by overprotecting the patient and may even sabotage treatment aimed at increasing physical activity.

During an interview, it is important to enter the patient's perspective (Table 4). Patients' beliefs about the cause of pain, its trajectory, and what treatments will benefit them appear to have an important influence on emotional adjustment and compliance with therapeutic interventions. A habitual pattern of maladaptive thought may contribute to a sense of hopelessness, dysphoria, and unwillingness to engage in activity. The psychologist attempts to determine both a patient's and a spouse's expectations and goals for treatment. Attention focuses on the patient's reports of specific thoughts, behaviors, affect, and physiologic responses that precede, accompany, and follow target behaviors, as well as the environmental conditions and consequences associated with the response. During the interview, the psychologist attends to the temporal association of these cognitive, affective, and behavioral events; their specificity versus generality across situations, the frequency of their occurrence, and so forth elucidate the topography of the target behaviors, including the controlling variables. The psychologist seeks information that will assist in the development of potential alternative behaviors, appropriate goals for the patient, and possible reinforcers for these alternatives.

The marital relationship is particularly important, as a spouse can be a major source of support, but it can also be an impediment to rehabilitation. It is important to examine the quality of the marital relationship. What would happen to the marriage if pain was alleviated? One component of the marital relationship frequently affected by pain is sexual activity. The psychologist will examine this aspect of the marital relationship to determine whether the pain has led to any significant dysfunction.

Many occupational MSD patients referred to pain clinics have problems with excessive alcohol, opioid, or sedative-hypnotic medication use. This complicates the assessment of the pain problem for a number of reasons. One is that patients may use their pain complaints to legitimize drug and/or alcohol use. Another reason is that patients may mislabel withdrawal symptoms as an increase in pain. Chronic use of opioid, barbiturate, and anxiolytic drugs can produce dysphoria and other symptoms that mimic depression, such as decreased energy, sleep disturbance, and appetite and weight changes. It is important to examine prior history of alcohol and drug use and to identify changes in the usual pattern that have evolved since the pain onset.

The psychologist will inquire about vocational history and identify factors that might impede return to work. The patient's satisfaction with his or her job, employer, and coworkers prior to pain onset is assessed. The patient is asked directly about specific plans, if any, for return to work and about potential barriers other than pain to returning to work. A patient may fear losing the financial support, particularly if the former job is unpleasant or no longer available, if vocational options appear limited, or if the patient fears reinjury or increased pain on return to work. These concerns may serve as disincentives to improvement.

If litigation is pending, the implications of improvement in pain and disability for the suit should be explored prior to making decisions about treatment. It has been suggested that pending litigation should constitute grounds for exclusion from a rehabilitation program if the suit appears to be an important factor in the promotion of continued disability. In some studies, however, litigation has not emerged as a significant predictor of outcome. Walsh and Dumitru (45) presented an excellent overview on research concerning pain, compensation, and litigation.

In addition to interviews, psychologists have developed a number of assessment instruments designed to evaluate patients' attitudes, beliefs, and expectations about themselves, their pain,

and the health care system (42). Standardized assessment instruments have a number of advantages over semistructured and unstructured interviews. Specifically, they are easy to administer, less time-consuming for psychologists and, most important, they can be submitted to analyses that permit determination of their reliability and validity (i.e., psychometric characteristics). They should be viewed not as alternatives but as supplements to interviews, as interviews permit more detailed examination and follow-up questioning. Space does not permit a detailed examination of all relevant instruments. Several review papers have examined these instruments in more detail (28,46–48). One specific instrument and approach is described later, as it illustrates a comprehensive strategy design to integrate assessment of psychologic and behavioral factors associated with reports of pain and disability with physical pathology and medical diagnoses.

Barriers to Recovery

Before leaving this discussion of important assessment issues, we should highlight the significance of barriers to recovery that need to be recognized to formulate an effective treatment plan for chronic pain disability patients. This has been reviewed elsewhere (28). Basically, Pilowsky (49) originally formulated the concept of "abnormal illness behavior" as a useful method for understanding and treating patients with physical symptoms or complaints for which there were unequivocally diagnosed organic underpinnings. This formulation stemmed from earlier "sick role" and "illness behavior" models that focused on aspects of behavior associated with being sick—what people do when they are sick. The sick role has both advantages and disadvantages. On the one hand, sick people are stigmatized with all the attendant social awkwardness and decreased attractiveness that being sick entails. On the other hand, they are excused from their normal responsibilities and obligations. Indeed, some people may be highly motivated to seek the protection that being sick provides. This may become a potent reinforcer for not becoming "healthy."

According to Pilowsky (49), a patient has a legitimate illness when he or she fulfills the requirements of an appropriate social group for admission to the sick role (usually the medical network or physician). However, a physician may begin to evaluate illness behavior as abnormal when a discrepancy exists between a patient's complaints or symptoms and observed disease or the patient's reaction to it. Because the determination of "abnormal" illness behavior is based on the judgment of the physician, considerable authority is obviously placed in the physician's hands. Unfortunately, because a lack of definitive information often exists about the range of normal illness behaviors and what is really "normal," this judgment can be subjective. The physician then has the difficult task of unraveling barriers to recovery or disincentives for becoming healthy again.

With the help of appropriate assessment materials, the clinician will be in a better position to determine such barriers to recovery. These barriers include psychologic, physical, financial, legal, social, and work-related issues that can significantly interfere with a patient's discarding the sick role and reassuming full functioning and a productive lifestyle. Psychologically, barriers include traditional concepts such as secondary gain (e.g., chronic disability may allow the individual to avoid an unpleasant job situation), symptom magnification (an increased sensitivity and concern about physical symptoms as a means of justifying continued disability), and resistance to change. At other times, real interfering circumstances may be used as a smokescreen or excuse for suboptimal performance and failure to adhere to the treatment regimen.

Treatment staff members must also be alert to potential secondary gains of continued disability—whether legal, financial, familial, or job-related. It is important that members of the treatment team are knowledgeable of all psychosocial issues while the patient is in rehabilitation. This knowledge allows staff members not only to better understand and serve the patient but also to be more effective in problem solving when the patient is not physically progressing as expected. Indeed,

failure to progress physically generally represents psychosocial barriers to recovery, because the muscles and joints will not fail to respond if they are exercised and trained appropriately as planned (unless rare denervation or ankylosis has occurred).

These barriers-to-recovery issues must be effectively assessed and brought to the attention of the entire treatment team. Steps can then be taken to understand their origins and avoid their interference with treatment goals. These issues involve the following:

- General psychologic issues,
- Compliance or resistance issues,
- Financial disincentives,
- Somatization or symptom magnification,
- General emotional reactions: depression, anxiety, fear, anger, and entitlement.

MULTIAXIAL ASSESSMENT OF PAIN PATIENTS

Although diverse assessment instruments can be used in the evaluation of patients with persistent pain, it is important to consider how the information gathered will be used. We suggest that the most appropriate use of psychologic evaluation for patients with persistent pain is to identify significant psychologic and behavioral contributors to pain and disability and use this information to assist decision making and guide treatment planning. One strategy for accomplishing these purposes has been proposed by Turk and Rudy (50,51), and will be described for illustrative purposes.

Turk and Rudy proposed a model of pain assessment that they labeled a *multiaxial assessment of pain* (MAP). The MAP approach postulates that three axes are essential for appropriate assessment of patients with persistent pain: biomedical, psychosocial, and behavioral. From this perspective, each of these general domains must be assessed with psychometrically sound instruments and procedures. Moreover, the results of the assessment of each axis should be combined into a meaningful taxonomy or classification system that can be of assistance in treatment decision making and planning. Table 5 lists the three

TABLE 5. *Multiaxial assessment of pain patients*

Axis I: biomedical
Laboratory and other diagnostic procedures
Physical examination
Mobility, strength, and flexibility
Axis II: psychosocial
Pain severity
Affective distress
Interference of pain with domains of life (e.g., social,
vocational, marital, recreational, physical)
Axis III: behavioral
Observable communications of pain and distress
Pain-related use of the health care system
Medication usage
Activity levels
Responses of significant others

axes of the MAP approach, with examples of the constructs incorporated within each axis.

Multidimensional Pain Inventory

In an attempt to assess the chronic pain experience in a comprehensive manner, Kerns et al. (52) developed the West Haven–Yale Multidimensional Pain Inventory (MPI). This assessment instrument was designed to assess the impact of pain from the patient's perspective. The MPI operationalizes psychologic reactions to chronic pain, perceived responses of significant others, and activities interfered with because of pain. It comprises three sections and 12 scales. The MPI has demonstrated good internal consistency, test–retest reliability, and convergent and discriminant validity; it can also be computer-scored (50–52).

Using the MPI, Turk and colleagues empirically identified three subgroups of patients (50–53):

• *Dysfunctional*, characterized by high levels of pain severity, life interference, and affective distress, and lower levels of life control;
• *Interpersonally distressed*, characterized by low levels of social support;
• *Adaptive copers*, characterized by lower levels of pain, life interference, and affective distress, and higher levels of life control.

Samples of headache, back pain, and temporomandibular joint disorder patients were classified within each of these three subgroups. These data indicate that certain modal patterns, based on the numeric integration of psychologic assessment data, recur in persistent pain patients, irrespective of physical diagnosis. Moreover, these patterns were not associated with age, sex, socioeconomic status, duration of pain, or number of surgeries. These subgroups have been replicated in several studies (54–56).

The tendency has been to provide all patients with much the same intervention and to compare the treatment outcome to pretreatment measures or a no-treatment comparison group. The unfortunate result of this type of research is that although patients with certain characteristics may benefit maximally from intervention, others with different sets of characteristics may be inappropriate for intervention. Combining both groups in a single study is likely to lead to results of modest success, at best, and subsequent hand wringing about the inability of pain treatment programs to demonstrate their efficacy. Classification of patients into more homogeneous groups should permit direct assessment of the relative effectiveness of different treatments for different patient groups on relevant characteristics and not just on the specific physical diagnosis or heterogeneous groups composed of generic "chronic pain syndrome."

Turk (57) suggested that consideration might be given to a dual-diagnostic approach, in which multiple classifications could be used simultaneously. For example, biomedical assessment and treatment could be directed toward the disease classification, and other treatments could focus on a psychosocial-behavioral taxonomy, such as the MPI classification that is complementary. For example, a persistent pain patient might be classified as suffering from a herniated disk and also be classified as dysfunctional on the MAP taxonomy. A second patient might also be diagnosed with a herniated disk but be classified as interpersonally distressed on the MPI classification. Conversely, patients might have quite different medical diagnoses but have identical MPI classification. The most appropriate treatment for these groups might vary, with different complementary components of treatment addressing both the biomedical and the psychosocial-behavioral diagnoses. The MPI taxonomy should enhance understanding of chronic pain, assist in evaluation and the prescription of specific therapeutic intervention, and further the ability to predict treatment outcome.

CONCLUSION

Because of the subjectivity inherent in pain, suffering, and disability, these constructs are difficult to prove, disprove, or quantify in a totally satisfactory fashion. Response to the question "How much does it hurt?" is far from simple. The experience and report of pain are influenced by many factors, including cultural conditioning, expectations, current social contingencies, mood states, and perceptions of control, among others. Physical pathology and the resulting nociception are only one, albeit a very important, contributor to the experience of pain. It is important to acknowledge the central role of patient self-reports along with behavior in pain assessment. It is highly unlikely that we will ever be able to evaluate pain without reliance on the individual's perceptions. Over the past two decades, a range of techniques has become available to improve the assessment process and should be of assistance in making the task of assessment more manageable. The central point to keep in mind is that it is the patient who reports pain, not the pain *per se*, that is being evaluated.

Physicians are frequently confronted with patients reporting persistent pain for whom evidence of nociceptive input is either absent or insufficient to account for the extent of suffering and disability reported by the patient. In addition, they are asked to care for patients who continue to report pain after having exhausted the traditional treatment modalities. It is incumbent on primary care physicians to make use of psychosocial evaluations for chronic pain patients on a regular basis, rather than only when they cannot find an adequate

cause for the reported pain or wish to choose from among the available treatment options. Moreover, physicians should take the time to explain to patients why a psychologic evaluation is being recommended. Psychologists and physicians should take the patient's perspective when they review the results, and then discuss with the patient the recommendations that follow from the psychosocial evaluation.

This chapter described the predominant perspectives on chronic musculoskeletal pain and how these perspectives guide referral questions. The lack of evidence regarding specific predictors of disability or treatment response was noted. A set of screening questions was proposed that should alert physicians to concerns about the role of psychologic and behavioral factors in their patients, and that might serve as the basis for a more thorough psychosocial assessment. The most common psychiatric diagnoses assigned to patients with persistent pain were summarized. Finally, a range of assessment strategies that follow from the different perspectives on complaints of persistent pain were described, and a comprehensive, multiaxial approach that integrates diverse information was presented.

It was our intention that this chapter should broaden the perspective concerning the potential use of psychologic evaluation with patients who have chronic pain in general. Psychologic consultation should be viewed as an important and useful adjunct to traditional medical evaluation; when treatment options for chronic pain patients are considered, psychologic evaluation should not be thought of as a last resort only.

ACKNOWLEDGMENT

Preparation of this manuscript was supported in part by grants from the National Institute of Arthritis and Musculoskeletal and Skin Diseases (AR/AI44724) and the National Institute of Child Health and Human Development (HD33989) awarded to the first author, and grant numbers R01 DE10713,

K02 MH01107, and 2R01 MH464-2-04A2 from the National Institutes of Health awarded to the second author.

REFERENCES

1. Deyo RA. The early diagnostic evaluation of patients with low back pain. *J Gen Intern Med* 1986;1:328–38.
2. Boden SD, Davis DO, Dina TS, Patronas NJ, Wiesel SW. Abnormal magnetic resonance scans of the lumbar spine in asymptomatic subjects. *J Bone Joint Surg Am* 1990;72:403–408.
3. Jensen MC, Brant-Zawadski MN, Obuchowski N, Modic MT, Malkasian Ross JS. Magnetic resonance imaging of the lumbar spine in people with back pain. *N Engl J Med* 1994;331:69–73.
4. Bigos S, Battie M, Spangler D, et al. A prospective study of work perceptions and psychosocial factors affecting the report of back injury. *Spine* 1991;16:1–6.
5. Turk DC. Transition from acute to chronic pain: role of demographic and psychosocial factors. In: Jensen TS, Turner JA, Wiesenfeld-Hallin Z, eds. *Proceedings of the 8th world congress on pain, progress in pain research and management.* Seattle, WA: IASP Press, 1997: 185–213.
6. Turk DC. Assess the person, not just the pain. Pain Clin Update 1993;1(3):1–4.
7. Turk DC, Meichenbaum D. A cognitive-behavioral approach to pain management. In: Wall PD, Melzack R, eds. *Textbook of pain,* 2nd ed. London: Churchill Livingstone, 1989:1001–1009.
8. Taylor VM, Deyo RA, Cherkin DC, Kreuter W. Low back pain hospitalization: recent United States trends and regional variations *Spine* 1994;19:1207–1212.
9. North RB, Campbell JN, James CS, et al. Failed back surgery syndrome: 5-year follow-up in 102 patients undergoing repeated operation. *Neurosurgery* 1991;28: 685–691.
10. Franklin GW, Haug J, Heyer NJ, McKeefrey L, Picciano JF. Outcome of lumbar fusion in Washington State workers' compensation. *Spine* 1994;19:1897–1904.
11. Hoffman RM, Wheeler KJ, Deyo RA. Surgery for herniated lumbar discs: a literature synthesis. *J Gen Intern Med* 1993;8:487–496.
12. Friedlieb O. The impact of managed care on the diagnosis and treatment of low back pain: a preliminary report. *Am J Med Qual* 1994;9:24–29.
13. Turk DC, Marcus DA. Comprehensive assessment of chronic pain patients. *Semin Neurol* 1994;14:206–212.
14. Block AR. *Presurgical psychological screening in chronic pain syndromes: a guide for the behavioral health practitioner.* Mahwah, NJ: Lawrence Erlbaum, 1996.
15. Nelson DV, Kennington M, Novy DM, Squitieri P. Psychological selection criteria for implantable spinal cord stimulators. *Pain Forum* 1996;5:93–103.
16. Main CJ, Spanswick CC. Personality assessment and the Minnesota Multiphasic Personality Inventory: 50 years on: do we still need our security blanket? *Pain Forum* 1995;4:90–96.
17. Love AW, Peck CL. The MMPI and psychological factors in chronic low back pain: a review. *Pain* 1987;28: 1–12.
18. Gatchel RJ, Polatin PB, Mayer TG. The dominant role of psychosocial risk factors in the development of chronic low back pain disability. *Spine* 1995;20:2702–2709.
19. Linton SJ, Hallden K. Can we screen for problematic back pain? A screening questionnaire for predicting outcome in acute and subacute back pain. *Clin J Pain* 1998;14:209–215.
20. Turk DC, Melzack R, eds. *Handbook of pain assessment.* New York: Guilford Publications, 1992.
21. Turk DC, Salovey P. Chronic disease and illness behaviors: a cognitive-behavioral perspective. In: Nicassio P Smith TW, eds. *Illness behavior: normal and abnormal.* Washington, DC: American Psychological Association Press, 1995:245–284.
22. American Psychiatric Association. *Diagnostic and statistical manual of mental disorders,* 4th ed. Washington, DC: American Psychiatric Association Press, 1994.
23. Social Security Administration, U.S. Department of Health and Human Services. *Report of the commission on the evaluation of pain.* Washington, DC: U.S. Government Printing Office, 1987. SSA publication 64031.
24. Sternbach RA. *Pain patients: traits and treatments.* New York: Academic Press, 1974.
25. Pincus T, Callahan LF, Bradley LA, Vaughn WK, Wolfe F. Elevated MMPI scores for hypochondriasis, depression, and hysteria in patients with rheumatoid arthritis reflect disease rather than psychological status. *Arthritis Rheum* 1986;29:1456–66.
26. Naliboff BD, Cohen MJ, Yellen AN. Frequency of MMPI profile types in three chronic illness populations. *J Clin Psychol* 1983;39:843–897.
27. Turk DC, Kerns RD. Conceptual issues in the assessment of clinical pain. *Int J Psychiatry Med* 1983;13:57–68.
28. Gatchel RJ. Psychosocial assessment and disability management in the rehabilitation of painful spinal disorders. In: TG Mayer, Mooney V, Gatchel RJ, eds. *Contemporary conservative care for painful spinal disorders: concepts, diagnosis and treatment.* Philadelphia: Lea & Febiger, 1991, pp. 441–454.
29. Melzack R, Wall PD. Pain mechanisms: a new theory. *Science* 1965;50:971–979.
30. Melzack R, Casey KL. Sensory, motivational and central control determinants of pain: a new conceptual model. In: Kenshalo D, ed. *The skin senses.* Springfield, IL: Charles C Thomas 1968:423–443.
31. Fordyce WE. *Behavioral methods for chronic pain and illness.* St. Louis, MO: Mosby, 1976.
32. Turk DC, Meichenbaum D, Genest M. *Pain and behavioral medicine: a cognitive-behavioral perspective.* New York: Guilford Publications, 1983.
33. Melzack R. The McGill Pain Questionnaire: major properties and scoring methods. *Pain* 1975;1:277–299.
34. Keefe FJ, Block AR. Development of an observation method for assessing pain behavior in chronic low back pain patients. *Behav Ther* 1982;13:365–378.
35. McDaniel LK, Anderson KO, Bradley LA, et al. Development of an observation method for assessing pain behavior in rheumatoid arthritis patients. *Pain* 1986;24: 165–173.
36. Keefe FJ, Caldwell DS, Queen KT, et al. Pain coping strategies in osteoarthritis patients. J Consult Clin Psychol 1987;55:208–219.
37. Keefe FJ, Wilkins RH, Cook, WA. Direct observation of pain behavior in low back pain patients during physical examination. *Pain* 1984;20:59–67.

38. Turk DC, Flor H. Pain > pain behaviors: utility and limitations of the pain behavior construct. *Pain* 1987;31: 277–295.

39. Flor H, Turk DC, Birbaumer N. Assessment of stress-related psychophysiological responses in chronic back pain patients. *J Consult Clin Psychol* 1985;53:354–364.

40. Keefe FJ, Brantley A, Manuel G, Crisson CL. Expectancies and functional impairment in chronic low back pain. *Pain* 1988;33:323–235.

41. Reesor KA, Craig KD. Medically incongruent chronic back pain: physical limitations, suffering, and ineffective coping. *Pain* 1988;32:35–45.

42. DeGood DE, Shutty MS. Assessment of pain beliefs, coping and self-efficacy. In: Turk DC, Melzack R, eds. *Handbook of pain assessment.* New York: Guilford Publications, 1992:214–234.

43. Turk DC, Rudy TE. Assessment of cognitive factors in chronic pain: a worthwhile enterprise? *J Consult Clin Psychol* 1986;54:760–768.

44. Bradley LA, Haile JM, Jaworski TM. Assessment of psychological status using interviews and self-report instruments. In: Turk DC, Melzack R, eds. *Handbook of pain assessment.* New York: Guilford Publications, 1992:193–213.

45. Walsh RE, Dumitru D. The influence of compensation on recovery from low back pain. *Occup Med* 1988;129: 89–116.

46. Karoly P, Jensen MP. *Multimethod assessment of chronic pain.* Elmsford, NY: Pergamon Press, 1987.

47. Keefe FJ, Williams DA. New directions in pain assessment and treatment. *Clin Psychol Rev* 1989;9:549–568.

48. Kerns RD, Jacob MC. Assessment of the psychosocial context in the experience of pain. In: Turk DC, Melzack R, eds. *Handbook of pain assessment.* New York: Guilford Publications, 1992:235–256.

49. Pilowsky I. Psychodynamic aspects of the pain experience. In: Sternbach RA, ed. *The psychology of pain.* New York: Raven Press, 1978:17–25.

50. Turk DC, Rudy TE. Toward a comprehensive assessment of chronic pain. *Behav Res Ther* 1987;25:237–249.

51. Turk DC, Rudy TE. Toward an empirically derived taxonomy of chronic pain patients: integration of psychological assessment data. *J Consult Clin Psychol* 1988; 56:233–238.

52. Kerns RD, Turk DC, Rudy TE. The West Haven-Yale Multidimensional Pain Inventory (WHYMPI). *Pain* 1985;23:345–356.

53. Turk DC, Okifuji A, Sinclair JD, Starz TW. Pain, disability, and physical functioning in subgroups of fibromyalgia patients. *J Rheumatol* 1996;23:1255–1262.

54. Etscheidt MA, Steger HG, Braverman B. Multidimensional Pain Inventory profile classifications and psychopathology. *J Clin Psychol* 1995;51:29–36.

55. Jamison RN, Rudy TE, Penzien DB, Mosley TH. Cognitive-behavioral classifications of chronic pain: replication and extension of empirically derived patient profiles. *Pain* 1994;57:233–239.

56. Lousberg R, Groenman N, Schmidt A. Profile characteristics of the MPI-DLV clusters of pain patients. *J Clin Psychol* 1996;52:161–167.

57. Turk DC. Customizing treatment for chronic pain patients: who, what, and why. *Clin J Pain* 1990;6:255–270.

Occupational Musculoskeletal Disorders
edited by T. G. Mayer, R. J. Gatchel, and P. B. Polatin.
Lippincott Williams & Wilkins, Philadelphia © 2000.

34

Job Analysis, Job Matching, and Vocational Intervention

Leonard N. Matheson

*Program in Occupational Therapy, Washington University School of Medicine, St. Louis,
St. Louis, Missouri 63108*

Active medical management of the worker who experiences an occupational musculoskeletal disorder should not conclude until the person has returned to work successfully or it becomes clear that a return to work is unlikely (1,2). This conclusion can be facilitated by interdisciplinary medical treatment that has a return-to-work focus (3). Such a focus is difficult to achieve without knowledge of the broad array of work demands facing the injured worker, but such knowledge is difficult to collect on more than a rudimentary level without a structured mechanism for collecting the data on which knowledge can be based. This is the value of job analysis, a formal appraisal of the demands imposed on the worker by the tasks that constitute the job. Job analysis provides the basic data to develop information about the work that is performed in specific organizations (4). This information is used for many purposes, including the following:

- Training: To determine the levels and types of skills necessary for work performance.
- Allocation of resources: To allocate an employer's human resources through identification of the demands placed on workers and to assist employers in allocating physical and financial resources so that these resources are adequate to the work undertaken.
- Recruitment of new workers: To provide meaningful and accurate information to recruit and select workers, matching workers' resources to job demands.
- Vocational counseling: To provide information about aspects of the job that vocational counselors can use to assist their clients in developing appropriate vocational goals.
- Job restructuring: To structure jobs to make the best use of the available workforce and, similarly, to modify job demands so that adequate work performance can be demonstrated by a wider variety of workers.
- Occupational safety: To provide the basic information to identify injury risks that are a consequence of job performance so that the job can be modified, thereby managing the risk of injury.

This chapter begins with an overview of three approaches to job analysis to focus on aspects of the job analysis process that are particularly important in the treatment of occupational musculoskeletal disorders. In addition to providing a structured mechanism for data collection, job analysis can be used by the health care professional to match the injured worker's resources to a target job's demands, using the techniques of job-match analysis presented later in this chapter. The chapter concludes with two case histories in which job-match analysis was used to assist injured workers with occupational musculoskeletal disorders in returning to work, including descriptions of tool and workstation modifications that were useful.

THREE APPROACHES TO JOB ANALYSIS

For the past 50 years, the predominant system of job analysis in the world was developed by the U.S. Department of Labor (DOL). The most recent version of this system is presented in the *Revised Handbook for Analyzing Jobs* (5). The structure and content of this process are based in part on the concept of functional job analysis (FJA), devised by Fine and Getkate (6), who developed a library of task descriptors that can be used to standardize the process of job analysis and to develop occupational descriptions that are consistent across employment sites and job analysts; these descriptors are used in the narrative occupational descriptions found in the *Dictionary of Occupational Titles* (7). Selection of the sentence structure and each of the verbs in the occupational description has been based carefully on the FJA taxonomy. An example of an occupational description from the *Dictionary of Occupational Titles* is presented in Table 1.

The job analysis on which the narrative in Table 1 is based considered many similar positions within the job, measuring and recording common tasks and their attendant elements. This process has a glossary that was developed to facilitate its standardized implementation. The basic terms and concepts of job analysis used in this system are presented in hierarchical order in Table 2.

It is important to recognize the difference between *occupation*, *job*, *position*, *task*, and *element*. The *Dictionary of Occupational Titles* presents short narrative descriptions of occupations that are based on job analyses that, in turn, are based on analyses of tasks found in similar positions. The tasks themselves are measured in terms of the elements that constitute the tasks. At the elemental level, task demands are considered in terms of five categories: exertion, posture, manipulation, sensory demand, and environmental de-

TABLE 1. *Dictionary of occupational titles narrative summary for the occupation of machine operator Code 616.360-018*

Sets up and operates metal fabricating machines, such as brakes, rolls, shears, saws, and heavy-duty presses to cut, bend, straighten, and form metal plates, sheets, and structural shapes as specified by blueprints, layout, and templates

Selects, positions, and clamps dies, blades, cutters, and fixtures into machine, using rule, square, shims, template, built-in gages, and hand tools

Positions and clamps stops, guides, and turntables

Turns hand wheels to set pressure and depth of ram stroke, adjustment rolls, and speed of machine

Locates and marks bending or cutting lines and reference points onto work piece, using rule, compass, straightedge, or by tracing from templates

Positions work piece manually or by hoist against stops and guides or aligns layout marks with dies or cutting blades

Starts machine

Repositions work piece and may change dies for multiple or successive passes

Inspects work, using rule, gauges, and templates

May set up and operate sheet-metal fabricating machines only and be designated sheet-metal-fabricating machine operator (any industry)

Department of Transportation (DOT) Code 616.360-018.

TABLE 2. *Hierarchical listing of terms and concepts of job analysis*

Occupation: A group of jobs, found at more than one establishment, in which a common set of tasks are performed or are related in terms of similar objectives, methodologies, materials, products, worker actions, or worker characteristics.

Job: A group of positions within an establishment which are identical with respect to their major or significant tasks and sufficiently alike to justify their being covered by a single analysis. There may be one or many persons employed in the same job.

Position: A collection of tasks constituting the total work assignment of a single worker. There are as many positions as there are workers in the country.

Task: One or more elements and one of the distinct activities that constitute logical and necessary steps in the performance of work by the worker. A task is created whenever human effort, whether physical or mental, is exerted to accomplish a specific purpose.

Element: An element is the smallest step into which it is practical to subdivide any work activity without analyzing separate motions, movements, and mental processes involved.

mand. The elements of these categories are presented in Table 3.

The *Dictionary of Occupational Titles* has been used by rehabilitation professionals for many years, providing a means for communication of information about job demands among health care professionals treating the person who has sustained an occupational musculoskeletal disorder.

This DOL process for analyzing jobs identifies categories of information that must be collected. The broadest categories involve information about the work performed and information about the worker's characteristics. Work performed includes the following information:

• Worker functions: The ways in which the job requires the worker to perform mental, interpersonal, and physical work
• Work fields: The technologies and socio-economic objectives that describe how the work gets done in terms of the purpose of the job
• Materials, products, subject matter, and services: The content of the work in terms of the raw materials used, the products produced, the information processed, and the services provided

The DOL system also analyzes jobs in terms of the worker characteristics that are required for minimum levels of work performance. This job analysis system includes the following worker characteristics:

• General educational development: The educational level of the worker in terms of reasoning, math, and language development

• Specific vocational preparation: The minimum level of training, skill development, and knowledge acquisition for acceptable performance on the job
• Aptitudes: The capacities that underlie abilities required of the worker to facilitate development of adequate levels of ability
• Temperaments: The ability of the worker to adapt to different situations at the job and worksite
• Interests: The types of preferences the worker has for work tasks and activities
• Physical demands: The demands placed on the worker in terms of lifting, carrying, handling, sitting, standing, walking, and other physical work tasks
• Environmental conditions: The ability of the worker to tolerate various environmental demands encountered in the typical environment in which the work is performed

The DOL system defines work performed in the job in gross functional terms. It falls short of providing the degree of specificity required to match the job to persons who have occupational musculoskeletal disorders, especially with regard to the strength demands of work. The five categories of strength, supplemented with ratings of typical energy expenditure, based on metabolic equivalents (MET) of work metabolic rate over basal metabolic rate (defined as the rate of energy expenditure requiring an oxygen consumption of 3.5 mL/02/kg body weight/minute) are (8,9):

• Sedentary work: Exerting up to 10 pounds of force occasionally or a negligible amount of force frequently or constantly to lift,

TABLE 3. *Elements of DOL task demands*

Exertion	Posture	Manipulation	Senses	Environment
Lift	Climb	Reach	See	Temperature
Carry	Balance	Handle	Hear	Wetness
Push	Stoop	Finger	Speak	Humidity
Pull	Crouch	Feel		Vibration
Stand	Kneel			Fumes
Walk	Crawl			Dust
Sit				Hazards

DOL, U.S. Department of Labor.

carry, push, pull, or otherwise move objects, including the human body. Sedentary work involves sitting most of the time, but it may involve walking or standing for brief periods. Jobs are sedentary if walking and standing are required only occasionally and all other sedentary criteria are met. Typical energy expenditure is 1.5 to 2.1 METS.

- Light work: Exerting up to 20 pounds of force occasionally, up to 10 pounds of force frequently, or a negligible amount of force constantly to move objects. Physical-demand requirements are in excess of those for sedentary work. Light Work usually requires walking or standing to a significant degree; however, if the use of arm or leg controls requires exertion of forces greater than that for sedentary work and the worker sits most of the time, the job is rated for Light Work. Typical energy expenditure is 2.2 to 3.5 METS.
- Medium work: Exerting 20 to 50 pounds of force occasionally or 10 to 25 pounds of force frequently or up to 10 pounds of force constantly to move objects. Typical energy expenditure is 3.5 to 6.4 METS.
- Heavy work: Exerting 50 to 100 pounds of force occasionally, 25 to 50 pounds of force frequently, or 10 to 20 pounds of force constantly to move objects. Typical energy expenditure is 6.0 to 6.4 METS.
- Very heavy work: Exerting in excess of 100 pounds of force occasionally, in excess of 50 pounds of force frequently, or in excess of 20 pounds of force constantly to move objects. Typical energy expenditure is 6.4 to 12.0 METS.

In this system, *occasionally*, *frequently*, and *constantly* describe activities or conditions that exist up to one-third of the time, from one-third to two-thirds of the time, and for two-thirds or more of the time, respectively.

The output from the DOL job analysis system is as broad as the tasks and elements found in the several positions within the job that have been analyzed. Therefore, a breadth of generalized information is produced that has many applications; however, the generality and breadth of this information create an absence of depth and specificity. Examples of three physical demands sections of a typical job analysis report that is based on the DOL system are presented as Tables 4, 5, and 6.

It is apparent that the physical demands of the job are presented in these excerpts in a

TABLE 4. *Physical demands report section of a typical job analysis report for the job of machine operator at XYZ lighting corporation*

	Strength and endurance position demand		
Position	Max minutes at 1 time	Total hours per day	Total % of workday
Sitting	0 min	0 h	0
Standing	150 min	7.0 h	88
Walking	10 min	0.5 h	6
Carrying	5 min	0.5 h	6
	Weight and force demand		
Task	None	Occasionally	Frequently
Lift: sheet stock		36 lb	9 lb
Carry: parts		36 lb	
Push: NA			
Pull: handles			3

Narrative description of strength demands: Reaches to raised pallet and retrieves sheet metal stock, lifts one piece to place in machine for cutting, bending, and stamping, depending on assignment. Retrieves machined part from machine and places on rack within arm's reach. May occasionally carry two machined parts in each hand short distance (15 to 50 ft) to place in rack at another machining station. Frequently pulls handles and levers on machine to actuate.

TABLE 5. *Physical demands characteristics level from a typical job analysis report for the job of machine operator at XYZ lighting corporation*

		Strength rating: Light		
Physical demand level	Occasional 0.33% of the workday	Frequent 34–66% of the workday	Constant 67–100% of the workday	Typical energy required
Sedentary	10 lbs	Negligible	Negligible	1.5–2.1 METS
Light	20 lbs	10 lbs and/or walk/stand/push/pull of arm/leg control	Negligible and/or push/pull of arm/leg control while seated	2.2–3.5 METS
Medium	20–50 lbs	10 to 25 lbs	10 lbs	3.6–6.3 METS
Heavy	50–100 lbs	25 to 50 lbs	10–20 lbs	6.4–7.5 METS
Very heavy	>100 lbs	>50 lbs	>20 lbs	>7.5 METS

manner that is not sufficiently precise to allow the health care professional to match an injured worker to the job. It would be difficult to use this information to identify mismatches between the injured worker's resources and the job demands on more than a rudimentary level.

One additional problem with the DOL job analysis system is that it is no longer supported by the U.S. DOL and is destined to be replaced (10–12). The O*NET system has been under development by the DOL for several years and eventually will replace the job analysis system on which the *Dictionary of Occupational Titles* is based. O*NET includes approximately 220 occupational-demand constructs, which are used to characterize approximately 1,100 occupations. The breadth of occupational demands extends far beyond those that normally must be considered with occupational musculoskeletal disorders.

Because the O*NET taxonomy is intended to focus on a full array of occupational demands without regard to impairment, it presents an excellent means to describe occupational demands. Use of O*NET, however, will require that linkages and crosswalks be made from the occupational-demand constructs to functional limitations that are a consequence

TABLE 6. *Physical demands ratings summary of a typical job analysis report for the job of machine operator at XYZ lighting corporation*

Demand	None	Occasional	Frequently
Climbing	X		
Balancing	X		
Stooping		X	
Kneeling	X		
Crouching		X	
Crawling	X		
Reaching			X
Handling			X
Fingering			X
Feeling	X		
Talking	X		
Hearing	X		
Tasting/smelling	X		
Near acuity	X		
Far acuity	X		
Depth perception	X		
Accommodation	X		
Color vision	X		
Field of vision	X		

of medical impairments. Thus, narrower focus will be required because the usual functional consequences of occupational musculoskeletal disorders are much more proscribed than the profiles of occupations in O*NET. An example of an item that might be developed to provide such a crosswalk is presented in Fig. 1.

Figure 1 is not currently an O*NET item; however, it is designed with similar characteristics, based on the model developed by Fleishman et al. (13–15). This model includes the seven-point rating scale that is used by all of the O*NET occupational-demand constructs. It also includes anchors at each end and behavioral descriptors positioned along the scale to provide calibration. It differs from the O*NET items in that it focuses on a particular component of performance: hand strength. Such a component is useful for health care professionals and could become part of a crosswalk from the O*NET occupational demands to impaired workers' resources.

Neither the DOL job analysis system nor the O*NET system were designed with the injured worker in mind. One method to measure job demands in light of the injured worker's abilities was the GULHEMP scale, developed soon after World War II by Leon Koyl, Med-

ical Director at deHavilland Aircraft Corporation in Canada (16). GULHEMP is an acronym:

G General physique
U Upper extremities
L Lower extremities
H Hearing
E Eyesight
M Mentality
P Personality

The original purpose of the GULHEMP scale was to match older workers and workers returning from medical leave to jobs according to their residual functional abilities. The scale allowed a convenient and general summary of the match between the worker's functional abilities and the job's demands. The GULHEMP system comprises the seven divisions represented by the acronym. Each division represents a functional area that is graded into seven levels of fitness, from completely competent (level 1) to completely incompetent (level 7). Application of the GULHEMP system requires assignment of the injured worker to one or another of the ordinal scale levels within each functional area. Examples of three of the divisions are presented in Table 7.

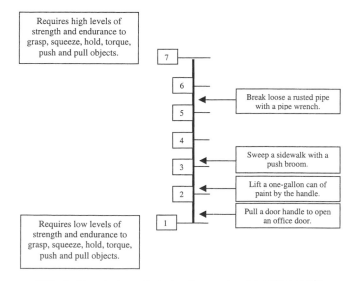

FIG. 1. Hand-strength behavior anchored rating scale.

TABLE 7. *Three GULHEMP measurement scales*

General physique
  G1 Fit for heavy manual work including digging, lifting, climbing regularly as main occupation
  G2 Fit for normal work including incidental or occasional heavy work as in G1. Can work changing shifts
  G3 Fit for all employment except-heavy labor, liable to deteriorate if meals are irregular, or if rest inadequate as with frequent shift changes
  G4 Fit for sedentary employment with regular hours and meals
  G5 Fit for restricted employment or part-time employment. The "handicapped worker" in home or out
  G6 Fit for self-care only
  G7 Bedfast; unable to care for self

Upper extremities
  U1 Fit to lift strongly to and above shoulder level, to dig, push or drag strongly as a main occupation, e.g., can drive heavy vehicle such as earth moving vehicles
  U2 Fit to lift strongly to and above shoulder, to dig, push or drag strongly; fit for manual work; fit for heavy work as in U1 incidentally or occasionally
  U3 Fit for moderately heavy lifting and loading, e.g., can drive light trucks and automobiles
  U4 Unilateral disability allowing efficient sedentary or clerical work or light labor
  U5 Bilateral disability or a complete unilateral disability allowing only a few gross or relatively ineffective movements and permitting restricted or part-time employment
  U6 Can give partial self-care. May be able to feed self
  U7 Unable to help self

Lower extremities
  L1 Able to run, climb, jump, dig and push with sustained effort as a main occupation, e.g., can drive heavy tractors and earth moving machinery
  L2 Fit for heavy labor. Able to stand, run, climb jump, push as in L1 incidentally or occasionally
  L3 Fit for moderately heavy labor including pushing and digging. Liable to tire if too long on feet, e.g., can drive light vehicles
  L4 Severe unilateral disability or lesser bilateral disability allowing efficient sedentary work or light labor
  L5 Bilateral or severe unilateral disability allowing a few relatively ineffective movements and permitting restricted employment; fit for sedentary work only
  L6 Unable to accept employment because of severity of disability
  L7 Bedfast

The GULHEMP system may be used to assess the worker's capacity in these seven divisions. The job analyst uses the same scale to evaluate the job's functional demand characteristics. Used in this way, a comparison between the worker's capacities and the job's demands can be accomplished easily. Although GULHEMP is attractive because of its simplicity, it is not sufficiently comprehensive to be useful in the process of assisting injured workers with occupational musculoskeletal disorders to return to work; it is too simple.

A HEALTH CARE ALTERNATIVE

Although the DOL job analysis system continues to be useful for introducing health care professionals to basic job analysis procedures, and the O*NET holds promise for the future, the Job Match Analysis system (17) presented in the following section is more suited to health care applications. It combines aspects of the DOL system and the GULHEMP system to facilitate standardized collection of job-task data in a manner that can be used by health care professionals to assist persons with occupational musculoskeletal disorders to return to work.

The process involved in job-match analysis considers only certain aspects of the demands of a specific job, because the intention is to facilitate the match between the residual functional capacity of a person with an occupational medical disorder and the demands of the job. The job-match analysis presented in this chapter focuses on job demands that are closely linked to occupational *musculoskeletal* disorders, namely those involving exertion (including strength), posture, and manipulation. Excluded are functional elements of work found in the DOL system, such as sensory and environmental demands, because these elements are likely to be less important in the case management of an injured worker who has an occupational musculoskeletal disorder. For example, a different job-match analysis model would be used with a population of persons who have occupational medical disorders as a result of traumatic brain injury.

NEED FOR JOB-MATCH ANALYSIS

Occupational musculoskeletal disorders and the impairments and disabilities to which they contribute often are due to a mismatch between the worker's resources and the demands of the job. Injured workers who do not return to their usual and customary jobs often fail to return to work because of such a mismatch. In terms of job demands, this mismatch can be in the force required for task performance, the frequency and duration of task performance, the physical environment within which the task is performed, or combinations of all three. In terms of worker resources, the mismatch can be in the strength, endurance, abilities, or skill required for task performance, the worker's value and interest in the job, the interpersonal environment within which the job is performed, or combinations of all three.

The process for determining the match between job demands and worker resources is *job-match analysis*. Based on information about the person's functional limitations that is collected in a functional-capacity evaluation and information about the job's demands that is collected in a compatible job analysis, the job-match analysis links the person with an occupational musculoskeletal disorder to the job in a manner that is designed to facilitate successful return to work. This chapter presents the process and techniques of job match analysis with a focus on occupational musculoskeletal disorders.

To Avoid Disability

Impairment that is precipitated by an occupational musculoskeletal disorder rarely results in chronic disability. If an early return to work is not effected, the incidence of chronic

disability rapidly increases. A return to work before healing has been completed often requires job matching to provide tool or workstation modifications or temporary light duty assignments. Without such accommodations, the impairment is more likely to become disabling. The following global causes of disability subsequent to an impairment precipitated by an occupational musculoskeletal disorder can be effectively avoided with job-match analysis:

1. Continuous trauma occupational musculoskeletal disorder gradually decreases residual functional capacity as the impairment is aggravated by the cumulative effect of job tasks that challenge the worker's functional capacity. The result is an accelerating mismatch between the worker's functional capability and the job's demands, which potentiates the impairment. Job-match analysis can be used to structure the job's demands so that they are within the injured worker's capacity.

2. Impairment worsens because of gradual physical deconditioning through inactivity; this inactivity results from the symptomatic response to activity as a consequence of a painful occupational musculoskeletal disorder. Assignment to light duty or rest may worsen the physical competence of the worker to withstand the rigors of the usual and customary job. Job-match analysis can be used to structure the job's demands so that they are less likely to exacerbate the injured worker's symptoms.

3. Functional limitations increase because of inappropriate adaptation. For example, impairment in one hand may lead to overuse of the other, which may cause new impairment; or impairment in one knee leads to a lower back cumulative trauma disorder. The secondary impairments occur because the accommodation of the worker is inappropriate. Job-match analysis can be used to assist the injured worker in effectively integrating the job's demands and appropriately adapting so that secondary impairment is avoided.

4. Functional limitations increase because of discouragement, loss of hope, sense of mis-

trust, and feelings of helplessness. Minor injuries for some workers who do not adapt well psychologically will lead to occupational musculoskeletal disability. Job-match analysis can be used to assist the injured worker to maintain occupational competence despite decreased functional capacity.

5. The interpersonal attention and interaction inherent in treatment of the impairment reinforce reports and displays of symptoms, which brings more attention, which further reinforces the injured worker's reports and displays of symptoms. Thus, an increasing spiral of symptoms occurs that itself becomes disabling. Job-match analysis presents an alternative approach to treatment that is work outcome oriented and designed to maintain a focus on preserving the injured worker's earning capacity.

The cost and delay in return to work after a severe occupational musculoskeletal disorder are closely related to job matching. Occupational musculoskeletal disorders that result in severe chronic impairment almost always require job-match analysis as a component of vocational intervention. This intervention can range from a return to the patient's usual and customary employment to vocational retraining to enter a new occupation, predicated on the appropriate matching of the biomechanical demands of the work to the musculoskeletal capacity of the worker. The more aggressive and skilled the job-match program, the more likely an early and inexpensive return to work will occur.

Aging Workforce

Another problem that can be addressed with job-match analysis is the interaction of age with an occupational musculoskeletal disorder, which can worsen the job-to-worker mismatch. Residual functional capacity decreases with age at different rates, depending on the body system and the individual (18–25). Occupational musculoskeletal injury can be worsened by the normal decremental effects of aging (26,27). Such injuries often produce decrements in functional capacity that potentiate and accelerate the normal changes that are found as workers age through middle adulthood to older adulthood. Although the general diminution in physically demanding work in the United States and Canada has somewhat attenuated this problem, this attenuation may be offset by more recent increases in the age of retirement. As the active workforce of the United States and Canada ages, it becomes increasingly likely that the aging workers' residual functional capacity will be inadequate to the jobs' demands. Job tasks themselves do not provide adequate opportunity to maintain adequate physical condition. In recent decades, the prevalence of occupational disability in American society has escalated among older workers. Only 26% of the American workforce is 45 years of age or older, but these workers experience 71% of the disabilities that last 5 months or longer (28). Approximately 59% of the workers in the disability support system are in the 55- to 64-year-old cohort, the age when the incidence of cumulative trauma disorder leading to chronic disability peaks (29). Job-match analysis is an effective approach to prevention of occupational musculoskeletal disorders among older workers who elect to remain in the workforce and to provide accommodations that will allow them to postpone retirement.

Risk Identification

The identification of job demands that increase the risk of injury is a useful component of job-match analysis, whether or not accommodation of the injured worker to the job is required. After an occupational musculoskeletal disorder has occurred and before the patient returns to work, it is useful to analyze the job's demands to identify the job-based risk factors that may have precipitated the original injury or that may increase the likelihood of reinjury. The job-match analysis procedures described in this chapter are intended to be used by health care professionals to analyze job demands in terms of the degree to which job tasks stress the musculoskeletal system. The human is considered as a system of levers, pulleys, and linkages through which force is channeled to move in three-dimensional space. The object of the movement is to perform work of a type and work levels of productivity that are acceptable to an employer. Although a biomechanical approach is somewhat simplistic, it can effectively identify risk factors for occupational musculoskeletal disorder to facilitate a return to work and minimize the likelihood of reinjury.

Process

The intent of the job-match analysis is to develop a good fit between the individual with an occupational musculoskeletal injury and a target job, with a focus on the interface between the biomechanical demands of the job and the musculoskeletal capacity of the worker. The job-match analysis guides the clinician in gathering information about the demands of the injured worker's job in such a way that the data about the demands of the job will complement information gathered in a subsequent functional-capacity evaluation, which is described in a subsequent chapter of this book (Chap. 40, Vocational Assessment and Retraining). Whereas the measurement of each musculoskeletal component in the functional-capacity evaluation is standardized to ensure safety, reliability, and validity, the aggregation of components in the evaluation is customized, based on information from the job-match analysis.

The process involved in job-match analysis comprises collection and recording of information about the physical demands of the job in terms of the demands on the worker for endurance, strength, and psychomotor ability. Data are recorded on the job-match analysis worksheet (Fig. 2). On the worksheet, basic information about the job and the employer is recorded. If possible, the code or the job is identified according to the *Dictionary of Occupational Titles*. The balance of the worksheet is completed at the job site through ob-

servation, measurement, and interviews with incumbent workers and supervisors. Tools and materials that usually are necessary include safety glasses, a hard hat, sturdy work shoes, a clipboard that holds the worksheet, a pencil, a 30-foot steel-rule tape measure, 20 feet of 1/4-inch woven nylon rope, and force-measuring devices, such as hand-held spring scales or hydraulic scales with up to 100 pounds of capacity and a floor scale with up to 200 pounds of capacity. A still camera and a video camera are both useful but not necessary. Photography is not accepted at many worksites and should be undertaken only with care and deliberation. The job match analysis procedure is begun by interviewing the incumbent worker and supervisor. It is important to develop an understanding of the workflow, developing a workflow diagram, as described in Fig. 3. This diagram need not be formal; a simple pencil drawing will suffice.

Referring to the workflow diagram, the most frequently encountered job tasks should be identified. The interview should focus on the process of the work from beginning to end, breaking each process into its component tasks and each task into its most significantly demanding elements. The worksheet allows recording of eight work tasks. It is likely that two or more worksheets will be required to record all of the significant job tasks. The selection of tasks and elements to record on the worksheet is determined by the complexity of the job. It is unusual for a job to have fewer than six or more than 30 pertinent tasks. Examples of jobs with few pertinent tasks include many machine-operation and equipment-control jobs. Jobs that have many more pertinent tasks include those in the skilled construction trades and most public safety occupations.

The identification of pertinent job tasks also can be influenced by knowledge of the musculoskeletal impairment of the worker. For example, a job-match analysis for an injured worker with an upper- extremity impairment would lead to a different focus than would the job-match analysis for an injured worker with a low back injury. The job tasks

Address: _____

City: _____

Phone: _____ Contact Person: _____

Worksite Visit Date: _____ D.O.T. Code Number: _____

Hours Per Day: _____ Days Per Week: _____

Overtime Hours per Week: _____ Scheduled Breaks: _____

Wage Structure: _____ Union Affiliation: _____

Vocational Preparation Requirements: _____

_____ _____ _____ _____

_____ _____ _____ _____

Brief Task Description

Task 1: _____

Task 2: _____

Task 3: _____

Task 4: _____

Task 5: _____

Task 6: _____

Task 7: _____

Task 8: _____

FIG. 2. Job match analysis worksheet.

that are more demanding on the musculoskeletal segments that have been impaired are those on which the job-match analysis should focus.

After the job tasks are listed on the worksheet, including brief descriptive statements, the duration of each job task is estimated, based on the number of hours per workshift that the worker is normally required to participate in each job task, performing each listed demand. This is specified to the one-tenth hour and is listed on the worksheet in that manner. After the duration of each job task is

recorded, the Psychomotor Ability Demands and Ergonomic Risk Demands are recorded. These ratings are based on the ordinal scale presented in Table 8.

Although risk factors such as those listed on the worksheet for both the upper extremities and spine are generally accepted as being significant, the presence of a risk factor does not necessarily mean that the particular individual performing the job task is at risk for injury. If fact, acceptable exposure levels to these risk factors have not yet been identified. These variables have been identified as risk

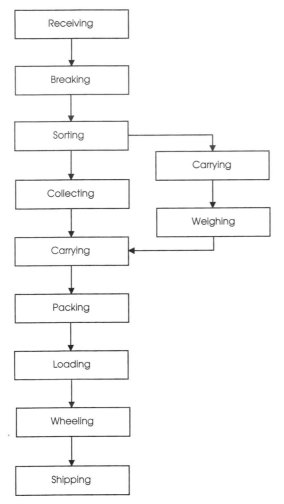

FIG. 3. Workflow diagram.

factors because they appear more frequently than would be expected in the postmortem of job tasks that have appeared to precipitate occupational musculoskeletal disorders.

Because of the central importance of lifting and lowering in occupational musculoskeletal

TABLE 8. *Psychomotor demands ranking scale*

Rating	Description
5	Constant, >90% of the task duration.
4	Frequent, 50% to 90% of the task duration.
3	Occasional, 10% to 49% of the task duration.
2	Rarely, <10% of the task duration.
1	Never

disorders, the job-match analysis includes a focus on these tasks. For occupational musculoskeletal disorders, lifting risk analysis is a necessary component of job-match analysis. Lifting risk analysis (LRA) is a process of identifying, depicting, and quantifying the relative risks in lifting and lowering elements of the job tasks. The LRA describes lifting in terms of range of motion under load (30) in graphic form. It provides sufficient specificity about the lifting and lowering demands of a job to compare job demands to the injured worker's functional limitations. The form for the lifting risk analysis is part of the job-match analysis form set. On the form, the following information is recorded:

• Object: The name of object being lifted or lowered.
• Load: The weight of the object being lifted or lowered.
• Horizontal displacement: The distance (in inches) between the center of the hands grasping the object to the center of the spine at the sacrum, measured horizontally. The center of the spine at the sacrum is directly above the midpoint between the lateral malleoli.
• Begin: The height (in inches) from the floor to the handholds at the start of the lift or lower.
• End: The height (in inches) from the floor to the handholds at the end of the lift or lower.
• Vertical displacement: The distance (in inches) that the hands travel from the start to the end of the lift or lower.
• Asymmetry: The number of degrees of angular rotation from the beginning to the end of the lift or lower.
• Frequency: The number of lift–lower cycles completed in 1 minute.
• Coupling: The classification of hand-to-object grasp. Good if the distal phalanges and metacarpals are flexed, fair if only the metacarpals are flexed, and poor if there is minimal flexion of the metacarpals.
• Recommended weight limit: The value calculated using the National Institute for Occupational Safety and Health (NIOSH) formula.

The lifting risk analysis is modeled after the procedure developed by NIOSH to identify the relative risk of lifting and lowering tasks in manual material handling jobs. This procedure is also useful in the management of occupational musculoskeletal injuries because it is simple and straightforward and lends itself to education of the employer and patient as well as modification of the work tasks. In 1981, NIOSH published the *Work Practices Guide for Manual Materials Handling* (31), which has been reissued under the same title by the American Industrial Hygiene Association. In 1991, NIOSH updated the procedure (32) as the recommended workload (RWL), which is the product of a mathematic formula based on the diminution of a lifting constant (LC) of 51 pounds by each of six variables' multipliers, depending on the degree to which the task caused each variable to diverge from an ideal model. The formula is presented in Fig. 4.

To facilitate the relative evaluation of risks from lifting, NIOSH developed a simple mathematic model, which included each domain's primary components, the lifting index (LI). The LI can be taken as a unifying concept that allows comparison of tasks. The data are collected with the LRA to derive the RWL values. The actual weight of the object is divided by the RWL, and the quotient (the LI) is used to compare tasks. Tasks with higher LI values are relatively more risky and should become the focus of attention in the job-match analysis. The following are the six variables in the RWL formula:

- Horizontal displacement (H): The first variable in the equation has the most potential impact. Horizontal displacement is primarily a biomechanical factor that rapidly increases the force of the load at each of the body joints by multiplying the value of the load by the distance the load is displaced from the fulcrum, taken to be the L5–S1 disc interspace. Within 6 inches from the spine, no discernible decrease in work capacity is seen, but there is a rapid decrease thereafter. It should be noted that objects that are grasped bilaterally in the sagittal plane will not be held closer than 6 inches from the spine, because to do so represents the minimum possible abdominal depth (Table 9).

- Vertical starting height of the lift (V): The second variable in the equation represents the effect of the vertical location of the hands at the origin of the lift. The optimal starting height of a lift is 30 inches from the floor, roughly comparable to knuckle height. Less than 30 inches from the floor will require that the worker begin to stoop and to flex the knees to retrieve the load, with an attendant decrease in safe work capacity. More than 30 inches from the floor will require additional upper-extremity involvement, with a similar though less pronounced decrease in safe work capacity (Table 10).

- Displacement of the load (D): The third variable in the equation represents the vertical travel distance from origin to destination of the worker's hands as they grasp the load. The vertical distance over which the load is lifted has a slight but significant impact on safe working capacity. Vertical displacement of a load that is less than 10 inches does not decrease safe work capacity. Beyond this lower limit, however, safe work capacity gradually decreases as the vertical displacement of the load increase (Table 11).

- Asymmetry of the load (A): The fourth variable in the equation represents the number of degrees of angular rotation from the beginning to the end of the lift or lower. Beyond 135 degrees of angular rotation, no load is considered safe. Although foot placement will vary from worker to worker, no foot movement is considered; that is, NIOSH assumes that the movement of the object will create as much rotation in the musculoskeletal system as there is angular displacement of the object (Table 12).

- Frequency (F): The average frequency in terms of lifts per minute has a direct and inverse relationship on safe work capacity. The primary factor affecting the extent of the decrement as a result of frequency is the posture in which the worker is performing the lift (Table 13).

$$RWL = LC \times HM \times VM \times DM \times AM \times FM \times CM$$

| Load Constant | Horizontal Multiplier | Vertical Multiplier | Distance Multiplier | Asymmetric Multiplier | Frequency Multiplier | Coupling Multiplier |

FIG. 4. National Institute for Occupational Safety and Health (NIOSH) workload recommended formula.

TABLE 9. *Horizontal displacement multiplier*

H (in.)	HM	H (in.)	HM
<=10	1.00	19	0.53
11	0.91	20	0.50
12	0.83	21	0.48
13	0.77	22	0.46
14	0.71	23	0.44
15	0.67	24	0.42
16	0.63	25	0.40
17	0.59	>25	0.00
18	0.56		

H, horizontal displacement of the center of the load from the center of the spine; HM, horizontal displacement multiplier.

TABLE 10. *Vertical start height multiplier*

V (inches)	VM	V (inches)	VM
0	0.78	40	0.93
5	0.81	45	0.89
10	0.85	50	0.85
15	0.89	55	0.81
20	0.93	60	0.78
25	0.96	65	0.74
30	1.00	70	0.70
35	0.96	>70	0.00

V, vertical start height of the hands on the object being lifted at the initiation of the lift. Measured in inches from the floor; VM, vertical start height multiplier.

TABLE 11. *Vertical displacement multiplier*

D (in.)	DM	D (in.)	DM
<=10	1.00	45	0.86
15	0.94	50	0.86
20	0.91	55	0.85
25	0.89	60	0.85
30	0.88	70	0.85
35	0.87	>70	0.00
40	0.87		

D, vertical displacement over the lift or lower as measured in inches; DM, vertical displacement multiplier.

TABLE 12. *Asymmetric multiplier*

A (degrees)	AM	A (degrees)	AM
0	1.00	90	0.71
15	0.95	105	0.66
30	0.90	120	0.62
45	0.86	135	0.57
60	0.81	>135	0.00
75	0.76		

A, asymmetric movement of the object being lifted. Measured in terms of rotation through the coronal plane; AM, asymmetric multiplier.

TABLE 13. *Frequency multiplier*

Frequency (lifts/min)	<1 h V< 30 in.	<1 h V >= 30 in.	1–2 h V< 30 in.	1–2 h V>= 30 in.	2–8 h V< 30 in.	2–8 h V >= 30 in.
<=0.2	1.00	1.00	0.95	0.95	0.85	0.85
0.5	0.97	0.97	0.92	0.92	0.81	0.81
1	0.94	0.94	0.88	0.88	0.75	0.75
2	0.91	0.91	0.84	0.84	0.65	0.65
3	0.88	0.88	0.79	0.79	0.55	0.55
4	0.84	0.84	0.72	0.72	0.45	0.45
5	0.80	0.80	0.60	0.60	0.35	0.35
6	0.75	0.75	0.50	0.50	0.27	0.27
7	0.70	0.70	0.42	0.42	0.22	0.22
8	0.60	0.60	0.35	0.35	0.18	0.18
9	0.52	0.52	0.30	0.30	0.00	0.15
10	0.45	0.45	0.26	0.26	0.00	0.13
11	0.41	0.41	0.00	0.23	0.00	0.00
12	0.37	0.37	0.00	0.21	0.00	0.00
13	0.00	0.34	0.00	0.00	0.00	0.00
14	0.00	0.31	0.00	0.00	0.00	0.00
15	0.00	0.28	0.00	0.00	0.00	0.00
>15	0.00	0.00	0.00	0.00	0.00	0.00

V, vertical start height of hand holds on the object being lifted at the initiation of the lift; h, hour.

TABLE 14. *Coupling multiplier*

Coupling type	V <30 in.	V >= 30 in.
Good	1.00	1.00
Fair	0.95	1.00
Poor	0.90	0.90

- Coupling (C): The fourth variable in the equation represents the classification of hand-to-object grasp: *Good* if the distal phalanges and metacarpals are flexed; *fair* if only the metacarpals are flexed; and *poor* if there is minimal flexion of the metacarpals (Table 14).

INTERVENTION

A comprehensive vocational rehabilitation program for occupational musculoskeletal injuries usually includes personnel and facilities to develop, test, and adapt effective tool and workstation modifications (33–36). Typically, this program begins with a job-match analysis that is conducted by program personnel at a target worksite. The job-match analysis information is used to design a job-matching functional-capacity evaluation that is subsequently administered to the injured worker. This type of functional-capacity evaluation usually requires 1 to 5 days and can range from a simple series of component-based tests to a more complex situational assessment (37). The latter assessment is more effective and is preferred in situations in which it is likely that tool and workstation modifications will be implemented. It is interesting to note that, although the situational assessment requires a much longer period for evaluation, it is not proportionally more expensive than the component-based functional-capacity evaluation. The cost of situational assessments is only slightly greater than the cost for a component-based functional-capacity evaluation, because the situational assessment with the injured worker normally is performed on a group basis, usually supervised by an evaluation technician who is supervised by a vocational evaluator, occupational therapist, or physical therapist. The functional-ca-

pacity evaluation, on the other hand, is performed on a one-to-one basis, usually by an occupational therapist or physical therapist.

Accommodations

One of the most effective and inexpensive vocational rehabilitation strategies is the development of accommodations based on an analysis of the job's biomechanical demands. Historically, these services have been provided by occupational therapists or physical therapists who have training in job analysis, functional capacity evaluation, and ergonomics. In recent years, professional ergonomists have become interested in this area and have sought training to develop similar skills (38).

Some types of accommodations are accepted more easily in the workplace than others. Typically, tool and workstation modifications are somewhat more difficult to develop, but they are transferred more easily from the rehabilitation setting to the work setting than are task modifications. Task modifications tend to be identified more easily, but usually they are much more difficult to implement in the work setting. Employers are more likely to embrace the former (especially if the tool and workstation modifications have been developed and paid for elsewhere) than the latter.

Job Task, Tool, and Workstation Modification

Modification of the job tasks, so that they are within the injured worker's functional limitations, is accomplished by modifying both the job tasks and the injured worker's approach to the job tasks. Both job modification and worker training must be undertaken with reference to the injured worker's specific job, usually beginning in a simulated work environment and proceeding to the actual workplace.

Tool and workstation modifications are often inexpensive and easily accomplished. A survey in California found that 81% of the job modifications that were used were either free or cost less than $500 (39). Another study of actual hardware costs found an average cost of $320, whereas 34% of the recipients required less than $50 worth of modifications (40). The following case scenarios present examples of effective workstation and tool modifications.

Case Scenario 1

Una J. is a 46-year-old woman who is a retail salesperson employed by a large department store. After 18 years of successful employment in this position, she experienced a slip-and-fall accident at work that resulted in a lumbar disk injury for which she received a decompressive laminectomy. The surgery was not altogether successful, and 2.5 years after the date of injury Una had not returned to employment because of chronic pain.

Una was referred to the vocational rehabilitation facility by the employer's workers' compensation insurance carrier. After consultation with Una and her physician, it became apparent that a return to her usual and customary employment was not likely, although another job with her employer in a capacity that provided a better match to her residual functional capacity was a possibility. Subsequent contact with the employer confirmed this possibility. The employer identified three positions that would be open to Una if she had the abilities and residual functional capacity to perform the jobs competently. Vocational testing (which will be described in Chap. 40) was performed. Job analyses that had been developed by the employer were reviewed. A position as an entry-level secretary was identified as the most appropriate job target. Subsequently, the occupational therapist and injured worker traveled to the potential worksite to meet the work supervisor and perform a brief job-match analysis to supplement the information contained in the employer's standardized job analysis.

Based on the information in the standardized job analysis and the information gathered from the worksite visit, a job-matching functional-capacity evaluation was designed. It consisted of a situational assessment that began with a standard clerical workstation. Una sat in a clerical chair at a desk on which there was a telephone, computer terminal, and various stacked file drawers. The office also contained a facsimile machine, computer printer, and four-drawer file cabinet.

The situational assessment began with a computerized keyboard tutorial program that was both engaging for Una and assisted her in improving her undeveloped keyboard skills. It also provided an opportunity for the evaluator to develop and implement various accommodations that improved the biomechanical match between Una and the workstation. Insofar as possible, the workstation in the evaluation facility was similar to the target workstation. The following accommodations were attempted:

- Elevated armrests on the clerical work chair
- Lumbar support on the clerical work chair
- Elevated footrest beneath the desk
- Telephone headset
- Wrist and forearm bolster pad in front of keyboard
- Lazy Susan for desktop trays
- Arrangement of file cabinet drawers so that the bottom drawer is used infrequently
- Elevation of the computer monitor
- Vertical copy holder

Within the first few hours of the situational assessment, it became apparent that Una was unable to sit in the clerical work chair more than 15 or 20 minutes at a time. She would typically sit for 15 to 20 minutes, stand for 10 minutes, and return to a seated position for another 15 to 20 minutes. On this basis, she was able to continue working for a target 2 hours before taking a scheduled work break. Given this pattern, it was determined that the standard clerical workstation would not be adequate. Accordingly, an elevated workstation was developed using an artist's adjustable worktable. The computer, monitor, keyboard, telephone, and desktop files were moved to the worktable, and a tall work stool was used to replace the standard clerical chair. These accommodations were successful, and Una returned to work as an entry-level secretary after a job training program.

Case Scenario 2

Neil E., a 53-year-old man, was an upholsterer and tentmaker who worked for a large amusement park. While repairing a tent as he stood atop a ladder one day, the ladder shifted and he fell approximately 20 feet. He sustained injuries to the lower extremities and spine. The lower-extremity injuries resolved without complication. The spinal injuries included three herniated lumbar disks with attendant musculoskeletal strain. Although surgery was recommended, Neil refused, citing concerns stemming from the recent death of a relative after a similar surgery.

Neil was referred to the vocational rehabilitation facility about three years after the injury. Neil was found to be chronically disabled because of pain and abusing narcotic analgesic medication and alcohol. He was depressed and reported suicidal ideation. When asked about his goals, Neil reported, "My work is all I have left. If I can't work, I don t have anything." Neil reported that he wanted to attempt to return to work as an upholsterer and tentmaker.

Contact with the employer found that Neil was welcome to return and likely would be well received; however, a subsequent job analysis identified spinal work demands that were likely to exacerbate his pain symptoms significantly. For example, many of the upholstery repair tasks required working in the car of an amusement ride. The configuration of most of these cars required the worker to extend, flex, and twist the spine fully to perform the repairs. Although about 50% of the work could be performed at a workbench in a manner that would allow spinal demands to be anticipated and, thus, worked around, the remainder of the work tasks was performed in a complex and nonpredictable environment. The employer expressed an interest in providing subcontract work to Neil that could be performed in a shop environment.

Neil had set up a small workshop at his home, where he had worked several hours per week before the injury. He had not been able to perform work, although he had made several attempts, since the injury. Thus, Neil chose to attempt to return to work at his home workshop and expand his business based on the promise of subcontracts from his previous employer. A job-match analysis at Neil's shop identified several demands that were likely to require modifications that were developed and tested in a subsequent situational assessment at the vocational rehabilitation facility, including the following:

1. Neil's industrial sewing machine used a treadle foot control in addition to a lever-action knee control. Both were necessary to facilitate movement of the material and regulate the stitch speed. The treadle control was not difficult for Neil to perform; however, the knee control quickly exacerbated symptoms in the low back and right leg that interfered with fine control as well as his ability to maintain a seated position. The knee-action lever was adapted by attaching a cable to the back of the lever, which was run through a sheath down to a foot-action automotive pedal placed on the floor next to the treadle. Thus, Neil used plantar flexion and extension of each foot to maintain control of the sewing machine.

2. Appurtenant to the sewing machine is a work surface 30 inches from the floor measuring 8 feet square. Neil spreads material on the work surface and moves it by tugging and spreading while leaning over the work surface. He works mostly with Naugahyde and leather or canvas. To minimize forward flexion, three semicircles 22 inches in diameter were cut into the work surface. Neil moves to these semicircles before flexing to reach and tug material on the table.

3. Neil's work stool provided no lumbar or arm support. Remaining seated for up to 30 minutes at a time while maintaining high levels of concentration is required in his job. A well-designed work stool with good lumbar support was selected. The armrests were

found to be inadequate. They were built up (with the upholstery performed by Neil) so that they provided elbow and forearm support in a position that allowed proper alignment of the spine, shoulders, and arms between the chair and the sewing machine.

4. Neil uses a heavy steel 5-gallon glue pot, which is constructed like a pressure cooker. It maintains glue under pneumatic pressure that can be sprayed through a nozzle attached to a hose coming from the pot. The glue is sprayed onto fabric, which is adhered to various surfaces. The pot must be lifted and carried infrequently. Opening and closing the pot are difficult; so Neil greatly prefers to fill it completely once it is open, resulting in a piece of equipment that weighs approximately 60 pounds that is lifted by a wire handle attached to its top. This quickly precipitates symptoms as Neil attempts to move it. He is able to drag the pot more easily but found that a plywood tray with caster wheels on each corner into which the glue pot was set made this task much easier; however, the apparatus would tip from time to time. Consequently, the size of the tray was increased by approximately 4 inches and was surrounded by a 3-inch-high lid. After the glue pot was set into the tray, concrete was poured around the glue pot for ballast. The glue pot still could be removed from the tray if the need should arise, but was firmly anchored for movement around the shop, typically accomplished by pulling on the hoses attached to the pot.

5. Neil used a mandrel press and a steel rule die to cut fabric into various shapes. A typical 3-inch round of fabric was necessary to be cut for coverage of buttons. Neil attempted to cut 10 to 15 layers of fabric at once by pulling down on the handle with as much force as he could generate. Although he was able to align himself well in this process, such a pull typically caused immediate aggravation and a significant increase in symptoms. Neil limited the layers of fabric to three or four to decrease the force required, this solution was not adequate. It was not uncommon for Neil to have to produce 200 button covers per day. A simple solution to this problem involved a

2-foot section of steel pipe with an interior diameter that was adequate to cover the mandrel handle. This extension of the lever greatly decreased the force Neil was required to pull.

These accommodations were successful, and Neil returned to work as a self-employed upholsterer.

SUMMARY

The job-match analysis process has its underpinnings in job-analysis systems that have been described in this chapter. These systems were not designed to be used to match the person who has an occupational musculoskeletal disorder to the job. The information that these systems provide is too general and not sufficiently oriented to the musculoskeletal system. The job-match analysis process, on the other hand, has been designed specifically to match the person who has an occupational musculoskeletal disorder to the job, focusing on the biomechanical demands of the job. The job-match analysis process is an effective strategy for analysis and intervention for occupational musculoskeletal disorders as health care professionals become more oriented to return to work as a valued medical treatment outcome.

REFERENCES

1. Matheson L. Work capacity evaluation. In: Tollison C, Kriegel M. *Interdisciplinary rehabilitation of low back pain.* Baltimore: Williams & Wilkins, 1989:323–342.
2. Shrey D. Worksite disability management and industrial rehabilitation: an overview. In: Shrey D, Lacerte M, eds. *Principles and practices of disability management in industry.* Winter Park, FL: GR Press, 1995:3–54.
3. Mayer T. Rehabilitative vs. conservative care: Patient selection criteria. In: Mayer T, Mooney J, Gatchel R, eds. *Contemporary conservative care for painful spinal disorders.* Philadelphia: Lea & Febiger, 1991, pp.433–441.
4. Otis J, Leukart R. *Job evaluation: a basis for sound wage administration,* 2nd ed. In: Yoder D. Prentice-Hall Industrial Relations and Personnel Series. Englewood Cliffs, NJ: Prentice-Hall, 1954:532.
5. *The revised handbook for analyzing jobs.* Washington, DC: United States Department of Labor, 1991.
6. Fine S, Getkate M. *Benchmark tasks for job analysis: a guide for functional job analysis,* 1st ed. In: Fleishman E, ed. Series in Applied Psychology, Mahwah, NJ: Lawrence Erlbaum Associates, 1995.
7. *Dictionary of occupational titles,* 4th ed. Vol I and II.

Washington, DC: United States Department of Labor, 1991.

8. Erb B. Applying work physiology to occupational medicine. *Occup Health Saf* 1981(June):20–24.

9. Matheson L. Safe limits: vocational potential of individuals with impaired myocardial function. In: Dye C, ed. *The cardiovascular system.* Los Angeles: Medical Rehabilitation Research and Training Center, University of Southern California School of Medicine, 1977, pp.162–178.

10. Peterson N, Mumford M, Borman W, Jeanneret P, Fleishman E. *Development of prototype occupational information system (O*NET) content model.* Utah Department of Employment Security, 1995.

11. Peterson NG, et al. *O*NET Final Techinical Report I,* 1997, Utah Department of Employment Security.

12. Peterson NG, Mumford M, Borman W, et al. *O*NET Final Technical Report II.* Utah Department of Employment Security, 1997.

13. Fleishman E, Reilly M. *Handbook of human abilities: definitions, measurements, and job task requirements.* Palo Alto, CA: Consulting Psychologists Press, 1992:127.

14. Fleishman E, Quaintance M. *Taxonomies of human performance: The description of human tasks.* Orlando, FL: Academic Press, 1984:461–464.

15. Fleishman E. Evaluating physical abilities required by jobs. *The Personnel Administrator* 1979(June):82–87.

16. Matheson L. *Work capacity evaluation for occupational therapists.* Rehabilitation Institute of Southern California, 1982.

17. Matheson L. *Work capacity evaluation: interdisciplinary approach to industrial rehabilitation.* Anaheim, CA: Employment and Rehabilitation Institute of California, 1984:146.

18. Astrand I, Astrand PO, Hallback I, Kilborn A. Reduction in maximal oxygen uptake with age. *J Appl Physiol* 1973;35:649–654.

19. Kallman D, Plato C, Tobin J. The role of muscle loss in the age-related decline of grip strength: cross-sectional and longitudinal perspectives. *J Gerontol* 1990;45:M82–M88.

20. Matheson L. Relationship among age, body weight, resting heart rate, and performance in a new test of lift capacity. *J Occup Rehabil* 1996;6:225–237.

21. Miles W. Correlation of reaction and coordination speed with age in adults. *Am J Psychol* 1931;43:377–391.

22. Nygård C, Suurnäkki T, Ilmarinen J. Effects of musculoskeletal work load and muscle strength on strain at work in women and men aged 44 to 58 years. *Eur J Appl Physiol* 1988;58:13–19.

23. Schaie K. The optimization of cognitive function in old age: Predictions based on cohort sequential and longitudinal data. In: Baltes P, Baltes M, eds. *Successful aging: perspectives from the behavioral sciences.* Cambridge: Cambridge University Press: Cambridge, 1990:94–117.

24. Stones M, Kozma A. Physical activity, age and cognitive motor performance. In: Howe M, Brainerd C, eds. *Cognitive development in adulthood: progress in cognitive development research.* Springer: New York, 1989, pp.101–117.

25. Birren J, Birren B. The concepts, models, and history of the psychology of aging. In: Birren J, Schaie K, eds. *Handbook of the psychology of aging.* San Diego: Academic Press: 1990:1–20.

26. Campbell M, Kemp B, Brummel-Smith K. *Later life effects of early life disability: comparisons of age-matched controls in indicators of physical, psychological and social status.* Rehabilitation Research and Training Center on Aging, Rancho Los Amigos Medical Center, University of Southern California, Downey, CA, 1990.

27. Krause J, Crewe N. Chronologic age, time since injury, and time of measurement: Effect on adjustment after spinal cord injury. *Arch Phys Med Rehabil* 1991;72:91–100.

28. Hester E, Decelles P, Hood C. *The relationship between age and physical disability among workers:* implications for the future. Topeka, Kansas: The Menninger Foundation, 1986.

29. Hester E, Decelles P. *The worker who becomes physically disabled: a handbook of incidence and outcomes.* Topeka, Kansas: The Menninger Foundation, 1985.

30. Matheson L, Ogden L. *Work tolerance screening.* Trabuco Canyon, CA: Rehabilitation Institute of Southern California, 1983.

31. *Work practices guide for manual lifting.* Cincinnati, OH: Division of Biomedical and Behavioral Science, NIOSH, 1981.

32. Waters T, Putz-Anderson V, Garg A, Fine LJ. Revised NIOSH equation for the design and evaluation of manual lifting tasks. *Ergonomics* 1993;36:749–776.

33. *Guidelines for work hardening programs.* Tuscon, Az: Commission on Accreditation of Rehabilitation Facilities, 1988.

34. Isernhagen S. Functional capacity evaluation and work hardening perspectives. In: Mayer T, Mooney J, Gatchel R, eds. *Contemporary conservative care for painful spinal disorders.* Philadelphia: Lea & Febiger, 1991:328–345.

35. Kornblau B. Work hardening. In: Tollison C, Kriegel M, eds. *Interdisciplinary rehabilitation of low back pain.* Baltimore: Williams & Wilkins, 1989:277–291.

36. Matheson L, Ogden LD, Violette K, Schultz K. Work hardening: occupational therapy in industrial rehabilitation. *Am J Occup Ther* 1985;39:314–321.

37. Ogden-Niemeyer L, Jacobs K. *Work hardening: state of the art.* Thorofare, NJ: SLACK, 1989.

38. Hart D, Isernhagen S, Matheson L. Refining the practice of ergonomics. Work 1993;3:69–72.

39. Gugerty J, Roshal A, Tradewell M, Anthony L. *Tools, equipment and machinery adapted for the vocational education and employment of handicapped people.* Madison, WI: Wisconsin Vocational Studies Center, 1981.

40. Britell C, McFarland S. Adaptive systems and devices for the disabled. In: Ja D, ed. *Rehabilitation medicine: principles and practice.* Philadelphia: JB Lippincott, 1988.372–388.

Occupational Musculoskeletal Disorders
edited by T. G. Mayer, R. J. Gatchel, and P. B. Polatin.
Lippincott Williams & Wilkins, Philadelphia © 2000.

35

Interdisciplinary Programs: Chronic Pain Management

*Martin Deschner and †Peter Barth Polatin

*Departments of Psychiatry and Anesthesiology and Pain Management, Eugene McDermott
Center for Pain Management; and †Department of Anesthesiology and Pain Management,
University of Texas Southwestern Medical School, Dallas, Texas 75235*

Interdisciplinary treatment programs evolved from a need to develop effective programs to treat the most challenging chronic pain syndromes, particularly those resulting from musculoskeletal injuries. Various philosophies of treatment have guided attempts to define and treat the needs of these patients. Some have maintained that pain relief is the ultimate goal of treatment. Others have emphasized the importance of extinguishing pain-related behaviors, and still others have focused on correcting structural instabilities or attempting to relieve pain through surgery. One group has maintained that improved physical function and the return to normal life and work, as opposed to subjective pain relief, are the true indices of patient improvement.

The professional strengths of each discipline often led to a focus on a single treatment approach; however, these single methods have generally failed to provide consistent and enduringly positive results with most chronic pain patients. In the last several years, professionals from different disciplines have realized that only by combining their strengths in interdisciplinary programs can they begin to address the complex treatment needs of chronic pain patients.

This chapter examines the salient issues concerning interdisciplinary programs: the separate elements, indications for use of such programs, and treatment objectives. The dif-fering philosophies of pain management as they affect treatment goals are discussed. Chronic pain management and functional restoration represent the two most highly evolved and staff-intensive manifestations of interdisciplinary treatment programs. Functional restoration is discussed in another chapter; here the focus is on pain management.

PAIN MANAGEMENT

Historically, chronic pain management predates functional restoration and is based on the emerging awareness in the 1950s that acute and chronic pain are different entities requiring different treatments (1). Bonica realized that the treatment of chronic pain required a comprehensive approach that would be fundamentally different from the traditional medical and surgical procedures used with acute pain. He recognized the importance of an interdisciplinary team led by a physician with specialized training in the management of chronic pain (2).

In the 1960s, important breakthroughs were made in the understanding of pain as a biopsychosocial phenomenon. Fordyce et al. (3,4) began to conceptualize chronic pain in terms of pain behaviors (complaints, grimaces, avoidance of physical activity, and the dependence on medications). These behaviors do not simply express medical pathology but also are the result of reinforcement based on operant learning principles that shape what a pain patient does for secondary gain rewards. Using these insights, Fordyce et al. at the University of Washington developed the first pain clinic to use a purely behavioral treatment program that emphasized the alteration of reinforcement patterns to encourage the opposite of sick behavior, that is, well behavior (5).

Melzack and Wall (6) were the first to integrate psychological with physiological perspectives of pain perception. They suggested that afferent pain impulses entering the spinal cord could be blocked or inhibited in the dorsal horn by pressure impulses carried by larger-diameter fibers. As a result of the balance between these two signals, the dorsal horn might function as a gate-control system, augmenting or diminishing pain impulses, and therefore the nociceptive experience. Other brain activities expressed as attention, emotion, and memories of prior experience might further modulate the sensory input through efferent impulses down the spinal cord to the dorsal horn. By this model, it was postulated that cognition and emotions could affect the subjective experience of pain (7).

Turk et al. (8) proposed a cognitive-behavioral model of pain that emphasized the importance of cognitive, affective, and behavioral elements in addition to the sensory input for the experience of pain. They suggested that a patient's attitudes and beliefs about illness, the ability to cope with stress, and interpersonal strengths and weaknesses would determine that patient's response to the primary nociceptive experience, particularly after pain had remained significant for a longer time.

Dworkin et al. (9) proposed a dynamic-ecologic perspective: physiological, psychological, and social components interact differently, depending on the duration of the pain. Therefore, there are chronological stages of pain as manifested by specific behaviors across time, which will be comparable between different patients.

Gatchel (10) also suggested behavioral and experiential stages of pain. In stage 1, a patient experiences fear and anxiety in response to an event causing pain. In stage 2, if the pain has continued for several months, there is worsening of emotional distress, as determined by premorbid personality and psychological characteristics. In stage 3, if pain has endured beyond 4 to 6 months, with accompanying emotional distress, the patient has now adopted the sick role, which excuses him or her from normal functioning and frequently will reinforce secondary-gain issues. At this point, there is very little motivation to recover, and both physical and psychological deconditionings have set in; an effective treatment program at this stage must address both these components.

INTERDISCIPLINARY PROGRAMS

The types of patients treated in interdisciplinary programs have complex needs and requirements. They represent the small minority but nevertheless a significant number of patients who have failed to benefit from a combination of spontaneous healing and short-term, symptom-focused treatment. They also have become financial burdens on their insurance carriers. In the case of injured workers, their prolonged disabilities have "saddled" their employers with increased insurance costs and loss of productivity. These patients have been treated with varying degrees of success at other facilities, usually by single-discipline practitioners, or with the consultative assistance of other professionals. They often have had repeated and extended contacts with several different physicians and other health care providers, but they have failed to experience significant pain relief. Physical and psychological deconditioning, secondary gain, and medication addiction may complicate their presentation. This stage of treatment is much more complex and demanding of health care professionals.

Components of
an Interdisciplinary Program

No single professional discipline is capable of adequately addressing the complex needs of chronic pain patients; therefore, an interdisciplinary treatment program is required. Effective communication and full participation in the treatment milieu require that team members be employed on site, preferably in a full-time capacity. Formally, communication takes place in the interdisciplinary treatment team meeting that occurs at least once a week, but the informal, daily contact with other team members, during which patient progress can be discussed, is equally important. Interdisciplinary treatment implies constant communication among treatment team members as well as a common understanding of the overall goals of the treatment program being offered to patients (11); so patients hear the same treatment philosophy from each member of the team. Patients who are themselves in conflict about their own future treatment may seek out any conflict between team members and use it to subvert treatment goals. In the face of a cohesive and united therapeutic plan, such patients are more likely to abandon such efforts and then participate fully in treatment. The Commission on Accreditation of Rehabilitation Facilities (CARF) requires a certified treatment team to include at least a physician, a specialized nurse, a physical therapist, and a clinical psychologist or psychiatrist (2). Although pain reduction figures prominently in CARF-defined program goals, other goals are equally important and are cited here to illustrate the multidimensional nature of effective chronic pain treatment. These include reducing the number of medications used, reducing current treatment costs and subsequent health care utilization for the present problem, encouraging a return to productivity, increasing physical activity, and increasing the ability to manage pain-related problems.

Physician

A physician serves as the medical director of the treatment team and must have a background in providing medical rehabilitation for the types of disorders frequently encountered in chronic pain programs. Formal training may vary from anesthesiology, orthopedic surgery, neurosurgery, psychiatry, physiatry, or occupational medicine to internal medicine or osteopathy. While taking charge of the overall treatment of the patient, the physician more specifically assumes a direct role in the medical management of the patient's pain, providing the medical history to the treatment team, and taking direct responsibility for medication management and for any medical interventions. Other team members and outside consultants may be involved in the medical treatment of the patient, but it is the physician's responsibility to coordinate these medical contributions to the patient's care. The physician also must evaluate and summarize the patient's progress at the end of treatment and relate improvements to the patient's future functioning by delineating an after-care plan and clarifying residual disability and secondary-gain issues. The physician has a strong educational role with each patient (5). Whether leading educational classes or interacting with patients more informally, the physician's position of authority facilitates the education of the patient about such subjects as ways of communicating more effectively with health care providers, the distinction between impairment and disability, the difference between cure and rehabilitation, and the importance of playing an active role in one's own rehabilitation (12)

Nurse

Not all programs use nursing services, but a pain-management program, which provides anesthesiology services involving injections, nerve blocks, and other medical procedures, requires a nurse. The nurse assists the physician in follow-ups or procedures, may interact with patients in the role of case manager, and may provide patient education. It is as physician extender and educator that the nurse has the most impact on the patient. It is frequently the nurse who maintains communication with the patient after hours by telephone, addressing urgent concerns that require education and reassurance. By emphasizing educational issues in the same way as other team members, the nurse is helping the patient to hear a consistent message from the treatment team, even though the message may be uncomfortable for the patient at the time of the call or unacceptable in light of preconceived notions regarding pain relief and cure.

Psychologist

Whereas the physician plays a major role in managing the physical status of a patient involved in an interdisciplinary treatment program, the psychologist plays the leading role in the day-to-day maintenance of the psychosocial aspects of the patient's care. As described by Gatchel (13), serious psychosocial barriers to a positive outcome to treatment develop as the patient progresses from acute through subacute to the chronic stage of a pain syndrome. A number of studies, such as the one by Polatin et al. (14), have highlighted clinical syndromes that include depression, anxiety, substance abuse, and somatoform pain disorders, which frequently are found with chronic pain patients.

At the beginning of treatment, the psychologist is responsible for performing a full psychosocial evaluation, which includes identification of psychosocial barriers and assessment of the patient's psychological strengths and weaknesses. This mass of psychosocial information must be reduced to the most relevant data, which is communicated to the treatment team in a formal staff meeting. It is in this meeting that all new patients are initially presented and then subsequently reviewed as treatment progresses.

Through individual treatment, group therapy, and—at times—marital or family therapy, the psychologist helps a patient to cope more adaptively with psychosocial barriers. A cognitive-behavioral approach will be used to address issues involving pain-related depression, anger, anxiety, and fear.

Cognitive-behavioral therapy combines elements of behavioral conditioning and cognitive therapy and focuses on the patient's long-term experience with pain. Whereas the acute patient is likely to experience pain as a simple response to the pathological pain generator, the chronic patient has learned pain behaviors that overlie the basic nociceptive experience. With the continued experience of pain occurring in the social context of the family and community, the patient learns to behave in ways that demonstrate that he or she is in pain. These behaviors frequently elicit responses from others that perpetuate the disability associated with chronic pain. Such operant behaviors may include grimaces, descriptions of pain, changes in gait, requests for medications, and retiring to bed (15). The patient's pain behaviors become barriers to recovery because they interfere with the patient's efforts to overcome the disability associated with the experience of pain.

From the cognitive perspective, the patient's perceptions and appraisal of pain and concurrent life circumstances determine the response to and ability to cope with pain. The manner in which the patient assesses the severity of the injury, the likelihood of its being effectively treated, and the perceived prospects for overcoming the injury strongly influence the affective state (depression, anxiety, fear, anger) and motivation to strive actively to recover.

Effective psychotherapy therefore needs to address both behavioral and cognitive elements of the patient's experience with pain to reduce barriers to recovery. As stated by Tollison et al. (15), therapy involves four main objectives: (a) to educate the patient about pain while correcting any misinformation or information deficits; (b) to teach the patient specific cognitive and behavioral coping skills to facilitate the reduction of pain, anxiety, and depression; (c) to encourage the patient to practice these skills in a safe therapeutic environment that provides accurate feedback and reinforcement of skills learned; and (4) to help the patient to generalize skills learned in therapy to the home and community environments.

In practice, the patient may fear that others do not understand his or her pain-related concerns. The psychologist should communicate that these concerns have been heard and that the treatment team will provide therapy that at first may be experienced as challenging but will help the patient to regain control over pain and the future course of his or her life. By providing training in relaxation techniques and biofeedback, more effective coping skills for managing stress and somatic anxiety may be acquired. Learning new techniques to control unpleasant symptoms encourages a sense of mastery, self-confidence, and autonomy.

The psychologist or support staff will also be responsible for the educational curriculum provided in interdisciplinary treatment, which includes such topics as differentiating between acute and chronic pain, coping with depression, developing problem-solving skills, reframing negative thoughts, and understanding return-to-work issues. A rehabilitation counselor, if part of the treatment team, will present additional topics about vocational issues.

Physical Therapist

The physical therapist interacts daily with the patient regarding his physical progression toward recovery. Psychosocial barriers in the chronic pain patient will be manifested as pain sensitivity, somatization, symptom magnification, and noncompliance during participation in physical therapy. The therapist must be familiar with psychosocial issues and basic psychological barriers that affect each individual patient. Effective communication with other team members is crucial. For example, the therapist must know when to work in coordination with the psychology staff to neutralize a particularly challenging psychosocial barrier or may coordinate efforts with the vocational therapist when a patient's fear of returning to work is interfering with an exercise program. When other behavioral symptoms arise in the course of physical therapy, the therapist first must be able to recognize and then to address these negative behaviors in a manner that is minimally disruptive to patient care and most conducive to physically progressing the patient.

The physical therapist also helps to educate the patient by addressing the physiological basis of pain and teaching ways of reducing the severity of pain episodes through the use of appropriate body mechanics. The patient is taught the importance of regaining and maintaining adequate physical conditioning to reduce the risk of reinjury and to function adequately in daily home, occupational, and recreational activities on completion of the program. At the completion of treatment, the physical therapist also may instruct the patient on home exercise to maintain the gains made in treatment.

Occupational Therapist

The occupational therapist is involved in both physical and vocational aspects of the patient's treatment. The vast majority of patients participating in an interdisciplinary program are likely not to be working because of their pain. Often they have become pessimistic about the prospect of returning to work and may have financial difficulties related to their temporary inability to earn an income. An occupational therapist addresses these vocational issues and the physical determinants underlying disability.

Whereas physical therapists emphasize the training of specific muscle groups to strengthen biomechanical weak links, the occupational therapist groups these musculoskeletal activities into coordinated whole-body activities that are close approximations of activities the patient is likely to perform in daily life. Job-simulation activities are a part of the occupational therapy training program and help the patient to strengthen coordinated movements required by his or her occupation. This activity serves not only to improve a patient's chances of returning to gainful employment but also improves his or her confidence in being able to do so. In treating a patient with primarily upper-extremity pain complaints, the occupational therapist is frequently the front-line therapist to direct mobilization and strengthening activities.

The occupational therapist also plays an important educational role. Teaching the patient techniques for managing pain on the job in ways that do not jeopardize the employment status and helping the patient to sharpen or learn new interviewing skills will assist him or her in returning to the workplace, even if the former job is not available.

Finally, the occupational therapist can play an important role as a case manager, that is, (a) to contact employers to obtain job descriptions and other information that would be beneficial in helping the patient to set goals for rehabilitation and (b) to contact employers near the time of patient discharge to facilitate the actual return-to-work process.

INDICATIONS FOR TREATMENT

Recently formulated algorithms of conservative care for pain disorders classify chronic pain management as either a tertiary or a palliative level of treatment (16–18).

Tertiary Care

Patients are at a minimum of 4 months postinjury and have been refractory to all other forms of intervention at a lesser intensity of health care utilization (i.e., primary and secondary levels of treatment). Tertiary care is seen as the final phase of nonoperative or postoperative treatment for severe and refractory pain. It is appropriate for patients who have demonstrated physical and psychosocial changes that are consistent with chronic disease with partial or complete disability. Tertiary-level care is medically directed, uses a high intensity of health care services, and is reserved for the most refractory patients. It employs individualized treatment protocols and interdisciplinary treatment services.

Chronic pain management and functional restoration are both tertiary care programs for chronic pain. The duration of treatment is 2 to 4 months, with the likely endpoint being a return to work, or at least the resumption of increased activities of daily living if work is not physically possible. Functional restoration is described fully in another chapter.

Palliative Care

Palliative level care is considered by Wong et al. (18) as the final phase of treatment, after all other treatments have been attempted or ruled out and have failed to help the patient to regain function or experience some degree of pain relief. The goal of intervention at this stage is to provide comfort in a cost-effective manner while maintaining maximum capacity for physical functioning. Patients are considered for palliative level care when all other forms of treatment have failed and psychological or psychosocial issues continue to be significant barriers to recovery. These patients may have persistent secondary-gain or socioeconomic issues. It is expected that after treatment, these patients will experience some decrease in symptoms, with partial return to adaptive functioning. It is also hoped that such patients will decrease their dependence on financial or health benefits and return to normalized activities of daily living.

Types of treatment consistent with palliative level care include medical maintenance procedures for episodic pain, reinstruction in fitness maintenance programs, relaxation training, coping and stress management techniques, injection procedures, behavioral programs, and limited passive modalities. For severe recurrence of pain, elements of secondary, tertiary, or surgical procedures may be tried or repeated. Socioeconomic interventions such as vocational rehabilitation and disability case management to resolve outstanding injury-related financial awards might also be pursued. For control of intractable pain, external devices such as a spinal cord stimulator, transcutaneous electric stimulator (TENS) unit, or analgesic pump might be tried as well as denervation procedures or long-term opioid maintenance.

Narcotics for the Long-term Treatment of Chronic Nonmalignant Pain

The opioids are the most effective pharmacologic agents for the relief of pain (19), but traditionally they have not been used with chronic pain of nonmalignant origin because of concerns about side effects, such as respiratory depression, impaired cognition, functional passivity, tolerance, and psychological and physical dependence. Additionally, clinicians have worried about potential liability and censure by regulatory agencies (20).

This clinical bias has been changing in recent years. Studies have shown that the risk of addiction in patients with opioid-responsive pain is low in the absence of such factors as a past history of substance abuse, experience of childhood traumatic events, or a severe personality disorder (21,22). It is now believed that pain physiologically antagonizes the central nervous system depressant effect of the opioids. Therefore, an addict or a control subject without clinical pain might demonstrate respiratory depression with the administration of narcotic medication, but a chronic pain patient will not experience this side effect (23,24).

Recently, there has been a public outcry for the humane treatment of patients with chronic nonmalignant pain, including the long-term prescription of narcotics. California drafted principles of responsible professional practice for such use of opioids in 1994 (25). These recommendations include a history, physical examination, formulated treatment plan, informed consent from the patient, periodic review, consultation as necessary, accurate record keeping, and compliance with controlled-substance regulations.

Preliminary guidelines now exist for such treatment. A prior trial of alternative analgesia is recommended as well as exclusion of patients with risk factors for dependence. A single physician should have primary medication responsibility, and the pain must be documented as responsive to opioids by clinical trial. Goals for functional improvement should be stipulated and agreed on to justify the regimen. Careful monitoring and documentation of degree of analgesia, side effects, functional status, and evidence of aberrant drug-seeking behavior should be carried out on a regular basis (26,27). The clinical challenge is to identify clearly the subpopulation

of chronic pain patients who will derive long-term partial analgesia from narcotic administration without the occurrence of intolerable side effects or aberrant drug-related behaviors (28).

Jamison et al. (29) conducted a randomized prospective study of oral opioid therapy in patients with chronic nonmalignant low back pain. The opioids clearly alleviated pain from a severe to a moderate level but rarely completely relieved it. Mood was frequently improved as well, but activity level was not consistently affected. Patients preferred a shorter-acting narcotic to a longer-acting one. Patients who varied their medication dose reported more sustained relief than those who adhered to a fixed dose. Younger patients tolerated the opioids better than the older group. Patients with limited support and greater physical impairment preferred this narcotic maintenance if they had previously exhausted other options and had to rely on "their own ability to function."

Oral methadone (30) and transdermal fentanyl (31) also have been found to be helpful in the treatment of chronic nonmalignant pain. Several studies reviewed the efficacy of long-term interspinal infusions of narcotics of such pain control (32–35).

From this preliminary research, it is clear that narcotics may be used safely over the long term in some patients with nonmalignant pain. Whether this therapy is palliative or actually leads to functional adaptation and true clinical improvement needs to be more rigorously studied in a larger number of cases and treatment settings.

CLINICAL SPECTRUM FOR THE TREAMENT OF CHRONIC PAIN

The increasing complexity and severity of chronic pain and the deteriorating physical, psychosocial, and economic factors affecting the patient (10) dictate a more comprehensive, interdisciplinary, programmatic approach to treatment. Clinicians and insurance carriers, among others, frequently experience the sense of time running out on the possibilities for helping the patient in any meaningful way. Failure to do so brings with it prospects of continued suffering for the patient and continued burdens on medical, economic, and emotional resources of the patient's family and community.

With a developing appreciation of the interrelationship of physiological and psychosocial factors in pain, a rapid growth in the number of pain clinics occurred, although not all of them were set up as interdisciplinary programs. In fact, a wide variety of pain-management programs now exists, ranging from single-modality pain clinics to interdisciplinary pain-management centers. Gatchel and Turk (5) cite the International Association for the Study of Pain (IASP) as delineating four levels of pain programs (36): (a) pain clinics treating single-diagnosis or specific body-region problems; (b) modality-oriented clinics providing specific types of treatment, such as biofeedback or nerve blocks; (c) multidisciplinary pain clinics; and (d) multidisciplinary pain centers. The latter two are similar in their inclusion of multiple disciplines on their staffs. The multidisciplinary pain center adds research and teaching activities to those specifically involving patient treatment and usually is affiliated with a major health science institution.

Parenthetically, the terms *multidisciplinary* and *interdisciplinary* are in this instance used interchangeably. Conceptually, however, these two terms have been differentiated in the degree of treatment, staff interaction, and coordination occurring in a given pain program. Accordingly, the term *interdisciplinary* refers to a more intensive and concerted effort on the part of the treatment team to communicate regularly about the care of the patients being treated and to coordinate their efforts consistently in addressing patient treatment issues and problems. The term *multidisciplinary* is used to refer to a less intensive, less coordinated treatment environment. Various disciplines, although present under one roof, are less invested in the full-court press of coordinated interdisciplinary focus on the care of each patient.

SUMMARY

At their best, interdisciplinary chronic pain treatment programs use the strengths of multiple disciplines working together to address complex issues confronting chronic pain patients, including education, stress reduction, disability management, physical reconditioning, emotional stabilization, and behavioral restructuring, as well as procedures and medications for the mitigation of pain. The therapeutic focus should be toward independence and autonomy while acknowledging those physical limitations that cannot be overcome. Adaptation does not mean defeat, and chronic pain patients can learn through the combined resources of an interdisciplinary program that it is possible to lead a successful and rewarding life in spite of chronic pain. Treatment programs that focus on a single modality may be successful in some cases but will not fully serve the spectrum of needs posed by this difficult patient group.

REFERENCES

1. Bonica J. *The management of pain*. Philadelphia: Lea & Febiger, 1980, vol. 1., p. 180.
2. Chapman S. Chronic pain. In: Sweet J, Rozensky R, Tovian S, eds. *Handbook of clinical psychology in medical settings*. New York: Plenum Press, 1991:38–70.
3. Fordyce W. *Behavioral methods for chronic pain and illness*. St. Louis: Mosby, 1976, pp. 11–99.
4. Fordyce W, Fowler R, Lehmann J, DeLateur B. Some implications in learning in problems of chronic pain. *Journal of Chronic Diseases* 1968;21:179–190.
5. Gatchel R, Turk D. Interdisciplinary treatment of chronic pain patients. In: WB Saunders ed. Psychosocial factors in pain: critical perspectives, New York: NY 1999, pp. 435–444.
6. Melzack R, Wall P. Pain mechanisms: a new theory. *Science* 1965;150:971–979.
7. Rudy T, Turk D. Psychological aspects of pain. *Int Anesthesiol Clin* 1991;29:9–21.
8. Turk D, Meichenbaum D, Genest M. *Pain and behavioral medicine: a cognitive-behavioral perspective*. New York: Guilford Press, 1983, pp. 145–173.
9. Dworkin S, Von Korff M, LeResche L. Epidemiologic studies of chronic pain: A dynamic-ecologic perspective. *Annals of Behavioral Medicine* 1992;14:3–11.
10. Gatchel R. Early development of physical and mental deconditioning in painful spinal disorders. In: Mayer T, Mooney V, Gatchel R, eds. *Contemporary conservative care for painful spinal disorders*. Philadelphia: Lea & Febiger, 1991:278–289.
11. Turk D, Stieg R. Chronic pain: the necessity of interdisciplinary communication. *Clin J Pain* 1987;3:63–167.

12. Turk D, Stacey B. Multidisciplinary pain centers in the treatment of chronic low back pain. In: Frymoyer J, ed. *The adult spine: principles and practice*, 2nd ed. Philadelphia: Lippincott-Raven, 1997, pp. 258–274.

13. Gatchel R. Psychological disorders and chronic pain: cause and effect relationships. In: Gatchel R, Turk D, eds. *Psychological approaches to pain management*. New York: The Guilford Press, 1996:33–52.

14. Polatin P, Kinney R, Gatchel R, Lillo E, Mayer T. Psychiatric illness and chronic low back pain: the mind and the spine—which goes first? *Spine* 1993;18:66–71.

15. Tollison C, Hinnant D, Kriegel M. Psychological concepts of pain. In: Mayer T, Mooney V, Gatchel R, eds. *Contemporary conservative care for painful spinal disorders*. Philadelphia: Lea & Febiger, 1991:133–142.

16. Mayer T, Polatin P, Smith B, et al. Contemporary concepts in spine care—spine rehabilitation. secondary and tertiary nonoperative care. *Spine* 1995;20:2060–2066.

17. Texas Workers' Compensation Commission Medical Review Division. Texas Workers Compensation Spine Treatment Guidelines. *Texas Register* March 28, 1995.

18. Wong D, Mayer T, Errico T, et al. *North American Spine Society phase III clinical guidelines for spine care specialists:* herniated disc. Draft June 30, 1998.

19. Polatin P. Integration of pharmacotherapy with psychological treatment of chronic pain. In: Gatchel R. Turk D, eds. *Psychological approaches to pain management:* a practitioner's handbook. New York: Guilford Press, 1996:305–328.

20. Joranson D. A new drug law for the states: An opportunity to affirm the role of opioids in cancer pain relief. *J Pain Symptom Manage* 1990;5:333–336.

21. Portnoy R, Foley K. Chronic use of opioid analgesics in nonmalignant pain: report of 38 cases. *Pain* 1986;25: 171–186.

22. Taub A. Opioid analgesics in the treatment of chronic intractable pain of non-neoplastic origin. In: Kitahata L, Collins J, eds. *Narcotics, analgesics in anesthesiology*. Baltimore, MD: Williams & Wilkins, 1982: 199–208.

23. Twycross R. Opioids. In: Wall P, Melzack R, eds. *Textbook of pain*, 3rd ed. 1994:943–962.

24. Walsh T, Baxter R, Bowman K, Leber B. High dose morphine and respiratory function in chronic cancer pain. *Pain* 1981;29(Suppl 1):539 (abst).

25. Medical Board of California. *Guidelines for prescribing controlled substances for intractable pain*. Sacramento: Medical Board of California, 1994, pp. 1–4.

26. Portnoy R. Opioid therapy for chronic nonmalignant pain: current status. In: Fields H, Liebeskind J, eds. *Progress in pain research and management*, vol 1. Seattle, WA: International Association for the Study of Pain Press, 1994:247–287.

27. Jamison R. Comprehensive pretreatment and outcome assessment for chronic opioid therapy in nonmalignant pain. *J Pain Symptom Manage* 1996;11:231–241.

28. Portnoy R. Opioid therapy for chronic nonmalignant pain: a review of the critical issues. *J Pain Symptom Manage* 1996;11:203–217.

29. Jamison R. Opioid therapy for chronic noncancer back pain. a randomized prospective study. *Spine* 1998;23: 2591–2600.

30. Gardner-Nix J. Oral methadone for managing chronic nonmalignant pain. *J Pain Symptom Manage* 1996;11: 321–328.

31. Jcal W, Benfield P. Transdermal fentanyl: a review of its pharmacological properties and therapeutic efficacy in pain control. *Drugs* 1997;53:109–138.

32. Nitescu P, Dahm P, Appelgren L, Curelaru I. Continuous infusion of opioid and bupivicaine by externalized intrathecal catheters in long-term treatment of refractory nonmalignant pain. *Clin J Pain* 1998;14:17–28.

33. Harvey S, O'Neil M, Pope C, Cuddy B, Duc T. Continuous intrathecal meperidine via an implantable infusion pump for chronic nonmalignant pain. *Ann Pharmacother* 1997;31:1306–1308.

34. Winkelmuller M, Winkelmuller W. Long term effects of continuous intrathecal opioid treatment in chronic pain of nonmalignant etiology. *J Neurosurg* 1996;85:458–467.

35. Paice J, Winkelmuller W, Butchiel K, Racz G, Piaget J. Clinical realities and economic considerations: efficacy of intrathecal pain therapy. *J Pain Symptom Manage* 1997;14(Suppl)514–526.

36. Loeser J. *Desirable characteristics for pain treatment facilities*. Washington, DC: International Association for the Study of Pain, 1990.

Occupational Musculoskeletal Disorders
edited by T. G. Mayer, R. J. Gatchel, and P. B. Polatin.
Lippincott Williams & Wilkins, Philadelphia © 2000.

36

Tertiary Nonoperative Interdisciplinary Programs

The Functional Restoration Variant of the Outpatient Chronic Pain Management Program

Tom G. Mayer and *Peter Barth Polatin

*Department of Orthopedic Surgery; *Department of Anesthesiology and Pain Management,
University of Texas Southwestern Medical School, Dallas, Texas 75235*

After the gamut of surgical and nonoperative primary and secondary treatment approaches have been used, most patients with occupational musculoskeletal disorders have returned to work and decreased their health utilization. Depending on the U.S. state or federal workers' compensation venue and musculoskeletal area, an average of about 10% of patients persist with workers' compensation disability 3 to 4 months postinjury. The range is from about 5% to 25%, with a smaller (but growing) group of patients persisting in *perpetual limited duty* (or *partial disability*) in conjunction with the recent advocacy for keeping patients on the job. In time, unless such patients are unable to return to full duty or significant modified jobs, they too go on to persistent work-adjustment problems with employers and increasing disability behaviors.

Certain musculoskeletal disorders have a particularly high likelihood of becoming chronic disabling problems. Spinal disorders, particularly those affecting the low back, usually beginning as sprains and strains, are more highly represented among chronic pain and disability work-related injuries than other musculoskeletal areas. Upper-extremity neurocompressive complaints, particularly those termed *repetitive motion* or *cumulative trauma disorders* (CTD), also have a higher rate of developing chronicity, and CTD claims are known to be 1.8 times more expensive than non-CTD claims (1–7). By contrast, lower-extremity injuries, particularly if they involve fractures, tend to resolve more completely within a usual tissue-healing period. In many ways, the more subjective the diagnosis and mechanism of injury, the greater the likelihood of symptom persistence.

Much controversy exists regarding the development of chronic pain and disability syndromes after work-related musculoskeletal injuries. A variety of psychosocial host factors, secondary gain, and socioeconomic predictors have been variably reported in the literature. Clinicians tend to focus on the nonphysiological aspects of pain persistence, regardless of the diagnosis, because of the reasonable assumption that bones, joints, and soft tissues have healed completely, even if imperfectly, in a finite period. Persistent bony malalignment, joint-degenerative arthritis, or soft-tissue scar may be present, and these changes are deemed "set in stone." They may result in some degree of *permanent impair-*

ment; however, whereas most injured workers (and a perceived greater percentage of patients without compensation) seem to recover in a timely fashion, a disturbingly large and costly group of chronic pain and disability patients remain disabled and refractory to treatment over a substantial period. These patients tend to demand a significant preponderance of indemnity and medical costs; follow-up in most federal social systems for 15 to 20 years shows that in every industrialized country they represent the greatest number of patients who become permanently disabled for the longest periods. The reason is that the average age of work-related musculoskeletal injury developing into permanent disability is in the mid-30s, much earlier than any other diagnostic entity producing such disability (with the possible exception of the much less common psychiatric disorders). For these chronic pain and disability patients, repeated passive therapy, manipulation, or surgical intervention have been tried commonly, but they have failed to relieve symptoms and overcome disability. These patients tend to produce the most significant cost to society in terms of medical care, disability payments, and loss of productivity. As such, they provoke a great deal of concern and interest. It is for this difficult group of patients, for whom *conservative care* or *surgery* have failed, that spinal functional restoration is intended.

As yet no one has managed to identify the unique structural pain generator in the chronic spinal disorder (CSD) patient. Description of such a site has eluded basic scientists, surgeons, internists, and psychologists and probably will continue to do so. The obvious reason is that pain is a subjective central experience of multifactorial origin. With the source of the pain deeply submerged and inaccessible to visual inspection (similar to headache and chronic abdominal pain), the spine is subject to diverse influences, such as psychological difficulty, social losses, and financial uncertainties. These secondary phenomena tend to be ignored by the physician and chiropractor who have no mechanism available to deal with these problems. As a consequence, a critical part of our understanding of spinal disability is lost. Because interdisciplinary experience is not usually part of most physician training, lack of conceptualization and resolution in the area of chronic spinal disability is to be anticipated.

Concepts of nonoperative care, particularly for work injuries, are changing rapidly. In the past, the term *physical therapy* was loosely applied to any nonoperative management not specifically performed by physicians. A multitude of developments over the past 2 decades, however, has permitted segmentation that permits definition of several levels of care tied to the time since injury. *Primary care* refers to care provided during the acute phases of injury and usually intended for symptom control, including but not restricted to the so-called passive modalities (e.g., electric stimulation, temperature modulation, manual techniques). A variety of early assisted mobilization and educational programs also may be included at this level. Customarily, treatment is provided by a single therapist, with a limited number of treatments generally applied to a large number of patients entering the medical system.

Secondary care refers to therapy provided to a smaller number of patients not responding to initial primary treatment. The long-standing symptoms pass into the post-acute or immediate postoperative period. In these cases, reactivation is the common need, with programs generally adapted to provide appropriate exercise and education as the primary modalities, but often these modalities are assisted by additional passive modalities still used for symptomatic control. In many cases, the secondary level of care lends itself to programmatic consolidation, particularly toward the end of the postacute period, in which interdisciplinary consultation might be available for specialized situations but will *not* be required on site or in most cases. The primary treaters in this phase usually involve physical and occupational therapists, with the available consultants including physicians, psychologists, social workers, disability managers, or chiropractors, depending on the venue or community standards.

In the small number of patients who do not respond to secondary care and whose pain becomes chronic or patients undergoing complex surgical procedures, *tertiary care* is the final option. Tertiary care involves *physician-directed, interdisciplinary team care with all disciplines on site and available to every patient*. The Commission for Accreditation of Rehabilitation Facilities (CARF) pain-management guidelines most closely identify common standards of some tertiary care programs, although such treatment may be diverse and eclectic. The picture is confused further by the fact that not all pain clinics provide tertiary care, just as not all work-hardening programs provide interdisciplinary consultative services needed to fulfill CARF definitions for this particular service. Specific programmatic terms are still in flux, but the concept of *levels of care* is becoming widely accepted. Thus, it is necessary to remain true to program definitions in understanding service provision to have hopes of achieving the goal of *quality of care*. It is with this in mind that a specific program, *functional restoration*, available at the Productive Rehabilitation Institute of Dallas for Ergonomics (PRIDE), will be discussed here as an example of tertiary care, mainly for work-related injury. The intent is to provide the reader a direct understanding of the roles of each member of the interdisciplinary team within this particular type of tertiary care (8,9).

Functional restoration involves several concepts not generally considered as part of nonoperative care. The first is the concept of *deconditioning*. From a physical point of view, disuse and immobilization lead to many deleterious effects on joint mobility, muscle strength, endurance, and soft-tissue homeostasis. There is a lack of visual feedback unique to complex spinal structures for both patient and physician, necessitating *quantification of function*. Such an approach is not specifically required in extremity rehabilitation.

The second major issue involves *psychosocial* and *socioeconomic* factors in disability, which often accompany chronic and postoperative spinal disorders. *Disability* refers to the inability to perform all the usual functions of daily living and is frequently linked to prolonged episodes of severe pain. Treatments of chronic pain derive from concepts about pain and methods of evaluation. Traditionally, doctors have focused on causes of pain, seeking the physiologic basis for pain that, once identified, could be eliminated or blocked. Assessment focused on identifying the physical basis. When no physical basis was identified, a psychological cause was assumed, hence the term *psychogenic pain*. The traditional view of persistent pain embraces a simple dichotomy: The pain is physical or psychological. This concept of a simple dichotomy is inadequate. Traditional medical approaches to chronic pain problems are ineffective, with long-term success rates below 30%. Physical factors do cause pain, and psychological factors contribute to symptoms; however, there is a range of psychosocial factors that occur secondary to an injury or disease.

The greatest assessment error for most clinicians is the failure to recognize socioeconomic factors in chronic pain patients. It has been well established over the years that patients being paid for remaining *disabled* and nonproductive will behave differently from patients who are uncompensated (10–13). Similarly, patients likely to receive a bonus settlement for permanent impairment, even if they are not receiving direct disability indemnity benefits, will likely demonstrate some illness behaviors. Major axis I psychiatric diagnoses [*Diagnostic and Statistical Manual of Mental Disorders* (DSM)-IV], such as substance use (often preexisting or iatrogenic, ally-abetted), or major depression, may strongly affect treatment progress and ultimate outcomes (14), particularly if the clinician fails to recognize or ignores these crucial issues by dealing only with the body and not the mind. Various treatment interventions have been designed to cope with the psychosocial and socioeconomic factors involved in total or partial disability.

Psychosocial assessment is often necessary to identify these factors and guide treatment.

In addition to psychosocial problems originating because of persistent pain and disability, latent psychopathology also may be activated by life disruption produced by pain and disability. As such, psychiatric interventions, including the use of psychotropic drugs and detoxification from narcotic and tranquilizer habituation, are helpful. Primary and secondary treatment alone may be ineffective to deal with these multifactorial chronic dysfunctions; so programmatic care delivered by an interdisciplinary team is desirable, if available.

QUANTIFICATION OF PHYSICAL DECONDITIONING

Whereas a normal soft tissue, joint, or bony healing period generally will have occurred by the time a patient enters a period of chronic pain or disability, progressive deterioration of physical and functional capacity still may be in an early stage. Deconditioning occurs as a consequence of disuse and fear-related inhibition. The quantitative assessment of function is a vital aspect of developing an effective treatment program for disabling spinal disorders. In the extremities, there is relatively good visual feedback to physical capacity. Joints are easily seen, and mobility is subject to goniometric measurements; the muscle bulk is subject to tape measurements. Right and left comparisons between a normal and abnormal side often can be made. In the spine, direct visual feedback as to physical capacity is inadequate. Yet this deficiency has not been generally recognized by clinicians, who often continue to rely on subjective self-report or physical measures that are either inaccurate or irrelevant. More accurate methods are necessary for objective quantification (9,15–17).

Deconditioning was recognized first in association with meniscal injuries of the knee during World War II and was further popularized by highly visible football players two decades later. Identification of deconditioning as a factor in limiting recovery led to a therapeutic revolution in combined surgical and rehabilitation treatment of the knee that goes on today. Although facilitated by easy visual access, the concepts translate nicely to spinal disorders. Inactivity leads to loss of general body functional performance, which is well recognized by any athlete, along with uniform loss of *functional capacity*. On the other hand, the injured area sustains more profound loss of paraarticular soft-tissue function, becoming progressively greater as the period of disuse and immobilization increases. These changes create a weak link in the localized extremity joint or spinal region, whose *physical capacity* must be measured separately.

In assessing low back function, we have drawn from experience with the extremities in identifying elements of performance that are of value in characterizing extremity physiologic *functional units*. Factors such as range of motion, strength, neurologic status, endurance combined with whole-body aerobic capacity, and activities of daily living measurements are traditionally assessed. In contrast, evaluation of extremity neurologic function (straight leg raising, lower-extremity strength, sensation and reflexes in dermatomal/myotomal patterns) still may be viewed by most neurologists as the most important objective spine examination components. In chronic low back pain, however, these neurologic findings may be irrelevant for several reasons. First, they are a measure of acute change when noted in relation to surgical pathology. In the chronic situation, the persistence of neurologic changes generally reflect epidural fibrosis or other permanent, noncorrectable anatomic abnormalities. In addition, the neurologic deficits, although emanating from spinal structures, are perceived by the patient as *extremity abnormalities* that produce pain, sensory changes, and weakness of the arms and legs. In sum, what the clinician currently views as standard objective functional tests may provide little useful information for treating spinal deconditioning. The answer is human performance testing to assess the debilitation cascade.

A critical principle of evaluating human performance is that measurements need to be *accurate*, *reliable*, and *discriminating*. They also need to be *relevant* to the physiology being measured. As an example of the latter, an isometric (National Institute of Occupational Safety and Health) (NIOSH) leg-lift strength test (performed with the back straight in a squatting position) probably says little about the strength of injured or deconditioned lumbar musculature. Physics-based principles must be used to evaluate quantitative measurement devices using terms such as *accuracy* and *precision*, much as would be used to evaluate the performance of a scale or speedometer (18). It is not sufficient to identify a device's measurement as reliable because accurate devices may give unreliable data as a result of normal human variability. This variability can be accounted for only by appropriate normative databases. Similarly, accurate devices may provide data incapable of being used clinically because of wide fluctuations in human performance caused by a variety of sources of error. These sources of error may include the human–device interface, training of test administrators, or a low signal output by the device relative to the noise in the system. Because of a variety of secondary-gain or fear issues, which may impede performance in the injured person, an effort-assessment capability is a desirable concomitant of an assessment protocol or device to be used in low back pain patients. The physicians, therapists, and technicians who use devices for indirect, objective measurement of spine function should have a basic understanding of the quantitative assessment science, which allows them to evaluate the merit of each system.

Objective, quantitative measurements of function provide the clinician with a baseline definition of a patient's physical capacity. Successive tests document changes in performance with treatment. Suboptimal effort demonstrates the degree to which barriers to recovery impede physical performance and lead to changes in psychosocial treatment interventions. Finally, at maximum medical recovery, the quantitative tests outline the patient's work capacity and the functional elements often required as part of impairment and disability evaluation.

Upper- and lower-extremity physical capacity is assessed by measuring mobility and strength about a specific extremity joint, usually corresponding to perception of a compensable area as a critical inclusion criterion for entering the workers compensation system. Because peripheral soft-tissue lesions, particularly the neurocompressive or sympathetically mediated syndrome, frequently produce a diffuse set of symptoms, the entire extremities are usually assessed in these cases. Although comparison to a contralateral side is often helpful, the fact that bilateral symptoms are not uncommon and inhibition of effort problems also may affect performance on the contralateral side. Therefore, normative databases are as important in the extremities as they are in the trunk. More detailed discussion of quantitative physical and functional capacity measurements takes place in an earlier chapter.

PSYCHOSOCIAL AND SOCIOECONOMIC ASSESSMENT

In a work environment, when injury is associated with compensation for disability, physical problems are rarely the only factor to be considered in organizing a treatment program. Many psychosocial and socioeconomic problems may confront the patient recovering from a spinal disorder, particularly if an inability to lead a productive lifestyle is associated with the industrial injury. The patient's inability to "see a light at the end of the tunnel" may produce a reactive depression, often associated with anxiety and agitation. The musculoskeletal injury itself may be associated with emotional distress as expressed by rebellion against authority or job dissatisfaction. Poor coping styles associated with reaction to stress or underlying personality disorders may be manifested in anger, hostility, and noncompliance directed at the therapeutic team. Organic brain dysfunction from age, alcohol, drugs, a supposedly minor head injury, or limited intelligence may produce cognitive dysfunctions that make patients difficult to manage and refractory to education.

Many chronic musculoskeletal disorders exist within an occupational "disability system." Workers' compensation laws initially were devised to protect workers' income and to provide timely medical benefits following industrial accidents. In return for providing these worker rights, employers were absolved of certain consequences of negligence, generally including cost-capped liability for any injury, no matter how severe, set by state or federal statute. Unfortunately, certain disincentives to recovery may emerge. One outcome of a guaranteed paycheck, while temporary total disability persists, is that there may be limited incentives for an early return to work. A casual approach to surgical decision making and rehabilitation may lead to further deconditioning, both mental and physical, making getting well more problematic. Complicating matters even further is the observation that no group (other than the employer) has a verifiable financial incentive to return patients to productivity rapidly. In consequence, an assortment of health professionals, attorneys, insurance companies, and vocational rehabilitation specialists are involved who have limited motivation to combat "footdragging" on the disability issue.

Early efforts to distinguish between *functional* (*nonorganic*) and *organic* pain did not meet with success. The complex nature of chronic pain makes it difficult to categorize component factors as purely physical or psychological. Chronic pain must be understood as an interactive, psychophysiological behavior pattern wherein the physical and the psychological overlap. The focus of psychological evaluation of the pain patient must shift away from functional versus organic distinctions to the identification of psychological behavioral motivators for each patient. These characteristics impact a patient's disability and his or her response to treatment efforts. Treatment planning and the prediction of favorable treatment outcome are facilitated by first identifying and then controlling these factors.

Specific assessment methods are covered in another chapter. The goal is to obtain a DSM-IV psychiatric diagnosis, particularly axis I or II, to assist the interdisciplinary treatment team in understanding and dealing with the preexisting and posttraumatic barriers to recovery. Depression, anxiety, substance use, and stress disorders frequently accompany chronic back pain, as do preexisting personality disorders and childhood abuse experiences. Socioeconomic factors related to compensation for the injury (or its premature cessation), may be factored in with the variety of problems associated with education, transferable skills, or family distress. Multidisciplinary medical treatment may include psychiatric interventions to detoxify and stabilize on psychotropic medication before the interdisciplinary team becomes involved in a treatment approach that requires education and counseling as significant components. Individualizing pain management, stress controls, and education as well as guidance toward future return to productivity is a vital outgrowth of the psychosocial assessment.

TERTIARY INTERDISCIPLINARY FUNCTIONAL-RESTORATION TREATMENT

Sports Medicine Concepts and Physical Training

The principles of sports medicine have come to be used generally to refer not merely to the rehabilitation of the competitive athlete. Instead, they have been modified to emerge as a conceptual and methodologic framework for actively treating all persons who wish to return to high levels of function. Its component parts are shown in Table 1. Much of the initial work was done with extremity injury, but these concepts now involve the spine as well.

An injury can be seen either as a massive overload that is generated exogenously or as a cumulative trauma that is generated endogenously. Whatever the source of the musculoskeletal insult, the initial phases following overload are characterized by hemorrhage and

TABLE 1. *Components of a functional restoration program*

Quantification of physical capacity and functional capacity
Quantification of psychological function
Reactivation for restoration of fitness
Reconditioning of the injured functional unit (weak link)
Retraining in multi-unit functional task performance
Work simulation in common generic tasks
Multimodal disability management program
Vocational/societal reintegration
Formalized outcome tracking
Posttreatment fitness maintenance program and monitoring

edema. After several days, cellular infiltration and enzymatic degradation of necrotic tissues occur, with involvement of prostaglandins, bradykinins, and kallikreins. A proliferative phase follows, with its timing and duration related to the quality of the blood supply in the area and other systemic factors, such as diabetes, cardiovascular and pulmonary disease, or cigarette smoking. Random deposition of collagen fibers takes place in the initial days of this phase. Subsequently, the collagen fibers align along lines of stress in a generalized form of Wolff's Law, termed the *Wolff's Law of mesothelial tissues*. This law basically states that tissue will align along lines of stress under conditions of both homeostasis and healing to produce the strongest, least adherent, and most efficient amounts of tissue. Clearly, a small amount of tissue injury with relatively good nutrition and low-grade stresses, such as might occur with a minor sprain or contusion, will proceed quickly through this process. Conversely, when extremely high stress, poor tissue nutrition (such as might involve the large, avascular discs), and substantial injury have occurred, considerably delayed and poorer quality healing may be anticipated. This is probably generally the case in the spine, just as it is in fractures of long bones. Finally, however, the injured area is left with a scar, visible or hidden, which has matured to fill the injured area but lacks the resilience, strength, and durability of the original tissue. If the scar is asymmetric in an ax-

ial structure, such as the spine, whether produced by injury, degeneration, or surgical trauma, one might anticipate severe disturbances of biomechanical performance in the critical spinal articulations as a secondary consequence of the healing process. Besides scar tissue, actual joint injury may occur in the spine or extremities, leading to misalignment and ultimately to development of *degenerative arthritis*. Posttraumatic degenerative changes are particularly common in occupational injuries associated with knee and discs or facets of the low back and midneck. Mechanical problems resulting from a combination of joint injuries and supporting mesothelial structures are also common in the foot and ankle, shoulder, and wrist.

A particular characteristic of the injured person is the tendency to splint and protect the injured area, which leads, in time, to delayed maturation of collagen (19,20), muscle atrophy (21), adhesions and deficits in joint lubrication (22), ligament atrophy (19), and bone loss (23). Subsequently, changes in endurance and aerobic fitness, discussed as the *deconditioning syndrome*, progress with declining physical capacity in which each pain episode increases patient fear, leading to more disuse and inactivity and declining physical capacity.

The physiologic approach to the deconditioning syndrome involves therapeutic exercise to address mobility, strength, endurance, cardiovascular fitness, and agility and coordination. The exercises must progress to involve simulation of customary physical activities to restore task-specific functions. Such exercises must be focused at the specific functional unit that has become deconditioned and ultimately must be generalized to whole-body functions.

Strength may be restored after injury in a variety of modes. Initially, soon after injury, when continued immobilization may be necessary, isometric exercise may be the only type that can be performed by the patient. This type of exercise involves exercising against fixed resistance without accompanying joint motion. These exercises may be done in a cast, splint, or brace, but the method has many drawbacks. First, it is the most fatiguing and least effective type of exercise (24). There is a specificity of strength training to the length of the muscle fibers at the time of exercise, with rapid fall-off in training efficiency at different muscle-fiber lengths. Additionally, there is limited translation of endurance and agility from isometric training to dynamic activities, although it can be used during the early rest phases to maintain muscle tone and produce relative resistance to atrophy. There is also some suggestion of the benefit of electric muscle stimulation in combination with isometric exercise, but some question has arisen of greater injury potential that may be associated with overvigorous contraction into a static pull (25).

Dynamic muscle training, which has been shown to be the most efficient method of training, also can be used. It involves three basic modes: isotonic, isokinetic, and psychophysical (free weights) (26). *Isotonic* exercises are those in which the same force is applied throughout the dynamic range and often is used inappropriately for exercises in which a changing lever arm actually alters the applied torque. This type of exercise most often is associated with the variable resistance devices, using a cam to equalize muscular demands throughout the dynamic range of motion.

Secondary effects of a functional restoration program are also critically important. Physical training appears to have a specific beneficial effect on pain (possibly through increased synthesis of specialized neurotransmitters) and has been demonstrated to prevent scarring and adhesions while improving cartilage nutrition. Mobility appears to be the key and can be done initially through passive and then subsequently through active means. Development of normal to supernormal strength and endurance in muscles acting around a joint may be of benefit in protecting a joint that has sustained cartilage damage or instability as a result of ligamentous incompetence. This development of protective muscular mechanisms is particularly important when a complete return to normal joint architecture can no longer be anticipated.

Thus, the specific exercise interventions involve stretching exercises, strengthening exercises, and exercises designed to improve cardiovascular fitness, endurance, and agility. Application of these exercises is individualized, based on quantitative testing of function, and the specificity and intensity of exercise change as repeated testing shows more rapid clearing of some deficits than others. A variety of weight equipment is used in such a program. A fitness maintenance program (FMP) must be established to build on the gains made during the intensive, supervised program.

Psychosocial Interventions in Functional Restoration

The patient undergoing musculoskeletal rehabilitation is customarily one who has issues of prolonged disability associated with long-standing pain. Traditional approaches have focused on pain management, which is intended to teach patients about coping with pain and modifying self-defeating behaviors. The essential flaw in this approach has been the continued focus on the patient's self-report of pain, which is ultimately self-serving and unmeasurable. In *functional restoration*, the physician emphasizes the return to function and the setting of specific goals to achieve this return, recognizing that improved physical capacity, decreased stress, and tension and return of self-esteem and self-confidence probably will reduce the patient's pain perception. The rehabilitation process itself may be a stressful and physically painful "spring training" experience for the physically and psychologically deconditioned person. One-half of the program is devoted to education and counseling, incorporating supportive and inspirational interventions to help the patient to complete rehabilitation successfully.

Individual and Group Counseling

Typically, patients are defensive during the initial psychological counseling and resist any interpretation of behavior that does not first acknowledge the validity of their physical complaints. Frustration regarding the pace of training inevitably occurs, making support during the difficult physical and psychologic tasks essential, and often takes place in one-on-one sessions. In group settings, discussion of difficulties with the process of rehabilitation are encouraged. The use of a "buddy system," pairing an advanced patient with one who is just getting started, can be helpful. There are group discussions of subjects such as psychologic testing, confidentiality, personal responsibility, the work ethic, concerns about returning to work, litigation, fear of pain, and medication or drug use. Depression is presented as a frequent component of chronic pain. Patients are encouraged to discuss their reactions to treatment staff and are given feedback about their behavior.

Behavioral Stress Management Training

Anxiety and accompanying physical tension clearly accentuate the psychophysiological experience of pain. Behavioral stress management is an important component of the treatment program. Biofeedback improves the patient's ability to relax physically and to gain better self-control over tight and painful muscles. Cognitive-behavioral training enables the patient to relax by gaining control over unwanted thoughts by directing attention away from stressors. Education in stress management teaches the patient to modulate stress by using properly controlled breathing. Group sessions provide discussion of the role of stress in sleep disturbance, stiff joints, tight muscles, and emotional distress; so patients understand more clearly the importance of a relaxation response when pain and tension increase.

Family Counseling

Families are an extremely important part of the disability process. They can encourage overprotectiveness and enable dysfunctional behavior, or they can act as instruments for recovery and return to independence. Involving spouses, parents, or children in treatment can be time consuming but is helpful. During counseling for families, a variety of topics are discussed. Permission and instruction must be given to family members to ignore illness behavior and encourage the patient to be more functional. Family members should encourage reactivation activities such as sports, exercise, and walks. The anger of family members at the patient for his lack of recovery should be diffused, and fear of reinjury should be realistically discussed. The secondary gains of being disabled (e.g., more time at home with spouse) should be acknowledged but placed in the proper perspective. The negative impacts of a chronic spinal pain syndrome on family health should be discussed. If the family supports rehabilitation, the patient is much more likely to be successful than if family members are suspicious of or in conflict with the goals of treatment.

OUTCOME MONITORING

Tertiary level nonoperative care almost always represents the final rehabilitative treatment prior to maximum medical improvement (MMI) for the most chronically disabled group of patients with work-related musculoskeletal disorders. As such, monitoring objective socioeconomic outcomes as well as more subjective self-report outcomes of pain and satisfaction is a vital part of program quality assurance. Although such outcome monitoring only recently has become a concern throughout the U.S. medical profession, its importance in work-related injuries has been recognized for some time. For more than 15 years, data on the functional restoration variant of chronic pain management have been collected (17,27,28). Details on the updated outcome collection method are summarized in Chapter 37.

The patient's ultimate socioeconomic outcomes depend on the maintenance of treatment goals. Under treatment supervision, patients generally achieve a much higher level of physical and functional capacities, which must be continued in an FMP. The patient is educated on an individualized FMP, based on the training level the patient has achieved at the program's conclusion. Repeated objective physical quantification leads to feedback to the patient on maintenance of physical capacity, which can be correlated with job demands. Relevant pieces of durable medical equipment or memberships in appropriately equipped fitness centers may be suggested. The repeated physical testing, usually performed at 3- and 6-month postintensive intervals on a voluntary basis, comprise both objective human-performance tests and self-report tests of pain, disability, depression, and treatment satisfaction as one aspect of outcome monitoring.

Combining follow-up interview information with preprogram demographic data on the same subjects can provide statistical comparisons of the ability of a comprehensive functional restoration program to deal with disability and cost. The CLBP patient accounts for 65% of the costs of degenerative musculoskeletal problems through a combination of medical treatment, lost productivity, indemnity, and government support. Irrespective of whether one is dealing with totally disabling compensation CLBP or episodic pain without significant disability, the monitoring of outcomes with objective means is essential to the discovery of what does or does not work (17,29–32).

Finally, just as the quantification of physical function and self-report provides feedback to the staff and patient on individual performance, follow-up outcome interviews provide objective statistical confirmation of success in achieving program goals on the most severely disabled patients. PRIDE's comprehensive program performs 1-year structured follow-up telephone interviews as a routine part of its ongoing quality assurance program at no additional cost to payors. The interview includes information on working status; additional surgical, medical, or chiropractic treatment; resolution of compensation issues (e.g., long-term disability, social security disability, permanent partial disability); and injury recurrence (27,33–37). It may be difficult to entice workers back for 1-year physical evaluations to obtain quantified physical capacity

and pain or disability self-report scores. With judicious attempts to maintain patient contact, a high percentage of success in performing follow-up structured phone interviews may be anticipated. The interviews must be performed while recognizing possible secondary-gain barriers to full disclosure by the patient, thus necessitating further investigation through contacts with employers, attorneys, family members, or third- party payors in some cases. Ultimately, a 98% to 99% acquisition rate for partial data and a 93% to 95% rate of actual patient contact can be anticipated. Actual outcomes may vary as a result of the disability system venue, degree of chronicity, occurrence of prerehabilitation surgery, age, compensation factors, and relevant legislation (33,34). The more subjective outcomes of pain and treatment satisfaction self-report should not be ignored.

In conclusion, the patient with chronic occupational musculoskeletal disorders represents the highest cost challenge to the medical provider. Both multidisciplinary medical assessment and interdisciplinary team programs have a place in treatment. Confusing terminology may provide the impression that secondary care is interdisciplinary, even though all participants, with the exception of physical therapists and technicians, are consultants only. Tertiary rehabilitation is not merely preventative for the development of the deconditioning syndrome but is designed to overcome its effect through quantification and education. Multiple psychosocial factors also lead to physical inhibition, complicating the physical rehabilitation process. Psychosocial assessment to help the treatment team deal with the patient on an individualized basis is essential. Recognition of vocational and socioeconomic factors in persistent disability is also vital. Such programs have demonstrated efficacy specific to the chronically disabled patient with occupational musculoskeletal disorders.

REFERENCES

1. Mayer T, Gatchel R, Polatin P, Evans T. Outcomes comparison of treatment for chronic disabling work-related upper extremity cumulative trauma to spinal disorders:

a prospective matched control trial. *J Occ Environ Med* (*in press*).

2. Vender M, Kasdan M, Truppa K. Upper extremity disorders: a literature review to determine work-relatedness. *J Hand Surg* 1995;20A:534–541.

3. Association of Schools of Public Health/National Institutes for Occupational Safety and Health. *Proposed national strategies for the prevention of leading work-related diseases and injures.* Part 1 Washington, DC: Association of Schools of Public Health, 1986:19.

4. Bureau of Labor Statistics. *Workplace injuries and illnesses in 1994.* Washington DC: U.S. Department of Labor, 1995. USDL Publication No. 95-508 WWW: http://www.bls.gov/osh/osnr0001.txt.

5. Bureau of Labor Statistics. *Workplace injuries and illnesses in 1996.* Washington, D.C., U.S. Department of Labor, 1997. USDL Publication No. 97-453. WWW: http://www.bls.gov/osh/osnr0005.txt.

6. Brogmus G, Sorock G, Webster B. Recent trends in work-related cumulative trauma disorders of the upper extremities in the United States: An evaluation of possible reasons. *J Occup Environ Med* 1996;38:401–411.

7. Webster B, Snook S. The cost of compensable upper extremity cumulative trauma disorders *J Occup Environ Med* 1994;36:713–727.

8. Hazard R. Spine update: functional restoration. *Spine* 1995;20:2345–2348.

9. Mayer T, Polatin P, Smith B, et al. Contemporary concepts in spine care: spine rehabilitation: secondary and tertiary nonoperative care. *Spine* 1995;18:2060–2066.

10. Rainville J, Sobel, Hartigan C, Wright A. The effect of compensation involvement on the reporting of pain and disability by patients referred for rehabilitation of chronic low back pain. *Spine* 1997;22:2016–2024.

11. Greenough C, Fraser R. The effects of compensation on recovery from low back injury. *Spine* 1989;14:947–955.

12. Hadler N, Carey T, Garrett J. The influence of indemnification by workers' compensation insurance on recovery from acute backache. *Spine* 1995;20:2710–2715.

13. Sanderson P, Todd B, Holt G, Getty C. Compensation, work status, and disability in low back pain patients. *Spine* 1995;20:554–556.

14. Polatin P, Kinney R, Gatchel R, Lillo E, Mayer T. Psychiatric illness and chronic low back pain: the mind and the spine—which goes first? *Spine* 1993;18:66–71.

15. Gatchel R, Mayer T, Hazard R, Rainville J, Mooney V. Functional restoration: pitfalls in evaluating efficacy [Editorial]. *Spine* 1992;17:988–995.

16. Hazard R, Fenwick J, Kalish S, et al. Functional restoration with behavioral support: a one-year perspective study of chronic low back pain patients. *Spine* 1989;14:157–165.

17. Mayer T, Gatchel R, Mayer H, Kishino N, Kelley J, Mooney V. A prospective two-year study of functional restoration in industrial low back injury: an objective assessment procedure. *JAMA* 1987;258:1763–1767.

18. Mayer T, Kondraske G, Beals S, Gatchel R. Spinal range of motion: accuracy and sources of error with inclinometric measurement. *Spine* 1997;22:1976–1984.

19. Akeson W, Amiel D, Woo S. Immobility effects on synovial joints: the pathomechanics of joint contracture. *Biorheology* 1980;17:95–100.

20. Gracovetsky S, Farfan H. The optimum spine. *Spine* 1986;11:543–573.

21. Montgomery J, Steadman J. Rehabilitation of the injured knee. *Clin Sports Med* 1985;4:333–343.

22. Salter R, Field P. The effects of continuous compression on living articular cartilage: an experimental study. *J Bone Joint Surg Am* 1961;43B:376–386.

23. Ruben C. Osteoregulatory mechanisms: Kappa Delta Award. In: *Transactions of Annual Meeting, American Academy of Orthopedic Surgeons*, New Orleans, LA, 1985

24. Hoshizaki T, Massey B. Relationships of muscular endurance among specific muscle groups for continuous and intermittent static contractions. *Res Q Exerc Sport* 1986;57:229–235.

25. Haggmark T. Comparison of isometric muscle training and electrical stimulation supplementing isometric muscle training in the recovery after major knee ligament surgery. *Am J Sports Med* 1979;7:169–171.

26. Eriksson E. Sports injuries of knee ligaments: their diagnosis, treatment, rehabilitation and prevention. *Med Sci Sports* 1976;8:133–144.

27. Mayer T, Gatchel R, Kishino N, et al. Objective assessment of spine function following industrial injury: a prospective study with comparison group and one-year follow-up. 1985 Volvo Award in Clinical Sciences. *Spine* 1985;10:482–493.

28. Mayer T, Gatchel R, Kishino N, et al. A prospective short-term study of chronic low back pain patients utilizing novel objective functional measurement. *Pain* 1986;25:53–68.

29. Brady S, Mayer T, Gatchel R. Physical progress and residual impairment quantification after functional restoration. Part 2: isokinetic trunk strength. *Spine* 1994;18:395–400.

30. Curtis L, Mayer T, Gatchel R. Physical progress and residual impairment after functional restoration. Part 3: isokinetic and isoinertial lifting capacity. *Spine* 1994;18:401–405.

31. Mayer T, Pope P, Tabor J, Bovasso E, Gatchel R. Physical progress and residual impairment quantification after functional restoration. Part I: lumbar mobility. *Spine* 1994;19:389–394.

32. Hazard R: Spine Update: Functional restoration. *Spine* 1995;20:2345–2348.

33. Mayer T, McMahon M, Gatchel R, Sparks B, Wright A, Pegues P. Socioeconomic outcomes of combined spine surgery and functional restoration in workers compensation spinal disorders with matched controls. *Spine* 1998;23:598–606.

34. Jordan K, Mayer T, Gatchel R. Should extended disability be an exclusion criterion for tertiary rehabilitation: socioeconomic outcomes of early vs. late functional restoration in compensation spinal disorders. *Spine* 1998;23:2110–2117.

35. Fishbain D, Rosomoff H, Goldbert M, et al. The prediction of return to the workplace after multidisciplinary pain center treatment. *Clin J Pain* 1993;9:3–15.

36. Garcy P, Mayer T, Gatchel R. Recurrent or new injury outcomes after return to work in chronic disabling disorders: tertiary prevention efficacy of functional restoration treatment. *Spine* 1996;21:952–959.

37. McMahon M, Gatchel R, Polatin P, Mayer T. Early childhood abuse in chronic spinal disorder patient: A major barrier to treatment success. *Spine* 1997;22:2408–2415.

Occupational Musculoskeletal Disorders
edited by T. G. Mayer, R. J. Gatchel, and P. B. Polatin.
Lippincott Williams & Wilkins, Philadelphia © 2000.

37

Objective Outcome Evaluation: Methods and Evidence

Tom G. Mayer, *J. Matthew Prescott, and †Robert J. Gatchel

*Department of Orthopedic Surgery, *Department of Case Management Services,
Productive Rehabilitation Institute of Dallas for Ergonomics (PRIDE); and
†Department of Psychiatry and Rehabilitation, University of Texas
Southwestern Medical School, Dallas, Texas 75235*

Changes in health policy and demands for improved allocation of health resources have placed great pressure on medical professionals to validate their use of resources. The focus is on cost containment because health care expenditures in the United States have exceeded 14% of the gross domestic product (GDP) and continue to grow faster than the inflation rate. Particular scrutiny has focused on health care utilization in the treatment of the prevalent musculoskeletal disorder, low back pain, and spinal disorders in general. This scrutiny results partly from its visibility as an extremely high-cost area of treatment (the most expensive benign condition in virtually all industrialized countries) and the rapid 14-fold increase in cost over a single recent decade (1). Additionally, low back pain is a condition involving quality of life rather than mortality and, as such, may be allocated a lower reimbursement priority by health planners, particularly in view of the difficulty in ascribing spinal disorders to specific anatomic diagnoses. In response to these challenges, great interest in health policy, treatment guidelines, and outcome monitoring emerged virtually overnight (2–7). Upper-extremity cumulative trauma disorders (CTD) now are projected to surpass low back disorders as the most frequent category leading to work disability in U.S. manufacturing plants

(8). Although a controversial topic, CTDs involving the upper extremity have at least quadrupled as a percentage of all state workers' compensation claims over the past decade (9–11). The average cost of an upper-extremity CTD case in 1992 was 80% higher than the average of all workers' compensation cases (12).

In a recent article, Turk and Rudy (13) presented an excellent overview of the critical issues to be considered when evaluating treatment-outcome studies, including statistical conclusion validity, internal validity, and treatment of outcome criteria. As part of that overview, they emphasized that in chronic pain and disability outcome research, follow-up periods of at least 1 year after treatment discharge are recommended. Moreover, when dealing with a complex problem such as pain, multiple measures should be used to tap the relevant demands of physical, psychosocial, behavioral, and functional indices. Indeed, although the demands for greater objectivity have been forthcoming from many sources, when a subjective construct, such as "pain," is being treated, considerable controversy exists over the appropriate mix of objective and subjective measurements to be used in outcome assessment (14). Whereas some commercially available products have come on the market for individual physician office computerization and data collection, including some specific to the musculoskeletal system, none is targeted specifically to the needs of health providers who deal primarily with occupational musculoskeletal disorders.

Over the past decade, innovative rehabilitation approaches for occupational musculoskeletal disorders have appeared. The methods of these approaches have placed greater emphasis on physical activation of patients and psychosocial attention to disability issues rather than on pain alone. It has been recognized over the years that patients being paid for remaining disabled and nonproductive will behave differently from patients who are uncompensated (15–21). As such, interest in spinal rehabilitation was spurred by recent attention to objective socioeconomic outcomes, such as return to work, as critical measures of treatment success (22). Subsequently, treatment efficacy was demonstrated for both early and late rehabilitation treatment for disabled low back pain patients in various environments (23–26). As might be anticipated, the attention elicited by positive return-to-work statistics in a previously recalcitrant chronic pain group (i.e., disability lasting longer than the natural history of soft-tissue healing) prompted other studies, some of which altered the outcome variables or treatment approach to permit comparison with previous outcome studies (27–29). The lack of a standardized outcome evaluation method prevents the reader of such articles from assessing the methodologic issues associated with comparison of different treatments.

Controversy and great variability continue to define the field of outcome evaluation for musculoskeletal disorders in general. It is the purpose of the present article to provide the reader with a standardized, structured interview instrument for assessing both objective and subjective outcomes of musculoskeletal treatment based on the model used for research purposes at the Productive Rehabilitation Institute of Dallas for Ergonomics (PRIDE) in Dallas, Texas. We propose the use of this standardized instrument to assist other surgeons and rehabilitation specialists in providing efficient, cost-

effective outcome monitoring and data collection. Although this method has been used primarily for publications on spinal disorders, it also can be used for other disabling musculoskeletal disorders (25,30—36).

EVALUATION OVERVIEW

Socioeconomic outcome variables specific to disabling musculoskeletal work injury relate to four major dimensions of societal functioning, each combining several important elements we chose to evaluate as vital 1-year socioeconomic outcomes as components of our outcome tracking and quality assurance systems Table 1.

Work return evaluates whether the patient ever returned to work after evaluation, whereas *work retention* defines whether the patient actually continues working at the 1-year outcome interview. *Health care utilization* is another important cost driver in the workers' compensation system and is evaluated by three separate elements from the perspective of disability and the use of health re-

TABLE 1. *Basic dimensions and elements of objective socioeconomic outcome monitoring for the PRIDE Model*

I. Return to work
  A. Work return
  B. Work retention (1 yr)
II. Health utilization
  A. Surgery to injured musculoskeletal area
  B. Percent patients visiting a new health provider (continued care—*and documentation*-seeking behaviors)
  C. Number of visits to new health providers
III. Recurrent (Same musculoskeletal area) or new (different area) injury claims
  A. Percent with recurrent or new injury claims
  B. Percent with injury claims involving work absence (lost time)
IV. Case closure
  A. Resolution of legal/administrative disputes over permanent partial/total impairment or disability resulting from occupational injury
  B. Resolution of related disputes (third party personal injury or product liability claims)
  C. Resolution of financial claims arising from perceived permanent disability (LTD, SSI, SSDI, etc.)

LTD, long term disability; SSI, supplemental security income; SSDI, Social Security Disability Income.

sources. *Additional surgery* to the same area of injury is potentially the most costly element; however, a person seeking attention from medical providers clearly identifies a treated subject who has not given up the role of patient. As such, we assess the *percentage of patients visiting health providers other than their referring and rehabilitation physicians*. We also assess the number of visits to such health providers. Another dimension of great importance that has achieved insufficient attention in recent years is *recurrent injury claims to the same musculoskeletal area* (or new injuries to other musculoskeletal areas). Fully reconditioned patients have shown remarkably low rates of recurrent injury in the year succeeding their preparation for return to work by optimum physical and mental reconditioning (35). In this outcome, we evaluate the percentage of patients who have made new or recurrent injury claims involving the musculoskeletal system and the separate issue of whether these injuries resulted in absence from work (*lost time*).

The final dimension of socioeconomic outcomes considered in the evaluation system for occupational musculoskeletal disorders is *case closure*. Not only is case closure a demonstrated major area of indemnity cost that generally represents 10% to 30% of workers' compensation claim costs, but in certain venues [e.g., the Federal Employers Liability Act (FELA)] and certain other federally mandated systems), the cost of case closure in some cases is well over 90% of total claims cost. Often certain related secondary costs must be considered tied to the occupational injury claim.

Thus, the elements we follow begin with the patients who have resolved the legal and administrative disputes tied to permanency claims (partial or total impairment or disability resulting from the original occupational injury). Not infrequently, a third-party claim is related to the occupational injury, such as when a subcontractor is considered to have performed a negligent act that led to the occupational injury. In these cases, resolution of third-party personal negligence or product li-

ability injury claims is tied to resolution of the original occupational injury. They also provide for subrogation of the occupational injury costs, often greatly affecting the behaviors of multiple stakeholders in the injury compensation system. Finally, for persons who continue to claim additional financial benefits from perceived permanent partial or total disability, other sources of payment may be tapped, including long-term disability (LTD) policies, federal sources within social security [Supplemental Security Income (SSI) or Social Security Disability Insurance (SSDI)], employer medical retirement options, and union disability pension benefits. This financial element also may include a variety of state and local welfare benefits available exclusively, or in greater measure, to claimants who have a demonstrable handicap or disability.

Although self-assessment of pain, disability, treatment satisfaction, and health status are all important factors in patient outcome evaluation, the nature of the indemnity, productivity, and health care components in workers' compensation makes more objective, quantitative, socioeconomic outcomes monitoring highly desirable and feasible. The present system, however, also assesses each of these more *subjective* self-reported dimensions of patient perception using simple, validated instruments or digital questions.

DATA-COLLECTION SYSTEM

Figure 1 (*A* and *B*) illustrates the data sheet used for pretreatment, posttreatment, and interval follow-up monitoring used in the PRIDE program. Space is provided for comments on the back of the sheet (Fig. 1*B*). In this way, all interview data, including 1-year outcome information (obtained in person or by telephone), can be provided on the same sheet. Data for the initial column (pretreatment) vary in certain respects from data collected during the posttreatment period. This data sheet is used as a supplement to the physical-capacity (and pain, disability, and depression self-report) test data sheets at the time of

MCM DATA SHEET QFE / PPQE
#4502-A   Page 4-A Rev Date -6/1/98

NAME:_____   CASE TYPE _____   Total Treatment Hours_____   D/C Date_____
                                 2 letter State   (_____)
*Code Required   Abbreviation
                                 (work comp cases only)   PPQE or DC/QFE

                                                    DC Dx Code*_____   DC Dx Code*_____ DC Dx Code*_____
                                                    DC Dx Code*_____   DC Dx Code*_____ DC Dx Code*_____

                    QFE

Interviewer's Initials   _____   Interviewer's Initials   _____   _____   _____   _____

DATE:	_____	**DATE:**	_____	_____	_____	_____
EMPLOYER at time of injury	_____	**EMPLOYER**	_____	_____	_____	_____
Job Title	_____	Job Title	_____	_____	_____	_____
Job Code*	_____	Job Code*	_____	_____	_____	_____
HRS PER DAY/DAYS PER WK	___/___	**HRS/DAY / DAYS/WK**	___/___	___/___	___/___	___/___
TIME AT JOB OF INJURY (mos.)	_____	**PRESENT JOB** (mos.)	_____		_____	_____
Lifting/Carrying Job Requirements	FRQ/OCC	Recent/Present Lifting/	FRQ/OCC	FRQ/OCC	FRQ/OCC	FRQ/OCC
for Job of Injury	___/___	Carrying Job Requirements	___/___	___/___	___/___	___/___
Job Demand of Job of Injury*	_____	Recent/Present Job Demand*	_____	_____	_____	_____
PRESENT WORK STATUS*	_____	**PRESENT WORK STATUS***	_____	_____	_____	_____
PRE-INJ JOB AVAILABILITY*	_____	**LIMITATIONS**	___/___	___/___	___/___	___/___
TOTAL YRS WORKING/		Temp. or Perm	_____	_____	_____	_____
TOTAL # EMPLOYERS	___/___	Release/RTW Date	_____	_____	_____	_____
UNION MEMBER Y or N	_____	**FIRST DAY ON JOB**	_____	_____	_____	_____
PRIOR WORK INJ.* Y or N	_____	**INCOME SOURCE***	_____	_____	_____	_____
TOTAL DISABILITY	_____	**CASE SETTLEMENT**				
(total months cumulative of TTD)		Original Injury-Work related*	_____			
Full Duty ____ (mos)		Date Settled (mo/dy/yr)	_____			
Partial Duty ____ (mos)		Open Medical (mos)	_____			
Light/Mod Duty ____ (mos)		**CASE SETTLEMENT**				
WEEKLY COMPENSATION RATE	$_____	3rd party/Personal Injury*	_____			
NET SALARY AT TIME OF INJURY	$_____	**HEALTH UTILIZATION:***				
(weekly)		Original Injury Y or N	_____			
INCOME SOURCE*	_____	**SURGERY: ORIG. INJ.***	_____			
CASE SETTLEMENT		Y or N				
Original Injury-Work related*	_____			Dx_____	Dx_____	Dx_____
Date Settled (mo/dy/yr)	_____			Surg_____	Surg_____	Surg_____
Open Medical (mos)	_____			Date_____	Date_____	Date_____
CASE SETTLEMENT						
3rd Party/Personal Injury*	_____			Dx_____	Dx_____	Dx_____
HEALTH UTILIZATION:*				Surg_____	Surg_____	Surg_____
Original Injury Y or N	_____			Date_____	Date_____	Date_____
SURGERY: ORIG. INJ.* Y or N	_____					

Dx_____   Dx_____   Dx_____   **NEW INJURY***
                                              Date of New Injury/   _____   _____   _____   _____
Surg_____   Surg_____   Surg_____   Number days lost time   ___/___   ___/___   ___/___   ___/___
Date_____   Date_____   Date_____   Musculoskeletal modifiers _____ _____   _____   _____

Dx_____   Dx_____   Dx_____
Surg_____   Surg_____   Surg_____
A   Date_____   Date_____   Date_____

FIG. 1. A. Outcome data sheet used by the Productive Rehabilitation Institute of Dallas for Ergonomics (*PRIDE*) and affiliates for in-person pretreatment and interim interviews and for posttreatment outcome monitoring. **B**. Outcome data sheet (back) with space for comments.

MCM DATA SHEET QFE / PPQE	
#4502-B	Page 4-B Rev Date -4/8/98

NAME:_____

			6-week	3-month	6-month	12-month

JOB SATISFACTION*
(Pre Injury/Post Injury)   Pre/Post __/__

HEALTH UTILIZATION New Injury*
Visits/Surgery   __/__   __/__   __/__   __/__

REPRESENTED BY ATTORNEY   Yes No

Dx_____   Dx_____   Dx_____

TELEPHONE NUMBER   _____

Surg____   Surg____   Surg____

WORK NUMBER   _____

Date____   Date____   Date____

Dx_____   Dx_____   Dx_____

Surg____   Surg____   Surg____

Date __   Date____   Date____

FMP-EQUIPT*   _____   _____   _____   _____

FMP-FREQ*   _____   _____   _____   _____

FMP-STATUS*   _____   _____   _____   _____

JOB SATISFACTION*
(most recent job)   _____   _____   _____   _____

RX SATISFACTION*   _____   _____   _____   _____

PAIN LEVEL *   _____   _____   _____   _____

? TELE. INTERVIEW ?   YES NO   YES NO   YES NO   YES NO

RECENT TELEPHONE #   _____   _____   _____   _____

WORK NUMBER   _____   _____   _____   _____

COMMENTS FROM QFE/PPQE INTERVIEWS

_____
_____
_____
_____
_____
_____
_____
_____
_____
_____
_____
_____
_____
_____
_____
_____
_____
_____
_____
_____

B

FIG. 1. Continued.

pretreatment testing, discharge, and postprogram quantitative evaluations customarily performed 1, 3, and 6 months after completion of the PRIDE comprehensive program. Physical-capacity testing (with an in-person interview) is optional at the 1-year follow-up. Failure to appear for testing at 1-year follow-up triggers the telephone interview process (using the identical outcome data form). Psychosocial data also are routinely collected prospectively (15,37–45). Forms can be used for interviews at any desired interview time and for certain projects have been used 2 and 5 years posttreatment.

Figure 2 (*A*, *B*, and *C*) illustrates the numeric and alphabetic codes used for the treatment evaluation assessment data sheet. Within each category, stringent efforts have been made to cover all possible eventualities likely to be encountered; however, certain positive findings trigger an automatic demand for a comment on the back of the data sheet (e.g., specifying the type of surgery performed or anatomic location of a new injury). Alphanumeric codes are chosen primarily for convenient insertion into a computerized database for subsequent analysis and comparison with demographic, historic, and physical-capacity data. A supplemental surgery code sheet delineates specific types of surgical procedures, and a diagnosis code sheet categorizes musculoskeletal diagnoses (Figs. 3 and 4). The remainder of this section details the use of the codes for optimal discrimination between patients for each outcome variable:

Pretreatment Data Collection

Job of Injury Data

The top portion of the first column (Fig. 1) deals with information about the job the patient was doing at the time of injury. After noting the appropriate case type [e.g., state workers' compensation, Federal Employees Compensation Act (FECA), FELA], the interviewer identifies the patient's original employer, job title, working hours, and number of months employed at the job (including time worked after the injury if the patient was not totally disabled). In most cases, pretreatment data are supplied by the patient. On admission to a comprehensive program, efforts are made to contact the employer to verify job information and date of injury. At the posttreatment interview, therapists obtain similar data about the patient's new job (if applicable).

The next two pieces of information are the lifting demands (frequently, occasionally), followed by the *job demand* category, which combines the lifting demands with the amount of significant vibration experienced on the job (e.g., truck driving, heavy equipment operation, or vibratory hand tools) into a four-point system. Vibration is a modifier that increases the level of work demands by one or more categories based on the hours of vibration per day and the lifting demands (Fig. 2*A*).

Patient report of present work status (e.g., light duty, not working) and impressions of job availability with the employer of injury are recorded next. Other job-related information sought includes reported total years in the workforce and total number of employers. These data provide the ability to assess job stability. Patient report of preinjury and postinjury job satisfaction is a significant factor relative to motivation for return to work. This information is used in planning and counseling the patient about vocational options.

Disability Income Data

To obtain a clear picture of the patient's disability history, several items provide useful information. Of particular interest is whether the patient has a history of work-related claims and, if so, the approximate number of claims. Also, specific to the injury for which the patient is being evaluated, the length of time (in months) performing full duty, partial duty, or light duty will provide needed background data to use in projecting employer receptivity to return to work at the original place of employment. The only other items unique to pretreatment data collection (located before "case settlement" items) are the two income items: the worker's weekly compensation rate (or short- and long-term disability payments) com-

---

MEDICAL CASE MANAGEMENT DATA CODE SHEET
#4518

Revised - 04/28/98

CASE TYPE [Write the corresponding code(s) for the appropriate Case Type(s) in the space provided] *Refer to State Code Supplement Sheet on all Workers' Compensation Cases (to be completed at the time of the QFE/Disability Assessment)*

1. Workers' Compensation Systems (2 letter state code required)
   A. Texas Workers' Compensation Case (post-January, 1991)
   B. Texas Workers' Compensation Case (pre-January, 1991)
   C. Non-Texas Workers' Compensation Case
   D. Other
2. Federal Workers' Compensation Systems
   A. FECA (Department of Labor)
   B. FELA (Railroad)
   C. Longshore Harbor Workers Act
   D. Maritime-Jones Act
   E. Other

3. Non-Subscriber
   A. Texas Non-Subscriber
   B. Occupational Health Policy/Owner Operator Rig
   C. Liability Policy Holder
   D. Other
4. Unregulated Compensation Systems
   A. Standard Personal Injury
   B. No Fault Personal Injury
   C. Longterm Disability (LTD)
   D. Private Insurance
   E. Other

EMPLOYER - Job Code (DOT)
1. Professional, Technical, and Managerial
2. Clerical and Sales
3. Service (food, housekeeping, health aides)
4. Agriculture
5. Chemical and Refining

6. Machine Trade (metal/wood processing, heavy manufacturing)
7. Light Manufacturing (assembly, repair)
8. Construction Trades
9. Miscellaneous (transportation, packaging, heavy equipment, natural resource extraction)

PRESENT OR MOST RECENT JOB DEMAND CATEGORY:

1. Sedentary/Light 0-15 lbs. lifting frequent
                    0-25 lbs. occasional

   No vibration present

2. Light/Medium 16-25 lbs. frequent
                 26-50 lbs. occasional

   If Vibration Present: Less than 2 hrs/day
                         with lifting demands in
                         Category 1 or 2

3. Medium/Heavy 26-50 lbs frequent
                 51-100 lbs. occasional

   If Vibration Present: More than 2 hrs/day with
                         lifting demands in Category 1 or 2
4. Heavy/Very Heavy More than 50 lbs frequent
                     More than 100 lbs occasional

   If Vibration Present: More than 2 hrs/day with
                         lifting demands in Category 3 or 4

WORK STATUS [When using working code(s), record the appropriate modifier(s) which may be more than one modifier.]

Current Employment Status?

WORKING CODES
1. Same employer/same job
2. Same employer/different job
3. Different employer/same job
4. Different employer/different job

5. Vocational training or school/retraining
6. Self-employed

WORK TIME MODIFIERS
A. 8 hrs. or more per day (Full Time)
B. 4-7 hrs. per day (Modified Work Schedule)
C. Less than 4 hrs per day ((Part Time)
D. Other (explain on back page)

NON-WORKING CODES

USED FOR PPQE'S ONLY

0. Presently Not Working (QFE)
   /Never returned to work after PRIDE (PPQE)
7. Denies work due to employment factors exclusively (i.e., laid off, seeking new job, moving family, seasonal fluctuations as nature of business, company went out of business, etc.)
8. Denies work but engages in activities that are or will be income producing (i.e., crafts, rental property, etc., or possible illicit activities, etc.)
9. Denies work but participating in non-income producing activity (i.e., retirement, housewife, volunteer work).
10. Returned to work, but not presently working because of new injury.
11. Returned to work, but not presently working because of original injury.

NOTE: For 12 month interview, if not 1,A –6,A, comments required.

JOB AVAILABILITY [Pre-injury job (QFE - patient report) (6WK PPQE - employer report)].
(Use any combination of code(s) and modifier(s))
0. No job available
1. Full Duty
2. Modified Duty (physical restrictions to pre-injury job)
3. Light Duty (less physically demanding job)

4. Transitional Return-To-Work (less than full-time hours)
5. Unknown

A. 8 hrs. or more per day
B. 4-7 hrs. per day
C. Less than 4 hrs. per day

PRIOR WORK INJURIES *(If Yes, select the appropriate # code)* [QFE Interview only]
0. No prior injuries
1. 1 prior injury
2. 2 prior injuries
3. 3 prior injuries
4. 4 prior injuries
5. 5 prior injuries
6. 6 or more prior injuries

INCOME SOURCE [Is the patient receiving any income, public assistance, etc...?] [Can be more than one choice] (PPQE only)
1. Personal Finances
   A. Salary
   B. Savings
   C. Loans
   D. Retirement Benefits
   E. Selling possesions
   F. Other
2. Family Assistance
   A. Cash
   B. Child Support
   C. Alimony
   D. Other

3. TTD Benefits
   A. TIBS
   B. Indemnity Payments/Wage Replacement
   C. Other
4. Impairment Disability Benefit/Insurance Settlement
   A. Ongoing (weekly, etc.) (IIBS)
   B. Lump Sum/Cash Settlement
   C. Supplemental Benefits (SIBS)
   D. Other

A

FIG. 2. A, B, C: Alphanumeric codes used with the outcome data sheet (*ODS*). The interviewer inserts the appropriate code on the data sheet, which is subsequently entered into a computerized database. Instructions demand additional detail on the back of the ODS (comment section) when necessary.

5. Private Disability Benefits
   A. STD
   B. LTD
   C. Disability Policy
   D. Other
6. Government Retirement/Disability Benefits
   A. SSDI
   B. SSI
   C. Military Retirement
   D. Veterans Benefits
   E. Other

7. Unemployment/Training Benefit
   A. Unemployment
   B. Vocational Stipend (TRC)
   C. Other
8. Welfare
   A. AFDC
   B. Foodstamps
   C. Section 8 Housing Assistance
   D. Other
9. Community Assistance Programs
   A. Charitable Programs
   B. Agency Assistance
   C. Churches
   D. Other

CASE SETTLEMENT: WORK RELATED INJURY

0. No Case
1. Case settled before PRIDE (if QFE, also PPQE)
2. Case settled after PRIDE (PPQE only)
3. Case settled, MIR in dispute
4. Case not settled
5. Case resolved, no settlement applicable

MODIFIERS:
A. Impairment/Schedule
B. Litigated
C. Negotiated

CASE SETTLEMENT: THIRD PARTY CLAIM [select as many letter/number combination codes as applies]

0. No case
1. Case settled before PRIDE
2. Case settled after PRIDE
3. Case dropped/terminated
4. Case still active

MODIFIERS:
A. Original
B. Intervening (Prior to PRIDE)
C. Subsequent (after PRIDE admission/discharge)

HEALTH UTILIZATION: ORIGINAL INJURY [Same injured musculoskeletal area(s) ONLY]
(If Yes, code the appropriate response)

0. No additional treatment (only standard recheck visits)
1. 1 to 5 Health Care Professional visits (not to PRIDE)
2. 6 to 10 visits (not to PRIDE)
3. 11 to 15 visits (not to PRIDE)
4. 16 to 20 visits (not to PRIDE)
5. 21 to 30 visits (not to PRIDE)
6. Greater than 30 visits (not to PRIDE)

NOTE: For 12 month interview, if # 2 through #6 above, comments required.

SURGERIES: ORIGINAL INJURY [Same injured musculoskeletal area(s) ONLY]
(If Yes, select the appropriate # code below and proceed with the appropriate coding from the DIAGNOSIS CODE SHEET AND SURGERY CODE SUPPLEMENT to be recorded in the appropriate space(s)).

0. No Surgery
1. 1 surgery
2. 2 surgeries
3. 3 surgeries
4. 4 surgeries
5. 5 surgeries
6. 6 or more surgeries

NOTE: For 12 month interview, if surgery, comments required.

NEW INJURY [Can be more than one choice, and modifier codes always required] Indicate lost time in space provided on MCM Data Sheet.
(PPQE only) if Yes, select appropriate choice(s) and modifier codes

1. Exacerbation of previous injury (on the job)
2. New injury same area (OTJ)
3. New injury, different muskulosketal area (OTJ)
4. New medical condition (non-muskuloskeletal - OTJ)
5. Exacerbation of previous injury (not OTJ)
6. New injury same area (not OTJ)
7. New injury, different muskuloskeletal area (not OTJ)
8. New medical condition (non-muskuloskeletal - not OTJ)

MUSCULOSKELETAL
(NEW INJURY) MODIFIERS

1. Cervical
2. Thoracic
3. Lumbar
4. Shoulder
5. Elbow
6. Wrist
7. Hand
8. Hip
9. Knee
10. Ankle
11. Foot
12. Other

EXTREMITY/JOINT
MODIFIERS
(must select for modifier items 4-1
A. Right
B. Left
C. Bilateral

HEALTH UTILIZATION: NEW INJURY - MUSCULOSKELETAL AREA(S) ONLY [Can be more than one choice]
(use only if 1,2,3,5,6 or 7 chosen above)   **(PPQE only)** (If YES to surgery, proceed with the appropriate coding from the DIAGNOSIS CODE SHEET and SURGERY CODES -SUPPLEMENT).

Health Visits:
0. No additional treatment
1. 1 to 5 health care professional visits (not to PRIDE)
2. 6 to 10 visits (not to PRIDE)
3. 11 to 15 visits (not to PRIDE)
4. 16 to 20 visits (not to PRIDE)
5. 21 to 30 visits (not to PRIDE)
6. Greater than 30 visits (not to PRIDE)

Surgery(s):
0. No surgery
A. 1 surgery
B. 2 surgeries
C. 3 surgeries
D. 4 surgeries
E. 5 surgeries
F. 6 or more surgeries

NOTE: For 12 month interview, if YES to surgery, and/or if health visits 4 or greater, comments required.

FITNESS MAINTENANCE PLAN (FMP) EQUIPMENT (Using the list below, select the patient response(s) to equipment recommended by PRIDE)
PPQE ONLY

1. Bricks
2. Free Weights (dumbbells)
3. Hand Gripper
4. Health Club

B

FIG. 2. Continued.

pared with the net salary at the time of injury. Additionally, space is provided to record any other sources of income received by the patient. These basic financial factors constitute only a small part of assembling a complete picture of the financial incentives and disincentives created by the patient's disability. Combined with other information, these data assist in developing a financially viable plan for future productivity.

5.	Health Rider		12.	Ski machine
6.	Heavy Job demands		13.	Stationery Bike
7.	Home gym		14.	Stretches
8.	Lifeline gym		15.	Treadmill
9.	Running/jogging		16.	Walking program
10.	Roman chair		17.	Weight boot
11.	Rowing machine		18.	Didn't receive anything
			19.	Other

FITNESS MAINTENANCE PLAN (FMP) FREQUENCY [Choose the most appropriate response (in the last month the maximum number of times exercised in one week)]

		PPQE ONLY	
0.	None	4.	4x/week
1.	1x/week	5.	5x/week
2.	2x/week	6.	6x/week
3.	3x/week	7.	7x/week

FITNESS MAINTENANCE PLAN (FMP) STATUS (Inquire of current participation in any exercise program learned at PRIDE)

(if Yes, code the appropriate response)

0. None
1. All
2. Stretching injured area
3. Aerobic activity (i.e. jogging, biking, swimming)
4. Functional work activities (i.e. lifting heavy work, climbing, etc)
5. Functional non-work activities (i.e. lifting bricks, climbing, heavy work)
6. Recreational/sports activities

JOB SATISFACTION (Have the patient select one choice only based on his/her opinion of job satisfaction for the job of injury (QFE) or most recent job (PPQE). (QFE - preinjury and post injury codes required).

1. Very satisfied	3. Neither satisfied nor dissatisfied	5. Very dissatisfied
2. Satisfied	4. Dissatisfied	

TREATMENT SATISFACTION [Have the patient select one choice only based on his/her opinion of treatment]   *(PPQE's only)*

1. Very satisfied	3. Neither satisfied nor dissatisfied	5. Very dissatisfied
2. Satisfied	4. Dissatisfied	

PAIN INTENSITY - [Have the patient select one choice only based on his/her pain (original injury) at the time of PPQE interviews]

C   No Pain   0   2   4   6   8   10 **Worst Possible Pain**

FIG. 2. Continued.

Data regarding the specifics of the status of a case settlement are collected on work-related injuries regardless of case type. In the event a third-party claim is associated with the work-related injury, this information is recorded in the specified space for third-party or personal-injury claims. For cases without a work-related injury and only a third-party claim, the appropriate codes would be reflected in the designated places. To complete the history of the patient's disability, the extent of utilization of medical treatment and surgical procedures performed is recorded.

Communication Sources

Two items, union and legal representation, serve to alert the interviewer to potential key persons or groups involved in communication on disability issues. In the United States,

a legal representative for the injured employee frequently is involved when chronic disability exists, and in some instances union representatives may provide guidance to injured members. Supplements to this section are the last items at the bottom of the page, with telephone numbers for home and work (if applicable) to allow careful monitoring of the patient's medical progress in the event of unanticipated absence. Additional marital, insurance, financial, and legal data are included in the standardized medical history obtained from each patient but are not routinely coded. The "psychology data sheet" may code some marital and financial data.

Interim and Posttreatment Data Collection

The remaining columns of the outcome data sheet refer to data obtained at postpro-

SURGERY CODES - SUPPLEMENT

rev 4/17/98

Basic Instructions :
There are three lines that need to be filled out with specific codes as follows:
    a. Diagnosis Code: The alpha numeric diagnosis code (from diagnosis code sheet) that with a diagnosis that is specific to
        the surgery performed (Example: 1e 0 for C5 ACF)
    b. Dates: Enter 2 digit month/4 digit year (if unknown: estimate month Example: 04/1994)
    c. Surgery Code: This will be a 3 digit surgery code described below

Each surgery performed for one of the compensable diagnosis should be laid out, preferably in chronological order. Because
the date will be correlated to the date of compensable injury, even *relevant* pre-injury surgery to the same body part can be
entered and should be recognized by the computer as surgery pre-existing versus surgery after the compensable injury. Multiple
surgeries for multiple compensable body parts can also be recorded with this system.

Specific Surgery Codes:
This system will have 3 digits based on the following:
    a. Digits 1/2: surgical procedure codes
    b. Digit 3: spinal surgical level modifier

Surgical Procedure Codes:

SPINAL DISCECTOMY
10 = Discectomy unspecified
11 = Microdiscectomy
12 = Percutaneous Discectomy
13 = Chemonucleolysis

SPINAL FUSION PROCEDURES
20 = Fusion unspecified
21 = Anterior fusion
22 = Posterior interbody fusion
23 = Posterior lateral fusion
24 = 360 Fusion
25 = Pseudoarthrosis repair
26 = Hardware removal
27 = Bone stimulator removal
28 = Discectomy+fusion
29 = Any decompression + fusion

NEURAL DECOMPRESSION PROCEDURES
30 = Neural decompression, spinal (foraminal/central)
31 = Neural decompression, carpal tunnel
32 = Neural decompression, cubital tunnel
33 = Neural decompression, thoracic outlet or
     brachial plexus
34 = Neural decompression, sympathectomy
35 = Neural decompression, miscellaneous

FRACTURE/DISLOCATION PROCEDURES
40 = Fracture/dislocation: Closed reduction
41 = Fracture/dislocation: Open reduction
42 = Pseudoarthrosis repair
43 = Hardware removal
44 = Amputation
45 = Repair nerve laceration
46 = Repair tendon laceration
47 = Repair, ligament tear

JOINT DERANGEMENTS
50 = Degenerative joint disease (DJD), unspecified
     procedure
51 = DJD: Arthroscopic joint decompression or
     chondroplasty, unspecified
52 = Soft tissue procedure, unspecified
     (Ex. patellar realignment)
53 = Arthroscopic meniscectomy
54 = Open meniscectomy
55 = DJD: Open arthroplasty
56 = Joint replacement
57 = Joint denervation (Ex. facet rhizotomy)

MISCELLANEOUS
60 = Herniorrhaphy
61 = Craniotomy
62 = Neurostimulator (Ex. SCS)
63 = Medication plump

70 = Other unspecified procedure

Spinal Surgical Level Modifier:
0 = No modifier
1 = 1 Level spine surgery

2 = 2 Level spine surgery
3 = 3 Levels spine surgery

Examples of coding for a particular surgery:
    • If a patient had a diagnosis of right wrist carpal tunnel syndrome and had a 7/93 surgery for a right carpal tunnel release
     the lines would be: 6dR   07/1993   310

FIG. 3. Supplement surgery code sheet delineating specific types of surgical procedures.

gram quantitative evaluation (PPQE) or during 1-year follow-up telephone interviews. For the PRIDE program, the first three columns are for the PPQE follow-up tests, in which physical capacity is measured objectively, and standardized pain, disability, and depression scales are provided (with standardized scoring), obviating the need for subjective data acquisition when these tests are performed (46–49). The second data column on the page (immediately after the second set of categories) is for the testing date, usually about a month after discharge from the intensive phase of the PRIDE program. Of course, if this form is used for other programs, the number of follow-up periods will

DIAGNOSIS CODE

rev 4/15/98

1 Cervical
- a fracture
- b dislocation
- c degenerative disc/facet disease
- d postoperative syndrome - discectomy
- e postoperative syndrome - fusion
- f radiculopathy/stenosis
- g other

2 Thoracic
- a fracture
- b dislocation
- c degenerative disc/facet disease
- d postoperative syndrome - discectomy
- e postoperative syndrome - fusion
- f radiculopathy/stenosis
- g other

3 Lumbar
- a fracture
- b dislocation
- c degenerative disc/facet disease
- d postoperative syndrome - discectomy
- e postoperative syndrome - fusion
- f radiculopathy/stenosis
- g spondylolysis/spondylolisthesis
- h other

note: all extremity diagnoses require a R (right) or L (left) trunk 3rd place is "O"

4 Shoulder
- a fracture
- b gleno-humeral dislocation
- c a.c. joint dislocation/arthritis
- d gleno-humeral joint arthritis
- e brachial plexus injury
- f impingement syndrome/ tendinitis (Supraspinatus/biceps)
- g other

5 Elbow
- a fracture
- b dislocation
- c arthritis
- d cubital tunnel syndrome
- e posterior interosseous nerve entrapment
- f lateral epicondylitis/tendinitis
- g medial epicondylitis/tendinitis
- h other

6 Wrist
- a fracture
- b dislocation
- c arthritis
- d Carpal Tunnel Syndrome (nerve)
- e de Quervains (tendinitis)
- f tendinitis (other)
- g Ligament sprain
- h Other

7 Hand
- a fracture
- b dislocation
- c arthritis
- d nerve laceration/entrapment
- e trigger joint
- f tendon laceration/dysfunction
- g tendinitis (other)
- h amputation
- i Ligament sprain
- j Other

8 Hip
- a fracture
- b dislocation
- c arthritis
- d femoral neuritis
- e meralgia paraesthetic (nerve)
- f trochanteric bursitis/tendinitis
- g piriformis syndrome/tendinitis
- h tendinitis (other)
- i other

9 Knee
- a fracture
- b dislocation
- c arthritis
- d peroneal or tibial nerve entrapment
- e patellofemoral dysfunction
- f Ligament injury (sprain)
- g meniscal injury/tear
- h tendinitis/bursitis (other)
- i other

10 Ankle
- a fracture
- b dislocation
- c arthritis
- d ligament injury (sprain)
- e tarsal tunnel syndrome (nerve)
- f tendinitis (other)
- g other

11 Foot
- a fracture
- b dislocation
- c arthritis
- d plantar fascitis
- e tendinitis (other)
- f Ligament sprain
- g Other

12 OTHER NON-JOINT

13 Head injury/concussion
- a Objective neurological injury
- b Subjective symptoms
- c Neurospychological dysfunction

14 Upper extremity (NOS)
- a long bone fracture
- b RSD/Causalgia
- c thoracic outlet syndrome
- d Peripheral nerve injury
- e Muscle strain
- f Other

15 Lower extremity (NOS)
- a long bone fracture
- b RSD/Causalgia
- c Peripheral nerve injury
- d Muscle strain
- e Other

16 Chest
- a fracture
- b dislocation
- c arthritis
- d costochondritis
- e Muscle/tendon strain
- f other

17 Abdomen
- a hernia
- b muscle strain
- c ligament sprain
- d other

Example: Lumbar spondylolysis/spondylolisthesis =3gO   (R) carpal tunnel syndrome = 6dR

FIG. 4. Supplement diagnosis code sheet categorizing musculoskeletal diagnoses.

be dictated by the needs of these particular programs.

The remainder of this section focuses on the posttreatment outcome measures, which differ from those obtained before treatment. The reader should assume, unless otherwise alerted, that the data supplied at each PPQE or telephone interview represent *time interval data*. Therefore, they document information received and events occurring since the most recent prior outcome assessment specified on the data sheet.

Present Work Status

This code, representing the patient's work status at the time of PPQE evaluation, is accompanied by the date on which the patient returned to work. We believe the alphanumeric categories (0–11, A–D) are sufficiently inclusive to categorize virtually all relevant vocational and avocational activities the patient is likely to engage in following treatment. These are summarized under six working and six nonworking codes. Each working code has an on-the-job time modifier (A–D) to characterize full-, limited-, or part-time work activities. Of the six working codes, a few explanations are in order. *Categories 2 and 4* apply to different jobs, distinguishing them from *categories 1 and 3*. This alternative job may be heavier or lighter (which can be identified by checking the job demand category and work-activity requirements). *Category 6* must be income-producing work (acknowledged by the patient), to contrast with nonworking *category 8*, in which gainful employment is denied by the patient. If sufficient proof of illegal or undocumented work activities is available (although they may be denied by the patient because of simultaneous illicit receipt of financial assistance, such as food stamps or SSDI), category 8 patients occasionally may be moved to the appropriate working status code.

In the nonworking status, *category 0* refers to workers who never returned to work post-treatment after becoming temporarily totally disabled from their original jobs. This category is in contrast to the other nonworking categories, all five of which suggest that the patient returned or attempted to return to gainful employment for at least a brief (minimum, 1 day) period during the 12-month period after program completion. *Category 7* includes those who are fired or laid off after a period of reemployment. Category 7 patients must be currently unemployed for lack of job availability rather than because of persistent symptoms from the original injury (*category*

11) or work disruption that results from a new injury (*category 10*). Finally, *category 9* is a nonworking status referring to those engaged in non–income-producing activities, such as retired persons, housewives, or those engaged in volunteer work. Categories 7, 8, and 9 non-working patients may have resumed active lifestyles, as distinguished from patients in categories 0, 10, and 11, who tend to remain inactive and disability focused, often with financial secondary gain motivating ongoing illness behaviors. Occasionally, more than one category is present simultaneously, as in the case of a patient in *category 5* (vocational rehabilitation) who also has a part-time job to supplement his or her income. Both alphanumeric codes are entered.

Limitations

At the time the patient reaches maximum medical recovery (or permanent and stationary status), a determination of a work-release date and appropriate limitations (based on objective tests of physical capacity individually compared with normative data) is made. Limitations generally involve frequent or occasional lifting restrictions, which may be temporary or permanent. The work-release date, when applicable, is also provided. Additional restrictions on generic job activities are appended to the "comments" section on the back of the page and are, of course, included in communication with the employer (e.g., no continuous walking, occasional squatting, bending, and stooping only; no overhead lifting or reaching).

Income Source

This section monitors the type of income, including public assistance, that a patient may be receiving. If the patient is not working, this information will indicate how he or she is able to subsist or thrive financially.

Case Settlement:
Work-related Original Injury

These data refer only to case settlement for the original workers' compensation injury (in venues where such settlements take place). The concept of *permanent partial disability* exists in most U.S. venues, resulting in the patient receiving a payment (either an ongoing weekly benefit or a lump sum) at the conclusion of an arbitrated administrative or legal process (28). Cases either are settled before pretreatment outcome monitoring (categories 1, 3, or 5), not settled yet (category 4), or settled following the PRIDE program (category 2). If no workers' compensation case is involved (noncompensation patient or personal injury), category 0 is used. The settlement financial date and length of post-settlement medical coverage (if applicable) are included to provide as concise a system for tracking nonmedical issues as possible.

Case Settlement: Third-party Claim

This category attempts to cover the gamut of personal injury settlements, with or without accompanying workers' compensation injuries, typically seen in a disabled population. It uses a similar numeric code (0–4) to identify various stages of personal injury litigation, with an alphabetic code to identify the type of injury. The injury may be an isolated initial personal injury (with or without concurrent workers' compensation injury), an intervening injury occurring after the original injury for which treatment is being provided (but before functional restoration treatment), or a subsequent injury occurring in association with a posttreatment new injury claim (see below).

Health Utilization: Original Injury

In this section, the number of visits, if any, made to health professionals for the original injury since the last outcome monitoring interview are listed. The interviewer makes clear that *all* health professionals should be included in the count (physicians, therapists, psychologists, chiropractors). More than ten visits will require a response in the "comments" section. The coding identifies patients continuing to seek additional health care following rehabilitation with new providers (other than their treating physician supervising PRIDE program participation). Thus, it excludes the small number of anticipated routine visits to return for postprogram testing or to renew medications in the posttreatment year.

Surgeries: Original Injury

This section refers only to surgeries performed on the original anatomic area(s) considered part of the original compensation injury. Any response other than "no" to this question requires identification of the date and type of appropriately coded procedure.

New Injury

Any new injury occurring after functional restoration completion or in the interval between outcome monitoring interviews is noted here. Any new injury claim requires the appropriate coding as to anatomic area. The date of injury and a count of the days off work are provided as part of the alphanumeric coding.

Health Utilization: New Injury

This self-explanatory section monitors the number of surgeries and health care professional visits for any new injury (with specification of the musculoskeletal area involved) based on alphanumeric coding. Any surgery, hospitalization, or more than ten health-professional outpatient visits requires comment.

Subjective Data

In each posttreatment column (applicable to all follow-up telephone interviews) is an entry for pain level. Pain ratings are necessitated when telephone interviews are being performed in the absence of the usual pain drawing. The other subjective report asked at all PPQEs is treatment satisfaction. Because pain intensity has been assessed throughout the program based on an analogue "pain intensity" 10-cm line, the pain intensity is judged on a scale of 10 to keep the overall ratings comparable (47).

Based on past research in the area, the treatment satisfaction rating uses a Likert scale from 1 to 5 (50). In addition, patients report present or most recent job satisfaction, also using the Likert scale. Other patients report items on fitness maintenance, including the equipment recommended (and received), the frequency of exercise during a peak exercise week, and present participation in a fitness-maintenance plan, are obtained in this section.

Information Source

Two items fall into this category. The term "TELE...INTERVIEW? (YES/NO)" asks the interviewer to identify the interview method. The information source (patient or employer) requests data on the present or most recent work activities (including job of injury if applicable). Usually, the first posttreatment column contains employer-supplied information on work activities in the original job of injury (to contrast with information previously provided by the patient). Subsequent columns contain information provided by the patient about jobs to which the patient has returned (whether currently employed or not).

Recent Phone Number

This critical portion of the interview form requires emphasis here. When dealing with a highly mobile, heterogeneous American workforce (particularly in states with large migrant populations, such as California and Texas), retaining patient contact for outcome monitoring can be a stupefying task. We have learned, through extensive experience, that contact can be maintained with a high percentage of patients only if the telephone numbers of patients, employers, and family members are updated at regular posttreatment interview times. With such precautions, 1-year contact rates greater than 90% can be anticipated, even in large U.S. cities such as Dallas.

Structured Clinical Interviewing Skills

The purpose of this structured interview format is to ensure that the same sequence of questions and information gathering is administered to each patient. All interviewers must be trained and totally familiar with the various outcome parameters to use the appropriate codes and modifiers. Not all persons, however, have the requisite clinical skills to be trained to become effective interviewers. Careful selection, training, and regular monitoring of interviewers are essential to guarantee reliability; regular reliability checks are essential. We found that psychologists, disability managers or counselors, and rehabilitation nurses have the best people skills to become potentially effective and competent interviewers. A small minority of patients, usually because of dissatisfaction or enmeshment with nonmedical compensation issues, may prove less than fully candid, or they may not be totally cooperative. The interviewer will need to be trained to become sensitive to this possibility and to seek out collateral sources (e.g., insurers, attorneys, family members, referring physicians) to verify any possible misinformation.

DISCUSSION

Treatment-outcome monitoring has assumed new importance in medical treatment. It is particularly vital in musculoskeletal pain research, which is currently targeted for attention by health planners because of its high cost and perceived inefficient care. A variety of health-policy initiatives are undergoing pilot implementation, such as second surgical opinion programs, fee-schedule reforms (with variable multiplier modifications to favor utilization of specific modalities), and 24-hour coverage (rolling group health and workers' compensation medical benefits into a single package). Currently, health planners have minimal data on which to base potentially massive interventions, a situation highly susceptible to abuse and revolutionary excess. When played against a backdrop of a total health care cost approximating 14% of the U.S. GDP, with nearly 15% of the American population underinsured or uninsured, pressure on health policy planners to "do something" to achieve increased access to primary care is substantial. Whether this "something" is rational or reactionary will depend to a great extent on data providing objective socioeconomic outcomes to evaluate treatment effectiveness on the basis of realistic social outcomes. As far as nonmedical professionals are concerned, these social concerns generally involve the patient's return to productivity and costs of disability (e.g., medical, legal, administrative), particularly in compensation injuries wherein a disability benefit accompanies medical treatment.

The present contribution presents a validated method of objective socioeconomic outcome evaluation that initially was used in PRIDE functional restoration programs (30–32,34,35,51,52). Similar information was obtained using the same instrument through an independent replication study at the University of Vermont (24). The reader will note the limited use of subjective data (usually thought of as quality-of-care information) obtained on pain report and treatment satisfaction. This limitation is intentional, based on our frequently discussed perception of the frailty of past outcome studies that have relied on self-report questionnaires as the sole source of data. Moreover, nonspecific self-reporting shows inherent variability, particularly in a somatizing, disabled group of patients with a high frequency of Diagnostic and Statistical Manual of Mental Disorders (DSM)-III-R axis I and II diagnoses (51,53–55). Some reviewers suggested that a generation of reliance on self-reported subjective information marred the reputation of behavioral therapy for chronic pain (56,57). We submit that whereas pain, disability, and satisfaction ratings may be useful in monitoring acute musculoskeletal trauma or interventions in noncompensation degenerative disease, their value as the primary outcome index in the multifactorial aspects of disabling, work-related, compensation musculoskeletal pain is questionable.

The reader should not be left with the impression that physical capacity (human performance) measures are of little consequence in functional restoration because of their omission in this chapter. Quantitative evaluations occur regularly for treatment monitoring and documentation of performance relative to normal subject data during the 6 months following discharge from an intensive program. These tests offer self-report scales of pain, disability, and depression, along with objective measures of mobility, strength, aerobic, and lifting capacity associated with effort ratings and a cumulative score (15,16,39,40,42, 43,45). These tests provide a multitude of benefits, including the following:

1. Initial levels of physical capacity to individualize initial physical training protocols
2. Evidence of low effort (due to excessive pain response leading to functional inhibition) guiding appropriate education and counseling to motivate and encourage patient participation and training as well as helping identify secondary gain and other barriers to functional recovery;
3. Interim testing leading to appropriate age-, gender-, and body weight-related progression of resistive exercise for optimal fitness maintenance training
4. Monitoring of physical capacities at maximum medical recovery, allowing objective determination of appropriate limitations for work release
5. Posttreatment monitoring of a home fitness maintenance program that uses specific equipment and exercise protocols to provide feedback to the patient on successful physical capacity maintenance or areas requiring additional attention

Each of these important results of quantification of function was impossible to perform before the advent of suitable technology and experience with normative databases for using these innovative methodologies with spinal and extremity disability patients. Such normative data will need to be collected for use with other specific musculoskeletal disorders. Thus, although it is not included in this report on socioeconomic outcomes, monitoring physical-capacity outcome is also vital for programmatic quality assurance and optimal patient training and education.

This chapter presents a system of data acquisition for monitoring socioeconomic outcomes of functional restoration; however, it can be used as an outcome evaluation method for other forms of treatment of various musculoskeletal disorders. Although no specific data are presented here, the system has been used in several outcome and predictor studies involving treatment in the U.S. states of Texas and Vermont. Objective socioeconomic outcomes will achieve greater importance in the allocation of health resources in the next decade, making standardization of outcome data collection and reporting beneficial to health care providers and policy planners. As such, the system presented here in detail, complete with reporting forms and alphanumeric coding system, lends itself well to documentation of treatment outcome for disabling musculoskeletal injuries. Prospective collection of quantitative physical, psychosocial function and objective socioeconomic data and the widespread implementation of this general format will allow development of large databases for standardized comparison of information from diverse medical treatment environments.

REFERENCES

1. Frymoyer J, Mooney V. Current concepts review: occupational orthopedics. *J Bone J Surg Am* 1986;68A:469.
2. American Academy of Orthopedic Surgeons, Committee on Outcome Studies. *Musculoskeletal outcome research register*. Park Ridge, Il: AAOS Press, 1991.
3. Russell G, ed. *American Academy of Orthopedic Surgeons clinical policies: low back musculoligamentous injury (sprain/strain)*. Park Ridge,IL: AAOS Press, 1991:3–6.
4. Deyo R. *Back pain outcome assessment team (spine surgery outcomes)*. Health Care Financing Administration Grant.
5. Deyo R, Tsui-Wu Y. Descriptive epidemiology of low back pain and its related medical care in the United States. *Spine* 1987;12:264–268.
6. Deyo R, Walsh N, Martin D, Schoenfeld L, Ramamurthy S. A controlled trial of transcutaneous electrical nerve stimulation (TENS) and exercise for chronic low back pain. *N Engl J Med* 1990;322:1627–1634.
7. Quebec Task Force on Spinal Disorders. Scientific approach to the assessment and management of activity-related spinal disorders: a monograph for clinicians. *Spine* 1987;12(Suppl):S22–S30.
8. Roughton J. Cumulative trauma disorders: The newest business liability. *Professional Safety* 1993;38:29–35.
9. Bureau of Labor Statistics. *Workplace injuries and illnesses in 1996*. Washington, DC: U.S. Department of Labor, 1997. USDL Publication No. 97-453. www: http://www.bls.gov/osh/osnr0005.txt

10. Brogmus G, Sorock G, Webster B. Recent trends in work-related cumulative trauma disorders of the upper extremities in the United States: An evaluation of possible reasons. *J Occup Environ Med* 1996;8:401–411.
11. Hales T, Bernard B. Epidemiology of work-related musculoskeletal disorders. *Orthop Clin North Am* 1997;27:679–709.
12. Webster B, Snook S. The cost of compensable upper extremity cumulative trauma disorders. *J Occup Med* 1994;36:713–727.
13. Turk D, Rudy T. Spine update methods for evaluating treatment outcomes: ways to overcome potential obstacles. *Spine* 1994;19:1759–1763.
14. Williams R. Toward a set of reliable and valid measures for chronic pain assessment and outcome research. *Pain* 1988;5:239–251.
15. Mayer T, Gatchel R. *Functional restoration for spinal disorders: the sports medicine approach*. Philadelphia: Lea & Febiger, 1988.
16. Mayer T, Mooney V, Gatchel R. *Contemporary care for painful spinal disorders: concepts, diagnosis and treatment*. Philadelphia: Lea & Febiger, 1991.
17. Waddell G. A new clinical model for the treatment of low back pain. *Spine* 1987;12:632–644.
18. Beals R, Hickman N. Industrial injuries of the back and extremities. Comprehensive evaluation—an aide in prognosis and management: a study of 180 patients. *J Bone J Surg Am* 1972;54A:1593–1611.
19. Greenough C, Fraser R. The effects of compensation on recovery from low back injury. *Spine* 1989;14:947–955.
20. Hadler N, Carey T, Garrett J. The influence of indemnification by workers' compensation insurance on recovery from acute backache. *Spine* 1995;20:2710–2715.
21. Sanderson P, Todd B, Holt G, Getty C. Compensation, work status, and disability in low back pain patients. *Spine* 1995;20:554–6.
22. Nachemson A. Work for all: for those with low back pain as well. *Clin Orthop* 1983;179:77–85.
23. Choler U, Nachemson A, et al. *SPRI Rapport 188*, Ont I Ryggen, ISSL0586-1691, 1988;1:100.
24. Hazard R, Fenwick J, Kalish S, et al. Functional restoration with behavioral support: a one-year perspective study of chronic low back pain patients. *Spine* 1989;14:157–165.
25. Mayer T, Gatchel R, Kishino N, et al. Objective assessment of spine function following industrial injury: a prospective study with comparison group and one-year follow-up: 1985 Volvo Award in Clinical Sciences. *Spine* 1985;10:482–493.
26. Mitchell R, Carmen G. Results of a multi-center trial using an intensive active exercise program for the treatment of acute soft tissue and back injuries. *Spine* 1990;15:514–521.
27. Gatchel R, Mayer T, Hazard R, Rainville J, Mooney V. Functional restoration: pitfalls in evaluating efficacy [Editorial]. *Spine* 1992;17:988–995.
28. Oland G, Tveiten G. A trial of modern rehabilitation for chronic low back pain and disability: vocational outcome and effect of pain modulation. *Spine* 1991;16:457–459.
29. Sachs B, David J, Olimpio D, Scala A, Lacroix M. Spinal rehabilitation by work tolerance based on objective physical capacity assessment of dysfunction: a prospective study with control subjects and 12-month review. *Spine* 1990;15:1325–1332.

30. Wright A, Mayer T, Gatchel R. Outcomes of disabling cervical spine disorders in compensation injuries: a prospective comparison to tertiary rehabilitation response for chronic lumbar spinal disorders. *Spine (in press)*.

31. Jordan K, Mayer T, Gatchel R. Should extended disability be an exclusion criterion for tertiary rehabilitation: socioeconomic outcomes of early vs. late functional restoration in compensation spinal disorders. *Spine* 1998;23;2110–2117.

32. Mayer T, McMahon M, Gatchel R, Sparks B, Wright A, Pegues P. Socioeconomic outcomes of combined spine surgery and functional restoration in workers' compensation spinal disorders with matched controls. *Spine* 1998;23:598–606.

33. Burton K, Polatin P, Gatchel R, Mayer T. Psychosocial factors and the rehabilitation of patients with chronic work-related upper extremity disorders. *J Occup Rehabil* 1997;7:139–153.

34. Mayer T, Gatchel R, Polatin P, Evans T. Outcomes comparison of treatment for chronic disabling work-related upper extremity cumulative trauma to spinal disorders: a prospective matched control trial. *J Occup Environ Med (in press)*.

35. Garcy P, Mayer T, Gatchel R. Recurrent or new injury outcomes after return to work in chronic disabling spinal disorders: tertiary prevention efficacy of functional restoration treatment. *Spine* 1996;21:952–959.

36. Mayer T, Gatchel R, Kishino N, et al A prospective short-term study of chronic low back pain patients utilizing novel objective functional measurement. *Pain* 1986;25:53–68.

37. Mayer T, Gatchel R, Mayer H, Kishino N, Keeley J, Mooney V. A prospective two-year study of functional restoration in industrial low back injury: an objective assessment procedure. *JAMA* 1987;258:1763–1767.

38. Gatchel R, Mayer T, Capra P, Diamond P, Barnett J. Quantification of lumbar function. Part 6: the use of psychological measures in guiding physical functional restoration. *Spine* 1986;11:36–42.

39. Keeley J, Mayer T, Cox R, Gatchel R, Smith J, Mooney V. Quantification of lumbar function. Part 5: reliability of range of motion measures in the sagittal plane and an *in vivo* torso rotation measurement technique. *Spine* 1986;11:31–35.

40. Kishino N, Mayer T, Gatchel R, et al. Quantification of lumbar function. Part 4: isometric and isokinetic lifting simulation in normal subjects and low back dysfunction patients. *Spine* 1985;10:921–927.

41. Kohles S, Barnes D, Gatchel R, Mayer T. Improved physical performance outcomes following functional restoration treatment in patients with chronic low back pain: early versus recent training results. *Spine* 1990;15:1321–1324.

42. Mayer T, Smith S, Kondraske G, Gatchel R, Carmichael T, Mooney V. Quantification of lumbar function. Part 3: preliminary data on isokinetic torso rotation testing with myoelectric spectral analysis in normal and low back pain subjects. *Spine* 1985;10:912–920.

43. Mayer T, Smith S, Keeley J, Mooney V. Quantification of lumbar function. Part 2: sagittal plane trunk strength in chronic low back pain patients. *Spine* 1985;10:765–772.

44. Polatin P, Kinney R, Gatchel R, Lillo E, Mayer T. Psychiatric illness and chronic low back pain: the mind and the spine—which goes first? *Spine* 1993;18:66–71.

45. Smith S, Mayer T, Gatchel R, Becker T. Quantification of lumbar function. Part 1: isometric and multi-speed isokinetic trunk strength measures in sagittal and axial planes in normal subject patients. *Spine* 1985;10:757–764.

46. Beck A, Steer R, Garbin W. Psychometric properties of the Beck Depression Inventory: twenty-five years of evaluation. *Clinical Psychological Review* 1988;8:77–100.

47. Capra P, Mayer T, Gatchel R. Adding psychological scales to your back pain assessment. *Journal of Musculoskeletal Medicine* 1985;2:41–52.

48. Million R, Haavik N, Jayson M, Balser R. Evaluation of low back pain and assessment of lumbar corsets with and without back support. *Ann Rheum Dis* 1981;40:449–545.

49. Mooney V, Cairns D, Robertson J. A system for evaluating and treating chronic back disability. *West J Med* 1976;24:370–376.

50. Gatchel R, Baum A, Krantz D. *Introduction to health psychology*. New York: McGraw-Hill, 1989.

51. Ward N. Tricyclic antidepressants for chronic low back pain: mechanisms of action and predictors of response (1986 Volvo Award in Clinical Science). *Spine* 1986;11:661–665.

52. Polatin P, Gatchel R, Barnes D, Mayer H, Arens C, Mayer T. A psychosociomedical prediction model of response to treatment by chronically disabled workers with back pain. *Spine* 1989;14:956–961.

53. Kinney R, Gatchel R, Mayer T. The SCL-90R: evaluated as an alternative to the MMPI for psychological screening of chronic low back pain patients. *Spine* 1991;8:940–942.

54. Wesley L, Gatchel R, Polatin P, Kinney R, Mayer T. Differentiation between somatic and cognitive/affective components in commonly used measures of depression in chronic low-back pain: let's not mix apples and oranges. *Spine* 1991;6S:S213–S215.

55. Gatchel R, Polatin P, Mayer T, Robinson R, Dersh J. Use of the SF-36 health status survey with a chronically disabled back pain population: strengths and limitations. *Spine (in press)*.

56. Fordyce W, Roberts A, Sternbach R. The behavioral management of chronic pain: a response to critics. *Pain* 1985;22:113–125.

57. Schmidt A. The behavioral management of pain: a criticism of a response. *Pain* 1987;30:285–291.

PART VII

Other Occupational Disorder Factors

Occupational Musculoskeletal Disorders
edited by T. G. Mayer, R. J. Gatchel, and P. B. Polatin.
Lippincott Williams & Wilkins, Philadelphia © 2000.

38

Impairment and Disability Evaluation

Mohammed I. Ranavaya and *Gunnar B.J. Andersson

*Appalachian Institute of Occupational and Environmental Medicine,
Chapmanville, West Virginia 25508; *Department of Orthopaedic Surgery,
Rush-Presbyterian-St. Luke's Medical Center, Chicago, Illinois 60612*

Impairment and disability evaluation is a process to which all physicians involved in musculoskeletal evaluation and care are exposed. It is not a process, however, that most physicians learn during their training. Indeed, many physicians are uncomfortable when asked to perform these evaluations. This chapter is the first of two in this book that address this topic. This chapter discusses history and definitions as well as possible alternative approaches to a disability evaluation and the 12 contemporary U.S. disability systems. The second chapter describes how to evaluate disability using the American Medical Association's (AMA) *Guides to the Evaluation of Permanent Impairment* (AMA Guides) (1).

HISTORY AND DEFINITIONS

Tolerance toward and care of the sick, injured, and disabled may be elemental components of our social fabric rooted in the very origins of human society (2). Anthropologic evidence (3) dates back to 60,000 years ago within the Neanderthal population and suggests that severe trauma was quite prevalent, that survival was indeed possible following catastrophic injury, and that the family group and society were developed enough to care for the injured and disabled.

The social justice system has existed since ancient times. As far back as more than 4,000 years ago, the Babylonians compensated for the loss of limb and life incurred in the service of the state. The Old Babylonian kingdom of Eshnunna's laws had an approach of economic compensation for the wrongdoing. These were a compilation of rules and monetary compensation schedules for bodily harm. For example, "If a man slaps another in the face— 10 shekels silver he shall weigh out. An eye—1 mina silver he shall weigh out. If a man bit and severed the nose of a man,—1 mina silver he shall weigh out. A tooth—1/2 mina; an ear—1/2 mina" (4). The Code of Hummarabi of 1750 BC as well as Mosaic laws decreed the punitive action against the person causing injury. The concept of Lex Talionis, an "eye for an eye and a tooth for a tooth," existed to compensate for wrongful injury.

The ancient Egyptians provided compensation for a wrongful act causing injury. Punitive damages were provided against physicians, such as amputation of a surgeon's hands, if a patient was blinded as a result of cataract removal. In ancient times, the Greeks also provided compensation for injured parties. The soldiers of Alexander the Great's army were compensated for the loss of limb or life. Ancient Romans provided compensation for both free men and slaves; however, social status determined the extent of compensation, with slaves receiving less than a free man for the same injury (5). The Roman masters also were required to care for the injured slaves.

Social justice was not always state sponsored; among the Western European Germanic and Nordic tribes (the Lombards), blood feud, which was the personal vengeance of the friends and family of the injured, was a traditional way of seeking justice. As these tribes became integrated in the Roman Empire, the blood feud eventually was replaced by state-administered justice between the injured and the accused. Compensation for injuries was based on a "whole person" concept. Each tribesman was considered to have an intrinsic monetary value, his "wergelt" or "man value," of 200 Roman solidi. This was the value of the tribesman's life or 100% whole-body impairment. There was a schedule for all sorts of injuries, from as trivial as an injury to a toe, to the loss of limbs, eyes, and life itself. The impairment values are extraordinarily similar to those used today. There was even compensation for cosmetic loss. Thus, if a molar tooth was knocked out, the compensation was four solidi (2% of the wergelt), but loss of a tooth that showed in a smile was equal to eight solidi (4% of the wergelt) (6).

In this regard, state-sponsored care for the poor and disabled who were without a responsible party (concept of social security) has a tradition in history as well. The first state-sponsored social security system was established by Muslims in 640 AD during the reign of the second *caliph omar.* The state treasury provided monthly benefits to blind people, widows, and orphans.

During the Middle Ages, various craft guilds provided sickness funds that were available to members who became sick or injured. Members of these craft guilds contributed to these funds. Another interesting twist in the history of compensation is that compensation of injured workers is not unique to civil societies. Even among pirates, a code existed whereby the greater share of the loot was given to pirates who lost an eye or limb during action.

In more recent times, contemporary disability management has escalated to new heights based on an explosion of medical and legal issues. Although many physicians have received specialty training in select areas (e.g., orthopedics or occupational medicine),

the various aspects of disability medicine cross specialty lines so frequently as to cause these borders to be blurred or, more often, not even present. Many times, individual physicians, no matter what their specialty, are asked by patients or others to provide a report of injury or disability for a workers' compensation agency, to fill out an insurance disability claim form, to write a note to support a request for accommodation, or to certify a medical condition causing disability.

Consequently, physicians who wish to practice disability medicine and to perform impairment evaluations need to know what disability or compensation system covers their patients and examinees, because each system has unique requirements and demands. Some systems may require physicians to perform the impairment rating and establish causality, whereas others may not need to establish causality of an impairment or disability (such as social security) and may require only that the physician perform the examination, make a diagnosis, and determine the severity of the illness but not rate the impairment. Yet other systems require a physician to comment on the disability, although disability determination traditionally is considered beyond the realm of the physician. Added to this are differences between states, which is beyond the discussion of this chapter.

In the Bible it is written, "If any would not work, neither shall they eat" (2 *Thessalonians* 3:10). Obviously, this ruling is not for those who are truly unable to be occupationally gainfully employed; rather, it is for those who choose not to be productive and attempt to fake disability. The question then arises of who determines disability. Hadler (7) noted that well into the eighteenth century the gentry decided who was "deserving poor" and therefore entitled to receive benefits and who was malingering. The person thought to be faking illness was beaten. Today the question still arises as to who is really disabled and who is malingering. There is a great concern that benefits not be given to someone who does not truly have serious problems; the issue is one of social justice.

One major problem in disability medicine is that the definition of exactly who is disabled, and therefore entitled to benefits, is imprecise and as such results in a considerable amount of litigation. For example, low back pain litigation costs at least five billion dollars a year (8). The decisions regarding disability usually are made administratively with the help of medical evaluations. At opposite ends of the health and disease continuum, these issues are relatively easy. For example, if a person is working full time and has no health problems, he or she usually is not considered disabled. On the other hand, a quadraplegic in a nursing home would be most likely regarded as totally disabled. Problems arise in cases where medical conditions are not so severe but may be disabling. For example, should a 56-year-old unemployed coal miner who has had back surgery and complains of chronic pain be considered disabled under the law and therefore entitled to social security benefits?

Many physicians do not completely understand the concept of economic or vocational disability. The type of medical problem causing an inability to be gainfully employed (i.e., to be vocationally disabled) depends not only on the severity and type of the illness itself but also on the age, education, previous work history, transferable skills, and local labor market. Snook and Webster reported that 16.5% of the U.S. population is disabled, of whom fewer than 20% are actually unable to work (9). More recently, Pope and Tarlov stated that about 35 million Americans (one in seven) have disabling conditions that interfere with their life activities (10).

In this regard, the concept of disability is related to that of *impairment*, defined as what is medically wrong with a body part or organ system and its functioning. According to the AMA *Guides*, *disability* is defined as "an alteration of an individual's capacity to meet personal, social, or occupational demands or statutory or regulatory requirements" (1). *Impairment*, on the other hand, is defined as "the loss, loss of use or derangement of any body part, system or function." Disability in this context can be regarded as a gap between what an individual can do and what he or she wants or is expected to do. For example, loss of the distal phalanx of the little finger of the right hand will impair the functioning of the digit and hand of both a concert pianist and a bank president; however, the pianist obviously will be much more occupationally disabled by this problem.

IMPAIRMENT EVALUATION SYSTEMS

For the musculoskeletal system, function is difficult to quantify. Different parts of the body interact differently, depending on requirements, and adaptation frequently occurs. To address this difficulty, three different impairment evaluation methods have evolved that sometimes are used separately and are sometimes combined (11).

Anatomic Systems
(Based on Examination)

The early anatomic approach to disability evaluation was to record amputation, ankylosis, and fixed deformity. Later weakness, loss of sensation, and measurement of range of motion (ROM) were included. Whereas amputation, ankylosis, and deformity can be accurately, reproducibly, and objectively determined, measurements of weakness, loss of sensation, and ROM have poorer reproducibility and are subjective in the sense that they all rely on the participation of the person to be evaluated. Further, it can be argued that weakness and ROM are indicators of function and therefore are, in fact, functional rather than anatomic measures. The reason these additional measures were included was that amputation, ankylosis, and deformity cover only a small part of impairment disorders. A pure anatomic system, therefore, would be useless in most evaluations. The AMA *Guides* initially used a modified anatomic approach, which included the measurement of ROM. In the most recent edition, diagnostic features were included for the lower extremity and the spine. This is an example of how impairment systems develop not along one methodologic principle only but by combining different evaluation principles.

Diagnostic Systems (Based on Pathology)

A diagnostic system is based on agreed-upon diagnostic groups to which impairment percentages are assigned. The advantages are simplicity and reproducibility (if the criteria for the groups are clear, objective, and enforced). Deciding on criteria appears simple on the surface, but consider the difficulty in diagnosing certain spinal conditions, such as a herniated disc or low back strain. Anatomic evidence of herniated discs is present in at least 25% of people who have never experienced back pain or sciatica and have no disability or impairment. For clinical (as distinct from anatomic or radiologic) diagnosis, a herniated disc seen on, for example, magnetic resonance imaging, is therefore not sufficient to make a diagnosis; appropriate symptoms and signs also must be present. Further, a narrow spinal canal accentuates the clinical syndrome of disc herniation but can be diagnosed equally correctly as spinal stenosis. Low back sprain, the most common back diagnosis, is a diagnosis by exclusion, which many physicians question. Any patient who complains of back pain can be fitted into this category if no other is applicable. It is not the difficulty in developing diagnostic criteria that is the main weakness of a diagnosis-based system, however; rather, it is the fact that the actual disability related to a diagnosis is highly variable. For these reasons, a diagnosis-based system often needs to be continued by using other measurements to differentiate within diagnostic categories. An expanded diagnosis-based system is currently used by the Social Security Administration (SSA) (12,13), and for Workers' Compensation disability evaluation in Minnesota (14). The SSA combines diagnosis with history, physical examination, and laboratory tests (as applicable), while the Minnesota Medical Association system combines diagnosis with history, physical examination, pain complaints, and radiographic evaluation. As mentioned, the fourth edition of the AMA *Guides* includes aspects of a diagnosis-based system.

Functional Systems

Currently, no pure functional system is in use, although conceptually this would be the best method to evaluate impairment and disability. The difficulty lies in measuring function. Several functional indicators can be measured, but their relationship to overall function remains uncertain. These functional indicators include ROM, the most frequently used functional estimate and the easiest to obtain, as well as strength, endurance, and coordination. The California Industrial Accident System includes functional parameters. These are patient estimates, however, without objective verification. The SSA attempts determine the claimant's ability to perform basic work activities and residual functional capacities for work but depends on medical reports for its review and rarely directly measures physical capacities. Requiring sophisticated objective measures of various functions is impractical and costly, and the methods still are not technically advanced to the level where function can be determined precisely.

THE DISABILITY PROCESS

The disability claims process usually begins with a person who decides that he or she can no longer work because of illness, at least not in his or her regular job. Indeed, these medical problems may be severe and functionally limiting, and this is probably the case most of the time; however, in some cases, the decision to apply for benefits under disability regulations is made after a person is laid off from work because for economic reasons. In this instance, the person attempts to use physical impairments that already existed and did not interfere with work capacity significantly in the past, hoping that he or she will be declared disabled and entitled to disability income. In other situations, the patient may not like his or her job and may attempt to use a minor medical problem to resolve an undesirable situation.

Most often, in the process for disability claims, the next step is to request a statement of disability from the physician, who may or may not agree that the person is disabled. The opinions of doctors regarding who is disabled vary a great deal. As such, a disability claimant can go "doctor shopping" to look for one who will support the claim. In some cases, a physician will certify the patient as disabled with little objective evidence of actual disability. It is therefore not unreasonable for third-party insurers to demand an independent medical examination. Relying on a treating or personal physician certification of their patient's alleged disability may mean relying on biased information.

U.S. COMPENSATION SYSTEMS

Physicians in the United States who wish to excel as independent medical examiners for impairment and disability evaluation need to understand fully the contemporary U.S. compensation systems. The following are the major players (15):

1. Tort Law/Common Law Liability
2. State Workers' Compensation Systems
3. Social Security Program
4. Veterans Administration Benefits Program
5. Federal Employees Compensation Act (FECA)
6. Longshore and Harbor Worker's Act
7. Federal Black Lung Program
8. Federal Employers Liability Act (FELA)
9. Jones Act (Merchant Marine Act)
10. Private insurances and other private organizations
11. Americans with Disability Act (ADA)
12. Family Medical Leave Act (FMLA).

Common Law Liability or Tort Law

The American College of Legal Medicine defines a *tort* as "a breech of duty that gives rise to an action for damages." Simply put, *tort* is a civil wrongdoing, and the concept of liability for tort is based on our common law, which is a colonial inheritance from England. English common law developed mostly in the past few centuries but has roots dating back to the reign of King Henry II in twelfth century, when the King delegated his judicial powers to various magistrates and divided the country into six circuits, with three judges to each circuit. These judges were charged to administer justice for civil claims based on previous decisions *(precedent)* and the common customs, hence the term *common law*. Essentially, common law is judge-made law. It is an evolving system and quite often reflects the contemporary values of the society. The aspect of common law that we actually come across in medical practice most often is tort law or tort liability. For a claim for compensation to be successful under the tort law, four facts must be shown or proven. First, a legal duty must exist. Second, there has to be a breach of duty. Third, harm or damage must have happened and must as a fourth be an approximate or direct result of that breach of duty.

Before various workers' compensation statutes were enacted around the turn of the century, tort or the common law was the only remedy available to the injured worker. It was difficult for the injured worker to collect because the employer's negligence needed to be proven in a court of law, which was time consuming and expensive. To prove negligence, a coworker might have to testify against the employer, placing the worker in a compromised position and making it difficult for injured workers to prove negligence and hence to collect compensation. As defendants, employers had powerful defenses available to them. The following three most powerful defenses were collectively called the "three wicked sisters": contributory negligence, assumption of risk, and the fellow servant doctrine.

First defense was *contributory negligence.* The employer would assert that it was not his or her fault that an employee sustained an injury. Rather, the person who sustained the injuries caused or contributed to it by his or her own negligence. For example, Joe fell off the ladder working on the roof. Actually, Joe did not set up the ladder correctly; so Joe's negligence caused the injury, and the employer was not responsible.

The second defense was *assumption of risk*, which meant that the employee knew about the potential risks involved in a certain job as much as the employer did, and therefore, by virtue of accepting employment, the worker assumed the risk. For example, an underground coal miner knows or should know that inherent in the coal-mining job is the risk of injury from roof falls, explosions, and accidents. Further, a worker could walk off the job to avoid the risk. Therefore, assumption of risk was a strong defense used by employers.

The third defense was the *fellow servant doctrine*, which meant that instead of the employer, another employee's negligence caused the injury. It is not surprising that before the workers' compensation laws evolved around the turn of the century, it was difficult for workers to collect under common law.

Larson (16) quotes statistics from the turn of the century reflecting on this difficulty. Causes of accidents in 1907 in Germany list "fault or negligence of the injured employee" at about 29%, "assumption of risk" about 42%, and "fellow employees fault" about 5%. The employer was responsible about 17% of the time. It is obvious that under the common law four of five employees could not prove that the employer was at fault, and hence the worker could not collect benefits for work-related injuries. It was stated that many injured workers became paupers as a result of injuries arising from employment, which led to social upheaval and labor unrest around the turn of the century, when various Workers' Compensation Statutes were enacted.

Workers' Compensation Statutes

The first such statute was enacted in Germany in 1887. Ten years later, a worker's compensation act was also introduced in England. In 1908 the first worker's compensation act was enacted in the United States, and it was a federal act. The first state workers' compensation statute was introduced in New York in 1910, but it was struck down by the U.S. Supreme Court a year later. The New York law was found to be unconstitutional on the grounds of depriving employers of property (premium for no-fault workers' compensation coverage) without due process. This legal challenge eventually was worked out, and the New Jersey law of 1911 was upheld. By 1949, Mississippi was the last state to enact a workers' compensation law.

Currently, workers' compensation laws exist in all 50 states. Workers' compensation is not one "system" *per se* but many state-based social insurance mechanisms enacted into legislation to compensate workers who are injured "on the job." Workers' compensation statutes therefore differ according to jurisdiction; however, some basic common principles exist. One of the key elements is the "no-fault" principle. All three "wicked sisters"— the assumption of risk, contributory negligence, and the fellow servant doctrine—are eliminated. Employees are entitled to certain benefits for injuries that "arise out of or in the course of employment," no mater what.

The benefits include wage replacement, which is usually about two-thirds of the worker's weekly wages, and medical and rehabilitation benefits. Wage replacement lasts as long as a temporary disability remains or until a predetermined maximum benefit level is exhausted. When maximum degree of medical improvement (MMI) is reached, if any residual deficit exists, permanent partial or permanent total disability benefits are paid based on the applicable laws. If the employee dies, the benefits are paid to the employee's dependents, including the funeral expenses. The state systems differ significantly in type, level, and duration of benefits.

Another common thread of all the workers' compensation statutes is that it is the exclusive remedy under the law for the employee against employer for personal injuries, diseases, or deaths "arising out of and in the course of employment." Under workers' compensation provisions, the employee and dependents give up the right to sue the employer for money damages for injury, even though the employer may have been negligent, except in extreme circumstances, usually defined as wanton neglect. The employee essentially must show that the employer intended to injure the employee, a heavy burden of proof. When obtaining workers' compensation insurance, the employer knows that liability will be limited. In return for premiums, the employer enjoys a certain immunity from third-party lawsuits. Therefore, it can be said that workers' compensation statues are a compromise for both employers and the employees.

Finally, common among all the workers' compensation statues is the provision that the employee retains the right to sue a third party. If, for example, the employer was using a product manufactured by a third party, and the employee was injured by using that product, the manufacturer of that product (third party) can be sued. A common example would be asbestos. Many employers used asbestos, and the injured employees successfully filed a third-party lawsuit against the asbestos manufacturers. Another example would be if a faulty machine malfunctioned, causing injury. The employee could sue the manufacturer of the machine as well as collect from workers' compensation.

PHYSICIAN'S ROLE IN WORKERS' COMPENSATION

What is the physician's role in a workers' compensation system? One key responsibility is to determine causality, that is, to identify the causal link between the job and the injury or disease. In obvious cases, such as an employee falling off a roof, thus fracturing a hip or leg, the cause is quite obvious. This situation does not need a physician to certify the causality. In cases in which questions arise about the cause of an injury, however, the physician often is asked to give an opinion about whether the job exposure that is claimed actually caused the injury. The required legal proof of such a causal relationship is not as strong as usually required in scientific research. Scientists usually require a p value of less than 0.05, which means being correct 95% of the time. The legal requirement is usually 51%.

Certainly, in a workers' compensation system, physicians are required to treat and coordinate rehabilitation. Once rehabilitation is completed, the physician helps the injured worker return to work, determining whether he or she is ready to go back to work and, if so, when the worker has reached the MMI. Further, the physician also determines whether any permanent partial impairments or work restrictions at the time of MMI. The most important skill for physicians to learn to be successful in the compensation arena is how to communicate medical facts to non-medical parties. Communicating scientific and medical facts succinctly and clearly, so that the information is useful to nonmedical persons, is a critical skill for the physician in the field of disability medicine.

SOCIAL SECURITY DISABILITY PROGRAM

The Social Security Disability Program is Public Law 74-271, "the Social Security Act." Although it is administered through the SSA as a national program, the initial process of disability determination occurs at the state level through the Social Security Disability Determination Services (Bureau of Disability Determination). The physician who would like to be involved in performing medical evaluations for social security can obtain referrals through the services at the state level.

A person does not qualify for social security disability (SSD) benefits merely because he or she cannot perform his or her usual occupation. SSD criteria require the worker to be unable to perform all past relevant work and any other work existing in the national economy. By contrast, workers' compensation programs (under individual state law, as opposed to the federal social security program) provide compensation for both total incapacity and partial incapacity. Workers' compensation typically considers marketability and whether the individual can secure work. Certain impairments have a scheduled length of incapacity. In contrast, SSD is not established for a finite number of weeks. The duration requirements pertain to impairment expected to be fatal or that already has lasted or can be expected to last at least 1 year. Although technically the duration requirement refers to the impairment(s), the prevalent position is that the disability (i.e., the inability to engage in substantial gainful activity) also must satisfy this criterion. Typically, unless the person has returned to work or has had significant medical improvement, he or she is considered continuously disabled for the indefinite future (17).

The SSA actually has two disability benefit programs: Social Security Disability Insurance Benefits and Supplemental Social Security Income (SSI). Disability Insurance is under Title II, which provides for disabled persons who have contributed to the program through Federal Insurance Contributions Act (FICA) payroll taxes. The minimum requirement is that the individual must have worked a requisite number of calendar quarters. Benefits are financed by a payroll tax. This benefit has risen from a rate of 2% at the inception of the program to more than 13% by the early 1980s. SSI is Title XVI and is funded through the general revenue. It provides benefits to eligible disabled persons who fall below a certain income or asset level.

Social security is the largest disability program in the United States. It assists between 33% and 50% of all people qualified as disabled. Physicians play an important role in the evaluation process. To begin, a statement by a treating physician that a person is disabled carries a great deal of weight. In addition, the agency hires physicians to do consultative examinations when there is insufficient medical evidence to make a decision. Other medical practitioners review records at the regional disability offices. According to social security law, *disability* is "the inability to engage in any substantial gainful activity by reason of a medically determinable physical or mental impairment that can be expected to result in death or can be expected to last for not less than 12 months." This definition is quite different from that of the AMA, which was provided earlier.

The original Social Security Act of 1935 provided retirement benefits only to retired workers themselves. In 1957 disability benefits were initiated that introduced a separate fund to provide money to workers over the age of 50 who were totally and permanently disabled. In later years, eligibility was expanded. Snook and Webster (9) reported in 1987 that SSD benefits were about $16.8 billion a year distributed to 4.5 million Americans. Each year, more than 1.5 million people file claims for SSD. It has been estimated that under the current "pay as you go" system with the increasing number of older people and less able and fewer workers, the combined expenditures for disability and Medicare might require a payroll tax of 22% by the year 2025; this is an obvious drive for reforms.

The claimant for SSD benefits has the burden of establishing, by credible evidence, that his or her impairments are indeed disabling. The person awarded these benefits must be found to be totally and permanently disabled. Under the social security criteria, there are no benefits for partial disability. The disabling conditions that are recognized under U.S. social security law include various orthopedic problems; visual, speech, and hearing impairments; cerebral palsy, heart and lung disease, cancer, mental retardation, specific learning disabilities, drug addiction and alcoholism, human immunodeficiency virus (HIV) infection, diabetes, and multiple sclerosis. Akermann found that the four most common causes of disability are accidents, coronary disease, diseases of the spine, and other orthopedic problems, accounting for 52.4% of all cases (18).

The first step for a person to receive social security disability benefits is to file an application. The case is reviewed at the state Bureau of Disability Determination. The adjudicator at this level may decide to refer the claimant, at the government's expense, to a physician for medical evaluation. The physician is asked to take a detailed medical history, perform an examination, and obtain tests (e.g., pulmonary function studies). The physician then should provide information regarding medical conditions suffered by the claimant and how they affect the activities of daily living; cause difficulties in maintaining social functioning; and result in deficiencies in concentration, persistence, or pace, causing failure to complete tasks and episodes of decompensation or deterioration. At the conclusion of the process, an initial determination of whether the person is totally and permanently disabled is made.

The initial determination can be appealed for reconsideration at the state level but by adjudicators other than the one involved in the initial determination. If disability again is denied, the claimant may request a hearing with an administrative law judge (ALJ), who reviews the evidence and can make a decision to grant benefits. Of the claims evaluated by an ALJ, about 60% are approved. At these hearings, testimony is taken from the claimant, physicians (medical experts), mental health practitioners, family members, vocational experts, and other involved parties. The ALJ considers the evidence in light of the law and makes a decision. A denial at the ALJ level can be appealed to the appeals council and then to federal district court and ultimately to the U. S. Supreme Court.

THE VETERANS ADMINISTRATION (VA) DISABILITY BENEFITS

Veterans Administration programs may provide both monetary and nonmonetary assistance to eligible veterans. Many of the currently 163 VA hospitals provide long-term residential care for those who are disabled. The disability often is psychiatric. Common diagnoses are substance abuse, posttraumatic stress disorder, and depressive illnesses. The VA has found that mental impairment constitutes the single largest category among veteran beneficiaries who receive benefits. The VA program is not based entirely on the inability to work. A "service-connected" veteran is paid *compensation*, and a nonservice-connected veteran is paid a *pension*. In addition, under present regulations, if a veteran meets certain income criteria, he or she is entitled to free medical care. This also occurs when the veteran has a service-connected disability.

Physician evaluators for the VA system find it unique. It does not require a physician to do any impairment or disability rating but only requires the medical evaluation, including making a diagnosis and describing the severity of the medical problem. The evaluation is submitted to a three-member board, who uses a manual to assign an impairment or disability rating. The three-member board comprises two VA officials and one physician, usually not the physician who originally examined the veteran. The VA system is generally regarded as more liberal than the AMA *Guides*. The evaluating physician need not be employed by the VA. Physicians interested in obtaining referrals for medical evaluation should contact the nearest VA Hospital for information.

FEDERAL WORKERS' COMPENSATION PROGRAMS

Three main U.S. federal workers' compensation program are administered through the various divisions of the Office of Worker's Compensation Programs (OWCP), located in Washington, D.C. The OWCP manages three federal workers' compensation acts: FECA, the Longshore and Harbour workers Compensation Act, and the Federal Black Lung Program. Physicians who wish to be involved as evaluators for these systems should contact the office of Worker's Compensation Programs, 200 Constitution Avenue, Room 53522, Washington, D.C. 20210.

Federal Employees Compensation Act (FECA)

Civilian employees of the federal government are provided compensation benefits under FECA. In addition, benefits may be provided to dependents if the condition results in death. The act covers civilian employees of the U.S. government, postal workers, Peace Corp workers, and others. A federal employee cannot sue the federal government or recover damages under any other statue for work-related injury and resulting disability. Benefits under FECA are the sole remedy against the

U.S. government for work-related injury or death. Unlike state compensation systems, FECA statutorily excludes disability benefit claims involving the brain, the heart, or back.

LaDou and Whyte (19) noted that in the federal workers' compensation system changes in the law in 1974 caused a dramatic increase in claims. At that time, it was decided that a continuation of pay would be mandated for any worker injured on the job. There is no time limit on wage loss or medical benefits, and there is no dollar limit on the coverage of medical benefits. Extensive vocational rehabilitation services are available. In addition, a worker could have any physician as a treating doctor; as such, a worker could go to different doctors in the hope of finding one who would fill out the forms by certifying that he or she is unable to work.

Longshore and Harbor Workers Act

This program is similar to FECA. It also excludes the disability benefits for the brain, heart, and back. It grants compensation benefits for disability or death to shoreside maritime employees, excluding administrative and clerical employees from coverage as well as others listed in the act. Mostly, this act covers any person engaged in maritime employment, including any longshoreman or other person engaged in longshoring operations and any harbor worker, including ship repairmen, builders, and breakers.

Employers responsible under this act include any employer whose employees work in maritime employment, in whole or in part, on the navigable waters of the United States, including any adjoining pier, wharf, dry dock, terminal, building way, marine railway, or other adjoining area customarily used by an employer in loading, unloading, repairing, or building a vessel (20).

Federal Black Lung Program

The 1977 Federal Mine, Safety and Health Act, or the Federal Black Lung Program, covers coal miners, whether they are surface or underground miners. It also covers railroad workers who hauled coal as well as other transportation workers, including coal truck drivers. This act provides monthly payments and medical treatment benefits to coal miners who are totally disabled from pneumoconiosis (black lung) arising from their employment in or around the nation's coal mines and monthly payments to eligible surviving dependents. Present and former coal miners (including certain transportation and construction workers exposed to coal mine dust) and their surviving dependents (including surviving spouses, orphaned children, totally dependent parents, brothers, and sisters) may file claims (20). The Federal Black Lung Program is administered through the U.S. Department of Labor, which processes claims.

The Federal Employers Liability Act

The Federal Employers Liability Act, or FELA, was enacted in 1908 and is the sole remedy for interstate railroad workers against their employers for job-related injury. It is quite an adversarial system. Railroad employees must bring a lawsuit to the state civil court or federal court against the railroad if they cannot reach a settlement for the disability claim with their employer without litigation. Physicians are required to examine the person, establish a diagnosis, do the rating, and in some cases comment on the disability. This area is one where a physician may be required to testify in a federal court.

In order for the employee to prevail, he or she must prove in court that the railroad was negligent. The railroad can assert a defense of contributory negligence. The jury then must decide whether the person was injured and whether there was any contributory negligence on the part of the employee. The jury may apportion the responsibility among parties. The injured railroad worker's recovery may be limited by his or her own contributory negligence unless the railroad was in violation of the Federal Safety Appliance Act or the Boiler Inspection Act. If the railroad is shown to be in noncompliance with these acts, the employee does not have to show or prove negligence on the part of the employer; railroad liability is automatically assumed. There are no limits to the amount of awards; however, most FELA cases are settled.

Jones Act (Merchant Marine Act)

This act is similar to FELA, and it covers civilian sailors while they are in the service of a ship or vessel in navigable waters. A sailor or a seaman who becomes sick on the ship is not covered by this law. Generally, the coverage for maintenance and cure of sickness and injuries is covered under the General Admiralty Law, including medical benefits and wage replacement. If the sailor is permanently injured, to collect, he or she must bring a lawsuit against the master or owner of the ship. Cases under the Jones Act usually are settled out of court, because courts are usually liberal toward the seamen, considering them a ward of the court.

Americans with Disabilities Act (ADA)

The ADA, enacted in 1992, prohibits employment discrimination based on disability. It compels employers to employ qualified persons with disabilities who meet the essential functions of the job, requiring the employer to make reasonable accommodations for a qualified person with a disability. The definition of *disability* under the ADA is liberal: "any physical or mental impairment that substantially limits one or more of the major life activities," which includes such functions as caring for oneself, performing manual tasks, walking, seeing, hearing, speaking, breathing, learning, and working.

This act requires employers to provide "a reasonable accommodation to the known physical or mental limitations of a qualified applicant or employee with a disability unless it can be shown that the accommodation would impose an undue hardship on the business." A *qualified* disabled employee (applicant) is one who with or without reasonable accommodation can perform the essential function of the position in question without posing a direct threat to the safety of himself or herself or others. *Essential* means fundamental, basic, necessary, or vital. *Accommodation* is defined as a modification of the job or the workplace that enables a disabled employee to meet the same job demand as other employees in the same job or a similar job. *Reasonable accommodation* means something that would not cause undue hardship to the employer, such as an accommodation, but does not impose significant difficulty or expense. The purpose of this legislation was, in part, to assist persons with disabilities to be employed. Recently, the *Washington Post* reported that in the first year since it was enacted, the ADA resulted in 12,000 cases of litigation, much more than the other civil rights acts. The costs of such litigation are obviously considerable. From July 26, 1992, to September 30, 1997, 17.4% of charges were back impairments.

Private Sector Disability Programs

In addition to the various compensation systems described in this chapter, physicians sometimes are asked to do a medical evaluation for private disability insurance companies and for various union and other private organizations' disability and retirement funds. Private disability insurance policies usually state that the policyholder need only have his or her personal physician certify the disability to start the benefits; however, this is not always true. Shernoff (21) described numerous cases in which insurance companies were assessed punitive damages for acting in "bad faith," when they refused payment of benefits under disability policies by asserting that no disability existed but the contrary was proven.

Family Medical Leave Act (FMLA)

As a basic law, the FMLA applies to employers of 50 or more employees. Employees must have worked for the employer for 12 months and at least 1,250 hours during the period before the leave request. Leave must be granted to both male and female employees for childbirth, adoption, care of immediate family, and the employee's own illness. Leaves are unpaid, but hospitalization and life insurance premiums must be continued while on leave. The employer may require a physician's certification to support the leave, and the employee can be required to give 30 days' notice (if possible).

The employer must designate the type of leave within 2 days of the leave request. That is, does it count toward the 12 weeks? It is regular sick leave or just time off? All such designations and limitations must be given to the employee in writing within 2 days of the leave. The employer must spell out in writing all the specific terms of the leave, including regular certification from the physician, whether the employer can substitute other leave plans, the method the employee must use to pay for medical coverage premiums, and under what conditions the employee will be restored to his or her original job. (Certain key employees may be permanently replaced during FMLA.)

For short-term leaves, the employer must ascertain each time whether the leave requested is under the FMLA. If the employee declines to so designate the leave, the employer may elect either to declare it FMLA or not. Notices of the FMLA must be posted in a form that can be easily read.

The base period for calculating the 12-month period must be stated in advance, such as the calendar year, fiscal year, employee's anniversary date, or a rolling 12-month period starting when the employee first uses the leave. The employee may be discharged properly if, following the 12 weeks of leave, he or she is unable to perform one or more essential functions of the job.

The ADA may be figured in here to require a reasonable accommodation. Light duty, if accepted by the employee, counts toward the 12 weeks but must be explained out front (22).

SUMMARY

Finally, the physician is considered the ultimate authority on dysfunctional status and overall work potential based on impairment (23). The problem is that many physicians often do not understand the issues involved in the practice of disability medicine, mainly because of a lack of experience or education in this field. Medical schools and residency trainings usually do not prepare physicians for this aspect of medical practice. Confronted with issues of impairment and disability evaluations and assisting administrators and adjudicators in making meaningful decisions, most physicians feel unprepared, uncomfortable, and sometimes inadequately trained. Decisions about work fitness and return to work often are based solely on the patient's symptoms or representations, resulting in claimants not being evaluated optimally or fairly. Physicians who deal with these issues on a regular basis need to familiarize themselves with various compensation systems in this country, the various impairment rating guides, and the medical legal issues involved in the specialty of disability medicine. Obtaining specialized training and credentials in this field would be most helpful.

The American Academy of Disability Evaluating Physicians, established in 1988, has about 1,500 members and fellows and provides comprehensive training programs in the assessment of disability and impairments. The institution of such training programs to reach and educate a wider number of physicians would help them to understand better the clinical and legal aspects of the disability evaluation process and would assist them to make more educated assessments.

REFERENCES

1. Doege T, ed. *Guides to the evaluation of permanent impairment,* 4th ed. Chicago: American Medical Association, 1993, pp. 7–12.
2. Ranavaya MI, Rondinelli RD. The major U.S. disability and compensation systems: origins and historical overview. In: Rondinelli, Katz, eds. *Impairment rating and disability evaluation.* Philadelphia: WB Saunders, Co 1998 (in press).
3. Trinkaus E, Zimmerman MR. Trauma among the Shanidar Neanderthals. *Am J Phys Anthropol* 1982;57: 61–76.
4. Yaron R. *The laws of Eshnunna.* Jerusalem-Leiden: The Magnes Press, The Hebrew University, 1988.

5. Johns RE. Compensation and impairment rating systems in the United States. *J Disabil* 1990;1:4.

6. Drew KF. *The Lombard laws*. Houston: University of Pennsylvania Press.

7. Hadler NM. Who should determine disability? *Semin Arthritis Rheum* 1984;14:45–51.

8. Hadler NM. Legal ramifications of the medical definition of back disease. *Ann Intern Med* 1978;89:992–999.

9. Snook SH, Webster BS. The cost of disability. *Clin Orthop* 1987;221:77–84.

10. Pope AM, Tarlov AR, eds. *Disability in America—toward a national agenda for prevention*. Washington, DC: National Academy Press, 1991.

11. Andersson GBJ. Disability evaluation. In: King PM, ed. *Sourcebook of occupational rehabilitation*, New York: Plenum Press, 1998:247–253.

12. U.S. Bureau of Disability Insurance. *Disability evaluation under social security: a handbook for physicians*. Washington, DC: U.S. Government Printing Office, 1970.

13. Social Security Administration. *Disability evaluation under social security*. Washington, DC: U.S. Government Printing Office, 1979, pp.1–22.

14. Minnesota Medical Association. *Workers' compensation permanent partial disability schedule*. Minneapolis, MN: Author, 1984.

15. Ranavaya MI. Impairment, disability and compensation in the United States: an overview. *Disability* 1996;5: 1–20.

16. Larson A. *The law of workmen's compensation*. New York: Matthew Bender, 1985;4.30, 1:26.

17. Zwecker H. Social security disability benefits: an overview. *J Disabil* 1991;2:2:135–140.

18. Akermann S. (Performance Spectrum in Occupational Disability. Causes—occupational groups—age—duration of insurance). *Versicherungsmedizin* 1990;42(6): 184–190. (In German).

19. LaDou J, Whyte AA. Workers' compensation: the federal experience. *J Occup Med* 1981;23:823–828.

20. Johns RE. Compensation and impairment rating systems in the United States. *J Disabil* 1990;1:4.

21. Shernoff WM. *How to make insurance companies pay your claim*. Mamaroneck, New York: Hastings House, 1990.

22. Holroyd FF. Business alert. *West Virginia State Journal*, July 3, 1995.

23. May R. Editorial comment. *Disability Evaluation and Rehabilitation Review* 1996;3:3.

24. Andersson GBJ. Disability evaluation. In: King PM, ed. *Sourcebook of occupational rehabilitation*, New York: Plenum Press, 1998:247–253.

Occupational Musculoskeletal Disorders
edited by T. G. Mayer, R. J. Gatchel, and P. B. Polatin.
Lippincott Williams & Wilkins, Philadelphia © 2000.

39

Current American Medical Association Techniques for Assessing Musculoskeletal Impairment and Maximum Medical Improvement

Robert H. Haralson III

*Department of Surgery, University of Tennessee Center for the Health Sciences,
Knoxville, Tennessee 37802*

The 4th Edition of the American Medical Association's (AMA) *Guides to the Evaluation of Permanent Impairment* (1) was published in June 1993. About 40 states either require or suggest the use of the AMA Guides for the evaluation of impairment. Most of these jurisdictions require the use of the 4th edition or the current edition. A few use the 3rd edition, revised. Significant differences exist between the 4th edition and the 3rd edition, revised, and the physician is encouraged to use the 4th edition for evaluations if at all possible. The most commonly used chapter is the "Musculoskeletal System" (Chap. 3). It has been estimated that this chapter is consulted 70% of the time that the AMA *Guides* is used. This chapter in this book deals only with that musculoskeletal chapter. The 5th edition will be an update of the 4th and is being written at this time.

IMPORTANT TIPS TO REMEMBER

Chapter 1 of the *Guides* discusses the philosophy of impairment rating, and Chapter 2 discusses the format of certain reports. Without an understanding of these two chapters, it is easy for the rater to make an error.

Read the Directions

Chapter 3 of the AMA *Guides* contains some specific "cookbook" directions for the evaluation of impairment, and the user should follow these directions.

The *Guides* is simply a guide; it is not "set in stone." The physician is free to stray from the guides if circumstances warrant. The only admonishment is that the rater needs to explain the departure in the report. An example is in the rating of rotator cuff dysfunction. The *Guides* does not provide a good way to rate rotator cuff disease if the patient has a full range of motion of the shoulder. In such a case, the rater must use other methods. The loss-of-strength index method can be used; because there are no normative values for shoulder strength, the rater must be somewhat innovative. However the rating is done, if the method does not follow the *Guides*, it is important to include a complete explanation of the method used and the reason for deviating from the *Guides*.

Understanding the Entire Section

The user should thoroughly understand the entire section being used, be it upper extremity, lower extremity, or spine. In many cases, a particular disease or injury can be rated several different ways, and the user must decide which of these different methods is best for a particular patient. Many of the mistakes we encounter when reviewing impairment ratings have come about by the rater merely turning to a particular area in the *Guides,* performing the rating from that limited area, and not understanding that there are other considerations that should be taken into account and that better methods may exist for rating that particular patient.

Range of Motion is Active

Range-of-motion measurements are of active range of motion. It is quite permissible for the evaluator to assist a patient gently when moving a joint to get a better idea of the difference in active and passive motion, but the final rating should be based on the active motion. For instance, if a flexor tendon in a finger is lacerated, a patient may have full passive motion of the finger, but the active motion is what is important to the function of that finger.

Hand Dominance

Hand dominance is not a factor in Chapter 3 of the *Guides*. There is an unfortunate inconsistency in the AMA *Guides*: Hand dominance is considered in the chapter on neurology (Chap. 4), but the authors of the musculoskeletal chapter elected not to penalize a patient just because the impairment was in the nondominant extremity.

Combined Values Tables

An understanding of the use of the combined values table found on pages 322 through 324 is important for proper use of the AMA *Guides*. Frequently, impairment ratings in different areas or body parts are not additive but are combined. The philosophy behind this concept is that if a patient deserves a rating in two body areas or two systems, the second rating is that of a patient who is already rendered less than 100% by an earlier rating.

Therefore, the second rating is multiplied by the first rating to give the combined value.

Pain

In general, pain is not considered when evaluating impairment in the musculoskeletal system. The authors assigned values to the impairment ratings that take into account the pain that usually accompanies the conditions causing the impairment. This is done because pain is not measurable in its quantity or quality, and therefore it is extremely difficult to assess impairment ratings based on the patient's interpretation of pain. Pain may be used in some instances to help the evaluator map out areas of neurologic damage or involvement in causalgia-like symptoms, but the amount of pain is not taken into account.

Round Off Joint Measurements

Because it is difficult to accurately measure joint motion within 10 degrees, the instructions are to round joint measurements to the nearest 10 degrees.

Condition Must Be Stable

Before a condition can be rated, it should be stable, meaning that no significant change in the patient's condition should be expected in the foreseeable future. If a surgical condition has a possibility of improving the patient's condition, but the patient elects not to undergo the surgical procedure, the rater should rate the patient based on the findings at that time. The rater may include a note in the report to the effect that improvement could be gained by use of a surgical procedure. The patient should not be rated as though he or she had undergone the surgical procedure.

The spine represents a special circumstance. In the lumbar spine, for instance, a ruptured disc that causes a significant radiculopathy would eventuate in a rating of 10% to the body as a whole. In the spine, the rating is the result of the injury, not the treatment. As a result, once a diagnosis of significant radiculopathy is made, the patient is stable in that the rating will not change despite possible improvement by the patient. Therefore, the patient can be rated as soon as the diagnosis of significant radiculopathy is made. This is true in the spine section only and does not hold true for the upper and lower extremity, where the results of treatment may affect the impairment rating.

Prepared Reports

There are prepared reports for the upper extremity, and the user is encouraged to use these reports. They force a complete, accurate evaluation and appear more officious than plain-text reports.

UPPER EXTREMITY

Fingers and Hand

The fingers are rated by combining ratings for amputation, sensory loss, and loss of range of motion. When evaluating a thumb or finger, all three of these impairments must be taken into consideration. The first step is to rate amputation. One merely compares the level of amputation to the appropriate figure in the *Guides* (Fig. 1). For the thumb (in the *Guides*, Fig. 7 on page 3/24; for the fingers,

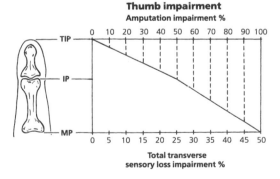

FIG. 1. Impairment of thumb resulting from amputation at various levels (**top scale**) or total transverse sensory loss (**bottom scale**). Total transverse sensory loss impairments correspond to 50% of amputation value. (From Swanson AB. Evaluation of impairment of function in the hand. *Surg Clin North Am* 1964, p. 927, Fig. 2.)

Fig. 17 on page 3/30), comparison is done of the level of amputation with the drawing in the figure; the impairment is read directly from the upper numeric scale. Note that the lower numeric scale is for total transverse sensory loss, which will be addressed later.

The next step is to assess loss of sensation. In a digit, loss of sensation can be either *transverse* (involving both digital nerves) or *longitudinal* (involving only one digital nerve). The rater first maps out the area involved and then assesses the degree of sensory loss, measured by determining two-point discrimination. This determination may be done using a paper clip, an electrocardiography (EKG) protractor, or one of the more sophisticated commercially available measuring devices. The rater determines whether the two-point discrimination is less than 7 mm (considered *normal*), 7 to 15 mm (considered *partial loss*), or greater than 15 mm (considered *total loss*). In the case of the thumb, if the sensory loss is transverse, the rater refers to the AMA *Guides*, Fig. 7 on page 3/24 (Fig. 1) and compares the length of the sensory loss with the numeric scale on the bottom of the figure. If the sensory loss is complete (i.e., greater than 15 mm), the impairment rating is read directly from the scale. If the sensory loss is transverse and partial (50%), the numeric value from the scale is halved. If the two-point discrimination is less than 7 mm, sensation is considered normal, and there is no impairment due to sensory loss.

In the case of longitudinal sensory loss, the rater refers to Table 4 on page 3/25 of the *Guides* for the thumb and little finger. Again, the degree of sensory loss is determined, and then the rating is read directly from Table 4. Note that the loss for the ulnar digital nerve of both the thumb and little finger is greater than the comparable loss of the radial digital nerve. In the case of the fingers, the procedure is similar; however, for transverse sensory loss, the rater refers to Fig. 17 on page 3/30 of the *Guides* and for longitudinal sensory loss, to Table 9 on page 3/31. Table 8 on page 3/31 is merely a reproduction of Table 4, mentioned earlier.

The next step in evaluating impairment of the fingers is to assess loss of range of motion in the various joints of the fingers. Range of motion of the fingers is measured using a goniometer, and several goniometers are commercially available. Those that are normally used to measure larger joints are sometimes difficult to use in the fingers; so I suggest the use of one of the commercially available finger goniometers (Fig. 2). In addition, modification of some of the goniometers obtained from hardware stores has been quite successful. The more active flexion and extension of each of the joints in the finger are measured. In the case of the thumb, the flexion and extension of the metaphalangeal (MP) and interphalangeal (IP) joints are measured. The measurements are rounded to the nearest 10 degrees, and then the rater refers to the appropriate pie chart and reads the impairment rating from the appropriate numeric scale (Fig. 3). As an example, we use the thumb IP joint and Fig. 10 on page 3/26 of the AMA *Guides*. If the rater measured flexion of the thumb IP joint to be 30 degrees (indicated by the letter *V* in the pie chart), the proper flexion impairment rating would be 4%, indicated by the scale headed by the letters *IF%*. Note that the possibility of an extension contracture is addressed in Fig. 10; if maximum flexion is −10 degrees of extension, the appropriate rating would be 11%. The rater then measures extension and refers to the scale marked *IE%*. In this case, the inability to extend the thumb past 0 results in no impairment; however, if the patient could not extend past 30 degrees of flexion, the proper rating would be impairment of 5%, read from the IE% scale. The *IA%* scale represents arthrodesis. If the patient has no mo-

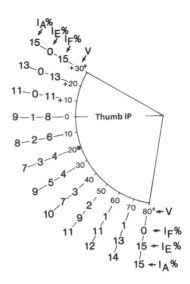

$I_A\%$ = Impairment due to ankylosis
$I_E\%$ = Impairment due to loss of extension
$I_F\%$ = Impairment due to loss of flexion
V   = Measured angles of motion
*   = Position of function

FIG. 3. Thumb Impairments due to abnormal motion at the interphalangeal (*IP*) joint. Relative value of functional unit is 15% of total thumb motion. (From Swanson AB, Goran-Hagert C, de Groot Swanson G. Evaluation of impairment of hand function. In: Hunter JM, Schneider LH, Mackin E, et al. *Rehabilitation of the Hand*. St. Louis, MO: CV Mosby Co., 1978. p. 62, Fig. 4-22.)

tion, then the angle of arthrodesis is measured, and the impairment rating is read from the arthrodesis, or IA%, scale. Note that the impairment rating for the IA% scale is the sum of the ratings for the IF% and IE% scales. Note also that the position of function (in the case of the thumb IP joint, 20 degrees of flexion) results in the smallest impairment rating. This procedure is repeated for the MP joint (in the *Guides*, referring to Fig. 13 on page 3/27).

In the case of the thumb, the rater must measure the motions in the carpometacarpal (CMC) joint. The thumb CMC joint has three motions: thumb adduction, thumb radial abduction, and thumb opposition. The rater refers to the appropriate tables on pages 3/28 and 3/29 and reads the impairment from the numeric scale. Explicit instructions for measuring these three motions in the thumb are found on pages 3/28 and 3/29 of the AMA *Guides*. A word of cau-

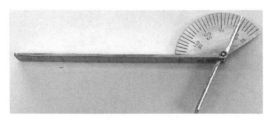

FIG. 2. A goniometer which is used to measure motion in single joints.

tion is needed. Many people cannot place their thumb pads over their fifth metacarpal heads when performing opposition, and that means that they would be given a rating according to the *Guides*. For this reason, comparison to the uninvolved side is appropriate, and the rating is adjusted accordingly. The impairment ratings for all three motions in the CMC joints then are added together to result in the total impairment rating for the loss of motion of the thumb CMC joint. If other joints of the thumb are involved, the impairment ratings for all the involved joints are added together, unlike the procedure in the fingers where the separate joint impairments are combined. This is because the thumb joint motions are so interrelated that the authors believed that addition rather than combination was more appropriate.

In the case of the fingers, flexion and extension of the distal interphalangeal (DIP), proximal interphalangeal (PIP), and metacarpophalangeal (MP) joints are similar to the thumb, and the rater refers to the appropriate pie chart and reads the impairment rating directly from the appropriate numeric scale. The rating for loss of flexion is added to the rating for the loss of extension to give the total loss for that joint. If more than one joint of the fingers is involved, the ratings from all the involved joints are combined to give the total impairment due to loss of motion of each finger.

The last step in rating impairment to a thumb or single finger is to combine the impairment ratings from amputation, sensory loss, and loss of motion to determine the final rating for impairment of each finger. Using Tables 1, 2, and 3 on pages 3/18, 3/19, and 3/20 of the *Guides*, the finger impairment can be related to impairment of the hand, to the upper extremity, and then to the body as a whole. If more than one finger is involved, the impairment of each finger is related to impairment of the hand, using Table 1 on page 3/18, and then the percents of hand impairment for each finger are added to give total hand impairment.

Wrist, Elbow, and Shoulder

The wrist, elbow, and shoulder joints usually are rated by assessing loss of range of motion. The ratings and the appropriate pie charts refer to impairments of the upper extremity.

The wrist has four motions: flexion, extension, radial deviation, and ulnar deviation; and the impairments for each of these four motions are added to determine total upper-extremity impairment resulting from loss of motion in the wrist. The elbow has four motions: flexion, extension, pronation, and supination. The impairment ratings for each of these four motions are added together to determine the impairment of the upper extremity for the elbow. In the case of a wrist injury that results in loss of wrist motion as well as pronation and supination, the rating must be a combination of the wrist and elbow ratings.

The shoulder has six motions: flexion, extension, adduction, abduction, internal rotation, and external rotation. Directions to obtain these measurements are specific in the AMA *Guides*. The rater refers to the appropriate pie charts, reads the impairment rating from the numeric scale, and adds the impairment ratings from each of the six motions together to obtain the total impairment of the upper extremity for loss of motion in the shoulder joint.

Peripheral Nerve Disorders

Peripheral nerve injuries and other disorders of nerves are fairly common in the upper extremity, and the impairment from these conditions can be determined through a stepwise procedure. The first step is to map out the area of the upper extremity that is involved and to make a determination as to which neurologic structures are involved. Figures 45 on page 3/50 and 48 on 3/55 will assist the rater in making this determination. There are three options: disorders of the cervical roots, disorders of the brachial plexus, or disorders of the peripheral nerves. Table 13 on page 3/51 of the *Guides* describes the percentage of impairment resulting from involvement of the roots (spinal nerves), and Table 14 on page 3/52 describes the percentage of impairment resulting from involvement of the brachial plexus and its individual trunks.

Table 15 on page 3/54 describes the impairments resulting from involvement of individual peripheral nerves.

The second step is to determine the magnitude of the sensory deficit and of the muscular weakness. Table 11 on page 3/48 describes the method of determining the magnitude of the sensory deficits and equates that to a percentage deficit. Table 12 on page 3/49 allows the rater to determine the percentage motor deficit of individual muscles groups.

Once the nerve structures involved are identified and the magnitude of the sensory and motor deficit determined, the rater refers to the tables appropriate for the particular nerve structure: Tables 13, 14, and 15. These tables give the percent of impairment attributable to 100% involvement of the sensory and motor component of each structure. The procedure is to multiply the magnitude of the sensory and motor components determined from Tables 11 and 12 by the of percent of impairment for total involvement found in Tables 13, 14, or 15 to determine the impairment for each component (sensory and motor). Then the impairments of the sensory component and the motor component are combined to calculate the total impairment for involvement of nerve structures in the upper extremity.

Entrapment Neuropathy

Entrapment neuropathy can be rated by using one of two methods. The preferred method is that described for evaluating other impairments of peripheral nerves. That is, the rater determines any loss of sensation and strength secondary to the nerve entrapment, determines the magnitude of the deficit from Tables 11 and 12, and then multiplies that figure by the proper number in Table 15 on page 3/54.

The alternative method is to use Table 16 on page 3/47. This table is controversial, however, and it is pointed out that no relationship exists between the magnitude of the delay of transmission of a nerve impulse and the magnitude of the symptoms. Therefore, a severe delay in nerve-conduction velocity across the

wrist does not necessarily mean the patient has severe carpal tunnel symptoms.

Vascular Disorders of the Upper Extremity

Table 17 on page 3/57 gives a detailed description of impairments resulting from vascular disorders, and the reader is referred to that table.

Other Disorders of the Upper Extremity

Many conditions are not rated well by loss of motion. Some conditions leave the joints with a full range of motion and yet render the patient significantly impaired. These are categorized as *bone and joint deformities* and *musculotendinous impairments*. Described under bone and joint deformities are joint crepitation with motion, joint swelling due to synovial hypertrophy, digital lateral deviation, digital rotational deformity, persistent joint subluxation or dislocation, joint instability, wrist and elbow joint radial and ulnar deviation, carpal instability, and arthroplasty. Under musculotendinous impairment are intrinsic tightness, constrictive tenosynovitis, extensor tendon subluxation at the MP joint, and other musculoskeletal system defects. These impairments can be determined by a stepwise procedure. Table 18 on page 3/58 of the *Guides* describes the impairment to the digit, hand, upper extremity, or whole person of a condition that renders that body area 100% impaired. The procedure is to determine the quantity of impairment of the individual condition by referring to the appropriate tables and then multiplying that percent by the impairment for 100% involvement of that particular structure. For instance, if impairment is from crepitation of a joint, the rater refers to Table 19 on page 3/59 and determines the magnitude of the impairments caused by the crepitation. If, for instance, there is moderate crepitation, constant during active range of motion, the impairment magnitude would be 20%. If the involvement was of the CMC joint of the thumb, the 20% impairment from Table 19 would be multiplied by 75% from Table 18, and the result would be a 15% impairment of the thumb.

Similarly, if the patient had impairment secondary to radial deviation of the elbow joint of a moderate degree, the result would be a 20% impairment of the joint, as indicated in Table 25 on page 3/60. That 20% then would be multiplied by the 70% from Table 18, with a resultant 14% of the upper extremity.

Musculotendinous impairments are determined in the same manner. For instance, if the patient had impairment secondary to intrinsic tightness, the severity would be determined from Table 28 on page 3/63. If moderate involvement were present, the result would be a 40% impairment of the digit, and if the involvement was of the ring or little finger PIP joint, the 60% impairment from Table 28 would be multiplied by the 80% impairment from Table 18, with a resultant 32% impairment of the ring or little finger.

In many sections, some italicized admonishments are listed, and it is important that the rater be familiar with these. For instance, in several sections, the instructions are to combine impairment from this section with impairment for loss of motion, and in other sections that is not done.

Strength Evaluation

The last method of determining impairment of the upper extremity to be discussed is *strength evaluation*. The strength-evaluation method can be used in one of two ways. If the rating physician does not believe the other methods of impairment rating adequately describe the patient's impairment, the rater may elect to combine impairment resulting from loss of strength with the previously determined impairment. This is an unusual circumstance, however. Usually, the rating from other areas of the upper-extremity section take into account the weakness that would accompany the loss of motion or other impairment. Occasionally, however, when the rater believes the weakness is not explained by the condition, the two methods can be combined.

Second, if the physician does not believe any of the previous methods can be used to determine impairment, this method can be used by itself. The normative values for grip and pinch strength listed in Tables 31, 32, and 33 on pages 3/64 and 3/65 of the *Guides* are gross measurements, and further research is necessary to give this method more validity. Nonetheless, this method is still useful in certain cases.

This method requires measuring strength by using a pinch gauge or measurement of grip strength with a Jamar dynamometer. When using the Jamar dynamometer, the second (4 cm) or third (6 cm) positions are used. The AMA *Guides* and the literature accompanying the Jamar dynamometer and the pinch gauge describe validity testing, including rapid exchange, repeated measures, and measurement of the uninvolved extremity as well as the involved extremity. The rater must be convinced that the patient is giving full effort. If all the criteria are met, this method can be used by determining the pinch and grip strength and inserting the measurements into the following formula: normal strength (from Tables 31, 32, or 33) minus abnormal strength (from the measurements of the patient), divided by normal strength. The quotient equals the percent of strength loss index. Impairment of the upper extremity secondary to loss of strength is read from Table 34 on page 3/65.

On pages 3/66 and 3/67 of the AMA *Guides* is a stepwise, detailed explanation of how to determine impairment in the upper extremity. On page 3/66 through 3/74 are some examples of impairment using the prepared upper-extremity chart with accompanying explanations. The reader is referred to those charts for review of the stepwise procedure.

LOWER EXTREMITY

General

Function in the upper and lower extremity varies considerably. The main function of the upper extremity is to place the hand in the proper position, and range of motion is therefore extremely important and, in general, the best way to rate the upper extremity. The function of the lower extremity, however, is to bear weight; as a result, certain conditions in the lower extremity that have little to do with range of motion become important in terms of impairment. For this reason, range of motion, although important in the lower extremity, has a lesser role, and the authors have supplied several other methods to rate impairment of the lower extremity. The user needs to be familiar with all the methods and should choose the best one. It is not uncommon to use several methods and then pick the one that most accurately reflects the impairment of that particular patient. The methods available are limb-length discrepancy, gait derangement, muscle atrophy, manual muscle testing, range of motion, joint ankylosis, arthritis, amputation, diagnosis-based estimates, skin loss, peripheral nerve injuries, causalgia and reflex sympathetic dystrophy, and vascular disorders. In general, only one method is used for each patient.

In the tables on the lower extremity, the impairment ratings frequently are listed in three forms. The number without parentheses or brackets is the rating to the body as a whole; the number with parentheses is a rating for the lower extremity, and the number with brackets is the rating of that particular area (i.e., foot). Under no circumstances should a rating exceed that for an amputation at the same level. The lower extremity is considered 40% of the body, and therefore no lower-extremity rating should exceed 40% of the body.

Leg-length Discrepancy

Leg-length discrepancy can be a significant impairment if it is greater than 2 cm. Impairments are described in Table 35 on page 3/75 of the *Guides*. In general, teleroentgenography should be used because measurement of the lower extremity using a tape measure can be inaccurate.

Gait Derangement

Gait derangements can be used to assess impairment if no better way to do so is known. Table 36 on page 3/76 describes a variety of gait derangements and assigns an impairment rating to each.

Muscle Atrophy

A number of conditions in the lower extremity can result in muscle atrophy and a significant impairment, even though they have healed. An example is a fracture of the tibia in an older person, which may heal in perfect alignment but renders the patient with an impairment because of the patient's inability to rehabilitate musculature. Therefore, the authors of the *Guides* included atrophy measurements as a way to assess impairment. Table 37 on page 3/37 lists impairments resulting from atrophies in the thigh and calf. The rater simply determines the amount of atrophy by comparing circumferential measurements of the thigh or calf with those of the sound extremity and reading the impairment from Table 37. This method cannot be used if there is bilateral lower-extremity involvement.

Manual Muscle Testing

Similar to muscle atrophy, the presence of weakness in the musculature can be used to assess impairment. Tables 38 and 39 on page 3/37 guide the reader in this method. The rater should note that there can be weakness associated with more than one motion about a joint, (flexion and extension). The most severe weakness should be used to determine impairment. For instance, if the patient's knee extension is grade IV but knee flexion is grade I, the rater should use the flexion impairment rating to determine the patient's impairment.

Range of Motion

In some cases, loss of range of motion is extremely important, as in the upper extremity. The authors of the *Guides* provided a number of tables on page 3/78 that describe impairments for loss of motion of the hip, knee, ankle, hindfoot (subtalar joint), and toes. To determine impairment resulting from loss of range of motion, the rater measures the active motion in the joint and refers to the corresponding Table on page 3/78. Rather than assessing impairment based on pie charts with a continuum of impairment ratings as in the upper extremity, in the lower extremity, impairments are grouped into *mild, moderate,* and *severe* categories. The rater should measure all the appropriate motions and select the impairment rating that is associated with the greatest loss. For instance, in the hip, if the patient has mild loss of internal rotation, external rotation, abduction, and adduction but severe loss of flexion, the rater would choose the severe category for impairment resulting from loss of hip range of motion. Note also that in certain deformities mentioned in Tables 41 and 44 on page 3/78 varus and valgus angulation of the knee and similar deformities of the hindfoot (subtalar joint) are associated with impairments. If the patient has both loss of motion and deformity, the two impairments are combined.

If there is loss of range of motion of multiple joints in the foot and ankle (toes, hindfoot, ankle), the ratings for loss of motion for each joint should be combined to determine the total impairment of the foot. Ratings for loss of motion of multiple lesser toe MP joints should be combined. There is no impairment for loss of motion of the IP joints of the lesser toes.

Joint Ankylosis

Sometimes injuries to joints result in complete loss of motion as a result of either a fibrous ankylosis or an actual bony arthrodesis. In these cases, the rater should refer to Tables 46-59 on pages 3/79 to 3/81 of the *Guides.* Note that ankylosis of any joint, even in the functional position, results in impairment. In the hip, ankylosis in the functional position, which is 25 to 40 degrees of flexion, neutral rotation, and neutral adduction–abduction, results in an impairment rating of 50% of the lower extremity or 20% of the body. In the knee, the functional position is 10 to 15 degrees of flexion and results in impairment of

67% of the lower extremity and 27% of the body. The functional position of the ankle is the neutral position and results in an impairment of 4% or the body, 10% of the lower extremity, and 14% of the foot. The optimal position of the hindfoot (subtalar joint) is neutral and results in an impairment of 4% of the whole person, 10% of the lower extremity, and 14% of the foot. When using this method, the rater determines whether there is a deviation of the joint from the optimal position and refers to Tables 46 through 59 to determine the amount of impairment that should be added to the impairment for ankylosis in the functional position (see instructions beneath each table). In the case of the hip, three possible deviations are possible: flexion, internal or external rotation, and adduction or abduction. If there is deviation from the optimal position of more than one measurement, the impairments of all of the measurements that deviate should be combined using the combined values tables; then the combined value is added to the impairment for ankylosis in the optimal position. In the knee, the rater must take into consideration flexion and extension, varus and valgus, and rotation. In the ankle, flexion and extension, varus and valgus, and internal and external rotation must be considered. In the subtalar joint, varus and valgus must be considered and the values are found in the ankle section (Tables 56 and 57 of the *Guides*).

In earlier printings of the 4th edition of the *Guides*, Table 60 lists impairments that result from the loss of Boehler's angle. In later printings, this was more appropriately called the *tibio-os calcis angle.* This is a radiographic finding on a lateral radiograph of the ankle, which is determined by measuring the angle between the long axis of the tibia and the long axis of the os calcis with the ankle in neutral. The impairment normally would be read from Table 60; however, there is a discrepancy between Table 60 and Boehler's angle in Table 64 on page 3/86. The rater should use the measurements in Table 64 because they portray the impairment more accurately because of loss of the tibio-os calcis angle. If loss of motion has occurred in the subtalar joint as well as in the tibio-os calcis angle, then the impairment from the loss of the tibio-os calcis angle should be added to the impairment for loss of motion. If there is loss of the tibio-os calcis angle and varus or valgus of the hind-foot, the impairment from the loss of the tibio-os calcis should be combined with the impairment for the varus or valgus and the combined value added to the impairment for loss of motion. The example of the calculation of ankle impairment at the bottom of page 3/81 is only partially correct. After combining the 7% impairment of ankle flexion and the 10% for ankle varus, the combined value of 16% should be added to the impairment for ankle fusion in optimal position (14% of the foot), for a final rating of 30% of the foot. Table 61 on page 3/82 is a "busy" table, but it describes impairment secondary to ankylosis of multiple toe combinations.

Arthritis

Not infrequently, patients with significant arthritic changes on radiography in joints of the lower extremity have significant impairment because of pain, but they have minimal loss of motion. Therefore, the authors introduced a method of rating based on the loss of joint space on standardized radiographs. Table 62 on page 3/83 of the *Guides* describes these impairments. This table describes impairment based on narrowing of particular joints compared with normative joint widths. It is important that the radiographs are taken in a standardized manner, that is, from a distance of 36 inches, with the x-ray beam parallel to the joint surface. The patellofemoral joint is assessed by a sunrise view, taken with the knee flexed 40 degrees and the beam tangential to the patellar articular surface. It should be noted that if the patient has a knee-flexion contracture, radiographic evaluation of narrowing of the knee joint space is difficult to perform, and these patients should be rated based on loss of motion.

Amputations

Amputations should be rated separately, and Table 63 on page 3/83 of the *Guides* lists

impairment that results from specific amputation levels. If a ratable condition is present proximal to an amputation, the impairment rating for the amputation should be combined with the impairment rating for the other conditions, but the total rating should not exceed the rating for amputation at the level of the most proximal condition.

Diagnosed-based Estimates

Several conditions are not rated particularly well by previous methods, and therefore the authors described the diagnosis-based estimates. Certain fractures, total joint replacement, ligamentous instability of the knee or ankle, Girdlestone arthroplasty, trochanteric bursitis, ischial tuberosity bursitis (Weaver's bottom), draining osteomyelitis, and certain foot deformities are examples. In Table 64 on page 3/86, there is a discrepancy in the listing for loss of Boehler's angle compared with the same listing in Table 60. The rater should use the rating that gives the patient the higher impairment. In later printings of the 4th edition, Table 60 is replaced by a measurement of the tibio-os calcis angle, but the discrepancy with Table 60 remains.

For hip arthroplasty, the rater uses Table 64 on page 3/85 and Table 65 on page 3/87. The functional results of the arthroplasty are categorized from Table 65 into a *good*, *fair*, or *poor* result. Table 64 then lists the impairments for the lower extremity and body as a whole based on these three categories. Unlike in the upper extremity, the impairment for loss of range of motion is not added to the impairment for the arthroplasty because loss of range of motion was accounted for in the determination of the functional result.

Similarly, knee arthroplasty functional result is categorized using Table 66 on page 3/88. Table 64 on page 3/85 lists the impairment for the three categories for knee arthroplasty.

Skin Loss and Chronic Draining Osteomyelitis

Full-thickness skin loss in certain weight-bearing areas of the body can lead to significant impairment, and Table 67 on page 3/88 lists impairment for those conditions. Note also that Table 67 lists impairment for chronic osteomyelitis with active drainage.

Peripheral Nerve Injuries

Impairment for peripheral nerve injuries are described on pages 3/88 and 3/99. Table 68 lists the impairments for total motor and sensory loss in the named peripheral nerves. The rater should refer to Table 11 on page 3/48 and Table 12 on page 3/49 in the section on the upper extremity to determine the percent of involvement of the motor and sensory component and multiply that by the rating for 100% involvement of a particular nerve. The motor and sensory values are added, and if there is dysesthesia in addition to motor and sensory involvement, the rater may add an additional impairment for the dysesthesia. This method differs from that for evaluating the upper extremity, in which the values from the two components of the nerve are combined, not added, and dysesthesia is not considered.

Causalgia and Reflex Dystrophy

Causalgia and reflex dystrophy in the lower extremity are handled similarly to the method in the upper extremity, and the user is referred to page 3/56.

Vascular Disorders

Table 69 on page 3/89 of the *Guides* describes impairment for certain vascular disorders, and the user is referred to that table for a detailed description.

SPINE

Two methods for determining impairment in the spine are described in the 4th edition of the AMA *Guides*; however, only the first (the DRE [Diagnosis Related Estimate] or injury model) is used to determine the final impairment rating. The range-of-motion method is used to adjudicate disagreements among physicians or to assist physicians in placing the patient in the proper DRE category.

The DRE method is based only on the presence of objective findings on physical examination sometime in the course of the patient's episode. Degenerative processes or radiographic changes attributable to aging do not enter into the assessment. Changes on imaging studies such as magnetic resonance (MR) imaging or computed tomography (CT)/myelogram may assist the physician in categorizing the patient; however, the diagnosis of degenerative disease on MR imaging does not necessarily mean that the patient has sustained an injury. Studies have shown that at least one-third of patients without a history of back pain will have abnormalities on MR imaging (2). Similarly, disc changes on MR imaging do not make the diagnosis of radiculopathy. The diagnosis of radiculopathy is made by the presence of objective physical signs of radiculopathy (see differentiators in the following). EMG studies can assist the physician in categorizing the patient but are not required. The presence of radiculopathy on EMG as defined in the *Guides*, however, makes a diagnosis of radiculopathy, which requires the presence of unequivocal evidence of acute nerve compromise (such as multiple positive sharp waves or fibrillation potentials or H-wave absence or delay greater than 3 mm per second) or evidence of chronic changes such as polyphasic waves in peripheral muscles. The absence of EMG changes does not mean that radiculopathy is not present.

Sciatic nerve tension signs are also helpful in making the diagnosis of radiculopathy. The literature suggests that crossed straight leg raising is the most reliable sign of a ruptured disc. To be interpreted as a positive tension sign, the straight leg raising should be done in both the sitting and the supine position. The pain elicited with straight leg raising should be in the extremity, not in the back, and it should be in the distribution of a nerve root. Internal rotation of the leg (because of tension on the piriformus muscle through or around which the sciatic nerve travels) or dorsiflexion of the foot (because of increased tension on the sciatic nerve) may increase the complaint of discomfort by the patient. External rotation of the leg and plantar flexion of the foot, on the other hand, should not increase the complaint of pain and in many cases will decrease it.

Several differentiators are defined as objective findings that may assist the physician in assigning the patient to a particular category. These differentiators, listed in Table 71 on page 3/109 of the *Guides*, are guarding, loss of reflexes, decreased muscle circumference, electrodiagnosis, lateral motion roentgenograms, loss of bowel or bladder control, bladder studies, and the range-of-motion model.

Guarding

Guarding, defined as paravertebral muscle guarding or spasm or nonuniform loss of motion (*dysmetria*), needs to have been observed and documented by a physician. With true muscle spasm, loss of lumbar lordosis or sciatic scoliosis is seen frequently. Radicular complaints that follow anatomic pathways but cannot be verified by neurologic findings (nonverifiable radiculopathy) also fit into this definition.

Loss of Reflex

If a reflex in the upper or lower extremities is absent or significantly reduced, this finding may signify radiculopathy. The rater must be certain that the loss of the reflex is secondary to the particular condition being evaluated, not secondary to prior difficulties. Reflexes that are lost because of previous episodes of radiculopathy often do not return.

Atrophy

Atrophy of musculature above or below the knee or elbow as measured by comparative circumferential measurements may suggest significant radiculopathy. Again, the rater must be convinced that it occurs secondary to the injury being assessed, not secondary to a previous injury. The *Guides* suggests that the atrophy should be greater than 2 cm to be significant. If it is early in the course of the patient's process, less than 2 cm may be significant.

Electrodiagnostic Evidence

This subject has been discussed earlier. If EMGs are done and meet the definition described in the *Guides*, the presence of radiculopathy is highly suggested; EMGs, however, are not required to make the diagnosis of radiculopathy.

Loss-of-Motion Segment Integrity

Loss-of-motion segment integrity, which is diagnosed on lateral flexion–extension radiographs, is determined by measuring the translation of one vertebra on another by 5 mm or more in the lumbar and thoracic spine or by 3.5 mm or more in the cervical spine. A second, less frequently used method, is to assess angular motion on lateral flexion–extension radiographs. Detailed descriptions of these two methods are listed on page 3/98 of the *Guides*. Flexion–extension radiographs are not necessary for every patient, however. Unless there is reason to believe that there is loss-of-motion segment integrity or if 5 mm (3.5 mm in the cervical spine) of translation is obvious on plain films, then the rater can forgo this examination. Loss-of-motion segment integrity is uncommon in the workers' compensation arena. It is most common in middle-aged women at the L4–5 level and is due to degenerative disease. The rater must ensure that the condition is due to the injury being rated (3).

Loss of Bowel or Bladder Control

Loss of bowel control can be confirmed on rectal examination by loss of sphincter tone. Loss of bladder control can be confirmed by the use of assistive devices such as catheters. Cystometrograms that show unequivocal neurologic compromise of the bladder, with resulting incontinence, suggest radiculopathy. Bladder studies are confirmatory but are not necessary if the physician rater is convinced that there is loss of bladder control.

Structural Inclusions

In addition to the differentiators, a number of conditions termed *structural inclusions*, are certain fractures of the vertebral bodies or posterior elements. The presence of a structural inclusion automatically places a patient into a particular category. If a patient can be categorized by the presence of structural inclusions, it is not necessary for the differentiators required for that particular category to be present. The following is a detailed description of the lumbosacral DRE categories and their impairment ratings. For a similar description of the cervicothoracic and thoracolumbar areas, the reader is referred to pages 3/103 to 3/107.

DRE Lumbosacral Category I:

Complaints or Symptoms

- Description and verification: The patient has no significant clinical findings, no muscle guarding or history of guarding, no documentable neurologic impairment, no significant loss of structural integrity on lateral flexion and extension roentgengrams, and no indication of impairment related to injury or illness.
- Structural Inclusions: None.
- Impairment: 0% Whole-person impairment.

DRE Lumbosacral Category II:

Minor Impairment.

- Description and verification: The clinical history and examination findings are compatible with a specific injury or illness and may include significant intermittent or continuous muscle guarding that has been observed and documented by a physician, nonuniform loss of range of motion (dysmetria, differentiator 1, Table 71, page 109), or nonverifiable radicular complaints. No objective sign of radiculopathy and no loss of structural integrity (Table 71, differentiator 1, page 109) are found.
- Structural inclusions: (a) Less than 25% compression of one vertebral body; (2) posterior-element fracture without dislocation (not developmental spondylolysis); the fracture is healed, and there is no los-of-motion segment integrity. A spinous or transverse process fracture with displacement without a vertebral body fracture is a category II impairment because it does not disrupt the spinal canal.
- Impairment: 5% Whole-person impairment.

DRE Lumbosacral Category III:
Radiculopathy

- Description and verification: The patient has significant signs of radiculopathy, such as loss of relevant reflex(es), or measured unilateral atrophy of greater than 2 cm above or below the knee, compared with measurements on the contralateral side at the same location. The impairment may be verified by electrodiagnostic findings. (See Table 71, page 109, differentiators 2, 3, and 4).
- Structural inclusions: (a) 25% to 50% compression of one vertebral body; (b) posterior element fracture but not fracture of transverse or spinous process, with displacement disrupting the spinal canal, healed without loss of structural integrity. Radiculopathy may or may not be present. Differentiation from congenital and developmental conditions may be accomplished by examining preinjury roentgenograms or a bone scan performed after onset of the condition.
- Impairment: 10% Whole-person impairment.

By far, the majority of patients being evaluated for workers' compensation or other third-party reasons will be included in the above three categories. The conditions in the categories below are uncommon except for the patient with the structural inclusions in DRE category IV. For this reason, the evaluator usually need make only two decisions. Did the patient have a significant injury, as evidenced by the presence of objective findings sometime in the course of the patient's condition, and did the patient have radiculopathy? With the answer to these two questions, most patients can be categorized.

DRE Lumbosacral Category IV:
Loss-of-Motion Segment Integrity

• Description and verification: The patient has loss-of-motion segment integrity (differentiator 5, Table 71, page 109). *Loss-of-motion segment* or *structural integrity* is defined as at least 5 mm of translation of one vertebra on another or angular motion at the involved motion segment that is 11 degrees more than that at an adjacent motion segment (Figs. 62 and 63, page 98). Loss of structural integrity at the lumbosacral joint is defined as at least 15 degrees more angular motion than at the L4—5 motion segment. A documented history of muscle guarding and pain is present. Neurologic abnormalities need not be present; if they are present, the examiner should consider using category V.
• Structural inclusions: (a) Greater than 50% compression of one vertebral body without residual neurologic compromise; (b) multilevel spine-segment structural compromise, as with fractures or dislocations, without residual neurologic motor compromise.
• Impairment: 20% Whole-person impairment.

DRE Lumbosacral Category V:
Radiculopathy and Loss of Motion Segment Integrity

• Description and verification: The patient meets the criteria of DRE lumbosacral categories III and IV; that is, both radiculopathy and loss of motion segment integrity are present (Table 71, differentiators 2, 3, 4, and 5, page 109). Significant lower-extremity impairment is indicated by atrophy or loss of reflex(es), numbness with an anatomic basis, or EMG findings as in lumbosacral category III and loss-of-motion spine-segment integrity as in lumbosacral category IV.
• Structural inclusions: Structural compromise is present, along with documented neurologic or motor compromise.
• Impairment: 25% Whole-person impairment.

DRE Lumbosacral Category VI:
Cauda Equina-like Syndrome without Bowel or Bladder Signs

• Description and verification: Patients in this category have a cauda equina-like syndrome with objectively demonstrated, permanent, partial loss of lower-extremity function bilaterally. They may or may not have loss-of-motion segment integrity. They do not have objectively demonstrated bowel or bladder impairment.
• Structural Inclusion: None.
• Impairment: 40% Whole-person impairment.

DRE Lumbosacral Category VII:
Cauda Equina-like Syndrome with Bowel or Bladder Impairment

• Description and verification: Cauda equina-like syndrome as defined in category VI is present, and the patient has bowel and bladder involvement requiring an assistive device. Evidence from EMG or other neurologic test or cystometrogram may be present, indicating spinal nerve compression.
• Structural inclusions: None.
• Impairment: 60% Whole-person impairment.

DRE Lumbosacral Category VIII:
Paraplegia, Total Loss of Lumbosacral Spinal Cord Function

• Description and verification: The patient has complete or nearly complete paraplegia because of neural compression in the lumbar spine region.
• Structural inclusions: None.
• Impairment: 75% Whole-person impairment.

Cervicothoracic and Thoracolumbar Spine

Impairment ratings for the cervicothoracic and thoracolumbar regions of the spine are similar to those of the lumbar spine. For a detailed definition of each category, refer to the AMA *Guides*, pages 3/103 through 3/107. There are several big differences in the cervicothoracic and thoracolumbar spine, however. In these two areas, there is the possibility of having both damage to the spinal cord, as evidenced by long-tract findings, as well as objective findings to suggest minor injury, radiculopathy, loss of structural integrity, or multiple-level neurologic involvement in the local area. In these cases, the rater must combine the findings of long track signs as described by categories VI, VII, and VIII in the cervicothoracic and thoracolumbar spine with the rating for the lower categories. For instance, if a patient had severe upper-extremity neurologic compromise, and therefore qualified for DRE cervicothoracic category V, and also had paraplegia and qualified for DRE cervicothoracic category VIII, the total impairment would be a combination of the 75% for category VIII and the 35% from category V. The result would be a total impairment of 80% of the body. In a patient with cervicothoracic categories II through V who does not qualify for categories VI, VII, or VIII and, yet, has a bowel or bladder impairment, the bowel and bladder impairment should be rated in the *Guides* chapters on the digestive or urinary and reproductive systems and then combined with the rating from cervicothoracic categories II through V.

In the thoracolumbar spine, categories II and III are separated into IIA and B, and IIIA and B. The B subcategories are for patients who qualify for the category because of the presence of structural inclusions. If a patient qualifies for thoracolumbar category II or III because of the presence of structural inclusions only and also has long-tract signs, the impairment from category II or III must be combined with the impairment from thoracolumbar category VI, VII, or VII. If a patient qualifies for thoracolumbar category IV for any reason and qualifies for thoracolumbar categories VI, VII, or VIII, the impairment from thoracolumbar category IV must be combined with the impairment from thoracolumbar categories VI, VII, or VIII. Impairment from thoracolumbar category V should not be combined with thoracolumbar categories VI, VII, or VIII because to do so will

result in an inappropriately high rating. In such a case, the leg signs should be considered in category IV and then combined with category VI, VII, or VIII. In regard to the thoracolumbar spine, if a patient qualifies for category II through V based on objective findings and also has bowel or bladder involvement but does not qualify for categories VI, VII, and VIII, the patient's bowel and bladder impairment should be rated from the *Guides* chapters on the digestive or urinary and reproductive systems and combined with the rating from DRE thoracolumbar category II, III, IV, or V.

Tables 72, 73, and 74 on pages 3/110 and 3/111 provide a summary description of the DRE method (Figs. 4–6). The user must consider the footnotes below the tables. For injuries at the dorsolumbar junction, the differentiation between thoracolumbar and lumbosacral is determined by the presence of cord involvement. If cord involvement is present, and thus long-tract signs, it is thoracolumbar. If there is no cord involvement, it is lumbosacral.

Procedure

To perform a spine rating, the rater should perform a thorough history and physical and review all the available records and imaging studies and other tests that have been performed. It is best to review the films directly, but if it is not possible to do so, the rater may rely on reports of imaging studies. In such a case, mention should be made in the evaluation report that the assessment of these studies was done by review of reports only. In the spine, treatment does not affect the final rating; therefore, the presence of objective findings anywhere in the patient's course qualify that patient for a particular category. In reviewing the records, the rater must be assured that observations of muscle spasm, dysmetria, and other conditions are accurate.

Patients who show no signs of significant injury will be classified as DRE category I and will have no impairment. Patients who have objective signs of significant injury but

DRE impairment category	Description	% Impairment of the whole person
I	Complaints or symptoms	0
II	Minor impairment: clinical signs of lumbar injury are present without radiculopathy or loss of motion segment integrity	5
III	Radiculopathy: evidence of radiculopathy is present	10
IV	Loss of motion segment integrity: criteria for this condition are described in Section 3.3b, p. 95	20
V	Radiculopathy and loss of motion segment integrity	25
VI	Cauda equina-like syndrome *without* bowel or bladder impairment	40
VII	Cauda equina syndrome *with* bowel or bladder impairment	60
VIII	Paraplegia	75

FIG. 4. DRE (diagnosis related estimate) lumbosacral spine impairment categories.

are without significant radiculopathy will be classified as DRE category II and will have 5% impairment. Patients with signs of significant lumbosacral radiculopathy, as evidenced by the presence of one or more differentiators or structural inclusions listed in the description of category III, will be placed in DRE category III and given 10% total body impairment in the lumbosacral spine and 15% in the cervicothoracic or thoracolumbar spine. In most cases, a straightforward categorization that is easily reproducible among evaluators can be made.

Range of Motion

If two physicians disagree about the proper category, or if a physician is having difficulty placing the patient into a category, the rater may turn to the range-of-motion model as the ultimate differentiator. If the range of motion model is used, it must be used in its entirety, which means that the impairment rating based

DRE impairment category	Description	% Impairment of the whole person	Impairment (%) with long-tract signs* combined		
			VI (40)	VII (60)	VIII (75)
I	Complaints or symptoms	0			
II	Minor impairment: clinical signs of neck injury are present without radiculopathy or loss of motion segment integrity	5	43	62	76
III	Radiculopathy: evidence of radiculopathy is present	15	49	66	79
IV	Loss of motion segment integrity or multilevel neurologic compromise	25	55	70	81
V	Severe upper extremity neurologic compromise: single-level or multilevel loss of function	35	61	74	84
VI	Cauda equina syndrome *without* bowel or bladder impairment	40	The 40% impairment for category VI must be combined with the impairment percent from the most appropriate cervicothoracic impairment category, II, III, IV, or V.		
VII	*Cauda equina* syndrome *with* bowel or bladder impairment	60	The 60% impairment for category VII must be combined with the impairment percent from the most appropriate cervicothoracic impairment category, II, III, IV, or V.		
VIII	Paraplegia	75	The 75% impairment for category VIII must be combined with the impairment percent from the most appropriate cervicothoracic impairment category, II, III, IV, or V.		

*If a patient has an impairment in cervicothoracic spine impairment category VI, VII, or VIII, the appropriate impairment percent should be *combined* (Combined Values Chart, p. 322) with the percent in cervicothoracic impairment category II, III, IV, or V that best reflects the patient's condition.

If the patient's bowel or bladder function is impaired and there is no cervicothoracic or lower-limb impairment that meets the criteria of categories VI, VII, or VIII, the impairment should be evaluated according to criteria in the *Guides* chapters on the digestive or urinary and reproductive systems.

FIG. 5. DRE (diagnosis related estimate) cervicothoracic spine impairment categories.

DRE impairment category	Description	% Impairment of the whole person	Impairment (%) with long-tract signs* combined		
			VI (35)	VII (55)	VIII (70)
I	Complaints or symptoms	0			
II	Minor impairment				
	A. Clinical signs of thoracolumbar injury are present without radiculopathy or loss of motion segment integrity	5			
	B. Structural inclusions are present, ie, less than 25% compression of vertebral body or posterior element fracture without dislocation	5	38	57	72
III	Radiculopathy				
	A. Neurologic evidence of limb impairment is present	15			
	B. Structural inclusions are present, ie, 25% to 50% compression fracture of 1 vertebral body or posterior element fracture disrupting spinal canal	15	45	62	75
IV	Loss of motion segment integrity or multilevel neurologic compromise	20	48	64	76
V	Radiculopathy and loss of motion segment integrity	25	Impairment percents in thoracolumbar category V are *not* combined with impairment percents representing long-tract signs for the thoracolumbar spine.		
VI	Cauda equina syndrome *without* bowel or bladder impairment	35	The 35% thoracolumbar category VI impairment must be combined with the impairment percent from the most appropriate thoracolumbar impairment category, II, III, or IV.		
VII	Cauda equina syndrome *with* bowel or bladder impairment	55	The 55% thoracolumbar category VII impairment must be combined with the impairment percent from the most appropriate thoracolumbar impairment category, II, III, or IV		
VIII	Paraplegia	70	The 70% thoracolumbar category VIII impairment must be combined with the impairment percent from the most appropriate thoracolumbar impairment category, II, III, or IV		

Note: If a patient has an impairment in thoracolumbar spine impairment category VI, VII, or VIII, the impairment percent for that category should be *combined* (Combined Values Chart, p. 322) with the percent in thoracolumbar category II, III, or IV (*not* V) that bests reflects the patient's condition.

Combining a thoracolumbar category II or category III impairment percent with an impairment percent representing long-tract signs (thoracolumbar categories VI, VII, VIII) is appropriate only if the patient qualifies for category IIB or category IIIB because of the presence of structural inclusions.

A thoracolumbar category V impairment should *not* be combined with a category VI, VII, or VIII impairment representing presence of long-tract signs.

If the patient's bowel or bladder function is impaired but the patient does not have thoracolumbar or lower extremity impairment that meets the criteria of categories VI, VII, or VIII, the bowel or bladder impairment should be evaluated according to criteria in the *Guides* chapters on the digestive or urinary and reproductive systems.

FIG. 6. DRE (diagnosis related estimate) thoracolumbar spine impairments.

on the range of motion is combined with impairments from Table 75 on page 3/113 and with impairments from Table 83 on page 3/130 if appropriate.

Method

An inclinometer is required for measuring motion in the spine; goniometers are not acceptable. When patients bend forward to touch their toes, about one-half of the motion is in the hips. The aim is to assess the motion of a particular spinal segment; because of the hip motion, use of the goniometer does not measure this motion accurately, and so an inclinometer must be used.

Several types of inclinometers are available. The flat-based type tends to rock on the spine of the patient, making accurate measurement difficult. The bipedal type gives much more satisfactory results (Fig. 7). The

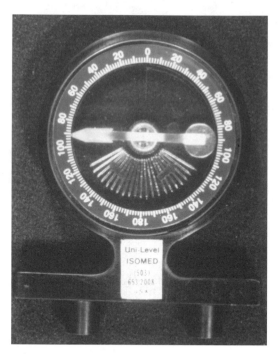

FIG. 7. An inclinometer which is used to measure motion in the spine.

Guides lists the addresses of distributors of inclinometers on page 130. Computerized models are convenient but expensive. A detailed description of the use of the one- and two-inclinometer methods in each of the three spinal areas is found in the AMA *Guides* on page 3/114 to page 3/130. The following is a detailed description of the method of determining range of motion in the lumbar spine using the two-inclinometer method. Determining range of motion in the cervical and thoracic areas is quite similar, and for a detailed explanation, the reader is referred to that section of the AMA *Guides*.

To measure motion of the lumbar spine, the patient must be in a gown with the back open so that the rater can observe the spine closely. Marks are placed on the spinous process of T-12 and S-1, and the two inclinometers are centered over these marks in the sagittal plane and zeroed. The patient is asked to bend forward as far as possible, and measurements from the upper and lower inclonometer are recorded. It is permissible for patients to rest their hands on their thighs if this position is more comfortable. Subtracting the measurement of the lower inclinometer from that of the upper inclinometer gives true lumbar flexion. Similarly, the patient is asked to extend as far as possible, and the readings from the two inclinometers are recorded. Subtraction of the lower inclinometer reading from the upper inclinometer reading gives true lumbar extension. These motions and measurements are repeated three times. The rater is looking for three consecutive measurements that are within five degrees or 10% of the mean of the three consecutive measurements of true lumbar flexion and true lumbar extension. If the first three measurements do not meet this criteria, the rater is instructed to obtain three more measurements so that there are three consecutive measurements that do meet the criteria. If, after six measurements, the rater cannot obtain three consecutive measurements that meet the criteria, the instructions are to invalidate that portion of the range-of-motion evaluation or to have the patient return at a later date for remeasurement. This validity check can be done in each of the three spinal segments. The largest of the three measurements is used to determine the true lumbar motion.

To obtain right and left lateral motion in the lumbar spine, the inclonometers are centered over the marks on T-12 and S-1 in the coronal plane and again zeroed. The patient is asked to bend first to the right and then to the left, and again the reading from the lower inclinometer is subtracted from the upper inclinometer to determine the true lumbar lateral motion. The validity criteria for consecutive measurements hold for lateral bending also. In the lumbar spine, motion in only two planes is measured: flexion–extension and right–left lateral bending. In the cervical spine, flexion–extension, lateral bending, and rotation are measured; and in the thoracic spine, flexion–extension and rotation are measured. Again, the reader is referred to the appropriate section of the AMA *Guides* for a detailed explanation of how to obtain these measurements.

A second validity check that can be used in the lumbar spine is the straight leg raising method. With the patient in the supine position, the inclinometer is placed on the tibial tubercle and zeroed. Straight leg raising is carried out, and the angle of maximum straight leg raising is recorded. This is repeated three times and, once again, the rater is seeking three consecutive measurements that fall within 5 degrees or 10% of the mean of the three measurements. The reading of the tightest straight leg raising angle is compared with the sum of the sacral flexion and extension angle. This is the sum of the flexion/extension measurements from the lower (S-1) inclinometer. This measurement is one of hip motion, not of back motion. If the tighter straight leg raising angle exceeds the sum of the sacral and flexion–extension angles by more than 15 degrees, the lumbosacral flexion test is ruled invalid. This validity test should not be used if the total sacral (hip) motion (flexion—-extension) exceeds 55 degrees for men or 65 degrees for women.

These two validity checks assess full effort by the patient. If the patient cannot reproduce the motion such that the rater can obtain three consecutive measurements that meet the validity criteria, it is assumed that the patient is not giving full effort. Similarly, if the straight leg raising measurement exceeds the sum of sacral flexion–extension (*hip motion*), the patient is considered not to be giving full effort when asked to bend forward.

If the measurements are considered valid, the rater refers to the appropriate table in the AMA *Guides*. For the lumbar spine, this would be Table 81 on page 3/128 for flexion–extension and Table 82 on page 3/130 for right and left lateral bending. Note that in Table 81, the rater must take into account the sacral flexion angle. Loss of hip flexion (*sacral flexion angle*) results in a higher rating for loss of true lumbar flexion because a patient who has a stiff hip is unable to compensate as well for a stiff back and therefore has a greater impairment. The procedure continues by referring to Table 75 on page 3/113 and determining whether any impairment is due for conditions listed in that table. Next, Table 83 on page 3/130 is consulted to determine whether any impairment

due to nerve-root involvement is present. The three impairments, if present, are combined to give total body impairment by the range-of-motion model for that area of the spine. If there is involvement of more than one area of the spine, the procedure is repeated for each of the involved areas, and then the impairment of each involved area is combined to give total body impairment.

Occasionally, the rater encounters a patient who has total ankylosis of a spinal segment. In this case, reference should be made to the ankylosis section of the appropriate table.

It is important to understand that the range-of-motion model is used only to assist physicians in placing the patient in the proper DRE category. The final rating should never be taken from the range-of-motion model. For instance, it is difficult to measure accurately the percent of compression of a compression fracture. If a patient has a compression fracture that was about 50%, the physician may have difficulty placing the patient in category III (less than 50%) or category IV (greater than 50%); yet, there is a 10% difference in the impairment rating. The physician then may use the range-of-motion model. If the range-of-motion model in its entirety, including Tables 75 and 83, resulted in an impairment rating of 20% or greater, then the patient would be placed in DRE lumbosacral category IV and given a rating of 20% whole-person impairment. If the range-of-motion model resulted in a rating of 10% or less, the patient would be placed in DRE lumbosacral category III and given a rating of 10% whole-person impairment. If the range-of-motion model resulted in a rating between 10% and 20%, the patient would be placed in the category with an impairment rating closer to the range-of-motion impairment rating.

Pelvis

Certain fractures in and around the pelvis result in impairment, and the rater is referred to the appropriate section on page 3/131 for a description of these impairments.

CONTROVERSIAL ISSUES

Carpal Tunnel Syndrome

The *Guides* discusses two ways to evaluate carpal tunnel syndrome. The preferred method is to use the peripheral nerve method, that is, to assess the sensory changes and muscular weakness according to Tables 11 and 12 and compare them to Table 15. The second method, which uses Table 16, has been controversial and confusing because "uninformed" persons tend to equate severe delay in transmission of electric impulse across the wrist to severe carpal tunnel syndrome. There is no evidence that the magnitude of delay is related to the magnitude of symptoms. In addition, the nerve-conduction velocity is rarely repeated after surgery (and there is no good reason to do so), and therefore the delay after treatment is usually unknown.

DRE Versus Range-of-Motion Method of Rating the Spine

In the 3rd edition and 3rd edition, revised, the range-of-motion method was the only way to rate spine impairment. Many physicians, however, believe that range of motion is not an acceptable method to determine impairment. In the spine, specifically, an article by Lowry et al. (4) suggested that significant impairment ratings in patients who denied having back pain was possible using the range-of-motion model, which does not take into account age-related changes in the spine, such as loss of motion and radiographic changes. For this reason, the authors suggested an alternative method, that being the DRE method. This method is the preferred method and should be used in almost every case. The range-of-motion model is to be used only to help place the patient in the proper DRE category. Thus, the rating always should come from the DRE method. The *Guides* suggests that a few conditions are best rated by the range-of-motion model. It may be that a patient who is being rated for administrative purposes, such as retirement, and one needs all possible injuries to the spine as well as age-related changes taken into account, may be better rated

by the range-of-motion model. Further research on the validity of both methods is ongoing.

Effect of Treatment on the Final Rating

In the spine, in contrast to the upper and lower extremity, the effect of treatment is not taken into account. If the patient has objective findings anytime during the course of the disease process, a rating according to those findings is appropriate. This means that if the patient has a ruptured disk with significant radiculopathy and subsequently, with or without surgery, has improvement of the symptoms, the patient still deserves a rating of 10% total body impairment. Some physicians believe this is inappropriate. On the other hand, there is ample evidence that once a patient sustains a ruptured disc, that patient is more likely to have future pain than the normal population. In addition, because the recurrence rate of ruptured disks is higher, the patient is not completely unimpaired, even though the symptoms may have temporarily disappeared. Similarly, if a patient sustains a ruptured disc and does not respond to conservative or surgical treatment, the rating is still the same (10% in the lumbar spine). At present, there is no way in the *Guides* to adjust ratings for a poor result that is due solely to the presence of pain. If the physician believes that the *Guides* does not adequately reflect the patient's impairment, it is always the rater's prerogative to adjust the rating appropriately with an explanation and justification for the adjustment.

Apportionment

The Guides allows apportionment throughout the musculoskeletal section. If a patient has a preexisting condition, and the impairment rating for the condition can be estimated, the new impairment rating is adjusted appropriately. If, for instance, the older impairment were in the same area as the new impairment, the older impairment would be subtracted from the newer impairment. If, on the other hand, it was in a different area, the newer impairment might be assessed against a person who was less than

100%, similar to the mathematics of the combined values tables. In the spine, this means that if a patient has a preexisting ruptured disc and a rating of 10%, a new ruptured disc (more radiculopathy) would not increase the rating. The patient certainly may have more pain, may have missed work, and deserves to be compensated for those events, but, from a pathophysiologic standpoint, the patient is no worse off. The quantity of radiculopathy cannot be measured. Radiculopathy is radiculopathy, and a second ruptured disc, whether it be another disc in the same spinal area, the same disc on the same side, or the same disc on another side, still results in a rating of 10%. This situation is similar to that of a patient with a sprained back and objective findings. The rating would be 5%. The patient does not get another 5% each time another sprain of the back occurs.

Controversy arises when a patient has a noncompensation ruptured disc, is treated with or without surgery, has a good result, and then has a second ruptured disc that is job related and is treated unsuccessfully with residual pain. The *Guides* does not provide a way to adjudicate this situation. The problem is left to the rater and the administrative process.

Hand Dominance

In the musculoskeletal chapter, hand dominance is not considered. The authors considered that because some patients are ambidextrous to varying degrees, it is not appropriate to penalize the patient because the injury was to the nondominant extremity. In Chapter 4 (The Nervous System), the opposite tack is taken, and the ratings for the dominant hand are greater than the ratings for the nondominant extremity. If the rating is carried out using Chapter 3 (The Musculoskeletal System), hand dominance is not considered.

REFERENCES

1. American Medical Association. *Guides to the evaluation of permanent impairment.* 4th ed. American Medical Association, Chicago, IL, 1993.
2. Boden SD, Davis DO, Dina TS, Patronas NJ, Wiesel SW. Abnormal magnetic-resonance scans of the lumbar spine in asymptomatic subjects: a prospective investigation. *J Bone Joint Srug Am* 1990;72:403–408.
3. Boden SD, Wiesel SW. Lumbosacral segmental motion in normal individuals. Have we been measuring instability properly? *Spine* 1990;15:571–576.
4. Lowery WD Jr, Horn TJ, Boden SD, Wiesel SW. Impairment evaluation based on spinal rage of motion in normal subjects. *J Spinal Disord* 1992;5:398–402.

Occupational Musculoskeletal Disorders
edited by T. G. Mayer, R. J. Gatchel, and P. B. Polatin.
Lippincott Williams & Wilkins, Philadelphia © 2000.

40

Vocational Assessment and Retraining

Leonard N. Matheson

*Program in Occupational Therapy, Washington University School of Medicine, St. Louis,
St. Louis, Missouri 63108*

This chapter presents the conceptual background and practical application of vocational assessment of persons with occupational musculoskeletal disorders (MSDs). It highlights some of the major vocational evaluation and rehabilitation approaches that are useful with this population.

CONTEXT OF TREATMENT

As treatment for an occupational MSD proceeds, it will become necessary to determine when and whether injured workers can return to their usual and customary employment. If a return to usual and customary employment is not possible, vocational assessment can be used to identify alternate occupations. If return to work is likely to be substantially delayed, vocational assessment can be used to assist in the identification and treatment of the psychologic and social factors that may be impeding a return to work.

ASSESSMENT TARGETS

Vocational assessment of injured workers is focused on factors that are of interest to employers. Most important, these include injured workers' work behavior, including productivity, safety, and interpersonal behavior. These factors address injured workers' acceptability as employees in the most general sense. They are the expectations that any employer in the competitive labor market has of any em-

ployee. Some of the questions asked include the following:

- Will the injured worker be productive?
- Will the injured worker be safe in the workplace?
- Can the injured worker get to work every day?
- Can the injured worker put in a full workday?
- Can the injured worker get along with his supervisors?

Employers consistently require acceptable responses to these questions whether they are considering hiring a clerical worker, a laborer, or an accountant. These issues pertain to all employers and to all employees in the competitive labor market.

In addition to concerns with the general acceptability of injured workers as employees, vocational assessment also addresses their ability to become employed within a particular occupation or a particular job. This has to do with the match between an injured worker's residual capabilities and the demands of the occupation or job. Some of the job demands will be within, and some will be beyond, the injured worker's work tolerances. Unless the mismatch is minimal or can be overcome through work hardening, training, or job and tool modification, the occupation or job will not be acceptable.

ASSESSMENT GUIDELINES

Vocational assessment is conducted with regard to professional guidelines and numerous state and federal laws. Guidelines for performance testing have been developed and published by the American Psychological Association (1), American Physical Therapy Association (2), and the American Academy of Physical Medicine and Rehabilitation (3). Federal guidelines for testing on which an employment decision is based are found in the *Uniform Guidelines on Employee Selection Procedures* (4). Because the testing procedure involves employment of a person with a disability, the Americans with Disabilities Act of 1990 is pertinent (5). Additional standards specific to testing of disabled people have been published (6). There is agreement among the various professional and governmental entities concerned with performance testing that selection of a test must be undertaken within the hierarchical context of safety, reliability, validity, practicality, and utility standards.

Safety

When used properly, a test should not be expected to lead to injury, given the known characteristics of the injured worker. Some tests that have been designed for employee selection, such as whole-body isometric strength testing, have the potential to cause harm to the person with an occupational MSD. Well designed tests provide exclusionary and performance guidelines and procedural rules that must be followed to minimize this likelihood. Safety is a function of the match between the performance demands placed on the injured worker and the injured worker's ability to limit performance appropriately. Determination of the injured worker's maximum safe and dependable performance level is a professional judgment made by the evaluator, based on the injured worker's performance during the evaluation (7). This judgment takes into account the signs, symptoms, and behaviors that indicate that the evaluation has progressed to a point at which its safety cannot be maintained with a reasonable degree of certainty. Thus, the professional evaluator's training and experience to utilize the test's maximum performance indicators are a necessary condition for functional testing.

Reliability

The test equipment and test protocol should produce a result that is stable within the test trial and across evaluators, injured workers, and the date or time of test administration. Reliability can be threatened both externally and internally. External threats are those over which the evaluator has control, such as equipment reliability, protocol reliability, and consistency of protocol application. Internal threats are those that reside within the injured worker, and include motivation, fear, and pain avoidance behavior. A vocational assessment requires that the injured worker put forth maximum voluntary effort in a meaningful task. The defined task may require full strength, full velocity, endurance, a target number of repetitions, a maximum rate of responding, or some other "full effort" performance. One characteristic distinguishing performance testing of persons with occupational MSDs from those who are not impaired is the importance of factors such as activity-related pain, fear of reinjury, test anxiety, and the cost-to-benefit ratio of task performance. While the effect of these factors is difficult to measure with precision, most clinicians agree that they are significant. The vocational assessment must be structured so that it is sensitive to these factors and can minimize their effects.

Validity

The interpretation of a test score should be able to predict or reflect the injured worker's performance in a target task. Whereas reliability has to do with the dependability of the measure, validity has to do with the adequacy of the measure to describe or predict performance. A valid vocational assessment that can be used with persons who have occupational MSDs must:

- Allow clinicians to gauge treatment effect by comparing an initial baseline level of performance with performance as treatment progresses;

- Make recommendations for return to work by comparing the injured worker's functional capacity to his or her job demands;
- Provide an estimate of disability for rating purposes by comparing the injured worker's performance to expected values.

Although there is a long history of validity testing of performance measures to predict productivity in fields such as industrial psychology (8,9), studies of the validity of functional tests to predict injury or disability are rare and often produce conflicting interpretations (10–13).

Practicality

The cost of a test should be reasonable. Cost is a function of the capital expenditure for the equipment, amortized over the life of the equipment, plus wage costs and overhead. Although "low-tech" approaches to vocational assessment are less expensive initially, if a more expensive "high-tech" system is able to provide similar results in less time or with lower-wage staff, a substantial portion of the additional expense for the latter approach may be offset.

Utility

The usefulness of a procedure is the degree to which it meets the needs of the injured worker, referrer, and payer. The first four factors in the hierarchy above must be adequately addressed for utility to be achieved. Without utility, the test is of no value and will not be supported by the users of the test information.

TEST SELECTION GUIDELINES

Beyond the legal framework for functional capacity evaluation, the evaluator must use tests that are *optimal*, given the injured worker and the evaluation circumstance. Tests must be selected to meet the unique needs of the person-to-job interface. In addition to these general guidelines, adherence to the following specific guidelines will insure an optimal balance of safety, reliability and validity:

Use only standardized test protocols that have all of the following characteristics:

Equipment has been demonstrated to be reliable with the level of maintenance that normally will be available;

Test protocol has been demonstrated to be reliable over time on an intrarater and interrater basis;

One or more means of intratest confirmation of consistency is available;

One or more means of intertest confirmation of consistency is available;

Multiple biomechanical or neuromusculoskeletal variations can be selected by the evaluator, based on the demands of the role;

Normative data or job demand data are available.

Become trained in the use of the test protocols, and formally demonstrate skill in the consistent application of the test protocols.

Select protocols from those identified above that meet the validity needs and practicality restrictions of the assessment process. Select each test in response to the demands of the target job. These demands should be derived from a job-match analysis, as described in Chapter 34.

After collecting the necessary pretest screening information about the injured worker to rule out contraindications for testing, administer the test in the standard manner.

Evaluate the *quality* of the data on the following basis:

Screen for intratest variability: If more variability exists than is reported to be normal for the protocol, retest;

Screen for intertest variability: If more variability exists than is reported to be normal for the protocol, retest.

Interpret the data and report the derived information in terms of the purpose of the vocational assessment.

This approach to vocational assessment will minimize problems with safety, reliability, and validity, thus improving utility. In the treatment of occupational MSDs, given the potential for problems in these areas that can harm the injured worker, practicality must be subordinate to these factors and should be included only with thoughtful administrative control.

STANDARDIZED VOCATIONAL ASSESSMENT

One example of a standardized vocational assessment designed to address all the basic requirements described above is the California Functional Capacity Protocol (Cal-FCP) (14). The Cal-FCP is a 120-minute, 11-part test of functional capacity designed to develop an estimate of lost work capacity to be used in a case management process and to address disability rating. An extended version of the Cal-FCP is used to perform the assessment to complement the job-match analysis procedures (see Chapter 34).

The Cal-FCP was designed to measure the work consequences of soft tissue musculoskeletal injuries. It allows measurement of an injured worker's work capacity by the treating physician or by other health care practitioners. It is administered 30 days after the injury if the injured worker either has not returned to work or continues in active treatment. Frequently, because of its low cost, it is administered on a serial basis, every 3 weeks, to measure response to treatment. This pattern of use addresses a concern of the treating physician to

maintain case control. Additionally, the involvement of the treating physician in interpreting the test results recognizes that he or she is the best professional to consider them in light of issues such as the injured worker's motivation, fears, and goals, and to integrate other medical findings. The information derived from the Cal-FCP is presented to the treating physician as a recommendation, along with all the data collected during the examination.

CAL-FCP TEST ORDER

The Cal-FCP evaluation tasks are grouped, and each task is presented to the injured worker in an invariant order to allow optimal observation of prolonged sitting and standing. Thus, the paper and pencil tasks combine to become a functional activity so that sitting tolerance can be assessed. The order in which each test is presented to the injured worker is listed in Table 1. The duration of each task will vary from injured worker to injured worker but has been shown in practice to conform to the general parameters in Table 1. The Cal-FCP test battery includes the evaluation tasks discussed in the following sections.

Structured Interview

Basic information concerning the injured worker's demographics and current status is collected through the use of a structured interview. This segment of the Cal-FCP test bat-

TABLE 1. *Order of testing in the California Functional Capacity Protocol*

Order	Task	Posture	Duration (min)	Cumulative Time (min)
1	Structured interview	Sitting	20	20
2	Health questionnaire	Sitting	5	25
3	Perceived physical capacity	Sitting	15	40
4	Pain and sensation drawing	Sitting	5	45
5	Job demands questionnaire	Sitting	5	50
6	Lateral pinch test	Sitting	5	55
7	Power grip test	Sitting	5	60
8	Standing range of motion	Standing	10	70
9	Lifting capacity test	Standing	35	105
10	Carrying test	Standing	5	110
11	Climbing test	Standing	5	115
12	Cool-down	Standing	5	120

TABLE 2. *Ordinal ability ranking scale for the California Functional Capacity Protocol*

Rank	Designation	Compared with ability prior to injury
1	Able	Evaluee can perform the activity with no difficulty
2	Slightly restricted	Evaluee can perform the task, but is slightly restricted
3	Moderately restricted	Evaluee can perform the task, but is moderately restricted
4	Very restricted	Evaluee can perform the task, but is very restricted
5	Unable	Evaluee cannot perform the activity at all

tery requires the use of a standard evaluation record. Questions are posed about current functional abilities compared with abilities prior to the injury. For example, the evaluator may ask the following:

• How would you rate your ability to sit in an office chair now as compared with prior to the injury? or

• How would you rate your ability to lift an object from waist to shoulder height with your right hand now as compared with prior to the injury?

• Based on the injured worker's response, the evaluator rates current ability on a 1 to 5 ordinal scale from "able" to "unable," compared with the injured worker's preinjury ability, using the criteria presented in Table 2.

Health Questionnaire

The most physically demanding aspect of the Cal-FCP is the lift capacity test. Because injured workers must be screened for cardiovascular risk factors prior to undertaking such a test, a health questionnaire is administered, and resting blood pressure and heart rate are recorded. After these items are completed, the health questionnaire is reviewed by the evaluator. Items that indicate medical instability or excess cardiovascular risk are noted and ex-

plored fully, and a determination is made whether or not the lift capacity test battery can be administered.

Perceived Physical Capacity

Perceived functional capacity is an important indicator of the effect of injury. To standardize collection of information concerning perceived functional capacity of persons with spinal impairment, the *spinal function sort* (SFS) is used (15). The injured worker is provided instructions and allowed to work on a self-paced basis. The evaluator is available for questions.

Pain and Sensation Drawing

Symptoms are an important indicator of injury, although the contribution of symptoms to the severity of an injury is not straightforward. To standardize collection of information concerning symptoms, a pain drawing form has been developed. The pain and sensation drawing is completed by the injured worker with the assistance of the evaluator. The pain drawing allows a record to be made of pain in terms of the following factors:

• *Location*: The injured worker uses a red pen or pencil to draw the location of the pain on the figure.

• *Type*: The injured worker draws on the figure the type of pain at each location. Adjectives commonly used to described symptoms are provided with a reference key.

• *Intensity of worst pain*: The injured worker draws an *X* on the 10-cm analogue scale at the bottom of each drawing with the red pen or pencil to describe the highest level of pain over the past week. The injured worker draws a line from the analogue scale to each pain location.

• *Frequency of worst pain*: After the injured worker has completed the intensity rating of each symptom area, the evaluator asks the injured worker about the frequency of this (these) symptom(s) and records the frequency of the drawing according to the rating scale in Table 3.

TABLE 3. *Pain frequency scale for the California Functional Capacity Protocol*

Rating	Interpretation
Constant	Most of waking and sleeping hours
Frequent	Most of waking hours
Intermittent	Several times during waking hours
Occasional	A few times during waking hours

- *Intensity of usual pain*: The injured worker draws an *O* on the analogue scale with the red pen or pencil to describe the usual level of pain over the past week, and a line from the analogue scale to each pain location.
- *Frequency of usual pain*: The evaluator asks the injured worker about the frequency of this (these) symptom(s) and records the frequency of the drawing according to the above rating scale.

Job Demands Questionnaire

A short questionnaire that structures input from the injured worker in terms of his or her job demands provides information about the perception of job demands against which the performance test measures can be compared. In addition, this activity extends seated-task duration. This information is not included in the disability rating but will be useful to the treating physician. Accordingly, it is included as an attachment to the Cal-FCP standard report form that is provided to the doctor at the conclusion of the evaluation.

Lateral Pinch Test

Isometric lateral pinch (also known as key pinch) strength is measured through the use of the *B&L Pinch Gauge* (B&L Engineering, Tustin, CA). This tests follows the protocol endorsed by the American Society of Hand Therapists (ASHT) because it has been shown to be reliable and normative data are based on it (16,17).

Power Grip Test

Grip strength is evaluated in a seated position through the use of the *JAMAR Hand Dy-*

namometer (Jamar, Bolinbrook, IL), following the protocol endorsed by the ASHT. Position no.2 on the dynamometer handle is utilized because normative data are based on testing with this span. The practice and test protocols are similar to those used for measurement of pinch strength.

Standing Range of Motion

The standing range-of-motion (ROM) test measures anthropometric ROM, that is, using the injured worker's own stature as a frame of reference. The evaluator begins each test session by explaining the purpose of the test to the injured worker. The injured worker stands in front of a solid wall at a distance, with arms outstretched so that hands can be comfortably placed on the wall. Feet are shoulder width apart. The injured worker is instructed to move from a standing position to each posture and to return to a standing position according to the heights listed in Table 4. Up to a 1-minute standing rest is allowed between postures. The evaluator counts down 15 seconds for the injured worker to hold each of the five postures.

Lift Capacity Test

An isoinertial measure of progressive lift capacity, the (Employment Potential Improvement Corporation) *EPIC lift capacity* test (ELC) is used in the Cal-FCP because of the availability of age-based normative data (18). In addition, the ELC test has been demonstrated to be safe and reliable, with low reactivity in use with persons who have medical impairments (19,20). In the Cal-FCP, the first three of the six subtests of the ELC test are administered following the standard procedures.

TABLE 4. *Stand-and-reach height and postures for the California Functional Capacity Protocol*

Height	Posture
Shoulder level	Standing
Eye level	Standing
Knee level	Stooping
Knee level	Crouching
Knee level	Kneeling

Carrying Test

The injured worker's ability to carry the loads that he or she was able to lift in ELC subtest 3 is assessed through the use of a structured task simulation. The injured worker is instructed to carry the ELC crate with each load that was used for each stage of ELC subtest 3 while walking on a 100-foot course over a flat and unobstructed surface at 3 miles per hour. The injured worker begins with the starting load for ELC subtest 3 and completes one cycle. After a 20-second standing rest, the load is increased by 10 lb and the injured worker completes another cycle. The test progresses in this manner until the maximum acceptable weight achieved in ELC subtest 3 is reached. After the injured worker completes the carrying task, the evaluator rates the injured worker's performance according to the criteria in Table 2.

Climbing Test

The injured worker's ability to climb while carrying the maximum load that he or she was able to lift in ELC subtest 3 is assessed through the use of a structured task simulation. This task simulates climbing up and down one 10-ft flight of stairs in an office building. The injured worker is instructed to carry the ELC crate with the maximum acceptable weight achieved in ELC subtest 3 while stepping up and down an 8-in high step for 15 cycles with a cadence of one-step per second. Cadence is counted by the evaluator. Alternately, a metronome can be used. The injured worker will require 60 seconds to complete this task. The injured worker's ability to complete this task is rated by the evaluator according to the five-point ability scale from able to unable. After the injured worker completes the climbing task, the evaluator rates the injured worker's performance according to the criteria in Table 2.

Effort Rating

Because the results of the Cal-FCP have important financial consequences for many injured workers, it is important to screen for less than full-effort performance. Four of the tests (SFS, pinch, grip, and ELC) have built-in indicators of effort. In addition, an evaluator's rating of effort is made in each case. The evaluator's rating of effort has been shown to be a reliable and useful indicator of full effort (21) and has been shown to be useful in both assessment and treatment of persons who are disabled due to spinal injury (22,23). Unlike the 10-point test performance scale used by Hazard et al. (23) or the four-point global scale used by Mayer (21,24), the Cal-FCP uses a three-level rating scale that focuses on effort during the ELC test. The scale ranges from "reliable effort" to "questionable effort" to "unreliable effort."

Feasibility Study

Once the Cal-FCP test protocol was developed, training of experienced health care clinicians was undertaken at five centers in various parts of California. A demonstration project was designed to evaluate the feasibility of implementation of the protocol across a broad spectrum (25). The duration of the Cal-FCP protocol in hands other than its developers, the internal consistency of the protocol, and its utility in measurement of work capacity were addressed.

Sixty-four subjects (32 women and 32 men) were studied. Subjects in the study included adults who were under treatment for work-related soft tissue musculoskeletal injuries as part of the California workers' compensation program. Lumbar spine patients predominated (n=46), with knee (n=5) and cervical patients (n=4) also represented. The remaining subjects had a variety of soft tissue injuries. Subjects reported onset of symptoms 1 month to 10 years prior to program entry, with a mean of 1.82 (standard deviation, 2.1) years. Only two of the subjects were tested within 30 days of injury onset, while an additional 23 subjects were tested within 1 year of injury. Subjects underwent Cal-FCP testing following the protocol described above. The test battery was administered by exercise physiologists, a registered nurse, physical therapists, and occupational therapists who had participated in a special 2-day training program that included a knowledge test and required demonstration of reliability on the ELC test with five test–retests of healthy subjects.

This study found no new injuries or exacerbations of current impairment. The mean duration of test administration was 84 minutes. This sample demonstrated a mean loss of lift capacity of 41%, with no significant difference between men and women. Seven of the subjects (four men and three women) had no loss of lift capacity. An additional 11 subjects (six men and five women) had a loss of lift capacity that was less than 25%, which is interpreted by the California disability determination model as indicating no residual disability. Twelve of the 64 subjects had effort ratings by the evaluator that were less than full effort. There were no significant differences between groups based on age, time since injury, duration of testing, pinch, or grip. Significant differences were found between the full-effort and less than full-effort groups for SFS score and loss of lift capacity. Interestingly, SFS score predicted both absolute lift capacity and capacity considered as a percentage of body weight on ELC test 3. The SFS score also predicted lost work capacity.

BEYOND BASIC ASSESSMENT

If the basic functional capacity of the injured worker will not allow return to work in a job or occupation for which the injured worker has adequate skills, plans must be made for retraining. The selection of a target occupation is based on a vocational assessment that considers the injured worker's goals, transferable skills based on work history, aptitudes, and interests within the context of the already established work capacity profile. This information is used to identify occupations that exist in the labor market that may be appropriate, often utilizing a computerized job-matching system. Transferable skills are the skills that remain after the effects of the chronic disability have been con-

sidered. Transferable skills are based on the injured worker's work history, training, and education. Transferable skills may be identified through the use of a computerized database to analyze the injured worker's work history or through the use of job analysis data supplied by the U.S. Department of Labor.

FORMAL VOCATIONAL ASSESSMENT

The following tests have been found to be useful in the vocational assessment of persons with occupational MSDs. Many others are also available.

General Reasoning

Raven's Standard Progressive Matrices (26) is a 60-item, paper-and-pencil, nonverbal test that measures abstract reasoning ability. In each problem, the injured worker is presented with a pattern or figure design that has a component missing. The injured worker's task is to select one of six to eight possible parts to complete the pattern.

Language Skills

The *Gates-MacGinitie Reading Test* is a paper-and-pencil test that measures reading achievement in the areas of vocabulary and reading comprehension (27). Six different levels of test difficulty allow appropriate evaluation of individuals in grades 1 through 12. Another excellent test in this area is the *Adult Basic Learning Examination* (ABLE), a measure of vocabulary, reading comprehension, spelling, arithmetic computation, and arithmetic problem solving (28).

Mathematics

In addition to the ABLE, the *Employee Aptitude Survey Test 2* (EAS-2) is quite useful (29). The EAS-2 is a 75-item, paper-and-pencil multiple choice test arranged in three parts (integers, decimals and percentages, and fractions) of 25 items each. This test measures basic arithmetic skill. The *Personnel Test for In-*

dustry—Numerical is a multiple-item paper-and-pencil test of mathematical competence that evaluates the ability to solve "word problems" that are common in the industrial environment (30).

General Aptitude

The *EAS* has 11 subtests that address verbal comprehension, numeric ability, visual pursuit, visual speed and accuracy, space visualization, numeric reasoning, verbal reasoning, word fluency, manual speed and accuracy, and symbolic reasoning. Normative data are provided for several occupational groups, as well as the general population. In a similar manner, the *Differential Aptitude Tests* are a measure of eight abilities that have application to industrial work (31). Abilities assessed include verbal reasoning, numeric ability, abstract reasoning, clerical speed and accuracy, mechanical reasoning, space relations, spelling, and language usage.

Temperament Factors

The *Sixteen Personality Factors Questionnaire* (16 PF)is a paper-and-pencil test of 105 to 187 items, depending on which of the five forms is used (32). This test measures 16 primary personality traits. Properly interpreted, the 16 PF can predict such items as probable length of employee tenure, tolerance for routine, and work efficiency. Occupational profile data based on 11,000 cases are available.

Interest Patterns

The *Career Assessment Inventory* (CAI) is a paper-and-pencil test that measures Holland's six occupational types, 22 basic occupational interest scales, and 91 specific occupational scales (33,34). The *Self-Directed Search* is a multiple-item, paper-and-pencil, self-guided assessment of Holland's six general occupational types (35). The *Strong-Campbell Interest Inventory* is a 325-item,

paper-and-pencil, multiple choice test that measures occupational interest in a wide range of career areas requiring advanced technical or college training (36). As does the CAI, the Strong-Campbell inventory yields scores on Holland's six general occupational types and 23 basic interest scales. The Strong-Campbell offers 162 specific occupational scales.

CASE EXAMPLE

Case Summary

Thomas Tamm[1] is a married, eighth-grade-educated automotive mechanic with a premorbid history of severe dyslexia leading to functional illiteracy. At age 46, he was injured in an automobile accident. A hospital discharge summary described a complex fracture–dislocation of the right hip, with a split of the femoral head and a bimalleolar fracture of the right ankle. Five months postdischarge, the right hip continued to be painful. He was not weight-bearing and was going to physical therapy. Aseptic necrosis of the femoral head and early indications of posttraumatic arthritis were found. Eight months postdischarge, Mr. Tamm had a mild antalgic gait with atrophy of the right lower extremity. He had fair ROM in the right hip, with pain, and limited ROM in the ankle. X-ray examination found avascular necrosis of the right hip and causalgia in the right foot with early osteoarthritis in the right ankle. Twelve months postdischarge, Mr. Tamm had trochanteric bursitis in the right hip, causalgia of the right foot, tenderness as a consequence of retained hardware in the right ankle, and possible posttraumatic degenerative joint disease in the right ankle. He was restricted to sedentary work only, using a crutch at all times while ambulating for the next 12 to 18 months. Fifteen months post-

---

[1]This case example of vocational assessment is a distillation of a much longer report based on an actual case. The injured worker's name has been changed to protect his privacy. All of the names in this document have been changed. The names do not refer to people who were involved with this case.

discharge, Mr. Tamm achieved maximum medical stability with an impairment rating of 20% of the whole person. His physician opined that he will have future problems with arthritis and was then suffering from avascular necrosis of the right hip, which may require a total hip arthroplasty. His prognosis was poor to fair. His ability to work as a mechanic had been impaired.

A functional capacity evaluation was recommended and performed by a physical therapist at 16 months postdischarge. In a work-simulation environment, Mr. Tamm was found to be capable of lifting 5 lb from floor to waist height, 10 lb from waist to shoulder height, and 5 lb over his head three to five times per day. He could not carry any weight while ambulating. He was able to lift 5 lb with the right hand and 10 lb with the left. Whole-body vertical isometric pushing was 50 lb and pulling was 70 lb maximum on an occasional basis. Standing appeared to be limited to 1 hour per day and no more than 5 minutes at one time. Mr. Tamm did not fully bear weight on the right side. He could walk 100 feet before he needed to stop and rest, and could ambulate 20 stairs without taking a break. He was able to crawl approximately 20 feet with difficulty. He was limited in kneeling, squatting, walking balance, straight-line ambulation, and standing with weightbearing on the right. He had approximately 3 minutes of tolerance for performing overhead work due to problems with weightbearing. He could perform work while seated for up to 30 minutes. Grip strength was normal and consistent. Subsequently, a vocational assessment as performed by an occupational therapist 19 months postdischarge.

Evaluation Findings of Vocational Assessment

Self-report

When asked about his difficulties with reading, Mr. Tamm reported that he had a reading problem since early childhood. He said, "I have learned to get around it. I am not interested in reading anymore. I have been so long without it, it's not like a handicap." Mr. Tamm provided the following self-report functional information:

- He is able to sit for 45 to 60 minutes, with a symptomatic response to this activity. (He consistently shifted and changed positions in the office armchair where he sat during the intake interview, rising to stand for 3 to 4 minutes after 35 to 40 minutes of seated activity. This pattern was repeated throughout the evaluation.)
- He is able to stand for approximately 60 minutes several times per day. He is able to walk approximately 50 yards at a time and notices that the type of shoes that he wears makes a difference. He finds ascending stairs worse than descending stairs due to increased symptoms in the right leg.
- His balance is impaired due to instability in his right lower leg. This is especially notable over snow or uneven terrain.
- He is able to stoop while extending his right leg. He avoids crouching or minimizes crouching due to difficulties with right leg flexibility. He is able to kneel slowly and has a substantial amount of difficulty arising from kneeling. He is unable to crawl due to problems with the right knee.
- He is able to reach overhead if he has no load. Attempting to retrieve a load during reaching produces right hip pain. He has a similar problem with forward reaching or lateral reaching.
- Pushing a shopping cart is an activity that he is able to do with more facility than walking unaided. He is able to pull open a heavy door.
- Lifting is limited to approximately 10 lb without a difference between his right and left hands. Carrying is limited to approximately 10 lb as well, with no side-to-side preference.
- Sensation in his right foot is disrupted. He reports that this is "like a TENS [transcutaneous electric nerve stimulation] unit." He describes the sensation, which is a frequent occurrence, as an "electrical shock."

Self-perception

The SFS was administered to evaluate Mr. Tamm's perception of his functional limitations as they may affect ability to work. His responses were questionable because of inconsistent responses on the validity check items. He had a rating of perceived capacity of 82, which places him at the 30th percentile for disabled men who are unemployed, well below the sedentary level of physical demand characteristics.

General Reasoning

Mr. Tamm's general reasoning and problem-solving abilities were evaluation using Raven's Standard Progressive Matrices. His performance resulted in placement at the 55th percentile compared with men of his age.

Verbal Skills

The ABLE was administered to evaluate Mr. Tamm's reading ability. His performance on this test placed him between the midfourth-grade the midfifth-grade instructional level for reading. He is a very slow and laborious reader.

Numeric Skills

To evaluate Mr. Tamm's abilities with arithmetic and numeric problem solving, the EAS-2 was administered. His performance placed him at the 15th percentile in terms of male draftsmen and at the 10th percentile in terms of male electronics technicians. Inspection of the test results indicates that Mr. Tamm has strong skills with addition, subtraction, multiplication, and division with integers but is much less skilled with decimals, percentages, and fractions.

Spatial Skills

The EAS-5 was administered to evaluate Mr. Tamm's abilities with three-dimensional spatial problem solving. His performance placed him at the 20th percentile in terms of both male draftsmen and male electronics technicians.

Symbolic Reasoning

Mr. Tamm's abilities with symbolic reasoning and problem solving were evaluated using the EAS-10. His performance placed him at the 15th percentile in terms of male draftsmen and at the 10th percentile in terms of male electronics technicians.

Manual Dexterity

The Crawford Small Parts Dexterity Test was utilized to evaluate Mr. Tamm's manual dexterity. His performance placed him at the 80th percentile for unilateral fine-dexterity assembly and the 50th percentile for bilateral fine-dexterity assembly.

Hand Strength

Evaluation of Mr. Tamm's hand strength was performed using isometric grip strength testing with the B&L Pinch Gauge and the JAMAR Hand Dynamometer. The scores, presented in terms of average pound of force, are detailed in Table 5. The coefficients of variation of these values are well within acceptable limits. The average force values place him within the normal range in terms of hand strength.

TABLE 5. *Scores for Mr. Tamm's isometric grip strength testing*

Test	Left (lb)	CV(%)	Right (lb)	CV(%)
Isometric key pinch	27.3	<5	28.5	<5
Isometric grip #2	126.5	<5	121.4	<5

Standing Range of Motion

Mr. Tamm's ability to stand and work with his hands in reaching activities was evaluated with the standing ROM test from the Cal-FCP battery. He had a significant symptomatic response to these activities and demonstrated a dependable degradation in function over the course of the test. He was unrestricted for reach forward, slightly restricted for reach to eye level, moderately restricted for reach while stooping, and unable to reach while crouching or kneeling.

Lift Capacity

To evaluate Mr. Tamm's lift capacity, the infrequent subtests from the ELC test were administered. His performance was significantly limited by his reported right hip pain. The values for bimanual lifts on the ELC test are detailed in Table 6. His heart rate was in an acceptable range, although it indicated deconditioning. His symptoms, as measured by the 10-cm horizontal Visual Analog Scale, dependably worsened and were his usual symptomatic response to similar activities. His symptoms diminished to level 6 after 15 minutes of seated distraction.

Vocational Interests

How Mr. Tamm's interests affect his occupational choices was evaluated with the CAI. His response percentages were negative in terms of activities, school subjects, and occupations. His highest general themes score was found in the "realistic" area. His basic interest scale score was highest in electronics and mechanical fixing. Reasonable occupations for Mr. Tamm to consider from an interests viewpoint include the following:

Holland code	Occupational title
R	Auto mechanic
R	Bus driver
RI	Camera repair technician
R	Carpenter
RI	Conservation officer
R	Janitor
RI	Radio/television repair
RI	Telephone repair
R	Truck driver

These occupations are those in which Mr. Tamm's profile of interests approximates the interests of people who are employed.

Vocational Planning

Once the injured worker's vocational profile is developed, a comparison between the occupation's demands and the profile is made. Computerized job-matching systems are widely available to assist with this task. Once an occupation is identified, a close comparison is made between its demands and the injured worker's goals and resources, with a special focus on functional tolerances. If the job meets the worker's goals and his or her resources provide an adequate match, a formal vocational rehabilitation program is developed. This may involve formal or on-the-job training and will usually require rehabilitation counseling support, job search and placement assistance, and postplacement follow-up to support job retention. A typical program of services, their duration, and cost is described in Table 7.

The vocational exploration process is supervised by a rehabilitation counselor using the vocational assessment results to identify occupations that the client will investigate. Use of materials such as the *Guide to Occupational Exploration* (37) and the *Occupational Outlook Handbook* (38) will be augmented by visits to work sites and interviews

TABLE 6. *Mr. Tamm's limitations for bimanual lifts on the lift capacity test*

Range	Maximum load (lb)	Heart rate	Pain response
Knuckle to shoulder	20	108	5 > 5
Floor to knuckle	10	124	5 < 8
Floor to shoulder	10	132	6 > 10

TABLE 7. *A typical program of vocational planning services*

Service	Duration	Units	Cost ($)
Vocational exploration	4 wk	12–16	1,500–2,000
Vocational training education	8–12 mo	NA	1,500–6,500
Work hardening	4–6 wk	20–30	3,500–5,500
Wage replacement on-the-job training	3 mo	NA	2,300–3,000
Workstation modification	NA	NA	1,200–3,500
Rehabilitation counseling	13–18 mo	20–32	1,700–3,200

NA, not available.

with incumbents workers. The vocational training and education process is also supervised by a rehabilitation counselor using the vocational exploration results to target the skill development that the client will need to become employed in his or her new occupation. Vocational training is available at community colleges and at private vocational technical schools. The former are inexpensive but usually require much more time to complete than the latter, which can be quite expensive. The work-hardening process is supervised by an occupational therapist using information provided by the rehabilitation counselor to identify necessary improvements in functional capacity. When shortfalls exist, the occupational therapist develops workstation modifications that are likely to be effective and acceptable to both the client and employer. These are implemented during work hardening to facilitate their adoption. Typical examples include the development of special armrests on work chairs and stools, elevated work-surface platforms that can be placed on standard workbenches, and modified hand and small power tools. In the final step in the return-to-work process, the rehabilitation counselor supervises the development and implementation of a wage-replacement on-the-job training program. It provides an identified employer with remuneration of the wage costs of the injured worker on a declining basis, beginning with 100% for the first one-third of the program and declining to 50% for the next one-third and to 25% for the final one-third. This facilitates identification of an available job and the final polishing of the injured worker's work-relevant skills.

CONCLUSION

This chapter has described a vocational assessment process that has both physical functional and general ability components. Along with description of several tests, an example of a vocational assessment report using an actual injured worker with an occupational MSD was presented. The vocational assessment process is necessary in circumstances in which injured workers cannot return to their usual and customary employment and must develop new occupational alternatives. This process provides injured workers and the professionals who work with them information that can be used to identify likely vocational targets. When combined with information about job demands, vocational assessment is useful in identifying injured workers' resources and thereby developing a job match.

REFERENCES

1. *Standards for educational and psychological testing.* Washington, DC: American Psychological Association, 1985:100.
2. Rothstein J, Campbell S, Echternach J, Jette A, Knecht H, Rose S. Appendix: standards for tests and measurements in physical therapy practice. In: Rothstein J, Echternach J, eds. *Primer on measurement.* Alexandria, VA: American Physical Therapy Association, 1993: 3–47.
3. Johnston M, Keith R, Hinderer S. Measurement standards for interdisciplinary medical rehabilitation. *Arch Phys Med Rehabil* 1992;73:S3–S23.
4. Equal Employment Opportunity Commission. Uniform guidelines on employee selection procedures (1978). *Federal Register* 1993 July 1:212–239.
5. *The Americans with disabilities act: title II technical assistance manual.* Washington DC: U.S. Department of Justice, 1992:52.
6. Hart D, Isernhagen S, Matheson L. Guidelines for func-

tional capacity evaluation of people with medical conditions. *J Orthop Sports Phys Ther* 1993;18:682–686.

7. Matheson L. Basic requirements for utility in the assessment of physical disability. *J Am Pain Soc* 1994;3: 193–199.

8. Fleishman E. On the relation between abilities, learning, and human performance. *Am Psychol* 1972;XX: 1017–1032.

9. Fleishman E. Evaluating physical abilities required by jobs. *Personnel Administrator* 1979(June):82–87.

10. Alpert J, Matheson L, Beam W, Mooney V. The reliability and validity of two new tests of maximum lifting capacity. *J Occup Rehabil* 1991;1:13–29.

11. Gibson L, Strong J. The reliability and validity of a measure of perceived functional capacity for work in chronic back pain. *J Occup Rehabil* 1996;6:159–175.

12. Matheson L, Mooney V, Caiozzo V, et al. Effect of instructions on isokinetic trunk strength testing variability, reliability, absolute value, and predictive validity. *Spine* 1992;17:914–921.

13. Lechner DE, Jackson JR, Roth DL, Straaton KV. Reliability and validity of a newly developed test of physical work performance. *JOM* 1994;36:997–1004.

14. Mooney V, Matheson L. *California functional capacity protocol (Cal-FCP) examiner's manual.* San Diego, CA: Orthomed Foundation, 1994.

15. Matheson L, Matheson M. *PACT spinal function sort.* Wildwood, MO: Employment Potential Improvement Corp, 1989.

16. Mathiowetz V, Weber K, Volland G, Kashman N. Reliability and validity of grip and pinch strength evaluations. *J Hand Surg [Am]* 1984;9:222–226.

17. Mathiowetz V, Kashman N, Volland G, Weber K, Dowe M, Rogers S. Grip and pinch strength: normative data for adults. *Arch Phys Med Rehabil* 1985;6:69–74.

18. Matheson L. Relationship among age, body weight, resting heart rate, and performance in a new test of lift capacity. *J Occup Rehabil* 1996;6:225–237.

19. Matheson L, Mooney V, Grant JE, et al. A test to measure lift capacity of physically impaired adults, 1. Development and reliability testing. *Spine* 1995;20:2119–2129.

20. Matheson L, Mooney V, Holmes D, et al. A test to measure lift capacity of physically impaired adults, 2. Reactivity in a patient sample. *Spine* 1995;20:2130–2134.

21. Mayer T, Gatchel RJ, Kishino N, et al. Objective assessment of spine function following industrial injury: a prospective study with comparison group and one-year follow-up. *Spine* 1985;10:482–493.

22. Mayer T. Using physical measurements to assess low back pain. *J Musculoskel Med* 1985;2(6):44–59.

23. Hazard R, Reeves V, Fenwick J. Lifting capacity: indices of subject effort. *Spine* 1992;17:1065–1070.

24. Mayer T. Physical assessment of the postoperative patient. *Spine* 1986;1:93–101.

25. Matheson L, Mooney V, Grant J, Leggett S, Kenney K. Standardized evaluation of work capacity. *J Back Musculoskel Rehabil* 1996;6:249–264.

26. Raven J. *Progressive matrices, standard.* San Antonio, TX: Psychological Corporation, 1960.

27. MacGinitie W. *Gates-MacGinitie reading tests*, 2nd ed. Riverside Publishing Co, Chicago, IL, 1978:8.

28. Karlsen B, Gardner E. *ABLE: adult basic learning examination*, 2nd ed. The Psychological Corporation/Harcourt Brace Jovanovich, New York, NY, 1986:71.

29. Grimsley G, Ruch F, Warren N, Ford J. *Employee aptitude survey: test 2—numerical ability.* Los Angeles: Psychological Services, 1956.

30. Doppelt J. *Personnel tests for industry: numerical test A, metricated version.* Windsor, UK: NFER—Nelson Publishing Co, 1976.

31. Bennett G, Seashore H, Wesman A. *Differential aptitude tests (DAT)*, 5th ed. The Psychological Corporation/Harcourt Brace Jovanovich, New York, NY, 1989.

32. Cattell R. *The sixteen personality factor questionnaire*, 5th ed. Champaign, IL: Institute for Personality and Ability Testing, 1993.

33. Johansson. *Career assessment inventory.* Minneapolis, MN: National Computer Systems, 1986.

34. Johansson C. Career assessment inventory, vocational version. RS, 2nd ed. In: Kramer J, Conoley MC, eds. *Mental measurements yearbook.* Lincoln, NE: University of Nebraska, Lincoln, Buros Institute of Mental Measurements, 1992.

35. Holland J. *Self-directed search (SDS) form E.* Odessa, FL: Psychological Assessment Resources, 1990.

36. Hansen J. *Strong-Campbell interest inventory, form T325 of the Strong vocational interest blank, revised.* Palo Alto, CA: Consulting Psychologists Press, 1985.

37. *Occupational Outlook Handbook: 1998–1999.* United States Department of Labor, Washington, D.C., 1998.

38. Farr J., ed. *the Complete Guide for Occupational Exploration,* 2nd ed. JIST Works, Indianapolis, IN, 1993.

Occupational Musculoskeletal Disorders
edited by T. G. Mayer, R. J. Gatchel, and P. B. Polatin.
Lippincott Williams & Wilkins, Philadelphia © 2000.

41

Developing Treatment Guidelines

David A. Wong

Department of Orthopedic Surgery, University of Colorado, Denver, Colorado 80218

Treatment guidelines help physicians address several issues in medical practice. Some of these are germane to the treatment of occupational musculoskeletal disorders, including the following:

- Incorporating evidence-based medicine into clinical practice,
- Addressing significant practice variations found throughout the country,
- Consolidating the concept of a continuous quality improvement (CQI) plan, or "best care," into the treatment of patients.

Since the 1970s, treatment guidelines have rapidly evolved from what was often a single physician's opinion or perspective on a particular clinical situation into more comprehensive documents with a more systematic, explicit methodology. This methodology generally evaluates and incorporates evidence-based medicine where possible. Treatment guidelines have at various times been known as practice guidelines, practice parameters, clinical policies, treatment protocols, care maps, critical pathways, clinical pathways, and treatment recommendations. Some have even been titled practice standards. This is a particularly bad term, with legal ramifications for the judicial "standards of care" concept. Establishing a standard of care is usually well beyond the scope of treatment guidelines (1–3).

The format of treatment guidelines generally falls into three categories:

- Narrative guidelines are descriptive, text-based guidelines.

- Matrix guidelines are most commonly known as clinical pathways. They have a time frame on one axis and goals of treatment on the other, with criteria for success specified in each box of the matrix.
- Algorithms are flowchart-based guidelines with branch points generally representing alternative treatment paths in a patient's clinical course.

Concerns have been expressed that treatment guidelines will result in "cookbook" medicine. In fact, nothing could be further from the truth. Implicit in medical practice is the requirement that clinical judgment be used in the evaluation of each patient. The appropriateness of any treatment (or guideline) in that specific clinical instance is ultimately the decision of the individual physician.

EVIDENCE-BASED MEDICINE

According to Sackett (4), evidence-based medicine is the "conscientious, explicit and judicious use of the current best evidence in making treatment decisions about the care of individual patients." Physicians' treatment decisions are generally based on knowledge from their training and experience. In the rapidly evolving medical world of today, reevaluation and updating of physicians' medical knowledge are essential to providing the best care. For individual physicians, updating their knowledge base in the musculoskeletal area is a daunting and time-consuming task. Dr. James Strickland (5), a past president of the American

Academy of Orthopaedic Surgeons (AAOS), has pointed out the explosion of articles in the musculoskeletal literature. In 1970, there were approximately 5,000 citations of published articles in *Orthopaedic Transactions*. In 1980, there were approximately 7,000 citations, and in 1990 approximately 12,700. Use of treatment guidelines, which have included evaluation of the literature in their methodology, helps busy practitioners incorporate evidence-based medicine into their practice without having to devote hours of time to individual review and evaluation of the literature. Sackett (4) succinctly summarized the relation between treatment guidelines and evidence-based medicine as follows:

> Because it requires a bottom-up approach that integrates the best external evidence with individual clinical expertise and patient choice, it [evidence-based treatment guidelines] cannot

result in slavish, cookbook approaches to individual patient care. External clinical evidence can inform, but can never replace, individual clinical expertise, and it is this expertise that decides whether external evidence applies to the individual patient at all, and if so, how it should be integrated into a clinical decision.

PRACTICE VARIATION

Some critics of treatment guidelines have suggested that such parameters are irrelevant, as they merely reflect the current practice of almost all physicians. This argument has been soundly refuted by studies indicating wide variation in medical practice. For example, a study of the rates of spinal surgery in Colorado showed seven-standard-deviations' difference in the rates of surgery among six geographic service areas (6) (Fig. 1). A nationwide analysis of practice variations in

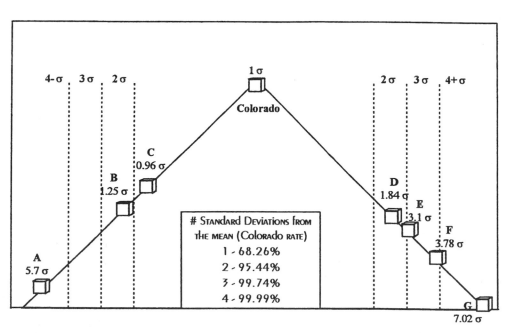

FIG. 1. Distribution of back and neck procedure rates. This graph shows the distribution of rates of spine surgery among six different geographic service areas in Colorado (*A–G*). The rate for geographic service area *A*, the lowest rate of spinal surgery, was still higher than the national rate. The highest surgical rate was in geographic service area *G*, which was more than seven standard deviations above the mean for the state of Colorado (at the apex of the distribution). The *square* below the curves shows the probabilities of variance resulting from chance alone. Variances of more than four standard deviations from the mean thus have a 99.99% probability of occurring secondary to factors other than chance.

multiple disciplines, including musculoskeletal care, was published by Wennberg (7). Studies have shown that in some musculoskeletal areas, clinical factors can be identified as a source of variation. Such evidence can then be incorporated into treatment guidelines. For example, Frymoyer (8) noted particular variation in the outcome of lumbar discectomy when pain and not a functionally significant neurologic deficit is the indication for surgery. He stated, "these variations appear to be driven less by the specific medical factors and more by the gender, occupation, income, education and the surgeon's preference." Balderston (9) asserted that inappropriate patient selection is the most common cause of failure after lumbar laminectomy. In work with the Maine Medical Assessment Foundation, Keller et al. (10) concluded that a significant reason for variation in the rates of lumbar discectomy was the lack of consensus among orthopedic surgeons and neurosurgeons about the management of herniated discs.

With appropriate patient selection and lack of consensus identified as key issues accounting for treatment variations, and with literature available specifying clinical factors associated with better outcomes, it would appear evident that the development of treatment guidelines is a reasonable approach to addressing the practice-variation issue.

QUALITY, COST-EFFECTIVE PATIENT CARE

Hand-in-hand with wide variation in clinical practice goes the concern to maintain quality yet cost-effective treatment for musculoskeletal problems. Practice guidelines represent a vehicle that may help physicians establish quality, effective musculoskeletal care (2,11,12). Cost effectiveness is an area of constantly ongoing review and controversy (2,13–16). Provision of quality musculoskeletal care should remain a cornerstone of the treatment philosophy of physicians, patients, insurance companies, and other third-party workers' compensation payers. Establishing the parameters to identify qual-

ity care (17–20) and the focus on improving quality of care (21) should be priorities in guideline development and methodology.

GUIDELINE DEVELOPMENT METHODOLOGY

Development of musculoskeletal treatment guidelines has undergone a significant evolution over the years. Initially, guidelines were commonly proposed by a single "expert" in the field. These were primarily based on opinion rather than specific evidence. Recognition of the wide variation in clinical practice throughout North America has driven a process of refining the methodology for the development of treatment guidelines. At present, quality musculoskeletal treatment guidelines are generally developed by a process combining (a) multidisciplinary expert consensus and (b) a literature review and evidence analysis. The study of musculoskeletal conditions does not lend itself to randomized, double-blind, controlled studies that would allow guideline treatment recommendations to be based on evidence analysis alone. Where many randomized, controlled clinical studies exist, more powerful evidence analysis techniques such as metaanalysis can be used. Such strength of evidence has not been found in the musculoskeletal literature. For the spine, for example, both the clinical practice guideline *Acute Low Back Problems in Adults*, developed by the federal Agency for Health Care Policy and Research (AHCPR) (22), and the clinical algorithms developed by the AAOS and the North American Spine Society (23), used a combined multidisciplinary expert consensus and literature review methodology.

Several components are key to the development of reasonable treatment guidelines. These include clinical decision-making analysis, consensus methodologies, and literature review methodologies.

Clinical Decision Making

Eddy (2,24–29) analyzed the components of clinical decision making, citing several important factors in the decision-making process.

The perspectives of both the physician and the patient weigh in the decision. Elements to be considered include the following:

- Evidence of treatment efficacy,
- Risk of treatment failure,
- Risk of treatment complications.

These factors need to be weighed against the option of no treatment and allowing the natural history of the problem to run its course. Value judgments on the acceptability of the various outcomes of treatment or nontreatment are weighed from the views of the patient and the physician in these judgments (2,12,30,31). Furthermore, societal values must also be factored in. These values generally revolve around a cost-effectiveness evaluation of treatment (2,32,33).

Consensus Methodologies

On the surface, it would seem straightforward and relatively simple to have a panel of experts convene and agree on the most appropriate way to treat a given clinical problem. In reality, however, experience has shown this to be anything but a simple exercise. Eddy (34) demonstrated the wide variation in expert physician responses to a given clinical situation. Variation is particularly noteworthy when the experts must respond to a question cold, based only on one's previous training and experience. Variation in responses narrows if the experts have had to review similar literature on the clinical question. This has led to the development of training protocols for physicians composing expert panels (35), as well as to the use of more specific consensus methodologies, such as the University of California, Los Angeles (UCLA)/Rand Appropriateness Method (36). In the UCLA/Rand methodology, for example, consensus of a panel of expert clinicians is evaluated through a review of responses elicited by various clinical scenarios. A mathematical scale and a statistical analysis of the responses are used to determine whether consensus exists on a given clinical problem.

Literature Review

A comprehensive literature review is generally performed as part of treatment guideline development. The most powerful literature review/evidence-weighing methodology is metaanalysis. Metaanalysis is a relatively new technique, proposed by Glass (37) in 1976 in an address to the American Educational Research Association. Unfortunately, metaanalysis is much misunderstood among physicians. Metaanalysis is *not* the equivalent of a comprehensive literature review. Rather, it is a technique based on *statistical analysis* of randomized, controlled clinical trials *only* (38). As such, it is a technique that is generally *not applicable* to the treatment of musculoskeletal problems. Sufficient randomized, controlled clinical trials of specific treatment alternatives simply do not yet exist.

The literature review methodology most commonly applied in quality treatment guidelines is a comprehensive literature review (using MEDLINE or a similar search engine) followed by grading of the articles by a group of physicians with content expertise. A simple grading scheme, such as that used for the AHCPR's (22) acute low back problems practice guideline, is commonly used. Evidence for treatment alternatives is graded and often evidence tables are constructed to help evaluate treatment recommendations. Because of the design constraints of available studies in the musculoskeletal literature, clinical recommendations for musculoskeletal treatment guidelines can only combine a formal literature review with consensus opinion from a multidisciplinary panel of experts.

TREATMENT GUIDELINES AND MEDICAL MALPRACTICE

First, it must be recognized by all parties involved—physicians, case managers, third-party payers, employers, and patients—that treatment guidelines do *not* represent standards of care. They are generally a reasonable approach to the evaluation and treatment of a clinical problem. The absence of well done definitive studies in the literature means that guidelines cannot be reviewed as "rigid standards" (39). Physicians have expressed the concern that treatment guidelines expose health care professionals to increased risk of malpractice suits. However, in a review of 259 malpractice claims from two insurance companies and responses of 578 malpractice attorneys to a mailed survey, Hyams (40) found infrequent use of guidelines in malpractice cases; in 259 malpractice suits, treatment guidelines were used in 17 cases (6.6%). Both plaintiff patients and defendant physicians sometimes included treatment guidelines in their arguments. The attorney survey indicated that guidelines that tended to exonerate a defendant physician induced attorneys not to bring malpractice suits. The state of Maine has passed legislation that allows defendant physicians to introduce guidelines in their defense. However, plaintiff patients are not allowed to use treatment guidelines as evidence in their arguments (41). Overall, it would appear that treatment guidelines represent a minor risk to physicians in the malpractice arena.

EVALUATION AND USE OF TREATMENT GUIDELINES

Not all guidelines are equally strong in their methodology or the evidence for recommendations on investigation and treatment. Several articles in the literature can help physicians evaluate these issues. Jaeschke et al. (42,43) focused on the evaluation of guidelines for diagnostic tests. Guyatt et al. (44,45) described a system to review articles on therapy or prevention. The issue of evaluating potential harm is described by Levine et al. (46), and the evaluation of patient prognosis by Laupacis et al. (47). The merits of a guideline's methodology and points to consider for clinical application to patients have been outlined by Oxman et al. (48), Richardson et al. (49,50), Hayward et al. (51), and Wilson et al. (52).

Despite similar methodologies and literature reviews, guidelines sometimes conflict. Eddy (53) discussed this issue and proposed methodology to resolve such conflicts. The AHCPR recently set up a guidelines clearing-

house on the World Wide Web (http://www.guideline.gov) (54). This web site allows viewing of guidelines, as well as generation of a side-by-side comparison of two or more guidelines on the same topic. A summary of the methodology used in development of the guideline is available, as well as details of the organization submitting it to the clearinghouse.

IMPLEMENTATION OF TREATMENT GUIDELINES IN OCCUPATIONAL MUSCULOSKELETAL DISORDERS

There has been a limited experience with implementation of musculoskeletal treatment guidelines in the occupational medicine arena. The state of Colorado developed treatment guidelines for low back pain, implementing them on January 1, 1994. Costs for a cohort of patients treated before implementation of the guidelines versus a cohort of patients treated under the guidelines were compared. Total medical costs after guideline implementation decreased significantly (55). Not all studies of guideline implementation have suggested cost savings. Suarez-Almazor et al. (56) retrospectively studied the records of 963 patients who had presented with a history of back pain of less than 3 months' duration. Of these patients, 127 (13%) had lumbar radiography during their first visit. After review of the patients' records, the authors concluded that if guidelines for acute low back pain from the AHCPR (22) had been used in evaluating this patient group, 426 (44%) of the patients would have had x-rays examinations. This would represent an increase of 238% in x-ray utilization.

TREATMENT GUIDELINES AND "BEST CARE"

The best care of patients is the ultimate goal of all health care professionals. A continuous CQI system incorporated into clinical practice will help make this ideal a reality. Treatment guidelines are an integral part of

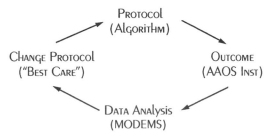

FIG. 2. Elements of a continuous quality improvement process. *1.* Treatment of patients by similar clinical protocols (treatment guideline or algorithm). *2.* Evaluation of patient clinical outcomes using a standard outcomes instrument. The American Academy of Orthopaedic Surgeons (AAOS) has instruments for various musculoskeletal conditions. *3.* Analysis of the data from the outcomes system. The AAOS has a computerized program (MODEMS) to assist with this. *4.* Changing treatment protocols based on the evidence gathered to promote "best care."

the best care/CQI process. The CQI process includes four steps (Fig. 2):

- Treatment of similar patients by a similar clinical protocol (treatment guideline/algorithm) so that patient outcomes can be reasonably compared;
- Evaluation of patient clinical outcomes using a standard outcomes instrument;
- Analysis of the data from the outcomes study, and identification of treatment factors associated with optimum patient outcomes;
- Changing treatment protocols based on the evidence gathered.

This process drives treatment guidelines toward the goal of providing the best care to patients.

CONCLUSION

Treatment guidelines in occupational musculoskeletal disorders are here to stay. Several states, including California (57), Colorado (58), Maine (59), Massachusetts (60), Minnesota (61), Oklahoma (62), Oregon (63), Rhode Island (64), Texas (65), Washington (66), and West Virginia (67), have incorporated musculoskeletal treatment guidelines into their workers' compensation systems. Musculoskeletal treatment guidelines have rel-

evance in the areas of quality patient care and CQI, incorporation of evidence-based medicine into clinical practice, cost effectiveness, and practice variation. However, to be effective, treatment guidelines must be developed using accepted consensus and literature review methodologies. They must be used and accepted by health care professionals, patients, and occupational health third-party payers.

REFERENCES

1. Bunt H, chair. *Legal issues related to clinical practice guidelines.* Washington, DC: National Health Trial Lawyers Association, 1995.
2. Eddy D. Practice policies: where do they come from? *JAMA* 1990;263:1265–1241.
3. Eddy D. Designing a practice policy: standards, guidelines, and options. *JAMA* 1990;263:3077–3084.
4. Sackett D. Evidence-based medicine. *Spine* 1998;23: 1085–1086.
5. Strickland J. Personal communication.
6. Wong DA, Waite D, Alexander W, Boymel C, Lenhart JM. Small area analysis of Medicare back and neck procedures in Colorado: breakdown of a seven standard deviation variance between the service areas. Presented at the tenth annual meeting of the North American Spine Society, Washington, DC; Oct 18–21, 1995.
7. Wennberg J. *Dartmouth atlas of health care.* Washington, DC: American Health Publishing, 1996.
8. Frymoyer JW. Lumbar disc disease: epidemiology. *Instr Course Lect.* 1992:41;217–223.
9. Balderston RA. Issues in the diagnosis and treatment of low back pain. *Health Policy Newsletter* 1990;3(2):5.
10. Keller RB, Soule DN, Wennberg JE, Hanley DF. Dealing with geographic variations in the use of hospitals. *J Bone Joint Surg [Am]* 1990;72:1286–1293.
11. Eddy D. What do we do about costs? *JAMA* 1990;264: 1161–1170.
12. Eddy D. Connecting value and costs: whom do we ask, and what do we ask them? *JAMA* 1990;264:1737–1739.
13. Eddy D. Cost-effective analysis: a conversation with my father. *JAMA* 1992;267:1669–1675.
14. Eddy D. Cost-effective analysis: is it up to the task? *JAMA* 1992;267:3342–3348.
15. Eddy D. Cost-effective analysis: will it be accepted? *JAMA* 1992;268:132–136.
16. Eddy D. Applying cost-effective analysis: the inside story. *JAMA* 1992;268:2575–2582.
17. Angell K, Kassirer JP. Quality and the medical marketplace—following elephants. *N Engl J Med* 1996;335: 883-885.
18. Blumenthal D. Quality of care: what is it? *N Engl J Med* 1996;335:891–894.
19. Brook RH, McGlynn EA, Cleary PD. Measuring quality of care. *N Engl J Med* 1996;335:966–970.
20. Blumenthal D. The origin of the quality-of-care debate. *N Engl J Med* 1996;335:1146–1149.
21. Chassin MR. Improving the quality of care. *N Engl J Med* 1996;335:1060–1063.
22. Agency for Health Care Policy and Research. *Acute low*

back problems in adults. Clinical practice guideline no 14. U.S. Department of Health and Human Services, Rockville, MD, 1994. AHCPR publication 95-0642.

23. Wong DA, Errico T, Saal J, Sims W, Watters W. Draft clinical algorithms on low back pain. In: Garfin S, Vaquero A, eds. Orthopaedic knowledge update: *spine.* Rosemont, IL: American Academy of Orthopaedic Surgeons, 1997:A26–A46.

24. Eddy D. The challenge. *JAMA* 1990;263:287–290.

25. Eddy D. Anatomy of a decision. *JAMA* 1990;263: 441–443.

26. Eddy D. Practice policies—what are they? *JAMA* 1990; 263:877–880.

27. Eddy D. Practice policies—guidelines for methods. *JAMA* 1990;263:1839–1841.

28. Eddy D. Guidelines for policy statements: the explicit approach. *JAMA* 1990;263:2239–2243.

29. Eddy D. Comparing benefits and harms: the balance sheet. *JAMA* 1990;263:2493–2505.

30. Eddy D. Rationing by patient choice. *JAMA* 1991;265: 105–108.

31. Eddy D. What care is essential? What services are basic? *JAMA* 1991;265:782–788.

32. Eddy D. The individual vs. society: is there a conflict? *JAMA* 1991;265:1446–1450.

33. Eddy D. The individual vs. society: resolving the conflict. *JAMA* 1991;265:2399–2406.

34. Eddy D. *Expert consensus in a manual for assessing health practices and designing practice policies: the explicit approach.* Philadelphia: American College of Physicians, 1992:14.

35. Schriger DL. Training panels in methodology. In: McCormick K, Moore S, Siegel R, eds. *Clinical practice guideline development methodology perspectives.* U.S. Department of Health and Human Services, Rockville, MD, 1994:115–121. AHCPR publication 95-0009.

36. Brook RH, Chassin MR, Fink A, Solomon DH, Kosecoff J, Park RE. A method for the detailed assessment of the appropriateness of medical technologies. *Int J Technol Assess Health Care* 1986;2:53–63.

37. Glass GV. Primary, secondary, and meta-analysis of research. *Educ Res* 1976;5:3–8.

38. Hedges LV. Combining estimates across studies: meta-analysis of research. In: McCormick K, Moore S, Siegel R, eds. *Clinical practice guideline development methodology perspectives.* U.S. Department of Health and Human Services, Rockville, MD, 1994:15–25. AHCPR publication 95-0009.

39. Hirshfeld EB. Practice parameters in the malpractice liability of physicians. *JAMA* 1990;236:379–382.

40. Hyams AL. Practice guidelines and malpractice Litigation: a two-way street. *Ann Intern Med* 1995;122: 450–455.

41. Smith GH. A case study in progress: practice guidelines in the affirmative defense in Maine. *J Quality Improve* 1993;19:355–368.

42. Jaeschke R, Guyatt GH, Sackett DL. Are the results of the study valid. *JAMA* 1994;271:389–391.

43. Jaeschke R, Guyatt G, Sackett Dl. What are the results and will they help me in caring for my patients? *JAMA* 1994;271:703–707.

44. Guyatt GH, Janeschke R, Sackett DL. Are the results of the study valid? *JAMA* 1993;270:2598–2601.

45. Guyatt GH, Jaeschke R, Sackett DL. What were the results and will they help me in caring for my patients? *JAMA* 1994;271:59–63.

46. Levine M, Walter S, Lee H, Haines T, Holbrook A, Moyer V. How to use an article about harm. *JAMA* 1994;271:1615–1619.

47. Laupacis A, Wells G, Richardson WS, Tugwell P. How to use an article about prognosis. *JAMA* 1994;272:234–237.

48. Oxman AD, Cook DJ, Guyatt GH. How to use an overview. *JAMA* 1994;272:1367–1371.

49. Richardson WS, Detsky AS. Are the results of the study valid? *JAMA* 1995;273:1292–1295.

50. Richardson WS, Detsky, AS. What are the results and will they help me in caring for my patients? *JAMA* 1995; 273:1610–1613.

51. Hayward RS, Wilson MC, Tunis SR, Bass EB, Guyatt G. Are the recommendations valid? *JAMA* 1995;274: 570–574.

52. Wilson MC, Hayward RS, Tunis SR, Bass EB, Guyatt G. What are the recommendations and will they help you in caring for your patients? *JAMA* 1995;274:1630–1632.

53. Eddy D. Resolving conflicts in practice policies. *JAMA* 1990;264:389–391.

54. Agency for Health Care Policy and Research. Invitation to submit guidelines to the National Guideline Clearinghouse. *Federal Register* 1998 Apr 13. pp. 63.

55. Mueller KL. Colorado Division of Workers' Compensation low back pain treatment guidelines: an analysis of CCI cases pre- and post-treatment guidelines. Proceedings of the Colorado spine symposium 8th annual meeting; Denver, CO, Nov 21, 1997:17–24.

56. Suarez-Almazor ME, Belserk E, Russell AS, Mackel JL. Use of lumbar radiographs for the early diagnosis of low back pain. *JAMA* 1997;277:1782–1786.

57. *Provisions of the California Code of Regulations. Article 7:* practice parameter for the treatment of common industrial injuries. San Francisco, CA: Department of Industrial Relations, Industrial Medical Council, 1997.

58. *Rule XVII:* exhibit A, *low back pain treatment guidelines; exhibit B, upper extremity treatment guidelines; and exhibit C, lower extremity treatment guidelines.* Denver, CO: Public Record Corporation, 1993.

59. Employment Rehabilitation. *Medical utilization review:* treatment protocols. Augusta, ME: Workers' Compensation Board, 1995.

60. *Information and application for 452 CMR 6.00. Utilization review and quality assessment program: audit instructions for use of treatment guideline and review criteria.* Boston, MA: Department of Industrial Accidents; Division of Health Affairs; Office of Health Policy, 1993.

61. *Permanent workers' compensation treatment parameter rules.* Minnesota Bookstore, St. Paul, MN, 1995.

62. *Physician advisory committee low back pain treatment guidelines, 1995.* Oklahoma City, OK: Medical Services Division, Oklahoma Workers' Compensation Court, 1995.

63. *Carpal tunnel syndrome:* diagnosis and treatment guideline [draft]. Salem, OR: Department of Consumer and Business Services, 1994.

64. Rhode Island Workers' Compensation Court. *Protocols 4, Edition 1.*

65. *Spine treatment guideline.* Austin, TX: Publications Office, Texas Workers' Compensation Commission, 1992.

66. *Provider bulletin.* Olympia, WA: Department of Labor and Industries, Health Services Analysis, Olympia, WA 1994.

67. *Workers' compensation protocols and guidelines.* Charlestown, WV: West Virginia Workers' Compensation Division, 1994.

Occupational Musculoskeletal Disorders
edited by T. G. Mayer, R. J. Gatchel, and P. B. Polatin.
Lippincott Williams & Wilkins, Philadelphia © 2000.

42

Managed Care:
Predictions for Future Medical Delivery

David W. Florence

Department of Occupational Medicine, Marshfield Clinic, Marshfield, Wisconsin 54449

GENERAL ISSUES

The difference between profit and nonprofit in health maintenance organizations (HMOs) is critical. It is apparent, especially in 1998, how for-profit health care organizations drain the system by ratcheting the payment schedules to providers in garroting proportions. This has occurred to the detriment of both providers and patients, with little return to the system. What do I mean when I refer to the "system" of health care? It relates to the multiple factors that have made health care in United States what it has been up to the present time: education, research, equipment replacement, technology upgrade, and indigent care plus the many other essential services that are unique to a particular community. By bleeding the system for investor profits, the for-profit sector, primarily HMOs, have appeared to stockholders to have a very enticing bottom line at the expense of the entire system, otherwise known as the short-term fix.

So what is next? The literature reflects that HMO premiums, which have been at rock-bottom levels in the last few years, will take a double-digit jump in 1999. Is the honeymoon over? I say, "Yes," but I will let you decide for yourself.

Are physicians satisfied in their relationship with HMOs? According to an article in *Medical Network Strategy Report* (1), in the process of contracting with HMOs, physicians have not been pleased with the short-term, insecure contracts with various plans and organizations. Such unhappiness leads to decreased productivity and ill will. Stability in the relationship between physicians and plans lies in trust and respect, factors not seen in most for-profit interfaces.

In an August 1998 article in *Healthcare Trends Report,* Stephanie Limb (2), associate editor, stated that "if a relationship between physicians and managed care ever existed, the current political climate indicates divorce." Such antimanaged-care emotions have reached the full spectrum—from patients, to providers, to medical organizations, to the public, to the media, and to the U.S. Congress. The tainted paintbrush has clouded many of the benefits of managed care, such as cost controls and accountability.

The Pew Research Center for the People and the Press noted in an August 1998 article that American voters ranked regulation of HMOs as the most important issue in the nation (3). In line with this is Les Gapay's (4) September 1998 article, "Showdown Looms on Patient Rights," pointing out that patients' rights have suddenly become one of the nation's hottest issues relating to whether or not there should be a strengthening of patient protections in managed health care organizations. Although both political parties have submitted several bills, none (at the time of this writing) has reached fruition in the U.S. Senate, although a compromise is very possible. Legislators are fully aware that there are 160 million voters under the age of 65 and these voters are primarily concerned about HMO limitations on choice of providers and services. Any constraints on HMOs by Congress could be just the straw to break the camel's back, since actuarial control is essential to the survival of HMOs and the free choice of provider and services would push actuarial controls and HMOs right out window.

Confusion on the part of the public is exemplified by average Americans' lack of knowledge about what exactly an HMO is and what all the fuss is about in Congress regarding managed care and the "patients' bill of rights." Nevertheless, average citizens do feel that additional regulations are needed to control HMOs, even though they do not know the difference between an HMO and a managed care entity (5). Irrespective of what Congress decides, average consumers will base their decision on physician choice on costs (5), even if this requires a change in plans. Affordability is a major factor for average families relative to any such change. However, the ability to choose one's own physician is also a key point at the top of the want list for families. Schmittdiel (6), in an article in the *Journal of the American Medical Association*, demonstrated that members of Kaiser-Permanente Northern California were much more satisfied if they could choose their own physician. It is of additional interest that the so-called popularity of the doctor had nothing to do with the level of satisfaction.

Just when there is such national anxiety over HMOs and managed care, Medicare bureaucrats are seeking to push Medicare beneficiaries into Medicare Plus Choice, a managed medical care program, and the endeavor is like walking on thin ice.

But what is fueling the public attention to and national anxiety about HMOs? Probably, individual experiences and the print and television media. Frustrated consumers have resorted to the media to get attention that they could not otherwise get. Because their physicians were not in a position to force changes (even for themselves), consumers have resorted to the media, which were quick to pick

up the opportunity for a good story. For example, a scathing March 1998 *Harper's Magazine* article stated that managed care "wasn't meant to care for sick people; it was meant to make and manage money" (7). Now that may be true for some of the for-profits outfits, but it is not true for the majority of the nonprofit organizations. The article even accused HMOs of hiding their abilities and potential so as not to attract costly sick patients, while at the same time seeking the enrollment of the young and healthy. All the legal protections and vices of HMOs will change drastically in the future, the article predicted, as consumers and buyers become more informed.

Although some studies have shown that some HMOs demonstrate as much quality of care as most fee-for-service systems, HMOs are on the hot seat with providers, the public, and legislators. One legislative change that has occurred, primarily at the state level, is the termination of the "gag clause" from HMO contracts, by which providers were restricted relative to the information that they could give to patients pertaining to treatment alternatives, particularly those that were more costly. Additional rights have been and will be given by law to patients in their relationship with providers. A comprehensive managed care outcome study conducted by the Institute for Clinical Outcomes Research demonstrated that "patients in systems with more restricted formularies used significantly more resources than those in systems in which physicians had a wider choice of agents" (8). Another complaint of patients and providers has been the lack of an appeals process. The report stated that these issues are changing, pointing out that, regretfully, it has taken legislation to accomplish this.

FOR-PROFIT VERSUS NONPROFIT

The question of whether for-profit or not-for-profit organizations offer the better medical care will continue to surface, but certain factors bear mentioning. Where does the health care dollar go in each? HMOs are required by law to maintain certain cash reserves. It is true that investor-owned HMOs can sell stock and raise capital for one purpose or another; however, if substantial profits in the system do not go to the stockholders, they will sell and there will be no HMO. So enters the stockholder in the decision-making process.

Stuart Altman (9), a health policy professor at Brandeis University, has stated that "the for-profits are generally nimble, quick and flexible," referring to the management end of managed care. Now this means quick decisions based on profits and losses, a very dangerous state for producing stability, not only in the system but among all the providers. For-profits are now the majority of all HMOs, and that in itself should strike fear into the hearts of consumers and providers. Nonprofits have been around longer and function more conservatively, deriving their operating monies from premiums and other benevolent sources, tarnished occasionally by commercial borrowing. Nonprofits have multiple other obligations (not respected by most for-profits) such as community needs, clinical research, medical education, and the continuous mandate to demonstrate quality (discussed later). Initially, many nonprofit HMOs were forced into for-profit status to raise needed capital. The for-profits functioned more as businesses, so they attacked the inefficiencies of the fee-for-service system during the early days of HMOs. The results offered early and high profits, and the investors bought. Of necessity, the nonprofits quickly learned efficiencies and cost cutting to remain competitive.

One should not get the idea that HMOs are the bad guys, because that is not the case. Both for-profits and not-for-profits have received high ratings under careful scrutiny. In the July 1998 *Medical Network Strategy Report*, the Sachs Group presented the "Honor Roll and Sachs Seal of Excellence" to 27 HMOs, based primarily on loyalty and member services (10). Both profit and nonprofit organizations were well represented. That same year the *American Medical News* rated West Coast HMOs the highest in quality and the lowest in cost, attributed primarily to the maturity of market and patient satisfaction (11). In fact, the satisfaction ratings for HMOs nationwide ranged from 84% to 89%, an enviable record. This demonstrates that HMOs can and do persist and do well in spite of the turbulence. Further, a summary from the *Economist* appearing in *Healthcare Trends Report* noted that HMOs have "drastically curbed the pace of health inflation while maintaining and sometimes improving U.S. medical standards; HMO enrollment growth remains strong; greater [HMO] consolidation is expected" (12). The well publicized Health Plan Employer Data and Information Set (HEDIS) rated not-for-profit HMOs as having higher consumer satisfaction, being better at providing preventive care, and spending and losing more money than for-profits (13). These differences could be expected, based on the respective missions of the profits versus the nonprofits.

One problem in comparing the HMO and the fee-for-service systems is that there are protective laws favoring HMOs at both the state and federal levels (14). For example, in some states HMOs are not legally responsible for paying physician claims, and if the HMO is in financial trouble, those physicians will probably get nothing. As an additional blow to physicians, the chief executive officer (CEO) of a large HMO management firm announced in 1998 that his organization would not be the last of its type to file Chapter 11 bankruptcy. In the business world, this is part of the process.

QUALITY

The term *quality* keeps creeping into the literature wherever HMOs are mentioned. Why is it so important? Quality is perceived to be a measuring device for the standards and performance of an HMO. What is interesting is that no one really knows what quality is. Some feel that quality is a solid rock on which an HMO rests, and in some cases that is true both literally and figuratively. Others perceive quality as an amorphous property that can be looked on through different-colored glasses, depending on what one wishes to see. However, in reality, quality is based on the level of satisfaction expressed by patients relative to access to health care and the level of services that they receive. Quality is not directly proportional to profit or nonprofit status, as it has an individual character in each organization, similar to the variations seen in the manufacturing world. Quality does suffer when the recycled profits are taken out of a system, and a system can only be bled so much before it bleeds to death. The guillotine is much sharper and faster in the for-profit sector, since a system's existence can be determined in a matter of hours by stockholders. That phenomenon can hardly be called stability and will be addressed later.

For HMOs to prosper, physician quality and productivity must be monitored and patient access to care carefully guided by some mechanism, usually a gatekeeper. This means restrictions on patients at a time when they are demanding greater and wider access to care, primarily based on being more astute and educated in health care matters. The gatekeeper is in direct conflict with consumers' desire for greater freedom of choice, especially relative to specialists, and consequently can hinder the growth and prosperity of an HMO, as well as spelling doom for a large segment of the system, especially if the Congress would make the requested changes. Since health care is now a business that must react to market forces, this will be a significant issue in both the present and the future. In her book on market-driven health care, Regina Herzlinger (15), a Harvard University business professor, pointed out that consumers are smarter and time-pressed and do not have the time to run all over town to see "approved doctors" in a health care plan. She stated that managed care will fail because it limits consumers' choice, and that could be the ticket to extinction. However, I believe that she is actually referring to HMOs and not managed care. She put HMOs on her list of "losers" that will not survive in a market-driven health care system. However, she agreed that comprehensive treatment sites or "focused factories," especially for chronic illnesses, will meet the needs of consumers, and this would fall under the aegis of disease management. Because of the tremendous expenditure relative to the treatment of chronic illnesses in the elderly with the present system, proper implementation and use of disease management could result in significant savings to any health care system. However, Herzlinger felt that any health care system that tries to do everything for everybody will lose out, and she put HMOs on that list.

Animosity toward the for-profits increased in 1998 from both patients and providers, not to mention the media (16). The blitz by the media brought the issues to the attention of Congress, and pending legislation on patients' rights is the result. The issue of profits received headlines, and consumers started to ask where the profits from the for-profits were going. Although the public is not privy to the amounts of cash in the for-profit reserves, it is obvious that most of the profits go to the stockholders or else they would not be stockholders. A major trigger of resentment was information in the media about exorbitant salaries and bonuses paid to higher executives of for-profit HMOs. For example, in 1996, for-profit CEO salaries averaged $6.2 million, with benefits averaging $13.5 million. One health plan's CEO received a $29 million salary plus $82.8 million in stock options (16). This money results from the exsanguination process of HMOs and returns nothing to patient care. Needless to say, a system like this cannot withstand the test of time.

Even some of the stellar for-profit HMOs have shown signs of collapse in recent months. For example, the Oxford Health Plan of Connecticut, founded in 1986, was considered a provider-friendly and kinder HMO. The softer profile was less intimidating to physicians. After the honeymoon, the image tarnished as delayed and denied payments became more prevalent. Second-quarter losses in 1998 of $500 million opened the eyes of the more than 50,000 providers. Losses in 1997 were $291 million plus $140 million in unpaid fees (17). Along with restructuring, Oxford plans to raise premiums. Is it possible that even some of the premier HMOs are in their death throes?

With regard to the quality issue, the definition is as yet undetermined, but this discussion has emphasized the importance of access and patient satisfaction in the formula. Other factors that have taken front stage are clinical outcomes, report cards, and costs. Actually, all of these are important for the viability of a quality HMO. According to Dr. Robert Wallen, Chair of the Mayo Foundation, Rochester, Minnesota, integrated delivery systems will continue to dominate in tomorrow's market (18), and this is probably true. However, if the integrated delivery system is causing havoc and increased costs in an area due to "managed competition," then as costs go up, the quality will go down, and the overall effort will be self-defeating. Regarding managed competition, is it still alive? Not according to Powers (19) writing in the *Kennedy Institute of Ethics Journal*. In his view, managed care has built-in incentives not to enroll the sickest population. Therefore, the lists of the sickest and the uninsured grow. He also pointed out that people switch employers and plans so frequently that long-term commitments (necessary in an HMO) are not realistic. As a result, both employers and consumers lack a long-term commitment, which defeats part of the concept of an HMO. An example of the cost-saving failure of managed competition can be seen in a small-sized city in the upper Midwest, where prior to managed competition the two hospitals shared services to reduce costs, and the physicians enjoyed mutual fellowship and community responsibility. However, a giant from an adjacent state moved into the area and purchased one of the hospitals and a large medical clinic. Consequently, the smaller health care organization was forced into a competing position, requiring the purchase of considerable equipment and personnel that were not needed prior to the managed competition. Not only greater expenditures occurred, but physicians also took sides and became opponents rather than a uniform, cooperative force.

In an article titled "Co-opetition," Coile (20) related that "when competitors reach a standoff in market advantage, they can switch to cooperation to increase their mutual strengths and benefits." That would be all well and good if the opposing parties had some common ground on which to negotiate, but I have seen situations where no such commonality existed. To cooperate for the mutual benefit of consumers and employers would in all probability require an external force to monitor and direct. Perhaps, an additional step is needed, namely, a regional control board that would determine how the integrated delivery system would function in a specific market. Integration does not preclude greed. Even high-quality not-for-profit organizations can be driven to becoming monsters if blinded to cost sharing or real community needs.

MANAGED CARE IN 1998

One might wonder whether I am an alarmist or a realist, but Jacobsen's (21) January 1998 *Managed Healthcare* article can help with this determination. In "Is the Managed Care Bubble About to Burst?" Jacobsen stated that "economics, quality and reform issues will force unprecedented changes in U.S. health care delivery." He recited the same litany of reasons previously described in this chapter, except that in his view antimanaged-care legislation will drive up health care costs and push small employers out of the market, thereby increasing the number of uninsured. Further, severe cuts in Medicare funding will drive most recipients to managed care. He feels that cookie-cutter HMO design is too inflexible to survive cost pressures and competition from alternate and emerging types of health plans. So it appears that both new and old forces stand ready to dismember HMOs, especially at a time when they are subject to criticism from all angles. The contenders in this competition are the corporate integrated care giants, physician group practices, employer groups, and coalitions.

What is a coalition? One progressive employer coalition in Minnesota, the Buyers' Health Care Action Group, gave consumers performance information relative to its health plan (22). One very prominent health care system was rated high on cost and low on quality. Such a report does and did effect enrollment in the plan, and subsequently major changes were made by providers to remedy the problems. Therefore, the coalition was effective in producing the desired changes.

"The prognosis for managed care companies is growing more grim" is a lead sentence that I am sure would induce readers to read on. Such a lead opened a *Business Week* article in which rapidly rising medical costs were given as the culprit, and managed care was accused of functioning as a "commodity business" (23). Direct negotiations of providers with employers was felt to be on the horizon and visible, with managed care plans fading. In reality, the author meant to say HMOs instead of managed care, as managed care truly has a role in the future of health care, corroborated by the fact that disease management— a form of managed care but not an HMO—is touted as a solid entity for the present and the future. At least these issues are receiving much public scrutiny.

1998: A DISASTROUS YEAR FOR THE HMOS

Quality does not guarantee survival. The August 1998 issue of *Modern Physician* had a front page captioned "Death of a Clinic," referring to the demise of the 78-year-old Thomas-Davis Medical Center in Tucson, Arizona (24). A medical management company that had acquired the clinic in December 1996 filed for Chapter 11 bankruptcy in the summer of 1998, setting a closure date for the center of August 31, 1998. The Thomas-Davis center consisted of 90 physicians in Tucson and 50 in Phoenix. The article described the ill will between physicians and the medical management company. There were even allegations of physicians' 401(k) retirement money being skimmed by the corporation.

For 78 years, the medical center had served the community of Tucson well. How could this possibly happen, and in such a short time? The claim by the management company of course was that the clinic was losing money. Could that have been a symptom of bad management? The demise started when the medical staff model, with a large HMO component, sold the entity for "stock" in November 1996. Thus, the machinations of profit tactics began, a disaster in itself. In December 1996, the remaining physicians unionized, and the owning management corporation announced closure on July 6, 1998. How is it possible that a 78-year-old quality, multispecialty clinic could spiral and crash in one and one-half years? The answer is that the ruthless tactics of the profit sector are no different from those in the remainder of the business world. The mission of providing quality medical care to the communities of Tucson and Phoenix was lost in the mayhem. And what about the stock that the physicians held as part of ownership? It was worthless.

Perhaps, one of the most dramatic and predictable collapses of a health care giant was that of the Allegheny System in Pennsylvania. At one time, this titan had a value of $5 billion. Facing a debt of $1.3 billion in the summer of 1998, the Allegheny Health, Education, and Research Foundation filed for Chapter 11 bankruptcy. The *Philadelphia Inquirer* reported that "this was the most visible symptom of a health care financing system that was out of control" (25).

Probably, the disaster that received the most attention in the national media was that of Columbia/HCA. Few parts of the nation were not affected by this debacle. It is important to note that an initial founder and physician was recalled to lead the organization down a more sane path.

The June/July 1998 issue of *Healthcare Leadership Review* contained an article that opened as follows: "Health care organizations seem to be self-destructing across the country. HMOs are generating huge losses" (26). Widespread physician unhappiness in major health care organizations was reported. Shouldn't statements like this be a cause for concern among physicians? It would appear that the system in general is out of control. In desperation, should physicians crawl on their hands and knees to Washington, DC, to plead for help—or should they stand up regionally and take control?

In this regard, many physicians may be pleased to know that they have a friend in the White House—at least according to Dr. Michael K. Rees (27). In an editorial in the March 1998 issue of *Modern Medicine*, Rees stated that "we as physicians have a chance to regain control of medicine, but—as humbling as this may be—we first have to prove that we are worthy of the responsibility." In his view, evidence-based medicine is the tool (discussed later).

Likewise, the list of physician practice management companies (PPMs), for-profit entities, going bankrupt, out of business, or reorganizing in 1998 was frightening. The list includes, for example, FPA Medical Management, Physicians Resource Group, Phy Matrix Corp, and several others. However, one cannot paint the canvas of PPMs solid red, as a few strong survivors have grown and prospered, for example, Pediatrix (headquartered in Texas), which specializes in neonatology and perinatology. Based on the stock market and my personal experience with Pediatrix, it is doing very well.

As more and more for-profit HMOs throughout the United States continue to gasp and die, or barely survive in a financial intensive care unit, FPA Medical Management declared bankruptcy in the summer of 1998, dropping 4,400 physicians and resulting in $170 million in health care plan losses for four well known HMOs. Bob Cook's (14) *Modern Physician* article alleged potential losses of "hundreds of millions of dollars in unpaid claims owed to physicians." At the same time, FPA Medical and its major creditors agreed to hefty pay raises for the company's executives. These were diverted monies that further deprived providers and consumers. Physicians were given the option of buying back their practice assets or locking their doors. Needless to say, any health care plan or system with this type of relationship with its physicians will not survive. Is there any question why even quality HMOs are getting a tainted name? In addition, the demise or bankruptcy of an organization the size of FPA

Medical Management does have a ripple effect. It was felt by Aetna/USHealthcare and Prudential Healthcare, both of which managed FPA Medical contracts in many states.

Aetna/USHealthcare is another for-profit managed-care Goliath that has tasted bitter gall in recent months (28). Physicians throughout the nation terminated contracts with Aetna/USHealthcare in 1998, primarily over contract disputes. This is just another sign of what is to come.

I have used the word *regional* a few times in this discussion, and for good reason. For example, an *American Medical News* article reporting on the "losing year" that New England HMOs had in 1997 pointed out that the larger national HMOs such as Kaiser-Permanente, Aetna/USHealthcare, and Foundation Health Systems all lost money in New England (29). However, the regional HMOs such as Harvard Pilgrim, Tufts, and Fallon made profits in 1997. The picture is coming into focus.

With regard to Aetna, additional proof of the shift of power to providers and purchasers was seen in the shift of focus by Aetna after its purchase of USHealthcare (30). The insurance giant awoke to the reality of higher medical care costs than anticipated plus the weakening HMO market. Another for-profit business venture was obviously shaky.

PREMIUM INCREASES FOR 1999

What is on the horizon for health benefit costs for 1999? Not good news, especially for managed care organizations. HMOs have bled providers to exsanguinated levels, research and education at the professional plane have essentially been ignored, high salaries have been paid to senior administrators, and the remaining profits have gone to stockholders. How can HMOs reestablish a workable financial base? Welcome to the return of the double-digit premiums in 1999. There is no other choice. Watson Wyatt Worldwide and the Washington Business Group on Health both reached that conclusion after surveying 527 employers and 1,286 health care organizations in major metropolitan markets nationwide (31). Similar concerns have been expressed by KPMG Peat Marwick after studying major health care plans. Although some prognosticators are stating that 4.5% to 8.5% increases will occur in 1999, double digits are certain for 2000.

Employers are simply not going to lie down and play dead as health care premiums increase significantly each year. Double-digit increases are really what is required to get many HMOs back on track. This could well be so for both the for-profits and the nonprofits, since the nonprofits have to be somewhat competitive in the premium price war. Employers do react and take action based on costs. For example, the Health Action Council of Northeast Ohio made an agreement with five hospitals in the greater Cleveland area (what happened to the other 25?) in July 1997 to provide services to patients with specific chronic problems (32). This encompassed 140 employers with more than 250,000 employees. These hospital cuts were based on data submitted to the Health Action Council but acted on by the employers. This is my first example of a regional control body acting in a way to control costs; it is a theme I return to repeatedly. So regional control bodies can act on submitted data, and at least this is a good-start effort.

An *American Medical News* article, "Employers Brace for Steep Premium Increases in 1999," oddly enough, predicted prescription highest increases would affect drug benefits followed by indemnity, with HMO increases last (33). The source of information was Watson Wyatt Worldwide. The alternative of direct contracting was again mentioned. The driving force behind the price increases was felt to be maturation of the managed care market, a strange way of describing the necessity of recouping losses after strangulation underpricing. The article admitted that there was no more fat left in the coffers. The carcass is bare, and the vultures have left. The real question is how high the premiums have to be to put flesh back on the bones?

Why has prescription drug usage hit an all-time high? Could it be successful television advertising by pharmaceutical companies? I ask, why should the average consumer pay the price for drug company advertising and exploitation? To solve this problem, I strongly recommend that any drug product advertised on television automatically *not* be covered by any form of health benefit or insurance. That scenario might change the picture over night.

Already accepting the fact that there will be substantial rises in health care premiums in 1999, providers and consultants of providers are drooling over potential elevations in capitation rates (34). However, they are overlooking the fact that such premium increases are necessary to keep many HMOs out of bankruptcy. The blood is out of the turnip, and a transfusion is urgently needed. Increased premiums are the only answer.

SURVIVAL TOOLS

Physicians are beginning to realize that third-party entities are taking a significant bite out of real and potential profits, and providers are banding together in highly organized groups to negotiate and deal directly with payers and the business world. As the phenomenon increases, it terrifies HMOs and third-party payers, which will be seen as unnecessary links in the chain, as well as a big black hole into which profits disappear. This can only have significance if physicians become knowledgeable, unite, implement state-of-the-art technology, and aggressively move forward, constantly monitoring quality and functioning in a cost-effective manner. Although alternative medicine choices will continue to increase, complementary health care systems will never prevail or reach a point to offset intelligent, research-based standard health care.

With regard to delivery systems, employers are now searching to find the ideal delivery system of the future, and in the view of *Managed Care Week*, the managed care product that combines consumer choice and flexibility is preferred provider organizations (PPOs) with tight management features and cost-effective efficiencies (35). So far PPOs appear to be the best kid on the managed care block, and greater patient choice is a major attraction. Morsels such as case management and billing management are most attractive attributes in the PPO system and of great interest to employers.

With managed care surfacing continuously, it will be important for physicians to shift their emphasis from procedures to solution-driven care. In the view of Timothy N. Troy (36), chief editor of *Managed Healthcare*, only when providers and plan members/consumers become part of the process will the necessary changes occur; only then will solutions be able to be measured and health care outcomes improved. The issue of consumer involvement is an important part of my ultimate recommendations in this chapter.

Revisiting the issue of survival tools, many physicians have found that they cannot negotiate or deal with HMOs to any reasonable degree of satisfaction. There are many options at that point: join a group, join a union, just give up fighting and give in, function independently and accept the consequences, or retire and fade away. Needless to say, the latter options are not feasible for younger physicians. Several of these ideas and more are well discussed in the June 15, 1998, issue of *Physician Financial News* (37). The article, "Doctors Find Life After Managed Care," is in depth and very informative. Location of practice and physician personality appear to be critical factors.

It is true that smaller provider groups have especially felt the squeeze of managed care. Low profits and high risks have necessitated the rush to either merge or be bought out. Likewise, smaller groups are being eliminated in the highly competitive marketplace, and survival has become the issue (38).

Two of physicians' more important tools for survival are direct contracting and disease management. Is direct contracting the next wave? In answer to this question, John D. Cochrane (39) in *Integrated Healthcare Report* described the action of the Buyers' Health Care Action Group in Minnesota (discussed earlier). The action of this group was precipitated by the perception that the three main health care providers in the Minneapolis/St. Paul were actually functioning as one entity or provider, as far as pricing and performance were concerned. It should be kept in mind that the payment system involved here was fee for service. Consumers then chose a case system in which to receive care. HMOs and the insurance companies were not included. Physicians should heed this example and set up a system to deal directly with employers, leaving out the money loss and overhead caused by intermediaries.

The other important survival tool, disease management, is a form of managed care, but not an HMO. It is a team approach to an illness or class of illnesses with a comprehensive concept rather than a bits-and-pieces approach seen in health care in the past. Decisions are communal, incorporating providers and patients. Those disease management entities that will be most successful will also involve the community, since many of the expenses for such care are of community-project origin. There is no room for arrogance or isolationism in that deck. Foreman and Friedman (40) stated that disease management models will be a formidable force, allowing physicians to be the clinical decision makers and allocators of resources.

Another important tool, which has met with mixed success in the past, is the use of practice guidelines. In the United States, there has been no opportunity to see how a national application of practice guidelines might effect society as a whole. Such controls are hardly available on a national basis when even some hospitals have not been able to implement guidelines. However, since 1994 in France, mandatory practice guideline have existed for 147 medical categories, and health care expenditures outside of hospitals have dropped significantly (41). Up to this point, the target has been outpatient only, but broader scopes are anticipated. Prescription guidelines were especially effective in reducing usage and costs. To give teeth to this effort, physicians violating the guidelines are actually fined. Is such an occurrence imaginable in the United States?

The relationship between physicians and patients is another factor that physicians can capitalize on. In "The Beginning of the End for HMOs," J. Daniel Beckham (42) very accurately pointed out the rising hostility toward HMOs from both consumers and providers. The essential point of the article, however, was the observation that patients have a stronger relationship with their physicians than they do with their health plan. Therefore, if patients can afford to make the change, they will do so. That is a point of leverage. In addition, patients will leave a health plan for other reasons, and physicians should know these reasons if they wish to regain some control in the system. In 1993 in California, it was found that 19% of enrollees of a health care plan would leave if they could (43). The reasons for wishing so included quality of care, problems with specialty access, inconvenience of care, doctor quality, and lack of access to hospital and emergency care.

The most critical nonmedical tool for physician survival is informatics, namely, the appropriate electronic accumulation of data and application of the same both from the medical care and business aspects. In fact, I will go so far as to say that without solid informatics, a health care entity will not survive in the future.

Joining a union was mentioned earlier, without elaboration. This chapter does not permit an elaborate discussion of unions; however, physicians are joining unions at an increasing rate. Although there are significant antitrust components, one can expect to see physician unions continue to increase in both size and comprehension in the future, primarily as a last-resort backlash by physicians against HMOs. Although more and more physicians are joining unions out of frustration with managed care, the federal antitrust laws still prevail in that only employed physicians can participate in collective bargaining. However, loopholes are possible. One approach is the third-party messenger model seen in some IPAs (independent practice associations), which are exempt from some antitrust regulations (44). The third-party messenger actually functions as an information exchanger rather than a negotiator.

Another survival tool for physician to remember is that local health care entities tend to be more successful than those from outside the region. A National Blue Cross/Blue Shield (BC/BS) Association survey found that a plan's being local was more critical to its success than its being for-profit or nonprofit. This reinforces my ultimate suggestion of regionally controlled health care entities. The BC/BS report would appear to be of significance, since true quality measurements of national HMOs, such as HEDIS, have been of questionable value. *Access* and *customer satisfaction* appear to be the essential words of the BC/BS report, and physicians should definitely emphasize these components in their practices, as they can win in the long run.

In my view, returning to basic values in medical practice is the key to success in the future, no matter which system prevails. The necessity of basic values centers on a strong patient–physician relationship. This concept was corroborated by Dr. Barry C. Dorn and Dr. Leonard J. Marcus (45) in an article in *American Medical News*. They stated that although technology will be an important factor in the future of health care, the basic values in medical practice will be critical. They accepted the premises of changing reimbursement systems and emerging technologies; nevertheless, they felt that new social mandates will surface and prevail. They emphasized keeping the individual needs of patients in balance with the collective needs of the population.

PHYSICIAN LEADERSHIP

In a striking lead article in *Healthcare Trends Report* in April 1998, Sylvia Fubini (46), editor, concluded that physicians will be the winners if managed care is out, based on their evidence-based decision-making abilities. Risk was felt to be an essential component in the new relationship between providers and consumers, and she used the Buyers' Health Care Action Group in Minneapolis/St. Paul as the example. The key for providers is a highly sophisticated information system that is used not only to record data but also to implement the information in outcome analysis and action plans.

Most physicians agree that restoring physicians to decision-making positions is necessary to reverse the tremendous outpouring of money from the systems and into stockholders pockets. However, one problem is that some of the greedy high-level administrators and stockholders are physicians. No matter what system is either initiated or restored, it must be consumer-oriented. Is such orientation feasible with any of the systems that we have today? Probably not. It will take outside forces working with physicians to mold the clay, and this must be accomplished with the focus on reasonable access and quality of care. There are high-quality physician leaders and administrators, but they will never overcome the market forces of a free-market society, where greed and profit prevail, unless some form of social community pressure or control mitigates these self-interests. This control must be a local or regional representative body that supervises in a reasonable fashion, shaping a multidirectional health care nonsystem into a rationally focused health care machine whose primary goals are community interests, reasonable access, and quality of care. Are physicians ready to accept such a system? Yes, if they can be part of the decision-making process.

In reality, some health care business leaders have expressed the opinion that physicians will never get their act together enough to work for the common good because of their independence and self-interests. I remember as a teenager (before the days of television), listening to the radio. One speaker, the president of a farmers union, had a message I will never forget (paraphrased): "There are two groups of people who are almost impossible to organize: doctors and farmers." Perhaps, that has started to change, as both groups struggle to survive in today's changing world. However, the change has started and will continue to be fueled by political-social and economic reality. Although competition will continue in one form or another, such competition must be under community control to avoid unnecessary duplication of services or expenses.

A legal argument will be made that HMOs do not practice medicine but merely facilitate health care, and consequently they would not be subject to such regional control. This is not true because HMOs do make health care and treatment decisions that directly affect patient care. Although the corporate practice of medicine has not been legal in certain states, such decisions by HMOs are protected rights to practice and restrict medical care, even when definitely needed. The practice of medicine must be given back to physicians, but it must be done in a responsible manner. Physicians must regain the decision-making powers that they have lost, but they must do so in a way that better meet the needs of patients and communities.

What does the guru of modern HMOs, Dr. Paul M. Ellwood Jr (47), have to say about this situation? In a May 1996 article in *Medical Economics*, he frankly stated that physicians have lost much of the control over health care, although he felt that much of this authority could be regained by "moving decisively and swiftly into a crucial new arena: quality of care." He warned physicians about being too pessimistic and doing nothing to make essential changes, endorsing the formation of smaller, physician-run organizations rather than dealing with the giants.

All agree that a new type of leadership is necessary if health care is to achieve the critical goals so far described. So who shall lead this daunting charge? Getting back to the basics calls for highly trained physicians to fulfill that role (48)—a position that I totally agree with. Many master's-level courses have sprung up around the country, but local or regional health-centered training is the most practical and applicable. Knowledge is needed, but a formal degree is a luxury, especially for physicians who cannot afford the time for travel or for subjects not directly applicable to their individual levels of responsibility. This pertains to the majority of physicians, who are saddled with additional administrative duties over and above their practice demands. An example of this practical application is the Sutter Health System in Sacramento, California. Sutter believed that physician leadership was key to the integrated delivery system's survival and consequently took aggressive steps, such as leadership laboratories, to achieve such leadership among its physicians (49).

Another example of education within a system was demonstrated by the American Academy of Orthopaedic Surgeons at its annual meeting in March 1998, where an instructional course, "Medical Practice Incentives: New Ways of Doing Business" was given (50). The panelists were all orthopedic surgeons who also happened to be recognized, accomplished businessmen. The counteroffensive presented alternative approaches, such as single-specialty IPAs, managed workers' compensation care, and case management, among others. Dr. William C. Mohlenbrock, medical director of Iameter in San Mateo, California, stated that "managed care knows nothing about managing care; it's about managing price." He stressed analyzing the variances in a practice that lead to cost increases. This is a critical point for leadership physicians to learn and apply if they are to be successful.

It would appear that physicians of leadership status in the future will be organized and business-minded, as well as on the offense in dealing with insurance carriers and health care plans. The goal should be to develop a seamless regional health care delivery system that is highly coordinated and could be perceived as a form of managed care. Quality and cost-effective health plans, both for-profit and nonprofit, will persist, but those in the profit category will gradually (or abruptly) decrease, with most dissolving after shareholders have milked the profits out of the system. When all the blood is out of the turnip, or if there is a variation in the market, the shareholders will sell abruptly, even if the problem is only perceived rather than real. When I say abruptly, I refer you to the proposed merger of United Healthcare Corporation and Humana Health Plans in the summer of 1998. The $5.5 billion stock swap was already reported in the medical publications as a done deal when overnight United Healthcare lost one-third of its stock value and the deal was not feasible.

Those HMOs that do survive will have knowledgeable physicians at the helm, directly involved in the day-to-day decision making (not after the fact), implementing state-of-the-art technology to drive cost savings and productivity in an infrastructure of knowledge, and utilizing management guidelines and incentives (51).

FUTURE OF HEALTH CARE

I was quite intrigued by a book review titled "The Economic Future of Health Care" in the June 18, 1998, issue of the *New England Journal of Medicine* (52). It concerned a book by Daniel Callahan, *False Hopes: Why America's Quest for Perfect Health is a Recipe for Failure.* Now those two titles should draw one's attention, and they did mine. The review's first sentence addressed the issue of the "seemingly intractable problems of our health care system." Acknowledging that both patients and physicians are not happy with the present system of competition and a price-driven market, the reviewer commented that such a market cannot be expected to keep costs down, and with this I wholeheartedly agree. He used three very appropriate words to describe the present system: expensive, dysfunctional, and inequitable.

Callahan opined that there can be no solution until expensive new technology is controlled, and that is certainly part of one aspect of the answer. However, it is clear that economics propels the technology front in medicine, and the doctor's pen is the start button. In my opinion, only when individual physicians' personal finances are affected will rational use of technology occur. Although I agree with Callahan's recommendations of preventive and public health, these two sectors are alien to most physicians because they lack the incentive of reimbursement. It may be true, as he believes, that technology has produced only marginal gains in general health care, but in reality the appropriate use of new technology can result in tremendous savings in life, time, and cost. While I agree with him that competitive market forces will not reduce or control costs, I part ways with him in his desperate cry for "more government regulation ... to protect the public interest." See what happens when physicians do not solve their own problems of public responsibility? The thought of an additional layer of incompetence being added to government is terrifying. Might I again suggest the reasonable compromise of regional health care control? Each part of the country has its own individual problems and needs, and the folks in Washington, DC, cannot see beyond their pocket books and the Beltway.

I had a similar smile when I read an article on health care industry outlook for 1998 in *Standard & Poor's Insurance Ratings* (53). In it, a recommendation was made to have the capital-rich insurance companies infuse money into underfunded managed care plans. The thought is wonderful, but what happens when the money runs out?

"*Health Trends' 1998* Guide to Managed Care Markets" provides an in-depth analysis (54). The report pointed out that managed care will grow because of needed changes in Medicare and Medicaid, and I agree with this, at least for growth in the public sector. However, the authors also added that the additional markets for growth will be in rural health, women's health, and alternative medicine. Rural health (with which I am involved) could well grow in managed care; however, the numbers are not huge to begin with and the pot is shrinking. Women's health has peaked in popularity in many parts of the nation and cannot be relied on to salvage HMOs. Alternative medicine is a mixed bag, since many of the users also use standard medical care and complementary medicine is just that; the situation is similar to what is seen with the use of more modern health care in areas of China. Only about 4% of Americans use alternative health care alone, and HMOs will not be saved by that entity. However, the authors pointed to consumer demands and stricter regulations as definite threats to the future of managed care (and again "HMOs" should be read for "managed care"). With these two points, I agree.

In "The Beginning of the End for HMOs," Beckham (42) predicted the elimination of the middleman in health care, similar to what was seen in industry. In his view, it is doubtful that HMOs have really produced cost reductions, although the overall literature would tend to dispute that opinion. However, he felt that the legal protections granted to HMOs will disappear in the future, and from what was happening in Washington in late 1998, that is probably true. He accurately pointed out that HMOs are designed for the young and healthy. But what happens when the young and healthy become old and decrepit? He envisioned provider-sponsored organizations as the mechanism for producing the needed changes from HMOs to managed care systems, and with this, I also agree.

So if HMOs are not part of the future, what is? I would vote for PPOs. It is important to point out that PPOs are a form of managed care, just as HMOs are a form of managed care. A health maintenance organization is just that, while managed care is any organized form of care that has a structure to create efficiency and quality in patient care. A PPO may have no maintenance factor such as preventive care because the structure of the organization may be for treatment only. That does not detract from its value. In 1998, PPOs accounted for about 50% of all managed care participants, and it can be anticipated that that percentage will increase significantly in the future.

Another way to bypass the HMOs for the PPOs is for employers to purchase services directly from providers. Similar to the coalition phenomenon in Minnesota (the Buyers' Health Care Action Group), another coalition, the Pacific Business Group on Health, was (at the time of this writing) beginning to develop, consisting of 35 corporations in the states of Arizona and California (55). It is a reflection of the times. Any such coalition does not occur overnight; extensive short- and long-term planning is critical to its success.

Some uninformed corporate executives believe that low cost and high quality are automatically seen in the same deck. It is not necessarily so, because the reasons for high costs and marginal quality (when identified) must each be examined separately. Employers, hospitals, physicians, and *community leaders* must all work together to define both the margins of reasonable costs and high quality for that respective region, as well as applying the same for the ultimate benefit of that community.

The potential of telecommunications for the future of health care is unlimited. I will not try to predict the distant future, but the present and near future are already a work in progress, especially as far as health care in rural and isolated areas is concerned. Use of consultants by primary care physicians not only will become a technical device (e.g., x-ray, electrocardiogram, cardiac monitoring, etc.) but also will grow precipitously in clinical areas such as dermatology, internal medicine, and musculoskeletal diseases. Instant communication among physicians and health care providers will result in greater efficiency and cost-effective health care for those who have been left out of the efficiency chain in the past. With the digitization of telecommunications, access to medical records, patient and provider education, and medical consultation is unlimited (56). Patient privacy will be a problem, but not an unsolvable one. Cost savings, both short- and long-run, will be the impetus.

In view of the title of this chapter, I would be remiss not to mention the 24-hour concept, which combines standard health care and workers' compensation health care. The problem with this blending is the indemnity factor in workers' compensation, but that does not mean that the health care factors of each cannot be isolated and then blended into a unique formula with a common mission. For some, the missions of the two are diverse, in that most nonworkers' compensation patients strive to get better or well and it is perceived that workers' compensation patients do not so strive. If this is the case, part of the problem results from our disconnected health care system, and not strictly from compensation, as alleged by some providers and employers. Although the latter factor does exist, newer methods of occupational medicine will do much to bridge the gap. There is even the pos-

sibility that both work-related and nonwork-related disability could be put under the same aegis. This chapter does not permit lengthy discussion of this issue. However, trial balloons can eventually be expected in select parts of the country, especially those not controlled by vested financial and insurance interests that now control the health care and disability markets in the majority of the country.

Finally, as to the future of managed care in Medicare and Medicaid, it is clear that these entities will need some rigid actuarial structure to properly disseminate and monitor appropriated funds. The capitation mechanism of HMOs or even PPOs could well be the only realistic answer. Highly organized PPOs can be expected to seek a piece of this action, and one of the essential tools will be disease management for chronic illnesses.

LOCAL BOARDS

So where are we headed? In an editorial in *Healthcare Forum Journal*, Ian Morrison (57) stated that "the backlash against managed care leads to laws implementing incentives for quality care rather than tighter federal regulations." He predicted that local communities will develop effective dialogue among managed care plans, hospitals, physicians, employers, and local government. I would take this concept a step further: Not only dialogue is needed, but mandatory regional regulatory boards should be set up to truly control the avarice of vested interests and serve to benefit all the community based on both the needs and the financial feasibility of the region.

A demonstration of the concept of regional health care control boards can be seen in a program of competition with regulation instituted in Arizona as a public health program for the poor. It is of interest that the article reporting on this development noted stated that "increased consolidation of the industry threatens to thwart competition" (58). That is exactly what precipitated the Buyers' Health Care Action Group in Minneapolis/St. Paul. Without competition, the game is over, and essentially there is a monopoly. However, with or without competition, regional regulatory powers and enforcement are necessary because the present systems are failing to meet community needs. And community need encompasses the uninsured and underinsured.

One factor to be considered in regional board supervision is the effect of for-profit "focused factories"in a region (59). This term refers to disease or health management specialty groups that treat or manage one particular health entity; examples include MedCath in cardiology and Pediatrix in neonatology, among many others. Although their services may be cost-effective and of quality, each of these specialty groups would be required to contribute financially to the community in which it functioned, since at present their profits arc free of the encumbrances of a general or nonprofit hospital, such as emergency room care, indigent care, education, and the uninsured and underinsured. In my view, focused factories should be subject to the rules and regulations of the regional control board in the same way as those permanently residing and functioning in the community. In other words, no health care provider would be exempt. This would help considerably to regulate the health care giants that tend to invade and control. The power of the board would also extend to telemedicine, for which medical licensure in that state would be required for a provider even to be considered. The assistance of each respective state legislature would be needed, and because of the cost savings to each state, such cooperation should not be difficult to obtain. However, it may take time because of the special interests that are certain to exert pressure at multiple levels, but such is the real world.

CONCLUSION

Contrary to much of the literature, managed care will not die but will prosper in the future. However, the subdivision of managed care called HMOs will see turbulent times. Payers from all sources will soon realize that fee for service in a well organized provider system—otherwise known as a PPO—will greatly exceed the benefits of HMOs in all measures, including quality and cost effectiveness. Payers will then gradually make the transition to either a quality PPO or a nonprofit HMO with a proven track record. Both for-profit HMOs and newer, nonprofit HMOs will probably not be able to cut the mustard in most situations. In addition, for-profit HMOs will be crippled by providers dealing directly with employers, which will drive down stock value, and the massive selling by stockholders will cascade, pushing for-profit HMOs over the brink into extinction. Very few will remain viable. Access, quality of care, and patient satisfaction will be the life rafts for the remaining HMOs, both profit and nonprofit. Medicare and Medicaid reform could be the island of rescue for the few remaining quality HMO providers. However, quality PPOs will be the benefactors.

A federal government takeover of the mess is likely to make things worse. Just think about the Social Security debacle if the thought lingers. Each state or region of the United States has its own individual needs and problems, and these cannot be solved at the federal level. Each state should legislatively determine its own system to meet its needs. Some states are so large that they have individual needs within regions. Therefore, regional boards of control make more sense, but they would have to be mandated by the state legislature to be effective. The needs of the people are at the center of this concept, and if this solution is to have any permanent value, it must be ongoing, not just hit-and-run. So my vision is one in which regional health care boards would control the services of health care organizations functioning in the region, introducing needed services, approving only those services that are needed, where and when they are needed, monitoring services, and eliminating redundancies.

Who would make up these regional boards? In addition to consumers, who would be at the top of the list of board members, boards would include employers, business leaders, professionals (medical, legal, and otherwise), and legislators. Physicians and health care administrators would fall into the above categories, but they would not be in the majority. All members would be paid a reasonable salary based on the abilities of the region and would be required to sign contracts clearly outlining the duties and obligations of the board. The board would meet at least 10 times per year but would have active subcommittees that would be required to perform to a pre-specified level based on specific guidelines. Board members would be paid because the duties and assignments would not be titular in nature and would be looked on as obligations. The scope of decision making would be broad, and appeals to major decisions could be taken to an appellate level consisting of two judges (one district and one state), a local legislator, and a physician-at-large chosen by the regional or county medical society. However, a two-thirds approval vote by the board would be required to activate the appeal. To prevent frivolous appeals, appellants would be fined a set amount if they lost the appeal. The money generated by fines would go toward support of the board. The size of a board would depend on a region's population. Its expenses and salaries of the members would come from a proportional assessment on all health care providers in the region.

As for the number of boards and where such should exist, such matters would be the responsibility of the legislature of each state, working with the providers and consumers of each region. An argument will be made that providers and health care organizations are already meeting community needs. However, the literature does not support that contention. Even the finest of nonprofit health care organizations have vested interests and individual agendas that can and do prevail over community needs. For example, for 6 years, I was the chairman of the board of health of a moderate-sized city that also happened to be the state capital. At no time in those 6 years did a representative of either of the two large hospitals in the city ask the board of health what the needs of the community were or how the hospitals could assist the board. The hospitals primarily based their functioning on business decisions rather than community needs. This scenario is not unusual, especially for a community without a county or city hospital. Somehow, the real needs of the citizens, especially the underprivileged, get lost in the shuffle, as the priorities of the health care institutions become paramount.

The regional board concept will probably not come to fruition in the near future for many reasons, some of which have been described in this chapter. However, down the road of repeated mistakes and misadventures, some region or state may say, "Let's give it a try." At that point, the health care system in the United States, which is now near collapse, will begin to change to meet the needs of the American people rather than those of the health care giants and for-profit corporations. In the meantime, out of desperation, physicians will rise to the cause, like a phoenix from the ashes, ready to participate in any system that makes more sense than the present. Can we really afford the expenditures and failures in the interim?

REFERENCES

1. Long-term contracts: hope behind the hype? *Medical Network Strategy Rep* 1998;7(7):1–5.
2. Limb S. "Physicians and managed care: a much–needed marriage of convenience." *Healthcare Trends Rep* 1998; 12(8):1–2.
3. Compared to 1994, voters not so angry, not so interested. *Healthcare Trends Rep* 1998;12(8):3.
4. Gapay L. Showdown looms on patient rights. *AARP Bull* 1998;39(8):1,18,19.
5. The illusion of managed care reform. *Healthcare Trends Rep* 1998;12(7):1–2.
6. Schmittdiel J. Choice of a personal physician and patient satisfaction in a health maintenance organization. *JAMA* 1997;278:1596–1599.
7. Glasser R. The doctor is not in. *Harper's Magazine.* 1998 March:35–41.
8. Anderson D. Who's calling the health care shots? *Business & Health* 1997 Oct:30–35.
9. Altman S. For profit or not: where's the best care? *Business & Health* 1998 July:46.
10. Who's been good and who's been really good? The Sachs Group says. *Medical Network Strategy Rep* 1998; 7(7):10.
11. Jacob J. West coast HMOs offer highest quality, lowest costs. *Am Med News* 1998 June 15/22:21,24.
12. Your money or your life. *Healthcare Trends Rep* 1998; 12(5):9. [From *The Economist* 1998 March 7:23–26.]
13. Blue skies or black eyes: HEDIS puts not-for-profit plans on top. *Healthcare Trends Rep* 1998;12(5):12. [From

Greene J. *Hospitals and Health Networks* 1998;72(8): 27–30.]

14. Cook B. Stormy weather. *Modern Physician* 1998 Sept: 2,8.

15. Cook B. A better spin. *Modern Physician* 1998 Feb: 76–78.

16. Altman S. For-profit or not: where's the best care? *Business & Health* 1998 July:51.

17. Tschida M. Healing process. *Modern Physician* 1998 Sept:56,58.

18. Top 10 quality trends. *Healthcare PR & Marketing News* 1998;7(6):6.

19. Powers M. Managed care: how economic incentive reforms went wrong. *Kennedy Inst Ethics J* 1997;7: 353–360.

20. Coile R. Co-opetition. *Healthcare Strategist* 1998 Jan: 1–6.

21. Jacobsen R. Is the managed care bubble about to burst? *Managed Healthcare* 1998 Jan:17.

22. Jossi F. A BHCAG update from the Twin cities. *Healthcare Leadership Rev* 1998;17(6):4.

23. Hammonds K. Hit where it hurts. *Business Week.* 1997 Oct 27.42–43.

24. Cook B. Closed book. *Modern Physician* 1998 Aug:2, 3,8.

25. Philadelphia Online, *The Philadelphia Inquirer.* Allegheny in turmoil: the causes, the diagosis, the treatment and the aftershocks. *Healthcare Trends Rep* 1998; 12(8):4–5.

26. Cochrane JD. What can go wrong and how to avoid it. *Healthcare Leadership Rev* 1998;17(6):6.

27. Rees M. A friend in the White House: let's seize the opportunity. *Modern Medicine* 1998;March;66:63–64.

28. Tschida M. Just say no. *Modern Physician* 1998 July:3.

29. 1997: a losing year for New England HMOs. *Am Med News* 1998 June 29:20.

30. Aetna's brave new world. *Healthcare Trends Rep* 1998; 12(5):5. [From Jackson S. *Business Week* 1998 March 30:180.]

31. The return of double digits. *Business & Health* 1998 July:13.

32. Moskowitz DB. Outcomes-based buying goes direct. *Business & Health* 1998;16(3):48.

33. Jacob J. Employers brace for steep premium increases in 1999. *Am Med News* 1998 June 29:21.

34. As premiums rise, will capitation rates follow suit? *Capitation Manage Rep* 1998;5(3):33–37.

35. PPO industry at a crossroads: toward a new model of delivery. *Healthcare Leadership Rev* Dec.1997. [From *Managed Care Week* 1997;7(38):6–7.]

36. Troy TN. Let's shift from procedures to solution-driven care. *Managed Healthcare* 1997;7(10):5.

37. Stevens S. Doctors find life after managed care. *Physician Financial News* 1998;16(8):1,28,29.

38. Feeling the squeeze. *Modern Physician* 1998 Feb:48.

39. Cochrane JD. Is direct contracting the next wave? *Integrated Healthcare Rep* 1997 Oct:1–7.

40. Foreman MS, Friedman S. Up and coming carve-outs. *Health Systems Rev* 1997;30(6):52–56.

41. Durand-Zaleski I, Colin C, Blum-Boisgard C. An attempt to save money by using mandatory practice guidelines in France. *BMJ* 1997;315:943–946.

42. Beckham JD. The beginning of the end for HMOs: providers have more clout than they think. *Healthcare Leadership Rev* 1998 March:3.

43. Kerr E. Does dissatisfaction with access to specialists affect the desire to leave a managed care plan? *Medical Care Res Rev* 1998;55(1):59–77.

44. Unions are not for everyone. *AAOS Bull* 1997:23.

45. Dorn BC, Marcus LJ. Model of the emerging medical leader. *Am Med News* 1998 June 15/22:18,20.

46. Fubini S. If managed care is out—who's in? *Healthcare Trends Rep* 1998;12(4):1,2.

47. Ellwood PM Jr. How doctors can regain control of healthcare. *Medical Economics* 1996 May 13:178–201.

48. Their S. Healthcare reform: who will lead? *Ann Intern Med* 1991;115:54–58.

49. Olson D. And a doctor shall lead them. *Healthcare Leadership Rev* Dec. 1997:6.

50. Panel advises surgcons: take back control. *Academy News [AAOS Bull]* 1998;6(3):14/A.

51. Limb S. Physicians & managed care: a much needed marriage of convenience. *Healthcare Trends Rep* 1998; 12(8):2.

52. Relman AS. The economic future of health care. In: Callahan D, ed. *False hopes: why America's quest for perfect health is a recipe for failure.* New York: Simon & Schuster, 1998:XXX–XXX.

53. Kumar A, Cohen J, Puccia M. 1998 health care industry outlook. In: *Standard & Poor's Insurance Ratings.* 1998. [From *Healthcare Trends Report* April 1998:6.]

54. Fubini S, Limb S, Morgan S. *Health Trends' 1998 guide to managed care markets.* Health Trends, Inc, 1998.

55. White JB, Rundle RL. Big companies fight health-plan rates. *Wall Street Journal* 1998 May 19.

56. Fubini S. The telecom revolution and health care—will there be a fit? *Healthcare Trends Rep* 1998; 12(6):1–2.

57. Morrison I, Schwartz P, Yankelovich D. Healthcare in the new millennium: the long boom meets the civil society. *Healthcare Forum Journal* 1998;41:18–22, 70–73.

58. Weil T, Battistella R. A blended strategy using competitive and regulatory models. *Health Care Manage Rev* 1998;23(1):37–45.

59. Focused factories. *Healthcare Trends Rep* 1998;12(5):6. [From Meyer H. *Hospitals and Health Networks* 1998; 72(7):25–30.]

Occupational Musculoskeletal Disorders
edited by T. G. Mayer, R. J. Gatchel, and P. B. Polatin.
Lippincott Williams & Wilkins, Philadelphia © 2000.

43

Workers' Compensation Systems and Benefits for Permanent Partial Disabilities

Peter S. Barth

Department of Economics, University of Connecticut, Storrs, Connecticut 06269-1063

This chapter describes the methods used by the states to compensate a worker for a work injury or illness that results in a permanent impairment. Compensating a worker who has sustained an occupational injury or illness can be a complex matter. Generalizing about the process is especially difficult in the United States because every state has its own approach to compensation. Indeed, coverage of employees varies from one state to another, and the conditions under which an injury is itself potentially compensable can vary significantly. In broad terms at least, the different state programs have many basic similarities; however, with respect to the compensation of permanent disabilities, significant differences in approach emanate from different perceptions about the underlying purposes of these programs.

PURPOSES OF WORKERS' COMPENSATION PROGRAMS

Most persons who are familiar with workers' compensation can agree with the five basic goals identified in 1972 by the National Commission on State Workmen's Compensation Laws. These goals identified the need for adequate and equitable benefits, broad coverage both of workers and of injuries and illnesses, full medical services, a scheme that encouraged positive health and safety practices, and efficient administration of the program. Another goal that should be added to this list is the need to ensure that there is a long-term, productive return to work. Experience appears to demonstrate that some elements of the workers' compensation systems are not difficult to adapt to be consistent with these goals. For example, where a worker has been injured at work and is unable to continue employment for sometime, the earnings loss associated with the injury is usually quite clear. Whether states actually replace a significant portion of the lost earnings is a separate matter, but the degree of loss to the worker is readily apparent. For some portions of these schemes, however, there has been consistent frustration in accomplishing widely accepted goals. Permanent partial disability (PPD) appears to be an area where the goal of the scheme itself is difficult to measure or even to define. A stereotypical PPD case in workers' compensation arises when a worker with a compensable injury or illness ceases to be eligible to receive temporary total or temporary partial disability benefits and is left with a permanent condition that is a result of the injury. At that point in every workers' compensation system, the worker is evaluated for purposes of determining whether there is an entitlement for any further indemnity (cash) benefits. The criteria used for such a determination vary considerably from one jurisdiction to another, which can reflect either different goals and objectives or simply different methods of accomplishing the same ends. It is probably accurate to say that more variation exists across jurisdictions in their approaches than in any other area of the scheme. Compounding this diversity, the language that the states use to describe elements of their programs is often inconsistent. In some instances, the same practice is described using different nomenclature, whereas in other instances, the same term does not refer to the same activity or method in different jurisdictions. The matter is complicated by the gap between what a law may describe as the method of compensation and the actual practices that have evolved that bear only a faint resemblance to prevailing practice.

Most observers agree that the general goals of a PPD program are to replace some portion of the income lost due to the worker's physiological or psychological loss. In so doing, the states are operating their PPD programs in a manner that is consistent with their treatment of other kinds of losses that workers or their survivors may incur because of work accidents or illnesses. How that loss can be measured and benefits delivered that are commensurate with those losses is the challenge that jurisdictions have not fully mastered. Furthermore, delivering those benefits can create certain incentives and disincentives that are not consistent with other goals of the program.

SCHEDULED BENEFITS

Most states deliver their PPD benefits in at least two distinct ways. More than 40 states pay benefits that are labeled as either *scheduled* or *specific*. Indeed, even those few that do not use scheduled benefits use a means that parallels this approach, and so its importance is even greater than first meets the eye. Scheduled benefits are those that appear in a statute or by rule and that specify what the benefit is to be for a specified loss. Most generally, the schedule covers losses of, or to, the extremities and to the eyes. In some jurisdictions, the losses that are so listed may include hearing loss, the genital organs, and various other body parts.

The determination that a worker has sustained a scheduled loss is made after the period of temporary disability has ended. This event typically occurs when one of three events occurs. First, if the worker has returned to employment or is found medically to be able to resume working, the temporary disability benefit is terminated by the insurer. Second, there may be a medical determination that the worker has reached maximum medical improvement (the terminology here varies; e.g., in California the person's condition is said to be permanent and stationary), and at that point the worker is evaluated. A third possibility, found in fewer states, is that the law limits temporary disability benefits to a fixed period, often 104 weeks from the date of injury, at which point the worker is evaluated.

A typical schedule might identify the loss of a hand, for example, as being valued at some amount, most commonly expressed as numbers of weeks of benefits. For example, the loss of a hand in Alabama entitles the worker to 170 weeks of benefits. The weekly benefit in that state, as in many others, is function of the worker's preinjury wage. For example, the loss of a hand in a compensable injury entitles the worker to a weekly benefit that is set at two-thirds of the worker's preinjury average weekly wage, with the benefit not to exceed $220 per week as of 1998. In early 1998, the average weekly wage of a worker in Alabama was $493. As such, the benefit actually bears little consistent relationship to the wages of those workers who earn more than $330 week.

The basis for placing this value on the loss of a hand is buried in some legislative accommodation made decades or generations ago. There appears to be no specific economic justification for the particular value of the hand, much less to explain why it might be valued more highly than a foot in some jurisdictions and not others. In large measure, the schedules have been retained in stable form for a considerable time, with the major change over time being in the maximum weekly benefit that a worker might receive.

Both a virtue and a shortcoming of the schedule can be seen as two sides of the same coin. On the one side, the schedule provides consistent treatment across workers who suffer the same impairment from a work injury. Two workers who have loss of a thumb will receive the same number of weeks of benefits and the same amount of money if their preinjury earnings are the same (I put aside any differences that workers may have from their temporary disability benefits). The consistency of benefits is even greater in those jurisdictions that pay the same benefit amounts to workers who have different preinjury wages. Idaho is an example of such a state.

The primary shortcoming, as perceived by some critics, is that the loss of a body part will have dramatically different economic results for different persons. In the case of a carpenter, the loss of a thumb may be immensely damaging to the worker's future earnings, whereas the same loss to a factory operative may be far less disabling. The scheduled loss is based on compensation for the degree of impairment, not for the disability that will result. Great consistency that assures equal indemnification for equal impairment can yield notably unequal treatment for persons who have vastly different levels of disability.

Although schedules have many structural similarities across the states, some interesting variations exist. For example, a few states differentiate between the loss of a body part by amputation and the loss of use of the body part. States that apply such a difference will simply add some proportion to the value of scheduled benefit for a loss by amputation.

A more common difference in treatment occurs in the situation in which the worker suffers a partial loss, or loss of use, of a scheduled body part. The hand may be valued at 200 weeks of benefits, but how can a worker who has suffered a loss of one-half of the hand be compensated? Two different methods exist: The most commonly used method is to evaluate the degree of (medical) impairment and set the benefit proportional to the value of the full body part. For example, if the total loss of the hand is shown in the schedule to be valued at 250 weeks of benefits, then the loss of one-half of the hand entitles the worker to 125 weeks of benefits. Just as the loss of the hand is compensated based on the impairment the worker has incurred, the loss of a portion of the body part also is evaluated based on the impairment, not on the basis of disability.

In a number of jurisdictions, however, the partial loss of the body part that is scheduled is evaluated for compensation based on the disability that the worker is expected to suffer. In such a jurisdiction, for example, a worker who suffers a loss of one-half of the hand, where the loss of the entire hand is valued at 250 weeks of benefits, may be able to be awarded up to 250 weeks of benefits for the partial loss. In these states, the degree of impairment usually sets the lower bound on the benefit that the worker may be able to be awarded. Thus, the worker will be certain to receive at least 125 weeks of benefits (for the impairment of one-half of the hand) and possibly up to 250 (for disability where the entire hand is valued at 250 weeks.)

States that compensate workers based on disability where there is partial loss of a scheduled body part add a dimension of flexibility to their program that does not exist where compensation is based entirely on the extent of impairment. The price of this flexibility is that there is more room for dispute over the value of the claim.

Another variation occurs when the size of the scheduled benefit, either in terms of dollars or weeks of benefits, can be reduced because of the time spent on temporary disability. Most states, however, do not alter the scheduled benefit because of the period over which temporary benefits were paid.

Yet another variation of the scheduled benefit can be found in a few states that permit workers to receive supplemental benefits over and above the benefits paid according to the schedule. Indeed, the presence of a supplement to the scheduled benefit, presumably where the disability is substantial, led some of these states to pay comparatively low benefits for the scheduled loss itself.

Two, or arguably three, states that use schedules adjust their scheduled benefit by some type of formula that takes into account factors such as the worker's age or occupation. Thus, these states have tried to build some variation into their benefits for a scheduled injury without leaving the door open to disputes over the value of a claim based on every possible measure of disability.

Earlier, it was noted that not all states used schedules, although in reality they used methods that were virtually the same. For example, Texas does not have a schedule *per se*. Instead, a worker with a permanent impairment is rated according to the American Medical Association's (AMA) *Guides to the Evaluation of Permanent Impairment* (AMA, 3rd Edition,). In Texas, a worker will be entitled to 3 weeks of benefits for every point of rated impairment. The *Guides* rate the loss of a hand as a 54% loss of the whole person. As such, the worker with a loss of a hand is entitled to 162 weeks of benefits at the rate of weekly compensation that is established by the statute. Essentially, that is precisely analogous to the state that employs a schedule and rates the hand at 162 weeks.

The schedule is so popular and so commonly used by the states (and in many jurisdictions outside the United States) because it is administratively simple and results in less wrangling over the size of any potential indemnity benefits, thereby assuring that the transactions costs of the system are not so high as in other elements of the program. Some may argue that the benefits provided by the schedule are too high or too low, overall, but the method itself has drawn relatively little fire from critics of the PPD system.

UNSCHEDULED BENEFITS

Virtually all states will provide a PPD benefit for a condition that is not in the state's schedule. Indeed, for many states, most PPD cases do not involve a scheduled loss. The fact that an unscheduled loss can be compensated differently from a scheduled one can create some problems for those who administer the system. Two examples may demonstrate this dilemma. First, in some cases, a worker may sustain both a scheduled and an unscheduled injury. In that event, how is the state to determine the appropriate level of benefits? This situation may be especially significant where thresholds exist in the law such that the greater the degree of disability, the greater the benefit *rate* will be. Another possible problem arises where the law provides more generous benefits under one type of condition, typically the unscheduled one, than for the other. In this situation, it is hardly surprising that the claimant will seek to have the condition evaluated under the more generous scheme. For example, an injury to the upper extremity is likely to be scheduled, and the maximum benefit is set in the schedule. If the worker can demonstrate that the condition has radiated into the shoulder (typically the shoulder is not scheduled), the worker's rating may be based on the unscheduled disability, which may lead to more generous benefits.

It is common for a worker to receive a lower weekly benefit for a PPD, scheduled or unscheduled, than for the temporary disability. In many states, the benefit formula provides a lower benefit rate for the permanent partial condition. Even where the formula appears to be the same, that is, where the worker is paid a typical compensation rate of two-thirds of the worker's average weekly wage for both the temporary and the permanent partial disability, the benefits are likely to be different. This situation occurs where the maximum weekly benefit for the PPD is set below the maximum allowable weekly benefit for the temporary disability. When the worker can anticipate a dropoff of benefits when being shifted from the temporary benefit to the PPD benefit, the worker may resist the change and seek to continue to receive the temporary benefit.

For unscheduled losses, states have developed four fundamental approaches to compensation. Each approach has certain strengths and weaknesses. The fact that the states have not converged on a single approach to so important a determination is probably a good indicator that dissatisfaction exists with elements of each of these approaches.

IMPAIRMENT BASIS FOR COMPENSATION

A number of the states as well as certain jurisdictions in other countries compensate workers based on the degree of their medical impairment. In such schemes, the benefit is determined by an evaluation done by a medical provider. Typically, but not necessarily, the evaluator is required or encouraged to rate the worker's loss according to a medical guide. The impairment rating then is transformed into a benefit determination. For example, if the worker's impairment is 20% and state law entitles the worker to 4 weeks of compensation benefits for every point of impairment, the worker is entitled to 80 weeks of benefits. Customarily, the compensation rate is associated with the employee's preinjury wage rate, although it need not be.

In some jurisdictions, the rating of an impairment is itself contentious and has given rise to a "dueling doc" syndrome. In these jurisdictions, it is not uncommon for the insurer to have the worker rated by a health care practitioner of its own choosing, one who is likely to avoid excessively high ratings. Similarly, workers in these jurisdictions often find their way to doctors or others who do ratings who have a reputation for giving generous, or worker-friendly, impairment ratings. Once these ratings are reconciled, or a decision is made by an adjudicator, the benefit is paid based on the rating.

The strength of the impairment approach is much the same as that of the schedule. If the determination can be made on a relatively objective basis, the likelihood of prolonged, expensive controversy is reduced. The process has some degree of certainty attached to it. Moreover, workers who have similar degrees of impairment are likely to receive similar benefits in terms of weeks of benefits, dollar amounts, or both. Because the impairment is unaffected by whether the worker has returned to work or is undergoing (vocational or other nonmedical) rehabilitation, the worker does not postpone or avoid these measures. In this way, the impairment approach has some of the same strengths as the scheduled approach.

Opposition to the impairment method comes from several corners. First, because this method does not consider disability, some workers who have relatively minor impairment will receive a relatively minor PPD benefit, even if the worker is seriously disabled. Another criticism comes from those who are suspicious of the medical impairment guides being used to rate impairment. A common concern on the part of those who represent workers is that the guides are often inadequate as they rate certain impairments (e.g., spine injuries). Indeed, most guides are hard pressed to explain the empirical grounds that form the basis for the specific rating of an impairment. This may be one of the reasons the AMA opposes the use of its *Guides* for the purpose of directly rating disability. Presumably, the AMA believes that the impairment rating should serve as only one of several inputs to be used in the rating of disability, although it is silent on precisely what is to be done.

Another criticism of the impairment approach is that it is occasionally used where it is obviously inappropriate. Specifically, some jurisdictions that limit temporary disability benefits to a certain time will require that the worker's impairment be rated at the time these benefits cease. Yet, in some instances, the worker has not reached a position of stability, and there is no legitimate way to rate the worker's impairment at that time. The problem is not unique to the impairment method of setting benefits, but it is likely to cause more problems than where other methods of rating are used.

Workers' attorneys tend to be highly critical of the impairment method for determining disability. Among other factors, it tends to move the argument over disability from the type of issues that attorneys are accustomed to using to strictly medical matters. Indeed, a number of jurisdictions have taken steps to limit disputes over medical matters by requiring that expert medical "neutrals" be used to settle any medical differences. In that case, there is less room for the attorneys to maneuver.

In a few jurisdictions that use the impairment method to determine disability for an unscheduled condition, the worker may be eligible to receive a supplemental benefit when the impairment benefit has ended. In such cases, some threshold may have been set below which no supplemental benefit can be paid. In Florida, a worker is ineligible for any benefit after the permanent impairment benefit has ended unless the worker has had an impairment rating of at least 20%. Among other requirements, the workers also must demonstrate that they continue to suffer an earning loss because of the compensable injury or illness.

LOSS OF WAGE-EARNING CAPACITY BASIS FOR COMPENSATION

A second approach to compensating workers who have an unscheduled PPD is to rate the worker based on the economic impact the permanent impairment will cause in the future. An essential characteristic of this approach is that once the worker has reached maximum medical improvement, the rating will determine what the lifetime impact of the condition is likely to be. Some states look to the worker's ability to compete in the labor market. Other laws appear to focus directly on the loss of earnings (in the future) or earnings power. I classify all of them in this category because they are all basically predictive. Also, because this method relies on predicting the future, this method is the most subjective, at least according to the critics of the approach. Others regard this approach simply as more flexible than the impairment method and possibly other methods as well.

The impact on a worker's capacity to earn in the future cannot easily be calculated by a formula, although several states attempt to do so. Factors that always seem to be considered in evaluating the loss, whether it be a result of a formula or otherwise, are the worker's age, education level, employment experience, language skills, and the regional or local labor market conditions. The degree of impairment often is used as well. Because the medically determined impairment rating is not the sole, or perhaps even a central, issue in rating the disability, the role of the medical evaluator is likely to be less significant than where the impairment method is used or where the loss is a scheduled one.

A concern with this method is that it may discourage the worker from seeking prompt, effective rehabilitation. The reason for this is that if the worker is anticipating being rated on the basis of the anticipated loss of future earnings, it is likely that the worker would prefer to be rated when his or her condition appears to be serious. It is not that the worker does not wish to be restored as closely as possible to the preinjury condition. Rather, if the worker's economic and health conditions are not good at the time of the rating, the worker is likely to receive a higher disability rating (i.e., a larger benefit).

Because of the room for differences in rating disability with the loss of wage earning capacity method, it appears that in many of these situations the parties settle with some form of compromise agreement. In most states, the agreement also is designed to release the employer or the insurer from any future liability. In most of these situations, the lump sum payment to the worker serves as the basis on which the attorney's fee is determined.

WAGE-LOSS BASIS FOR COMPENSATION

A third method used to compensate workers with an unscheduled PPD is to base benefits on the actual—as distinct from the predicted—loss of earnings. In this approach, which is used in a handful of states, the worker can continue to receive benefits for an extended period as long as the worker has some degree of earnings loss attributable to the compensable condition. In this approach, the worker is not likely to have full earnings loss replaced but, instead, is entitled to some fraction of the loss to be made up.

Almost without exception, if a worker suffers an unscheduled permanent impairment in a wage loss state, and the worker is able to return to work at or near to the preinjury earnings level, the worker is not entitled to a PPD benefit. The sole basis for a PPD benefit is the loss of earnings and, as such, the worker who can overcome the impairment will not receive the PPD indemnity benefit. Undoubtedly, this will appear to be harsh to some critics of the wage loss approach. It suggests that the worker with a strong work ethic may be penalized economically, even when the impairment is serious.

The most serious difficulty with the wage loss approach is that it is difficult to administer well. Suppose a worker with an impairment returns to work briefly but then loses his or her job. Was the reason for the job loss the impairment, which may have prevented the worker from successfully doing the work? Is any prolonged unemployment a result of the impairment that the worker sustained, or is it attributable to conditions in the labor market generally? Is the worker's loss of earnings a result of the worker's lack of motivation in the presence of the opportunity to receive compensation benefits when not employed? What must workers do to prove that they have been actively seeking employment? How frequently can the insurer seek to have the state workers' compensation agency or a court terminate or reduce the worker's benefit on the grounds that the income loss is due to the worker's lack of motivation and not to the condition? In reality, these issues can give rise to frequent and regular disputes arising in the same case. The costs to the parties can be substantial. As a result, it is common for these potential controversies to be avoided by settling the case and ending the insurer's or employer's future liability.

An incentive that may be generated by the wage loss approach is that the employer may save on future workers' compensation costs by continuing to employ the injured or sick worker. To the extent that the employer's future insurance premiums are likely to rise as a result of the experience rating formula, the employer may find it advantageous to retain the worker. The self-insured employer is also likely to find that rehiring the worker can save on workers' compensation costs. Whereas the possibility must exist that this situation will occur, there is simply little evidence to assess how frequent this practice is. There is a good deal of anecdotal wisdom regarding the efforts that some employers will expend to avoid rehiring former employees who have used the workers' compensation system. The efforts to avoid rehiring such employees seem to be greatest when the employee has not been a long-term employee of the company, when the employer fears that further injury is more likely to occur, and in smaller establishments.

BIFURCATED BASIS FOR COMPENSATION

In the light of some of the difficulties with each of these approaches, some states use more than one approach to compensating an unscheduled PPD. Specifically, the approach depends on the working status of the injured employee at the time that the PPD is rated. If the worker is employed and earning a wage equal to or near the preinjury earning level, the worker will be entitled to a PPD benefit based on the degree of impairment. In such a situation, the benefit is similar to the method used in the impairment-based states. The worker is rated, probably based on a medical guide, and the benefit is a direct consequence of the impairment rating.

If the injured or sick worker has not returned to work or has done so but is earning below some threshold rate of preinjury earnings, the worker is rated according to the loss of wage-earning capacity. As such, in the light of postinjury earnings, if any, and the worker's age, impairment, education, occupation, and such factors, the worker will be rated for disability. The impairment benefit that the worker would have received had the person been reemployed at preinjury earnings is likely to be the base amount the worker will receive. In practice, the worker will receive a larger benefit.

Unlike the wage-loss approach, the worker in a state using the bifurcated method for an unscheduled loss will receive a PPD benefit, even when no earnings loss has occurred. Also unlike the wage-loss method, the decision regarding disability benefits is made at or near the time the worker's health condition has reached maximum medical improvement. It is not the source of a long-term, continuing assessment of the worker's earning level and the reasons for its changes, if any. The bifurcated method provides the same incentive to the employer to reemploy the injured employee as does the wage-loss approach.

Most importantly, the bifurcated method of compensating an unscheduled PPD is that it has the advantages of the impairment method (i.e., greater consistency of evaluation, fewer grounds for controversy in cases in which the employee has been able to return to work). Further, it does not have the most serious shortcoming that the impairment method has (i.e., that a worker with a disability that is substantially greater than the impairment rating measures can be greatly undercompensated).

DEVELOPMENTS

During the latter part of the 1980s and into the early 1990s, several states considered their workers' compensation program to be in crisis. Essentially, employers were finding the costs of their insurance rising unacceptably rapidly. In turn, this situation created certain problems for insurers, particularly where the costs of claims were rising and the states that regulated insurance rates did not permit them to recover those costs fully. Certainly, some states experienced problems with their systems, which led to changes in state laws. Not surprisingly, one area that received considerable attention is the permanent disability portion.

It seems apparent that in this period of change, the states tended to move in the direction of the impairment method of compensating PPD claims. Texas may have been the initiator of the movement when it moved from loss of earning capacity to impairment in 1989 (Texas is one of the impairment states that enables the worker to receive supplemental benefits after the impairment benefit has ended, at least under certain circumstances). Shortly thereafter, Colorado made a similar shift. In 1993 Florida changed its law, replacing the wage-loss method that it adopted in 1979 with the impairment approach (with a possibility of a supplemental benefit). Two years ago, Minnesota abandoned the bifurcated method that it had long used to become an impairment-method state.

Unfortunately, there is a dearth of hard evidence as to the actual outcomes that result from the different PPD approaches. For a number of reasons, workers' compensation is a program that has been barely studied rigorously. The advantages of one method over another may be more mythical than actual. Some systematic evidence from multiple jurisdictions covering some reasonable period is needed for policy makers to make informed decisions on the alternative ways to deliver these PPD benefits.

Occupational Musculoskeletal Disorders
edited by T. G. Mayer, R. J. Gatchel, and P. B. Polatin.
Lippincott Williams & Wilkins, Philadelphia © 2000.

44

Profile of Workers' Compensation Administration

Judith Greenwood

Department of Community Medicine, Institute of Occupational and Environmental Health, University of West Virginia, Morgantown, West Virginia 26506

The initial experiences of many health care providers who have had to deal with workers' compensation administrative agencies are often negative. They object to the paperwork requirements that may seem unnecessarily complicated and endless. They do not like claims administrators or adjusters questioning or second guessing the diagnostic and treatment opinions they submit in their reports. Moreover, when disputes arise over issues in a workers' compensation claim and formal litigation ensues, the decisions that adjudicators make may seem at variance with medical experience. The premise of this chapter is that with some basic understanding of workers' compensation administration, medical providers can treat occupational injuries and illnesses more effectively and even deal more comfortably with adjudication when disputes in a claim occur.

An opening caveat for readers is to be aware that there is a great deal of variation in workers' compensation administration in the United States. It begins with how the state administrative agency itself is known. It may be called a *board*, a *commission*, an *office*, a *bureau*, or a *division* within another state agency. In the Canadian provinces, more consistency exists, with the administrative agency known as either a *board* or *commission*. A second caveat is that in the United States, the medical provider is usually in a communication pattern that includes the insurer of a claim as well as the administrative agency. In Canada, the insurer and administrative agency are one and the same.

Whereas the historical narrative in this chapter focuses on workers' compensation in the United States, the description of the administrative functions are similar in Canada. Dispute resolution and adjudication as described herein, again, reflect experience in the United States. Other countries, of course, have programs that compensate occupational injuries and illnesses, but administration and adjudication practices vary.

OVERVIEW

In the United States, the movement to compensate workers injured on the job was advanced by the Progressive Party of Theodore Roosevelt and the American Association for Labor Legislation at the end of the first decade of the twentieth century. Because interpretation of constitutional law precluded any federal program for compensating workers injured on the job, this first social insurance program in the United States was left to the states. The states turned largely to private insurance carriers to provide coverage for employers and their employees through a premium tax on their payrolls. In contrast, the Canadian provinces established publicly financed provincial funds similar to the European model of social insurance to provide coverage for occupational injuries.

By 1920, 45 states had enacted workers' compensation legislation based on the principles of no fault and limited liability. These state laws replaced tort law, fashioned after British common law, which often exonerated employers through three strong defenses: contributory negligence on the part of the injured worker, a coworker's negligence, and the worker's acceptance of a risky job assignment. By midcentury, all states and the District of Columbia had workers' compensation legislation along with laws for territories, federal workers, railroad workers, longshore and harbor workers. Some Indian tribes formed separate jurisdictions.

The multijurisdictional complexity of the U.S. workers' compensation system is compounded by the various ways employers finance their coverage: mostly through private insurance carriers as noted, but also through state or mutual funds, or through meeting state bonding requirements for self-insuring their losses. Not all are available in every state. Private insurance coverage is available in all but five states that have exclusive state funds: Washington, West Virginia, Wyoming, Ohio, and North Dakota. (Originally there were seven, but Oregon and Nevada now also allow private insurance.) In these five states, the exclusive state funds function not only as the insurers, but also as the administrative equivalent of boards and commissions in Canada and administrative agencies in other states. Two states (Wyoming and North Dakota) do not allow self-insurance. More than a third of the states have public or quasi-public state or nonprofit mutual funds that compete with private carriers and also provide coverage to employers placed in assigned risk pools when their losses exceed the maximum allowable premium rate set by the state's insurance commissioner.

The core commonality among administrative agencies is to ensure that employers secure their financial basis for providing wage replacement and medical benefits to injured workers under jurisdictional law and then to ensure the equitable delivery of benefits to injured workers. Although workers' compensa-

tion programs grew and improved slowly during the midpart of the century, variations in benefit levels, occupational disease coverage, and other administrative issues caused concerns among policy makers. In 1970, Congress passed the Occupational Safety and Health Act and, within that act, established the National Commission on State Workmen's Compensation Laws [sic]. That act introduced a period of nationwide reforms that brought about more standardization among state-run programs; even now, nomenclature differs, benefit structures differ, and administrative databases differ.

BRIEF HISTORY

This development and maturation of workers' compensation in the United States is within the context of the twentieth century (1). The movement to compensate injured workers originally was joined to the early Progressive Party movement for compulsory health care insurance to cover entire families to relieve poverty. Data from the period indicate that when a worker lost wages because of an occupational injury, wage losses were two to four times greater than medical costs related to the injury. Total family losses, however, were more severe because additional medical costs related to the needs of dependents resulted in overall medical losses approximating the wage losses (2). After World War I, by the end of the decade, national health insurance had lost its constituency among a number of leading physicians who had for a few years supported it. Employers and private insurance companies always had been opposed, and the general public did not appear to care much.

In contrast, workers' compensation grew out of the publicly recognized need for workers to have economic relief following injury at the workplace and for their dependents to have some protection, particularly in the event of a worker's premature work-related death. At the same time, employers wanted the ability to predict risk rather than to take the chance of losing an adverse tort suit against them, even though the odds were that they would not. When an adverse judgment was made, often the damages were high. Limited liability meant employers would be able to reserve the dollar amount needed to pay wage and medical benefits. Thus, the famous *quid pro quo* was born. That is, in return for limited liability, employers agreed to pay premiums for workers' compensation insurance and, in return for quickly delivered benefits, employees gave up the right to sue their employers for punitive damages. The state-by-state process of legislating workers' compensation laws has been called "the most dramatic event in the twentieth-century history of social justice...." (3).

After the rapid decade of development of workers' compensation programs that were intended to be administered on a no-fault basis, the 1920s saw the aspirations and ideals of the early reformers in decline. Although early proponents of the new programs had envisioned that they would be run by specialists and experts in dealing with industrial problems, it was not long before appointments to administrative agencies were made politically rather than on the basis of experience. A labor/management dichotomy emerged and, with it, litigation and a trial bar of attorneys. Loopholes in state laws encouraged litigation. The original no-fault concept was weakened, and the fledging state programs, adapting to entrenched state political processes, became truncated versions of tort law rather than its no-fault replacement.

Administrative subtleties arose, such as legitimate proof that an injury arose out of and during the course of an employee's job. Simple cause-and-effect concepts of accident and injury yielded to technological and medical concepts of predisposing, precipitating, and aggravating factors. Challenges arose regarding prolonged exposures to toxic substances in the workplace, thus introducing occupational diseases. Challenges were made as to whether the injury resulted in some permanent impairment that had economic consequences in terms of job performance and job opportunity. Challenges also were made over the necessity and appropriateness of medical

care. Benefit levels varied greatly from jurisdiction to jurisdiction, and challenges arose regarding equity and fairness.

Reforms began in state workers' compensation programs in the latter part of the twentieth century after passage of the Occupational Safety and Health Act in 1970, as noted earlier. The 1972 *Report of the National Commission on State Workmen's Compensation Laws* [sic] brought with it the threat of abolishment of deficient state-run programs in favor of some form of federalization. State administrative agencies were scrutinized. In turn, they began to improve administrative functions related to the payment of wage replacement, or temporary total disability benefits, and benefits for permanent disability and the provision of appropriate medical care to injured workers. The goal has been to make workers' compensation programs as self-executing as possible in terms of delivering timely and equitable benefits and returning injured workers to work through appropriate medical and rehabilitation services.

MEDICAL NEXUS FOR ADMINISTRATION

Reforms have depended on improvements in reporting and monitoring the treatment of occupational injuries and illness. Injuries in the early part of the century were amputations and loss of limb function and were observed to have occurred in the workplace by fellow workers. Commonly, they were covered by an administrative schedule of compensation benefits; that is, benefit rates for various injuries had been established before occurrence of the injury. These schedules remain as part of state workers' compensation statutes today; however, scheduled injuries now, although they do occur, are not the ones that cause friction within the system. Today, musculoskeletal injuries and occupational diseases are common workers' compensation claims. They are not the observable traumatic events of earlier years and must be related to the workplace and work activity by medical reports, known as *first reports of injury*. These reports provide the injured workers entry to the workers' compensation system after a claim has been filed with the employer. With these reports, physicians take on an administrative financial responsibility, as the reports are the basis for the delivery of monetary benefits over a given period.

Whether musculoskeletal injury, occupational disease, or acute trauma, successful recovery from an occupational injury or illness often requires continuous treatment over time and may involve medical rehabilitation toward the end of this period. With occupational injuries, the acute-care period can be up to 3 months, which is long compared with an acute-care episode in general health. At the end of the course of treatment, commonly referred to as *maximum medical improvement*, compensation for any permanent physical impairment often depends on a physician's evaluation and rating, not on a neutral schedule. Again, when making impairment ratings, the physician takes on an administrative financial responsibility because the amount of benefits awarded are based wholly, or in part, on the rating, depending on the jurisdiction's law.

At the outset of an occupational disability claim, insurance claims adjusters receive and then must act on the first reports of injury or illness in concert with workers' compensation administrators. A diagnosis must be made for the medical treatment given, and a probable duration of that treatment must be estimated. The reports should be clear and concise, written to be understood by nonmedical personnel who are agents of the employer and the insurer. Later in the course of the claim, other parties may be interested in these reports of occupational injury or illness: union representatives, attorneys, case managers, rehabilitation providers, and adjudicators. These first reports of injury and subsequent or interval reports on continued occupational disability and medical status are the basis of all communication among the parties involved in the claim. Subsequent reports must document any change in diagnosis, what medical progress has been made, if any work limitations seem likely, and if any medical or vocational rehabilitation may be needed. When maximum medical improvement is reached, physicians must report any residual impairment and whether any job functions will be compromised. A complete chapter describing what and how physicians need to communicate, along with sample report forms, appears in a 1997 Mosby Year Book publication (4). It must be emphasized that the entire course of medical communication regarding an occupational injury or illness is an administrative "open book" with legal implications..

The administrative function in workers' compensation clearly has evolved over the century into a complicated medicolegal process for which few policy makers, administrative decision makers, adjudicators, and physicians have been trained and cross trained adequately at the outset of their experience. Whereas this evolution has brought about some mutual antagonism, it has also created the absolute need to resolve differences and to develop mutual respect. Managed care has drawn workers' compensation administrators and physicians into a closer relationship with regard to developing treatment guidelines, methods of utilization review, and fee schedules, which have become part of many workers' compensation administrative programs. Progress has been made in achieving more self-executing programs, but disputes do arise, and litigation may ensue.

DISPUTE RESOLUTION AND ADJUDICATION

Most U.S. jurisdictions have some form of informal dispute resolution with the goal of avoiding formal hearings. Informal dispute resolution may be known as *mediation, arbitration, pretrial conferences*, or *informal hearings*. These conferences may address multiple issues, such as compensability, medical treatment, medical bills, utilization review, amount of wage loss benefits, and others. Issues also may be identified ahead of time and addressed in specialized conferences. In informal dispute resolution, there are few or no procedural rules and no sworn testimony or cross examination of witnesses.

A recent publication from the Workers' Compensation Research Institute in Cambridge, Massachusetts, is an excellent resource on describing informal dispute-resolution processes as well as formal dispute adjudication (5).

When disputes cannot be settled informally, a prehearing conference is held in most jurisdictions before a formal hearing occurs. Commonly, some specific preparation is required, such as the exchange of reports. If a settlement cannot be reached in the conference, formal hearings take place with sworn testimony, cross examination of witnesses, a formal record of the proceeding, and a written decision by the adjudicator. Generally, the formal hearing takes place as a single session, but more sessions may occur. In a few jurisdictions, multiple sessions are common. There is much wider variation among jurisdictions in the length of any one formal session. Some can be as short as 15 minutes and others as long as several hours, even an entire day, depending on the issue or issues being litigated. Medical evidence usually is introduced by report, but also may be given as a deposition. Physicians are less commonly asked or required to appear at a formal hearing in person.

When physicians are asked to give depositions or to appear at a formal hearing, they may think their testimony must be at least 90% accurate. In legal terminology, this is analogous to the level of proof of "beyond a reasonable doubt" required in criminal trials. When an adjudicator renders a formal hearing decision, however, it is on the basis of the level of proof required in a civil trial, more probable than not meaning 51% probability or greater. The different expectations with regard to level of proof can be the basis for why a medical provider may not understand the reasoning behind a particular decision and thus disapprove it.

A criticism of decision making in workers' compensation is that adjudicators make decisions based on politics. It is true that many adjudicators are politically appointed or hold civil service positions because of a higher-level political appointee. Politics is less meaningful to a good adjudicator's decision, how-

ever, than the precision and clarity of the original reports of injury, follow-up reports, any independent medical examination reports, and depositions or formal-hearing testimony of physicians introduced as evidence in the case.

In all jurisdictions, there is a process for appealing the decision of the formal hearing to a specially appointed appeal board, review authority, or state court and, ultimately, to the jurisdictional supreme or superior court. Most adjudicators are attorneys bound by the ethical standards set by state bar associations governing their professional practice. Whether the dispute is over causation and compensability, medical treatment and reimbursement, return to work, or permanent impairment rating, the adjudicator renders a decision based on the medical evidence submitted by the plaintiff and defense attorneys. No adjudicator likes to render a decision and then have it appealed to a higher level. Thus, there is a professional self-interest in determining the factual situation in any case and following established precedent when possible.

What has been described here represents only the general structure of dispute resolution found in the United States. The handling of litigation and dispute resolution is the area in which jurisdictions probably differ most. Not mentioned so far is the dispute resolution that can take place outside the workers' compensation administrative program itself. Some states allow private mediation and arbitration. Since the early 1990s, a few jurisdictions have allowed labor and management to experiment with resolving disputes involving workers' compensation issues as part of collective bargaining. The construction industry especially has been involved in this alternative method. It is likely that policy makers will become more interested in evaluating the methods and outcomes of dispute resolution both within and outside administrative programs as more information becomes available.

MOVING INTO THE FUTURE

As workers' compensation administration moves into the twenty-first century, new challenges will arise, such as improving dispute resolution and reducing litigation. Resources available to state agencies will make advancements easier. One new resource that is becoming widely used is the Internet. All state jurisdictions now have web sites that at minimum provides information about their services and can extend to offering full transactions, such as allowing employers to purchase coverage on line.

Important national organizational resources exist. The oldest affiliate organization is the International Association of Industrial Accident Boards and Commissions (IAIABC), formed in 1914. Until 1990, it had only a part-time director, but it now has a full-time director and a professional staff that has increased since 1995. A mid-1940s offshoot of the IAIABC is the American Association of State Compensation and Insurance Funds (AASCIF) that, as the name implies, represents the exclusive and competitive state insurance funds. The National Symposium on Workers' Compensation has developed annual in-depth educational programs since the mid-1970s, following the *Report of the National Commission on State Workmen's Compensation Laws* [sic]. Finally, a premiere resource the Workers' Compensation Research Institute (WCRI) was incorporated in 1983 and has had a growing professional staff since then. These organizational resources have become robust, both singly and in concert.

On the technological front, the IAIABC is the lead organization in developing and maintaining electronic data interchange (EDI) for the entire workers' compensation industry. EDI allows insurance carriers and state administrative agencies to exchange standardized first and subsequent reports of injury electronically, thereby eliminating paper, reducing clerical error, and decreasing processing and action time. Other administrative transactions are possible through EDI. Employers can submit proof of coverage on electronic forms to insurance carriers and administrative agencies. Likewise, medical providers may submit data on diagnosis, procedures performed, and billing costs. Also, rehabilitation data and return-to-work

data may be collected on standard forms and exchanged. Some administrative agencies will be able to use EDI to transmit forms related to litigation and receive outcome results.

The educational front is important to the future of administration. The annual National Symposium of Workers' Compensation has already been mentioned. The IAIABC is also a prominent educational resource, having sponsored since 1973 an intensive 5-day course of study on medical and legal issues and administrative procedures. Since 1992 it has added a specialized concurrent 5-day course for workers' compensation adjudicators.

In the area of workers' compensation research, the WCRI is the obvious leader. The Institute has numerous publications, many devoted to administrative inventories of the state-run program and others focusing on how benefit and medical costs are driven in the different programs. An important annual publication is on managed care and medical cost containment (6). In the late 1990s, WCRI launched two major initiatives: The first is designed to measure and benchmark system performance on outcomes such as cost containment, return to work, and the promptness and adequacy of benefit payments. Researchers will gather data from 15 to 25 of the largest state programs. Policy makers in state legislatures and decision makers in administrative agencies will be able to engage in continuous improvement of the administrative functions of workers' compensation, based on analysis of internal practices and external constraints (such as market economy) among diverse states.

A second initiative addresses disability management and benefit integration in response to the growth of managed care, and the probability that medical care and benefits provided under workers' compensation will come into a closer relationship with general health care. To support this effort, as well as other WCRI research, a claims database will contain detailed data on about half of the workers' compensation disability claims in the nation. Along with claims data supplied by private insurance carriers and state insurance funds, the database will have outcome measures from employee surveys and data measuring the effects of health networks on cost and medical outcomes in occupational disability.

Whereas about two-thirds of all benefit payments in workers' compensation are made in the permanent partial disability category, administrative agencies have not had the necessary tools to calibrate these benefits equitably. There is variance for similar disabilities from one jurisdiction to another. For example, there is about a $100,000 difference for the scheduled loss of an arm at the shoulder between Pennsylvania and New York (7). Even within the single court-administrated jurisdiction of Tennessee, there is marked inconsistency in awarding permanent partial disability benefits over time, by region, and by type of injury (8).

The American Medical Association has published *Guides to the Evaluation of Permanent Impairment* since 1961, when the 1st edition appeared. Since then, three more editions have appeared. The latest as of this writing is the 4th edition and before that a revised 3rd edition. Consensus panels of physician specialists have developed all editions to date. A steering committee for the upcoming 5th edition, has advised that this edition should include scientific studies that support the ratings to increase their validity and consistency among the different body systems. The steering committee is of the strong opinion that physicians should use the *Guides* to rate only permanent impairment, but it also recommends that the new edition include a chapter or appendix on how administrators and adjudicators can better understand the consequences of permanent impairment and gather evidence that would be relevant to move from permanent impairment and determine work disability. It is likely, however, that the more complex and controversial issues related to impairment rating and determining how impairment relates to permanent disability will not be addressed until a planned 6th edition.

THE BROAD VIEW

To this point, the workers' compensation administration has been profiled in a histori-cal context, in a functional context, and in a context of national resources. Workers' compensation administration also may be viewed in the context of the broader disability system. I have written on this topic elsewhere (9,10) and will provide here a summary from the cited writings.

The basic tenet of any disability compensation—workers' compensation, social security, or other—is that monetary resources, rather than being distributed according to individual work and output, are distributed based on some definition of need and proof of that need. In workers' compensation, proof was discussed earlier in terms of causation: proof that an injury arose out of and in course of an employee's job performance. In theory, the definitions of need that underpin disability programs are assumed to be neutral, and proof is assumed to be clear. The reality is that any disability program is highly dynamic and malleable because the popular concept of disability is broader than the official statements or definitions of disability. Thus, the basic legal construct of disability becomes socially manipulated, becoming a *de facto* economic construct with an inherent tendency to expand. Proof of disability is therefore not so clear.

Noted earlier was the idea that the scientific method in which physicians are trained demands accuracy of at least 90%. This high demand for accuracy, however, has not limited medically sanctioned disabilities. On the contrary, greater diagnostic specification and increased technology have put medicine in the forefront of expanding disability categories. The discovery in the mid-1930s of ruptured disc as the diagnosis for inguinal herniation legitimized the concept of back pain as trauma. Current epidemiologic research identifies workers at risk of becoming disabled because of certain occupational functions they perform. As one author noted, it is not hard to imagine the process by which epidemiologic research makes possible the identification of potentially disabled people who are then disadvantaged in the labor market (11).

Whereas occupational disability has been and, in all likelihood, will remain an expanding concept, the bureaucratization and medicalization of disability that has occurred in the twentieth century probably will subside in favor of a more *particularized* model. By this term, I mean that disability is now understood not only as a condition involving medical impairment but also one involving attitudinal, behavioral, and situational factors. Whereas bureaucratic services for monetary compensation and medical services for diagnosis and treatment always will be needed, a variety of disability prevention and management services also must be provided if the complexity of disability is to be addressed.

Administrators, insurers, and employers for the better part of the twentieth century accepted the premise that the disability process begins when an injured employee files a claim, an act that employers often regard as negative behavior. Particularizing the process of disability shifts the focus from claim filing to the actual occurrence of an injury or illness episode. This shift brings with it a heightened safety consciousness along with early and later disability management efforts. These efforts concentrate on what is needed for a satisfactory, timely return to work beyond medical treatment itself. First is the quality communication between employers and employees. Psychological factors and perceptions of work have been found to be more predictive of occupational disability from back pain than physical factors (12,13). Just as job satisfaction is important in preventing occupational disability, satisfactory return to work when a disabling condition is present may call for a temporarily modified work assignment or work schedule or a modified workstation or other job accommodation.

Administration of workers' compensation is evolutionary, responding to changes in both its social and economic environment. Medical cost containment, for example, became a focus with the rapid rise of medical costs in the late 1980s and has remained an administrative responsibility. The challenge for workers' compensation agencies is to continue to broaden their role in cost containment through promoting safety and disability management practices

among employers, insurers, physicians, and all others who constitute the workers' compensation system. Prevention of occupational injuries and illnesses and active disability management can begin to balance the expansion of accepted disability and its socioeconomic effects of lost productivity and costs. One could argue that it is the fiduciary responsibility of workers' compensation administrative agencies to become safety and disability management proponents.

SUMMARY

The twentieth century saw the beginning of state-administered workers' compensation programs in the United States and provincial programs in Canada. In the states, the programs experienced some decline after their idealistic start and rapid expansion in the second decade of the century. Subtleties emerged in state laws that were not anticipated by the early reformers, and challenges arose from medical and technological advances in diagnosis and treatment. By midcentury, state programs lacked consistency, and questions arose over the adequacy and fairness of the laws and their administration. In the 1970s, states undertook serious and comprehensive reforms. By the end of the century, the state programs had recourse to sound national resources that could provide research and information for advancing improvements.

An overall administrative goal is to achieve as self-executing a program as possible, delivering benefits to injured and ill workers from the outset of disability and providing medical treatment and disability management for a safe return to work. The administrative process in workers' compensation revolves around medical reports from beginning to end. Physicians bear a financial responsibility in terms of the duration of benefits as well as a medical responsibility in managing a workers' compensation claim. In most instances, the course of a disability claim goes relatively smoothly.

The result of intertwining medicine and the administration of a social insurance program to compensate occupational disability provides the opportunity for contention and disputes, however. What is the cause of an occupational disability? What is the appropriate medical treatment? Is there any permanent impairment? How does the permanent impairment affect return to work, future job opportunities, and income? These questions and other issues are raised and settled in various formats: informal conferences, formal hearings, private mediation and arbitration, even collective bargaining between labor and management. Workers' compensation dispute resolution is a new area of research and information. As the processes and outcomes of dispute resolution become clearer, disputes in workers' compensation may lessen even while medical advances may lead to new occupational disabilities.

REFERENCES

1. Greenwood JG. A historical perspective on workers' compensation in the context of national health policy debate. In: Greenwood J, Taricco A, eds. *Workers compensation health care cost containment.* Horsham, PA: LRP. Publications, 1992:1–26.
2. Starr P. *The social transformation of American medicine.* New York: Basic Books, Harper Collins Publishers, 1982:245.
3. Darling-Hammond L, Kneisner TJ. *The law and economics of workers' compensation.* Santa Monica, CA: Rand Publications, 1980:v.
4. Greenwood J, Wyman ET Jr. The workers' compensation system. In: Nordin, M, Andersson, GBJ, Pope, MH. eds. *Musculoskeletal disorders in the workplace.* St. Louis, MO: Mosby Year Book, 1997:599–609.
5. Ballantyne DS. *Dispute prevention and resolution in workers compensation: a national inventory.* Cambridge, MA: The Workers' Compensation Institute, 1998:3–229
6. Tanabe RT. *Managed care and medical cost containment in workers' compensation: a national inventory, 1998–1999.* Cambridge, MA: The Workers Compensation Institute, 1999:3–309.
7. *Analysis of Workers' Compensation Laws.* Washington, DC: U.S. Chamber of Commerce, 1998:43.
8. Gardner JA, Telles CA, Moss GA. *Cost drivers and system performance in a court based system.* Cambridge, MA: The Workers' Compensation Institute, 1998:65–69.
9. Greenwood J. Socioeconomic factors in back pain and compensation systems. In: Mayer TG, Mooney V, Gatchel RJ. eds. *Contemporary conservative care for painful spinal disorders.* Philadelphia: Lea & Febiger, 1991:155–166.
10. Greenwood J. History of disability as a legal construct. In: Demeter SL, Andersson GBJ, Smith GM. eds. *Disability evaluation.* St. Louis, MO: Mosby Year Book, 1996:5–12.
11. Stone D. *The disabled state.* Philadelphia: Temple University Press, 1984:179.
12. Battie MC, Bigos S. Industrial back pain: a broader perspective. *Orthop Clin* 1991;22:273–282.
13. Bigos S, Battie MC, Spengler DM, et al. A prospective study of work perceptions and psychological factors affecting the report of back injury. *Spine* 1991;16:1–6.

Occupational Musculoskeletal Disorders
edited by T. G. Mayer, R. J. Gatchel, and P. B. Polatin.
Lippincott Williams & Wilkins, Philadelphia © 2000.

45

The Politics of Health Care Delivery in the Workers' Compensation System

Alfred Taricco

113 Kimberly Drive, Manchester, Connecticut 06040

In discussing the history and evolution of the workers' compensation system in the United States, the previous chapter coherently points out that there is a process that needs to be followed to administer the system; that the process, although basically the same in the 51 jurisdictions (50 states plus Washington, D.C.) for the purpose of assuring that health care as well as compensation benefits are provided, differs in how those benefits (both medical and compensation) are managed and delivered. The concept of providing medical care for the injured worker, as well as compensation benefits, represents a significant and noble responsibility taken on by society at large for its members.

This chapter presents the argument that, over time, this noble concept has become tainted by those who regard the system not as a venue to benefit the injured worker and his or her family but as one that can benefit them either politically or financially. As a result, the nobility of the concept has suffered, and with it, society, in some measure. This argument is based on personal observations coupled with those of others who have noted the abusive activities of persons working in the arena of workers' compensation, including both employers and employees; the providers of health care whether they be physicians, surgeons, chiropractors, and therapists of various specialties; attorneys; legislators; administrators of the system; and finally the commissioners and their appointed adjudicators.

Suffice it to say that although many talented and dedicated people are working in the system, the process of running the system at times can become twisted, to the detriment of the injured worker while benefiting the provider or attorney. It is the adjudicator's responsibility to maintain a level playing field. Because the adjudicator who has a legal but not a medical background is asked to make medical decisions based on the process established by law, the determinations made can run counter to sound medical principles and sometimes are considered to challenge the sanity of reason. Based on the activities of one (the author) who not only has been on the provider end, but also on the payor end evaluating claims, and finally, simply as an observer of the system while working as a consultant in the field, this chapter attempts to point out certain weaknesses in the system that relate to the medical aspects of the claim. These weaknesses need to be addressed and corrected to strengthen the system on behalf of workers, weaknesses that seem to be related primarily to politics of the system as related to the law but also related to those of the medical academic arena.

WHERE TO BEGIN

The adjudicator in any hearing is the representative of the commissioner. Therefore, decisions rendered by the adjudicator reflect on the commissioner. Consequently, a discussion regarding the performance of the workers' compensation agencies, boards, and commissions clearly invites the rendered opinion to be based on, and biased by, an individual's experiences with the adjudicators. An attorney's opinion is apt to be tempered by the outcome of his or her representation of the plaintiff or the defense. An insurance representative will have another opinion and the claimant still another. Physicians can be expected to have still another opinion. Finally, the commissioners and their appointed adjudicators may have differing views. More often than not, adjudicators are considered to be professionals by persons who agree with their decisions and political pawns when they render a negative decision.

Adjudicators are in a unique position. They must uphold the law but have considerable latitude in their decision-making processes. All they need to rule in favor of the claimant is that the issue at hand needs only a 51% chance of it being more probable than not. The question, then, is why the law allows the adjudicator to make such a simple statistically based decision when science requires a much greater preponderance of evidence to conclude probability? (More about this later.) It is here that payors have difficulty accepting decisions, whereas attorneys can accept them readily. Further difficulties arise when decisions are rendered based on faulty analyses of causation.

Additionally, it needs to be pointed out that one of the major reasons for the wide latitude is that currently inherent in the decision-making process is the basic difficulty in validly measuring three important factors used in determining the degree of work incapacity due to some injury: pain, impairment, and disability. The term *impairment* refers to the physical or psychological limitations of normal functioning resulting from disease or injury. Such impairment, determined by a physician, is a quantifiable anatomic or functional loss, either temporary or permanent. On the other hand, *disability* refers to the reduction of the capacity to perform activities of daily living or employment due to the impairment. Disability, the determination of which is usually an administrative decision, is a more complex phenomenon, reflecting

the interaction between impairment and socioeconomic factors. Finally, pain is an experiential psychophysiological phenomenon that usually is assessed by the patient and therefore represents the subjective interpretation of the level of the patient's discomfort. Waddell astutely noted that there is often a discordance or low correlation among these three factors (1). One therefore cannot assume that these factors will be highly correlated with one another. High impairment does not necessarily translate into high disability; there also can be a high rate of self-reported pain with little impairment. Physicians, insurance adjusters, and adjudicators need to be aware of this fact in their decision-making processes. Because of the 51% rule, which allows the adjudicators such wide latitude, conflicts arise between them and the payors (insurance carriers) and employers (as self-insurers). The latter two want to see a preponderance of evidence as the basis for a final decision.

WHAT IS THE THINKING PROCESS USED: EMPIRICISM OR LOGIC?

When dealing with the adjudicators of various workers' compensation agencies, boards, and commissions, it soon becomes clear that most have no concept of the scientific method. Too often, they are ready to accept someone's word that an injury or illness is directly related to the job. The application of causation analysis (2) to evaluate the veracity of a claim is usually bypassed. Some adjudicators, however, by experience, are able to make the right connection, but it would seem those connections are more intuitive than based on a rational examination of the facts.

Commissioners usually have a legal background. By virtue of this background, they are on a collision course when dealing with medical professionals, whose background is built on the principle of the scientific method. In presenting a case at trial, it is common for the lawyer to begin with what he or she believes to be the conclusion. This is done to build a case, up to and including conspiracies, if necessary. The science of medicine begins its quest for the facts by making repeated observations that, over time, eventually lead to a consensus. That consensus is never absolute and is subject to change should new observations justify a change. In other words, lawyers start at the end and build toward the beginning, whereas physicians begin at the beginning and work forward. Some adjudicators reveal this reverse thinking in rendering their decisions, which too often demonstrate the folly of those decisions because of their limited knowledge of the pathophysiology necessary to make a rational, valid decision based on sound medical principles. They pay little or no attention to causation analysis but will accept a claim of causation even when there is no factual basis to support the relationship between the job and the injury or illness. Emotions often play a more important role than common sense. In fairness to adjudicators, however, the providers can and do add to the confusion by not properly establishing causation, providing incomplete documentation and, finally, even providing fraudulent data in some cases.

Perhaps it will help to understand the approach used by some adjudicators (and by some attorneys) if one uses the demise of TWA Flight 800 as an example. From the moment the plane blew up and dropped to earth in a fireball, the conclusion as to what happened had already been determined by everyone, even though there was no evidence yet. (Insert the nonscientific approach here.) The assumption was that a terrorist had planted a bomb on the plane. Why else would a plane blow up just after taking off, especially one with such an air-worthy record as the 747? An attempt was made to prove this but to no avail. The investigation of the incident included a follow-up of 3,000 leads, interviews of more than 7,000 people, and the sophisticated forensic examination of about a million pieces of debris. After 15 months, the Federal Bureau of Investigation arrived at a consensus. (Insert the use of the scientific approach.) The conclusion was that no evidence of foul play was found. They were ready, however, to examine any new in-

formation that might justify a change in their opinion. (Once again, insert the scientific approach.) This is an example of how emotions ran ahead of the facts, leading to an inappropriate conclusion.

VALUE OF ANECDOTAL EVIDENCE TO REVEAL PROCESS PROBLEMS

Clearly, the use of anecdotal evidence can be considered a weak approach in an attempt to persuade another person to accept one's opinion regarding the subject being discussed. Nonetheless, it must also be said that if enough anecdotal evidence is accumulated, it becomes necessary to evaluate individual instances as symptoms of an overall problem, which seems the case with the workers' compensation system. It is also clear that because there are 51 jurisdictions dealing with workers' compensation, their autonomy lends them not to a list of similar problems but to a list of dissimilar problems related to what is considered to be work related and what is not, as well as how the process of distributing benefits is managed. Therefore, not being able to present examples from all quarters of the United States, only a few are presented. Furthermore, these examples can demonstrate the difficulties that may arise when medical evaluation decisions are made by adjudicators whose training is oriented to the law and lacking in the direction of medicine. Although attempts at educating adjudicators and others on medical matters have been made, such as provided by the Workers' Compensation College, these attempts have proved inadequate and are further complicated by virtue of the autonomy of each state. This topic is discussed more fully later. These examples should demonstrate that a diversity of difficulties are related to the politics of each jurisdiction and also suggest that a more uniform system would serve society better, especially because society pays for its costs.

One of the most illogical decisions made by an adjudicator was the conclusion that a claimant suffered from bulimia and that this was a work-related condition. As mentioned in

Taricco's "Medical issues of fraud and abuse in workers' compensation," *Dorland's Medical Dictionary* defines *bulimia* as "a mental disorder occurring...with onset usually in adolescence or early adulthood, characterized by episodes of binge eating that continue until terminated by abdominal pain, sleep, or self-induced vomiting" (2). This seems to be another extension of the ever-widening panorama of diagnoses that are incorrectly accepted as work-related conditions. With this kind of liberal acceptance and misapplication of the criteria of causation analysis regarding what is work related, one should not be surprised if a pregnancy resulting from conception during a business trip is deemed to be work related. Facetiousness aside, one might ask why such an ill-conceived decision regarding bulimia was allowed to stand. More to the point, how can professionals who are trained to seek the truth make such an erroneous decision? After much observation and many dealings with various agencies, boards, and commissions, it is evident that the chief factor of influence is *politics*: the politics of appointments, the politics of legislation, the politics of labor, the politics of litigation, and the politics of health care providers who treat injured workers. All contribute to the escalating costs of workers' compensation through the agenda each espouses for personal financial or political gain. Yet, with all these players trying to "gain an edge," one would hope that the adjudicator would be above the fray and use logic rather than expediency to reach a conclusion. Many do, but it is no easy task.

MORE REAL-WORLD EXAMPLES

Not all problems with the workers' compensation system can be laid at the feet of the adjudicators; many others work in the system and share in the lack of probity to maintain the level of quality society intended when it established the workers' compensation system. One colleague (L. Wise, personal communication) described a civil servant working for a workers' compensation board in a midwestern state. Apparently, this example is one of a bureaucrat given too much autonomy by the state. The result is that arbitrary and irrational regulatory interpretations are dispensed. When requests are made for clarification of this individual's unilateral decisions, the responses are such that they could be considered punitive. These decisions also include the micromanagement of issues that are widely accepted in other states.

In another example (L. Wise, personal communication) of what might be called legislative confusion is the midwestern state that has been attempting to implement Managed Care Organization legislation for at least 2 years. A series of what were considered by many to be unreasonable and sophisticated requirements were issued. The vendors in that state were forced to "jump through the hoops" of certification, only to be told subsequently that the state was not ready to accept the required information. The confusion left in the wake of such a regulatory *faux pas* is to be considered the result of faulty, perhaps even uninformed, thinking processes motivated by the politics of that jurisdiction. At this writing, the state is apparently more than 2 years behind the legislated deadlines.

Another example of confusion that can be labeled commission confusion occurred in a southern state (L. Wise, personal communication). The issue had to do with the hospital inpatient *per diem* fee schedule. The workers' compensation commission set these rates with little or no factual basis and supported their application long after they were outdated. The hospital charges were reduced so dramatically by these *per diem* rates that the hospital association took the commission to court and won.

The appellate court held that the *per diem* rates were invalid because they could not be supported by data and, further, that hospitals should be paid the "usual and customary" rate. Yet, lawyers for the commission sent a notice to all carriers and third-party administrators that they should continue to use the invalidated *per diem* rates. Many questioned the authority and validity of the directives issued by the commission's lawyers (as opposed to those of the commission itself or the appellate court). Most likely, this dispute will be litigated well into the future.

In one eastern seaboard state (L. Wise, personal communication), the insurance department appears to be "held hostage" by physicians. There, at a minimum, the state medical society has successfully lobbied the state's insurance department. The reason for such a conclusion is that the state's reimbursement regulations are based on usual and customary language; notwithstanding such a regulation, the insurance department does not tolerate *any* reductions of providers' fees. This position is untenable if cost controls are to be valid. Furthermore, regardless of how statistically sound reduction methods may be or how inflated the charges may be, it places restrictions on adjudicators who recognize that such manipulations are improper.

In the past few years, another eastern seaboard state (L. Wise, personal communication) demonstrated how politically appointed adjudicators can be either pawns or demagogues. In this state, the rulings handed down by the various adjudicators were not consistent in the interpretation of similar facts. A conservative ruling may be presented by an adjudicator appointed by a former conservative governor, whereas a similar case may result in a liberal decision from an adjudicator appointed by a former liberal governor. The net result is that one can find multiple diametrically opposed precedents to support any claim. Such a lack of uniformity is detrimental to the overall success of any system and makes the state, the commission, and its adjudicators appear inconsistent in the handling of claims.

An area of health care that adjudicators seem to not understand has to do to with the management of chronic pain. The experience of providers indicates that adjudicators sometimes demonstrate a lack of the medical knowledge necessary to make an informed decision centering around the issue of pain management. Too often, a request for pain management, whether appropriate or not, ends in becoming a referral by the adjudicator to a pain clinic instead of a multidisciplinary pain center. Often, this is done because the sense is that the treating physician is lacking in the ability to care for the injured claimant. This being the case, the doctor is "damned" and the claimant sent to the local pain clinic (3). No clear data are necessary to justify such an approach, nor are any outcome data used to determine which or where the best institutions are located for a proper referral. Compounding the problem is the fact that should the referral result in no benefit to the claimant, the adjudicator runs the risk of helping to create a "psychic cripple," who probably never will return to work or to a functional lifestyle (2).

Finally, one of the most egregious cases handled by an adjudicator centers around a patient who was being "held hostage" by the treating surgeon because of a conflict with the state's fee schedule. The case involved a reconstruction procedure that, according to the claimant's original surgeon, required the services of another surgeon located in a different part of the country. It was to be a multistaged procedure. The treating surgeon tried to obtain approval for the charges before the first operative procedure. The carrier informed the surgeon that payment would be made based on the state's fee schedule.

The first stage was performed, and the charges were submitted to the carrier. The fee charged was far in excess of what the state fee schedule allowed (and considered by many to be excessive even for private health care insurance carriers). Four physicians reviewed the case and the charges that had been submitted. Each independently concluded that the procedure was miscoded and therefore was not in accordance with the fee schedule. Even after the carrier stated that the charges would be reviewed and paid based on the prevailing state fee schedule, the surgeon refused to proceed with the second stage of the operation unless the initial charges were paid in full. This case was one of flagrant patient abuse by the surgeon for monetary gain.

The charges were contested, and the case was heard before an adjudicator from the claimant's home state. Two physicians were asked to testify, one on the inappropriateness of the procedure and the other on the state fee schedule codes that precluded such an exorbitant fee. The adjudicator had the opportunity to uphold the state fee schedule and to force the surgeon to respect the state law in this regard; but he did not. What he did do was bounce the case back to the office of the original adjudicator in another part of the state, thereby delaying further surgery and prolonging the mental agony of the patient. Eventually, because of mass confusion on the part of the carrier, the astronomic charge was paid, and the patient had his second operation. Ironically, he was no better and even sustained complications.

Having made the comment regarding mass confusion, one should not be left with the impression, however, that the sometimes "mass confusion" phenomenon is experienced only by carriers, lawyers, or adjudicators. It also may be experienced by physicians, especially when dealing with the measurement of pain, impairment, and disability, discussed earlier in this chapter. For example, in one of the numerous studies of its kind, Brand and Lehmann (4) reported a great deal of variability (a form of confusion) in impairment ratings among orthopedists in Iowa when the same spine condition was rated. Andersson (5) summarized other such studies that prompted him to highlight "...the difficulty inherent in an impairment rating based on patient history and physical examination. Value judgments result in variation and contribute to measurement errors." Again, more confusion and, again in deference to the adjudicators, such confusion on the part of providers does not make the adjudicator's job easier. At the same time, this confusion should emphasize the fact that before rendering any decisions, it is incumbent on the adjudicator to explore, in depth, the facts of the case in the attempt to provide a satisfactory resolution to the issues at hand. A resolution that can be said to have been arrived at with a foundation that exhibits some sense of reason on which that decision is made and, therefore, justified.

THE POSITIVE SIDE

As obvious in these examples, adjudicators often are "caught between a rock and a hard place" when dealing with the array of parties involved in compensation disputes. Even so, good outcomes can be obtained. For example, an adjudicator in a southern state was dealing with a claimant who had suffered a traumatic brain injury. The claimant, his wife, and his attorney had agreed to a settlement fee proposed by the carrier; however, the adjudicator did not accept the fee, saying that, in the event the couple ever divorced, the funds available for the claimant were insufficient to care for the claimant. He requested that a higher allowance be determined before he would approve it (J. Urso, personal communication). In this instance, the concern of the adjudicator for the future of the claimant is to be applauded.

POLITICS OF SURVIVAL

The decisions of the commissioners and their appointed adjudicators sometimes place them in "harm's way," jeopardizing their jobs. Here are four examples: two commissioners (as opposed to their appointed adjudicators) of quality who were dismissed; one who hangs on not knowing his future; and one who formed a "sick peace" with a governor to survive for another term. The first two dismissed commissioners are of interest for different, but also for the same, reasons. They came from two distinctly different areas of the country. One had been a commissioner for several years and had run an effective commission with conservative leanings. The other came to the job with a liberal labor background and outstanding credentials and was making progress but had not been in the job long. The reason both lost their jobs had to do with the election of a new governor of the opposite political party. It is difficult to develop an organization into an effective instrument of government if its leader survives only if the governor so wishes.

In another state, workers' compensation was a major problem for a variety of reasons. The governor decided that this situation was going to change; and change it did, with the appointment of a new commissioner who surrounded himself with capable personnel. In time, the governor decided to leave office. What will happen after the next election depends on what the collegial relationship will be between the next governor and the commissioner as well as the political party differences, if any.

Finally is a case in which the new governor was left with a commissioner of the same political party but with whom he had differences. What to do? It became clear to the governor that the commissioner enjoyed the backing of the business community, and therefore it was necessary for the governor to retain the commissioner if he wanted to avoid conflicts with the business community. Hence, what has been described as a "sick peace" between the governor and the commissioner was the resolution.

IS THERE A BETTER WAY?

Might a better, more honest, or apolitical approach to selecting adjudicators be possible to prevent many of the external pressures that can be brought to bear on them? One is proposed by Spence in his book, *O.J., The Last Word* (6). Although he was not discussing the adjudication of workers' compensation claims, his suggestion has merit. Spence suggests that lawyers be selected at random, by the drawing of lots, to serve as judges (substitute the term *adjudicators* for the workers' compensation system) for a prescribed period, after which they would return to their law practices. In the event a claim is up for appeal, only attorneys who have already served as judges (adjudicators) would be considered to serve as an appellant judge (adjudicator). Once again, the random selection of a judge (adjudicator) would be based on lot drawings. With such a system, attorneys would have the opportunity to see what it is like to be on both sides of the bar and, as a result, become more rational in their decisions as attorneys and in their duties as judges (adjudicators).

WORKERS' COMPENSATION ADJUDICATORS AS MANAGERS OF HEALTH CARE

An interesting fact that is rarely, if ever, considered by the adjudicators is that al-though they have no training in the pathophysiology and care of injuries or illnesses and only limited understanding of managed care systems, they are "big players" in both arenas. Managed care in the United States covers about three-quarters of all persons who have health care insurance. Only in recent years has managed care come into the arena of workers' compensation. Although it is a common complaint that there is a two-tier system of health care in the United States, in reality there is a three-tier system if we consider the health care delivery systems involved in liability issues. Because workers' compensation is one of those liability issues, it is here that the medical issues of workers' compensation can come under the aegis of the workers' compensation adjudicator.

When reading or listening to adjudicators' medical decisions, it becomes clear that the impact of those decisions often are not in concert with prevailing medical science or managed care practices. Some examples include the acceptance of "junk science" as the basis for many of those decisions, especially in toxic tort cases; the lack of attention paid to cost constraints imposed in a managed care environment, such as utilization management or capitated contracts; the difference between a health maintenance organization (HMO) and a point-of-service HMO; that payment from the first dollar for whatever is medically reasonable and necessary can be the "mantra" by which many decisions are made; that, by virtue of the authority vested in them by the state, they are in fact health care managers; and, finally, that because of these (and more) reasons, they are not qualified to rule on the medical issues of a claim in a rational, scientific, and unbiased point of view. Too often, adjudicators appear incapable of separating the "wheat from the chaff," namely, what is appropriate and necessary from what is not. In deference to the adjudicators again, it also must be stated that providers too often do not supply adequate information on their submitted forms, and, as a result, the adjudicator cannot even make an "educated guess" as to what is appropriate. More confusion comes into play from health care providers who are looking for profit and attorneys who request test after test to build their case, also for monetary gain. Added to these is the attempt by the state legislatures to establish managed care organizations for the purpose of controlling costs, which then begs the question, What qualifies adjudicators to make these cost-effective (read as medical quality) decisions while assuring that the claimant is receiving optimal care?

COST OF CARE IN WORKERS' COMPENSATION: HOW, WHERE, AND WHY IT DIFFERS

Payors, through their claims adjusters, always seem to be in a battle with providers as to why certain studies are performed, especially if there does not seem to be a correlation with the claimed injury, and why the providers' charges are seemingly so outrageous at times. In some instances, the type of injury and manner of care are so standardized that the differences between the costs of care in workers' compensation differs little from costs related to private health insurance. On the other hand, the costs for the care of certain injuries are excessively high and bear no relationship to the same care provided if that injury were treated under the aegis of a private health insurance policy. As a demonstration, two examples are discussed, the first having to do with a fractured humerus, the second with a back injury.

Let us suppose we are asked to determine the appropriate care to be given a person who sustains a fracture of the humerus at the midshaft level. Whether this fracture occurs in Maine or California, on or off the job, the methods of treatment are well established, and their use will result in an expected outcome. Payment for the services rendered will be based on the standards of the payor's accrued payment data, whether it be Health Care Financing Administration (HCFA) for medicare, private health insurance carriers, the contracted fee schedule of a managed care organization, a usual and customary fee schedule, or

perhaps a state fee schedule as in the case of some workers' compensation jurisdictions. The criteria used are specific, although in many instances they will be proprietary.

Remember, a fractured arm is a fractured arm. How it is treated and how much reimbursement should be allowed for the necessary treatment should be essentially the same, accounting for regional differences as in the Resource Based Relative Value Scale fee schedule. In the case of a fracture, the standard of care is such that the differences in the charges rendered for care are relatively small, whether to a workers' compensation or a private health insurance carrier. This standard was demonstrated in a study by the Minnesota Department of Labor and Industry that compared costs between workers compensation and Blue Cross for comparable injuries (7).

In the case of back pain, 90% of these cases represent nothing more than a backache (2); however, because of the abusive activities of some providers and attorneys, excessive numbers of unnecessary and inappropriate tests are requested and performed. Added to these are the unnecessary and inappropriate operations that too often lead to poor results and the "failed back syndrome" (2). The fees to be paid for the care of a back injury will vary based on whether an excessive number of tests were done, the billing codes that were used, whether those codes were unbundled or upcoded, the use of a state fee schedule or the use of a usual and customary fee database, or the use of an excessive number of consultants. Additional variations occur when a fee is challenged by the carrier or a physician. Under such circumstances, the commissioner can see fit to accept, reduce, or augment the fee at will.

Another report, by Johnson et al. (8), compared the Minnesota data with data from California. The findings were essentially the same, namely, that the cost of care for a back injury was higher in a workers' compensation setting compared with that of a non-workers' compensation setting (i.e., available private health insurance coverage). The conclusion of that study begins with the statement that "Price discrimination contributed to the excess costs of treatment for work related injuries in Minnesota," whereas in California "overutilization of health care services and a more expensive combination of providers explain the high costs of treating work-related injuries." Adjudicators are in a position to protect claimants from their unscrupulous advocates by forcing them to justify the need for such procedures and the use of additional providers, especially when dealing with common injuries. One wonders whether the U.S. Supreme Court's requirement (based on *Daubert v Merrill Dow Pharmaceuticals*) that judges learn how to approach scientific questions (9) is given any consideration by the adjudicators of workers' compensation claims.

Consider this for a moment: If adjudicators do not control the abusive activities affecting costs, and they get no effective leadership from the legislatures in how to deal with the problem, then it will be a nightmare of logistics when and if a 24-hour health care policy (simply stated, a coupling of group health care and workers' compensation management protocols and their fee schedules under one policy) becomes the standard. How will the adjudicators explain that the care delivered in the workers' compensation setting exceeds the accepted standard of care in the other areas of health care if they continue to allow inappropriate, unnecessary, expensive tests and treatments without the benefit of statistically proven better outcomes?

Backaches occur across the country. Therefore, the question of why so many operations on the spine are performed in the West as opposed to the East? The answer may well be that the compensation health managers (the adjudicators) have not developed an educational process to establish a uniformity of process for their decisions. State autonomy and politics are the first two thoughts that come to mind and are the primary causes for what can be seen as major a weakness in the workers' compensation system: a lack of adequate knowledge regarding the pathophysiology of injury and disease in the workplace, a weakness that is not germane to the adjudicators alone but to all who work in the system. To overcome this weakness, let us turn to the important issue of adjudicator (or commissioner) education.

EDUCATION IS KEY

In the attempt to overcome this weakness, courses are provided by the workers' compensation organizations. The volume of information provided, however, tends to be directed toward the legal and procedural aspects of workers' compensation and little to the fundamentals of the pathophysiology of injury and disease, let alone any education on the tenets of causation analysis. Some states have established medical guidelines for all who work in the workers' compensation system. The physicians and the adjudicators are expected to know those guidelines. The former may be assisted by the protocols of managed care organizations that are incorporated into their software. It is unlikely, however, that the commissions have such stop-gap measures in place for the adjudicators.

Commissioner Education

At a national meeting of commissioners, this author was asked by a commissioner from a western state if a program could be designed to educate commissioners (adjudicators) in that state about medical facts germane to workers' compensation. The intent was to assist the adjudicators in determining what facts were important and what was considered appropriate management of typical workers' compensation cases. Unfortunately, on follow-up, the state's chief commissioner decided against proceeding with the request. This was a lost opportunity to upgrade the quality of the commissioners' (adjudicators') medical decision-making processes and their managerial skills in the third tier of health care insurance. There are usually two sides to every story, however. What follows is a discussion of how the medical profession has defaulted in the education of its students and residents regarding the practice of medicine in the real world, including issues related to workers' compensation as well as the legal and contractual issues they will confront in the day-to-day management of patients.

Education Regarding Workers' Compensation and Medical Costs

A universal problem for young physicians entering private practice is the lack of knowledge and experience necessary to deal with the yearly fusillade of health care legislative changes. Among these changes are those that pertain to workers' compensation. Because of the autonomy of each state, the respective legislatures can write the laws as they see fit. As a result, confusion can reign supreme as these young physicians attempt to separate state from federal health-related legislation. The idea that a nonphysician, such as an adjudicator, an attorney, or a managed care organization, may control the way doctors practice medicine is often repugnant to these young physicians. Furthermore, they are not prepared to deal with these issues appropriately. Hence, it is incumbent on the medical profession to intervene and to begin to incorporate into its teaching programs concepts that prepare these future physicians to deal with those nonphysicians in a way that protects the patient. The following section demonstrates that this is not so easy as it may seem.

THE ATTEMPT

Several years ago, as a medical director for a major carrier, I realized that too many physicians had a poor grasp of the interconnections between the law and the economics of health care delivery systems. How physicians dealt with the legal and cost-control aspects of Medicare, Medicaid, private health care insurers, workers' compensation, auto liability, and general liability made it obvious that they lacked an understanding of the developing cost-containment practices and how the law affected them in each of the different delivery systems. Their approaches implied that what worked in one system applied to all systems.

Based on this observation, a teaching program was assembled for the purpose of bringing the realities of the law and economics to the halls of medical education. Included in the program were issues related to workers' compensation to demonstrate the impact of the law in the management of care and how, in workers' compensation, care could differ because of the law. The carrier supported my efforts, paying for the printing costs involved; the making of a tape, which included an insurance representative, an attorney, and a physician; and travel expenses incurred for the project. Not only were the issues related to workers' compensation presented but also topics covering cost-containment practices.

The program had initial success that soon disappeared despite the interest of some medical schools. The reason for the lack of interest in promoting this program was made clear by a professor at one northeastern medical school who pointed out that professors were reluctant to give up 15 or 30 minutes of their allotted teaching time for a course designed to educate students on the vicissitudes of the practice of medicine, especially for something that was going to disappear, namely, managed care. It must be emphasized that, at that time, managed care was in its infancy and was seen primarily in the group health side of care and being spearheaded in California and the West. It had limited exposure in the arena of workers' compensation. Well, managed care did not disappear but gained a stronger foothold. The attitude demonstrated by members of the "ivory towers" made it clear that they were unaware of the vicissitudes of the real world or were engaging in denial; they were selfishly interested in their careers and were not preparing their students for the rigors of private practice. Much of this situation has changed because the impact of managed care has affected how medical institutions now practice medicine to maintain viability. Residents and students are aware of managed care and its impact on these institutions, but they are not necessarily aware of the impact on private practice.

Although it should be clear from the foregoing that the world of the workers' compensation system is not perfect, it should also be clear that medical educators bear some responsibility for some of the difficulties. Preparation for the practice of medicine outside the academic arena is a responsibility of medical educators. Numerous resources from the business world can be called on to assist in the education of medical students regarding the practical and legal aspects of the practice of medicine. It is important to learn from the mistakes of medical educators of the past. In not providing adequate preparation of their students for the rigors of private practice, they "left a hole" in the formal education of each student. The politics of medical educators need to be left outside the classroom doors.

It is especially important for the directors of those training programs dealing with musculoskeletal disorders that it be made clear to their residents that they will be confronted with claims of work-related injuries or illnesses once they enter private practice. Therefore, it should be incumbent on the directors of those programs to ensure that the residents are schooled in causation analysis, appropriate diagnostic algorithms, and an understanding of the meaning and intent of medically reasonable and necessary. This plea is made because it is clear after reviewing the files of physicians replete with non–work-related diagnoses, inappropriate treatments, miscodings, or false codings, that loss costs can be reduced not only for the carrier but also for the physician, an important issue in these days of managed care. Moreover, appropriate care will be delivered because the physician trained in the issues of workers' compensation will be better prepared to deal with the politics of the commissions and the law while providing the care required.

century. Having said that, it is also clear that the workers' compensation system has been the target of abuse. Because the system supports the autonomy of the 51 jurisdictions, the system is prey to unscrupulous persons, including employers, employees, union leaders, health care providers, attorneys, legislators, commission administrators, and, finally, adjudicators. This autonomy is a weakness of the system because the process is fractionated and uniformity of the decision-making process is hindered. Furthermore, not all claims are universally accepted in all jurisdictions or, if they are, conditions of applicability can vary.

The claim for a work-related condition should rest solidly on the foundation of causation analysis, which clearly establishes that the claim in fact can and does have a relationship to the job of the claimant. Educating all participants in the system, especially the adjudicators, regarding the pathophysiology of workplace injury and disease is necessary if an accurate analysis is to be performed and will insure that there is a better chance scientific proof will be used to establish causation rather than having it left to a guess of probability. In other words, application of the scientific method would be more appropriate to the system instead of the continued use of the 51% rule of probability.

Inadequate education of those who have the greatest impact on the system, especially as they relate to the medical topics germane to the injured worker, is one of the system's greatest weaknesses. No matter how great the educational attempts, however, if the politics of the system (the greatest weakness) are not overcome, then the educational benefits will be lost.

SUMMARY

The concept of workers' compensation as a social contract to protect the injured worker by having the costs of medical care and salary compensation covered by the employer is an honorable one that represents one of the great forward social leaps of the twentieth

REFERENCES

1. Waddell G. Clinical assessment of lumbar impairment. *Clin Orthop Res* 1987;221:110.
2. Taricco A. Medical issues of fraud and abuse in workers' compensation. Horsham, PA: LRP Publications, 1995:1–11, 15.
3. Taricco A. Perils of payors: a pain center paradigm. In: Cohen MJM, Campbell JN, eds. *Pain treatment centers at a crossroads: a practical and conceptual reappraisal,*

vol 7. *Progress in pain research and management.* Seattle: ISAP Press, 1996:112–115.

4. Brand RA, Lehmann TJ. Low back impairment rating of orthopaedic surgeons. *Spine* 1093;8:75.

5. Andersson GBJ. Impairment evaluation issues and the disability system. In: Mayer TG, Mooney V, Gatchel RJ, eds. *Contemporary conservative care for painful spinal disorders.* Philadelphia: Lea & Febiger, 1991.

6. Spence G. *O.J., The Last Word.* New York: St. Martin's Press, 1997:248–249.

7. Minnesota Department of Labor and Industry. *Report to the legislature: health care cost containment in Minnesota workers' compensation.* Minneapolis: Minnesota Department of Labor and Industry, 1980.

8. Johnson WG, Baldwin MJ, Marcus SC, Burton JF. *The Zenith Project: the excess costs of health care for work-related injuries, an executive summary.* Report no. 1.

9. Angell M. *Science on trial.* New York: WW Norton, 1996:127–132.

Occupational Musculoskeletal Disorders
edited by T. G. Mayer, R. J. Gatchel, and P. B. Polatin.
Lippincott Williams & Wilkins, Philadelphia © 2000.

46

Workers' Compensation: In Search of Perfection

John H. Jones, Jr.

Nationwide Insurance Companies, Wausau, Wisconsin 54402-8017

The search for perfection in state workers' compensation systems makes the implicit assumption that both the author and the reader would recognize perfection when or if we found it. To increase the difficulty of this challenge, the question that naturally follows is, From whose perspective should judgment of perfection emanate?

To illustrate the difficulty in defining perfection in a workers' compensation system, let us examine the traditional tension that exists in all workers' compensation systems between injured workers and employers. Injured workers view system performance in terms of the ease in which they can enter a workers' compensation benefit delivery system and the generosity of wage replacement and medical benefits. Employers, however, view system satisfaction from the perspective that costs associated with the system are affordable and sufficient system incentives exist to ensure prompt return to work by injured workers.

Because there is little likelihood of agreement, let alone recognition of perfection in any one state workers' compensation system by both workers and employers, the question remains as to what information we can glean to assist health care providers who want to see evidence of systems at work, albeit perhaps not perfectly.

Several state workers' compensation systems have improved their performance in managing costs, providing reasonably adequate and equitable benefits to injured work-

ers, and providing incentives to encourage prompt return to work. One state system that has achieved high marks is Wisconsin.

Wisconsin's workers' compensation system is often mentioned as one that has achieved a high level of success. In fact, the Wisconsin system is often considered the system to study by states seeking to improve the performance of the workers' compensation program. When other states consider reform of their workers' compensation systems, often they send a delegation to Wisconsin to learn about a system that achieves outcomes that other states want: reasonable benefits, a good delivery system, and affordable, stable costs (1). The focus of this chapter is to identify four major features of a workers' compensation system that provide opportunities to improve the system:

- Agency oversight: Interaction
- Return to work: Performance outcomes
- Dispute resolution: Getting along with each other
- Advisory council: Reform advocacy

Before beginning with the first system feature, credit should be given to the Workers' Compensation Research Institute for significant contributions to the body of knowledge about state-based workers' compensation systems. This organization, whose members include employers, insurers, unions, and state workers' compensation agencies, is devoted to researching public policy issues embraced within state-based workers' compensation systems.

The institute is a nonpartisan, not-for-profit research organization founded in 1983 and located in Cambridge, Massachusetts. The institute does not take positions on the issues it selects to research and publish. It provides to its many audiences objective and empirical information that addresses significant public policy issues impacting state-based workers' compensation systems. This chapter relies heavily on their many published contributions to a better understanding of where system performance can be enhanced and alternatives identified to achieving that end.

To the extent that the Wisconsin system has addressed those opportunities, the details of how it did so are provided to illustrate the technique or strategy. Finally, each system feature is be viewed from the health care provider perspective. Given the diverse constituencies and their views as to what is "in it for them," this perspective can provide the practical day-to-day improvements that could be expected from the health care provider's perspective.

AGENCY OVERSIGHT: INTERACTION

Workers' compensation is a form of social insurance that is based on a no-fault principle. The employer accepts responsibility for providing injured workers with wage loss and medical benefits. In exchange, the worker accepts benefits defined in the law and surrenders the right to pursue a civil action against the employer for monetary damages. All states have passed laws providing for workers' compensation benefits, and no two states have adopted identical statutory frameworks.

Whereas workers' compensation laws differ, all states use public agency(ies) to provide administrative support and a degree of oversight to their system. To the extent that this is a similarity in all states, it is equally true that no two states exercise the same level of administrative support or oversight. This can be explained by differences in state philosophy about the level of needed regulation of workers' compensation as well as the adequacy of funding for the agency.

Active agency supervision and involvement in the delivery of benefits to injured workers are important system features in well-performing state workers' compensation systems. Workers' compensation is a statutorily defined benefit delivery system; however, often this view is not shared by all the participants. In particular, some refer to injured workers and their opportunity to pursue benefits in a workers' compensation system as a "tradition claim process" with the view that the injured worker must establish entitlement, as a claimant would have to establish in a tort claim.

Agency supervision is intended to provide the state and its citizens a workers' compensation system in which benefits are delivered in a timely fashion, as required by law or regulation, and in as efficient a manner as possible. In discharging this role, the agency seeks to ensure that all participants, employees, employers, insurance carriers, health care providers, attorneys, and others behave in a responsible manner in providing value-added services to their constituents and to the beneficiaries of the workers' compensation system. To that end, supervision will encompass a level of regulation to achieve these administrative goals and day-to-day involvement to provide the most efficient and effective system of benefit possible.

Wisconsin is noted both for its active and involved administrative agency. The Department of Work Force Development has delegated to the Workers' Compensation Division the assignment to achieve the public policy goals of efficient benefit delivery and to facilitate cooperation between labor and management through day-to-day involvement with the participants in the workers' compensation system (2). In this role, the division monitors the performance of participants and gathers statistical information from all insurance carriers and self-insured employers on the timeliness of the initial payment of wage loss benefits. Chapter Ind 80.02(3)(a) of the Wisconsin Administrative Code provides that, in an undisputed case, the initial compensation payment must be made within 14 days of the report of injury

(3). Although other states have similar approaches to timeliness of initial compensation, Wisconsin makes the most of the importance of the information it gathers to ensure high levels of insurance carrier and self-insured employer performance.

The division tracks all initial payment performance and establishes a benchmark at 80% or more of all initial compensation payments. The results are gathered, and performance reports are sent to insurers and employers. For insurers, the report is generally sent to the chief executive officer, and for the self-insured employers it is sent to the president or chief operations officer.

Chronic nonperformance or behavior exhibiting "hardball" tactics of denial without just cause may well require an insurer or self-insured employer to appear before the division to explain this behavior and to document initiatives to improve performance. Making the "short list" of substandard performance in Wisconsin is not something either to dismiss or take lightly. Division efforts to raise performance levels are both prompt and effective. If the power of persuasion fails, some provisions within the law assess penalties for substandard performance (4).

In addition to monitoring initial payments, the division underscores its role in the day-to-day oversight by tracking the delivery of benefits to injured workers. This tracking process begins with the receipt of the required notice of injury (3). This notice usually is provided by the injured worker's employer or its insurance carrier. This information triggers the active case management of virtually all claims for benefits under the Workers' Compensation Act. This monitoring process continues until the case is closed.

The division has assigned to the Public Services Unit the important role as information provider for those seeking information about workers' compensation. Persons in this unit estimate that they receive between 120 to 200 telephone calls in an average day (1). In addition to receiving requests for information and help, they generate on their own dialogue with employers, insurers, and health care providers in an effort to resolve misunderstandings or disputes.

As active as this involvement by the Workers' Compensation Division appears to be, there is room for improvement to enhance system performance. A more comprehensive information strategy should be undertaken to raise the awareness of all participants about the need to achieve a self-executing system of benefit delivery (5). In addition, far more must be done in measuring performance and outcomes in workers' compensation cases to lay the foundation for system changes that will improve system performance for all participants. These two recommendations are applicable not only to Wisconsin but to all state systems seeking substantially improved performance.

A meaningful information strategy would focus on improving participant understanding of workers' compensation and developing a self-executing philosophy for benefit delivery. The first focus should be the needs of the injured worker.

Typically, the injured worker will receive an initial briefing about workers' compensation as part of an orientation process with the employer. It is safe to assume that unless injury occurs in a relatively short time after orientation, little knowledge about workers' compensation is retained by the worker. Few actually plan or expect to be injured on the job, and it is certainly not as interesting as the employer options in a 401K benefit package. It is probably accurate to say that an injured worker receives information about the workers' compensation system from a number of sources, some reliable and some not. In a workers' compensation system that is a high-performing system, the injured worker should receive accurate information describing the workers' compensation benefit-delivery system at the earliest opportunity.

The report of injury, when received by the agency, is an excellent trigger for the dissemination of valuable and needed information to the injured worker. No assurances or assumptions should be made about employer or insurer education of workers about the role of workers' compensation and their lives. The impartial provider of important information essential to understanding workers' compensation is a unique role that the state agency is qualified to fulfill.

In addition, this information opportunity can serve not only to educate the injured worker about his or her rights but also to emphasize the corresponding responsibilities that are part of the law as well. Injured workers need to know what is expected of them in terms of maintaining their eligibility for benefits, participating in medical examinations, and the reasons for answering legitimate inquiries seeking information necessary to ensure that benefits are paid for work-related injuries. This information opportunity should define for the worker the reasonable expectations from a workers' compensation system at the various stages of involvement, including an understanding of how disputes are resolved.

The explanation of workers' compensation law and procedure must not be left to chance or to interpretation from those who may have other agendas. Disputes that arise from erroneous information, misunderstandings, or unfounded expectations can and should be reduced to the lowest possible level by the timely delivery of accurate and easily understood information from the agency. Information sharing is an investment in the effort to provide benefits in an efficient and effective manner and to prevent unnecessary disputes based on ignorance.

A comprehensive information strategy was identified in the publication entitled *Dispute Prevention and Resolution of Workers' Compensation: A National Inventory*, published by the Workers' Compensation Research Institute. This recommended information strategy draws from the experiences of all the states in addressing the issue of information dissemination. It is interesting that only 7 of the 50 states incorporate all the suggested strategies (5):

- The communication process should be automatically initiated by the state agency on receipt of the notice of injury.

- All participants, workers, employers, and medical providers should be included in the information strategy.
- Multilingual written communication should address the diversity of the workplace.
- Communication material should explain the rights, responsibilities, and expectations of participants.
- Multimedia communication should include written, telephone, and computer access to knowledgeable agency personnel.
- Agency should have access to employer or insurer claims and electronic mail systems (5).

The importance of this communication strategy from the health care provider's perspective is simple. If you improve the understanding of system participants, explain rights and responsibilities, and inject reality into participant expectations, their assessment of system performance will be enhanced. By providing information at the earliest opportunity and making agency oversight focus on participant performance, disputes, when and if they arise, will not be based on misunderstanding or ignorance. This strategy complements other efforts to create a high-performing workers' compensation system by minimizing the opportunity for disputes, delays, and the attendant expense and disruption that follow.

The health care provider's role is not just to treat injured workers but to provide information to other participants in the worker's compensation system. In this role, the health care provider is the essential communicator of invaluable information. No one but the health care provider can answer the important questions involving causation and the nature and the extent of disability as well as the need for future medical care and rehabilitation. The failure to communicate vital information or delays in communication may well interrupt the delivery of benefits to the patient, that is, the injured worker. Medical opinions as to causation, length of healing period, the need for future medical treatment, and the nature and extent of permanent partial disability are critically important pieces of information without which benefits cannot be paid, cases resolved, and prompt return to work accomplished for the injured worker.

The ability of the health care provider to supply accurate and timely information about the patient will be enhanced by knowing what the agency communication protocols are and, in designing administrative support function, to complement those protocols to ensure the prompt and accurate sharing of information. As a stakeholder in the workers' compensation system, health care provider satisfaction is important to the public policy debates on how to improve system performance. To raise that level of satisfaction, health care providers should welcome the opportunity to be involved in the development of appropriate health care provider information strategies and communication protocols to eliminate unnecessary delays, expense, and inconvenience to all participants.

The second issue is the need to establish performance and outcome measurement in workers' compensation, which not only will establish benchmarks of current system performance but also provide solid information from which system performance can be improved.

When it comes to measuring system performance and outcome results of workers' compensation cases, the information currently available is limited. These limitations are not driven only by the availability of agency resources and statistical information. Limitations are in essence self-imposed because states have neglected to expand their role in the measurement of system performance, especially from the perspective of the injured worker. The absence of reliable information on system performance and of the ability to compare the performance of one state with another has been recognized for years. The state should promptly undertake, under expert guidance, the establishment of a permanent, scientific, uniform system of compensation statistics (6). Unfortunately, no systematic effort has been undertaken to achieve this laudable goal since it was first recognized in 1917.

Despite the presence of some systems performance data, vital aspects of systems behavior and impact on injured workers are simply missing. Little information is available to measure the levels of satisfaction experienced by injured workers who have received benefits. Second, little information is available to measure the impact of medical cost containment strategies on worker return-to-work rates and total-benefit delivery cost per case. Finally, there is a dearth of information with which to examine the long-term impact on injured workers after cases have been closed on their subsequent functional and wage loss experience and employment history.

The importance of having these elements of information for performance measurement and outcome analysis is that workers' compensation is an important part of the public policy-making process. Legislative and administrative rule making is a process in forming public policy, driven in part to improve system performance. How can an effective debate for improved system performance be ensured if no systematic evaluation is made of how a system performs from the perspective of the intended beneficiary, the injured worker?

Measures of cost and return-to-work outcomes are routinely the basis of much of the public policy debate in various states looking at system performance or anticipating reform and changes to the workers' compensation system. Whereas this information is valuable, it is not enough to ensure complete understanding of how a workers' compensation system currently performs or should perform in an enriched environment. To attempt to drive system performance toward higher goals of satisfaction, the views of injured workers must be part of that public policy debate.

Systematic sampling methods can be made available to measure worker satisfaction levels and to assess how various participants performed in that environment. The process certainly would be more complicated than a simple satisfaction survey. A process for measuring worker satisfaction can be developed and data gathered that will provide a more complete view of how a system performs and where system performance can be significantly improved.

In addition, more needs to be done from the agency perspective to follow up with workers to determine how they fare once cases are closed. Data gathering and analysis of worker functional performance as well as wage and employment history are a few meaningful areas that should be considered in any public policy debate, especially one focusing on the adequacy and equity of workers' compensation benefits. This is especially true in efforts to solve the perpetual problem of permanent partial disability benefits and their relationship to the wage and employment histories of workers who receive those benefits. This historical information must be factored into the public policy debate to determine the adequacy and equity of benefits as related to specific injuries and specific employees who may be adversely affected later in life because the benefits they received were not adequate for the injuries sustained.

Agency involvement should seek to achieve these broader measures of satisfaction and performance outcome measurement. State agencies must redefine their mission as not only a "watch dog" of participant behavior but as the organization that can accept responsibility for maintaining a high level of stakeholder satisfaction with the workers' compensation system. This role necessarily expands the perspective of measurement of our workers' compensation systems beyond traditional data to seek evidence of levels of satisfaction that can provide additional vital information about system performance.

System satisfaction cannot be based on antidote or perception. Criteria must be established to lay a broad foundation for the development of best practices that can redefine the levels of expected performance by participants in any workers' compensation system, complemented by the establishment of levels of benchmark performance as it relates to specific best practices and a systematic measure of performance by the participants in achieving those goals. To achieve recognized best practices for system participants, guidelines should be established

to hold stakeholders accountable for their actions within the system. The agency can assist in defining reasonable expectations and the needs of various constituents and focus participant performance on achieving these higher levels of performance in a sustained high-performance environment. The measurement and publication of these results will go a long way to ensuring all participants that the workers' compensation system is focused on achieving higher levels of satisfaction and outcome results on a "go-forward" basis by the continuous measurement of quality, cost, and productivity.

To achieve a meaningful assessment of any workers' compensation system and how it serves its constituents, this multidimensional analysis must be applied on a continuous basis to the performance of the system. Specifically, measurements must be established that will shed information, that is, reliable information, on the quality, cost, and efficiency of a state workers' compensation system. No one or two of these measures in this multidimensional analysis will be sufficient to identify successful system performance. The agency must serve as the stimulus for the development of performance measurement that truly identifies the important measures of quality, cost, and efficiency.

From the perspective of the health care provider, this is a meaningful strategy to support. Health care providers are now locked in debates with insurers, employers, and state agencies over the costs of providing health care benefits to injured workers. The reforms established in many states to decrease the rapid escalation of health care costs in workers' compensation have achieved some cost-containment success; however, the costs of achieving that success have not been fully measured. What you want—what you need—is *efficient* health care, not *cheap* health care. Medical providers have furnished health care appropriate to the injury, and that focus on assisting the injured worker to reach maximum recovery as quickly as possible will be, in the end, less expensive. These providers not only will generate less medical expense overall but also will save indemnity dollars (7).

The relationship between avoiding unnecessary and unreasonable medical interventions and costs always has been appropriate as a strategy to contain health care costs and improve outcomes in workers' compensation. The elimination of unnecessary or ineffective medical care is something about which all involved probably agree because it improves the quality of outcome while decreasing expenditures (7). What has not been thoroughly studied is the cost of some traditional nonoccupational health care strategies, such as later rather than sooner, less rather than more on issues such as return-to-work rates by injured workers impacted by this strategy and the results on the total cost per case of rationing health care for certain injured workers with specific injuries.

Health care providers must insist that system performance evaluations move beyond the issue of cost and cost containment to meaningful performance and outcome measurement. Through this broader measurement of results, health care providers can play a role in the debate over the reasonableness and necessity of medical care in the treatment of specific injuries to establish the best outcomes for injured workers. In some injury situations, *more* rather than less and *sooner* rather than later may be the desired protocol for treatment by health care providers for injured workers to achieve the best possible outcomes. Without this broader measurement process, health care providers will continue to struggle in the public policy debate over the issue of "cost" rather than outcome.

RETURN TO WORK: PERFORMANCE OUTCOMES

Although no uniformity exists among state workers' compensation laws, agreement does exist on the importance of returning injured workers to the workplace. In an important study published by the Workers' Compensation Research Institute, *What Are the Most Important Factors Shaping Return to Work? Evidence From Wisconsin*, that consensus was reaffirmed. "One of the most important functions of the workers' compensation systems is returning injured workers to productive employment in a timely manner" (8).

The benefits of an effective implementation of incentives and strategies to facilitate proper return to work by injured employees inure to the benefit of injured workers and employers alike. For the employee, delayed return to work puts at risk the opportunity to return to a preinjury employer, especially if the employer has a small workforce. In today's economy, few employers can hold positions open for an indefinite period while awaiting return of an injured employee. The pressures to reduce cost, improve productivity, and raise the quality of goods and services are never more evident than they are in the current economy.

In addition, the worker is always at risk in attempting to maintain appropriate physical fitness, workplace habits, and job necessary skills, all value-added attributes but unique to each worker, to be successful in returning to work. Workers' compensation benefits are a partial wage replacement to virtually all injured workers, and prolonged absence from the job and attendant regular earnings represent an economic risk few can ignore. These potential negative effects are often cumulative and can be detrimental in the injured worker's return to meaningful employment.

For the employer, workers' compensation benefits are a cost of doing business. Normally, this cost is incorporated in the price of goods and services sold to the public. Employers who experience high costs associated with workers' compensation may find their goods and services uncompetitive compared with employers who exercise greater efforts to contain and reduce the costs of workers' compensation injuries.

Employers can insure against their exposure to workers' compensation costs in many states; however, workers' compensation insurance is experience rated, and higher premiums go hand in hand with higher losses. Although the employer may qualify for self-insurance, if compensation costs increase, the result is obvious: larger out-of-pocket expenditures for work-related injuries. Employers who aggressively seek opportunities to expedite the return of injured workers to their employment are taking control of the future in terms of mitigating workers' compensation costs. Employers who exhibit this aggressive response to on-the-job injuries can enhance their competitive posture through their efforts at reducing costs associated with workers' compensation.

Employers can mitigate or eliminate other costs not often thought about in terms of the issue of return to work. These are costs associated with vacancies resulting from injured workers not returning to work, costs associated with replacement workers, costs associated with activities to alter or modify the work processes to adjust for the unfilled position. Finally, if the worker fails to return, costs normally are incurred in recruiting, training, and nurturing a replacement worker to a position of a trained and productive employee.

On paper, it is simple. Efforts undertaken by injured workers, employers, the supervising agency, and workers' compensation laws to motivate and enable prompt return to work find this strategy to be purely and simply a "silver bullet" when it comes to achieving the socially desirable objective of returning injured workers to work. In reality, there are lessons to learn to make return to work a critical success factor for all workers' compensation systems and outcome and performance measurement that desires more attention.

Wisconsin uses several distinct strategies to fulfill its objective to return injured workers to the workplace promptly. Initially, the wage-loss replacement-benefit structure establishes wage-replacement rates for temporary total disability at 66.6% of the state's average weekly wage (9). This rate is periodically reviewed and adjusted to reflect changes in the wages of employees in the state. Temporary total wage-loss benefits are paid for the duration of the healing period or, as some states call it, maximum medical improvement. The wage-loss benefit does not match actual wage loss because to do so would create disincentives to prompt return to work by injured workers.

If the worker sustains some degree of permanent partial disability, benefits are paid by stated maximum weekly amounts for a given number of weeks up to 1,000 weeks. Each percentage point of disability translates to 10 weeks of benefits paid on a monthly basis. The permanent partial disability payment is approximately one-third of the temporary total disability benefit. Again, the benefit level is intended to compensate the injured worker as well as to motivate the worker to return to work.

No representation is advanced here that this strategy of benefit levels is the ideal. It is offered simply to illustrate the public policy objective of benefit levels that do not act as disincentives to injured workers to return to work. It must be remembered that wage-loss benefits must be sufficiently high to prevent injured workers from becoming destitute either during the healing period or in compensating them for permanent partial or total disability.

In addition to the benefit structure, two important additional statutory provisions contribute to direct incentives to employers to accept injured workers back to their employment. Section 102.44(6) of the Wisconsin statutes provides that workers who sustain nonscheduled injuries, back injuries, for example, will receive only permanent partial disability benefits for functional impairment, not loss of wage-earning capacity, if the injured worker is reemployed by the preinjury employer at more than 85% of the preinjury average weekly wage. If the employer offers the employment at the wage provided in the statute and the employee unreasonably refuses to accept the offer of reemployment, the injured worker's benefits are limited to functional impairment as well. This "carrot" has appealed to employers as a way of permitting them to participate in an affirmative way their efforts to control costs.

To ensure an employer's good faith in acting under this statute, the law provides that the claim for loss of earning capacity remains open and is not barred by a statute of limitations. This law inhibits an employer from reemploying the worker and subsequently terminating the worker as a strategy to defeat loss of wage-earning capacity claims associated with some functional injuries and disability.

The second significant incentive for employers in Wisconsin is a statute that penalizes employers for unreasonably failing to rehire injured workers. The employer may be responsible for paying a penalty of up to a year's wages to the injured worker in such a circumstance (10).

A third incentive is not quite as obvious as the previously described two incentives in its ability to influence injured workers to return to work. It deals with the concept of lump-sum payments as part of an award for benefits under a workers' compensation claim. Any effort to compromise and close a disputed claim in Wisconsin puts the agency in a position to oversee the compromise and resolution process actively. For example, workers' compensation benefits that were originally denied and subsequently found as a matter of either agreement or of an order now due the injured worker are impacted by this oversight. Only the sums that were incurred and not paid may be "lump-summed" for the injured worker (11). Future workers' compensation benefits are not "lump-summed." Future payments of permanent partial disability, for example, act as a positive incentive to return to work because the future payments are not intended to match the preinjury earnings of the worker.

For health care providers, return to gainful employment of any patient injured in the workplace is a desirable outcome whether the provider is a treating physician or a vocational or physical rehabilitation specialist. Additional information coming out of ongoing research may give health care providers better insight into the opportunities for prompt return to work and ways to elevate such successes as a true outcome measurement of the positive role that health care providers play in workers' compensation.

Often the credit for prompt return to work is attributed, appropriately, to the worker and employer. The health care provider can and should play a prominent role in this effort as well. Some findings from new research on return to work and some factors that can improve efforts and results in returning injured workers to gainful employment should be examined. In the publication entitled *What Are the Most Important Factors Shaping Return to Work? Evidence From Wisconsin*, the authors expend the body of knowledge about challenges of returning injured workers to work and point to the need for better outcome measurement.

This study essentially had two objectives. The first was to provide information about worker characteristics that can and do impact on return-to-work success rates. The second objective was to identify the consequences of delayed reentry into the workplace to stimulate readers and public policy makers to explore creative new incentives to encourage workers and employers to work more aggressively in their efforts at early return to work.

The authors selected Wisconsin as the state to study because of Wisconsin's reputation as having a good workers' compensation system that incorporates benefits and incentives to motivate workers and employers to execute return-to-work strategies. So caution must be exercised to temper findings by following the authors' caveat: "Some findings probably are affected by special features of the Wisconsin system. Still, our results are often applicable to other states that have different systems because they derive from human nature, from economic incentives, or from other economic factors people face wherever they live" (8).

The study focused heavily on workers who sustained injury and were absent from the workplace for at least 30 days, the period selected because it represented 52% of the 118,965 workers who were a part of the study and 98% of the lost time from work generated by those injuries. In addition, 94% of the wage replacement benefits were paid for injuries to workers occurring during calendar years 1989 and 1990. For the authors, this group of workers represented those whose injuries contributed to more than 30 days of lost time and represented the largest population in which positive change in return-to-work behavior would bring the greatest impact.

The study identified four major factors that influence success in returning workers who were off from work for more than 30 days. The first factor was returning the worker to the preinjury employer. Simply put, success begins at home. The study points out that preinjury employment with this employer is an important qualification. The greater length of time of preinjury employment, the greater the success in predicting a successful return to work with this employer. Equally important, if reemployment did not occur, the duration of time off increased by a factor of twofold to threefold. A worker with a profile of 1 or more years with the preinjury employer is a significant characteristic for a health care provider to consider in beginning to predict successful outcomes for return to work.

The second major factor, although intuitively well known, focused on the attitudes and behavior of injured employees in the preinjury workplace. Specifically, factors such as age, education, skill level, and employment history are significantly important in predicting a successful return to work. A worker who has little education, low job skills, a "checkered" employment history, especially with employers whose operations are seasonal or intermittent, are more troublesome candidates for successful reemployment with the preinjury employer as well as reemployment with any future employer.

The third major factor are the characteristics of the preinjury employer. To begin with, small employers have more difficulty in preserving open positions or in making changes in work assignments or providing even light or modified work for someone seeking return to work. Whereas generalizations are dangerous, there are exceptions to these observations: employers of fewer than 50 employees who have a decided bias toward workers who are longer-term employees. Larger employers, that is, those who have 1,000 workers or more, have advantages in implementing aggressive return-to-work strategies, which can include light duty, modified work, and other assistance programs to ease a worker back into gainful employment. Even in union shops, there is strong evidence that labor management through appropriate negotiations and collective bargaining can implement strategies to set aside or modify seniority rules to the advantage of workers who need limited, modified, or light-duty employment.

The last major feature developed in the study was consideration of certain economic factors facing the injured worker. The study included that higher wage earners tend to return to work faster than lower wage earners and, according to the research, the reason may not be so much the benefit level, which is correspondingly lower than actual wages, but that the worker knows that workers' compensation benefits will end, and there is a strong desire to maintain high on-the-job wages in the future.

Other economic factors are perhaps more subtle but deserve mention. In families with two wages, the effect of an injury to either worker on early return to work can be influenced by such issues as whether the husband or wife is the injured worker. Although the researchers come close to political incorrectness, one observation from the data indicates that if the wife, in addition to employment, is also the major player in the house, time off from work may be viewed differently than if her husband was the injured employee. A significant additional consideration in the two-wage-earners family is the tax code in the particular state as well as the federal tax provisions. State and federal taxes treat workers' compensation wage-replacement benefits as exempt from taxation. If a husband and wife file a joint return with one taxable wage and the other income is tax-free workers' compensation benefits, after-tax income realized by that family will increase because the only taxable income is now divided between husband and wife. This can be a telling disincentive to early return to work.

For the health care provider, the message is clear. Outcome measurement in terms of prompt return to work is a critical success factor in workers' compensation. Many factors, including injury severity, play various roles in predicting successful return to work. It is clear that having more information available early in the treatment phase is critically important to tailor both treatment regimens and vocational services to ensure a decided bias toward successful return-to-work outcomes.

Specifically, more information must be obtained from the injured worker to develop a sufficiently detailed profile that takes into consideration many of the issues raised in the study. Worker history should include education, skill, work history, wage history, length of employment, worker attitudes about employment, employer characteristics and future employment interests, as well as other economic factors that mgiht shed light on the terms of prediction of the likelihood of prompt return to work. This information must be made available to health care providers earlier in the relationship with the injured worker to assess outcome potential.

For the health care provider, the laudable goal of return to work as quickly as possible may be frustrated by the advent of managed care strategies in workers' compensation. If the managed care strategies take on the similarity of those strategies used in nonoccupational injury and disease settings, the introduction of this type of strategy may frustrate early return to work. For example, delayed treatment and prolonged periods between appointments, even broadening a theory that less is better than more and later is better than earlier, conflict strongly with the message in the research study. The longer an individual is off work, the more difficult reemployment, even with the preinjury employer, becomes. Much more research needs to be done, but what is known now is that for some injuries aggressive treatment early on, which results obviously in higher immediate medical costs, may well prove to be a lower total-cost solution over the long term. Simply put, more spent with health care providers, both treating medical practitioners as well as vocational and physical rehabilitation specialists, may bring about a lower cost in terms of both medical and indemnity than strategies devoted solely containing and reducing medical expenditures.

Workers' compensation always must be understood as a discipline that involves issues dealing with both medical costs and wage-loss benefits. The two issues in many cases are inseparable. Exercising prudent restraint on unnecessary and unreasonable medical expenditures is always an appropriate public policy goal. Much more needs to be done, however, in terms of outcome measurement so that we can determine what the appropriate protocols should be for specific injuries to ensure the best outcome, not simply the lowest medical cost.

DISPUTE RESOLUTION

Disputes can and do occur between some injured workers and their employers and insurance carriers over the many issues impacting the eligibility for and the extent of medical and indemnity benefits. These disputes can involve issues of whether an injury or disease is related to the workplace, the length of the healing period, the need for future medical care, the nature and extent of permanent partial disability, timeliness of the payment of benefits, the need for and extent of physical or vocational rehabilitation, the existence and significance of scarring or disfigurement, whether or not future expected wage loss results from a work-related injury, and in some states bad faith practices of self-insured employers or insurance carriers.

For a no-fault social insurance mechanism in which concepts such as negligence are immaterial, this can appear as a daunting list of opportunities for claim payers to deny, delay, or discount benefits to injured workers. The number of disputed claims will vary from state to state, but most workers injured on the job have their medical costs paid and their indemnity payments made without dispute.

The Workers' Compensation Research Institute developed a compendium of state workers' compensation dispute prevention and resolution approaches (5). The significance of this effort is that it gathered together in one study the breadth of strategies currently used by states and laid a foundation for future research into benchmarks to enable state comparisons in terms of outcomes. In this work, the author identifies the public policy goals that motivate state agencies in their efforts to create a self-executing workers' compensation program. These following are the public policy goals:

- Entitled benefits are delivered and terminated in a timely manner, thus minimizing economic and social hardships for workers and providing reasonable costs to employers.
- Disputes are resolved with a minimum of friction cost (including attorney fees, medical and legal costs, and claims handling cost).
- Workers return to work faster (5).

A previous section of this chapter deals with the benefits of efforts made to prevent as many disputes as possible among the workers' compensation stakeholders. These efforts are investments intended to create the self-executing delivery of benefits to eligible injured workers at affordable cost to employers. Affordability improves when friction costs, those incurred by all parties in the disputes process, are not spent.

Strategies to improve communication, to monitor and benchmark performance to best practices, and to facilitate interactive exchanges with the public agency are intended to filter out all but the most important disputes, which can be sent to informal or formal dispute resolution. The study characterized the dispute-resolution process as comprising both informal and formal approaches. An understanding of the concept of *informal* can be aided by defining the characteristics of this approach:

- There are no or few rules.
- There are no rules governing the admissibility of evidence.
- There is no sworn testimony or cross-examination of witnesses.
- No transcript or other formal hearing record is kept (5).

The most important part of dispute resolution for the health care provider is the formal process, which varies widely from state to state. It is important because, although health care providers are sometimes comfortable with patient advocacy, the great majority find it to be a less attractive role in their chosen discipline. Although some physicians specialize in occupational medicine or compensation medicine, many others seem to want as little contact as possible with the workers' compensation system. Some physicians find such processes unacceptably time consuming. No doubt, many doctors have little taste for the adversary process wherein their professional views are challenged openly by attorneys and other physicians (12). Formal dispute resolution generates medical and legal costs, inconvenience, delays, and adversarial relationships that most health care providers would choose to avoid whenever possible. Health care providers, however, are critically important participants in determining the eligibility and the nature and extent of benefits associated with work-related injuries and diseases. Whereas this role is critically important in the proper functioning of any workers' compensation system, the challenge is to make the contribution by health care providers as efficient and hassle-free as possible.

Some system features can provide relief from the usual delays and transaction costs normally associated with the formal dispute-resolution process in workers' compensation. Wisconsin has crafted a mutually reinforcing set of system features for assessing the extent of disability in resolving disputes about permanent partial disability (1). There are four specific system features that reduce disputes and attorney involvement that are worth mentioning. No one feature, standing alone, is a significant driver in Wisconsin's ability to reduce significantly litigation rates. This interdependency is described in detail in the Workers' Compensation Research Institute's publication, *Workers' Compensation in Wisconsin.*

The first system feature is a schedule of minimum permanent partial impairment ratings for a specific list of injuries that normally result in impairment of bodily function. Section Ind 80.32 of the Wisconsin Administrative Code provides a schedule for back and neck injuries that establishes minimum permanent partial disability ratings. The schedule was prepared by a panel of orthopedic surgeons for the Workers' Compensation Division. The schedule provides the following:

- Laminectomy, no undue symptomatic complaints or any objective findings: 5%
- Spinal fusion L5–S1, good results: 10%
- Spinal fusion L4–S1, good results: 10%
- Cervical fusion, successful: 5%
- Compression fractures of vertebrae of such degree to cause permanent disability, 5% and graded upward (3)

Greater disability may be present, and physicians are not inhibited by the schedule in assessing a greater degree of disability based on the outcome of treatment. The schedule provides a "floor" in terms of the extent of disability for the enumerated injuries and resulting outcomes. This schedule assumes no preexisting disability to the affected body parties. If there is preexisting disability, the physician must provide an estimate and a reduction to the schedule minimums if appropriate.

The second and third system features can be appreciated best by examining them together. The agency places great credibility on medical opinions rendered by treating physicians, especially in the challenging arena of the nature and extent of permanent partial disability.

In Wisconsin, the agency requires the treating physician, at the conclusion of the healing period, to render a written opinion on the nature and extent of any permanent partial disability. The opinion is entered on a state-approved form and sent to the agency. The agency in turn informs the self-insured employer or its insurance carrier that, absent evidence rebutting the treating physician's opinion, voluntary payment of benefits is expected.

This feature is important in the system because the burden shifts to the employer or the employer's insurance carrier to unseat the bias that favors opinions of the treating physician and marshals contrary evidence. Such evidence generally requires an investment of expense to secure a contrary medical opinion. Normally, an independent medical examination is limited by a case where the cost is justified as an expenditure to establish a meritorious position that calls into doubt the medical opinion of the treating physician. Absent such a case, voluntary payment is expected in Wisconsin.

The fourth system feature is the concept of final-offer adjudication (1). Section 102.18(1)(d) of the Wisconsin statutes provides that, when an administrative law judge is faced with two expert medical opinions in a functional impairment case, the judge must select one or the other opinion. The only statutory latitude available to the judge is to increase the lowest rating by no more than 5% or to decrease the highest rate by no more than 5% (13).

This system feature demonstrates the agency's determination to avoid case decisions by a split-the-difference rationale. The agency has made a determination that it is in the best interest to avoid, to the extent possible, the concept of dueling doctors. This system feature, found in many states, encourages disputing participants to seek medical opinions that unnecessarily inflate and deflate impairment ratings so that a compromise is inevitable and splitting the difference is the outcome. Perhaps put in a slightly different perspective, 0% ratings from nontreating physicians obtained to compromise financial responsibility for benefits for an injured worker do not "play well" in Wisconsin.

Another unique approach instituted by Wisconsin currently plays a limited but potentially larger role in dispute prevention and resolution. Section 102.13(3) of the Wisconsin statutes details a procedure to expedite the resolution of a difference of opinion between two physicians about the end of the healing period, the need for additional or specific medical care, and the ability of an injured worker to return to work (14). The statute provides for a tiebreaker medical examination. The insurer or self-insured employer must pay for the examination, and the examining physician is one of a panel of physicians established by the agency. If the injured worker is receiving temporary total disability benefits, these benefits will continue until the agency concludes its review of the examining physician's report.

Whereas this procedure is restricted to limited and specific issues, there is an opportunity to expand this approach to other workers' compensation issues if Wisconsin has the "appetite for change" and a consensus among the stakeholders can be achieved. It would be possible to develop physician panels by speciality and, in cases of physician dispute on such difficult issues as occupational disease causation and the extent of permanent partial disability, to allow a panel physician to cast the deciding vote.

If a difference of medical opinions exist between a treating physician and a physician that examines an injured worker for an employer or its insurance carrier, referral to a physician panel established by the agency for a third binding opinion would be a bold approach to reducing disputes. While due process protections must be observed such as notice to and agreement by the disputing participants, the agency would assure responsibility for the competency and independence of the panel participants. The agency would establish an expedited process for examination and report submission as well as geographic panel representation to avoid unnecessary travel costs and delays.

In addition to the specific strategies to reduce disputes and the involvement of attorneys in resolving disputed workers' compensation claims, certain other statutory and administrative rules go far in minimizing friction costs when disputes cannot be resolved without a formal hearing. Section 102.17(d) of the Wisconsin statutes provides a cost-effective way to submit medical testimony and other expert testimony in a workers' compensation proceeding (15). Special forms prepared by the agency are used with the only caveat that the verification, the signature of the physician, creates the *prima facie* status of the opinion contained in the report and the report will be received into evidence so long as the physician will consent, should a request be made, to appear for cross examination.

Section Ind 80.21 of the administrative code specifically empowers the agency to require all parties to submit all available medical and vocational reports as well as to exchange them (16). Although the rule is seldom formally invoked in Wisconsin, it is because the state has

embraced the concept that concealing evidence before a hearing is detrimental not only to the parties involved but to the system itself. It is not uncommon for an administrative law judge who finds that a party has concealed important evidence either before or during a hearing to grant the opposing party an opportunity for a second hearing to recover from the surprise or ambush.

In Wisconsin the use of depositions is strongly discouraged, and strict limits are placed on their use. Section 102.17(1)(f) of the Wisconsin Statutes sets forth the only permitted uses of depositions, and in all other instances they are forbidden without the specific authorization of the agency (17). Essentially, in Wisconsin, there is no need for discovery depositions. This public policy substantially reduces the medical and legal costs associated with dispute resolution experienced in many other states that do not limit discovery procedures in workers' compensation matters.

For the health care provider, there are ways to achieve both the prevention and expedited resolution of workers' compensation claims in a cost-effective manner. Articulating a bias for treating physician opinions, agency efforts to improve system performance include expediting voluntary payments of benefits; inhibiting disputing participants from gaming the system; strictly limiting the use of discovery in workers' compensation proceedings; and reducing the time, expense, and inconvenience of physician involvement are all strategies that can improve system performance.

ADVISORY COUNCIL: REFORM ADVOCACY

"The ultimate social philosophy behind compensation liability is belief in the wisdom of providing, in the most efficient, most dignified, and most certain form, financial and medical benefits for the victims of work-connected injuries which an enlightened community would feel obligated to provide in any case in some less satisfactory form, and of allocating the burden of these payments to the most appropriate source of payment, the consumer of the product" (18). The first state to pass a workers' compensation law that was upheld as constitutional was Wisconsin in 1911 (19). Other states followed with laws of their own, each an expression of the state's perspective of what was needed to address the needs of injured workers and what could be afforded by employers. What can be said about the state-based approach to workers' compensation is that each system evolved at its own pace. "The historical evolution of workers' compensation systems can be characterized by significant policy surges taking place after alterations in the industrial and economic processes of the United States" (20). No significant "groundswell" of support for the need for state consistency in workers' compensation occurred until 1970.

In that year, Congress passed the Occupational Safety and Health Act of 1970 (21). Contained within this important legislation was a provision urging the president to appoint a national commission on state workers' compensation laws. The legislation called for a 15-member commission to examine the state workers' compensation approach in addressing the legitimate needs of injured workers and to issue a report on their findings that also should address whether there was a need to substitute a federal statutory approach to workers' compensation.

The commission was created in part as a response to the emergency of occupationally related diseases and the ability of state-based workers' compensation laws to address worker needs adequately. The report urged states to expand eligibility for coverage to more workers, raise wage loss benefits to reflect the economic needs of workers for income replacement, include coverage for occupational disease claims, expand medical benefits to include rehabilitation benefits, and other significant recommendations.

The not-so-subtle threat for the state-based approach to workers' compensation was the call for federal legislation incorporating standards or, alternatively, to replace state workers' compensation acts with a fed-

eral legislation to provide consistency in treatment of injured workers.

Efforts by states to address deficiencies in the state laws, particularly wage replacement of benefit levels, triggered not only dramatic change in benefits provided to injured workers but also a significant increase in employer costs in many states. Some states were particularly enthusiastic in their effort and upset the previous equilibrium between benefit levels and affordability. Because the cost of workers' compensation is to be borne by the purchasers of goods and services, employers in some states found the cost to be too great to continue operation. Employers made business decisions that resulted in migrating operations to less costly states.

It was this flurry of state-initiated legislative activity and reform that laid a foundation for the partisan legislative battles that have impacted state workers' compensation laws since 1970. It is the search for adequate and equitable benefits at affordable cost that is at the root of this issue. For many states, the direct legislative process was the only choice as a forum for debating workers' compensation reform, but was the legislative arena a preferred choice for this debate, or did other ways exist that could have produced reform in a less partisan fashion?

It can be said that "Workers' compensation was not invented; it evolved. It developed out of a series of social adjustments to meet a social need" (22). The report of the National Commission was just such a social adjustment.

In all states, reform of workers' compensation is ultimately a legislative activity that usually requires some consensus that change is required and a legislative majority to enact remedial legislation into law. On its face, this process would appear to be relatively straightforward. After all, how could elected legislators be anything but sympathetic and support enhanced workers' compensation system performance?

In the past several years, many states have passed workers' compensation reform legislation intended to address system performance. Policy formulation has become more conflict driven, however, as more special-interest groups have formed and have intensified their participation in the legislative process (23). Whereas the experience in legislative change initiatives differs from state to state, certain observations can be made.

Absent a crisis in the performance of a state workers' compensation system, legislators have an inherent reluctance to enact workers' compensation legislation. This is true, in part, by the tension that exists in all workers' compensation systems between the desires of workers and the demands of employers. Simply put, workers' compensation issues are viewed by many legislators as being politically high risk. In addition, workers' compensation is a complex subject that requires effort by legislators both to analyze the issues and to craft appropriate legislative solutions to address system performance improvement. If the workers' compensation system is not in crisis but is functioning without significant constituent complaint, the attitude by legislators is generally to "leave well enough alone."

What can be said of the direct legislative effort is that workers' compensation is not a matter of sustained interest for most politicians. The exception occurs when a real or perceived crisis appears. Absent broad constituent demand for change, workers' compensation remains simply too complex, too esoteric, and for all a potentially politically divisive issue. The result for many states is simply a crisis, reform in crisis strategy.

When legislators are energized to action, the experience in many states has been disappointing. Workers' compensation systems in general suffer from a lack of statistical information to quantify clearly for a legislator the nature and extent of the problem and what the appropriate proposals for change may be. In the absence of good analysis and information, reform tends to be driven by other strategies. Far too often, reform is driven by antidote rather than fact, heat rather than light. If reform emerges from such an environment, there is often little appetite for legislators to follow up to determine the impact of the corrective legislation for fear that they

will be brought back into another public policy debate, this time with a demonstrative failure to address the system-performance concerns properly.

Several states developed a better strategy: to empower an oversight group representing various stakeholders in the workers' compensation system who have the luxury of taking a longer-term view of the process of change and appreciate and share an understanding of the complexity and interrelationship of the various aspects of workers' compensation.

The Workers' Compensation Research Institute recently prepared a study on one such type of oversight group, commonly referred to as an *advisory council*. In their publication, *Workers' Compensation Advisory Councils: A National Inventory, 1997–1998*, they defined the concept of an advisory council as "...organized groups that are composed of key system stakeholders and that provide input to policy makers on a broad range of worker's compensation policy issues" (24).

This informative study developed a list of states where advisory councils have been created. Thirty-four states have advisory councils, but no two state advisory councils function in the same fashion. Some have become standard features in their state workers' compensation systems and primary players in the process of the development of public policy debates and subsequent workers' compensation system reform. In this work, the institute has identified a number of highly desirable advisory council objectives:

- Facilitating mutual cooperation and coordination among various system participants
- Increasing system participant awareness and education about workers' compensation issues and policies
- Serving as a forum wherein workers' compensation system stakeholders may raise issues, identify problems, and propose solutions
- Acting as a vehicle for giving system stakeholders input into the policy-making process
- Improving workers' compensation systems by advising policy makers, recommending

improvements, and monitoring the implementation of changes (24)

The most successful advisory councils have developed an appreciation that workers' compensation laws and regulations should not, in the first instance, be "held hostage" to the political fortunes of partisan politics in the state legislature. A system's comprehensive and interrelated features, which are intended to provide adequate and equitable as well as affordable benefits, should be the provenance of stakeholders who ultimately would bear the responsibilities as well the benefits of a successful workers' compensation system.

If such a process is to succeed, the advisory council must be responsible for its actions and accountable to a legislature or administrative agency in a particular state. The more successful advisory councils play major roles in defining issues and recommending proposals to enhance system performance.

Wisconsin is credited with one of the most successful workers' compensation advisory councils. This council can trace its roots to the original Workers' Compensation Act passed in 1911 (19). It was initially introduced as a committee, but little is known of the early history. It has now become a feature of the workers' compensation system and an institutionalized organization for the citizens of Wisconsin. Section 102.14(2) of the Wisconsin statutes establishes the advisory council as an essential feature in its workers' compensation law by providing the following:

- Advice to the Department of Industry, Labor, and Human Relations (now the Department of Work Force Development) in carrying out the purposes of the Workers' Compensation Act
- Recommendations to the legislature in each regular session with respect to amendments to the Workers' Compensation Act
- Views on any bill pending before the legislature with respect to amendments to the Workers' Compensation Act
- At the request of the chairpersons of the Senate and Assembly Labor Committees, meeting and discussion of any matters of

legislative concern related to the Workers' Compensation Act (25)

An additional goal of the council, although not specifically mentioned in the statute, is "to maintain the overall stability of the workers' compensation system without regard to partisan changes in the legislature or the governor's office" (2). The goal perhaps can be more simply stated by an anecdote "... while the stock market appreciates bulls and bears, it hates hogs!" Political shift in some stakeholder constituencies may prosper temporarily, but long-term high performance in a workers' compensation system cannot be sustained if the balance achieved by consensus is more times than not out of balance.

Workers' compensation system performance can be elevated above the fray of partisan politics if an advisory council earns and sustains a reputation as a deliberative body exercising enlightened stewardship. Such an organization understands its mission to oversee the evolution of workers' compensation laws and regulations intended to address constituent needs. Such an environment is nurtured when consensus is valued and stakeholders are focused on deal making, not deal breaking.

The Wisconsin Advisory Council historically has provided a deliberative body wherein the primary stakeholders, labor and business, can influence the development and formulation of proposed legislation to institute evolutionary changes to the Workers' Compensation Act. Creators of the Wisconsin Workers' Compensation Law believe that business and labor are the parties most concerned with workers' compensation issues, and therefore the council is structured so that these are the primary interests represented in this council (23).

To reflect this legislative intent, labor and management each have five members who have the power of the vote. One additional member, the head of the Workers' Compensation Division, presides and also has one vote. Historically, this position vote has been cast only rarely, in favor of a consensus process rather than majority rule.

In practice, the council has expanded its membership to include three nonvoting representatives from the Wisconsin workers' compensation insurer community. The role of the council is to provide insight and information on the potential impact, from their perspective, of changes to the law.

Recently, the council expanded its membership by creating room at the table for additional stakeholders. Three liaisons from the diverse medical community joined the council. This expansion was driven, in part, by the impact of medical cost inflation and medical cost-containment strategies that recently significantly impacted the debate over affordability of workers' compensation. Whereas representation of the medical community always has been a part of the development of workers' compensation legislation and regulation in Wisconsin, this role was largely behind the scenes or by special *ad hoc* committee formation. Now they have a seat at the table but unfortunately no vote.

The makeup of the council today "...suggests that the council plays a role in facilitating coalition formulation, byproduct of which may be policy proposals that are closer to the policy preferences of the "median" interest rather than the extremes. This may help to reduce the pendulum effect present in other states" (23). In addition, this deliberative process of diverse viewpoints gives an early alert opportunity to provide input into the process of change. This can reduce the risk of important interest groups from being blindsided and resorting to the legislature for special treatment because of perceived or real unfairness in the process.

For health care providers, the path to sustaining performance improvement in workers' compensation is challenging if the result is solely a lobbying effort in state legislatures. For those familiar with workers' compensation and the various efforts to improve it in the past, there is a recognition that the toughest "nut to crack" may well be defined as a technique to implement and enforce proposed reforms (12).

Such a technique is available in the 34 states that have adopted an advisory council

process; however, these advisory councils must step up to the higher expectation of participation and performance demonstrated by the advisory council in Wisconsin to be effective. The simple presence of an advisory council may only be cosmetic unless it is prepared to address the issues energetically to improve system performance by inviting a broad group of constituents and stakeholders to the table.

CONCLUSION

Although the search for perfection is futile, the opportunity for enhanced workers' compensation system performance is available in every state. The prescription for change is simple: involvement. Individual involvement, provider associations, or teaming up with other like-minded constituencies is a desirable strategy to influence the effort to improve, from the health care provider perspective, system performance. No more persuasive argument can be made for involvement than to learn from the history of the evolution of workers' compensation "...an examination of the history of [worker's] compensation reveals that workers' compensation gained momentum after the industrial changes of the late 19th and early 20th century (mine) only *after* powerful nongovernmental groups recognized the importance of workers' compensation and supported its establishment. It is not surprising that these groups are still involved in the promulgation of workers' compensation programs" (20).

REFERENCES

1. Ballantyne DS, Telles TA. *Workers' Compensation in Wisconsin:* Administrative Inventory. Cambridge, MA: Workers' Compensation Research Institute, 1992:xv; 61–99.
2. Council on Workers' Compensation. *Report to the Lieutenant Governor on functions of workers' compensation advisory council.* Madison, WI: Workers' Compensation Division, 1995:3–4.
3. *Wisconsin Administrative Code*, Chapter Ind 80, Workers' Compensation 1998.
4. *Wis. Stat.* § 102.22.
5. Ballantyne DS. *Dispute prevention and resolution in*

workers' compensation: a national inventory, 1997–1998. Cambridge, MA: Workers' Compensation Research Institute, 1998:3,8–9.

6. National Industrial Conference Board. *Summary of report on workmen's compensation acts in the United States—the legal phase.* Boston: NICB, 1917:6.

7. DeMoss DL. Medical outcomes data: road map to quality. In: Kimpon K, ed. *Workers' compensation medical care: effective measurement of outcomes.* Cambridge, MA: Workers' Compensation Research Institute, 1996: 4,58.

8. Galizzi M, Boden LI. *What are the most important factors shaping return to work? Evidence from Wisconsin.* Cambridge, MA: Workers' Compensation Research Institute, 1996:3,5.

9. *Wis. Stat.* § 102.11.

10. *Wis. Stat.* § 103.35(3).

11. *Wis. Stat.* § 102.32(6).

12. Barth, Peter S., and Hunt, Allan H. Workers' Compensation and Work-Related Illnesses and Diseases, p. 275.

13. *Wis. Stat.* § 102.18(1)(d).

14. *Wis. Stat.* § 102.13(3).

15. *Wis. Stat.* § 102.17(d).

16. *Wisconsin Administrative Code.* Chapter Ind 80.21, 1994.

17. *Wis. Stat.* § 102.17(1)(f).

18. Larson A. Workman's Compensation Law Desk Edition (New York: Matthew Bender) §2.20,1–5.

19. Chapter 50, Law of 1911.

20. Thompson J. Outputs and Outcomes of State Workers' Compensation Laws. Journal of Politics, 43: 1129–1131.

21. 29 U.S.C. § 27 (1970).

22. Somers H, Somers A. Workmen's Compensation: Prevention, Insurance, and Rehabilitation of an Occupational Disability. New York: John Wiley, p. 131.

23. Fox S. The Role of Advisory Councils in Workers' Compensation Systems: Observations From Wisconsin (Cambridge MA: Workers Compensation Research Institute) p. 8–9.

24. Fox S. Workers' Compensation Advisory Councils: A National Inventory (Cambridge, MA: Workers Compensation Research Institute) p. 3–13.

25. *Wis. Stat.* § 102.14(2).

Subject Index

Note: Page numbers followed by f indicate figures; those followed by t indicate tables.